CALCULATE with CONFIDENCE

Seventh Edition

Deborah C. Gray Morris, RN, BSN, MA, LNC
Chairperson
Department of Nursing and Allied Health Sciences
Bronx Community College of the City University of New York (CUNY)
Bronx, New York

ELSEVIER

ELSEVIER

3251 Riverport Lane
St. Louis, Missouri 63043

CALCULATE WITH CONFIDENCE

ISBN: 978-0-323-39683-7

Notices

Knowledge and best practice in this field are constantly changing. As new research and experience broaden our understanding, changes in research methods, professional practices, or medical treatment may become necessary.

Practitioners and researchers must always rely on their own experience and knowledge in evaluating and using any information, methods, compounds, or experiments described herein. In using such information or methods, they should be mindful of their own safety and the safety of others, including parties for whom they have a professional responsibility.

With respect to any drug or pharmaceutical products identified, readers are advised to check the most current information provided (i) on procedures featured or (ii) by the manufacturer of each product to be administered, to verify the recommended dose or formula, the method and duration of administration, and contraindications. It is the responsibility of practitioners, relying on their own experience and knowledge of their patients, to make diagnoses, to determine dosages and the best treatment for each individual patient, and to take all appropriate safety precautions.

To the fullest extent of the law, neither the Publisher nor the authors, contributors, or editors, assume any liability for any injury and/or damage to persons or property as a matter of products liability, negligence or otherwise, or from any use or operation of any methods, products, instructions, or ideas contained in the material herein.

Library of Congress Cataloging-in-Publication Data

Names: Morris, Deborah C. Gray, author.
Title: Calculate with confidence / Deborah C. Gray Morris.
Description: Seventh edition. | St. Louis, Missouri : Elsevier, [2018] |
Includes bibliographical references and index.
Identifiers: LCCN 2017015434 | ISBN 9780323396837 (pbk. : alk. paper)
Subjects: | MESH: Drug Dosage Calculations | Nursing Care--methods |
Pharmaceutical Preparations--administration & dosage | Mathematics |
Problems and Exercises
Classification: LCC RS57 | NLM QV 18.2 | DDC
615/.1401513--dc23 LC record available at
https://lccn.loc.gov/ 2017015434

Senior Content Strategist: Yvonne Alexopoulos
Content Development Manager: Lisa Newton
Senior Content Development Specialist: Danielle M. Frazier
Publishing Services Manager: Jeff Patterson
Senior Project Manager: Tracey Schriefer
Design Direction: Ashley Miner

Printed in Canada

Last digit is the print number: 9 8 7 6 5 4

To my children, Cameron, Kimberly, Kanin, and Cory, thanks for your love and support. You light up my life. To my mother, your love, support, guidance, and nurturing helped me to become the person I am today. To my husband, Reggie, thank you for all the hard work you did in helping me with this edition. Your support and encouragement throughout this project kept me on track and focused.

To the two special additions and loves of my life, my two grandsons, Ryan and Eison, you touch my life more than you know.

Thank you to friends, nursing colleagues, and students past and present. To future and current practitioners of nursing, I hope this book will be valuable in teaching the principles of dosage calculation and reinforcing the importance of safety in administration of medications to all clients regardless of the setting.

Reviewers

Lou Ann Boose, RN, BSN, MSN
Professor
Department of Nursing
Harrisburg Area Community College
Harrisburg, Pennsylvania

Jessica Gonzales, ARNP, RN, MSN
Psychiatric Mental Health Nurse Practitioner
Harborview Medical Center
Seattle, Washington;
The Evergreen Clinic
Kirkland, Washington

Jane C. Parish, BBA, PhD, RN, CPN, CNE
Professor of Nursing
Walters State Community College
Morristown, Tennessee

Bobbi Steelman, BS, Ed, M.A.Ed, CPhT
Director of Education
Pharmacy Technician Program Director
Daymar College
Bowling Green, Kentucky

Anne S. Van Landingham, RN, BSN, MSN
Instructor
Orange Technical College - OCPS
Apopka High School
Apopka, Florida

Preface to the Instructor

INTRODUCTION

Safety is a priority in the delivery of health care. To advance client safety and its importance in health care delivery worldwide, several organizations are involved in reinforcing the promotion of client safety in health care, which includes emphasis on improving safety in medication administration. These organizations include the Institute of Medicine (IOM), the Institute for Safe Medication Practices (ISMP), and The Joint Commission (TJC).

The Quality and Safety Education for Nurses (QSEN) looks at six competencies, two of which are relevant to medication administration: safety and informatics. *Safety* refers to reducing the risk of harm to clients, and *informatics* refers to technology used to mitigate errors. Safety and informatics will be referred to in this text where applicable. The text uses the term *client* to denote one who is the recipient of nursing care and can also be referred to as *patient, resident,* and *health care consumer.*

The seventh edition of ***Calculate with Confidence*** not only teaches the aspects of dosage calculation; it also emphasizes the importance of safety in medication administration. ***Calculate with Confidence*** is written to meet the needs of nursing students as well as nurses returning to the workforce after being away from the clinical setting. It is also suitable for courses within nursing curricula whose content reflects the calculation of dosages and solutions. The text can generally be used as a reference by any health care professional whose responsibilities include safe administration of medications and solutions to clients in diverse clinical settings.

***Calculate with Confidence,* seventh edition,** has incorporated feedback from users of previous editions, including students, instructors, and reviewers. This edition has maintained a style similar to previous editions. The text presents three methods of dosage calculation—dimensional analysis, formula method, and ratio and proportion. Each method is illustrated, empowering students to choose the method that suits their learning style and works for them. It also enables the instructor to teach a preferred method or multiple methods to students.

The new edition responds to changes in the health care field and includes the introduction of new medications, discussion of new methods for medication administration, and an emphasis on clinical reasoning in prevention of medication errors. Principles of QSEN have been incorporated where applicable. An ample number of practice problems that include the shading of syringes where indicated continues to be featured to allow for visualization of dosages, reinforcement of clinical thinking skills, and prevention of medication errors. Safety alerts are also incorporated throughout the chapters to further reinforce the importance of error prevention in medication administration. Despite technological advances in equipment, health care professionals must continue to use clinical reasoning skills and have a consistent focus on safety to minimize the risk of harm to clients. Answers to practice problems include rationales to enhance understanding of principles and answers related to dosages. Answers have been placed at the end of chapters to allow for immediate feedback.

In response to the increased need for competency in basic math as an essential prerequisite for dosage calculation, practice problems in the basic math section are provided to allow the student to identify his or her strengths and weaknesses in basic math areas that provide the foundation for math skills applied in dosage calculation.

The once controversial use of calculators is now a more accepted practice, and they are used on many nursing examinations, including the NCLEX; however, their use is individualized. Many health care agencies have policies that require the use of calculators to verify calculations (e.g., critical care calculations) to avoid medication errors. A basic handheld calculator that has functions of addition, subtraction, multiplication, division, and a square root key is usually sufficient for medical dosage calculation, and students should know how to use such a calculator.

ORGANIZATION OF CONTENT

The seventh edition continues to be organized in a progression from simple topics to more complex ones, making content relevant to the needs of the student and using realistic practice problems to enhance learning and make material clinically applicable.

The 25 chapters are arranged into 5 units.

Unit One includes Chapters 1 through 5. This unit provides a review of basic arithmetic skills, including roman numerals, fractions, decimals, ratio and proportion, and percentages. A pre-test and post-test are included. This unit allows the student to determine his or her weaknesses and strengths in arithmetic and provides a review of basic math, which includes fractions, decimals, and ratio and proportion. Ample practice problems as well as word problems are included in the basic math sections.

Unit Two includes Chapters 6 through 9. Chapters 6 through 8 introduce the student to the three systems of measurement: metric, household, and apothecary. The metric system is emphasized, and some aspects relating to household measures are discussed because of their implications for care at home. Apothecary measures are not emphasized because they are outdated and not recommended for use. Apothecary measures have been placed in Appendix A. Chapter 9 provides conversions relating to temperature, length, weight, and international time. Calculation of completion times for IV therapy is also discussed.

Unit Three includes Chapters 10 through 16. This unit provides essential information that is needed as a foundation for dosage calculation and safe medication administration. Chapter 10 includes an expanded discussion of medication errors; routes of medication administration; equipment used in medication administration; the six basic rights of medication administration, as well as additional rights to be considered when administering medications; and the nursing role in preventing medication errors. Chapter 11 presents the abbreviations used in medication administration and interpretation of medication orders. Chapter 12 introduces students to medication administration records and has been updated to include the various medication distribution systems. Chapter 13 provides the student with the skills necessary to read medication labels to calculate dosages. Medication labels include medications in current use as well as some of the newer medication labels on the market. The important skill of reading labels is developed by providing practice with identification of information on labels. Resources that include TJC's official "Do Not Use" list and ISMP's list of Error-Prone Abbreviations, Symbols, and Dose Designations are emphasized and have been included in the appendices, along with other resources. Emphasis is placed on the nurse's responsibility to stay abreast of standards regarding medication orders to ensure client safety and prevent errors in medication administration. Chapters 14 through 16 introduce the various methods used for dosage calculation (ratio and proportion, formula method, and dimensional analysis). Practice problems are provided for each method, giving the student the opportunity to practice the various methods and choose the one preferred.

Unit Four includes Chapters 17 through 20. In Chapter 17, the student learns the principles and calculations related to oral medications (solid and liquids). In Chapter 18, the student learns about the various types of syringes and the skills needed for calculating injectable medications. Chapter 19 introduces concepts of solutions. Calculations associated with reconstituted solutions for injectable and oral medications are discussed. Calculations associated with preparation of noninjectable solutions, including nutritional feedings, determining the strength of solutions, and calculation of solutions, are also included. Chapter 20 introduces the student to insulin types, the addition of U-500 insulin, and calculations involving U-500 insulin. The chapter has also been expanded to include discussion of insulin pens and current information on the use of the sliding scale and basal prandial insulin therapy. Three methods of dosage calculation are illustrated in the chapters (ratio and proportion, formula method, and dimensional analysis), and practice problems are provided in each chapter.

Unit Five includes Chapters 21 through 25. Chapters 21 and 22 provide a discussion of intravenous (IV) fluids and associated calculations related to IV therapy. Content includes focus on safety with IV administration and recalculating IV flow rate with an alternative method of determining the percentage of variation. IV labels have been added throughout the chapter, with a discussion of additives to IV solutions. Chapter 23 presents a discussion of heparin and has been updated to include the new heparin labels. Heparin weight-based protocol has been expanded to include adjusting IV heparin based on activated partial thromboplastin time (APTT). Chapter 24 provides the student with the skills necessary to calculate critical care IV medications. Titration of IV flow rates for titrated medications is explained, as well as how to develop a titration table. Additional practice problems have also been added to the chapter. Chapter 25 provides the student with the skills and principles for calculation of pediatric and adult dosages, with emphasis on calculation based on body weight and verification of safe dosages. Calculation of daily fluid maintenance for children has also been included, with practice problems.

Safety Alerts, Practice Problems, Clinical Reasoning scenarios, and Points to Remember are included throughout the text. A Comprehensive Post-Test is included at the end of the text and includes practice problems covering content from all 25 chapters.

NEW FEATURES TO THE SEVENTH EDITION

- Update of the insulin chapter (Chapter 20)
- Addition of new medication labels
- Additional practice problems throughout the text
- Continual integration of QSEN principles and competencies in text to alert the student to the importance of client safety and reduction of medication errors
- Expansion of content relating to medication errors, including the use of tall man lettering and in-depth discussion of the six basic rights of medication administration and additional rights of medication administration
- Addition of appendices that include the apothecary system, TJC's official "Do Not Use" list, ISMP standards, and a medication label index that includes labels found in the text
- Calculation of daily fluid maintenance
- Updating of section on intake and output to include basic and complex
- Updating of the IV chapter to include content on the Dial-A-Flow IV infusion device
- Addition of new heparin labels
- Increased discussion on preventing medication errors in chapters dealing with high-alert medications (heparin and insulin)
- Additional Safety Alert boxes to direct the student to common errors that can be made

ANCILLARIES

Evolve Resources for ***Calculate with Confidence*, seventh edition,** are available to enhance student instruction. These online resources can be found at http://evolve.elsevier.com/GrayMorris/.

These resources correspond with the chapters of the main book and includes the following:

- Student Review Questions and Sample NCLEX Review Questions
- NEW! Elsevier's Interactive Drug Calculation Application, version 1: This interactive drug calculation application provides hands-on, interactive practice for the user to master drug calculations. Users can select the mode (Study, Exam, or Comprehensive Exam) and then the category for study and exam modes. There are eight categories that cover the main drug calculation topics. Users are also able to select the number of problems they want to complete and their preferred drug calculation method. A calculator is available for easy access within any mode, and the application also provides history of the work done by the user. There are 750 practice problems in this application.

It is my hope that this book will be a valuable asset to current and future practitioners. May it help you calculate dosages accurately and with confidence, using calculation and critical thinking skills to ensure that medications are administered safely to all clients regardless of the setting. This is both a priority and a primary responsibility of the nurse.

Deborah C. Gray Morris

Acknowledgments

I wish to extend sincere gratitude and appreciation to my family, friends, and colleagues at Bronx Community College of the City University of New York (CUNY) for their support and encouragement during the writing of the seventh edition. A special thanks to my daughter-in-law who we call Marcy (Marcella Willis-Gray, MD) for taking the time out of her busy schedule to answer questions relating to medication orders and researching information for me regarding specific dosages of medications and calculations when indicated. A special thanks to Professor Lois Augustus, former chairperson of the Department of Nursing and Allied Health Sciences, for all of her encouragement. A special thank you to my colleague, Mr. Clarence Hodge (Lecturer), who currently teaches Pharmacology Computations with me; your feedback, suggestions, and validation of answers while revising this text were invaluable. Thank you to Professor Helen Papas-Kavalis for your help with questions regarding pediatrics. Special thanks also to the reviewers of this text; your comments and suggestions were invaluable. Particular thanks to the math reviewers. A special thanks to Dr. Andrew McInerney, Professor in the Department of Mathematics and Computer Science at Bronx Community College, for your help with checking my mathematical answers and the suggestions you made when indicated.

Thanks to past students at Bronx Community College who brought questions regarding basic math and calculations and helped me have an appreciation for the problems that students encounter with basic math and calculation of medication dosages. Thanks for your valuable feedback.

I am particularly grateful to former colleagues who provided me with the encouragement and nurturing I needed to consider publication. Who would have thought this book would now be in its seventh edition? Thank you to Professor Germana Glier, former chairperson of Mathematics and Computer Science at Bronx Community College; your mathematical expertise was invaluable. Thanks to former Chairpersons of The Department of Mathematics and Computer Sciences at Bronx Community College, Professor Germana Glier and the late Dr. Gerald S. Lieblich, whose mathematical expertise was invaluable.

I am especially grateful to the staff at Elsevier for their support and help in planning, writing, and producing the seventh edition of this text. A special thanks to Danielle M. Frazier for her time, support, patience, and understanding with this revision; thanks for your encouragement and sincere concern at the times when I needed them most. Thanks also to Tracey L. Schriefer, whose help was invaluable in revising this text.

To Anna Nunnally, my dearest friend who is like a sister, thanks for all of your support and encouragement. To my friend the late Frank A. Rucker, your encouragement, inspiring words, and admiration for me as an author will always remain with me. A special note of thanks to Professor Ellen Hoist, a colleague and friend who has given me encouragement and support from the beginning with the first edition of this text. You could see the potential for this text beyond the first edition even when I expressed doubt.

Thank you to all!

Deborah C. Gray Morris

Contents

Unit One Math Review 1

Pre-Test 2

1 Roman Numerals 6

2 Fractions 11
- Types of Fractions 12
- Converting Fractions 13
- Comparing Fractions 13
- Reducing Fractions 15
- Adding Fractions 16
- Subtracting Fractions 17
- Multiplying Fractions 19
- Dividing Fractions 20

3 Decimals 28
- Reading and Writing Decimals 29
- Comparing the Value of Decimals 31
- Adding and Subtracting Decimals 32
- Multiplying Decimals 34
- Dividing Decimals 35
- Rounding Off Decimals 37
- Changing Fractions to Decimals 39
- Changing Decimals to Fractions 39

4 Ratio and Proportion 44
- Ratios 44
- Proportions 45
- Solving for x in Ratio and Proportion 46
- Applying Ratio and Proportion to Dosage Calculation 48

5 Percentages 55
- Converting Percentages to Fractions, Decimals, and Ratios 56
- Percentage Measures 59
- Comparing Percents and Ratios 60
- Determining the Percent of a Quantity 61
- Determining What Percent One Number Is of Another 61
- Calculating the Percent of Change 63

Post-Test 69

Unit Two Systems of Measurement 73

6 Metric System 74
Particulars of the Metric System 74
Rules of the Metric System 77
Units of Measure 78
Conversions Between Metric Units 80

7 Apothecary and Household Systems 85
Apothecary System 85
Household System 86
Other Medication Measurements Used in Dosage Calculation 88

8 Converting Within and Between Systems 92
Equivalents Among Metric and Household Systems 92
Converting 92
Methods of Converting 93
Converting Within the Same System 96
Converting Between Systems 97
Calculating Intake and Output 100

9 Additional Conversions Useful in the Health Care Setting 111
Converting Between Celsius and Fahrenheit 111
Formulas for Converting Between Fahrenheit and Celsius Scales 112
Metric Measures Relating to Length 113
Conversions Relating to Weight 115
Military Time 117
Calculating Completion Times 119

Unit Three Methods of Administration and Calculation 125

10 Medication Administration 126
Medication Errors 126
Critical Thinking and Medication Administration 130
Factors That Influence Medication Dosages and Action 130
Special Considerations for the Elderly 131
The Rights of Medication Administration 132
Medication Reconciliation 137
Client Education 138
Home Care Considerations 139
Routes of Medication Administration 140
Equipment Used for Medication Administration 142
Equipment for Administering Oral Medications to a Child 144

11 Understanding and Interpreting Medication Orders 149
Verbal Orders 150
Transcription of Medication Orders 151
Writing a Medication Order 152
Components of a Medication Order 153
Interpreting a Medication Order 156

12 Medication Administration Records and Medication Distribution Systems 164
Medication Orders 164
Medication Administration Record 165
Essential Components on a Medication Record 167
Documentation of Medications Administered 168
Explanation of Medication Administration Records 169
Use of Computers in Medication Administration 169
Medication Distribution Systems 170

Advantages and Disadvantages of Technology 173
Scheduling Medication Times 174
Military Time 174

13 Reading Medication Labels 179
Reading Medication Labels 179

14 Dosage Calculation Using the Ratio and Proportion Method 219
Use of Ratio and Proportion in Dosage Calculation 219

15 Dosage Calculation Using the Formula Method 248
Formula for Calculating Dosages 248
Using the Formula Method 249

16 Dosage Calculation Using the Dimensional Analysis Method 270
Understanding the Basics of Dimensional Analysis 270
Dosage Calculation Using Dimensional Analysis 273

Unit Four Oral and Parenteral Dosage Forms and Insulin 291

17 Oral Medications 292
Forms of Solid Medications 292
Calculating Oral Liquids 317
Measuring Oral Liquids 318

18 Parenteral Medications 359
Parenteral Medication Packaging 359
Syringes 362
Reading Parenteral Labels 371
Medications Labeled in Percentage Strengths 376
Solutions Expressed in Ratio Strength 377
Parenteral Medications Measured in Units 377
Parenteral Medications in Milliequivalents 378
Calculating Parenteral Dosages 379
Calculating Injectable Medications According to the Syringe 380
Calculating Dosages for Medications in Units 384
Mixing Medications in the Same Syringe 386

19 Reconstitution of Solutions 427
Basic Principles for Reconstitution 428
Reconstituting Medications with More Than One Direction for Mixing (Multiple Strength) 438
Reconstitution from Package Insert Directions and Medications with Different Reconstitution Directions Depending on Route of Administration 441
Medications with Instructions to "See Accompanying Literature" (Package Insert) for Reconstitution and Administration 441
Calculation of Dosages 443
Reconstitution of Noninjectable Solutions 445

20 Insulin 482
Types of Insulin 483
Labels 483
Insulin Action Times 484
Appearance of Insulin 487
Insulin Administration 488
Insulin Orders 496
Current Recommendations for Use of the Sliding Scale Protocol 497
Preparing a Single Dosage of Insulin in an Insulin Syringe 497
Measuring Two Types of Insulin in the Same Syringe 498

Unit Five Intravenous, Heparin, and Critical Care Calculations and Pediatric and Adult Calculations Based on Weight 513

21 Intravenous Solutions and Equipment 514
IV Delivery Methods 515
IV Solutions 515
Administration of IV Fluids 521

22 Intravenous Calculations 536
IV Flow Rate Calculation 536
Manually Regulated IVs 539
Calculating Flow Rates in Drops Per Minute Using a Formula 543
Calculating IV Flow Rates When Several Solutions Are Ordered 554
Calculating IV Flow Rates Using a Dial-A-Flow Controller 556
Calculating Intermittent IV Infusions Piggyback 556
Determining the Amount of Medication in a Specific Amount of Solution 560
Determining Infusion Times and Volumes 562
Steps to Calculating a Problem with an Unknown with the Formula Method 562
Recalculating an IV Flow Rate 565
Calculating Total Infusion Times 570
Calculating Infusion Time When Rate in mL/hr Is Not Indicated for Large Volumes of Fluid 572
Calculating Infusion Time for Small Volumes of Fluid 574
Charting IV Therapy 575
Labeling Solution Bags 575
Administration of Medications by IV Push 576

23 Heparin Calculations 603
Heparin Errors 603
Heparin Dosage Strengths 604
Reading Heparin Labels 605
Calculation of Subcutaneous Dosages 606
Calculation of IV Heparin Solutions 607
Calculating Heparin Dosages Based on Weight 609

24 Critical Care Calculations 629
Calculating Rate in mL/hr 630
Calculating Critical Care Dosages per Hour or per Minute 631
Medications Ordered in Milligrams per Minute 632
Calculating Dosages Based on mcg/kg/min 633
IV Flow Rates for Titrated Medications 634
Developing a Titration Table 636

25 Pediatric and Adult Dosage Calculations Based on Weight 657
Pediatric Medication Dosages 659
Principles Relating to Basic Calculations 659
Calculation of Dosages Based on Body Weight 659
Converting Pounds to Kilograms 660
Converting Kilograms to Pounds 662
Converting Grams to Kilograms 664
Adult Dosages Based on Body Weight 676
Calculating Pediatric Dosages Using Body Surface Area 681
Reading the West Nomogram Chart 683
Calculating Body Surface Area Using a Formula 684
Dosage Calculation Based on Body Surface Area 687
Calculating Using a Formula 688
IV Therapy and Children 690
Calculating IV Medications Using Volume Control Set 692
Determining Whether an IV Dose Is Safe for Children 695
Calculation of Daily Fluid Maintenance 696
Pediatric Oral and Parenteral Medications 698

Comprehensive Post-Test 720

References 742
Appendix A: Apothecary System 744
Appendix B: FDA and ISMP Lists of Look-Alike Drug Names with Recommended Tall Man Letters 745
Appendix C: TJC's "Do Not Use" List of Abbreviations 751
Appendix D: ISMP's List of Error-Prone Abbreviations, Symbols, and Dose Designations 752
Appendix E: ISMP List of High-Alert Medications in Acute Care Settings 754
Appendix F: ISMP List of High-Alert Medications in Community/Ambulatory Healthcare 755
Index 756
Drug Label Index 766

UNIT ONE

Math Review

An essential role of the nurse is providing safe medication administration to all clients. To accurately perform dosage calculations, the nurse must have knowledge of basic math, regardless of the problem-solving method used in calculation. Knowledge of basic math is a necessary component of dosage calculation that nurses need to know to prevent medication errors and ensure the safe administration of medications to all clients, regardless of the setting. Serious harm to clients can result from a mathematical error during calculation and administration of a medication dosage. The nurse must practice and be proficient in the basic math used in dosage calculations. Knowledge of basic math is a prerequisite for the prevention of medication errors and ensures the safe administration of medications.

Although calculators are accessible for basic math operations, the nurse needs to be able to perform the processes involved in basic math. Controversy still exists among educators regarding the use of calculators in dosage calculation. Calculators may indeed be recommended for complex calculations to ensure accuracy and save time; the types of calculations requiring their use are presented later in this text. However, because the basic math required for less complex calculations is often simple and can be done without the use of a calculator, it is a realistic expectation that each practitioner should be competent in the performance of basic math operations without its use. Performing basic math operations enables the nurse to think logically and critically about the dosage ordered and the dosage calculated.

Pre-Test

Chapter 1 Roman Numerals

Chapter 2 Fractions

Chapter 3 Decimals

Chapter 4 Ratio and Proportion

Chapter 5 Percentages

Post-Test

PRE-TEST

This test is designed to evaluate your ability in the basic math areas reviewed in Unit One. The test consists of 72 questions. If you are able to complete the pre-test with 100% accuracy, you may want to bypass Unit One. Any problems answered incorrectly should be used as a basis for what you might need to review. The purposes of this test and the review that follows are to build your confidence in basic math skills and to help you avoid careless mistakes when you begin to perform dosage calculations.

Express the following in Roman numerals.

1. 9 ______________
2. 16 ______________
3. 23 ______________
4. $10\frac{1}{2}$ ______________
5. 22 ______________

Express the following in Arabic numbers.

6. $\overline{\text{xiss}}$ ______________
7. $\overline{\text{xii}}$ ______________
8. $\overline{\text{xviii}}$ ______________
9. $\overline{\text{xxiv}}$ ______________
10. $\overline{\text{vi}}$ ______________

Reduce the following fractions to lowest terms.

11. $\frac{14}{21}$ ______________
12. $\frac{25}{100}$ ______________
13. $\frac{2}{150}$ ______________
14. $\frac{24}{30}$ ______________
15. $\frac{24}{36}$ ______________

Perform the indicated operations; reduce to lowest terms where necessary.

16. $\frac{2}{3} \div \frac{3}{9} =$ ______________
17. $4 \div \frac{3}{4} =$ ______________
18. $\frac{2}{5} + \frac{1}{9} =$ ______________
19. $7\frac{1}{7} - 2\frac{5}{6} =$ ______________
20. $4\frac{2}{3} \times 4 =$ ______________
21. $3\frac{5}{6} + 5\frac{2}{3} =$ ______________
22. $5\frac{6}{7} + 3\frac{5}{7} =$ ______________
23. $2\frac{1}{6} - 1\frac{1}{4} =$ ______________
24. $9 - \frac{3}{5} =$ ______________
25. $4\frac{1}{4} - 1\frac{3}{4} =$ ______________
26. $7\frac{1}{5} - 1\frac{3}{4} =$ ______________
27. $7 - \frac{9}{16} =$ ______________
28. $3\frac{3}{10} - 1\frac{7}{10} =$ ______________

Change the following fractions to decimals; express your answer to the nearest tenth.

29. $\frac{6}{7}$ ______________________

30. $\frac{6}{20}$ ______________________

31. $\frac{2}{3}$ ______________________

32. $\frac{7}{8}$ ______________________

Indicate the largest fraction in each group.

33. $\frac{3}{4}, \frac{4}{5}, \frac{7}{8}$ ______________________

34. $\frac{7}{12}, \frac{11}{12}, \frac{4}{12}$ ______________________

Perform the indicated operations with decimals. Provide the exact answer; do not round off.

35. $20.1 + 67.35 =$ ______________________

36. $0.008 + 5 =$ ______________________

37. $4.6 \times 8.72 =$ ______________________

38. $56.47 - 8.7 =$ ______________________

Divide the following decimals; express your answer to the nearest tenth.

39. $7.5 \div 0.004 =$ ______________________

40. $45 \div 1.9 =$ ______________________

41. $84.7 \div 2.3 =$ ______________________

Indicate the largest decimal in each group.

42. 0.674, 0.659 ______________________

43. 0.375, 0.37, 0.38 ______________________

44. 0.25, 0.6, 0.175 ______________________

Solve for *x*, the unknown value.

45. $8:2 = 48:x$ ______________________

46. $x:300 = 1:150$ ______________________

47. $\frac{1}{10}:x = \frac{1}{2}:15$ ______________________

48. $0.1:1 = 0.2:x$ ______________________

Round off to the nearest tenth.

49. 0.43 ______________________

50. 0.66 ______________________

51. 1.47 ______________________

Round off to the nearest hundredth.

52. 0.735 ______________________

53. 0.834 ______________________

54. 1.227 ______________________

Complete the table below, expressing the measures in their equivalents where indicated. Reduce to lowest terms where necessary.

	Percent	Decimal	Ratio	Fraction
55.	6%	______	______	______
56.	______	______	7:20	______
57.	______	______	______	$5\frac{1}{4}$
58.	______	0.015	______	______

Find the following percentages. Express your answer to the hundredths place as indicated.

59. 5% of 95 ______________

60. $\frac{1}{4}$% of 2,000 ______________

61. 2 is what % of 600 ______________

62. 20 is what % of 100 ______________

63. 30 is what % of 164 ______________

64. A client is instructed to take $1\frac{1}{2}$ teaspoons of a cough syrup three (3) times a day. How many teaspoons of cough syrup will the client take each day?

____

65. A tablet contains 0.75 milligrams (mg) of a medication. A client receives three (3) tablets a day for five (5) days. How many mg of the medication will the client receive in five (5) days? ______________

66. A client took 0.44 micrograms (mcg) of a medication every morning and 1.4 mcg each evening for five (5) days. What is the total amount of medication taken?

____

67. Write a ratio that represents that every tablet in a bottle contains 0.5 milligrams (mg) of a medication. ______________

68. Write a ratio that represents 60 milligrams (mg) of a medication in 1 milliliter (mL) of a liquid. ______________

69. A client takes 10 milliliters (mL) of a medication three (3) times a day. How long will 120 mL of medication last? ______________

70. A client weighed 275 pounds (lb) before dieting. After dieting, the client weighed 250 lb. What is the percentage of change in the client's weight? ______________

71. A client was prescribed 10 milligrams (mg) of a medication for a week. After a week, the health care provider reduced the medication to seven (7) mg. What was the percentage of decrease in medication? ______________

72. A client received 22.5 milligrams (mg) of a medication in tablet form. Each tablet contained 4.5 mg of medication. How many tablets were given to the client? ______________

Answers on p. 5

ANSWERS

1. ix, $\overline{\text{ix}}$, IX
2. xvi, $\overline{\text{xvi}}$, XVI
3. xxiii, $\overline{\text{xxiii}}$, XXIII
4. xss, $\overline{\text{xss}}$
5. xxii, $\overline{\text{xxii}}$, XXII
6. $11\frac{1}{2}$
7. 12
8. 18
9. 24
10. 6
11. $\frac{2}{3}$
12. $\frac{1}{4}$
13. $\frac{1}{75}$
14. $\frac{4}{5}$
15. $\frac{2}{3}$
16. 2
17. $5\frac{1}{3}$
18. $\frac{23}{45}$
19. $4\frac{13}{42}$
20. $18\frac{2}{3}$
21. $9\frac{3}{6} = 9\frac{1}{2}$
22. $8\frac{11}{7} = 9\frac{4}{7}$
23. $\frac{11}{12}$
24. $8\frac{2}{5}$
25. $2\frac{2}{4} = 2\frac{1}{2}$
26. $5\frac{9}{20}$
27. $6\frac{7}{16}$
28. $1\frac{6}{10} = 1\frac{3}{5}$
29. 0.9
30. 0.3
31. 0.7
32. 0.9
33. $\frac{7}{8}$
34. $\frac{11}{12}$
35. 87.45
36. 5.008
37. 40.112
38. 47.77
39. 1,875
40. 23.7
41. 36.8
42. 0.674
43. 0.38
44. 0.6
45. $x = 12$
46. $x = 2$
47. $x = 3$
48. $x = 2$
49. 0.4
50. 0.7
51. 1.5
52. 0.74
53. 0.83
54. 1.23

	Percent	Decimal	Ratio	Fraction
55.	6%	0.06	3:50	$\frac{3}{50}$
56.	35%	0.35	7:20	$\frac{7}{20}$
57.	525%	5.25	21:4	$5\frac{1}{4}$
58.	1.5%	0.015	3:200	$\frac{3}{200}$

59. 4.75
60. 5
61. 0.33%
62. 20%
63. 18.29%
64. $4\frac{1}{2}$ teaspoons
65. 11.25 milligrams (mg)
66. 9.2 micrograms (mcg)
67. 0.5 mg : 1 tablet
68. 60 mg : 1 mL
69. 4 days
70. 9%
71. 30%
72. 5 tablets

CHAPTER **1**

Roman Numerals

Objectives

After reviewing this chapter, you should be able to:

1. Recognize the symbols used to represent numbers in the Roman numeral system
2. Convert Roman numerals to Arabic numbers
3. Convert Arabic numbers to Roman numerals

The Roman numeral system dates back to ancient Roman times and uses letters to designate amounts. Although it appears that Roman numerals are obsolete, they are still in use in the modern times. There are no commas or zeros in this system. Roman numerals are arranged and combined in a specific order to represent numbers.

Box 1-1 lists the common Arabic equivalents for Roman numerals (review them if necessary). They are often expressed with lowercase letters. Review this list before proceeding to the rules pertaining to Roman numerals. You will most commonly see Roman numerals up to the value of 30 when they are used in relation to medications. Larger Roman numerals, such as L(l) = 50, C(c) = 100, and larger, are usually not used in relation to medications. It is recommended to use uppercase letters when smaller numbers are part of a number over 30, for example, 60 = LX not lx.

BOX 1-1 Arabic Equivalents for Roman Numerals

Arabic Number	Roman Numeral	Arabic Number	Roman Numeral
½	ss or $\overline{ss}$	9	ix or $\overline{ix}$, IX
1	i or $\overline{i}$, I	10	x or $\overline{x}$, X
2	ii or $\overline{ii}$, II	15	xv or $\overline{xv}$, XV
3	iii or $\overline{iii}$, III	20	xx or $\overline{xx}$, XX
4	iv or $\overline{iv}$, IV	30	xxx or $\overline{xxx}$, XXX
5	v or $\overline{v}$, V	50	L(l)
6	vi or $\overline{vi}$, VI	100	C(c)
7	vii or $\overline{vii}$, VII	500	D(d)
8	viii or $\overline{viii}$, VIII	1,000	M(m)

Although the Roman numerals for 50, 100, 500, and 1,000 are not used in relation to medications, a well-known mnemonic: "**L**ovely **C**ats **D**on't **M**eow," can help you to remember the order and value of the Roman numerals (L, C, D, M) for 50, 100, 500, and 1,000 (Box 1-2).

BOX 1-2 Mnemonic Device: Note the pattern:

50-100-500-1,000

L = 50	**Lovely**
C = 100	**Cats**
D = 500	**Don't**
M = 1,000	**Meow**

RULE

Rules Relating to the Roman System of Notation

1. The same Roman numeral is never repeated more than three times.
   a. Example: Convert the Arabic number 4 to a Roman numeral.
      i. Right: 4 = iv
      ii. Wrong: 4 = iiii
   b. Example: Convert the Arabic number 9 to a Roman numeral.
      i. Right: 9 = ix
      ii. Wrong: 9 = viiii
2. When a Roman numeral of a lesser value is placed **after** one of equal or greater value, the numerals are **added.**
   a. Example: Convert the Arabic number 25 to a Roman numeral.
      i. Right: 25 = xxv (10 + 10 + 5 = 25)
   b. Example: Convert the Roman numeral xvi to an Arabic number.
      i. Right: xvi = 16 (10 + 5 + 1 = 16)
3. When a Roman numeral of a lesser value is placed **before** a numeral of greater value, the numerals are **subtracted.**
   a. Example: Convert the Roman numerals ix and xxiv to Arabic numbers.
      i. Right: ix = 9 (10 − 1 = 9)
      ii. Right: xxiv = 24 [10 + 10 + (5 − 1) = 24]
   b. Example: Convert the Arabic numbers 19 and 14 to Roman numerals.
      i. Right: 19 = xix [10 + (10 − 1) = 19]
      ii. Right: 14 = xiv [10 + (5 − 1) = 14]

Roman numerals are still used today. An example of their current use is hour marks on time pieces (e.g., watches, clocks). In this context, inconsistencies can be seen. Some clock faces that use Roman numerals show IIII for four o'clock (as opposed to IV) but IX for nine o'clock. The clock on the Palace of Westminster in London (also known as "Big Ben") uses IV to indicate four o'clock. Other uses include names of monarchs and popes (e.g., Louis XIV, Pope Benedict XVI); Super Bowl XXVII, sequels of movies (e.g., *Rocky IV*); generational suffixes, particularly in the United States, for people sharing the same name across generations (e.g., Robert Griffin III); car styles (e.g., Mach V); and Mach V computers.

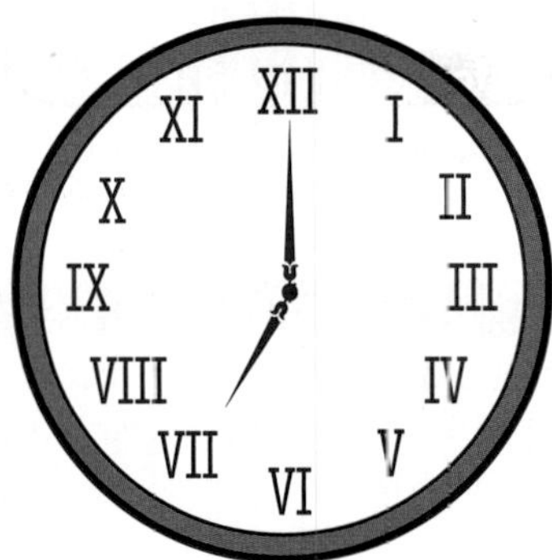

Roman numerals are used in the apothecary system of measurement for writing medication dosages.

Example:

gr x

Apothecary measure (unit of weight) ← → Roman numeral (Arabic equivalent 10)

Roman numerals are also seen on the labels of medications to designate Drug Enforcement Administration (DEA) schedules for controlled substances (medications that can lead to abuse or dependence). Controlled substances can be readily recognized by a large "C" (control) on the medication label. A Roman numeral (I–V), written as a capital letter, is inserted in the center of the "C" to indicate the potential for abuse, as shown in Figures 1-1 and 1-2. This will be discussed in more detail in Chapter 13, Reading Medication Labels.

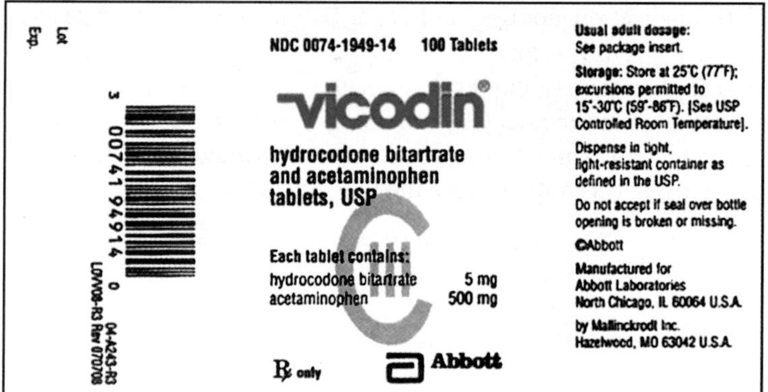

Figure 1-1 Vicodin (hydrocodone bitartrate and acetaminophen) is a controlled substance schedule III medication as indicated by CIII on the label.

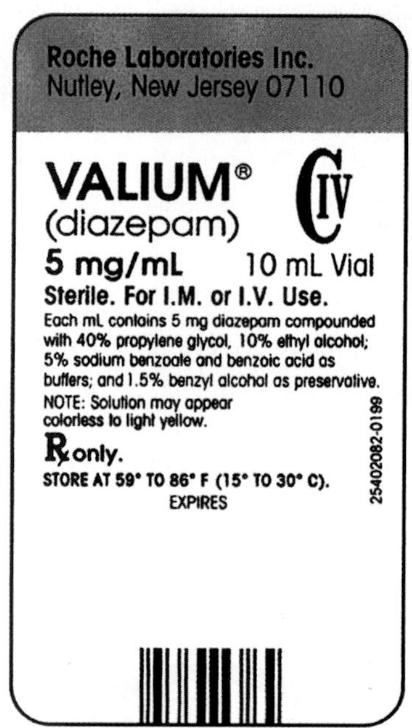

Figure 1-2 Valium (diazepam) is a controlled substance schedule IV as indicated by CIV on the label.

SAFETY ALERT!

Use caution when interpreting the controlled substance schedule. Misinterpretation of the symbol for a controlled substance can lead to a medication error. For example, Schedule IV can be misinterpreted for intravenous (IV) route (how the medication is administered).

Roman numerals are also used to identify different clotting factors found in a person's blood. For example, Factor I (Fibrinogen) and Factor III (Thromboplastin).

Each of the 12 cranial nerves has a name and corresponding Roman numeral (e.g., I is the olfactory nerve [sense of smell] and VII is the facial nerve). In chemistry, Roman numerals are often used to denote the groups of the periodic table (e.g., Group IIA denotes elements that have two valence electrons).

In the Arabic system, numbers, not letters, are used to express amounts. The Arabic system also uses fractions ($\frac{1}{2}$) and decimals (0.5).

Most medication dosages are ordered using metric measurements (e.g., 1 gram [g], 500 milligrams [mg]) and Arabic numbers; however, on rare occasions, medication orders may include a Roman numeral.

Example: Aspirin gr x, which is correctly interpreted as aspirin 10 grains

To calculate medication dosages and assist in the prevention of medication errors, nurses need to know both Roman numerals and Arabic numbers. Lowercase letters are usually used to express Roman numerals in relation to medications. The Roman numerals you will see most often in the calculation of dosages are built on the basic symbols *i*, *v*, and *x*. To prevent errors in interpretation, a line is sometimes drawn over the symbol. If this line is used, the lowercase "i" is dotted above the line, not below.

Example 1: 10 grains = gr x

Example 2: 2 = $\overline{\text{ii}}$

SAFETY ALERT!

Correctly identifying Roman numerals will assist in preventing medication errors. According to the Institute for Safe Medication Practices (ISMP), abbreviations increase the risk for occurrence of medication errors. Although some health care providers may still use Roman numerals and the apothecary system, the ISMP recommends using the metric system.

RULE

As illustrated in the example, with apothecary measures, the label *grains* when abbreviated (*gr*) precedes the Roman numeral.

When the symbol for $\frac{1}{2}$ (ss) is used in conjunction with Roman numerals, the symbol is placed at the end.

Example 1: $3\frac{1}{2}$ = $\overline{\text{iii}}$ss or $\overline{\text{iiiss}}$

Example 2: $1\frac{1}{2}$ = grains = gr $\overline{\text{i}}$ss or gr $\overline{\text{iss}}$

PRACTICE **PROBLEMS**

Write the following as Roman numerals.

1. 15 ______
2. 13 ______
3. 28 ______
4. 11 ______
5. 17 ______
6. 65 ______
7. 1,001 ______
8. 69 ______

Write the following as Arabic numbers.

9. xiv ______
10. xxix ______
11. iv ______
12. xix ______
13. xxxiv ______
14. CC ______
15. MVIII ______
16. MCMIV ______

Answers on p. 10

CHAPTER REVIEW

Write the following Arabic numbers as Roman numerals.

1. 6 ____________
2. 30 ____________
3. $1\frac{1}{2}$ ____________
4. 27 ____________
5. 12 ____________
6. 18 ____________
7. 20 ____________
8. 3 ____________
9. 21 ____________
10. 26 ____________
11. 150 ____________
12. 999 ____________
13. 400 ____________

Write the following Roman numerals as Arabic numbers.

14. $\overline{\text{viiss}}$ ____________
15. $\overline{\text{xix}}$ ____________
16. $\overline{\text{xv}}$ ____________
17. $\overline{\text{xxx}}$ ____________
18. $\overline{\text{ss}}$ ____________
19. $\overline{\text{iii}}$ ____________
20. $\overline{\text{xxii}}$ ____________
21. $\overline{\text{xvi}}$ ____________
22. $\overline{\text{v}}$ ____________
23. $\overline{\text{xxvii}}$ ____________
24. XC ____________
25. LXXV ____________
26. DXIV ____________
27. LXIII ____________
28. MCMXVI ____________
29. CCVII ____________
30. MLXVI ____________

Answers below

ANSWERS

Chapter 1

Answers to Practice Problems

1. xv, $\overline{\text{xv}}$, XV
2. xiii, $\overline{\text{xiii}}$, XIII
3. xxviii, $\overline{\text{xxviii}}$, XXVIII
4. xi, $\overline{\text{xi}}$, XI
5. xvii, $\overline{\text{xvii}}$, XVII
6. LXV
7. MI
8. LXIX
9. 14
10. 29
11. 4
12. 19
13. 34
14. 200
15. 1,008
16. 1,904

Answers to Chapter Review

1. vi, $\overline{\text{vi}}$, VI
2. xxx, $\overline{\text{xxx}}$, XXX
3. iss, $\overline{\text{iss}}$, iss
4. xxvii, $\overline{\text{xxvii}}$, XXVII
5. xii, $\overline{\text{xii}}$, XII
6. xviii, $\overline{\text{xviii}}$, XVIII
7. xx, $\overline{\text{xx}}$, XX
8. iii, $\overline{\text{iii}}$, III
9. xxi, $\overline{\text{xxi}}$, XXI
10. xxvi, $\overline{\text{xxvi}}$, XXVI
11. CL
12. IM
13. CD
14. $7\frac{1}{2}$
15. 19
16. 15
17. 30
18. $\frac{1}{2}$
19. 3
20. 22
21. 16
22. 5
23. 27
24. 90
25. 75
26. 514
27. 63
28. 1,916
29. 207
30. 1,066

CHAPTER 2
Fractions

Objectives

After reviewing this chapter, you should be able to:

1. Compare the size of fractions
2. Add fractions
3. Subtract fractions
4. Divide fractions
5. Multiply fractions
6. Reduce fractions to lowest terms

Health care professionals need to have an understanding of fractions. Fractions may be seen in medical orders, client records, prescriptions, documentation relating to care given to clients, and literature related to health care. Nurses often encounter fractions when converting metric to household measures in dosage calculation.

Fractions may be used occasionally in the writing of a medication order or used by the pharmaceutical manufacturer on a medication label (which usually includes the metric equivalent). According to *Medication Errors,* abridged edition (2010), edited by Michael R. Cohen, president of the Institute for Safe Medication Practices (ISMP), "Occasionally using fractions instead of metric designation could help prevent errors (Figure 2-1). For example, the dosage embossed on 2.5 mg Coumadin tablets is expressed as '$2\frac{1}{2}$ mg' to prevent confusion with 25 mg."

Coumadin is an anticoagulant. An overdose of Coumadin (example: 25 mg instead of $2\frac{1}{2}$ mg) can result in a serious adverse effect, such as a severe hemorrhage.

As you will see later in the text, some methods of solving dosage calculations rely on expressing relationships in a fraction format. Therefore, proficiency with fractions can be beneficial in a variety of situations.

A fraction represents a part of a whole (Figure 2-2). It is written as two quantities: an upper number referred to as the **numerator** (parts of the whole) and a **denominator,** the bottom part of the fraction that represents the whole. The numerator and denominator are separated by a horizontal line. The horizontal line above the denominator is a division sign; therefore a fraction may also be read as the numerator divided by the denominator.

$$\frac{\text{numerator}}{\text{denominator}} \leftarrow \text{horizontal bar (division sign)}$$

Examples: Suppose you have to administer a medication that is scored (marked) for division into four parts to a client and you must administer one part of the tablet. The denominator represents the whole tablet and the numerator represents the amount you administer. The fraction, or part, of the tablet you administer is written as:

$$\frac{\text{Numerator}}{\text{Denominator}} = \frac{1 \text{ part}}{4 \text{ parts}} = \frac{1}{4}$$

This number is read as one-fourth. The denominator is 4 because 4 parts make up the whole. If you administer one part, you administer $\frac{1}{4}$ of the tablet.

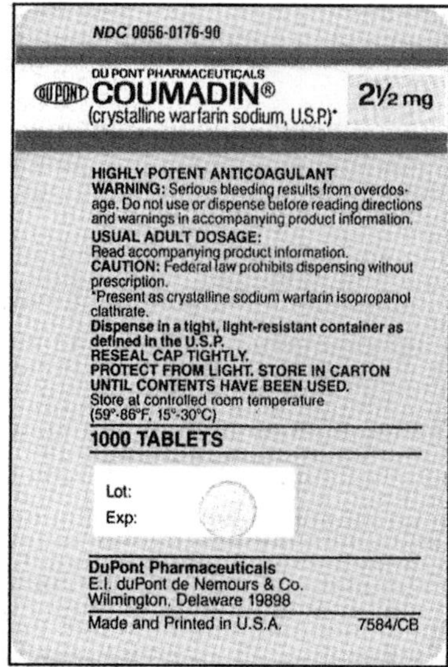

Figure 2-1 Coumadin label.

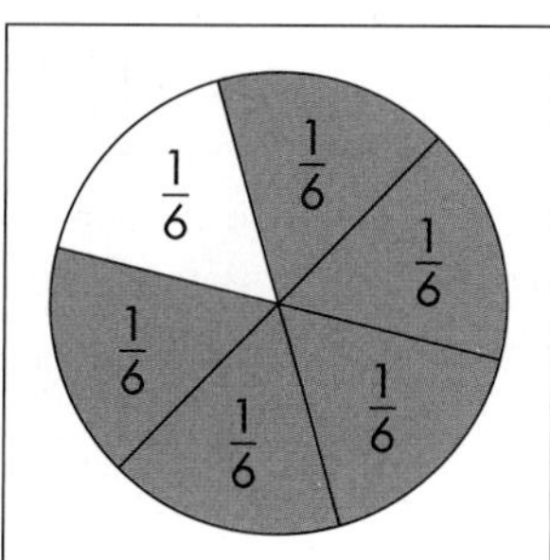

Figure 2-2 The shaded part of the circle, which is 5 parts, reflects the numerator, and the total number of parts (6) is the denominator. Therefore $\frac{5}{6}$ means 5 of 6 equal parts.

Occasionally fractions may be used to show the relationship between part of a group and the whole group. For example, you are working on a surgical unit, and in a group of 18 clients who had surgery, 7 developed infections. The number of clients in the full group, 18, is the whole, or the denominator. You write the fraction of clients who developed infections as:

$$\frac{\text{Part (numerator)}}{\text{Whole (denominator)}} = \frac{\text{clients who developed infections}}{\text{whole group}} = \frac{7}{18}$$

Types of Fractions

There are various types of fractions:

Proper Fraction: Numerator is less than the denominator, and the fraction has a value of less than 1.

Examples: $\frac{1}{8}, \frac{5}{6}, \frac{7}{8}, \frac{1}{150}$

Improper Fraction: Numerator is larger than, or equal to, the denominator, and the fraction has a value of 1 or greater than 1.

Examples: $\frac{3}{2}, \frac{7}{5}, \frac{300}{150}, \frac{4}{4}$

Mixed Number: Whole number and a proper fraction in which the total value of the mixed number is greater than 1.

Examples: $3\frac{1}{3}, 5\frac{1}{8}, 9\frac{1}{6}, 25\frac{7}{8}$

Complex Fraction: Numerator, denominator, or both are fractions. The value may be less than, greater than, or equal to 1.

Examples: $\frac{3\frac{1}{2}}{2}, \frac{\frac{1}{3}}{\frac{1}{2}}, \frac{2}{1\frac{1}{4}}, \frac{2}{\frac{1}{150}}$

Whole Numbers: Have an unexpressed denominator of one (1).

Examples: $1 = \frac{1}{1}, 3 = \frac{3}{1}, 6 = \frac{6}{1}, 100 = \frac{100}{1}$

Converting Fractions

An improper fraction can be changed to a mixed number or whole number by dividing the numerator by the denominator. If there is a remainder, that number is placed over the denominator, and the answer is reduced to lowest terms.

Examples: $\frac{6}{5} = 6 \div 5 = 1\frac{1}{5}, \frac{100}{25} = 100 \div 25 = 4, \frac{10}{8} = 10 \div 8 = 1\frac{2}{8} = 1\frac{1}{4}$

A mixed number can be changed to an improper fraction by multiplying the whole number by the denominator, adding it to the numerator, and placing the sum over the denominator.

Example: $5\frac{1}{8} = \frac{(5 \times 8) + 1}{8} = \frac{41}{8}$

Comparing Fractions

Comparing the size of fractions is important in the administration of medications. It helps the new practitioner learn the value of medication dosages early on. Fractions can be compared if the numerators are the same by comparing the denominators or if the denominators are the same by comparing the numerators. These rules are presented in Box 2-1.

BOX 2-1 Rules for Comparing Size of Fractions

Here are some basic rules to keep in mind when comparing fractions.

1. If the numerators are the same, the fraction with the smaller denominator has the greater value.

Example 1: $\frac{1}{2}$ is larger than $\frac{1}{3}$

Example 2: $\frac{1}{150}$ is larger than $\frac{1}{300}$

2. If the denominators are the same, the fraction with the larger numerator has the greater value.

Example 1: $\frac{3}{4}$ is larger than $\frac{1}{4}$

Example 2: $\frac{3}{100}$ is larger than $\frac{1}{100}$

Two or more fractions with different denominators can be compared by changing both fractions to fractions with the same denominator (see Box 2-1). This is done by finding the lowest common denominator (LCD), or the lowest number evenly divisible by the denominators of the fractions being compared.

Example: Which is larger, $\frac{3}{4}$ or $\frac{4}{5}$?

Solution: The lowest common denominator is 20, because it is the smallest number that can be divided by both denominators evenly. Change each fraction to the same terms by dividing the lowest common denominator by the denominator and multiplying that answer by the numerator. The answer obtained from this is the new numerator. The numerators are then placed over the lowest common denominator.

For the fraction $\frac{3}{4}$: $20 \div 4 = 5; 5 \times 3 = 15$; therefore $\frac{3}{4}$ becomes $\frac{15}{20}$.

For the fraction $\frac{4}{5}$: $20 \div 5 = 4; 4 \times 4 = 16$; therefore $\frac{4}{5}$ becomes $\frac{16}{20}$.

Therefore $\frac{4}{5}\left(\frac{16}{20}\right)$ is larger than $\frac{3}{4}\left(\frac{15}{20}\right)$.

Box 2-2 presents fundamental rules of fractions.

BOX 2-2 Fundamental Rules of Fractions

In working with fractions, there are some fundamental rules that we need to remember.

1. When the numerator and denominator of a fraction are both multiplied or divided by the same number, the value of the fraction remains unchanged.

Examples:

$$\frac{1}{2} = \frac{1 \times (2)}{2 \times (2)} = \frac{2}{4} = \frac{2 \times (25)}{4 \times (25)} = \frac{50}{100}, \text{ etc.}$$

$$\frac{50}{100} = \frac{50 \div (10)}{100 \div (10)} = \frac{5}{10} = \frac{5 \div (5)}{10 \div (5)} = \frac{1}{2}, \text{ etc.}$$

As shown in the examples, common fractions can be written in various forms, provided that the numerator, divided by the denominator, always yields the same number (quotient). The particular form of a fraction that has the smallest possible whole number for its numerator and denominator is called the *fraction in its lowest terms.* In the example, therefore, $^{50}/_{100}$, $^{5}/_{10}$, or $^{2}/_{4}$ is $^{1}/_{2}$ in its lowest terms.

2. To change a fraction to its lowest terms, divide its numerator and its denominator by the largest whole number that will divide both evenly.

Example: Reduce $\frac{128}{288}$ to lowest terms.

$$\frac{128}{288} = \frac{128 \div 32}{288 \div 32} = \frac{4}{9}$$

Note: When you do not see the largest number that can be divided evenly at once, the fraction may have to be reduced by using repeated steps.

Example:

$$\frac{128}{288} = \frac{128 \div 4}{288 \div 4} = \frac{32}{72} = \frac{32 \div 8}{72 \div 8} = \frac{4}{9}$$

Note: If both the numerator and denominator cannot be divided evenly by a whole number, the fraction is already in lowest terms. Fractions should always be expressed in their lowest terms.

3. LCD (lowest common denominator) is the smallest whole number that can be divided evenly by all of the denominators within the problem.

Example: $\frac{1}{3}$ and $\frac{5}{12}$: 12 is evenly divisible by 3; therefore 12 is the LCD.

$\frac{3}{7}, \frac{2}{14},$ and $\frac{2}{28}$: 28 is evenly divisible by 7 and 14; therefore 28 is the LCD.

PRACTICE PROBLEMS

Circle the fraction with the least value in each of the following sets.

1. $\frac{6}{30}$ $\frac{4}{5}$

2. $\frac{5}{4}$ $\frac{6}{8}$

3. $\frac{1}{75}$ $\frac{1}{100}$ $\frac{1}{150}$

4. $\frac{6}{18}$ $\frac{7}{18}$ $\frac{8}{18}$

5. $\frac{4}{5}$ $\frac{17}{85}$ $\frac{3}{5}$

6. $\frac{4}{8}$ $\frac{1}{8}$ $\frac{3}{8}$

7. $\frac{1}{40}$ $\frac{1}{10}$ $\frac{1}{5}$

8. $\frac{1}{300}$ $\frac{1}{200}$ $\frac{1}{175}$

9. $\frac{4}{24}$ $\frac{5}{24}$ $\frac{10}{24}$

10. $\frac{4}{3}$ $\frac{1}{2}$ $\frac{1}{6}$

Circle the fraction with the greater value in each of the following sets.

11. $\frac{6}{8}$ $\frac{5}{9}$

12. $\frac{7}{6}$ $\frac{2}{3}$

13. $\frac{1}{72}$ $\frac{6}{12}$ $\frac{1}{24}$

14. $\frac{1}{10}$ $\frac{1}{6}$ $\frac{1}{8}$

15. $\frac{1}{75}$ $\frac{1}{125}$ $\frac{1}{225}$

16. $\frac{2}{5}$ $\frac{6}{5}$ $\frac{3}{5}$

17. $\frac{1}{8}$ $\frac{4}{6}$ $\frac{1}{4}$

18. $\frac{7}{9}$ $\frac{5}{9}$ $\frac{8}{9}$

19. $\frac{1}{10}$ $\frac{1}{50}$ $\frac{1}{150}$

20. $\frac{2}{15}$ $\frac{1}{15}$ $\frac{6}{15}$

Answers on p. 26

Reducing Fractions

Fractions should always be reduced to their lowest terms.

RULE

To reduce a fraction to its lowest terms, the numerator and denominator are each divided by the largest number by which they are both evenly divisible.

Example 1: Reduce the fraction $\frac{6}{20}$.

Solution: Both numerator and denominator are evenly divisible by 2.

$$\frac{6}{20} \div \frac{2}{2} = \frac{3}{10}$$

$$\frac{6}{20} = \frac{3}{10}$$

Example 2: Reduce the fraction $\frac{75}{100}$.

Solution: Both numerator and denominator are evenly divisible by 25.

$$\frac{75}{100} \div \frac{25}{25} = \frac{3}{4}$$

$$\frac{75}{100} = \frac{3}{4}$$

PRACTICE PROBLEMS

Reduce the following fractions to their lowest terms.

21. $\frac{10}{15}$ = ______________

22. $\frac{7}{49}$ = ______________

23. $\frac{64}{128}$ = ______________

24. $\frac{100}{150}$ = ______________

25. $\frac{20}{28}$ = ______________

26. $\frac{14}{98}$ = ______________

27. $\frac{10}{18}$ = ______________

28. $\frac{24}{36}$ = ______________

29. $\frac{10}{50}$ = ______________

30. $\frac{9}{27}$ = ______________

31. $\frac{9}{9}$ = ______________

32. $\frac{15}{45}$ = ______________

33. $\frac{124}{155}$ = ______________

34. $\frac{12}{18}$ = ______________

35. $\frac{36}{64}$ = ______________

Answers on p. 26

Adding Fractions

RULE

To add fractions with the same denominator, add the numerators, place the sum over the denominator, and reduce to lowest terms.

Example 1: $\frac{1}{6} + \frac{4}{6} = \frac{5}{6}$

Example 2: $\frac{1}{6} + \frac{3}{6} + \frac{4}{6} = \frac{8}{6}$

$$\frac{8}{6} = \frac{4}{3} = 1\frac{1}{3}$$

NOTE

In addition to reducing to lowest terms in Example 2, the improper fraction was changed to a mixed number.

RULE

To add fractions with different denominators, change fractions to their equivalent fraction with the lowest common denominator, add the numerators, write the sum over the common denominator, and reduce if necessary.

Example 1: $\frac{1}{4} + \frac{1}{3}$

Solution: The lowest common denominator is 12. Change to equivalent fractions.

$$\begin{array}{r} \frac{1}{4} = \frac{3}{12} \\ +\frac{1}{3} = \frac{4}{12} \\ \hline \frac{7}{12} \end{array}$$

Example 2: $\frac{1}{2} + 1\frac{1}{3} + \frac{2}{4}$

Solution: Change the mixed number $1\frac{1}{3}$ to $\frac{4}{3}$. Find the lowest common denominator, change fractions to equivalent fractions, add, and reduce if necessary. The lowest common denominator is 12.

$$\frac{1}{2} = \frac{6}{12}$$
$$\frac{4}{3} = \frac{16}{12}$$
$$+\frac{2}{4} = \frac{6}{12}$$
$$\frac{28}{12} = 2\frac{4}{12} = 2\frac{1}{3}$$

Subtracting Fractions

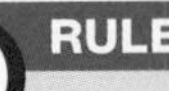

RULE

To subtract fractions with the same denominator, subtract the numerators, and place this amount over the denominator. Reduce to lowest terms if necessary.

Example 1: $\frac{5}{4} - \frac{3}{4} = \frac{2}{4} = \frac{1}{2}$

Example 2: $2\frac{1}{6} - \frac{5}{6}$

Solution: Change the mixed number $2\frac{1}{6}$ to $\frac{13}{6}$

$$\frac{13}{6} - \frac{5}{6} = \frac{8}{6} = \frac{4}{3} = 1\frac{1}{3}$$

RULE

To subtract fractions with different denominators, find the lowest common denominator, change to equivalent fractions, subtract the numerators, and place the sum over the common denominator. Reduce to lowest terms if necessary.

Example 3: $\frac{15}{6} - \frac{3}{5}$

Solution: The lowest common denominator is 30. Change to equivalent fractions, and subtract.

$$\frac{15}{6} = \frac{75}{30}$$
$$-\frac{3}{5} = \frac{18}{30}$$
$$\frac{57}{30} = 1\frac{27}{30} = 1\frac{9}{10}$$

Example 4: $2\frac{1}{5} - \frac{4}{3}$

Solution: Change the mixed number $2\frac{1}{5}$ to $\frac{11}{5}$. Find the lowest common denominator, change to equivalent fractions, subtract, and reduce if necessary. The lowest common denominator is 15.

$$\begin{array}{r} \frac{11}{5} = \frac{33}{15} \\ -\frac{4}{3} = \frac{20}{15} \\ \hline \frac{13}{15} \end{array}$$

Subtracting a Fraction from a Whole Number

RULE

To subtract a fraction from a whole number, follow these steps:

1. Borrow 1 from the whole number, and change it to a fraction, creating a mixed number.
2. Change the fraction so it has the same denominator as the fraction to be subtracted.
3. Subtract the fraction from the mixed number.
4. Reduce if necessary.

Example 1: Subtract $\frac{7}{12}$ from 6

$$\begin{array}{r} 6 = 5 + \mathbf{\frac{1}{1}} = 5\frac{\mathbf{12}}{12} \\ -\frac{\mathbf{7}}{12} = \frac{7}{12} \\ \hline 5\frac{\mathbf{5}}{\mathbf{12}} \end{array}$$

Subtracting Fractions Using Borrowing

RULE

To subtract fractions using borrowing, use the following steps:

1. Change both fractions to the same denominator if necessary.
2. Borrow 1 from the whole number and change it to the same denominator as the fraction in the mixed number. Add the two fractions together.
3. Subtract the fractions and the whole numbers.
4. Reduce if necessary.

Example 2: $5\frac{1}{4} - 3\frac{3}{4}$

In the above example, because $\frac{3}{4}$ is larger than $\frac{1}{4}$, subtraction of the fractions is not possible. Both fractions have the same denominator; no changes need to be made. Therefore, borrow 1 from the whole number part (5), and add the 1 to the fractional part $\left(\frac{1}{4}\right)$.

This results in $5\frac{1}{4} = 4 + \frac{1}{1} + \frac{1}{4} = 4 + \frac{4}{4} + \frac{1}{4} = 4\frac{5}{4}$

$$
\begin{array}{r}
5\frac{1}{4} = 4\frac{5}{4} \\
-3\frac{3}{4} = 3\frac{3}{4} \\
\hline
1\frac{5-3}{4} = 1\frac{2}{4} = 1\frac{1}{2}
\end{array}
$$

Example 3: Subtract $4\frac{3}{4}$ from $9\frac{2}{3}$

Both fractions need to be changed to the same denominator of 12:

$$9\frac{2}{3} = 9\frac{8}{12} \text{ and } 4\frac{3}{4} = 4\frac{9}{12}$$

Subtraction of the fractions is not possible because $\frac{9}{12}$ is larger than $\frac{8}{12}$.

Therefore, borrow 1 from 9.

$9\frac{8}{12} = 8 + \frac{1}{1} + \frac{8}{12} = 8 + \frac{12}{12} + \frac{8}{12} = 8\frac{20}{12}$

Now subtract:

$$
\begin{array}{r}
9\frac{2}{3} = 9\frac{8}{12} = 8\frac{20}{12} \\
-\ 4\frac{3}{4} = 4\frac{9}{12} = 4\frac{9}{12} \\
\hline
4\frac{11}{12}
\end{array}
$$

Multiplying Fractions

RULE

1. Cancel terms if possible.
2. Multiply the numerators, multiply the denominators.
3. Reduce the result (product) to the lowest terms, if necessary.

Notice in this example the numerator and denominator of any of the fractions involved in multiplication may be cancelled when they can be divided by the same number. (cross-cancellation)

Example 1:

$$\frac{3}{\cancel{4}_2} \times \frac{\cancel{2}^1}{5} = \frac{3}{10}$$

Example 2:

$$\frac{2}{4} \times \frac{3}{4}$$

Solution: Reduce $\frac{2}{4}$ to $\frac{1}{2}$ and then multiply.

$$\frac{1}{2} \times \frac{3}{4} = \frac{3}{8}$$

Example 3:

$$6 \times \frac{5}{6}$$

$$\frac{\cancel{6}^1}{1} \times \frac{5}{\cancel{6}_1} = 5$$

or

$$\frac{6 \times 5}{6} = \frac{30}{6} = 5$$

Example 4:

$$3\frac{1}{3} \times 2\frac{1}{2}$$

Solution: Change mixed numbers to improper fractions. Proceed with multiplication.

$$3\frac{1}{3} = \frac{10}{3};\ 2\frac{1}{2} = \frac{5}{2}$$

$$\frac{10}{3} \times \frac{5}{2} = \frac{50}{6} = 8\frac{2}{6} = 8\frac{1}{3}$$

or

$$\frac{\cancel{10}^5}{3} \times \frac{5}{\cancel{2}_1} = \frac{25}{3} = 8\frac{1}{3}$$

Dividing Fractions

RULE

1. To divide fractions, invert (turn upside down) the second fraction (divisor); change ÷ to ×.
2. Cancel terms, if possible.
3. Multiply fractions.
4. Reduce where necessary.

Example 1:

$$\frac{3}{4} \div \frac{2}{3}$$

Solution:

$$\frac{3}{4} \times \frac{3}{2} = \frac{9}{8} = 1\frac{1}{8}$$

Example 2: $1\frac{3}{5} \div 2\frac{1}{10}$

Solution: Change mixed numbers to improper fractions. Proceed with steps of division.

$$1\frac{3}{5} = \frac{8}{5}; 2\frac{1}{10} = \frac{21}{10}$$

$$\frac{8}{\cancel{5}_1} \times \frac{\cancel{10}^2}{21} = \frac{16}{21}$$

Example 3: $5 \div \frac{1}{2}$

Solution: $5 \times \frac{2}{1} = \frac{10}{1} = 10$

or

$$\frac{5}{1} \times \frac{2}{1} = \frac{10}{1} = 10$$

When doing dosage calculations that involve division, the fractions may be written as follows: $\frac{1/4}{1/2}$. In this case, $\frac{1}{4}$ is the numerator and $\frac{1}{2}$ is the denominator. Therefore, the problem is set up as: $\frac{1}{4} \div \frac{1}{2}$, which becomes $\frac{1}{\cancel{4}_2} \times \frac{\cancel{2}^1}{1} = \frac{1}{2}$.

PRACTICE PROBLEMS

Change the following improper fractions to mixed numbers, and reduce to lowest terms.

36. $\frac{18}{5} =$ __________

37. $\frac{60}{14} =$ __________

38. $\frac{13}{8} =$ __________

39. $\frac{35}{12} =$ __________

40. $\frac{112}{100} =$ __________

Change the following mixed numbers to improper fractions.

41. $1\frac{4}{25} =$ __________

42. $4\frac{2}{8} =$ __________

43. $4\frac{1}{2} =$ __________

44. $3\frac{3}{8} =$ __________

45. $15\frac{4}{5} =$ __________

Add the following fractions and mixed numbers, and reduce fractions to lowest terms.

46. $\frac{2}{3} + \frac{5}{6} =$ __________

47. $2\frac{1}{8} + \frac{2}{3} =$ __________

48. $2\frac{3}{10} + 4\frac{1}{5} + \frac{2}{3} =$ __________

49. $7\frac{2}{5} + \frac{2}{3} =$ __________

50. $12\frac{1}{2} + 10\frac{1}{3} =$ __________

Subtract and reduce fractions to lowest terms.

51. $\frac{4}{3} - \frac{3}{7} =$ ______

52. $3\frac{3}{8} - 1\frac{3}{5} =$ ______

53. $\frac{15}{16} - \frac{1}{4} =$ ______

54. $2\frac{5}{6} - 2\frac{3}{4} =$ ______

55. $\frac{1}{8} - \frac{1}{12} =$ ______

56. $14 - \frac{5}{9} =$ ______

57. $3\frac{3}{10} - 1\frac{7}{10} =$ ______

Multiply the following fractions and mixed numbers, and reduce to lowest terms.

58. $\frac{2}{3} \times \frac{4}{5} =$ ______

59. $\frac{6}{25} \times \frac{3}{5} =$ ______

60. $\frac{1}{50} \times 3 =$ ______

61. $2\frac{5}{8} \times 2\frac{3}{4} =$ ______

62. $\frac{5}{12} \times \frac{4}{9} =$ ______

Divide the following fractions and mixed numbers, and reduce to lowest terms.

63. $2\frac{6}{8} \div 1\frac{2}{3} =$ ______

64. $\frac{1}{60} \div \frac{1}{2} =$ ______

65. $6 \div \frac{2}{5} =$ ______

66. $\frac{7}{8} \div \frac{7}{8} =$ ______

67. $3\frac{1}{3} \div 1\frac{7}{12} =$ ______

Answers on p. 26

CHAPTER REVIEW

Change the following improper fractions to mixed numbers, and reduce to lowest terms.

1. $\frac{10}{8} =$ ______

2. $\frac{30}{4} =$ ______

3. $\frac{67}{10} =$ ______

4. $\frac{11}{4} =$ ______

5. $\frac{64}{15} =$ ______

6. $\frac{100}{13} =$ ______

Change the following mixed numbers to improper fractions.

7. $7\frac{3}{8} =$ ______

8. $8\frac{4}{10} =$ ______

9. $3\frac{1}{5} =$ ______

10. $12\frac{3}{4} =$ ______

11. $6\frac{5}{7} =$ ______

Add the following fractions and mixed numbers. Reduce to lowest terms.

12. $\frac{2}{5} + \frac{1}{3} + \frac{7}{10} =$ ____________

13. $\frac{1}{4} + \frac{1}{6} + \frac{1}{8} =$ ____________

14. $6\frac{1}{4} + \frac{2}{9} + \frac{1}{36} =$ ____________

15. $10\frac{1}{6} + 12\frac{4}{6} =$ ____________

16. $1\frac{4}{5} + 7\frac{9}{10} + 3\frac{1}{2} =$ ____________

Subtract the following fractions and mixed numbers. Reduce to lowest terms.

17. $2\frac{1}{4} - 1\frac{1}{2} =$ ____________

18. $\frac{4}{5} - \frac{1}{6} =$ ____________

19. $\frac{4}{5} - \frac{1}{4} =$ ____________

20. $4\frac{1}{6} - 1\frac{1}{3} =$ ____________

21. $\frac{8}{5} - \frac{1}{3} =$ ____________

22. $\frac{5}{6} - \frac{7}{12} =$ ____________

23. $48\frac{6}{11} - 24 =$ ____________

24. $39\frac{11}{18} - 8\frac{3}{6} =$ ____________

Multiply the following fractions and mixed numbers. Reduce to lowest terms.

25. $\frac{1}{3} \times \frac{4}{12} =$ ____________

26. $2\frac{7}{8} \times 3\frac{1}{4} =$ ____________

27. $36 \times \frac{3}{4} =$ ____________

28. $\frac{5}{4} \times \frac{2}{4} =$ ____________

29. $\frac{10}{25} \times \frac{5}{3} =$ ____________

30. $\frac{1}{2} \times \frac{3}{4} \times \frac{3}{5} =$ ____________

31. $\frac{3}{5} \times 3\frac{1}{8} =$ ____________

32. $2\frac{2}{5} \times 4\frac{1}{6} =$ ____________

33. $2 \times 4\frac{3}{8} =$ ____________

34. $\frac{2}{5} \times \frac{5}{4} =$ ____________

Divide the following fractions and mixed numbers. Reduce to lowest terms.

35. $2\frac{1}{3} \div 4\frac{1}{6} =$ ____________

36. $25 \div 12\frac{1}{2} =$ ____________

37. $\frac{7}{8} \div 2\frac{1}{4} =$ ____________

38. $\frac{4}{6} \div \frac{1}{2} =$ ____________

39. $\frac{3}{10} \div \frac{5}{25} =$ ____________

40. $3 \div \frac{2}{5} =$ ____________

41. $\frac{15}{30} \div 10 =$ ____________

42. $\frac{3}{4} \div \frac{3}{8} =$ ____________

43. $12 \div \frac{2}{3} =$ ____________

44. $\frac{7}{8} \div 14 =$ ____________

45. $\frac{15}{8} \div 5 =$ ____________

Arrange the following fractions in order from largest to the smallest.

46. $\frac{3}{16}, \frac{1}{16}, \frac{5}{16}, \frac{14}{16}, \frac{7}{16}$

47. $\frac{5}{12}, \frac{5}{32}, \frac{5}{8}, \frac{5}{6}, \frac{5}{64}$

Apply the principles of borrowing, and subtract the following:

48. $2 - \frac{10}{21} =$ ____________________

49. $9\frac{1}{4} - \frac{3}{4} =$ ____________________

50. $5\frac{1}{2} - 3\frac{3}{4} =$ ____________________

51. A client is instructed to drink 20 ounces of water within 1 hour. The client has only been able to drink 12 ounces. What portion of the water remains? (Express your answer as a fraction reduced to lowest terms.) ____________________

52. A child's oral Motrin Suspension contains 100 milligrams per teaspoonful. 20 milligrams represents what part of a dosage? ____________________

53. A client is receiving 240 milliliters of Ensure by mouth as a supplement. The client consumes 200 milliliters. What portion of the Ensure remains? (Express your answer as a fraction reduced to lowest terms.) ____________________

54. A client takes $1\frac{1}{2}$ tablets of medication four times per day for 4 days. How many tablets will the client have taken at the end of the 4 days? ____________________

55. A juice glass holds 120 milliliters. If a client drinks $2\frac{1}{3}$ glasses, how many milliliters did the client consume? ____________________

56. On admission a client weighed $150\frac{3}{4}$ lb. On discharge the client weighed $148\frac{1}{2}$ lb. How much weight did the client lose? ____________________

57. How many hours are there in $3\frac{1}{2}$ days? ____________________

58. A client consumed the following: $2\frac{1}{4}$ ounces of tea, $\frac{1}{3}$ ounce of juice, $1\frac{1}{2}$ ounces of Jello. What is the total number of ounces consumed by the client?

____

59. One tablet contains 200 milligrams of pain medication.

How many milligrams are in $3\frac{1}{2}$ tablets? ____________________

60. A bottle of medicine contains 30 doses. How many doses are in $2\frac{1}{2}$ bottles. ____________________

61. The nurse gave a client $\frac{3}{4}$ tablespoons (tbs) of medication with breakfast, $\frac{1}{2}$ tbs at lunch, $\frac{1}{2}$ tbs at dinner, and $1\frac{1}{4}$ tbs at bedtime. How much medication did the nurse administer? ____________________

62. A client weighed $160\frac{1}{2}$ lb at the previous visit to the doctor. At this visit, the client weighs $2\frac{3}{4}$ lb more. How many lb does the client weigh? ____________________

63. At the beginning of a shift there are $5\frac{1}{4}$ bottles of hand sanitizer available. At the end of the shift, $3\frac{1}{2}$ bottles are left. How much was used? ____________________

64. A client was given a 16-ounce container of water to drink throughout the day. If the client drank $\frac{7}{8}$ of the container, how many ounces did the client drink? ____________________

65. How many $1\frac{1}{2}$-ounce doses of medication are there in a 24-ounce bottle?

____

66. A bottle contains 36 tablets. If a client took $\frac{1}{3}$ of the tablets, how many tablets are left? ____________________

67. A client drank $4\frac{3}{4}$ ounces of juice, $5\frac{1}{2}$ ounces of coffee, and $4\frac{1}{4}$ ounces of water. How much fluid did the client drink? ____________________

68. One tablet contains 400 milligrams of medication. A client was given $1\frac{1}{2}$ tablets for 5 days. How many milligrams of medication did the client receive in 5 days? ____________________

69. An order is written for a client to receive $1\frac{1}{2}$ ounces of a powdered medication dissolved in water. The client drank $\frac{3}{4}$ ounces of the medication. How much more medication must be given to the client? ____________________

70. An infant grew $\frac{3}{4}$ inch in the first month, $\frac{1}{2}$ inch in the second month, $\frac{7}{8}$ inch in the third month, and $1\frac{1}{8}$ inches in the fourth month. How many inches has the infant grown? ____________________

71. For 4 days a client received $2\frac{1}{2}$ ounces of medication 4 times per day. How many ounces did the client receive over 4 days? ____________________

72. A bottle contains 24 ounces of a liquid pain medication. If a typical dose is $\frac{3}{4}$ ounce, how many doses are there in the bottle? ____________________

73. A nurse worked $9\frac{3}{4}$ hours on Monday, $11\frac{1}{2}$ hours on Tuesday, and $10\frac{3}{4}$ hours on Wednesday. How many hours did she work for the 3 days? ____________________

74. A nurse needs $\frac{1}{2}$ hour to complete an intake interview form on each new client. How many intake interview forms can the nurse complete in $2\frac{1}{2}$ hours?

____

75. A client drinks $\frac{3}{4}$ of a glass of juice that contains 180 milliliters. How many milliliters of juice did the client drink? ____________________

76. A client is instructed to drink the equivalent of 8 glasses of water daily. How many times will the client need to drink $\frac{1}{2}$ glass of water? ____________________

77. One tablet contains 150 milligrams of medication. How many milligrams are in $3\frac{1}{2}$ tablets? ____________________

78. A client at home was instructed to take $\frac{3}{4}$ ounce of medication with meals. The nurse learns that the client took $\frac{2}{3}$ ounce. Did the client take too little, too much, or just the right amount? ____________________

79. A client has taken $\frac{3}{4}$ of a bottle of tablets that contained 100 tablets. How many tablets has the client taken? ____________________

80. A client drank $3\frac{1}{2}$ cups of water from a cup that held 210 milliliters. How many milliliters did the client drink? ____________________

Answers on p. 27

ANSWERS

Chapter 2

Answers to Practice Problems

1. LCD = 30; therefore $\frac{6}{30}$ has the lesser value.
2. LCD = 8; therefore $\frac{6}{8}$ has the lesser value.
3. $\frac{1}{150}$ has the lesser value; the denominator (150) is larger.
4. $\frac{6}{18}$ has the lesser value; the numerator (6) is smaller.
5. $\frac{17}{85}$ has the lesser value; reduced to $\frac{1}{5}$; the numerator (1) is smaller.
6. $\frac{1}{8}$ has the lesser value; the numerator (1) is smaller.
7. $\frac{1}{40}$ has the lesser value; the denominator (40) is larger.
8. $\frac{1}{300}$ has the lesser value; the denominator (300) is larger.
9. $\frac{4}{24}$ has the lesser value; the numerator (4) is smaller.
10. LCD = 6; therefore $\frac{1}{6}$ has the lesser value.
11. LCD = 72; therefore $\frac{6}{8}$ has the higher value.
12. LCD = 6; therefore $\frac{7}{6}$ has the higher value.
13. LCD = 72; therefore $\frac{6}{12}$ has the higher value.
14. $\frac{1}{6}$ has the higher value; the denominator (6) is smaller.
15. $\frac{1}{75}$ has the higher value; the denominator (75) is smaller.
16. $\frac{6}{5}$ has the higher value; the numerator (6) is larger.
17. LCD = 24; therefore $\frac{4}{6}$ has the higher value.
18. $\frac{8}{9}$ has the higher value; the numerator (8) is larger.
19. $\frac{1}{10}$ has the higher value; the denominator (10) is smaller.
20. $\frac{6}{15}$ has the higher value; the numerator (6) is larger.
21. $\frac{10 \div 5}{15 \div 5} = \frac{2}{3}$
22. $\frac{7 \div 7}{49 \div 7} = \frac{1}{7}$
23. $\frac{64 \div 32}{128 \div 32} = \frac{2}{4} = \frac{1}{2}$
24. $\frac{100 \div 50}{150 \div 50} = \frac{2}{3}$
25. $\frac{20 \div 4}{28 \div 4} = \frac{5}{7}$
26. $\frac{14 \div 14}{98 \div 14} = \frac{1}{7}$
27. $\frac{10 \div 2}{18 \div 2} = \frac{5}{9}$
28. $\frac{24 \div 12}{36 \div 12} = \frac{2}{3}$
29. $\frac{10 \div 10}{50 \div 10} = \frac{1}{5}$
30. $\frac{9 \div 9}{27 \div 9} = \frac{1}{3}$
31. $\frac{9 \div 9}{9 \div 9} = \frac{1}{1} = 1$
32. $\frac{15 \div 15}{45 \div 15} = \frac{1}{3}$
33. $\frac{124 \div 31}{155 \div 31} = \frac{4}{5}$
34. $\frac{12 \div 6}{18 \div 6} = \frac{2}{3}$
35. $\frac{36 \div 4}{64 \div 4} = \frac{9}{16}$
36. $3\frac{3}{5}$
37. $4\frac{2}{7}$
38. $1\frac{5}{8}$
39. $2\frac{11}{12}$
40. $1\frac{3}{25}$
41. $\frac{29}{25}$
42. $\frac{34}{8}$
43. $\frac{9}{2}$
44. $\frac{27}{8}$
45. $\frac{79}{5}$
46. $1\frac{1}{2}$
47. $2\frac{19}{24}$
48. $7\frac{1}{6}$
49. $8\frac{1}{15}$
50. $22\frac{5}{6}$
51. $\frac{19}{21}$
52. $1\frac{31}{40}$
53. $\frac{11}{16}$
54. $\frac{1}{12}$
55. $\frac{1}{24}$
56. $13\frac{4}{9}$
57. $1\frac{3}{5}$
58. $\frac{8}{15}$
59. $\frac{18}{125}$
60. $\frac{3}{50}$
61. $7\frac{7}{32}$
62. $\frac{5}{27}$
63. $1\frac{13}{20}$
64. $\frac{1}{30}$
65. 15
66. 1
67. $2\frac{2}{19}$

Answers to Chapter Review

1. $1\frac{2}{8} = 1\frac{1}{4}$
2. $7\frac{2}{4} = 7\frac{1}{2}$
3. $6\frac{7}{10}$
4. $2\frac{3}{4}$
5. $4\frac{4}{15}$
6. $7\frac{9}{13}$
7. $\frac{59}{8}$
8. $\frac{84}{10}$
9. $\frac{16}{5}$
10. $\frac{51}{4}$
11. $\frac{47}{7}$
12. LCD = 30; $1\frac{13}{30}$
13. LCD = 24; $\frac{13}{24}$
14. LCD = 36; $\frac{234}{36} = 6\frac{18}{36} = 6\frac{1}{2}$
15. $22\frac{5}{6}$
16. LCD = 10; $13\frac{2}{10} = 13\frac{1}{5}$
17. LCD = 4; $\frac{3}{4}$
18. LCD = 30; $\frac{19}{30}$
19. LCD = 20; $\frac{11}{20}$
20. LCD = 6; $\frac{17}{6} = 2\frac{5}{6}$
21. LCD = 15; $\frac{19}{15} = 1\frac{4}{15}$
22. LCD = 12; $\frac{3}{12} = \frac{1}{4}$
23. $24\frac{6}{11}$
24. LCD = 18; $31\frac{1}{9}$
25. $\frac{4}{36} = \frac{1}{9}$
26. $9\frac{11}{32}$
27. 27
28. $\frac{10}{16} = \frac{5}{8}$
29. $\frac{50}{75} = \frac{2}{3}$
30. $\frac{9}{40}$
31. $1\frac{7}{8}$
32. 10
33. $8\frac{3}{4}$
34. $\frac{1}{2}$
35. $\frac{42}{75} = \frac{14}{25}$
36. 2
37. $\frac{7}{18}$
38. $1\frac{1}{3}$
39. $1\frac{25}{50} = 1\frac{1}{2}$
40. $7\frac{1}{2}$
41. $\frac{15}{300} = \frac{1}{20}$
42. 2
43. 18
44. $\frac{1}{16}$
45. $\frac{3}{8}$
46. $\frac{14}{16}, \frac{7}{16}, \frac{5}{16}, \frac{3}{16}, \frac{1}{16}$
47. $\frac{5}{6}, \frac{5}{8}, \frac{5}{12}, \frac{5}{32}, \frac{5}{64}$
48. $1\frac{11}{21}$
49. $8\frac{2}{4} = 8\frac{1}{2}$
50. $1\frac{3}{4}$
51. $\frac{2}{5}$ of water remains
52. $\frac{1}{5}$ the dosage
53. $\frac{1}{6}$ of Ensure remains
54. 24 tablets
55. 280 milliliters
56. $2\frac{1}{4}$ lb
57. 84 hours
58. $4\frac{1}{12}$ ounces
59. 700 milligrams.
60. 75 doses.
61. 3 tbs.
62. $163\frac{1}{4}$ lb
63. $1\frac{3}{4}$ bottles.
64. 14 ounces
65. 16 ($1\frac{1}{2}$ ounce doses in the bottle)
66. 24 tablets
67. $14\frac{1}{2}$ ounces
68. 3,000 milligrams
69. $\frac{3}{4}$ ounce
70. $3\frac{1}{4}$ inches
71. 40 ounces
72. 32 ($\frac{3}{4}$ ounce doses in the bottle)
73. 32 hours
74. 5 interview forms
75. 135 milliliters
76. 16 times
77. 525 milligrams
78. too little
79. 75 tablets
80. 735 milliliters

CHAPTER 3
Decimals

Objectives

After reviewing this chapter, you should be able to:

1. Read decimals
2. Write decimals
3. Compare the size of decimals
4. Convert fractions to decimals
5. Convert decimals to fractions
6. Add decimals
7. Subtract decimals
8. Multiply decimals
9. Divide decimals
10. Round decimals to the nearest tenth
11. Round decimals to the nearest hundredth

Medication dosages and other measurements in the health care system use metric measures, which are based on the decimal system. An understanding of decimals is crucial to the calculation of dosages. In the administration of medications, nurses calculate dosages that contain decimals (e.g., levothyroxine 0.075 mg).

Decimal points in dosages have been cited as a major source of medication errors. A misunderstanding of the value of a dosage expressed as a decimal or the omission of a decimal point can result in a serious medication error. Decimals should be written with great care to prevent misinterpretation of a value. A clear understanding of the importance of decimal points and their value will assist the nurse in the prevention of medication errors.

Example 1: Digoxin 0.125 mg

Example 2: Coreg 3.125 mg

A decimal is a fraction that has a denominator that is a multiple of 10. A decimal fraction is written as a decimal by the use of a decimal point (.). The decimal point is used to indicate place value. Some examples are as follows:

Fraction	Decimal Number
$\frac{3}{10}$	0.3
$\frac{18}{100}$	0.18
$\frac{175}{1,000}$	0.175

The decimal point represents the center that separates whole and fractional amounts. The position of the numbers in relation to the decimal point indicates the place of value of numbers.

- The whole number is placed to the **left** of the decimal point. These numbers have a value of one (1) or greater.
- Decimal fractions are written to the **right** of the decimal point and represent a value that is less than one (1) or part of one. The words for all decimal fractions end in *-th(s)*.

The easiest way to understand decimals is to memorize the place values (Box 3-1).

BOX 3-1 Decimal Place Values

The decimal value is determined by its position to the right of the decimal point.

(100,000)	(10,000)	(1,000)	(100)	(10)	(1)	Decimal point	(0.1)	(0.01)	(0.001)	(0.0001)	(0.00001)
Hundred-thousands	Ten-thousands	Thousands	Hundreds	Tens	Ones (Units)	↓	Tenths	Hundredths	Thousandths	Ten-thousandths	Hundred-thousandths
6	5	4	3	2	1	.	1	2	3	4	5

Whole Numbers to the Left — **Decimal Numbers to the Right**

Example 1: 0.3 = three tenths

Example 2: 0.03 = three hundredths

Example 3: 0.003 = three thousandths

SAFETY ALERT!

When there is no whole number before a decimal point, place a zero (0) to the left of the decimal point to emphasize that the number is a decimal fraction and has a value less than 1. This will emphasize its value and prevent errors in interpretation and avoid errors in dosage calculation. This zero does not change the value of the number. This has been emphasized by the Institute for Safe Medication Practices (ISMP) and is a requirement of the accrediting body for health care organizations, The Joint Commission (TJC), when writing decimal fractions in medical notation and is part of TJC's official "Do Not Use" list (2016).

The source of many medication errors is misplacement of a decimal point or incorrect interpretation of a decimal value.

Reading and Writing Decimals

RULE

To read the decimal numbers, read:

1. The whole number,
2. the decimal point as "and," and then
3. the decimal fraction by naming the value of the last decimal place.

Notice that the words for all decimal fractions end in th(s).

Example 1: The decimal number 1.125 is read as "one and one hundred twenty-five thousandths"

Example 2: The number 12.5 is read as "twelve and five tenths"

Example 3: The number 10.03 is read as "ten and three hundredths"

RULE

When reading decimal numbers where a zero is placed before the decimal such as in a decimal fraction (whose value is less than 1), the number is read alone, without stating the zero.

Example 1: 0.4 is read as "four tenths"

Example 2: 0.175 is read as "one hundred seventy-five thousandths"

TIPS FOR CLINICAL PRACTICE

An exception to this is in an emergency situation when a nurse must take a verbal order over the phone from a prescriber. When repeating back an order for a medication involving a decimal, the zero should be read aloud to prevent a medication error.

Example: "Zero point 4" would be the verbal interpretation of Example 1 and zero point 175 of Example 2. In addition to repeating the order back, the receiver of the order should write down the complete order or enter it into a computer, then read it back, and receive confirmation of the order from the individual giving the order.

RULE

To write a decimal number, write the following:

1. The whole number (If there is no whole number, write zero [0] to the left of the decimal.)
2. The decimal point to indicate the place value of the rightmost number
3. The decimal portion of the number to the right of the decimal

Example 1: Written, seven and five tenths = 7.5

Example 2: Written, one hundred twenty-five thousandths = 0.125

Example 3: Written, five tenths = 0.5

RULE

When writing decimals, placing a zero after the last digit of a decimal fraction does not change its value and is not necessary.

Example: 0.37 = 0.370

SAFETY ALERT!

When writing decimals, trailing zeros should not be placed at the end of the number to avoid misinterpretation of a value. This is also a recommendation of the Institute for Safe Medication Practices (ISMP) and is a part of The Joint Commission (TJC) official "Do Not Use" List (2016). TJC forbids the use of trailing zeros for medication orders or other medication-related documentation. Omitting trailing zeros decreases the potential for giving a client 10 times the ordered dose or more. Exception: A trailing zero may be used only when required to demonstrate the level of precision of the value being reported, such as for laboratory results, imaging studies that report the size of lesions, or catheter/tube sizes.

Because the last zero does not change the value of the decimal, it is not necessary. For example, the required notation is 0.37, not 0.370, and 30, not 30.0, which could be interpreted as 370 and 300, respectively, if the decimal point is not clear or is missed.

Example 4: 1.6×0.05

$$\begin{array}{r l} 1.6 & \text{(1 decimal place)} \\ \times 0.05 & \text{(2 decimal places)} \\ \hline 080. & \end{array}$$

Answer: $0.080 = 0.08$

In Example 4, three decimal places are needed (1.6 has one number after the decimal and 0.05 has two), so a zero has to be placed between the decimal point and 8 to allow for enough places. The unnecessary zero is eliminated in the final answer, and a zero is placed before the decimal point.

Multiplication by Decimal Movement

RULE

This method may be preferred when doing metric conversions because it is based on the decimal system. Multiplying by 10, 100, 1,000, and so forth can be done by moving the decimal point to the right the same number of places as there are zeros in the number by which you are multiplying.

When multiplying by 10, move the decimal one place to the right; by 100, two places to the right; by 1,000, three places to the right; and so forth.

Example 1: $1.6 \times 10 = 16$ (The multiplier 10 has 1 zero; decimal point moved 1 place to the right.)

Example 2: $5.2 \times 100 = 520$ (The multiplier 100 has 2 zeros; decimal point moved 2 places to the right.)

Example 3: $0.463 \times 1{,}000 = 463$ (The multiplier 1,000 has 3 zeros; decimal point moved 3 places to the right.)

Example 4: $6.64 \times 10 = 66.4$ (The multiplier 10 has 1 zero; decimal point moved one place to the right.)

SAFETY ALERT!

When multiplying decimals, be sure the decimal is placed in the correct position in the answer (product). Misplacement of decimal points can lead to a critical medication error.

PRACTICE **PROBLEMS**

Multiply the following decimals.

27. $3.15 \times 0.015 =$ ____________

28. $3.65 \times 0.25 =$ ____________

29. $9.65 \times 1{,}000 =$ ____________

30. $8.9 \times 0.2 =$ ____________

31. $14.001 \times 7.2 =$ ____________

Answers on p. 43

Dividing Decimals

Division of decimals is done in the same manner as division of whole numbers except for placement of the decimal point. Incorrect placement of the decimal point changes the numerical value and can cause errors in calculation. Errors made in the division of decimals are commonly caused by improper placement of the decimal point, incorrect placement of numbers in the quotient (answer), and omission of necessary zeros in the quotient.

The parts of a division problem are as follows:

$$\text{Divisor}\overline{)\text{Dividend}}^{\text{Quotient}}$$

The number being divided is called the **dividend,** the number being divided into the dividend is the **divisor,** and the answer is the **quotient.**

Symbols used to indicate division are as follows:

1. $\overline{)\quad}$

Example: $9\overline{)27}$ Read as 27 divided by 9.

2. ÷

Example: $27 \div 9$ Read as 27 divided by 9.

3. The horizontal bar with the dividend on the top and the divisor on the bottom

Example: $\frac{27}{9}$ Read as 27 divided by 9.

4. The slanted bar with the dividend to the left and the divisor to the right

Example: $^{27}/_{9}$ Read as 27 divided by 9.

Dividing a Decimal by a Whole Number

RULE

To divide a decimal by a whole number, place the decimal point in the quotient directly above the decimal point in the dividend. Proceed to divide as with whole numbers.

Example: Divide 17.5 by 5

$$\begin{array}{r} 3.5 \\ 5\overline{)17.5} \\ -15 \\ \hline 25 \\ -25 \\ \hline 0 \end{array}$$

Answer: 3.5

Dividing a Decimal or a Whole Number by a Decimal

RULE

To divide by a decimal, the decimal point in the divisor is moved to the right until the number is a whole number. The decimal point in the dividend is moved the same number of places to the right, and zeros are added as necessary. Proceed to divide as with whole numbers.

Example: Divide 6.96 by 0.3

Step 1: $6.96 \div 0.3 = 0.3\overline{)6.96}$

$3\overline{)69.6}$ (after moving decimals in the divisor the same number of places as the dividend)

Step 2:

$$
\begin{array}{r}
23.2 \\
3\overline{)69.6} \\
\underline{-6} \\
9 \\
\underline{-9} \\
6 \\
\underline{-6} \\
0
\end{array}
$$

Answer: 23.2

Division by Decimal Movement

> **RULE**
> To divide a decimal by 10, 100, or 1,000, move the decimal point to the **left** the same number of places as there are zeros in the divisor.

Example 1: 0.46 ÷ 10 = 0.046 (The divisor 10 has 1 zero; the decimal point is moved 1 place to the left.)

Example 2: 0.07 ÷ 100 = 0.0007 (The divisor 100 has 2 zeros; the decimal point is moved 2 places to the left.)

Example 3: 0.75 ÷ 1,000 = 0.00075 (The divisor 1,000 has 3 zeros; the decimal point is moved 3 places to the left.)

Rounding Off Decimals

The determination of how many places to carry your division when calculating dosages is based on the equipment being used. Some syringes are marked in **tenths** and some in **hundredths.** As you become familiar with the equipment used in dosage calculation, you will learn how far to carry your division and when to round off. To ensure accuracy, most calculation problems require that you carry your division at least **two decimal places (hundredths place)** and **round off to the nearest tenth.**

> **NOTE**
> In some instances, such as critical care or pediatrics, it may be necessary to compute decimal calculations to thousandths (three decimal places) and round to hundredths (two decimal places). These areas may require this accuracy.

> **RULE**
> To express an answer to the nearest tenth, carry the division to the hundredths place (two places after the decimal). If the number in the hundredths place **is 5 or greater,** add one to the tenths place. If the number **is less than 5,** drop the number to the right of the desired decimal place.

Example 1: Express 4.15 to the nearest tenth.

Answer: 4.2 (The number in the hundredths place is 5, so the number in the tenths place is **increased by one.** 4.1 becomes 4.2.)

Example 2: Express 1.24 to the nearest tenth.

Answer: 1.2 (The number in the hundredths place is less than 5, so the number in the **tenths place does not change.** The 4 is dropped.)

Example 3: Express 0.98 to the nearest tenth.

Answer: 1.0 = 1 (The number in the hundredths place is 8, so the number in the tenths place is **increased by one.** 0.9 becomes 1. The zero at the end of this decimal is dropped, because it is unnecessary and can cause potential confusion).

RULE

To express an answer to the nearest hundredth, carry the division to the thousandths place (three places after the decimal). If the number in the thousandths place is **5 or greater,** add one to the hundredths place. If the number **is less than 5,** drop the number to the right of the desired decimal place.

Example 1: Express 0.176 to the nearest hundredth.

Answer: 0.18 (The number in the thousandths place is 6, so the number in the hundredths place is **increased by one.** 0.17 becomes 0.18.)

Example 2: Express 0.554 to the nearest hundredth.

Answer: 0.55 (The number in the thousandths place is less than 5, so the number in **the hundredths place does not change.**) The 4 is dropped.

Example 3: Express 0.40 to the nearest hundredth.

Answer: 0.4 (There is a 0 in the hundredths place, when this is rounded to the hundredths, the final zero should be dropped. It is not necessary to clarify the number and can cause potential confusion.)

PRACTICE **PROBLEMS**

Divide the following decimals. Carry division to the hundredths place where necessary. Do not round off.

32. 2 ÷ 0.5 = ____________

33. 1.4 ÷ 1.2 = ____________

34. 63.8 ÷ 0.9 = ____________

35. 39.6 ÷ 1.3 = ____________

36. 1.9 ÷ 3.2 = ____________

Express the following decimals to the nearest tenth.

37. 3.57 ____________

38. 0.95 ____________

39. 1.98 ____________

Express the following decimals to the nearest hundredth.

40. 3.550 ____________

41. 0.607 ____________

42. 0.738 ____________

Divide the following decimals.

43. 0.005 ÷ 10 = ____________

44. 0.004 ÷ 100 = ____________

Multiply the following decimals.

45. 58.4 × 10 = ____________

46. 0.5 × 1,000 = ____________

Answers on p. 43

Changing Fractions to Decimals

RULE

To change a fraction to a decimal, divide the numerator by the denominator and add zeros as needed. If the numerator doesn't divide evenly into the denominator, carry division three places.

Example 1: $\frac{2}{5} = 5\overline{)2} = 5\overline{)2.0}$ (quotient 0.4)

Example 2: $\frac{3}{8} = 8\overline{)3} = 8\overline{)3.000}$ (quotient 0.375)

Changing fractions to decimals can also be a method of comparing fraction size. The fractions being compared are changed to decimals, and the rules relating to comparing decimals are then applied. (See Comparing the Value of Decimals, p. 31.)

Example: Which fraction is larger, $\frac{1}{3}$ or $\frac{1}{6}$?

Solution: $\frac{1}{3} = 0.333\ldots$ as a decimal

$\frac{1}{6} = 0.166\ldots$ as a decimal

Answer: $\frac{1}{3}$ is therefore the larger fraction.

Changing Decimals to Fractions

RULE

To convert a decimal to a fraction, write the decimal number as a whole number in the numerator of the fraction, and express the denominator of the fraction as a power of 10. Place the number 1 in the denominator of the fraction, and add as many zeros as there are places to the right of the decimal point. Reduce to lowest terms if necessary. (See Reading and Writing Decimals, p. 29.)

Example 1: 0.4 is read "four tenths" and written $\frac{4}{10}$, which $= \frac{2}{5}$ when reduced.

Example 2: 0.65 is read "sixty-five hundredths" and written $\frac{65}{100}$, which $= \frac{13}{20}$ when reduced.

Example 3: 0.007 is read "seven thousandths" and written $\frac{7}{1{,}000}$.

Notice that the number of places to the right of the decimal point is the same as the number of zeros in the denominator of the fraction.

PRACTICE **PROBLEMS**

Change the following fractions to decimals, and carry the division three places as indicated. Do not round off.

47. $\frac{3}{4}$ ______________________

48. $\frac{5}{9}$ ______________________

49. $\frac{1}{2}$ ______________________

Change the following decimals to fractions, and reduce to lowest terms.

50. 0.75 ________

51. 0.0005 ________

52. 0.04 ________

Answers on p. 43

POINTS TO REMEMBER

- Read decimals carefully.
- When the decimal fraction is **not** preceded by a whole number (e.g., .12), **always place a "0"** to the left of the decimal (0.12) to avoid interpretation errors and to avoid overlooking the decimal point.
- Never follow a whole number with a decimal point and zero. This could result in a medication error because of misinterpretation (e.g., 3, not 3.0).
- Add zeros to the right as needed for making decimals of equal spacing for addition and subtraction. These zeros do not change the value. Eliminate unnecessary zeros at the end in the final answer.
- Adding zeros at the end of a decimal (except when called for to create decimals of equal length for addition or subtraction) can result in error (e.g., 1.5, not 1.50).
- Adding zeros before the decimal point can change the value (e.g., 1.5 is not equal to 1.05, nor is it the same number).
- To convert a fraction to a decimal, divide the numerator by the denominator.
- To convert a decimal to a fraction, write the decimal number as a whole number in the numerator and the denominator as a power of 10. Reduce to lowest terms (e.g., $0.05 = \frac{5}{100} = \frac{1}{20}$).
- Double-check work to avoid errors.

CHAPTER REVIEW

Identify the decimal with the largest value in the following sets.

1. 0.4, 0.44, 0.444 ________
2. 0.8, 0.7, 0.12 ________
3. 1.32, 1.12, 1.5 ________
4. 0.1, 0.05, 0.2 ________
5. 0.725, 0.357, 0.125 ________

Arrange the following decimals from smallest to largest.

6. 0.5, 0.05, 0.005 ________
7. 0.123, 0.1023, 1.23 ________
8. 0.64, 4.6, 0.46 ________
9. 5.15, 5.05, 5.55 ________
10. 0.73, 0.307, 0.703 ________

Perform the indicated operations. Give exact answers.

11. $3.005 + 4.308 + 2.47 =$ ________
12. $20.3 + 8.57 + 0.03 =$ ________
13. $5.886 - 3.143 =$ ________
14. $8.17 - 3.05 =$ ________
15. $3.8 - 1.3 =$ ________

Solve the following. Carry division to the hundredths place where necessary.

16. $5.7 \div 0.9 =$ ________
17. $3.75 \div 2.5 =$ ________
18. $1.125 \div 0.75 =$ ________
19. $0.15 \times 100 =$ ________
20. $15 \times 2.08 =$ ________
21. $472.4 \times 0.002 =$ ________

Express the following decimals to the nearest tenth.

22. 1.75 ____________________ 23. 0.13 ____________________

Express the following decimals to the nearest hundredth.

24. 1.427 ____________________ 25. 0.147 ____________________

Change the following fractions to decimals. Carry division three decimal places as necessary.

26. $\frac{8}{64}$ ____________________ 28. $6\frac{1}{2}$ ____________________

27. $\frac{3}{50}$ ____________________

Change the following decimals to fractions, and reduce to lowest terms.

29. 1.01 ____________________ 30. 0.065 ____________________

Add the following decimals.

31. You are to give a client one tablet labeled 0.15 milligram (mg) and one labeled 0.025 mg. What is the total dosage of these two tablets? ____________________

32. If you administer two tablets labeled 0.04 milligram (mg), what total dosage will you administer? ____________________

33. You have two tablets, one labeled 0.025 milligram (mg) and the other 0.1 mg. What is the total dosage of these two tablets? ____________________

34. You have just administered 3 tablets with dose strength of 1.5 milligrams (mg) each. What was the total dosage? ____________________

35. If you administer two tablets labeled 0.6 milligram (mg), what total dosage will you administer? ____________________

Multiply the following numbers by moving the decimal.

36. $0.08 \times 10 =$ ____________________ 37. $2.34 \times 10 =$ ____________________

Divide the following numbers, and round to the nearest hundredth.

38. $0.13 \div 0.25 =$ ____________________ 40. $5 \div 14.3 =$ ____________________

39. $4 \div 4.1 =$ ____________________

Round the following decimals to the nearest thousandth.

41. 4.2475 ____________________ 43. 7.8393 ____________________

42. 0.5673 ____________________ 44. 5.8333 ____________________

45. A client's water intake is 1.05 liters (L), 0.65 L, 2.05 L, and 0.8 L. What is the total intake in liters? ______

46. A client's creatinine level on admission was 2.5 milligrams per deciliter (mg/dL). By discharge the creatinine level dropped 0.9 mg. What is the client's current creatinine level? ______

47. A baby weighed 4.85 kilograms (kg) at birth and now weighs 7.9 kg. How many kilograms did the baby gain? ______

48. A client is taking $\frac{1}{15}$ of a liquid medication containing 0.375 milligram (mg) of medication every day. How many milligrams will the client take in 4 days? ______

49. A client's sodium intake at one meal was the following: 0.002 gram (g), 0.35 g. How many grams of sodium did the client consume? ______

50. True or False? 2.4 grams (g) = 2.04 g. ______

51. 0.7 milligrams (mg) of a medication has been ordered. The recommended maximum dosage of the medication is 0.35 mg, and the minimum recommended dosage is 0.175 mg. Is the dosage ordered within the allowable limits? ______

52. A client weighed 186.4 pounds (lb) before getting sick. After a lengthy recovery period, the client weighed 167.6 lb. How much weight did the client lose? ______

53. If a dosage of medication is 2.5 milliliters (mL), how much medication is needed for 25 dosages? ______

54. A client received 17.5 milligrams (mg) of a medication in tablet form. Each tablet contained 3.5 mg of medication. How many tablets were given to the client? ______

55. A client received a total of 4.5 grams (g) of a medication. If the client received the total over a 3-day period and was given 3 doses per day, what was the strength of each dose? ______

56. A client is brought to the emergency room with a body temperature of 95.3° F. If the normal body temperature is 98.6° F, how far below normal was the client's temperature? ______

57. A vial holds a total of 7.5 milliliters (mL) of medication. If two injections are withdrawn from the vial (1.6 mL and 0.8 mL), how much medication is left in the vial? ______

58. One dose of flu vaccine is 0.5 milliliter (mL). How much vaccine is needed to vaccinate 30 walk-ins at a clinic? ______

59. A client's hemoglobin was 13.8 grams (g) before surgery. During surgery, the hemoglobin dropped 4.5 g. What was the hemoglobin value after it dropped? ______

60. For a certain medication, the safe dosage should be greater than or equal to 0.7 gram (g) but less than or equal to 2 g. Which of the following dosages fall within the range? (More than one answer is correct.)

    0.8 g, 0.25 g, 2.5 g, 1.25 g

61. In a 24-hour period, a premature infant drank 5.5 milliliters (mL), 15 mL, 5.25 mL, 15 mL, 6 mL, and 12.5 mL. How many mL did the infant drink in 24 hours? ______

62. A baby weighed 3.7 kilograms (kg) at birth. The baby now weighs 5.65 kg. How many kg did the baby gain? ______________

63. A client receives a dosage of 5.5 milliliters (mL) of medication 4 times a day. How much medication would the client receive in 7 days? ______________

64. A client received 17.5 milligrams (mg) of medication in tablet form. Each tablet contains 2.5 mg of medication. How many tablets were given to the client? ______________

65. The doctor prescribed 1.5 tablets of a medication to be administered to a client 4 times a day for 7 days. How many tablets were prescribed? ______________

Answers below

ANSWERS

Chapter 3

Answers to Practice Problems

1. eight and thirty-five hundredths
2. eleven and one thousandth
3. four and fifty-seven hundredths
4. five and seven ten thousandths
5. ten and five tenths
6. one hundred sixty-three thousandths
7. 0.4
8. 84.07
9. 0.07
10. 2.23
11. 0.05
12. 0.009
13. 0.5
14. 2.87
15. 0.375
16. 0.175
17. 7.35
18. 0.087
19. 18.4
20. 40.449
21. 3.95
22. 3.87
23. 2.92
24. 43.1
25. 0.035
26. 5.88
27. 0.04725
28. 0.9125
29. 9,650
30. 1.78
31. 100.8072
32. 4
33. 1.16
34. 70.88
35. 30.46
36. 0.59
37. 3.6
38. 1
39. 2
40. 3.55
41. 0.61
42. 0.74
43. 0.0005
44. 0.00004
45. 584
46. 500
47. 0.75
48. 0.555
49. 0.5
50. $\frac{3}{4}$
51. $\frac{1}{2000}$
52. $\frac{1}{25}$

Answers to Chapter Review

1. 0.444
2. 0.8
3. 1.5
4. 0.2
5. 0.725
6. 0.005, 0.05, 0.5
7. 0.1023, 0.123, 1.23
8. 0.46, 0.64, 4.6
9. 5.05, 5.15, 5.55
10. 0.307, 0.703, 0.73
11. 9.783
12. 28.9
13. 2.743
14. 5.12
15. 2.5
16. 6.33
17. 1.5
18. 1.5
19. 15
20. 31.2
21. 0.9448
22. 1.8
23. 0.1
24. 1.43
25. 0.15
26. 0.125
27. 0.06
28. 6.5
29. $1\frac{1}{100}$
30. $\frac{13}{200}$
31. 0.175 mg
32. 0.08 mg
33. 0.125 mg
34. 4.5 mg
35. 1.2 mg
36. 0.8
37. 23.4
38. 0.52
39. 0.98
40. 0.35
41. 4.248
42. 0.567
43. 7.839
44. 5.833
45. 4.55 L
46. 1.6 mg/dL
47. 3.05 kg
48. 0.1 mg
49. 0.352 g
50. False
51. No, 0.7 mg is outside the allowable limits of the safe dosage range of 0.175 mg to 0.35 mg. It is twice the allowable maximum dosage.
52. 18.8 lb
53. 62.5 mL
54. 5 tablets
55. 0.5 g per dose
56. 3.3° F
57. 5.1 mL
58. 15 mL
59. 9.3 g
60. 0.8 g, 1.25 g
61. 59.25 mL
62. 1.95 kg
63. 154 mg
64. 7 tablets
65. 42 tablets

CHAPTER 4
Ratio and Proportion

Objectives

After reviewing this chapter, you should be able to:

1. Define ratio and proportion
2. Define means and extremes
3. Calculate problems for a missing term (*x*) using ratio and proportion

Ratio and proportion is one logical method for calculating medications. It can be used to calculate all types of medication problems. Nurses use ratios to calculate and to check medication dosages. Some medications express the strength of the solution by using a ratio. Example: An Epinephrine label may state 1:1,000. Ratios are used in hospitals to determine the client-to-nurse ratio. Example: If there are 28 clients and 4 nurses on a unit, the ratio of clients to nurses is 28:4 or "28 to 4" or 7:1. As with fractions, ratios should be stated in lowest terms. Like a fraction, which indicates the division of two numbers, a ratio indicates the division of two quantities. The use of ratio and proportion is a logical approach to calculating medication dosages.

Ratios

A ratio is used to indicate a relationship between two numbers. These numbers are separated by a colon (:).

Example: 3:4

The colon indicates division; therefore a ratio is a fraction.

RULE

The numbers or terms of the ratio are the numerator and the denominator. The numerator is always to the left of the colon, and the denominator is always to the right of the colon. Like fractions, ratios should be stated in lowest terms.

Example 1: 3:4 (3 is the numerator, 4 is the denominator, and the expression can be written as $\frac{3}{4}$).

Example 2: In a nursing class, if there are 25 male students and 75 female students, what is the ratio of male students to female students? 25 male students to 75 female students = 25 male students per 75 female students = $^{25}/_{75} = {^1}/_{3}$. This is the same as a ratio of 25:75 or 1:3.

Ratio Measures in Solutions

Some medications express the strength of the solution by using a ratio. Ratio measures are commonly seen in solutions. Ratios represent parts of medication per parts of solution, for example, 1:10,000 (this means 1 part medication to 10,000 parts solution).

Example 1: A 1:5 solution contains 1 part medication in 5 parts solution.

Example 2: A solution that is 1 part medication in 2 parts solution would be written as 1:2.

Ratio strengths are always expressed in lowest terms.

TIPS FOR CLINICAL PRACTICE

The more solution a medication is dissolved in, the less potent the strength becomes. For example, a ratio strength of 1:1,000 (1 part medication to 1,000 parts solution) is more potent than a ratio strength of 1:10,000 (1 part medication to 10,000 parts solution). A misunderstanding of these numbers and what they represent can have serious consequences.

Proportions

A proportion is an equation of two ratios of equal value. The terms of the first ratio have a relationship to the terms of the second ratio. A proportion can be written in any of the following formats:

Example 1: 3:4 = 6:8 (separated with an equals sign)

Example 2: 3:4::6:8 (separated with a double colon)

Example 3: $\frac{3}{4} = \frac{6}{8}$ (written as a fraction)

The examples above are read as follows: 3 is to 4 equals 6 is to 8; 3 is to 4 as 6 is to 8; or, as a fraction, three fourths equals six eighths.

Proving that ratios are equal and that the proportion is true can be done mathematically.

Example:

5:25 = 10:50

or

5:25::10:50

The terms in a proportion are called the *means* and *extremes.* Confusion of these terms can result in an incorrect answer. To avoid confusion of terms in proportions, remember **m** for the middle terms **(means)** and **e** for the end terms **(extremes)** of the proportion. Let's refer to our example to identify these terms.

The extremes are the outer or end numbers (previous example: 5, 50), and the means are the inner or middle numbers (previous example: 25, 10).

Example:

means

5:25 = 10:50

extremes

RULE

In a proportion, the product of the means (the two inner, or middle, numbers) equals the product of the extremes (the two outer, or end, numbers). To find the product of the means and extremes, you multiply.

In other words, the answers obtained when you multiply the means and extremes are equal.

NOTE

The product of the means, 250, equals the product of the extremes, 250, proving the ratios are equal and the proportion is true.

Example:

$$5:25 = 10:50$$

$$\underbrace{25 \times 10}_{\text{means}} = \underbrace{50 \times 5}_{\text{extremes}}$$

$$250 = 250$$

Because ratios are the same as fractions, the same proportion can be expressed as a fraction like this:

$$\frac{5}{25} = \frac{10}{50}$$

The fractions are equivalent, or equal.

The numerator of the first fraction and the denominator of the second fraction are the extremes. The denominator of the first fraction and the numerator of the second fraction are the means.

Example:

$$\frac{5\ (\text{extreme})}{25\ (\text{mean})} = \frac{10\ (\text{mean})}{50\ (\text{extreme})}$$

Cross-multiply to find the equal products of the means and extremes.

$$\frac{5}{25} = \frac{10}{50}$$

$$5 \times 50 = 10 \times 25$$

$$250 = 250$$

Solving for *x* in Ratio and Proportion

Because the product of the means always equals the product of the extremes, if three numbers of the two ratios are known, the fourth number can be found. The unknown quantity may be any of the four terms. In a proportion problem, the unknown quantity is represented by x. After multiplying the means and extremes, the unknown x is usually placed on the left side of the equation. Begin with the product containing the x, which will result in the x being isolated on the **left** and the answer on the **right.**

Example: $12:9 = 8:x$

Steps:

$12x = 72$

1. Multiply the extremes and then the means. (This results in x being placed on the left side of the equation.)

$$\frac{12x}{12} = \frac{72}{12}$$

$$x = \frac{72}{12}$$

$$x = 6$$

2. Divide both sides of the equation by the number preceding the x, in this instance 12, without changing the relationship. The number used for division should always be the number preceding the unknown (x), so that when this step is completed, the unknown (x) will stand alone on the left side of the equation.

Proof: Place the answer obtained for x in the equation, and multiply to be certain that the product of the means equals the product of the extremes.

$$12:9 = 8:6$$
$$9 \times 8 = 12 \times 6$$
$$72 = 72$$

Solving for x with a proportion in a fraction format can be done by cross-multiplication to determine the value of x.

Example: $\frac{4}{3} = \frac{12}{x}$

Steps:

$4x = 36$

1. Cross-multiply to obtain the product of the means and extremes.

$\frac{4x}{4} = \frac{36}{4}$

2. Divide both sides by the number preceding x (in this example, 4) to obtain the value for x.

$x = \frac{36}{4}$

$x = 9$

Proof: Place the value obtained for x in the equation; the cross-products should be equal.

$$\frac{4}{3} = \frac{12}{9}$$
$$4 \times 9 = 12 \times 3$$
$$36 = 36$$

Solving for x in proportions that involve decimals in the equation can be done by the same process.

Example: $25:5 = 1.5:x$

Steps:

$25x = 5 \times 1.5$

1. Multiply the extremes and then the means. (The x will be placed on the left side of the equation.)

$\frac{25x}{25} = \frac{7.5}{25}$

2. Divide both sides by the number preceding x (in this example, 25) to obtain the value for x.

$x = \frac{7.5}{25}$

$x = 0.3$

Proof:

$$25:5 = 1.5:0.3$$
$$25 \times 0.3 = 5 \times 1.5$$
$$7.5 = 7.5$$

Solving for x in proportion that involve fractions in the equation can be done by the same process.

Example: $\frac{1}{2}:x = \frac{1}{5}:1$

Steps:

$\frac{1}{5} \times x = \frac{1}{2} \times 1$

1. Multiply the means and then the extremes. (The x will be placed on the left side of the equation.)

$\frac{1}{5}x = \frac{1}{2}$

$\frac{\frac{1}{5}x}{\frac{1}{5}} = \frac{\frac{1}{2}}{\frac{1}{5}}$

$x = \frac{1}{2} \div \frac{1}{5}$

$x = \frac{1}{2} \times \frac{5}{1}$

2. Divide *both* sides by the number preceding x (in this example, $\frac{1}{5}$). Division of the two fractions becomes multiplication, and the second fraction is inverted. Multiply numerators and denominators.

$x = \frac{5}{2} = 2.5 \text{ or } 2\frac{1}{2}$

3. Reduce the final fraction to solve for x.

Proof:

$$\frac{1}{2}:2\frac{1}{2} = \frac{1}{5}:1$$

$$1 \times \frac{1}{2} = 2\frac{1}{2} \times \frac{1}{5} = \frac{5}{2} \times \frac{1}{5}$$

$$\frac{1}{2} = \frac{5}{10} = \frac{1}{2}$$

$$\frac{1}{2} = \frac{1}{2}$$

RULE

Note: If the answer is expressed in fraction format for x, it must be reduced to **lowest terms.** Division should be carried **two decimal places** when an answer does not work out evenly and may have to be **rounded to the nearest tenth** to prove the answer correct.

Applying Ratio and Proportion to Dosage Calculation

Now that we have reviewed the basic definitions and concepts relating to ratio and proportion, let's look at how this might be applied in dosage calculation.

In dosage calculation, ratio and proportion may be used to represent **the weight of a medication that is in tablet or capsule form.**

Example 1: $1 \text{ tab}:0.125 \text{ mg } or \ \frac{1 \text{ tab}}{0.125 \text{ mg}}$

This may also be expressed by stating the weight of the medication first:

$$0.125 \text{ mg}:1 \text{ tab } or \ \frac{0.125 \text{ mg}}{1 \text{ tab}}$$

This means that 1 tablet contains 0.125 mg or is equal to 0.125 mg of medication.

Example 2: If a capsule contains a dosage of 500 mg, this could be represented by a ratio as follows:

$$1 \text{ cap}:500 \text{ mg } or \ \frac{1 \text{ cap}}{500 \text{ mg}}$$

This may also be expressed stating the weight of the medication first:

$$500 \text{ mg}:1 \text{ cap } or \ \frac{500 \text{ mg}}{1 \text{ cap}}$$

Another use of ratio and proportion in dosage calculation is to express liquid medications used for oral administration and for injection. When stating a dosage of a liquid medication, a ratio expresses the **weight (strength) of a medication in a certain volume of solution.**

Example 1: A solution that contains 250 mg of medication in each **1 mL** could be written as:

$$250\text{ mg}:\mathbf{1\ mL}\ \textit{or}\ \frac{250\text{ mg}}{\mathbf{1\ mL}}$$

1 mL contains 250 mg of medication

Example 2: A solution that contains 80 mg of medication in each **2 mL** would be written as:

$$80\text{ mg}:\mathbf{2\ mL}\ \textit{or}\ \frac{80\text{ mg}}{\mathbf{2\ mL}}$$

2 mL contains 80 mg of medication

SAFETY ALERT!

When using ratio and proportion in dosage calculation, do not forget the units of measurement. Including units in the dosage strength will help you avoid some common errors. For example, if you have two solutions of a medication, one of the solutions contains 1 gram (g) of the medication in 25 milliliters (mL); the other contains 1 milligram (mg) of the medication in 25 milliliters (mL). Notice that although both of these solution strengths have a ratio of 1 : 25, they are obviously different from each other. To clearly distinguish between them and avoid error, the unit of measurement should be included. The first solution should be written as 1 g : 25 mL. The second solution is written as 1 mg : 25 mL.

Proving mathematically that ratios are equal and the proportion is true is important with medications. This can be illustrated by using the previous medication strength examples.

Example 1: 1 cap : 500 mg = 2 cap : 1,000 mg

If 1 cap contains 500 mg, 2 cap will contain 1,000 mg

extremes

1 cap : 500 mg = 2 cap : 1,000 mg

means

$$500 \times 2 = 1{,}000 \times 1$$

$$1{,}000 = 1{,}000$$

Example 2: 2 mL : 80 mg = 1 mL : 40 mg

$$80 \times 1 = 2 \times 40$$

$$80 = 80$$

POINTS TO REMEMBER

- Proportions represent two ratios that are equal and have a relationship to each other.
- When three values are known, the fourth can be easily calculated.
- When solving for the unknown (*x*), regardless of which term of the equation is the unknown, the unknown value (*x*) is usually placed on the left side. Begin with the product containing *x*, so *x* can be isolated on the left side and the answer on the right side.
- Proportions can be stated using an equal (=) sign, a double colon (::), or a fraction format.
- Ratio can be used to state the amount of medication contained in a volume of solution, tablet, or capsule. When using ratio and proportion in dosage calculation, include the units of measurement in the dosage strength.
- Proportions are solved by multiplying the means and extremes.
- Ratios are always stated in their lowest terms.
- Double-check work.

PRACTICE PROBLEMS

Express the following solution strengths as ratios.

1. 1 part medication to 100 parts solution ____________
2. 1 part medication to 3 parts solution ____________

Identify the strongest solution in each of the following:

3. 1 : 2, 1 : 20, 1 : 200 ____________
4. 1 : 1,000, 1 : 5,000, 1 : 10,000 ____________
5. Assume that the ratio of clients to nurses is 15 to 2. Express the ratio in fraction and colon form. ____________

Express the following dosages as ratios. Include the unit of measurement and the numerical value.

6. An injectable liquid that contains 100 mg in each 0.5 mL ____________
7. A tablet that contains 0.25 mg of medication ____________
8. An oral liquid that contains 1 g in each 10 mL ____________
9. A capsule that contains 500 mg of medication ____________

Determine the value for x in the following problems. Express your answer to the nearest tenth as indicated.

10. $12.5 : 5 = 24 : x$ ____________
11. $1.5 : 1 = 4.5 : x$ ____________
12. $750/3 = 600/x$ ____________
13. $1/300 : 3 = 1/120 : x$ ____________
14. $x : 12 = 9 : 6$ ____________

Answers on p. 53

CHAPTER REVIEW

Express the following fractions as ratios. Reduce to lowest terms.

1. $\frac{2}{3}$ ____________
2. $\frac{1}{9}$ ____________
3. $\frac{6}{8}$ ____________
4. $\frac{1}{5}$ ____________
5. $\frac{5}{10}$ ____________
6. $\frac{2}{10}$ ____________

Express the following ratios as fractions. Reduce to lowest terms.

7. 3 : 7 ____________
8. 4 : 6 ____________
9. 1 : 7 ____________
10. 8 : 6 ____________
11. 3 : 4 ____________

Solve for x in the following proportions. Carry division two decimal places as necessary.

12. $20:40 = x:10$ ________

13. $\frac{1}{4}:\frac{1}{2} = 1:x$ ________

14. $0.12:0.8 = 0.6:x$ ________

15. $\frac{1}{250}:2 = \frac{1}{150}:x$ ________

16. $x:9 = 5:10$ ________

17. $\frac{1}{4}:1.6 = \frac{1}{8}:x$ ________

18. $\frac{1}{2}:2 = \frac{1}{3}:x$ ________

19. $125:0.4 = 50:x$ ________

20. $x:1 = 0.5:5$ ________

21. $\frac{2.2}{x} = \frac{8.8}{5}$ ________

22. $0.5:0.15 = 0.3:x$ ________

23. $\frac{16}{40} = \frac{22}{x}$ ________

24. $20:40 = x:15$ ________

25. $\frac{x}{26} = \frac{10.1}{13}$ ________

26. $12:1 = x:5.5$ ________

27. $\frac{60}{1} = \frac{x}{2\frac{1}{4}}$ ________

Set up the following problems as a proportion and solve. Include labels in the set up and on the answer.

28. If 150 milligrams (mg) of medication is in 2 capsules (caps), how many mg of medication is in 10 caps? ________

29. If 60 milligrams (mg) of a medication is in 500 milliliters (mL), how many mL of solution contain 36 mg of medication? ________

30. If 1 kilogram (kg) equals 2.2 lb, how many kg are in 61.6 lb? ________

31. If one glass of milk contains 280 milligrams (mg) of calcium, how many mg of calcium is in $2\frac{1}{2}$ glasses of milk? ________

32. The prescriber orders 0.25 milligram (mg) of a medication. The medication is available in 0.125 mg tablets. How many tablets will you give? ________

Express the following dosages as ratios. Be sure to include the units of measure and numerical value. Do not reduce the ratio.

33. A capsule that contains 250 mg of medication ________

34. An oral solution that contains 125 mg in each 5 mL ________

35. An injectable solution that contains 40 mg in each mL ________

36. An injectable solution that contains 1,000 mcg in each 2 mL ________

37. An injectable solution that contains 1 g in each 3.6 mL ________

38. A tablet that contains 0.4 mg of medication ________

39. A capsule that contains 1 g of medication ________

40. An oral liquid that contains 0.5 mg in each milliliter ________

Express the following strengths as ratios.

41. 1 part medication to 2,000 parts solution ______________________

42. 1 part medication to 400 parts solution ______________________

43. 1 part medication to 50 parts solution ______________________

Identify the weakest solution in each of the following:

44. 1:50, 1:500, 1:5,000 ______________________

45. 1:3, 1:6, 1:60 ______________________

Set up the following word problems as proportions and solve. Include labels in the set up and on the answer.

46. The prescriber orders 15 milligrams (mg) of a medication for every 10 lb of a client's weight. How many mg of medication will be given for a person who weighs 120 lb? ______________________

47. 15 grams (g) of a medication is dissolved in 300 milliliters (mL) of solution. If 45 g of the medication is needed, how many mL of the solution are needed? ______________________

48. The ratio of male to female clients in a nursing facility is 3 to 5. If there are 40 women in the facility, how many men are there? ______________________

49. If 3 ounces (oz) of medicine must be mixed with 7 oz of water, how many ounces of water are needed for 12 oz of medicine? ______________________

50. At an assisted living facility, the resident-to-nurse ratio is 7 to 1. If there are 84 residents, how many nurses work at the facility? ______________________

51. If 100 grams (g) of ice cream contains 20 g of fat, how many g of fat are in 275 g of ice cream? ______________________

52. A survey indicates that 8 out of 10 people suffer from colds each year. If there are 48,000 people in the area, how many people will suffer from colds? ______________________

53. A nurse counts a client's pulse at 19 beats in 15 seconds. If the nurse counts the client's pulse for 1 minute, how many beats would there be in 1 minute? (1 minute = 60 seconds) ______________________

54. A low-fat cheese has 80 calories per ounce (oz). A client that is having their caloric intake measured has eaten $1\frac{1}{4}$ ounces of the low-fat cheese. How many calories has the client eaten? ______________________

55. A client receives 275 milligrams (mg) of medication given evenly over $5\frac{1}{2}$ hours. How many mg of the medication does the client receive per hour? ______________________

56. A client is receiving an intravenous medication at a rate of 6.25 milligrams (mg) per minute. After 50 minutes, how many mg of medications has the client received? ______________________

57. A label on a dinner roll wrapper reads, "2.5 grams (g) of fiber per $\frac{3}{4}$ ounce (oz) serving." If a client eats $1\frac{1}{2}$ ounces of dinner rolls, how many g of fiber will the client consume? ______________________

58. If 100 milliliters (mL) of solution contains 20 milligrams (mg) of medication, how many mg of the medication will be in 650 mL of the solution? ________

59. The label on a bag of popcorn reads, "140 calories per serving; one serving is 4 cups." If you consume $1\frac{1}{2}$ cups, how many calories did you consume? ________

60. If 40 vitamin tablets (tabs) contain 5,000 milligrams (mg), how many tabs are needed for a dosage of 375 mg? ________

Answers below and on p. 54

ANSWERS

Chapter 4

Answers to Practice Problems

1. 1:100
2. 1:3
3. 1:2
4. 1:1,000
5. $\frac{15}{2}$, 15:2
6. 100 mg:0.5 mL, 0.5 mL:100 mg,
7. 0.25 mg:1 tab, 1 tab:0.25 mg,
8. 1 g:10 mL, 10 mL:1 g,
9. 500 mg:1 cap, 1 cap:500 mg,
10. $x = 9.6$
11. $x = 3$
12. $x = 2.4$
13. $x = 7.5$
14. $x = 18$

Answers to Chapter Review

1. 2:3
2. 1:9
3. 3:4
4. 1:5
5. 1:2
6. 1:5
7. $\frac{3}{7}$
8. $\frac{2}{3}$
9. $\frac{1}{7}$
10. $1\frac{1}{3}$
11. $\frac{3}{4}$
12. $x = 5$
13. $x = 2$
14. $x = 4$
15. $x = 3.33$
16. $x = 4.5$
17. $x = 0.8$
18. $x = 1.33$ or $\frac{4}{3}$
19. $x = 0.16$
20. $x = 0.1$
21. $x = 1.25$
22. $x = 0.09$
23. $x = 55$
24. $x = 7.5$
25. $x = 20.2$
26. $x = 66$
27. $x = 135$
28. 150 mg:2 caps = x mg:10 caps *or*

    $$\frac{150 \text{ mg}}{2 \text{ caps}} = \frac{x \text{ mg}}{10 \text{ caps}}$$

    $x = 750$ mg
29. 60 mg:500 mL = 36 mg:x mL *or*

    $$\frac{60 \text{ mg}}{500 \text{ mL}} = \frac{36 \text{ mg}}{x \text{ mL}}$$

    $x = 300$ mL
30. 1 kg:2.2 lb = x kg:61.6 lb *or*

    $$\frac{1 \text{ kg}}{2.2 \text{ lb}} = \frac{x \text{ kg}}{61.6 \text{ lb}}$$

    $x = 28$ kg
31. 1 glass:280 mg = $2\frac{1}{2}$ glass:x mg *or*

    $$\frac{1 \text{ glass}}{280 \text{ mg}} = \frac{2\frac{1}{2} \text{ glass}}{x \text{ mg}}$$

    $x = 700$ mg
32. 0.125 mg:1 tab = 0.25 mg:x tab *or*

    $$\frac{0.125 \text{ mg}}{1 \text{ tab}} = \frac{0.25 \text{ mg}}{x \text{ tab}}$$

    $x = 2$ tabs
33. 250 mg:1 cap *or* 1 cap:250 mg
34. 125 mg:5 mL *or* 5 mL:125 mg
35. 40 mg:1 mL *or* 1 mL:40 mg
36. 1,000 mcg:2 mL *or* 2 mL:1,000 mcg
37. 1 g:3.6 mL *or* 3.6 mL:1 g
38. 0.4 mg:1 tab *or* 1 tab:0.4 mg
39. 1 g:1 cap *or* 1 cap:1 g
40. 0.5 mg:1 mL *or* 1 mL:0.5 mg
41. 1:2,000
42. 1:400
43. 1:50

44. 1 : 5,000
45. 1 : 60
46. 15 mg : 10 lb = *x* mg : 120 lb *or*
    $\frac{15 \text{ mg}}{10 \text{ lb}} = \frac{x \text{ mg}}{120 \text{ lb}}$
    $x = 180$ mg
47. 15 g : 300 mL = 45 g : *x* mL *or*
    $\frac{15 \text{ g}}{300 \text{ mL}} = \frac{45 \text{ g}}{x \text{ mL}}$
    $x = 900$ mL
48. 3 males : 5 females = *x* males : 40 females *or*
    $\frac{3 \text{ males}}{5 \text{ females}} = \frac{x \text{ males}}{40 \text{ females}}$
    $x = 24$ males
49. 3 oz medicine : 7 oz water = 12 oz medicine : *x* oz water *or*
    $\frac{3 \text{ oz medicine}}{7 \text{ oz water}} = \frac{12 \text{ oz medicine}}{x \text{ oz water}}$
    $x = 28$ oz
50. 7 residents : 1 nurse = 84 residents : *x* nurses *or*
    $\frac{7 \text{ residents}}{1 \text{ nurse}} = \frac{84 \text{ residents}}{x \text{ nurses}}$
    $x = 12$ nurses
51. 100 ice cream : 20 g fat = 275 g ice cream : *x* g fat *or*
    $\frac{100 \text{ g ice cream}}{20 \text{ g fat}} = \frac{275 \text{ g ice cream}}{x \text{ g fat}}$
    $x = 55$ g
52. 8 cold sufferers : 10 people = *x* cold sufferers : 48,000 people *or*
    $\frac{8 \text{ cold suffers}}{10 \text{ people}} = \frac{x \text{ cold sufferers}}{48{,}000 \text{ people}}$
    $x = 38{,}400$ people
53. 19 beats : 15 seconds = *x* beats : 60 seconds *or*
    $\frac{19 \text{ beats}}{15 \text{ seconds}} = \frac{x \text{ beats}}{60 \text{ seconds}}$
    $x = 76$ beats
54. 80 calories : 1 oz = *x* calories : $1\frac{1}{4}$ oz *or*
    $\frac{80 \text{ calories}}{1 \text{ oz}} = \frac{x \text{ calories}}{1\frac{1}{4} \text{ oz}}$
    $x = 100$ calories
55. 275 mg : $5\frac{1}{2}$ hours = *x* mg : 1 hour *or*
    $\frac{275 \text{ mg}}{5\frac{1}{2} \text{ hours}} = \frac{x \text{ mg}}{1 \text{ hour}}$
    $x = 50$ mg
56. 6.25 mg : 1 minute = *x* mg : 50 minutes *or*
    $\frac{6.25 \text{ mg}}{1 \text{ minute}} = \frac{x \text{ mg}}{50 \text{ minutes}}$
    $x = 312.5$ mg
57. 2.5 g : $\frac{3}{4}$ oz = *x* g : $1\frac{1}{2}$ oz *or*
    $\frac{2.5 \text{ g}}{\frac{3}{4} \text{ oz}} = \frac{x \text{ g}}{1\frac{1}{2} \text{ oz}}$
    $x = 5$ g
58. 20 mg : 100 mL = *x* mg : 650 mL *or*
    $\frac{20 \text{ mg}}{100 \text{ mL}} = \frac{x \text{ g}}{650 \text{ mL}}$
    $x = 130$ mg
59. 140 calories : 4 cups = *x* calories : $1\frac{1}{2}$ cups *or*
    $\frac{140 \text{ calories}}{4 \text{ cups}} = \frac{x \text{ calories}}{1\frac{1}{2} \text{ cups}}$
    $x = 52.5$ calories or $52\frac{1}{2}$ calories
60. 5,000 mg : 40 tabs = 375 mg : *x* tabs *or*
    $\frac{5{,}000 \text{ mg}}{40 \text{ tabs}} = \frac{375 \text{ mg}}{x \text{ tabs}}$
    $x = 3$ tabs

CHAPTER 5
Percentages

Objectives

After reviewing this chapter, you should be able to:

1. Define percent
2. Convert percents to fractions
3. Convert percents to decimals
4. Convert percents to ratios
5. Convert decimals to percents
6. Convert fractions to percents
7. Convert fractions to ratios
8. Determine the percent of numbers

Percents, as decimals and fractions, is a way to express the relationship of parts to a whole. Percent (%) means parts per hundred. A percentage is the same as a fraction in which the denominator is 100, and the numerator indicates the part of 100 that is being considered.

The symbol used to indicate a percent (%) is placed after the number, as in 40%. The example 40% (40 percent) means 40 out of 100. Percents can be more than 100% (such as 200%) or less than 1% (0.1%). A percent may also contain a decimal (0.6%), a fraction ($\frac{1}{2}$%), or a mixed number ($14\frac{1}{2}$%).

Example: $4\% = 4 \text{ percent} = \frac{4}{100} \text{ (4 per 100)} = 0.04$

Health care professionals see percentages written with medications (e.g., magnesium sulfate 50%, lidocaine 2%). Solutions for the eye and topical (for external use) ointments, lotions, and creams use percentages to express dosage strength. For example, hydrocortisone cream is available in 1% and 2.5%. Timolol ophthalmic solutions are available in 0.25% and 0.5%.

In addition, nurses and other health professionals frequently administer solutions with the concentration expressed as a percent, such as intravenous (IV) solutions (e.g., 5% dextrose in water). IV means directly into a person's vein.

Percents may also be used by nurses when it is required to calculate percentages of partial quantities (e.g., to determine the percentage of a diet of fluids that a client consumed).

In current practice, percentage solutions are prepared by the pharmacy, and people can purchase solutions or components of the solutions over the counter. Some institutions require nurses to prepare solutions in house (in the hospital) as well as in home care for clients being cared for at home. Understanding percentages provides the foundation for preparing and calculating dosages for medications that are ordered in percentages.

Percentages are also used in the assessment of burns. The size of a burn (percentage of injured skin) is determined by using the rule of nines in an adult. The basis of the rule is that the body is divided into anatomical sections, each of which represents 9% or a multiple of 9% of the total body surface area (BSA). The total BSA is represented by 100%. Another method used is the age-specific burn diagram or chart. Burn size is expressed as a percentage of the total BSA. In children, age-related charts are used because their body proportions differ from those of an adult.

Let's get an understanding of the relationship of ratios, percents, fractions, and decimals by showing how to convert from one to another.

Converting Percentages to Fractions, Decimals, and Ratios

RULE

To convert a percent to a fraction:

1. Drop the percent sign.
2. Write the number as the numerator (top number in a fraction).
3. Write 100 as the denominator (bottom number in a fraction).
4. Reduce the fraction to lowest terms.

Example 1: $8\% = \frac{8}{100}$, reduced is $\frac{2}{25}$

Example 2: $\frac{1}{4}\% = \frac{1}{4} \div 100 = \frac{1}{4} \times \frac{1}{100} = \frac{1}{400}$

RULE

To convert a percent to a decimal:

1. Drop the percent sign.
2. Divide the number by 100; this is the same as moving the decimal point two places to the left (add zeros as needed).

Example 1: $25\% = \frac{25}{100} = 25 \div 100 = .25 = 0.25$

Example 2: $1.4\% = \frac{1.4}{100} = 1.4 \div 100 = .014 = 0.014$

Example 3: $75\% = \frac{75}{100} = \frac{3}{4}$ (lowest terms). Divide the numerator of the fraction (3) by the denominator (4).

$$4\overline{)3.00}\text{ (quotient } 0.75) = 0.75$$

Example 3 is an alternative method. Drop the percent sign. Write the remaining number as the numerator. Write "100" as the denominator. Reduce the result to lowest terms. Divide the numerator by the denominator to obtain a decimal.

RULE

To convert a percent to a ratio:

1. Drop the percent sign.
2. Write the number as a fraction (place it in the numerator).
3. Write 100 as the denominator.
4. Reduce the fraction to lowest terms.
5. Place the numerator as the first term of the ratio and the denominator as the second term.
6. Separate the two terms with a colon (:).

Example 1: $10\% = \frac{10}{100} = \frac{1}{10} = 1:10$

Example 2: $80\% = \frac{80}{100} = \frac{4}{5} = 4:5$

RULE

To convert a fraction to a percent:

1. Multiply the fraction by 100.
2. Reduce if necessary.
3. Add the percent sign (%).

OR

1. Convert the fraction to a decimal.
2. Multiply decimal by 100, which is the same as moving the decimal point two places to the right.
3. Add the percent sign (%).

Example 1: $\frac{3}{4}$ changed to a percent is *or* $\frac{3}{4}$ changed to a decimal is

$\frac{3}{4} \times \frac{100}{1} = \frac{300}{4} = \frac{75}{1} = 75$

Add percent sign: 75%

$4\overline{)3.00}$ = 0.75

$0.75 \times 100 = 0.75 = 75\%$

Add percent sign: 75%

Example 2: $5\frac{1}{2}$ changed to a percent is

Change to an improper fraction: $\frac{11}{2}$

$\frac{11}{2} \times \frac{100}{1} = \frac{1{,}100}{2} = \frac{550}{1} = 550$

Add percent sign: 550%

or Change to an improper fraction: $\frac{11}{2}$

$2\overline{)11.0}$ = 5.5

$5.5 \times 100 = 5.50 = 550$

Add percent sign: 550%

RULE

To convert a decimal to a percent:

1. Multiply the decimal number by 100, which is the same as moving the decimal point two places to the right. Add zeros if necessary.
2. Add the percent sign (%).

Example 1: Change 0.45 to %.

Move the decimal point two places to the right.

Add the percent sign:

0.45. = 45%

Example 2: Convert 2.35 to %.

Move the decimal point two places to the right.

Add the percent sign:

2.35 = 235%

Another method that can be used to convert a decimal to a percent can be done as follows:

RULE

To convert a decimal to a percent:

1. Change the decimal to a fraction, then follow the steps to convert a fraction to a percent.
2. If the percent does not end as a whole number, express the percent with the remainder as a fraction, to the nearest whole percent, or to the nearest tenth of a percent.

Example: $0.625 = \frac{625}{1{,}000} = \frac{5}{8} = 62\frac{1}{2}\%$, 63%, or 62.5%

$$\frac{625}{1{,}000} = \frac{5}{8}; \frac{5}{8} \times \frac{100}{1} = \frac{500}{8} = 62.5\%$$

RULE

To convert a ratio to a percent:

1. Convert the ratio to a fraction, and proceed with the steps for changing a fraction to a percent.

OR

1. Convert the ratio to a fraction.
2. Convert the fraction to a decimal.
3. Convert the decimal to a percent.

Example: $1:4 = \frac{1}{4}; \frac{1}{4} \times \frac{100}{1} = 25$ *or* $1:4 = \frac{1}{4}$

$$4\overline{)1.00} = 0.25$$

$0.25 \times 100 = 0.25. = 25\%$

Add percent sign: 25%   Add percent sign: 25%

PRACTICE PROBLEMS

Change the following percents to fractions, and reduce to lowest terms.

1. 1% ______
2. 2% ______
3. 50% ______
4. 150% ______
5. 3% ______

Change the following percents to decimals. Round to two decimal places, as indicated.

6. 10% ______
7. 35% ______
8. 50% ______
9. 14.2% ______
10. $\frac{6}{7}\%$ ______

Change each of the following percents to a ratio. Express in lowest terms.

11. 25% ______
12. 11% ______
13. 75% ______
14. 4.5% ______
15. $\frac{2}{5}\%$ ______

Change the following fractions to percents.

16. $\frac{2}{5}$ ______________________

17. $\frac{11}{4}$ ______________________

18. $\frac{1}{2}$ ______________________

19. $\frac{1}{4}$ ______________________

20. $\frac{7}{10}$ ______________________

Convert the following decimals to percents.

21. 1.32 ______________________

22. 0.02 ______________________

23. 0.8 ______________________

24. 2.3 ______________________

25. 0.013 ______________________

Change the following ratios to percents.

26. 1:25 ______________________

27. 3:4 ______________________

28. 1:10 ______________________

29. 1:100 ______________________

30. 1:2 ______________________

Answers on p. 68

Percentage Measures

As previously stated, **intravenous (IV) solutions are ordered in percentage strengths, and nurses need to be familiar with their meaning (e.g., 1,000 milliliters [mL] 5% dextrose in water). Percentage solution means the number of grams (g) of solute per 100 mL of diluent.**

Example 1: 1,000 mL IV of 5% dextrose and water contains 50 g (grams) of dextrose

$$\% = \text{g per 100 mL; therefore } 5\% = 5 \text{ g per 100 mL}$$

$$5\text{ g}:100\text{ mL} = x\text{ g}:1{,}000\text{ mL}$$

$$x = 50\text{ g dextrose}$$

Example 2: 250 mL IV of 10% dextrose contains 25 g (grams) of dextrose

$$\% = \text{g per 100 mL; therefore } 10\% = 10 \text{ g per 100 mL}$$

$$10\text{ g}:100\text{ mL} = x\text{ g}:250\text{ mL}$$

$$x = 25\text{ g dextrose}$$

PRACTICE **PROBLEMS**

Determine the number of grams of medication and dextrose as indicated in the following solutions.

31. How many grams of medication will 500 mL of a 10% solution contain?

____

32. How many grams of dextrose will 1,000 mL of a 10% solution contain?

____

33. How many grams of dextrose will 250 mL of a 5% solution contain?

____

34. How many grams of medication will 100 mL of a 50% solution contain?

____

35. How many grams of dextrose will 150 mL of a 5% solution contain?

____

Answers on p. 68

Comparing Percents and Ratios

Nurses as well as other health care professionals administer solutions that may be expressed as percents or ratios. Intravenous solutions come in varying percentages. Example: 0.45%, 5%. It is important to be clear on the numbers and quantities they represent. An IV solution that is 5% is more potent or concentrated than a 0.45% solution. Converting percentages and ratios to equivalent decimals can clarify values so professionals can compare concentrations.

Like IV fluids, ointments, creams, and lotions can be available in different percentage strengths, and nurses need to be clear on the quantities they represent as well. A 0.025% ointment is more potent or concentrated than one that is 0.02%.

Example 1: $0.45\% = \dfrac{0.45}{100} = 0.45 \div 100 = .00.45 = = 0.0045$

Example 2: $5\% = \dfrac{5}{100} = 5 \div 100 = .05. = 0.05$ (greater value, stronger concentration than 0.0045)

Compare solution concentrations expressed as a ratio, such as 1 : 1,000 and 1 : 10,000.

Example 1: $1:1{,}000 = \dfrac{1}{1{,}000} = 0.001$ (1 : 1,000 is a stronger concentration than 1 : 10,000)

Example 2: $1:10{,}000 = \dfrac{1}{10{,}000} = 0.0001$

> **SAFETY ALERT!**
>
> The higher the percentage strength, the stronger the solution or ointment. A misunderstanding of these numbers (%) can have serious consequences.

Example: 10% IV solution is more potent than 5%. A solution of 5% is more potent than 0.9%. **Always check the percentage of IV solution prescribed.**

PRACTICE **PROBLEMS**

Identify the strongest solution, ointment, or cream in each of the following:

36. Ophthalmic solution 0.1%, 0.5%, 1% ______________________________

37. Ointment 0.025%, 0.3%, 0.5% ______________________________

38. Cream 0.02%, 0.025%, 0.25% ______________________________

39. Solution 1:30, 1:300, 1:3 ______

40. Solution 0.33%, 0.9%, 0.45% ______

Answers on p. 68

Determining the Percent of a Quantity

Nurses may find it necessary to determine a given percentage or part of a quantity.

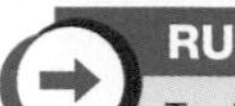

RULE

To determine a given percent of a number:

1. First convert the percent to a decimal or fraction.
2. Multiply the decimal or fraction by the number.

Example 1: A client reports drinking 25% of an 8-ounce cup of tea. Determine what amount 25% of 8 ounces is.

Solution: Change the percentage to a decimal:

$$25\% = \frac{25}{100} = .25 = 0.25$$

Multiply the decimal by the number:

$$0.25 \times 8 \text{ ounces} = 2 \text{ ounces}$$

Therefore 25% of 8 ounces = 2 ounces

Determining the percent of a quantity may also be solved using a ratio and proportion written in colon or fraction format. For example, using the above problem:

$$25:100 = x:8 \quad or \quad \frac{25}{100} = \frac{x}{8}$$

Either one of these formats would net the same answer.

Example 2: 40% of 90

Solution:

$$40\% = \frac{40}{100} = .40 = 0.4$$

$$0.4 \times 90 = 36$$

Therefore 40% of 90 = 36

Determining What Percent One Number Is of Another

RULE

To determine what percent one number is of another, it is necessary to make a fraction with the numbers.

1. The **denominator** (bottom number) of the fraction is the number following the word "of" in the problem.
2. The other number is the **numerator** (top number) of the fraction.
3. Convert the fraction to a decimal, and then convert to a percentage.

Example 1: 12 is what percentage of 60? *or* What percentage of 60 is 12?

Solution: Make a fraction using the two numbers:

$$\frac{12}{60}$$

Convert the fraction to a decimal:

$$60\overline{)12.0}\quad 0.2$$

Convert the decimal to a percentage:

$$0.2 \times 100 = 0.20. = 20\%$$

Therefore 12 = 20% of 60 or 20% of 60 = 12

Example 2: 1.2 is what percentage of 4.8? *or* What percentage of 4.8 is 1.2?

Solution: Make a fraction using the two numbers:

$$\frac{1.2}{4.8}$$

Convert the fraction to a decimal:

$$4.8\overline{)1.200}\quad 0.25$$

Convert the decimal to a percentage:

$$0.25 \times 100 = 0.25. = 25\%$$

Therefore, 1.2 = 25% of 4.8 *or* 25% of 4.8 = 1.2

Example 3: $3\frac{1}{2}$ is what percentage of 8.5? *or* What percentage of 8.5 is $3\frac{1}{2}$?

Solution: Make a fraction using the two numbers:

$$\frac{3\frac{1}{2}}{8.5} = \frac{3.5}{8.5}$$

Convert the fraction to a decimal:

$$\begin{array}{r} 0.4117 \\ 8.5\overline{)3.50000} \\ -340 \\ \hline 100 \\ -85 \\ \hline 150 \\ -85 \\ \hline 650 \\ -595 \\ \hline 55 \end{array}$$

Convert the decimal to a percentage:

$$0.412 \times 100 = 0.412 = 41.2\%$$

Therefore $3\frac{1}{2}$ = 41.2% of 8.5 or 41.2% of 8.5 = $3\frac{1}{2}$

PRACTICE **PROBLEMS**

41. A client drinks 30% of a bowl of broth that holds 200 milliliters (mL). How many mL did the client drink? ______

42. A client drinks 80% of a 5-ounce (oz) cup of ginger ale. How many oz did the client drink? ______

Perform the indicated operations. Round decimals to the hundredths place.

43. 60% of 30 ______
44. 20% of 75 ______
45. 2 is what percentage of 200? ______
46. 50 is what percentage of 500? ______
47. 40 is what percentage of 1,000? ______
48. 3% of 842 ______
49. 0.7% of 60 ______
50. 75% of 165 ______
51. 25 is what percentage of 40? ______
52. 1.3 is what percentage of 5.2? ______
53. $\frac{1}{4}$% of 68 ______
54. What percentage of 8.4 is $3\frac{1}{2}$? ______

Answers on p. 68

Calculating the Percent of Change

It may be useful to determine a percent of change (increase or decrease). For example, you might want to know if an increase or decrease in a client's weight is a significant increase or decrease.

RULE

To determine the percent of change

1. Make a fraction of change $= \frac{\text{change}}{\text{old}}$
2. Multiply the fraction by 100 to change the fraction to a percent OR change the fraction to a decimal and multiply decimal by 100, which is the same as moving the decimal point two places to the right.
3. Add the percent sign.

Example 1: A client's weight before surgery was 176 lb. Following 2 weeks of bed rest, the client's weight was 184.8 lb. What was the percent of increase in the client's weight?

Solution: The increase = 184.8 lb − 176 lb = 8.8 lb.

Fraction of change $= \frac{8.8}{176}$

$$\frac{8.8}{176} \times 100 = \frac{880}{176} = 5\%$$

or

Change fraction to a decimal, multiply by 100.

Fraction of change $= \frac{8.8}{176}$

$$\frac{8.80}{176} = 0.05 \qquad 0.05 \times 100 = 0.05. = 5\%$$

The percent of increase in the client's weight was 5%.

Example 2: A client was drinking 40 ounces of water per day, but this was reduced by 10 ounces per day. What is the percent of change?

Solution: The decrease = 40 ounces − 30 ounces = 10 ounces.

$$\text{Fraction of change} = \frac{10}{40} = 25\%$$

$$\frac{10}{40} \times 100 = \frac{1{,}000}{40} = 25\%$$

or

Change fraction to a decimal, multiply by 100.

$$\text{Fraction of change} = \frac{10}{40}$$

$$40\overline{)10.00} = 0.25 \times 100 = 0.25. = 25\%$$

0.25; -80; 200

PRACTICE **PROBLEMS**

55. A client's weight before dieting was 300 lb. After one month of dieting, the client's weight was 240 lb. What was the percent of decrease in the client's weight? ________

56. A client was taking 400 milligrams (mg) of a pain medication. The doctor increased the dosage to 600 mg. What is the percent of increase in the dosage? ________

57. Physical therapy increases a client's pulse rate. The client's rate before the physical therapy was 60 beats per minute. At the completion of physical therapy, the rate is 75 beats per minute. What is the percent of increase in the pulse rate? ________

58. The number of nurses on the night shift has increased from 4 to 6. What is the percent of increase? ________

59. The population at a small assisted-living facility dropped from 150 to 135 residents. What was the percent of decrease in population? ________

60. In February, 2,500 cases of flu were reported. In June of the following year, 900 cases of flu were reported. What is the percent decrease in reported cases of flu? ________

Answers on p. 68

POINTS TO REMEMBER

- Fractions, decimals, ratios, and percents are related equivalents.
- Express ratios to lowest terms.
- **To convert a percent to a fraction,** drop the % sign and place the remaining number as the numerator, write 100 as the denominator, and reduce the fraction to lowest terms.
- **To convert a percent to a decimal,** drop the % sign and divide by 100.
- **To convert a percent to a ratio,** first convert the percent to a fraction in lowest terms. Then, place the numerator as the first term of the ratio and the denominator as the second term. Separate the two terms with a colon (:).
- **To convert a fraction to a percent,** multiply the fraction by 100, reduce if necessary, and add the % sign. **OR** convert the fraction to a decimal, multiply the decimal by 100, and add the % sign.

- **To convert a decimal to a percent,** multiply the decimal by 100 and add the % sign **OR** change the decimal to a fraction, then follow the steps to convert a fraction to a percent. If the percent does not terminate as a whole number, express the percent with the remainder as a fraction to the nearest whole percent, or to the nearest tenth of a percent.
- **To convert a ratio to a percent,** convert the ratio to a fraction and proceed with the steps for changing to a fraction to a percent **OR** convert the ratio to a fraction, convert the resulting fraction to a decimal and then to a percent.
- Percentage solutions means the number of grams of solute per 100 milliliters of diluent.
- The higher the percentage strength, the stronger the solution, ointment, or cream.
- To determine the given percent or part of a quantity, convert the percent to a decimal or fraction. Multiply the decimal or fraction by the number. This can also be done using any of the formats for ratio and proportion.
- **To calculate the percent of change,** make a fraction of the change $= \frac{\text{change}}{\text{old}}$ and multiply the fraction by 100 to change the fraction to a percent. **OR** change the fraction to a decimal, multiply by 100, and add the % sign.

CHAPTER REVIEW

Complete the table below. Express each of the following measures in their equivalents where indicated. Reduce fractions and ratios to lowest terms; round decimals to hundredths.

	Percent	Ratio	Fraction	Decimal
1.	52%	______	______	______
2.	71%	______	______	______
3.	______	______	$\frac{7}{100}$	______
4.	______	1:50	______	______
5.	______	______	______	0.06
6.	______	______	$\frac{3}{8}$	______
7.	______	______	$\frac{61}{100}$	______
8.	______	7:1,000	______	______
9.	5%	______	______	______
10.	2.5%	______	______	______

Perform the indicated operations.

11. A client reports drinking 40% of a 12-ounce can of ginger ale. How many ounces did the client drink? ______________________________

12. 40% of 140 ______________

13. 100 is what percentage of 750? ______

14. $\frac{1}{2}$ is what percentage of 60? ________ 15. 15% of 250 ________

16. What percentage of 6.4 is 1.6? ________

17. Which of the following solutions is strongest: 0.0125%, 0.25%, 0.1%? ________

Change each of the following percentages to a ratio, and reduce to lowest terms.

18. 16% ________ 19. 45% ________

20. A client is on a 1,000 mL fluid restriction per 24 hours. At breakfast and lunch the client consumed 40% of the fluid allowance. How many milliliters did the client consume? ________

21. A client drank 75% of a 12 ounce can of ginger ale. How many ounces did the client drink? ________

22. A client consumes 55% of a bowl of chicken broth at lunch. The bowl holds 180 mL. How many milliliters did the client consume? ________

23. In a class of 30 students, 6 students did not pass an exam. What percentage of the students did not pass the exam? ________

24. At the first prenatal visit a client weighed 140 pounds. At the second visit the client had a 5% weight increase. How many pounds did the client gain? ________

25. An infant consumed 55% of an 8 ounce bottle of formula. How many ounces of formula did the infant consume? ________

26. In a portion of turkey that is 100 g (grams), there are 23 g of protein and 4 g of fat.

    What percentage of the portion is protein? ________

    What percentage of the portion is fat? ________

27. A nursing review test has 130 questions, and you answer 120 correctly. What is your score, as a percentage? ________

28. A client's intake for the day was 2,000 calories, and 600 of the calories came from fat. What percentage of the client's intake came from fat? ________

29. A client began receiving 325 mg (milligrams) of a medication. The prescriber increased the dosage of medication by 10%. What will the new dosage be?

    ________ mg

30. The recommended daily allowance (RDA) of a vitamin is 14 milligrams (mg). If a multivitamin provides 55% of the RDA, how many mg of the vitamin would the client receive from the multivitamin? ____________

31. A client's pulse rate decreases from 80 beats per minute to 72 beats per minute. What is the percent of decrease? ____________

32. A client's medication is increased from 400 milligrams (mg) to 500 mg. What is the percent of increase in the dosage? ____________

33. A client's weight increased from 120 lb to 132 lb. What was the percent of increase in body weight? ____________

34. A client's intake decreased from 2,500 milliliters (mL) per day to 2,000 mL per day. What was the percent of decrease? ____________

35. The number of capsules a client received each day has decreased from 3 capsules each day to 2 capsules per day. What is the percent of decrease? ____________

36. If a client ate 400 calories at breakfast, what percentage of a 2,000-calorie diet was consumed? ____________

37. A newborn weighed 3,751 grams (g) at birth and 3,352 g prior to discharge. What is the percentage of weight loss? ____________

38. In August of one year, 15 cases of heat stroke were treated in the emergency room. In August of the next year, 12 cases of heat stroke were treated. What is the percent of decrease in cases of heat stroke? ____________

39. A client is on a 2,000-calorie-per-day diet. If lunch accounts for 45% of a client's daily calories, how many calories can the client have for lunch? ____________

Convert the following percents to decimals.

40. 4.4% ____________ 41. 103% ____________

Convert the following decimals to percents.

42. 0.32 ____________ 43. 0.06 ____________

Identify the strongest in each of the following.

44. 1:10, 1:100, 1:200 ____________ 45. 1:25, $\frac{1}{5}$, 0.02% ____________

Answers on p. 68

ANSWERS

Chapter 5

Answers to Practice Problems

1. $\frac{1}{100}$
2. $\frac{1}{50}$
3. ½
4. 1½
5. $\frac{3}{100}$
6. 0.1
7. 0.35
8. 0.5
9. 0.14
10. 0.0086
11. 1:4
12. 11:100
13. 3:4
14. 4.5:100
15. 0.4:100
16. 40%
17. 275%
18. 50%
19. 25%
20. 70%
21. 132%
22. 2%
23. 80%
24. 230%
25. 1.3%
26. 4%
27. 75%
28. 10%
29. 1%
30. 50%
31. 50 g
32. 100 g
33. 12.5 g
34. 50 g
35. 7.5 g
36. 1%
37. 0.5%
38. 0.25%
39. 1:3
40. 0.9%
41. 60 mL
42. 4 oz
43. 18
44. 15
45. 1%
46. 10%
47. 4%
48. 25.26
49. 0.42
50. 123.75
51. 62.5%
52. 25%
53. 0.17
54. 41.67%
55. 20%
56. 50%
57. 25%
58. 50%
59. 10%
60. 64%

Answers to Chapter Review

	Percent	Ratio	Fraction	Decimal
1.	52%	13:25	$\frac{13}{25}$	0.52
2.	71%	71:100	$\frac{71}{100}$	0.71
3.	7%	7:100	$\frac{7}{100}$	0.07
4.	2%	1:50	$\frac{1}{50}$	0.02
5.	6%	3:50	$\frac{3}{50}$	0.06
6.	37.5%	3:8	$\frac{3}{8}$	0.38
7.	61%	61:100	$\frac{61}{100}$	0.61
8.	0.7%	7:1,000	$\frac{7}{1,000}$	0.007
9.	5%	1:20	$\frac{1}{20}$	0.05
10.	2.5%	1:40	$\frac{1}{40}$	0.03

11. 4.8 oz
12. 56
13. 13.3%
14. 0.83%
15. 37.5
16. 25%
17. 0.25%
18. 4 : 25
19. 9 : 20
20. 400 mL
21. 9 oz
22. 99 mL
23. 20%
24. 7 lb
25. 4.4 oz
26. 23% protein, 4% fat
27. 92.3%
28. 30%
29. 357.5 mg
30. 7.7 mg
31. 10%
32. 25%
33. 10%
34. 20%
35. 33.3% or $33\frac{1}{3}\%$
36. 20%
37. 10.6%
38. 20%
39. 900 calories
40. 0.044
41. 1.03
42. 32%
43. 6%
44. 1:10
45. ⅕

POST-TEST

After completing Unit One of this text, you should be able to complete this test. The test consists of a total of 75 questions. If you miss any questions in any section, review the chapter relating to that content.

Express the following in Roman numerals.

1. 5 ______
2. 17 ______
3. 27 ______
4. 29 ______
5. 30 ______

Express the following in Arabic numbers.

6. $\overline{\text{viss}}$ ______
7. $\overline{\text{xxiv}}$ ______
8. $\overline{\text{xix}}$ ______
9. $\overline{\text{XXV}}$ ______
10. $\overline{\text{XV}}$ ______

Reduce the following fractions to lowest terms.

11. $\frac{8}{6}$ ______
12. $\frac{22}{33}$ ______
13. $\frac{27}{63}$ ______
14. $\frac{10}{15}$ ______
15. $\frac{16}{10}$ ______

Perform the indicated operations with fractions; reduce to lowest terms where needed.

16. $\frac{5}{6} \div \frac{7}{10} =$ ______
17. $5\frac{1}{2} \div 4\frac{1}{2} =$ ______
18. $6\frac{1}{3} \times 4 =$ ______
19. $5\frac{1}{5} - 3\frac{4}{7} =$ ______
20. $\frac{5}{4} + \frac{2}{9} =$ ______
21. $\frac{4}{9} + \frac{7}{9} =$ ______
22. $1\frac{1}{3} + \frac{5}{7} =$ ______
23. $7\frac{1}{2} \times \frac{3}{4} =$ ______
24. $7\frac{1}{4} - 2\frac{1}{3} =$ ______
25. $2 - \frac{10}{21} =$ ______

Change the following fractions to decimals; express each answer to the nearest tenth.

26. $\frac{8}{7}$ ______
27. $\frac{1}{8}$ ______
28. $\frac{1}{15}$ ______
29. $\frac{12}{13}$ ______

Indicate the largest fraction in each group.

30. $\frac{1}{2}, \frac{2}{3}, \frac{5}{9}$ ______
31. $\frac{3}{4}, \frac{7}{10}, \frac{5}{8}$ ______

Perform the indicated operations with decimals. Provide exact answers.

32. $16.7 + 21 =$ ______

33. $0.007 + 17.4 =$ ______

34. $10.57 \times 10 =$ ______

35. $36.8 - 3.86 =$ ______

Divide the following decimals; express each answer to the nearest tenth.

36. $67.8 \div 0.8 =$ ______

37. $9 \div 0.4 =$ ______

38. $5.01 \div 10 =$ ______

Indicate the largest decimal in each group.

39. 0.85, 0.085 ______

40. 3.002, 0.39, 0.399 ______

41. 0.478, 0.445, 0.493 ______

Solve for x, the unknown value.

42. $10:20 = x:8$ ______

43. $500:x = 200:1$ ______

44. $0.3:x = 1.8:0.6$ ______

45. $\frac{1}{4}:x = \frac{1}{8}:2$ ______

Round off to the nearest tenth.

46. 0.57 ______

47. 0.99 ______

48. 1.42 ______

Round off to the nearest hundredth.

49. 0.677 ______

50. 0.832 ______

51. 1.222 ______

Complete the table below. Express each of the measures in their equivalents where indicated. Reduce fractions and ratios to lowest terms; round decimals to hundredths.

	Percent	Decimal	Ratio	Fraction
52.	______	______	1:10	______
53.	60%	______	______	______
54.	$66\frac{2}{3}\%$	______	______	______
55.	25%	______	______	______

Find the percentage.

56. 9% of 200 ______

57. 2.5% of 750 ______

58. 30 is what percent of 45? ______

59. 5 is what percent of 2,000? ______

60. 25 is what percent of 65? ______

Express the following solution strengths as ratios.

61. 1 part medication to 80 parts solution ________________

62. 1 part medication to 300 parts solution ________________

63. 1 part medication to 20 parts solution ________________

Identify the strongest solution in each of the following:

64. 1 : 80, 1 : 800, 1 : 8,000 ____________ 65. 1 : 1,000, 1 : 2,000, 1 : 5,000 ________

66. A client who weighed 81.5 kilograms (kg) lost 3.75 kg. How much does the client weigh now? ________________

67. A client's weight increased from 175 pounds (lb) to 210 lb. What was the percent of increase in the client's weight? ________________

68. A client is receiving 0.6 milligrams (mg) of a medication four (4) times a day. How many mg would the client receive after $2\frac{1}{2}$ days? ________________

69. If 6 oz of medication must be mixed with 15 oz of water, how many oz of water is needed for four (4) oz of medication? ________________

70. A client is taking two (2) tablets twice a day for 14 days. The tablet contains 2.2 mg. How much medication did the client receive? ________________

71. A client should have received 3.25 grams (g) of medication. In error the nurse administered 32.5 g. How much more medication did the client receive? ________________

72. Write a ratio that represents 20 milligrams (mg) of a medication in 100 milliliters (mL) of liquid. ________________

73. A client's weight decreased from 150 pounds (lb) to 132 lb. What is the percent of decrease in the client's weight? ________________

74. A client receives a total of 13.5 milligrams (mg) from nine (9) tablets. What is the dosage strength of each tablet? ________________

75. Write a ratio that represents every capsule in a bottle contains 0.75 milligram (mg).

____

Answers on p. 72

ANSWERS

1. v, $\overline{\text{v}}$, V
2. xvii, $\overline{\text{xvii}}$, XVII
3. xxvii, $\overline{\text{xxvii}}$, XXVII
4. xxix, $\overline{\text{xxix}}$, XXIX
5. xxx, $\overline{\text{xxx}}$, XXX
6. $6\frac{1}{2}$
7. 24
8. 19
9. 25
10. 15
11. $1\frac{1}{3}$
12. $\frac{2}{3}$
13. $\frac{3}{7}$
14. $\frac{2}{3}$
15. $1\frac{3}{5}$
16. $1\frac{4}{21}$
17. $1\frac{2}{9}$
18. $25\frac{1}{3}$
19. $1\frac{22}{35}$
20. $1\frac{17}{36}$
21. $\frac{11}{9} = 1\frac{2}{9}$
22. $2\frac{1}{21}$
23. $5\frac{5}{8}$
24. $4\frac{11}{12}$
25. $1\frac{11}{21}$
26. 1.1
27. 0.1
28. 0.1
29. 0.9
30. $\frac{2}{3}$
31. $\frac{3}{4}$
32. 37.7
33. 17.407
34. 105.7
35. 32.94
36. 84.8
37. 22.5
38. 0.5
39. 0.85
40. 3.002
41. 0.493
42. $x = 4$
43. $x = 2.5$ *or* $2\frac{1}{2}$
44. $x = 0.1$ *or* $\frac{1}{10}$
45. $x = 4$
46. 0.6
47. 1
48. 1.4
49. 0.68
50. 0.83
51. 1.22

	Percent	Decimal	Ratio	Fraction
52.	10%	0.1	1:10	$\frac{1}{10}$
53.	60%	0.6	3:5	$\frac{3}{5}$
54.	$66\frac{2}{3}$%	0.67	67:100	$\frac{67}{100}$
55.	25%	0.25	1:4	$\frac{1}{4}$

56. 18
57. 18.75
58. 66 2/3% *or* 66.7% *or* 67%
59. 0.25%
60. 38.46% *or* 38.5% *or* 38%
61. 1:80
62. 1:300
63. 1:20
64. 1:80
65. 1:1,000
66. 77.75 kilograms (kg)
67. 20%
68. 6 milligrams (mg)
69. 10 oz
70. 123.2 milligram (mg)
71. 29.25 gram (g)
72. 20 mg:100 mL *or* 1 mg:5 mL
73. 12%
74. 1.5 milligram (mg)
75. 0.75 mg:1 capsule

UNIT TWO

Systems of Measurement

In order for the nurse to be competent in the administration of medications, the nurse must be knowledgeable in the measurement system used to order, measure, and administer medications. The metric system is the preferred system of measurement used in health care. Because the metric system is preferred, we will begin with the discussion of the metric system.

Chapter 6 Metric System

Chapter 7 Apothecary and Household Systems

Chapter 8 Converting Within and Between Systems

Chapter 9 Additional Conversions Useful in the Health Care Setting

CHAPTER 6
Metric System

Objectives

After reviewing this chapter, you should be able to:

1. Express metric measures correctly using rules of the metric system
2. State common equivalents in the metric system
3. Convert measures within the metric system

To administer medications safely to clients, it is important to have a thorough knowledge of the system of measurements used in medication administration. Understanding common equivalents and the systems of measurement used in medication administration will help in the prevention of **medication errors** related to incorrect dosages.

Historically, there were three different systems of measure used in medication administration: the apothecary, household, and metric systems. As stated, the metric system is the preferred system of measurement for medications and measurements used in the health care setting. For example, newborn weights are recorded in grams (g) and kilograms (kg); centimeters (cm) are used in obstetrics to express fundal height (upper portion of the uterus) and to measure incisions.

The metric system is an international decimal system of weights and measures that was introduced in France in the late seventeenth and eighteenth centuries. It is also referred to as the *International System of Units.* The International System of Units, universally abbreviated SI (from the French Le Systéme International d Unités), is the modern metric system of measurement. The abbreviations of this system of metric notations are the most widely accepted. The benefit of the metric system lies in its simplicity and accuracy because it is based on the decimal system. The nurse will find that medication calculation and administration skills involve familiarity and accuracy with the metric system to administer medications safely.

Prescribers should use the metric system for prescribing medications to prevent medication errors. The Joint Commission (TJC), Food and Drug Administration (FDA), and Institute for Safe Medication Practices (ISMP) concur that the metric system should be used to prevent medication errors. This includes writing prescriptions in the metric system, and all US FDA-approved prescription medication labels provide metric dosage.

Particulars of the Metric System

1. The metric system is based on the decimal system, in which divisions and multiples of 10 are used. Therefore, a lot of math can be done by decimal point movement.
2. Three basic units of measure are used in the metric system, as shown in Table 6-1.

Dosages are calculated by using metric measurements that relate to weight and volume. Meter (m), which is the base unit used for linear (length) measurement, is the least used measurement for dosage calculations but is important in the health care setting. Linear

TABLE 6-1 Basic Units of Metric Measurement

Table of Measure	Basic Unit	Abbreviation
Weight (solid)	Gram	g
Volume (liquid)	Liter	L
Length	Meter	m

measurements are commonly used to measure the height of an individual, for serial abdominal girth (the circumference of the abdomen, usually measured at the umbilicus), the circumference of an infant's head, length of an amount of medicated ointment or paste, and for pressure ulcer measurements. These are examples of important measures that can be seen in the health care setting. Most length measurements seen in the health care setting are millimeters (mm) and centimeters (cm).

3. Common prefixes in this system denote the numerical value of the unit being discussed. Memorization of these prefixes is necessary for quick and accurate calculations. The prefixes in bold in Table 6-2 are the ones used most often in health care for dosage calculations. However, some of the prefixes may be used to express other values, such as laboratory values. *Kilo* is a common prefix used to identify a measure larger than the basic unit. The other common prefixes used in medication administration are smaller units: *centi, milli,* and *micro.*

Let's look at the following example to see how the prefixes may be used.

Example: 67 milligrams

Prefix—*milli*—means measure in thousandths of a unit.
Gram is a unit of weight.
Therefore 67 milligrams = 67 thousandths of a gram.

4. Regardless of the size of the unit, the name of the basic unit is incorporated into the measure (see Table 6-1). This allows easy recognition of the unit of measure.

Example 1: milli**liter**—The word *liter* indicates you are measuring volume (*milli* indicates 1/1,000 of that volume).

Example 2: kilo**gram**—The word *gram* indicates you are measuring weight (*kilo* indicates 1,000 of that weight; 1 kilogram = 1,000 grams).

Example 3: kilo**liter**—The word *liter* indicates you are measuring volume (*kilo* indicates 1,000 of that volume; 1 kiloliter = 1,000 liters).

Example 4: deci**liter**—The word *liter* indicates that you are measuring volume (*deci* indicates 0.1 of that volume [liter], or 100 milliliters). "Female's normal hemoglobin is 12 to 16 g/dL," means there are 12 to 16 grams of hemoglobin contained in 100 milliliters of blood.

Example 5: cubic milli**meter** (mm^3)—cubic millimeter is a unit of volume of three-dimensional space (length × width × height). In a normal individual the white blood cell count ranges between 5,000 and 10,000 cells per cubic millimeter of blood. Therefore, 1 mm^3 of blood contains between 5,000 and 10,000 white blood cells (5,000/mm^3 and 10,000/mm^3).

SAFETY ALERT!

Do not confuse units of measure in the metric system for weight, volume, and length that have similar names. Milligram is a unit of weight; milliliter is a unit of volume; and millimeter is a unit of length.

TABLE 6-2 Common Prefixes Used in Health Care

Prefix	Numerical Value	Meaning
Kilo*	1,000	one thousand times
Hecto	100	one hundred times
Deka	10	ten times
Deci	0.1	one tenth
Centi*	0.01	one hundredth part of
Milli*	0.001	one thousandth part of
Micro*	0.000001	one millionth part of

*Prefixes used most often in medication administration.

POINTS TO REMEMBER

It is important to memorize the prefixes and the amounts they represent. A mnemonic to help remember the important metric prefixes order from largest measurement to smallest is: **K**itty **H**awk **D**oesn't **D**rink **C**anned **M**ilk **M**uch.

kilo, hecto, deka, deci, centi, milli, micro.

5. The abbreviation for a unit of measure in the metric system is often the first letter of the word. Lowercase letters are used more often than capital letters.

Example 1: g = gram

Example 2: m = meter

The exception to this rule is liter, for which a capital letter is used.

Example 3: liter = L

6. When prefixes are used in combination with the basic unit, the first letter of the prefix and the first letter of the unit of measure are written together in lowercase letters.

Example 1: Milligram—abbreviated as *mg.* The *m* is taken from the prefix *milli* and the *g* from *gram,* the unit of weight.

Example 2: Microgram—abbreviated as **mcg.** Microgram is also abbreviated using the Greek symbol (μg). Use of this symbol for micrograms (μg) should not be used for communicating medical information, including medication orders. It can be misinterpreted as mg (milligrams), resulting in a thousandfold overdose.

SAFETY ALERT!

The abbreviation μg for microgram is listed on the Institute for Safe Medication Practice (ISMP) list of Error-Prone Abbreviations, Symbols, and Dose Designations (2013). Confusion of the symbol used for microgram with the abbreviation for milligram could cause a critical error in dosage calculation. These units differ from each other in value by 1,000.

Example 3: Milliliter—abbreviated as **mL.** Note that when *L (liter)* is used in combination with a prefix, it **remains capitalized.** Milliliter (mL) is a small volume, it is one-thousandth of a liter, and commonly used in dosage calculation.

SAFETY ALERT!

You may see gram abbreviated as Gm or gm, liter as lowercase l, or milliliter ml. These abbreviations are outdated and can lead to misinterpretation. Use only the standardized SI abbreviations. Use g for gram, L for liter, and mL for milliliter. Cubic centimeter, abbreviated cc, was used interchangeably for mL. Using cc for mL should not be done and has been misinterpreted for zeros (00) or units (U). In addition, cc is not a measure of volume; it is the amount of space occupied by a milliliter (mL). The use of the abbreviation U is prohibited and must be spelled out (unit). It has been mistaken for zero (0) and the number 4 (four). When in doubt about an abbreviation being used, never assume; ask the prescriber for clarification.

SAFETY ALERT!

It is critical to differentiate between the SI abbreviations for milligram (mg) and milliliter (mL). At a quick glance these abbreviations appear similar; however, confusing these two units can result in lethal consequences for a client.

Box 6-1 lists the common metric abbreviations.

BOX 6-1 Common Metric Abbreviations

gram = g
microgram = mcg
milligram = mg
kilogram = kg
liter = L
*deciliter = dL
milliliter = mL

*Seen in the expression of laboratory values (e.g., hemoglobin, creatinine levels).

Rules of the Metric System

Certain rules specific to the metric system are important to remember (Box 6-2). **These rules are critical to the prevention of errors and ensure accurate interpretation of metric notations when used in medication orders. [Never assume.]** Ask for clarification if you are not sure of the abbreviation or notation to prevent an error.

SAFETY ALERT!

As part of the National Patient Safety Goals, TJC set up specific guidelines for the use of leading and trailing zeros. This is also a recommendation of ISMP. A zero should always be placed in front of the decimal when the quantity is less than a whole number (leading zero). When the quantity expressed is preceded by a whole number, zeros are not placed after the number (trailing zeros). This rule is critical to preventing misinterpretation and medication errors. Always double-check the placement of decimals and zeros.

Example 1: .52 mL is written as 0.52 mL to **reinforce the decimal** and avoid being misread as 52 mL. Lack of a leading zero before the decimal point could result in the decimal point being missed and cause a critical error in dosage interpretation.

Example 2: 2.5 mL is written as 2.5 mL, not 2.50 mL. **Addition of unnecessary zeros can lead to errors in reading;** 2.50 mL may be misread as 250 mL instead of 2.5 mL. Unnecessary zeros can also result in the decimal point being missed and cause a critical error in dosage interpretation.

BOX 6-2 Metric System Rules

1. Use Arabic numbers to express quantities in this system.

   Example: 1, 1,000, 0.5

2. Express parts of a unit or fractions of a unit as decimals.

   Example: 0.4 g, 0.5 L $\left(\text{not } \frac{2}{5} \text{ g}, \frac{1}{2} \text{ L}\right)$

3. Always write the quantity, whether in whole numbers or in decimals, before the abbreviation or symbol for a unit of measure.

   Example: 1,000 mg, 0.75 mL (not mg 1,000, mL 0.75)

4. Use a full space between the numeral and abbreviation.

   Example: 2 mL, 1 L (not 2mL, 1L)

5. Always place a leading zero to the left of the decimal point if there is no whole number. Eliminate trailing zeros to the right of the decimal point.

   Example: 0.4 mL, 2 mg (not .4 mL, 2.0 mg)

6. Do not use the abbreviation μg for microgram; it might be mistaken for mg. Remember mg is 1,000 times larger.
7. Do not use the abbreviation *cc* for mL. This abbreviation can be misinterpreted as zeros. mL is the acceptable unit for volume.

   Example: 2 mL (not 2 cc)

8. Avoid periods after the abbreviation for a unit of measure to avoid the possibility of it being misread for the number 1 in a poorly handwritten order.

   Example: mg (not mg.)

9. Place commas in values at 1,000 or above. ISMP recommends this to improve readability.

   Example: 100,000 units (not 100000 units)

10. Do not add "s" on a unit of measure to make it plural; this could lead to misinterpretation.

    Example: mg (not mgs)

PRACTICE **PROBLEMS**

Applying the guidelines relating to the use of leading and trailing zeros, express the following values correctly.

1. .750 g ____________
2. 1.70 mL ____________
3. .68 L ____________
4. 7.0 kg ____________
5. .002 mg ____________

Answers on p. 84

Units of Measure

Understanding common equivalents in the metric system can assist the nurse in preventing medication errors related to incorrect dosage.

Weight

The gram is the basic unit of weight. Medications may be ordered in grams or fractions of a gram, such as milligram or microgram.

1. The milligram is 1,000 times smaller than a gram:

$$1 \text{ g} = 1{,}000 \text{ mg}$$

2. The microgram is 1,000 times smaller than a milligram and 1 million times smaller than a gram. The word *micro* also means tiny or small. Micrograms are tiny parts of a gram (i.e., 1,000 mcg = 1 mg). A milligram is 1,000 times larger than a microgram. It takes 1 million mcg to make 1 g.
3. The kilogram is very large and is not used for measuring medications. A kilogram is 1,000 times larger than a gram (i.e., 1 kg = 1,000 g). This measure is often used to denote weights of clients, on which medication dosages are based. This is the only unit you will see used to identify a unit larger than the basic unit.

Volume

1. The **liter** is the basic unit.

   1 L = 1,000 mL

2. The **milliliter** is 1,000 times smaller than a liter. It is abbreviated as mL.

   1 mL = 0.001 L

3. As previously stated, **cubic centimeter** (cc) should not be used because of misinterpretation. The cubic centimeter is the amount of space that 1 mL of liquid occupies. Remember, mL is the correct term for volume. The use of cc for mL is currently prohibited by many health care organizations. TJC has also suggested that institutions prohibit the use of the abbreviation cc and add it to their "Do Not Use" List. ISMP also includes cc as an abbreviation that should not be used. Figure 6-1 shows metric measures that may be seen on a medication cup. Note: mL indicated on the medicine cup indicating a capacity of 30 mL.

Although pint and quart are not metric measures, they have metric equivalents. For example, a quart is approximately the size of a liter: 1 quart ≈ 1,000 mL and 1 pint ≈ 500 mL. Although pint and quart are not measures used in medication administration, you may need them to calculate a solution, especially in home care. For pharmacological purposes, the equivalents stated for pint and quart are used.

Box 6-3 presents the metric units of measure used most often for dosage calculations and measurement of health status. This text will use the standardized abbreviations for metric units throughout.

BOX 6-3 Metric Equivalents to Memorize

Weight
1 kilogram (kg) = 1,000 grams (g)
1 gram (g) = 1,000 milligrams (mg)
1 milligram (mg) = 1,000 micrograms (mcg)

Volume
1 liter (L) = 1,000 milliliters (mL)
1 milliliter (mL) = 0.001 liter (L)

Length
1 meter (m) = 100 centimeters (cm) = 1,000 mm
1 millimeter (mm) = 0.001 meter (m) = 0.1 cm

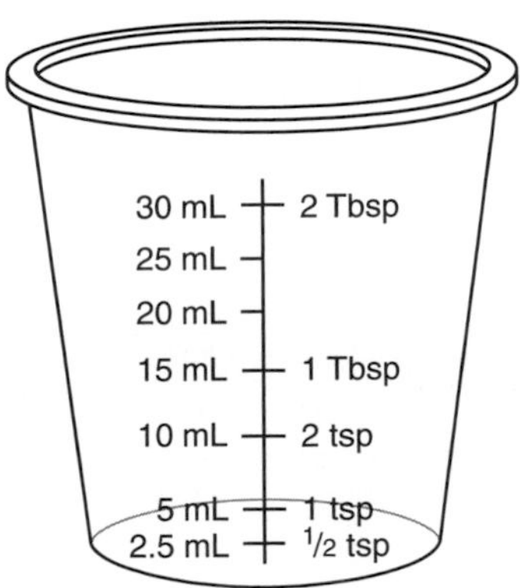

Figure 6-1 Medicine cup showing volume measure in milliliters (mL).

Conversions Between Metric Units

Because the metric system is based on the decimal system, conversions between one metric system unit and another can be done by moving the decimal point. The number of places to move the decimal point depends on the equivalent. In health care, each unit of measure in common use for purposes of medication administration differs by 1,000. In the metric system the most common terms used are the kilogram, gram, milligram, microgram, liter, milliliter, and centimeter. To **convert** or make a **conversion** means to change from one unit to another. This converting can be simply changing a measure to its equivalent in the same system. Changing from grams to milligrams illustrates a metric measure changed to another metric measure. Each metric unit in common use for *medication administration* differs from the next by a factor of 1,000. Metric conversions can therefore be made by dividing or multiplying by **1,000.** Knowledge of the size of a unit is important when converting by moving the decimal because this determines whether division or multiplication is necessary to make the conversion.

Nurses often make conversions within the metric system when administering medications, for example, grams to milligrams.

To make conversions within the metric system, remember the common conversion factors (1 kg = 1,000 g, 1 g = 1,000 mg, 1 mg = 1,000 mcg, and 1 L = 1,000 mL) and the following rules:

RULE

To convert a **smaller** unit to a **larger** one, **divide** by moving the decimal point **three places to the left.**

Example 1: 100 mL = ___ L (conversion factor: 1,000 mL = 1 L)
(smaller) (larger)

100 mL = .100 = 0.1 L **(Placing zero in front of the decimal is important.)**

Example 2: 50 mg = ___ g (conversion factor: 1,000 mg = 1 g)
(smaller) (larger)

50 mg = .050 = 0.05 g **(Placing zero in front of the decimal is important.)**

RULE

To convert a **larger** unit to a **smaller** one, **multiply** by moving the decimal **three places to the right.**

NOTE

Answers to conversions should be labeled with the unit of measure.

Example 1: 0.75 g = ___ mg (conversion factor: 1 g = 1,000 mg)
(larger) (smaller)

0.75 g = 0.750 = 750 mg

Example 2: 0.04 kg = ___ g (conversion factor: 1 kg = 1,000 g)
(larger) (smaller)

0.04 kg = 0.040 = 40 g

SAFETY ALERT!

When converting quantities in the metric system from one unit of measure to another within the metric system, pay close attention to the decimal point. Moving the decimal point incorrectly (in the wrong direction) can result in a dangerous error.

PRACTICE PROBLEMS

Convert the following metric measures by moving the decimal.

6. 300 mg = ______________ g
7. 6 mg = ______________ mcg
8. 0.7 L = ______________ mL
9. 180 mcg = ______________ mg
10. 0.02 mg = ______________ mcg
11. 4.5 L = ______________ mL
12. 4.2 g = ______________ mg
13. 0.9 g = ______________ mg
14. 3,250 mL = ______________ L
15. 42 g = ______________ kg
16. 529 mg = ______________ g
17. 645 mcg = ______________ mg
18. 347 L = ______________ mL
19. 238 g = ______________ mcg
20. 3,500 mL = ______________ L
21. 0.04 kg = ______________ g
22. 658 kg = ______________ g
23. 51 mL = ______________ L
24. 1.6 mg = ______________ mcg
25. 28 mL = ______________ L

Answers on p. 84

POINTS TO REMEMBER

- The liter and the gram are the basic units used for medication administration.
- Conversion factors must be memorized to do conversions. The common conversion factors in the metric system are 1 kg = 1,000 g, 1 g = 1,000 mg, 1 mg = 1,000 mcg, and 1 L = 1,000 mL (mL is the correct term to use in relation to volume, not cc).
- Express answers using the following rules of the metric system:
  1. Fractional metric units are expressed as a decimal.
  2. Place a leading zero in front of the decimal point when the quantity is less than a whole number to prevent potential dosage error.
  3. Omit trailing zeros to avoid misreading of a value and potential error in dosage.
  4. The abbreviation for a measure is placed after the quantity.
  5. Place a full space between the numeral and abbreviation.
  6. Use standard SI abbreviations.
- Converting common metric units used in medication administration from one unit to another is done by multiplying or dividing by 1,000.
- Answers should be stated with the unit of measure as the label.
- Place commas in amounts of 1,000 or above.
- Never guess at the meaning of a metric notation, ask for clarification.

CHAPTER REVIEW

1. List the three units of measurement used in the metric system.

   a. ______________ c. ______________

   b. ______________

2. Which is larger, kilogram or milligram? ______________________

3. 1 mL = ______________ L

4. What units of measure are used in the metric system for:

   a. liquid capacity? ______________ b. weight? ______________

5. 1,000 mg = ______________ g

6. 1 L = ______________ mL

7. 1,000 mcg = ______________ mg

8. 1,000 mL = ______________ L

Using the rules of the metric system, state the acceptable abbreviations for the following units of measure.

9. liter ______________

10. microgram ______________

11. milliliter ______________

12. gram ______________

13. kilogram ______________

Provide the meaning for the following prefixes

14. kilo ______________

15. milli ______________

Using abbreviations and the rules of the metric system, express the following quantities correctly.

16. Six tenths of a gram ______________

17. Fifty kilograms ______________

18. Four tenths of a milligram ______________

19. Four hundredths of a liter ______________

20. Four and two tenths micrograms ______________

21. Five thousandths of a gram ______________

22. Six hundredths of a gram ______________

23. Two and six tenths milliliters ______________

24. One hundred milliliters ______________

25. Three hundredths of a milliliter ______________

Convert the following metric measures by moving the decimal.

26. 950 mcg = ______________ mg

27. 58.5 L = ______________ mL

28. 130 mL = ______________ L

29. 276 g = ______________ mg

30. 550 mL = ______________ L

31. 56.5 L = ______________ mL

32. 205 g = ______________ kg

33. 0.025 kg = ______________ g

34. 1 L = ______________ mL

35. 0.015 g = ______________ mg

36. 250 mcg = ______________ mg

37. 8 kg = ______________ g

38. 2 kL = ______________ L

39. 5 L = ______________ mL

40. 0.75 L = ______________ mL

41. 0.33 g = ______________ mg

42. 750 mg = ______________ g

43. 6.28 kg = ______________ g

44. 36.5 mg = ______________ g

45. 2.2 mg = ______________ g

46. 400 g = ______________ kg

47. 0.024 L = ______________ mL

48. 100 mg = ______________ g

49. 150 g = ______________ mg

50. 85 mcg = ______________ mg

51. 1.25 L = ______________ mL

52. 0.05 mg = ______________ mcg

53. 120 mg = ______________ g

54. 475 mL = ______________ L

55. 4.5 g = ______________ mg

56. 8.6 mg = ______________ mcg

57. 250,000 mcg = ______________ mg

58. 40 mg = ______________ g

59. 0.65 kg = ______________ g

60. 37.5 mcg = ______________ mg

61. 0.026 mg = ______________ mcg

62. 36,000 mg = ______________ g

63. 0.125 g = ______________ mg

64. 5,524 g = ______________ kg

65. 8,500 mcg = ______________ mg

Which of the following is stated correctly using metric abbreviations and rules?

66. .5 g, 0.5 gm, .5 gm, 0.5 g ______________

67. 4 KG, 4.0 Kg, Kg 04, 4 kg ______________

68. 1500.0 mg, 1,500 MG, 1,500 mg, 1500 mg

69. 1.5 mm, 1.50 mm, 1½ mm, 1.5 Mm

70. cm 2, 2.0 cm, 2 cm, 0.2 cm

71. 80.0 mcg, 080 mcg, 80 mcg, mcg 80

72. mL .7, .7 mL, mL 0.7, 0.7 mL

73. Lasix 20.0 mg, Lasix 20 mg, Lasix 20 MG, Lasix mg 20 ______________

74. Gentamicin 1½ mL, gentamicin 1.5 ml, gentamicin 1.5 mL, gentamicin 1½ ml ______________

75. Ampicillin 500 mg, ampicillin 500.0 mg, ampicillin 500 MG, ampicillin mg 500 ______________

Answers on p. 84

evolve

For additional practice problems, refer to the Conversions and Equivalents section of the Elsevier's Interactive Drug Calculation Application Version 1 on Evolve.

ANSWERS

Chapter 6

Answers to Practice Problems

1. 0.75 g
2. 1.7 mL
3. 0.68 L
4. 7 kg
5. 0.002 mg
6. 0.3 g
7. 6,000 mcg
8. 700 mL
9. 0.18 mg
10. 20 mcg
11. 4,500 mL
12. 4,200 mg
13. 900 mg
14. 3.25 L
15. 0.042 kg
16. 0.529 g
17. 0.645 mg
18. 347,000 mL
19. 238,000,000 mcg
20. 3.5 L
21. 40 g
22. 658,000 g
23. 0.051 L
24. 1,600 mcg
25. 0.028 L

Answers to Chapter Review

1. gram (g), liter (L), meter (m)
2. kilogram (kg)
3. 0.001 L
4. a. L (liter), mL (milliliter)
   b. g (gram), mg (milligram), mcg (microgram), kg (kilogram)
5. 1 g
6. 1,000 mL
7. 1 mg
8. 1 L
9. L
10. mcg
11. mL
12. g
13. kg
14. one thousand times
15. the thousandth part of
16. 0.6 g
17. 50 kg
18. 0.4 mg
19. 0.04 L
20. 4.2 mcg
21. 0.005 g
22. 0.06 g
23. 2.6 mL
24. 100 mL
25. 0.03 mL
26. 0.95 mg
27. 58,500 mL
28. 0.13 L
29. 276,000 mg
30. 0.55 L
31. 56,500 mL
32. 0.205 kg
33. 25 g
34. 1,000 mL
35. 15 mg
36. 0.25 mg
37. 8,000 g
38. 2,000 L
39. 5,000 mL
40. 750 mL
41. 330 mg
42. 0.75 g
43. 6,280 g
44. 0.0365 g
45. 0.0022 g
46. 0.4 kg
47. 24 mL
48. 0.1 g
49. 150,000 mg
50. 0.085 mg
51. 1,250 mL
52. 50 mcg
53. 0.12 g
54. 0.475 L
55. 4,500 mg
56. 8,600 mcg
57. 250 mg
58. 0.04 g
59. 650 g
60. 0.0375 mg
61. 26 mcg
62. 36 g
63. 125 mg
64. 5.524 kg
65. 8.5 mg
66. 0.5 g
67. 4 kg
68. 1,500 mg
69. 1.5 mm
70. 2 cm
71. 80 mcg
72. 0.7 mL
73. Lasix 20 mg
74. Gentamicin 1.5 mL
75. Ampicillin 500 mg

CHAPTER 7
Apothecary and Household Systems

Objectives

After reviewing this chapter, you should be able to:

1. Differentiate apothecary and household system of measurement
2. Identify reasons for non-use of apothecary measures and symbols
3. State the common household equivalents
4. State specific rules that relate to the household system
5. Identify measures in the household system
6. Define other measures used in medication administration:
   - milliequivalent (mEq)
   - international units
   - unit

Apothecary System

The apothecary system of measurement is an English system and considered to be one of the oldest systems of measure. It is also referred to as the *fraction system* because parts of units are expressed by using fractions, with the exception of the fraction one half, which is expressed as ss or $\overline{ss}$. The notations are unusual and can be confusing. The recent trend is to eliminate apothecary measures from use and to use the metric system. The Institute for Safe Medication Practices (ISMP) has recommended that all medications be prescribed and calculated with metric measures. The unusual notations and inclusion of fractions and Roman numerals have caused concern about the use of the apothecary system.

Although apothecary measurements such as grains are disappearing from many medication labels, some medication labels may still include both apothecary and metric measure. For example, the label shown in (Figure 7-1), Nitrostat (nitroglycerin) indicates that 1/150 grain (gr) is equivalent to 0.4 milligrams (mg). Milligrams are the metric measure and grains (in parentheses) are the apothecary measure. At a quick glance grains could be easily misread and confused with grams.

Always use the metric measure on labels for dosage calculations that include both apothecary and metric measures. However, many of the newer labels include metric measures only.

Although the metric system is the preferred system, you may still see remnants of the apothecary system on syringes (minim), and medication cups (dram). Although ounce, which is apothecary, is still used today as part of the household system, the apothecary symbol for ounce (℥) should not be used. Many of the newer syringes in use today do not have the minim scale on them because of its inaccuracy.

Because of the difficulty encountered with using the apothecary system, the medication errors resulting from its use, and the recommendations of TJC, ISMP, and the Food and Drug Administration (FDA or USFDA), the apothecary system measures and rules will not be focused on. See Appendix A for a discussion of apothecary units and their metric equivalents. The FDA is often referred to as the "consumer watchdog." The FDA is responsible for protecting and promoting public health through regulation and supervision of products that include food and prescription and over-the-counter medications. The United

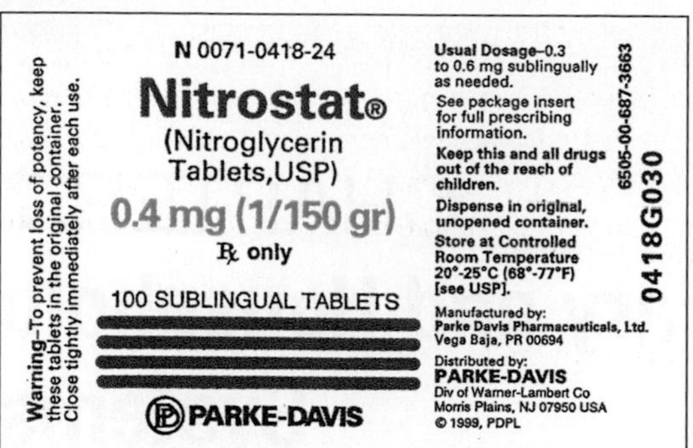

Figure 7-1 Medication label showing apothecary (gr) and metric (mg) measures.

States Pharmacopeia (USP) also does not recognize the apothecary system as an official system for measurement of medication dosages. There are symbols and abbreviations in this system that have been identified as error prone and should not be used.

SAFETY ALERT!

Do not use the following error-prone abbreviations and symbols. Always differentiate them from acceptable units of measure if they are used. Always clarify to be safe and prevent error before proceeding with any order using them. **The use of error-prone abbreviations and symbols can cause harm!**

DO NOT USE

gr (grains, apothecary unit of weight) confused with metric gram.
m (minim) mistaken for mL.
ʒ (dram, apothecary drop) mistaken for 3.
℥ (ounce, apothecary symbol) obsolete.
ss, $\overline{\textbf{ss}}$ (one half, apothecary symbol for ½) mistaken for 55.

Household System

The household system is an old system and the **least accurate** of the three systems of measure. It is a modified system designed for everyday use at home and includes approximate equivalents. Many of the household measures originated as apothecary measures. Conversions between household and metric measures are based on approximate equivalents, as can be seen with pints and quarts. For example, there are 32 ounces in a quart, which is generally accepted to be 1 liter (1,000 mL). Nurses need to be familiar with household measures because clients often use utensils in the home to take prescribed medications. Capacities of utensils such as a teaspoon, a tablespoon, and a cup vary from one house to another; therefore liquid measures are approximate. Because of the increase in nursing care provided at home (home care, visiting nurse), it is imperative that nurses become adept at converting from one system to another. When calculating doses or interpreting the health care provider's instructions for the client at home, the nurse must remember that household measures are used. Consequently, the nurse must be able to calculate equivalents for adaptation in the home, even though medication administration spoons, droppers, and medication measuring cups (Figure 7-2) are available.

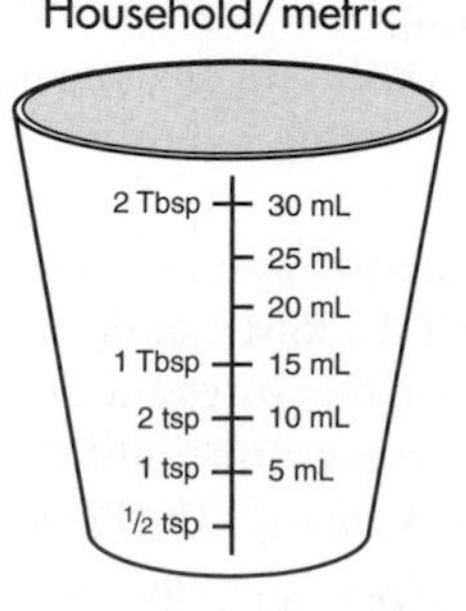

Figure 7-2 Medicine cup showing household/metric measurements.

SAFETY ALERT!

Although household utensils may be most familiar to clients, they may invite inaccuracies with medication dosages. Using ordinary household utensils may constitute a safety risk because ordinary household utensils do not come in standard sizes. Therefore, clients and their families should be advised to use the measuring device provided with the medication or purchase calibrated devices from the pharmacy as opposed to using their kitchen teaspoon for example.

Common household measures to memorize are the following:
1 teaspoon (t, tsp) = 5 mL
1 tablespoon (T, tbs) = 15 mL
1 measuring cup = 8 oz

NOTE

Anything less than a teaspoon should be measured in a syringe-type device that has no needle, not in a measuring cup.

SAFETY ALERT!

To ensure accurate dosages at home, utensils used should be marked or calibrated. Determine what kind of measuring devices the client is using at home and teach their proper use. Review the household equivalents and abbreviations, be extremely cautious, and do not confuse the abbreviations for teaspoon (t) and tablespoon (T). 1 teaspoon equals 5 mL, and 1 tablespoon equals 15 mL; confusing the abbreviations and their equivalents could result in a threefold error.

Particulars of the Household System

1. Some of the units for liquid measures are the same as those in the apothecary system, for example, pint and quart.
2. There are no standard rules for expressing household measures, which accounts for variations in their use.
3. Standard cookbook abbreviations are used in this system.
4. Arabic numerals and fractions are used to express quantities.
5. The smallest unit of measure in the household system is the drop (gtt).
6. The unit ounce used to measure liquid is sometimes referred to as fluid ounce.

SAFETY ALERT!

Drops should never be used as a measure for medications because the size of drops varies according to the diameter of the utensil and therefore can be inaccurate. When drops are used as a measure for medications, they should be calibrated or used only when associated with a dropper size, as in intravenous (IV) flow rates. When drops are ordered, the dropper often comes with the medication and should be used only for that medication.

See Box 7-1 for the household measures and metric equivalents.

It is important for the nurse providing care in the home to remember that clients need specific instructions for measuring accurately at home. Sometimes solutions may have to

BOX 7-1 Household/Metric Equivalents

Unit	Abbreviation	Equivalent	Metric Equivalent
teaspoon	t (tsp)	-----------	5 mL
tablespoon	T (tbs)	1 T = 3 t	15 mL
ounce (fluid)	oz	1 oz = 2 T	30 mL
cup (standard measuring	C	1 cup = 8 oz	240 mL
pint	pt	1 pt = 2 cups (16 oz)	500 mL*
quart	qt	1 qt = 4 cups = 2 pt = 32 oz	1,000 mL*
pound (weight)	lb	1 lb = 16 oz	2.2 lb = 1 kg (1,000 g)

NOTE: The unit "ounce," which is used to measure liquid volume, is sometimes referred to as fluid ounce.
*Approximate equivalent in the metric system.

be made at home with household measures. Some examples illustrating solutions made in the home using household devices are listed.

1. Normal saline solution (0.9%)—2 teaspoons of salt to 4 cups of water
2. Acetic acid solution (0.25%)—3 tablespoons of white vinegar to 4 cups of water for wound/dressing care and cleaning equipment

Household measures are most commonly used in the home care setting and less frequently in the clinical setting. With medication errors being one of the most common causes of client harm, it is quite possible that these measures may be eliminated in the near future because of the goal within health care to improve medication labeling and recommendations of organizations such as TJC and ISMP regarding abbreviations and use of metric measures in relation to medications to decrease medication errors.

Other Medication Measurements Used in Dosage Calculation

Other measurements that may be used to indicate the strength or potency of certain medications include unit, international unit, milliunit, and milliequivalent (mEq). The quantity or amount is expressed using Arabic numbers, with the unit of measure following.

Units express the amount of medication present in 1 milliliter (mL) of solution and are specific to the medication for which they are used. Units measure a medication in terms of its action. Medications such as heparin, insulin, and penicillin are measured in the United States Pharmacopeia unit (USP unit). USP unit has been standardized between manufacturers and has been determined by the United States Pharmacopeia (USP). USP is a government agency that sets standards for medications.

International unit represents a unit of potency used to measure things such as vitamins and chemicals. These International units represent the amount of medication needed to produce a certain effect and are standardized by international agreement.

Milliunit is 1/1,000 of a unit. 1 unit is equal to 1,000 milliunits. Nurses may need to convert units to milliunits. For example, oxytocin (Pitocin) is available in units (10 USP units per 1 mL). Very small doses of oxytocin may be ordered in milliunits. When oxytocin is used to augment labor, the intravenous infusion rate can be 0.5 to 2 milliunits per minute (0.0005 = 0.002 USP units).

Milliequivalents (mEq) are used to measure electrolytes (e.g., potassium) and the ionic activity of a medication. The milliequivalent is one thousandth (1/1,000) of the equivalent weight of an ion. The chemist or pharmacist defines milliequivalents as an expression of the number of grams of medication contained in 1 mL of normal solution. Other electrolytes measured in mEq include calcium, magnesium, and sodium.

The nurse does not have to memorize conversions for the international unit, USP unit, or milliequivalent, because medications that are ordered in these measurements are also prepared and administered in the same system. For example, medications that are ordered in units (such as insulin) will be available in units. Potassium is ordered in milliequivalents and available in milliequivalents. Figure 7-3 shows sample labels of medications in milliequivalents and units.

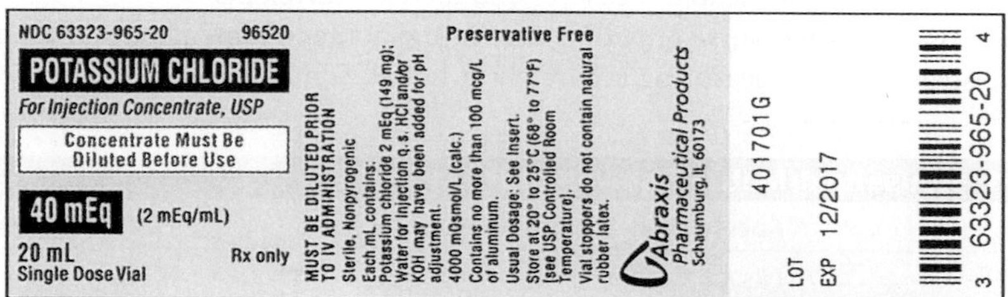

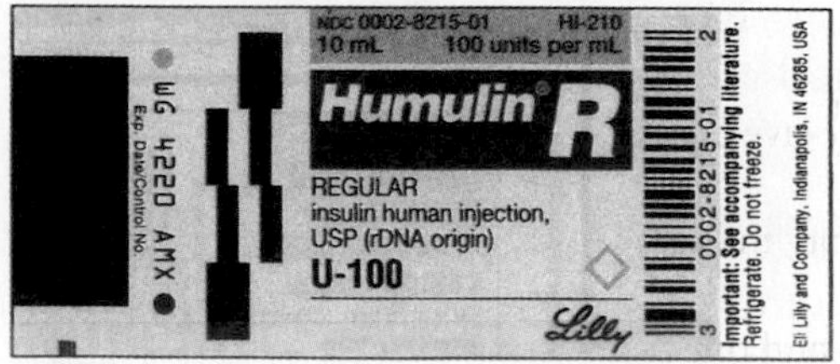

Figure 7-3 Medication labels showing milliequivalents and units.

SAFETY ALERT!

The abbreviations U and IU are prohibited and must be written out (units and international units). The abbreviation U and IU are included on TJC's official "Do Not Use" List (2016) and ISMP's list of Error-Prone Abbreviations, Symbols, and Dose Designations.

POINTS TO REMEMBER

- Teaspoon and tablespoon are common measures used in the household system.
- For safety, encourage clients to use the measuring device that comes with the medication or a measuring device purchased from the pharmacy.
- There are no rules for stating household measures.
- The household system uses fractions and Arabic numerals.
- Conversions between metric and household measures are approximate equivalents.
- Dosages less than a teaspoon should be measured with a syringe-type device that does not have a needle attached.
- When possible, convert household measures to metric measures.
- When in doubt about an unfamiliar unit or one that is not used often, consult a reference or an equivalency table.
- No conversion is necessary for unit, international unit, and milliequivalent. Medications prescribed in these measures are available in the same system.
- 1 unit = 1,000 milliunits. Nurses may have to convert units to milliunits.

PRACTICE **PROBLEMS**

Write the abbreviations for the following measures.

1. ounce ______
2. tablespoon ______
3. pint ______
4. teaspoon ______
5. pound ______
6. quart ______

Use Box 7-1 to determine the following equivalents.

7. $\frac{1}{2}$ oz = ______ mL
8. 2 tsp = ______ mL
9. 45 mL = ______ tbs
10. $\frac{1}{2}$ pt = ______ oz
11. 90 mL = ______ oz
12. 8 oz = ______ cup
13. 1 oz = ______ T
14. 3 tbs = ______ mL
15. 3 pt = ______ mL

Write the following amounts correctly using numerals and abbreviations.

16. 10 ounces ______
17. fifteen units ______
18. sixty-five pounds ______
19. twenty milliequivalents ______
20. two and one half teaspoons ______

21. three quarts ____________________

22. fourteen and one quarter ounces ________

23. ten tablespoons ____________________

24. What household measure might be used to give $\frac{1}{2}$ ounce of cough syrup?

____

25. The nurse encouraged a client with diarrhea to drink 40 ounces of water per day.

How many cups does this represent? ____________________

26. Medications such as penicillin and insulin are commonly measured in ________.

27. The unit used to measure the concentration of serum electrolytes such as potassium and sodium is the __________ and is abbreviated __________.

Answers on p. 91

CHAPTER REVIEW

Express the following using numerals and abbreviations:

1. one-third ounce ____________
2. three million units ____________
3. five and one-quarter teaspoons ____________
4. ten thousand units ____________
5. three and one-half quarts ____________
6. forty-five milliequivalents ________
7. five ounces ____________

Complete the following:

8. Pound is a unit of ____________.
9. The abbreviation for drop is ______.
10. T is the abbreviation for ________.
11. The abbreviation t is used for ____________________.
12. 1 t = ____________ mL
13. 1 oz = ____________ mL
14. 1 cup = ____________ oz
15. 1 tbs = ____________ mL
16. 1 pt = ____________ oz
17. 1 qt = ____________ oz

Express the following notations in words:

18. $8\frac{1}{4}$ oz ____________
19. 30 mEq ____________
20. 2 pt ____________
21. $15\frac{1}{2}$ lb ____________
22. 8 tbs ____________

23. True or False? The household system of measurement is commonly used for client dosages at home. ______________

24. True or False? Units can be abbreviated as U. ______________

25. True or False? Household measures are approximate equivalents. ______________

Answers below

evolve

For additional information, refer to the Conversions and Equivalents section of the Elsevier's Interactive Drug Calculation Application, Version 1 on Evolve.

ANSWERS

Chapter 7

Answers to Practice Problems

1. oz
2. T, tbs
3. pt
4. t, tsp
5. lb
6. qt
7. 15 mL
8. 10 mL
9. 3 tbs
10. 8 oz
11. 3 oz
12. 1 cup
13. 2 T
14. 45 mL
15. 1,500 mL
16. 10 oz, oz 10
17. 15 units
18. 65 lb
19. 20 mEq
20. $2\frac{1}{2}$ t, $2\frac{1}{2}$ tsp (varies)
21. 3 qt, qt 3
22. $14\frac{1}{4}$ oz, oz $14\frac{1}{4}$
23. 10 T, 10 tbs (varies)
24. 1 T, 1 tbs (varies)
25. 5 cups
26. units
27. milliequivalent; mEq

Answers to Chapter Review

1. $\frac{1}{3}$ oz, oz $\frac{1}{3}$
2. 3,000,000 units
3. $5\frac{1}{4}$ t, $5\frac{1}{4}$ tsp (varies)
4. 10,000 units
5. $3\frac{1}{2}$ qt, qt $3\frac{1}{2}$
6. 45 mEq
7. 5 oz, oz 5
8. weight
9. gtt
10. tablespoon
11. teaspoon
12. 5 mL
13. 30 mL
14. 8 oz
15. 15 mL
16. 16 oz
17. 32 oz
18. eight and one quarter ounces
19. thirty milliequivalents
20. two pints
21. fifteen and one half pounds
22. eight tablespoons
23. True
24. False
25. True

CHAPTER 8
Converting Within and Between Systems

Objectives

After reviewing this chapter, you should be able to:

1. State the equivalent metric and household approximate equivalents
2. Convert a unit of measure to its equivalent within the same system
3. Convert a unit from one system of measurement to its equivalent in another system of measurement

Equivalents Among Metric and Household Systems

As noted in earlier chapters dealing with the systems of measure, some measures in one system have equivalents in another; however, equivalents are not exact measures, and there are discrepancies. Several tables have been developed illustrating conversions/equivalents. Sometimes drug companies use different equivalents for a measure.

In the health care system, it is imperative that nurses be proficient in converting among the different systems of measure. Nurses are becoming increasingly responsible for administration of medications to clients and teaching clients and family outside of the conventional hospital setting (e.g., home care). Nurses have become more involved in discharge planning and are responsible for ensuring that the client can safely self-administer medications in the correct dosage. Table 8-1 lists some of the equivalents. You may need to convert between systems. Memorize these common equivalents!

Converting

The term *convert* means to change from one form to another. Converting can mean changing a measure to its equivalent in the same system or changing a measurement from one system to another system, which is called *converting between systems.* The measurement obtained when converting between systems is **approximate, not exact.** Thus, certain equivalents have been established to ensure continuity.

One of the most important skills needed for calculating dosages is the nurse's ability to make conversions when necessary to administer the ordered amount of medication. The

TABLE 8-1 Approximate Equivalents to Remember

1t = 5 mL
1 T = 3 t = 15 mL
1 oz = 30 mL (2 T)
1 pt = 16 oz (500 mL)
1 qt = 32 oz (2 pt), (1,000 mL)
1 cup (measuring) = 8 oz
16 oz = 1 lb
2.2 lb = 1 kg (1,000 g)
1 in = 2.5 cm

Note: Equivalents in the table are those used most often. The preferred and accurate unit for liquid measurements is milliliter (mL).

nurse therefore must understand the system of measurement and be able to convert within the same system and from one system to another with accuracy.

Before beginning the actual process of converting, the nurse should learn the approximate equivalents in the Equivalents to Remember in Table 8-1 and apply the following important points to make converting simple.

POINTS TO REMEMBER

1. Memorization of the equivalents/conversions is essential.
2. Think of memorized equivalents/conversions as essential conversion factors, or as a ratio.

Example: 1,000 mg = 1 g is called a conversion factor.
1,000 mg : 1 g is a ratio.

3. Follow basic math principles, regardless of the conversion method used.
4. Answers should be expressed by applying specific rules that relate to the system to which you are converting.

Example: The metric system uses decimals; the household system uses fractions.

5. THINK CRITICALLY—select the appropriate equivalent to make conversions (see Table 8-1).

Methods of Converting

Moving the Decimal Point

Moving the decimal point is discussed in Chapter 6. Because the metric system is based on the decimal system, conversions within the metric system can be done easily by moving the decimal point. This method cannot be applied in the household system because decimal points are not often used in the system (with the exception of pounds). **Remember the two rules for moving decimal points:**

RULE

To convert a smaller unit to a larger one in the metric system, divide or move the decimal point three places to the left.

Example: 350 mg = ______ g
(smaller) (larger)

Solution: After determining that mg is the smaller unit and that you are converting to a larger unit (g), recall the conversion factor that allows you to change milligrams to grams (1 g = 1,000 mg). Therefore, 350 is divided by 1,000 by moving the decimal point three places to the left, indicating 350 mg = 0.35 g.

350mg = .350 = 0.35 g

Note: The final answer is expressed in decimal form. Remember to always place a zero (0) in front of the decimal point to indicate a value that is less than 1.

RULE

To convert a larger unit to a smaller one in the metric system, multiply or move the decimal point three places to the right.

Example: 0.85 L = ______ mL
(larger) (smaller)

Solution: After determining that L is the larger unit and you are converting to a smaller unit (mL), recall the conversion factor that allows you to change liters to milliliters (1 L = 1,000 mL). Therefore, 0.85 is multiplied by 1,000 by moving the decimal point three places to the right, indicating 0.85 L = 850 mL.

$$0.850 \text{ L} = 0.\underbrace{850}. = 850 \text{ mL}$$

Note the addition of a zero here to allow movement of the decimal point the correct number of places.

PRACTICE **PROBLEMS**

For additional practice in converting by decimal movement, convert the following metric measures to the equivalent units indicated.

1. 600 mL = ______________ L
2. 0.016 g = ______________ mg
3. 4 kg = ______________ g
4. 3 mcg = ______________ mg
5. 0.3 mg = ______________ g
6. 0.01 kg = ______________ g
7. 1.9 L = ______________ mL
8. 0.5 g = ______________ kg
9. 0.07 mg = ______________ mcg
10. 650 mL = ______________ L

Answers on p. 110

Using Ratio and Proportion

Using ratio and proportion is one of the easiest ways to make conversions, whether within the same system or between systems. The basics on how to state ratios and proportions and how to solve them when looking for one unknown are presented in Chapter 4. To make conversions using ratio and proportion, a proportion that expresses a numerical relationship between the two systems must be set up. A proportion may be written in colon format or as a fraction when making conversions. Regardless of the format used, there are some basic rules to follow when using this method.

RULE

Rules for Ratio and Proportion

1. State the known equivalent first (memorized equivalent).
2. Add the incomplete ratio on the other side of the equals sign, making sure the units of measurement are written in the same sequence.

Example: mg : g = mg : g

3. Label all terms in the proportion, including *x*. (These labels are not carried when multiplying or dividing.)
4. Solve the problem by using the principles for solving ratios and proportions. (The product of the means equals the product of the extremes.)
5. The final answer for *x* should be labeled with the appropriate unit of measure or desired unit.

When using the method of ratio and proportion to make conversions, as with any method used, the known equivalents must be memorized. Stating the proportion in the fraction format may be a way of avoiding confusion with the terms (means and extremes). However, regardless of the format used, the terms must correspond to each other in value and have a relationship. Division should always be carried at least two decimal places to ensure accuracy.

Example: 8 mg = _____ g

Solution: State the known equivalent first, then add the incomplete ratio, making sure the units are in the same sequence. Label all the terms in the proportion, including x.

$$1{,}000 \text{ mg} : 1 \text{ g} = 8 \text{ mg} : x \text{ g}$$

(known equivalent) = (unknown)

Read as "1,000 mg is to 1 g as 8 mg is to x g."

Once the proportion is stated, solve it by multiplying the means (inner terms) and then the extremes (outer terms). Place the "x" product on the left side of the equation.

Result:

means: 1 g and 8 mg

$$1{,}000 \text{ mg} : 1 \text{ g} = 8 \text{ mg} : x \text{ g}$$

extremes: 1,000 mg and x g

$$1{,}000 \times x = 1 \times 8$$

$$\frac{1{,}000\,x}{1{,}000} = \frac{8}{1{,}000}$$

$$x = \frac{8}{1{,}000}$$

$$x = 0.008 \text{ g}$$

Because the measure you are converting to is metric, the fraction is changed to a decimal by dividing 8 by 1,000 to obtain an answer of 0.008 g. However, because the measures are metric in this example, perhaps moving the decimal point would be the preferred method as opposed to actual division.

An alternate way of stating the problem illustrated in the previous example would be stating it as a fraction and cross multiplying to solve for x.

$$\frac{1{,}000 \text{ mg}}{1 \text{ g}} \times \frac{8 \text{ mg}}{x \text{ g}}$$

$$1{,}000\,x = 8$$

$$\frac{1{,}000\,x}{1{,}000} = \frac{8}{1{,}000}$$

$$x = 0.008 \text{ g}$$

Another way of writing a ratio and proportion to eliminate errors is to set up the conversion problem in a fraction format.

Place the conversion factor first (numerator), and place the problem underneath matching up the units (the denominator); then cross multiply to solve for x.

Example: 8 mg = _____ g

$$\frac{1{,}000 \text{ mg}}{8 \text{ mg}} \times \frac{1 \text{ g}}{x \text{ g}}$$

$$1{,}000\,x = 8$$

$$\frac{1{,}000\,x}{1{,}000} = \frac{8}{1{,}000}$$

$$x = 0.008 \text{ g}$$

The remainder of this chapter will show examples of the methods used in converting within the same system and between systems.

Converting Within the Same System

Converting within the same system is often seen with metric measures; however, it can be done using the household system of measurement, such as one household measure being converted to an equivalent within the household system. Any one of the methods discussed can be used, but movement of decimal points is limited to the metric system as shown in previous examples. Ratio and proportion can be used for all systems set up in a fraction or colon format as illustrated..

Dimensional Analysis Dimensional analysis is a conversion method that has been used in chemistry and other sciences and will be discussed in more detail in Chapter 16. Dimensional analysis involves manipulation of units to get the desired unit. This method can be used for conversion in all systems. As with other methods discussed, you must know the conversion factor (equivalent).

Steps for Converting Using Dimensional Analysis:

1. Identify the desired unit you are converting to.
2. Write the conversion factor (equivalent) in fraction format, so that the desired unit is in the numerator of the fraction. This is written first in the equation, followed by a multiplication sign (×). (Notice the unit in the numerator is the same as the unit you desire.)
3. Write the unit in the successive numerator to match the unit of measure in the previous denominator.
4. Cancel the alternate denominator/numerator units to leave the unit desired (being calculated).
5. Perform the mathematic process indicated.

Example:

(metric) (metric)

0.12 kg to g

Solution: You want to cancel the kilograms and obtain the equivalent amount in grams. Begin by identifying the unknown, in this case, g. Because 1 kg = 1,000 g, the fraction that will allow you to cancel kg is $\frac{1{,}000\text{ g}}{1\text{ kg}}$.

$$x\text{ g} = \frac{1{,}000\text{ g}}{1\text{ kg}} \times \frac{0.12\text{ kg}}{1}$$

Note: The unit you want to cancel is always written in the denominator of the fraction. Then proceed by placing as the next numerator the same label as the first denominator, in this case, kg.

Note: Placing a 1 under a number does not change its value.

$$\text{Cancel the units } x\text{ g} = \frac{1{,}000\text{ g}}{1\ \cancel{\text{kg}}} \times \frac{0.12\ \cancel{\text{kg}}}{1}$$

$$1{,}000 \times 0.12 = 120\text{ g}$$

$$x = 120\text{ g}$$

Answer: 0.12 kg is equivalent to 120 g.

PRACTICE PROBLEMS

Convert the following measures to the equivalent units indicated.

11. 500 mL = ________________ L

12. 4 kg = ________________ g

13. 1.4 L = ________________ mL

14. 45 mL = ________________ oz

15. 4.5 mg = ________________ mcg
16. $3\frac{1}{2}$ oz = ________________ mL
17. 6.5 L = ________________ mL
18. 60 g = ________________ kg
19. 600 mg = ________________ g
20. 0.736 mg = ________________ mcg
21. 1,600 mL = ________________ L
22. 0.015 L = ________________ mL
23. 0.18 g = ________________ mg
24. 25 mcg = ________________ mg
25. 5.2 g = ________________ kg

Answers on p. 110

Converting Between Systems

The methods presented previously can be used to change a measure in one system to its equivalent in another, or the conversion factor method can be used. This method requires that you consider the size of units. To convert from a larger unit to a smaller unit of measure, you multiply by the conversion factor as shown in Example 1. To convert from a smaller to a larger unit of measure, you must divide by the conversion factor.

Example 1:

(household) (metric)

4 oz = _____ mL

(large) (small)

✓ Solution Using Conversion Factor Method

Equivalent: 1 oz = 30 mL

Conversion factor is 30.

An ounce is larger than a milliliter.

Multiply 4 by 30 to obtain 120.

Answer: 120 mL

Alternative: Express the conversion in proportion format and solve for x. (One way to remember this method is to remember that it is the known or have : want to know or have.)

✓ Solution Using Ratio and Proportion

$$1\text{ oz} : 30\text{ mL} = 4\text{ oz} : x\text{ mL}$$

$$x = 30 \times 4 = 120$$

$$x = 120\text{ mL}$$

or

$$\frac{1\text{ oz}}{30\text{ mL}} = \frac{4\text{ oz}}{x\text{ mL}}$$

$$x = 4 \times 30 = 120$$

$$x = 120\text{ mL}$$

or

$$\frac{1\text{ oz}}{4\text{ oz}} = \frac{30\text{ mL}}{x\text{ mL}}$$

✓ Solution Using Dimensional Analysis

Here you want to cancel oz to find the equivalent amount in mL. Because 1 oz = 30 mL, the fraction you desire so you can cancel oz is:

$$\frac{30 \text{ mL}}{1 \text{ oz}}$$

Therefore:

$$x \text{ mL} = \frac{30 \text{ mL}}{1 \cancel{\text{oz}}} \times 4 \cancel{\text{oz}}$$

$$x = 30 \times 4 = 120$$

$$x = 120 \text{ mL}$$

120 mL is equivalent to 4 oz

Example 2: (household) (metric)

110 lb = _____ kg

✓ Solution Using Conversion Factor Method

Equivalent: 1 kg = 2.2 lb

Conversion factor is 2.2.

A pound is smaller than a kilogram; 110 is divided by 2.2.

Answer: 50 kg

✓ Solution Using Ratio and Proportion

$$1 \text{ kg} : 2.2 \text{ lb} = x \text{ kg} : 110 \text{ lb}$$

$$\frac{2.2x}{2.2} = \frac{110}{2.2}$$

$$x = 50 \text{ kg}$$

or

$$\frac{1 \text{ kg}}{2.2 \text{ lb}} = \frac{x \text{ kg}}{110 \text{ lb}}$$

or

$$\frac{1 \text{ kg}}{x \text{ kg}} = \frac{2.2 \text{ lb}}{110 \text{ lb}}$$

✓ Solution Using Dimensional Analysis

Here you want to cancel lb to find the equivalent amount in kg. Because 1 kg = 2.2 lb, the fraction you desire so you can cancel lb is:

$$\frac{1 \text{ kg}}{2.2 \text{ lb}}$$

Therefore:

$$x\text{ kg} = \frac{1\text{ kg}}{2.2\cancel{\text{lb}}} \times \frac{110\cancel{\text{lb}}}{1}$$

$$x = \frac{110}{2.2}$$

$$x = 50\text{ kg}$$

Example 3: (metric) (household)

55 cm = ______ in.

✓ Solution Using Conversion Factor Method

Equivalent: 1 in = 2.5 cm

Conversion factor is 2.5

A cm is smaller than an inch (in); 55 is divided by 2.5.

Answer: 22 in

✓ Solution Using Ratio and Proportion

$$2.5\text{ cm} : 1\text{ in} = 55\text{ cm} : x\text{ in}$$

$$\frac{2.5x}{2.5} = \frac{55}{2.5}$$

$$x = 22\text{ in}$$

or

$$\frac{2.5\text{ cm}}{1\text{ in}} = \frac{55\text{ cm}}{x\text{ in}}$$

or

$$\frac{2.5\text{ cm}}{55\text{ cm}} = \frac{1\text{ in}}{x\text{ in}}$$

✓ Solution Using Dimensional Analysis

Here you want to cancel cm to find the equivalent amount in inches (in). Because 2.5 cm = 1 in, the fraction you desire so you can cancel cm is:

$$\frac{1\text{ in}}{2.5\text{ cm}}$$

Therefore:

$$x\text{ in} = \frac{1\text{ in}}{2.5\cancel{\text{cm}}} \times \frac{55\cancel{\text{cm}}}{1}$$

$$x = \frac{55}{2.5}$$

$$x = 22\text{ in}$$

Answer: 22 in is equivalent to 55 cm

Calculating Intake and Output

The nurse often converts between systems to calculate a client's **intake and output.** Intake and output is abbreviated **I&O.** Intake refers to the monitoring of fluid a client takes orally (p.o.), by feeding tube, or parenterally. Oral intake includes fluids and solids that become liquid at body and room temperature, such as gelatin and Popsicles. Intake also includes water, broth, and juice. Intake does not include solids, such as bread, cereal, or meats. Liquid output refers to fluids that exit the body, such as diarrhea, vomitus, gastric suction, and urine. A client's intake and output are usually recorded on a special form called an intake and output flow sheet (or I&O flow sheet or record) (Figure 8-1), which varies from institution to institution. In some institutions where the charting is computerized, the I&O may be recorded in the computer. A variety of clients require I&O monitoring, such as those whose fluids are restricted and those who are receiving diuretic or intravenous (IV) therapy.

Intake and output may still be recorded at some institutions using cubic centimeters or milliliters. The preferred term for volume is milliliters. Milliliters will be used throughout this text. When measuring output, the nurse uses a graduated receptacle calibrated in metric measures (mL), and conversions are not necessary. Oral intake usually must be converted from household measures to metric measures before it can be recorded. Each time a client takes oral liquids, even those administered with medications, the amount and time are recorded on the appropriate form. The total intake and output are recorded at the end of each shift and also totalled for a 24-hour period.

Conversion of a client's intake is usually required when recording measurements such as a bowl or coffee cup. Each agency usually has an I&O sheet with a ledger that indicates the standard measurement for the utensils used in its facility. For example, it may indicate that a standard cup is 6 oz or a coffee cup is 180 mL. A client's oral intake is calculated in the same manner as other conversion problems. After each item is converted, the items are added together for the total intake. Intake and output are based on the conversion factor 1 oz = 30 mL.

Juice glass	– 180 mL	Jello cup	– 150 mL
Water glass	– 210 mL	Ice cream	– 120 mL
Coffee cup	– 240 mL	Creamer	– 30 mL
Soup bowl	– 180 mL		
Small water cup	– 120 mL		

Date October 30, 2017

Addressograph with Client Information

INTAKE						OUTPUT				
ORAL			IV						OTHER	
TIME	TYPE	AMT	TIME	TYPE	AMOUNT ABSORBED	TIME	URINE	STOOL		
8A	Juice	60 mL								
	Coffee	120 mL								
	Milk	250 mL								

Figure 8-1 Sample I&O flow sheet.

Example 1: Calculate the client's intake for breakfast in milliliters. Assume that the glass holds 6 oz and the cup holds 8 oz. The client had the following for breakfast at 8 AM:

Items	Conversion Factors
⅓ glass of apple juice	1 oz = 30 mL
2 sausages	1 pint = 500 mL
1 boiled egg	1 cup = 8 oz
½ cup of coffee	1 glass = 6 oz
½ pint of milk	

*The 2 sausages and one boiled egg are not part of fluid intake.

Solution:

1. ⅓ glass of apple juice

$$1 \text{ glass} = 6 \text{ oz}; \frac{1}{3} \text{ of } 6 \text{ oz} = 2 \text{ oz}$$

Therefore, 1 oz = 30 mL, 2 oz × 30 mL = 60 mL

✔ Solution Using Ratio and Proportion

1 oz : 30 mL = 2 oz : x mL, x = 60 mL (ratio and proportion)

✔ Solution Using Dimensional Analysis

$$x \text{ mL} = \frac{30 \text{ mL}}{1 \cancel{\text{oz}}} \times \frac{2 \cancel{\text{oz}}}{1}$$

2. ½ cup of coffee

$$1 \text{ cup} = 8 \text{ oz}; \frac{1}{2} \text{ of } 8 \text{ oz} = 4 \text{ oz}$$

Therefore, 4 oz × 30 = 120 mL

✔ Solution Using Ratio and Proportion

1 oz : 30 mL = 4 oz : x mL, x = 120 mL

✔ Solution Using Dimensional Analysis

$$x \text{ mL} = \frac{30 \text{ mL}}{1 \cancel{\text{oz}}} \times \frac{4 \cancel{\text{oz}}}{1}$$

3. ½ pint of milk

$$1 \text{ pint} = 500 \text{ mL}; \frac{1}{2} \text{ of } 500 \text{ mL} = 250 \text{ mL}$$

4. Total mL = 60 mL + 120 mL + 250 mL = 430 mL

Another solution would be to total the number of ounces (6 oz in this example). Convert ounces to milliliters, and add the half pint of milk (expressed in milliliters).

✔ Solution Using Ratio and Proportion

$$1 \text{ oz} : 30 \text{ mL} = 6 \text{ oz} : x \text{ mL}$$

$$x = 180 \text{ mL}$$

$$180 \text{ mL} + 250 \text{ mL} = 430 \text{ mL}$$

✔ Solution Using Dimensional Analysis

$$x \text{ mL} = \frac{30 \text{ mL}}{1 \cancel{\text{oz}}} \times \frac{6 \cancel{\text{oz}}}{1}$$

The conversions are recorded on an I&O flow sheet (or record) next to the time ingested. The I&O sheet in Figure 8-1 is filled out with the data for this sample problem.

8:00 AM juice, 60 mL coffee, 60 mL milk, 250 mL

Let's look at a more complex I&O calculation. This can be done applying the same principles and methods shown in the previous example:

A client receives 75 mL/hr of IV fluid from 7 AM to 3 PM. The client also consumes the following:

Breakfast	3 oz juice
	$1\frac{1}{2}$ cups coffee (cup = 8 oz)
Lunch	$\frac{3}{4}$ bowl of broth (bowl = 6 oz)
	4 oz gelatin dessert

At 3 PM the client's foley catheter is emptied of 800 mL of urine and a surgical drain emptied of 75 mL.

(a) How many milliliters will you record for the intake? ________________

(b) How many milliliters will you record for the output? ________________

Solution

1. 75 mL/hr of IV fluid from 7 AM to 3 PM

   7 AM to 3 PM = 8 hr   75 mL × 8 = 600 mL/8 hr

2. **Oral intake:**
   - 3 oz juice, 1 oz = 30 mL, 3 oz × 30 mL = 90 mL
   - $1\frac{1}{2}$ cups coffee, 1 cup = 8 oz; $1\frac{1}{2}$ × 8 oz = 12 oz; therefore, 1 oz = 30 mL = 12 × 30 = 360 mL
   - $\frac{3}{4}$ bowl of broth, 1 bowl = 6 oz; $\frac{3}{4}$ of 6 oz = $4\frac{1}{2}$ oz 1 oz = 30 mL, $4\frac{1}{2}$ × 30 = 135 mL
   - 4 oz gelatin, 1 oz = 30 mL, 4 × 30 = 120 mL

3. Add the milliliters to get the total intake

   600 mL IV fluid + 705 mL oral intake (90 mL + 360 mL + 135 mL + 120 mL)

   Total intake is: 600 mL (IV)
   + 705 mL (oral)
   1,305 mL

Note: This could have also been done using any of the methods shown in the previous example. Here you could have also gotten the total ounces, which is $23\frac{1}{2}$ in this example (then converted ounces to milliliters and added the IV solution in milliliters to get the total).

4. The output is in milliliters; no conversion is needed.
   Add the mL: 800 mL (urine) + 75 mL (surgical drain) = 875 mL
   Total intake recorded = 1,305 mL
   Total output recorded = 875 mL

In addition to oral intake, if a client is receiving IV therapy, the amount of IV fluid given is also recorded on the I&O flow sheet (or record). When an IV bottle or bag is hung or added, the nurse indicates the time and the type and amount of fluid in the appropriate column on the sheet (or record). When the IV fluid has infused or the IV is changed, the nurse records the actual amount of fluid **infused,** or **absorbed.**

In a situation in which a bag or bottle of IV fluid is not completed by the end of the shift, the nurse beginning the next shift is informed of how much fluid is left in the bag. At some institutions, the amount is also indicated on the I&O flow sheet (or record) with the abbreviation LIB (left in bag or bottle).

Example: The nurse hangs a 1,000-mL bag of D5W at 7 AM. At 3 PM, 150 mL is left in the bag. The nurse records 850 mL was absorbed and indicates 150 mL is LIB. Refer to the sample I&O form in Figure 8-2, which shows how this example is charted.

I&O flow sheets usually have a place for recording p.o. intake and IV intake and a column or columns for output. Figure 8-3 shows a sample 24-hour I&O flow sheet illustrating the charting of intake.

As discussed, output is also recorded on the I&O form. The most commonly measured output is urine. After a client's output is recorded, sometimes the nurse needs to compute an average. The most important average nurses compute in most health care settings is the hourly urine output. The **hourly** urine output for an adult to maintain proper renal function is 30 mL/hr to 50 mL/hr. Usually, the hourly amount is more significant than each

Juice glass – 180 mL
Water glass – 210 mL
Coffee cup – 240 mL
Soup bowl – 180 mL
Small water cup – 120 mL
Jello cup – 150 mL
Ice cream – 120 mL
Creamer – 30 mL

Client information

Date: September 21, 2017

INTAKE						OUTPUT			
Time	Type	Amt	Time	IV/ blood type	Amount absorbed	Time	Urine	Stool	Other
			7A	D5W 1,000 mL	850 mL				
8 hr total					850 mL				
			3P	D5W 150 mL LIB					

Figure 8-2 Charting IV fluids on an I&O flow sheet. *LIB,* Left in bag.

Juice glass – 180 mL	Small water cup – 120 mL		Client information
Water glass – 210 mL	Jello cup – 150 mL		
Coffee cup – 240 mL	Ice cream – 120 mL		
Soup bowl – 180 mL	Creamer – 30 mL		

Date: September 21, 2017

INTAKE						OUTPUT			
Time	Type	Amt	Time	IV/ blood type	Amount absorbed	Time	Urine	Stool	Other
8A	juice	240 mL	7A	D5W 1,000 mL	850 mL	8A	300 mL		
	milk	120 mL				10A	200 mL		
	coffee	200 mL				1³⁰/P	425 mL		
9³⁰/A	water	60 mL							
12P	broth	180 mL							
	juice	120 mL							
1P	water	120 mL							
8 hr total		1,040 mL			850 mL		925 mL		
5P	tea	100 mL	3P	D5W 150 mL LIB	150 mL	4p	425 mL		
	broth	360 mL	5P	D5W 1,000 mL	750 mL	7p	350 mL		
	ice-cream	120 mL				9³⁰/P	200 mL		
9 P	water	240 mL							
8 hr total		820 mL			900 mL		975 mL		
1A	water	120 mL	11P	D5W 250 mL LIB	250 mL				
5A	tea	200 mL	3A	D5W 1,000 mL	600 mL	2A	350 mL		
						5A	150 mL		
8 hr total		320 mL			850 mL		500 mL		
24 hr total		2,180 mL			2,600 mL		2,400 mL		

Total intake 24 hr: (4,780 mL) (2,180 mL + 2,600 mL)

Total output 24 hr: (2,400 mL) (925 mL + 975 mL + 500 mL)

Figure 8-3 I&O flow sheet (completed 24 hours). *LIB,* Left in bag.

voiding. To find the hourly average of urinary output, take the total and divide by the number of hours.

Example: $\frac{400 \text{ mL of urine}}{8 \text{ hr}} = 50 \text{ mL of urine/hr}$

The charting of I&O varies at each institution. Always check the policies to ensure compliance with a particular institution.

PRACTICE **PROBLEMS**

Convert the following to the equivalent measures and express answer to two decimal places as indicated.

26. 60 lb = ________________ kg
27. 187.5 cm = ________________ in
28. 66 lb = ________________ kg
29. $3\frac{1}{2}$ pt = ________________ oz
30. 7 oz = ________________ mL
31. 250 mL = ________________ qt
32. 45 mL = ________________ tbs
33. 10 cm = ________________ in
34. 178.2 lb = ________________ kg
35. 20 mL = ________________ tsp
36. 3 oz = ________________ T
37. 4 qt = ________________ mL
38. 72 kg = ________________ lb
39. 3 in = ________________ cm
40. 2.4 L = ________________ mL

Compute how much IV fluid you would document on an I&O form as being absorbed from a 1,000 mL bag if the following amounts remain.

41. 300 mL ________________
42. 450 mL ________________
43. 100 mL ________________

Compute the average hourly urinary output in the following situations (round to nearest whole number).

44. 650 mL in 8 hr ________________
45. 250 mL in 8 hr ________________
46. 1,000 mL in 24 hr ________________
47. 1,240 mL in 24 hr ________________

48. A client's output for the 3 to 11 PM shift was as follows:
    325 mL of urine at 4:00 PM
    75 mL of vomitus at 7:00 PM
    225 mL of urine at 8:00 PM
    200 mL of nasogastric (NG) drainage at 11:00 PM
    50 mL of wound drainage at 11:00 PM
    What is the total output in milliliters? ________________

49. What is the client's output in liters in question 48? ________________

50. If 375 mL of a 500 mL bag of IV solution were absorbed on the 3 to 11 PM shift, the nurse records that 375 mL was absorbed. How many milliliters are recorded as left in bag (LIB)? ____________

51. A client had the following during an 8-hour shift

- 125 mL/hr of IV fluid from 7 AM to 1 PM
- 250 mL of packed red blood cells from 1 PM to 3 PM

Breakfast	$2\frac{1}{2}$ cup of coffee (cup = 6 oz)
	$\frac{1}{2}$ glass of juice (glass = 4 oz)
Lunch	$1\frac{1}{2}$ bowls of broth (bowl = 6 oz)
	3 oz milk

The client voided four times during the shift:

350 mL, 275 mL, 450 mL, and 300 mL of urine

Calculate the I&O for the 8-hour shift in milliliters

a) Intake mL ____________

b) Output mL ____________

Answers on p. 110

POINTS TO REMEMBER

- Regardless of the method used for converting, **memorizing equivalents** is a necessity.
- Answers stated in fraction format should be **reduced** as necessary.
- When more than one equivalent is learned for a unit, use the **most common equivalent** for the measure or use the number that divides equally without a remainder.
- Division should be carried to the hundredths place or two decimal places to ensure accuracy, and it is not rounded.
- Decimal point movement as a method for converting is limited to the metric system; ratio and proportion, dimensional analysis, and conversion factor method can be used for all systems of measure.
- Oral intake is converted before placing data on an I&O flow sheet (or record). The amount is usually recorded in cubic centimeters at some institutions; however, milliliter is the correct unit for volume. Conversion factor for I&O is 1 oz = 30 mL.
- Always check the policy of the institution regarding I&O and the charting of it.
- The most common units of measure used to calculate dosages are metric units of measurement.

CHAPTER **REVIEW**

Convert the following to the equivalent measures indicated.

1. 0.007 g = ____________ mg
2. 1 mg = ____________ g
3. 6,000 g = ____________ kg
4. 5 mL = ____________ L
5. 0.45 L = ____________ mL
6. 75 mL = ____________ oz
7. 1.8 mg = ____________ mcg
8. 23 g = ____________ kg
9. 6.5 mcg = ____________ mg
10. $1\frac{1}{2}$ qt = ____________ mL
11. 1,200 mL = ____________ oz
12. 1.6 L = ____________ mL

13. 47 kg = ______________ lb
14. 3 mL = ______________ L
15. 75 lb = ______________ kg
16. 0.008 g = ______________ mg
17. $4\frac{1}{2}$ pt = ______________ mL
18. 0.25 mg = ______________ mcg
19. 82 kg = ______________ g
20. 6,172 g = ______________ kg
21. 200 mL = ______________ tsp
22. 102 lb = ______________ kg
23. 204 g = ______________ kg
24. 1.5 L = ______________ mL
25. 200 mcg = ______________ mg
26. 48.6 L = ______________ mL
27. 0.7 L = ______________ mL
28. $6\frac{1}{2}$ oz = ______________ mL
29. 4 tsp = ______________ mL
30. 1.8 mg = ______________ g
31. 2 tbs = ______________ mL
32. 67.5 mL = ______________ t
33. 66.25 cm = ______________ in
34. 16 t = ______________ mL
35. 20 oz = ______________ mL
36. 16 mcg = ______________ mg
37. 75 tsp = ______________ mL
38. 255 mL = ______________ oz
39. 4 kg = ______________ lb
40. 3.25 mg = ______________ mcg

Calculate the fluid intake in milliliters. Use the following equivalents for the problems below: 1 cup = 8 oz, 1 glass = 4 oz.

41. Client had the following at lunch:
4 oz fruit cocktail
1 tuna fish sandwich
$\frac{1}{2}$ cup of tea
$\frac{1}{4}$ pt of milk

Total mL = ______________

42. Calculate the following individual items and give the total number of milliliters:
3 Popsicles (3 oz each)
$\frac{1}{2}$ qt iced tea
$1\frac{1}{2}$ glasses water
12 oz soft drink

Total mL = ______________

43. Client had the following:
8 oz milk
6 oz orange juice
4 oz water with medication

Total mL = ______________

44. Client had the following:
10 oz of coffee
8 oz water
6 oz vegetable broth

Total mL = ______________

45. Client had the following:
$\frac{3}{4}$ glass of milk
4 oz water
2 oz beef broth

Total mL = ______________

46. A client had the following at lunch:
$\frac{1}{4}$ glass of apple juice
8 oz chicken broth
6 oz gelatin dessert
$1\frac{3}{4}$ cups of coffee

Total mL = ______________

Convert the following amounts of fluid to milliliters.

47. $3\frac{1}{2}$ oz = ________________ mL

48. $\frac{3}{4}$ C (8 oz cup) = ____________ mL

Compute how much IV fluid you would document on an I&O form as being absorbed from a 1,000 mL bag if the following amounts are left in the bag.

49. 275 mL ________________

50. 550 mL ________________

51. 75 mL ________________

Compute the average hourly urinary output in each of the following situations (round to nearest whole number).

52. 500 mL in 8 hr ____________

53. 640 mL in 24 hr ____________

54. 700 mL in 8 hr ____________

Compute how much IV fluid you would document on an I&O form as being absorbed from a 500 mL bag if the following amounts are left in the bag.

55. 125 mL ________________

56. 225 mL ________________

57. A client received 1,750 mL of IV fluid. How many liters of IV fluid did the client receive? ________________

58. A client has an order for 125 mcg of digoxin. How many milligrams will you administer to the client? ________________

59. The prescriber directs a client to take 15 oz of the laxative agent GoLYTELY. The cup holds 6 oz. How many cups will the client have to drink? ________________

60. A client has an order for 1,500 mL of water by mouth every 24 hours. How many ounces is this? ________________

61. A client had an output of 1.1 L. How many milliliters is this? ________________

62. The prescriber orders 2 ounces of a liquid medication for a client. How many tablespoons should the client take? ____________ tbs

63. A client is given a prescription for 7.5 mL of a cough suppressant every four hours. The client will be using a measuring device that is calibrated in teaspoons. How much medication should the client take for each dose? ____________ tsp

64. A client weighed 95 kg on the initial visit to the clinic. When the client reported for the subsequent visit the client reported losing 11 lb. What is the client's current weight in kg? ____________ kg

65. A client is instructed to drink 2,500 mL of water per day. How many quarts of water should the client be instructed to drink? ____________ qt

66. An infant's head circumference is 45 cm. The parents ask for the equivalent in inches. You tell the parents their infant's head circumference is ____________ in

67. A client drank 24 ounces of water. How many cups did the client drink? ____________ cups

68. A client needs to drink $1\frac{1}{2}$ ounces of an elixir per day. How many tablespoons would this be equivalent to? ____________ tbs

69. A client consumed $2\frac{1}{2}$ pints of water in a day. How many cups of water is this equivalent to? ____________ cups

70. An infant drinks 4 ounces of a ready to feed formula every 3 hours during the day and night. The formula comes in a quart container. How many quarts of formula should the mother buy for a 7 day supply? ____________ qt

71. Calculate the total fluid intake in mL for 24 hours.

Breakfast: 5 oz milk
2 oz orange juice
4 oz water with medication

Lunch: 12 oz gingerale

Snack: 10 oz hot tea
2 oz gelatin dessert

Dinner: 4 oz water
6 oz apple juice
3 oz chicken broth

Snack: 3 oz jello
8 oz ice-tea
6 oz water with medication

Total = ____________ mL

72. Calculate the client intake for 12 hours (7 AM to 7 PM)
The client receives intravenous fluids at 100 mL/hr from 7 AM to 3 PM, 300 mL of packed red blood cells from 3 PM to 5 PM, and 50 mL/hr of IV fluid from 5 PM to 7 PM. The client consumed 4 oz of orange juice, 8 oz of hot tea at breakfast, 8 oz milk for lunch, and 4 oz of hot tea with dinner. How many milliliters will you record on the I&O for the intake? ____________

73. A client's intake and output was the following for 8 hours:

Intake:
1.2 L of IV fluid

Breakfast: 1½ cups of tea (cup = 6 oz)
Lunch: 1 can ginger ale (can = 12 oz)
Dinner: 1 bowl chicken broth (bowl = 6 oz)

Output:
Foley catheter: 1,200 mL of urine
Surgical drain: 100 mL
Calculate the I&O in milliliters.

a) Total intake ____________

b) Total output ____________

Answers on p. 110

ANSWERS

Chapter 8

Answers to Practice Problems

1. 0.6 L
2. 16 mg
3. 4,000 g
4. 0.003 mg
5. 0.0003 g
6. 10 g
7. 1,900 mL
8. 0.0005 kg
9. 70 mcg
10. 0.65 L
11. 0.5 L
12. 4,000 g
13. 1,400 mL
14. oz $1\frac{1}{2}$, $1\frac{1}{2}$ oz
15. 4,500 mcg
16. 105 mL
17. 6,500 mL
18. 0.06 kg
19. 0.6 g
20. 736 mcg
21. 1.6 L
22. 15 mL
23. 180 mg
24. 0.025 mg
25. 0.0052 kg
26. 27.27 kg
27. 75 in, in 75
28. 30 kg
29. 56 oz, oz 56
30. 210 mL
31. 1/4 qt, qt 1/4
32. 3 tbs, tbs 3
33. 4 in, in 4
34. 81 kg
35. 4 tsp, tsp 4
36. 6 T, T 6
37. 4,000 mL
38. 158.4 lb *or* $158\frac{2}{5}$ lb, lb 158.4 *or* lb $158\frac{2}{5}$
39. 7.5 cm
40. 2,400 mL
41. 700 mL
42. 550 mL
43. 900 mL
44. 81 mL/hr
45. 31 mL/hr
46. 42 mL/hr
47. 52 mL/hr
48. 875 mL
49. 0.875 L
50. 125 mL
51. a) 1,870 mL
    b) 1,375 mL

Answers to Chapter Review

1. 7 mg
2. 0.001 g
3. 6 kg
4. 0.005 L
5. 450 mL
6. oz $2\frac{1}{2}$, $2\frac{1}{2}$ oz
7. 1,800 mcg
8. 0.023 kg
9. 0.0065 mg
10. 1,500 mL
11. 40 oz, oz 40
12. 1,600 mL
13. 103.4 lb, $103\frac{2}{5}$ lb
14. 0.003 L
15. 34.09 kg
16. 8 mg
17. 2,250 mL
18. 250 mcg
19. 82,000 g
20. 6.172 kg
21. 40 tsp, tsp 40
22. 46.36 kg
23. 0.204 kg
24. 1,500 mL
25. 0.2 mg
26. 48,600 mL
27. 700 mL
28. 195 mL
29. 20 mL
30. 0.0018 g
31. 30 mL
32. $13\frac{1}{2}$ t, t $13\frac{1}{2}$
33. $26\frac{1}{2}$ in, in $26\frac{1}{2}$
34. 80 mL
35. 600 mL
36. 0.016 mg
37. 375 mL
38. $8\frac{1}{2}$ oz, oz $8\frac{1}{2}$
39. 8.8 lb, $8\frac{4}{5}$ lb
40. 3,250 mcg
41. 245 mL
42. 1,310 mL
43. 540 mL
44. 720 mL
45. 270 mL
46. 870 mL
47. 105 mL
48. 180 mL
49. 725 mL
50. 450 mL
51. 925 mL
52. 63 mL/hr
53. 27 mL/hr
54. 88 mL/hr
55. 375 mL
56. 275 mL
57. 1.75 L
58. 0.125 mg
59. $2\frac{1}{2}$ cups
60. 50 oz, oz 50
61. 1,100 mL
62. T 4, 4 T
63. t $1\frac{1}{2}$, tsp $1\frac{1}{2}$, $1\frac{1}{2}$ t, $1\frac{1}{2}$ tsp
64. 90 kg
65. qt $2\frac{1}{2}$, $2\frac{1}{2}$ qt
66. 18 in, in 18
67. 3 cups
68. tbs 3, T 3, 3 tbs, 3 T
69. 5 cups
70. qt 7, 7 qt
71. 1,950 mL
72. 1,920 mL
73. a) 2,010 mL
    b) 1,300 mL

evolve

For additional information, refer to the Conversions and Equivalents section of the Elsevier's Interactive Drug Calculation Application, Version 1 on Evolve.

CHAPTER 9
Additional Conversions Useful in the Health Care Setting

Objectives

After reviewing this chapter, you should be able to:

1. Convert between Celsius and Fahrenheit temperature
2. Convert between units of length: inches, centimeters, and millimeters
3. Convert between units of weight: pounds and kilograms, pounds and ounces to kilograms
4. Convert between traditional and international time

Converting Between Celsius and Fahrenheit

Most health care facilities use electronic digital temperature thermometers, which instantly convert between the two scales, rather than mercury thermometers. However, such devices do not eliminate the need for the nurse to understand the important difference between Celsius and Fahrenheit. In addition, it may be necessary for the nurse to explain to clients or families how to convert from one to the other.

Another factor is the recognition that all persons involved in client care do not have a "universal" measurement for temperature; therefore, Fahrenheit or Celsius may be used. Let's look first at some general information that will help you understand the formulas used.

Differentiating Between Celsius and Fahrenheit

To differentiate which scale is being used (Fahrenheit or Celsius), the temperature reading is followed by an *F* or *C*. *F* indicates Fahrenheit, and *C* indicates Celsius. (*Note:* Celsius was formerly known as *centigrade.*)

Examples: 98° F
36° C

The freezing point of water on the Fahrenheit scale is **32° F**, and the boiling point is **212° F.** The freezing point of water on the Celsius scale is **0° C**, and the boiling point is **100° C.**

The difference between the freezing and boiling points on the Fahrenheit scale is **180°**, whereas the difference between these points on the Celsius scale is **100°.**

The differences between Fahrenheit and Celsius in relation to the freezing and boiling points led to the development of appropriate conversion formulas. Figure 9-1 shows two thermometers reflecting the relationship of pertinent values between the two scales.

The **32° difference** between the freezing point on the scales is used for converting temperature from one scale to the other. There is a **180°** difference between the boiling and freezing points on the Fahrenheit thermometer and **100°** between the boiling and freezing points on the Celsius scale. These differences can be set as a ratio, 180:100. Therefore, consider the following:

$$180:100 = \frac{180}{100} = \frac{9}{5}$$

The fraction $\frac{9}{5}$ expressed as a decimal is 1.8; therefore, you will see this constant used in temperature conversions.

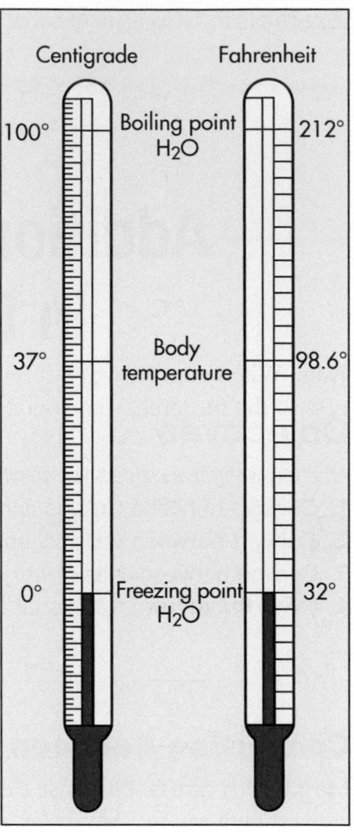

Figure 9-1 Celsius and Fahrenheit temperature scales. (From Clayton BD, Willihnganz M: *Basic pharmacology for nurses,* ed. 17, St. Louis, 2017, Mosby.) *Note:* Glass thermometers pictured here are for demonstration purposes only. Electronic digital temperature devices are more commonly used in health care settings.

Formulas for Converting Between Fahrenheit and Celsius Scales

RULE

To convert from Celsius to Fahrenheit, multiply by 1.8 and add 32.

$$°F = 1.8(°C) + 32$$

or

$$°F = \frac{9}{5}(°C) + 32$$

Example: Convert 37.5° C to ° F.

$°F = 1.8(37.5) + 32$ *or* $°F = \frac{9}{5}(37.5) + 32$

$°F = 67.5 + 32$ *or* $°F = 67.5 + 32$

$°F = 99.5°$ *or* $°F = 99.5°$

RULE

To convert from Fahrenheit to Celsius, subtract 32 and divide by 1.8.

$$°C = \frac{°F - 32}{1.8} \quad or \quad °C = (°F - 32) \div \frac{9}{5}$$

Example: Convert 68° F to ° C.

$$°C = \frac{68 - 32}{1.8} \qquad °C = (68 - 32) \div \frac{9}{5}$$

$$°C = \frac{36}{1.8} \qquad °C = 36 \div \frac{9}{5}$$

$$°C = (36) \times \frac{5}{9}$$

$$°C = 20° \qquad °C = 20°$$

Note: When converting between Fahrenheit and Celsius, if necessary carry the math process to the hundreds and round to tenths.

PRACTICE **PROBLEMS**

Convert the following temperatures as indicated (round your answer to tenths).

1. 4° C = ________________ ° F
2. 101° F = ________________ ° C
3. 38.1° C = ________________ ° F
4. 101.3° F = ________________ ° C
5. 37.5° C = ________________ ° F

Change the given temperatures in the following statements to their corresponding equivalents in ° C or ° F (round your answer to tenths).

6. Store medication at room temperature: 20° to 25° C. ________________ ° F
7. Notify health care provider for temperature greater than 101° F. ________________ ° C
8. Store vaccine serum at 7° F. ________________ ° C
9. Normal adult body temperature is 37° C. ________________ ° F
10. Do not store IV solutions at less than 46° F. ________________ ° C

Answers on p. 123

In addition to temperature conversions, other measures that may be encountered in the health care setting relate to linear measurement. As with temperature conversion, even though there are devices that instantly convert these measures, nurses need to understand the process. For the purpose of this chapter, we will focus on millimeters (mm) and centimeters (cm).

Metric Measures Relating to Length

In health care settings, metric measures relating to length include the following:

- Diameter of the pupil of the eye may be described in millimeters (mm); the normal diameter of pupils is 3 to 7 mm. Charts may show pupillary size in millimeters.
- Accommodation of pupils is tested by asking a client to gaze at a distant object (e.g., a far wall) and then at a test object (e.g., a finger or pencil) held by the examiner approximately 10 centimeters (cm) (4 in) from the bridge of the client's nose.
- A baby's head and chest circumference are expressed in centimeters.
- Gauze for dressings is available in different size squares measured in centimeters. Example: 10 × 10 cm (4 × 4 in); 5 × 5 cm (2 × 2 in).
- Length of an incision may be expressed in measures such as centimeters.

Refer to the conversions in Box 9-1.

BOX 9-1 Conversions Relating to Length

1 cm = 10 mm
1 in = 2.54 cm*

*The approximate conversion of 1 in = 2.5 cm is used for conversions.

Now let's try some conversions using these equivalents.

Example 1: A client's incision measures 25 mm. How many centimeters is this?

Conversion factor: 1 cm = 10 mm

Solution: Think: mm is smaller and cm is larger. Divide by 10, or move the decimal point one place to the left.

$$25 \div 10 = 2.5 \text{ cm } \textit{or } 2\underset{\smile}{5}. = 2.5 \text{ cm}$$

Answer: 2.5 cm

Example 2: Convert 30 cm to inches (in).

Conversion factor: 1 in = 2.5 cm

Solution: Think: smaller to larger (divide).

$$30 \div 2.5 = 12 \text{ in}$$

Answer: 12 in

Example 3: An infant's head circumference is 35.5 cm. How many millimeters is this?

Conversion factor: 1 cm = 10 mm

Solution: Think: larger to smaller (multiply). Multiply by 10, or move the decimal point one place to the right.

$$35.5 \times 10 = 355 \text{ mm } \textit{or } 35.\underset{\smile}{5} = 355 \text{ mm}$$

Answer: 355 mm

*Any methods presented in previous chapters may be used for converting. Decimal movement, however, is limited to conversions of one metric measure to another.

PRACTICE **PROBLEMS**

Convert the following to the equivalent indicated.

11. A gauze pad for a dressing is

    10 cm ______________ in

12. A client's incision measures

    45 mm ______________ cm

13. An infant's head circumference is

 37.5 cm ______________ mm

14. A newborn is $20\frac{1}{2}$ in long

 ______________ cm

15. 14.8 in = ______________ cm

16. 6.5 cm = ______________ in

17. 100 in = ______________ cm

18. An infant's chest circumference is

 32 cm ______________ in

19. An infant's head circumference is

 38 cm ______________ in

20. A newborn is 20 in long

 ______________ cm

Answers on p. 123

Conversions Relating to Weight

Determination of body weight is important for calculating dosages in adults, children, and, because of the immaturity of their systems, even more so in infants and neonates. This chapter focuses on converting weights for adults and children. Medications such as heparin are more therapeutic when based on weight in kilograms. The most frequently used calculation method for pediatric medication administration is milligrams per kilogram. Some medications are calculated in micrograms per kilogram.

Because medication dosages in drug references are usually based on kilograms, it is essential to be able to convert from pounds to kilograms. However, the nurse also needs to know how to do the opposite (convert from kilograms to pounds). In addition, because a child's weight may be in pounds and ounces, conversion of these units to kilograms is also important. Knowledge of weight conversions is an important part of general nursing knowledge.

Converting Pounds to Kilograms

RULE

Equivalent: 2.2 lb = 1 kg

To convert lb to kg, divide by 2.2 (think smaller to larger).

The answer is rounded to the nearest tenth.

Example 1: A child weighs 65 lb. Convert to kilograms.

$$65 \div 2.2 = 29.54 = 29.5 \text{ kg}$$

Example 2: An adult weighs 135 lb. Convert to kilograms.

$$135 \div 2.2 = 61.36 = 61.4 \text{ kg}$$

Converting Weight in Pounds and Ounces to Kilograms

Step 1: Convert the ounces to the nearest tenth of a pound, and **add** this to the total pounds.

Equivalent: 16 oz = 1 lb

Step 2: Convert the total pounds to kilograms, and round to the nearest tenth.

Equivalent: 2.2 lb = 1 kg

Example 1: A child's weight is 10 lb, 2 oz.

Think: smaller to larger.

2 oz ÷ 16 = 0.12 = 0.1 lb

10 lb + 0.1 lb = 10.1 lb

Think: smaller to larger.

10.1 ÷ 2.2 = 4.59 = 4.6 kg

Example 2: A child's weight is 7 lb, 4 oz.

4 oz ÷ 16 = 0.25 = 0.3 lb

7 lb + 0.3 lb = 7.3 lb

7.3 ÷ 2.2 = 3.31 = 3.3 kg

PRACTICE **PROBLEMS**

Convert the following weights to kilograms (round to the nearest tenth).

21. 6 lb, 5 oz = ______________ kg
22. 12 lb, 2 oz = ______________ kg
23. 10 lb, 4 oz = ______________ kg
24. 7 lb, 12 oz = ______________ kg

Convert the following weights in pounds to kilograms (round to the nearest tenth where indicated).

25. 20 lb = ______________ kg
26. 64 lb = ______________ kg
27. 22 lb = ______________ kg
28. 121 lb = ______________ kg
29. 85 lb = ______________ kg

Answers on p. 123

Converting Kilograms to Pounds

RULE

Equivalent: 2.2 lb = 1 kg
To convert kilograms to pounds, multiply by 2.2. (Think: larger to smaller.)
Answer is expressed to the nearest tenth.

Example 1: A child weighs 24.7 kg. Convert to pounds.

(24.7) × 2.2 = 54.34 = 54.3 lb

Example 2: An adult weighs 72.2 kg. Convert to pounds.

(72.2) × 2.2 = 158.84 = 158.8 lb

Any of the methods presented in Chapter 8 can be used for converting pounds to kilograms and kilograms to pounds, except decimal movement. Remember, pounds can be expressed using a decimal.

PRACTICE PROBLEMS

Convert the following weights in kilograms to pounds (round to the nearest tenth where indicated).

30. 20 kg = ________________ lb
31. 46 kg = ________________ lb
32. 98.2 kg = ________________ lb
33. 10.4 kg = ________________ lb
34. 34.9 kg = ________________ lb
35. 5.8 kg = ________________ lb

Answers on p. 123

Military Time

Another conversion that is necessary for the nurse to know is the conversion of traditional time using the 24-hour clock. The 24-hour clock is commonly referred to as military time, international time, or 24-hour time. Although some watches are manufactured with traditional time and military time visible on the face of the watch to eliminate confusion, learning the conversion of time is the best method for avoiding errors.

The traditional 12-hour clock provides a source for error in medication administration. On the traditional 12-hour clock, each time occurs twice a day. For example, the hour 7:00 is recorded as both 7:00 AM and 7:00 PM. The abbreviation: "AM" means ante meridian or before noon; "PM" means post meridian or after noon. The times 7 AM and 7 PM may look very similar if the A and P are not clear; the client could receive the medication at the wrong time.

Military time (international time) is a 24-hour clock (Figure 9-2). The main advantage of using military time is that it prevents errors in documentation and medication errors because numbers are not repeated. Each time occurs once per day. In military time, 7:00 AM is written as 0700, whereas 7:00 PM is written as 1900.

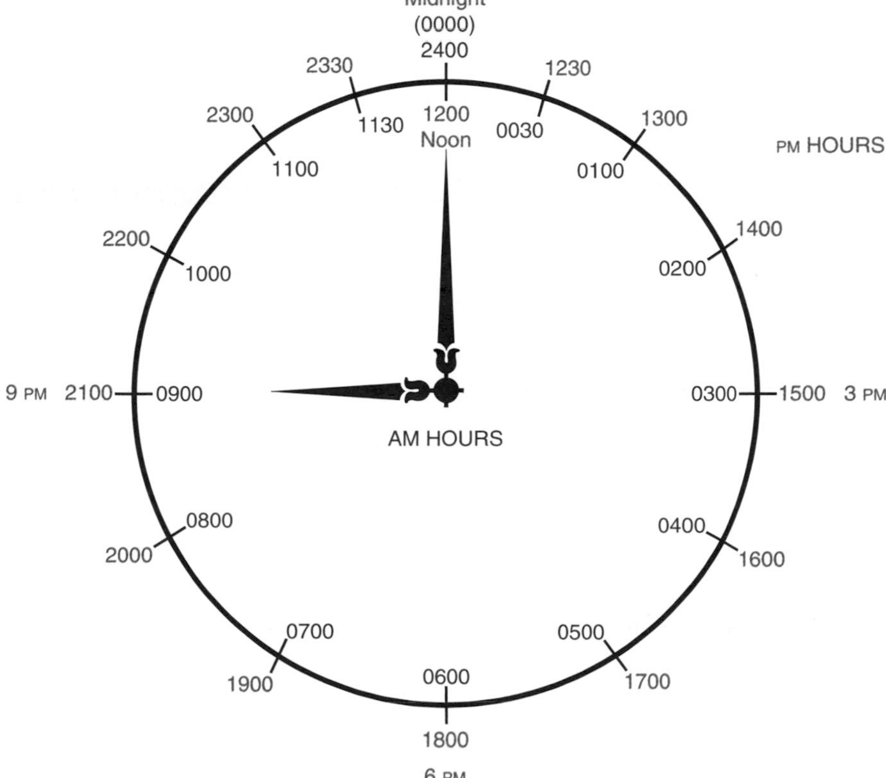

Figure 9-2 24-Hour clock.

In military time, you write a four-digit number without the colon and AM and PM are omitted. The first two digits represent the hour; the last two digits, the minutes. The AM or PM notations are the only things that differentiate traditional time.

The day begins after 0000 (midnight); the first minute of the day is 0001, and the day ends at 2400 (midnight). The minutes between 2400 (midnight) and 0100 (1:00 AM) are written as 0001, 0002 . . . 0058, 0059. Midnight can be written as 0000 or 2400. The time 0000 is commonly used by the military and read as "zero hundred"; 2400 is read as "twenty-four hundred." Although still referred to as military time, a more accurate term is "international time."

Many health care facilities are using military time in documentation such as nursing notes, medication administration records and to document treatments. Use of military time prevents misinterpretation about when a therapeutic measure is due, such as medications, and is less problematic.

Rules for Conversion to Military Time (International Time)

RULE

To convert AM time: omit the colon and AM and ensure that a 4-digit number is written, adding a zero in the beginning as needed.

Example: 8:45 AM = 0845

RULE

To convert PM time: omit the colon and PM; add 1200 to time.

Example: 7:50 PM = 750 + 1200 = 1950

Rules for Converting to Traditional Time

RULE

To convert AM time: insert the colon, add AM, and delete any zero in front of number.

Example: 0845 = 8:45 AM

RULE

To convert PM time: subtract 1200, insert the colon, and add PM.

Example: 1950 = 1950 − 1200 = 7:50 PM

PRACTICE PROBLEMS

Convert the following traditional times to military (international) time.

36. 7:30 AM = ____________
37. 10:30 AM = ____________
38. 8:10 PM = ____________
39. 5:45 PM = ____________
40. 12:16 AM = ____________
41. 6:20 AM = ____________
42. 1:30 PM = ____________
43. 11:45 AM = ____________
44. 11:58 PM = ____________
45. 2:10 AM = ____________

Convert the following military (international) times to traditional (AM/PM) time.

46. 0207 = ______________________
47. 1743 = ______________________
48. 0004 = ______________________
49. 0240 = ______________________
50. 1259 = ______________________
51. 0525 = ______________________
52. 1620 = ______________________
53. 1050 = ______________________
54. 1830 = ______________________
55. 1200 = ______________________

Answers on p. 123

Calculating Completion Times

As you will see in Chapter 22, the nurse can determine the time an IV (intravenous) bag will be completed or empty using military time (international time) or traditional time depending on institutional policy. Now that we have discussed the conversion of time, let's briefly look at how the addition of times (traditional and military) can be used. This will be discussed in more detail in Chapter 22.

Military (International) Time Calculations

Example 1: An IV started at 0300 is to be completed in 3 hr 30 min. Determine the completion time.

- Add the 3 hr 30 min infusion time to the 0300 start time.

$$\begin{array}{r} 0300 \\ +\,330 \\ \hline 0630 \end{array}$$

- The completion time is 0630.

Example 2: An IV started at 0650 is to be completed in 4 hr 10 min. Determine the completion time.

- Add the 4 hr 10 min infusion time to the 0650 start time.

$$\begin{array}{r} 0650 \\ +\,410 \\ \hline 1060 \end{array}$$

- Change the 60 min to 1 hr, and add to 1000 to equal 1100.

Traditional Time Calculations

Example 1: An IV medication will infuse in 30 minutes. It is now 6:15 PM. Determine the completion time.

- Add the 30-min infusion time to the 6:15 PM start time.

6:15 PM + 30 min = 6:45 PM

- The completion time is 6:45 PM.

Example 2: An IV with an infusion time of 12 hr is started at 2:00 AM. Determine the completion time.

- Add the 12-hr infusion time to the 2:00 AM start time.

$$\begin{array}{r} 2{:}00 \text{ AM} \\ +\,12{:}00 \\ \hline 14{:}00 \end{array}$$

- Subtract 12 hr to make the time 2:00 PM.

PRACTICE **PROBLEMS**

Calculate the following completion times in military (international) time.

56. An IV started at 0215 to infuse in 2 hr 30 min ________________

57. An IV started at 0250 to infuse in 5 hr 10 min ________________

Calculate the following completion times in traditional time.

58. An IV started at 6:30 AM that has an infusion time of 45 min ________________

59. An IV started at 9:00 AM that has an infusion time of 6 hr 30 min ________________

60. An IV started at 7:05 PM that has an infusion time of 8 hr ________________

Answers on p. 123

POINTS TO REMEMBER

Use these formulas to convert between Fahrenheit and Celsius temperature.

- To convert from ° C to ° F: ° F = 1.8 (° C) + 32 *or* $\frac{9}{5}$(° C) + 32.
- To convert from ° F to ° C: ° C = $\frac{°\text{F} - 32}{1.8}$ *or* (° F − 32) ÷ $\frac{9}{5}$.
- When converting between Fahrenheit and Celsius, carry math to hundredths and round to tenths.

Conversions Relating to Length

- Conversions can be made by using any of the methods presented in the chapter on conversions; however, moving of decimals is limited to converting between metric measures.

1 cm = 10 mm

1 inch = 2.5 cm

Conversions Relating to Weight

2.2 lb = 1 kg

16 oz = 1 lb

- Weight conversion of pounds to kilograms is done most often because many medications are based on kilograms of body weight.
- Body weight is **essential** for determining dosages in infants and neonates.
- To convert pounds to kilograms, divide by 2.2. Round answer to the nearest tenth.
- To convert pounds and ounces to kilograms, convert the ounces to the nearest tenth of a pound; add this to the total pounds. Convert the total pounds to kilograms and round answer to the nearest tenth.
- To convert kilograms to pounds, multiply by 2.2. Round answer to the nearest tenth.

Conversions Relating to Time

- The 24-hour clock is also referred to as military time, international time, or 24-hour time.
- To change traditional AM time to military time, omit the colon and AM and make sure that a 4-digit number is written, adding a zero in the beginning as needed.
- To change traditional PM time to military time, omit the colon and PM, and add 1200 to the time.
- To convert military time to traditional AM time, insert a colon and add AM. Delete any zero in front of numbers.
- To convert military time to traditional PM time, subtract 1200, insert the colon, and add PM.
- Military time (International time) decreases the possibility of error in administering medications or misinterpretation of when a therapy is due or actually was done because no two times are expressed by the same number.

CHAPTER **REVIEW**

For each of the following statements, change the given temperature to its corresponding equivalent in ° C or ° F. (Round to the nearest tenth.)

1. Notify health care provider for temperature greater than 101.4° F. __________ ° C
2. Store medication at room temperature, 77° F. __________ ° C
3. Store medication within temperature range of 15° C to 30° C. __________ ° F
4. An infant has a body temperature of 36.5° C. __________ ° F
5. Store vaccine at 6° C. __________ ° F
6. A nurse reports a temperature of 37.8° C. __________ ° F
7. Do not expose a medication to temperatures greater than 84° F. __________ ° C
8. A medication contains a crystalline substance with a melting point of about 186° C. __________ ° F
9. Store vaccine at 4° C. __________ ° F
10. Do not expose medication to temperatures greater than 88° F. __________ ° C

Convert temperatures as indicated. Round your answer to the nearest tenth.

11. −10° C = __________ ° F
12. 0° F = __________ ° C
13. 102.8° F = __________ ° C
14. 29° C = __________ ° F
15. 106° C = __________ ° F
16. 70° F = __________ ° C
17. 39.6° C = __________ ° F
18. 64.4° F = __________ ° C
19. 35° C = __________ ° F
20. 50° F = __________ ° C
21. 39.8° C = __________ ° F
22. 86° F = __________ ° C
23. 41° C = __________ ° F

Convert the following to the equivalent indicated. Do NOT round off.

24. 18 in = ________________ cm

25. 31 cm = ________________ in

26. 44.5 cm = ________________ mm

27. 32 in = ________________ cm

28. 3 cm = ________________ mm

29. 7.9 cm = ________________ mm

30. 4 in = ________________ cm

31. 36.6 cm = ________________ mm

32. 6.2 in = ________________ cm

33. 350 mm = ________________ in

34. $21\frac{1}{2}$ in = ________________ cm

35. 2 in = ________________ mm

Convert the following weights in pounds to kilograms (round to the nearest tenth where indicated).

36. 63 lb = ________________ kg

37. 150 lb = ________________ kg

38. 78 lb = ________________ kg

39. 81 lb = ________________ kg

40. 27 lb = ________________ kg

Convert the following weights in kilograms to pounds (round to the nearest tenth of a pound).

41. 77.3 kg = ________________ lb

42. 7 kg = ________________ lb

43. 4.5 kg = ________________ lb

44. 9 kg = ________________ lb

45. 56.1 kg = ________________ lb

46. A child weighs 70 lb during a pediatric clinic visit. How many kilograms does the child weigh? (Round to the nearest tenth.) ________________

47. A client's wound measures 41 mm. How many centimeters is this? __________ cm

48. A client weighs 99.2 kg. How many pounds does the client weigh? (Round to the nearest tenth.) __________ lb

49. An infant's head circumference is 40 cm. How many inches is this? __________ in

50. An infant's head circumference is 40.6 cm. How many millimeters is this? _____ mm

Convert the following weights to kilograms. (Round to the nearest tenth.)

51. 7 lb, 1 oz = ________________ kg

52. 9 lb, 3 oz = ________________ kg

53. 10 lb, 12 oz = ________________ kg

54. 8 lb, 10 oz = ________________ kg

55. 5 lb, 5 oz = ________________ kg

Convert the following military (international) times to traditional times (AM/PM).

56. 0032 = ________________

57. 0220 = ________________

58. 1650 = ________________

59. 1345 = ________________

60. 2122 = ________________

Convert the following traditional times to military (international) times.

61. 5:20 AM = ____________

62. 12:00 midnight = ____________

63. 12:05 AM = ____________

64. 4:30 PM = ____________

65. 1:35 PM = ____________

State whether AM or PM is represented by the following times.

66. 0154 ____________

67. 1450 ____________

68. If a client had IV therapy for 8 hours, ending at 1100, when on the 24-hour clock was the IV started? ____________

State the following completion times as indicated.

69. An IV started at 11:50 PM with an infusion time of 3 hr 30 min ____________ (traditional time).

70. An IV started at 0025 with an infusion time of 1 hr 15 min ____________ (military time).

Answers on p. 124

ANSWERS

Chapter 9

Answers to Practice Problems

1. 39.2° F
2. 38.3° C
3. 100.6° F
4. 38.5° C
5. 99.5° F
6. 68° F to 77° F
7. 38.3° C
8. −13.9° C
9. 98.6° F
10. 7.8° C
11. 4 in
12. 4.5 cm
13. 375 mm
14. 51.25 cm
15. 37 cm
16. 2.6 in
17. 250 cm
18. 12.8 in
19. 15.2 in
20. 50 cm
21. 2.9 kg
22. 5.5 kg
23. 4.7 kg
24. 3.5 kg
25. 9.1 kg
26. 29.1 kg
27. 10 kg
28. 55 kg
29. 38.6 kg
30. 44 lb
31. 101.2 lb
32. 216 lb
33. 22.9 lb
34. 76.8 lb
35. 12.8 lb
36. 0730
37. 1030
38. 2010
39. 1745
40. 0016
41. 0620
42. 1330
43. 1145
44. 2358
45. 0210
46. 2:07 AM
47. 5:43 PM
48. 12:04 AM
49. 2:40 AM
50. 12:59 PM
51. 5:25 AM
52. 4:20 PM
53. 10:50 AM
54. 6:30 PM
55. 12:00 PM (noon)
56. 0445
57. 0800
58. 7:15 AM
59. 3:30 PM
60. 3:05 AM

evolve

For additional information, refer to the Conversions and Equivalents section of the Elsevier's Interactive Drug Calculation Application, Version 1 on Evolve.

Answers to Chapter Review

1. 38.6° C
2. 25° C
3. 59° F to 86° F
4. 97.7° F
5. 42.8° F
6. 100° F
7. 28.9° C
8. 366.8° F
9. 39.2° F
10. 31.1° C
11. 14° F
12. −17.8° C
13. 39.3° C
14. 84.2° F
15. 222.8° F
16. 21.1° C
17. 103.3° F
18. 18° C
19. 95° F
20. 10° C
21. 103.6° F
22. 30° C
23. 105.8° F
24. 45 cm
25. 12.4 in
26. 445 mm
27. 80 cm
28. 30 mm
29. 79 mm
30. 10 cm
31. 366 mm
32. 15.5 cm
33. 14 in
34. 53.75 cm
35. 50 mm
36. 28.6 kg
37. 68.2 kg
38. 35.5 kg
39. 36.8 kg
40. 12.3 kg
41. 170.1 lb
42. 15.4 lb
43. 9.9 lb
44. 19.8 lb
45. 123.4 lb
46. 31.8 kg
47. 4.1 cm
48. 218.2 lb
49. 16 in
50. 406 mm
51. 3.2 kg
52. 4.2 kg
53. 4.9 kg
54. 3.9 kg
55. 2.4 kg
56. 12:32 AM
57. 2:20 AM
58. 4:50 PM
59. 1:45 PM
60. 9:22 PM
61. 0520
62. 2400 (0000 used in military)
63. 0005
64. 1630
65. 1335
66. AM
67. PM
68. 0300
69. 3:20 AM
70. 0140

UNIT THREE

Methods of Administration and Calculation

Note: The safe and accurate administration of medications to a client is an important and primary responsibility of a nurse. Being able to read and interpret an order correctly and calculate medication dosages is necessary for accurate administration.

Chapter 10 Medication Administration

Chapter 11 Understanding and Interpreting Medication Orders

Chapter 12 Medication Administration Records and Medication Distribution Systems

Chapter 13 Reading Medication Labels

Chapter 14 Dosage Calculation Using the Ratio and Proportion Method

Chapter 15 Dosage Calculation Using the Formula Method

Chapter 16 Dosage Calculation Using the Dimensional Analysis Method

CHAPTER 10
Medication Administration

Objectives

After reviewing this chapter, you should be able to:

1. State the consequences of medication errors
2. Identify the causes of medication errors
3. Identify the role of the nurse in preventing medication errors
4. Identify the role of the Institute for Safe Medication Practices (ISMP) and The Joint Commission (TJC) in the prevention of medication errors
5. State the basic six "rights" of safe medication administration
6. Identify factors that influence medication dosages
7. Identify the common routes for medication administration
8. Define *critical thinking*
9. Explain the importance of critical thinking in medication administration
10. Identify important critical thinking skills necessary in medication administration
11. Discuss the importance of client teaching
12. Identify special considerations relating to the elderly and medication administration
13. Identify home care considerations in relation to medication administration

Medication Errors

Medications are therapeutic measures aimed at improving a client's health and are a primary form of treatment for most illnesses. Medication administration is one of the most critical functions of nursing practice and has an essential role in preparing and administering medications. Therefore, it is critical and required that nurses be vigilant in embracing safe administration practices. When medications are administered carelessly and incorrectly, errors can be made, and the consequences can be harmful and threatening to the life of a client. According to the National Coordinating Council for Medication Error Reporting and Prevention (NCCMERP), a medication error is defined as follows:

> A medication error is any preventable event that may cause or lead to inappropriate medication use or patient harm while the medication is in the control of the health care professional, patient, or consumer. Such events may be related to professional practice, health care products, procedures, and systems, including prescribing, order communication, product labeling, packaging, and nomenclature, compounding, dispensing, distribution, administration, education, monitoring, and use.

Outcomes from medication errors include increased hospital stay, increased health care costs, acute or chronic disability, and even death. Additional, indirect consequences can affect the nurse involved both emotionally and professionally and could result in loss of position, legal consequences, or loss of license to practice.

With the increased focus on client safety, there is no surprise that medication safety is linked to a health organization's ability to attract clients, meet the requirements of accreditation, and obtain reimbursement for services. Publications regarding the numerous medication errors have caused astonishment among members of the health care profession and society as a whole. According to current literature, despite technological advances, preventive strategies, systematic methods of reporting errors, and definitions of what constitutes error, medication errors continue to be one of the most prevailing causes of client injury.

According to the landmark 2006 report *Preventing Medication Errors,* from the Institute of Medicine (IOM, 2006), these errors injure 1.5 million Americans each year and could have been prevented. According to *Quality and Safety in Nursing: A Competency Approach to Improving Outcomes,* medication errors account for over 7,000 deaths annually (Sherwood Given & Jan Barnsteiner, 2017). On average, in-patients may experience at least one medication error per day. Almost 2% of Americans experience a preventable adverse event, which increases hospital costs by $4,700 per admission, or about $2.8 million annually for a 700-bed hospital; multiplied, this would amount to $12 billion nationally. The national cost for preventable adverse events ranges between $17 billion and $29 billion.

Information concerning medication errors has serious implications for health and safety of clients and warrants a collaborative approach with numerous strategies to prevent errors. A focus on safety has implications for those involved in the education of nurses as well, with safety being a central concept. The critical role that nurses play in medication safety is a primary focus of this text and is based on the knowledge and understanding of careful, correct, and safe medication administration.

The reporting of significant or sentinel events that result in client harm has become an expectation from those involved in the delivery of health care. Promotion of a culture of safety has become a priority in health care.

Organizations Involved in Safe Medication Practices

The IOM became involved in the promotion of client safety and published reports that included data relating to medication errors and preventing them. According to the IOM report *Identifying and Preventing Medication Errors (2006),* which presented a national agenda for reducing medication errors, changes across the health care industry require collaboration among doctors, nurses, pharmacists, the Food and Drug Administration, other government agencies, hospitals and other health care organizations, and patients to prevent medication errors.

To advance client safety worldwide, several organizations have become involved. The Institute for Safe Medication Practices (ISMP) and the United States Pharmacopeia (USP) are just two organizations actively involved in monitoring medication error reports and the development of strategies aimed at correcting the problem and educating personnel involved in the administration of medications. The Joint Commission (TJC), which provides accreditation to U.S. hospitals and health care facilities, is also working to achieve high standards in the U.S. health care system. One of its goals has been in the area of medication errors; TJC implemented National Patient Safety Goals, one of which is aimed at assisting health care facilities in the prevention of devastating medication errors.

The U.S. Food and Drug Administration (FDA) recognized the potential of barcoding to improve client safety. In 2004, the FDA issued a regulation that requires all new pharmaceuticals to be barcoded upon launch into the market (FDA, 2006). The barcodes are used with a barcode-scanning system and computerized database. The barcode must contain the drug's National Drug Code as a minimum. Hospitals have barcode scanners that are linked to a hospital's electronic medical records. The barcoding allows the health care provider to scan the client's barcode prior to administering medications, which allows access to the client's medication record. Each medication is scanned prior to administration to the client, letting the computer know what medication is being administered. The information is then compared with the client's database and alerts the health care provider if there is a problem requiring investigation. The FDA is also responsible for the placement of the "black box" warning on certain medications to alert the health care providers to certain risks associated with the medication.

The Quality and Safety Education for Nurses (QSEN) project has the goal of preparing student nurses with the knowledge, skills, and attitudes (KSAs) that are needed to improve the quality and safety of client care. QSEN looks at six competencies, one of which is relevant to medication administration: safety. Another is informatics, which relates to technology to mitigate errors. Many nursing curriculums have integrated the QSEN competencies into the curriculum. QSEN will be referred to in areas in which it is applicable in this text.

Another important organization wherein patient safety is a core component of its mission is the National Quality Forum (NQF) (http://www.qualityforum.org). NQF is a nonprofit, voluntary, consensus standard-setting organization that was established in 1999. To ensure that all patients are protected from injury while receiving care, NQF developed and endorsed a set of Serious Reportable Events (SREs) in 2002. According to NQF, SREs are a compilation of serious, largely preventable, and harmful clinical events, designed to help the health care field assess, measure, and report performance in providing safe care.

The purpose of this endorsed list of SREs, according to NQF, is to facilitate uniform and comparable public reporting to enable systematic learning across health care organizations and systems and to drive systematic national improvements in patient safety based on what is learned both about the events and about how to prevent recurrence. Originally endorsed in 2002 for adverse events that occur in hospitals, SREs now go beyond the hospital setting and address patient safety across a range of settings in which patients receive care, including office-based settings and ambulatory surgery centers.

In the NQF's *Serious Reportable Events in Health Care—2011 Update: A Consensus Report* (2011), 29 events were recommended (4 new and 25 updated) for endorsement as voluntary consensus standards suitable for public reporting. NQF considers SREs to be unambiguous; largely, if not entirely, preventable; and serious. The list of SREs includes injuries during case management (rather than underlying disease) and errors in patient safety, and aims to prevent future adverse events. SREs focus on areas that include: Surgical or Invasive Procedure Events, Product or Device Events, Potential Criminal Events, and Care Management Events.

An SRE that has particular relevance to this text, listed under the area of Care Management Events, is indicated as 4A, patient death or serious injury associated with a medication error (e.g., errors involving the wrong drug, wrong dose, wrong patient, wrong time, wrong rate, wrong preparation, or wrong route of administration). Notice this SRE includes the "rights" of medication administration, which has been cited as one of the reasons for medication error when they are not consistently followed by nurses in medication administration. This SRE has application in any area in which patients receive care.

Discussion of these organizations helps further reinforce the importance of safety in medication administration and the avoidance of harm to clients in our care across the health care settings.

Technological advances in terms of medication administration (e.g., use of barcoding, computerized unit dose medication carts) have been instituted in many facilities as a means of preventing and decreasing medication errors; however, computer technology cannot replace human intellect or negate the need to follow various steps in medication administration to ensure client safety.

Medication errors can occur anywhere in the medication process, including administration, dispensing, and prescribing. The causes of medication errors can involve multiple factors, including lack of information about the medication, lack of information about the client to whom the medication is being administered (e.g., allergies, other medications the client is taking, the reason for the medication being administered), and confusing medication names (look-alike or sound-alike).

Other causes of medication errors include errors in mathematical calculation of dosages, incomplete orders, failure to observe "rights" of medication administration when administering medications, failure to identify a client accurately, and miscommunication of orders.

Miscommunication of medication orders can involve poor handwriting, misuse of zeros and decimal points, confusion of metric and other dosing units, inappropriate abbreviations, and errors in computer order entry.

Other contributing factors to medication errors include failure to educate clients properly about medications they are taking, administration of medications without critical thought, and failure to comply with the required policy or procedure related to medication administration. With the shortage of nursing personnel, factors such as shift changes, floating staff, double shifts, and workload increases have contributed to errors.

Distractions and interruptions as contributory factors to medication errors have been found to be plausible in the literature. Distraction was identified as a key reason for error during medication administration in 2010. In 2010, a bulletin from the United States Pharmacopeial Convention titled *Physical Environments That Promote Safe Medication Use* identified the work environment as one of the most commonly reported factors contributing to medication errors. In addition, studies have shown that interruption of nurses during the medication process increases the chances of error, and as the number of distractions increases, so do the number of errors and the risk to client safety. According to the ISMP newsletter *ISMP Medication Safety Alert, Acute Care Edition* (November 29, 2012) in an article titled "Side Tracks on the Safety Express. Interruptions Lead to Errors and Unfinished. . . . Wait, What Was I Doing?" a study indicated that "the risk of any medication error increases 12.7% with each interruption, and the risk of harmful medication error is doubled when nurses are interrupted 4 times during a single drug administration and tripled when interrupted 6 times. Thus distractions and interruptions have major consequences in healthcare."

It is not possible to completely eliminate distractions and interruptions in health care facilities. However, actions have been taken in some facilities, including designating the medication area as a "No Interruption Zone" and educating staff on the importance of avoiding interruption of the nurse administering medications.

SAFETY ALERT!

Focus solely on the task at hand, medication administration (when the actual act of medication administration occurs). Distractions can result in error during medication administration, jeopardize the client's safety, and may cause harm.

Certain medications, referred to as *high-alert medications,* have also been identified as contributing to harmful errors. The medications on this list include concentrated electrolyte solutions, such as potassium chloride. Other medications that are associated with harmful errors include heparin, insulin, morphine, neuromuscular drugs, and chemotherapy drugs.

Although advances in technology such as automatic dispensing cabinets (ADC), computer prescriber order entry (CPOE), and barcode medication administration have decreased the number of medication errors, it has been stressed that these advances are useful only if they are properly applied and if the systems are effective and efficient.

The reasons for medication errors are not limited to those presented and are not nursing errors alone. The best solution to the problem of medication errors is prevention. To prevent medication errors, personnel involved in the administration of medications must do meticulous planning and implement the task properly, paying close attention to detail.

The administration of medications is more than just giving the medication because it is what is ordered. The prescriber orders the medication; the nurse is accountable for being knowledgeable about the action, uses, side effects, expected response, contraindications, and range of dosage for the medication being administered. The nurse should not hesitate to consult a valid and current drug reference about any medication that is unfamiliar.

Medication administration involves using the nursing process, which includes assessment, nursing diagnosis/nursing problem, planning, implementation, and evaluation.

SAFETY ALERT!

Failure to think about what you are doing and why you are doing it and failure to assess a client can result in errors. You are accountable for your actions.

Critical Thinking and Medication Administration

There are numerous definitions for *critical thinking.* The best way to define critical thinking is as a process of thinking that includes being reasonable and rational. Thinking is based on reason. Critical thinking is important to all phases of nursing but is particularly relevant in the discussion of medication administration. Critical thinking is necessary to the development of clinical reasoning skills and clinical judgment.

Critical thinking encompasses several skills relevant to medication administration. One such skill is the ability to identify an organized approach to the task at hand. For example, in medication administration, calculating dosages in an organized, systematic manner (formula, ratio and proportion, dimensional analysis) decreases the likelihood of errors.

A second skill characteristic of critical thinking is the ability to be an autonomous thinker—for example, challenging a medication order that is written incorrectly rather than passively accepting the order. Critical thinking also involves the ability to distinguish irrelevant information from that which is relevant. For example, when reading a medication label, the nurse is able to decipher from the label the information necessary for calculating the correct dosage. Critical thinking involves reasoning and the application of concepts—for example, choosing the correct type of syringe to administer a dosage, and using concepts learned to decide the appropriateness of a dosage. Critical thinking also involves asking for clarification of what is not understood and not making assumptions. Clarifying a medication order and dosage indicates critical thinking. Checking the accuracy and reliability of information decreases the chance of medication errors. The ability to validate information requires a high level of thinking and decreases the chance of medication errors that could be harmful to the client.

Critical thinking is essential to the safe administration of medications. This process allows a nurse to think before doing, translate knowledge into practice, and make appropriate judgments. To safely administer medication, the nurse must base decisions on rational thinking and thorough knowledge of medication administration. Proper medication administration involves evaluation of the client and the medication's effects, which requires critical thinking and skills of assessment. A nurse who administers medication in a routine manner, rather than with thought and reasoning, is not using critical thinking skills.

SAFETY ALERT!

Remember that the nurse who administers a medication is legally liable for the medication error regardless of the reason for the error occurrence.

Factors That Influence Medication Dosages and Action

Several factors influence medication dosages and the way they act, including the following:

1. Route of administration
2. Time of administration
3. Age of the client
4. Nutritional status of the client
5. Absorption and excretion of the medication
6. Health status of the client
7. Gender of the client
8. Ethnicity and culture of the client
9. Genetics

All these factors affect how clients react to a medication and the dosage they receive, and all must be considered when medications are prescribed and administered. Because of differences in the actions and types of medications, clients respond in various ways, and therefore dosages must be individualized. No two clients will respond to a medication in the same manner. Nurses must keep these factors in mind when administering medications. These factors can account for individuals responding differently to the same medication.

Special Considerations for the Elderly

Elderly individuals can be considered high-risk medication consumers. Approximately two-thirds of older adults use both prescription and nonprescription medications, and one-third of all prescriptions are written for older adults. With the number of individuals over the age of 65 rapidly increasing, the use of medications in this age group will also increase. According to the Administration on Aging (AOA) (http://www.aoa.acl.gov/Aging statistics/index.aspx), the older population (persons 65 years or older) numbered 44.7 million in 2013 (the latest year for which data is available). By 2060, there will be about 98 million older persons in the United States, more than twice the number in 2013. Americans 65 years or older represented 14.1% of the population in the year 2013 but are expected to be 21.7% of the population by 2040.

People are now living longer, and older people tend to use health care services more often. As with children (see Chapter 25), special consideration should be given to the client who is over 65 years of age. With the aging process come physiological changes that have a direct effect on medications and their action in the elderly individual. Aging causes the slowing down of the body's functions. Other physiological changes include a decrease in circulation, slower absorption, slower metabolism, a decrease in excretory functions, and a decrease in the ability to respond to stress such as the stress of medications on the system. Other changes with aging include a decrease in body weight, which can affect the dosage of medications, and changes in mental status, possibly caused by the effects of physical illness or physiological changes in the neurological system that can occur with aging. These physiological changes can cause unexpected medication reactions and make the elderly person more sensitive to the effects of many medications.

According to Clayton and Willihnganz (*Basic Pharmacology for Nurses,* 2017), although people who are older than 65 years represent about 14% of the U.S. population, they consume more than 25% of all prescription medicines and 33% of all nonprescription medicines sold. A study of the U.S. noninstitutionalized adult population has indicated that more than 90% of persons 65 years or older use at least one medication per week. More than 40% use five or more medications, and 12% use 10 or more different medications per week. Because the elderly are often taking more than one medication (polypharmacy), problems such as medication interactions, severe adverse reactions, medication and food interactions, and an increase in medication errors occur. The Beers criteria is a list of medications that are used to evaluate quality and safety in nursing homes. According to Clayton and Willihnganz (2017), these medications are considered to be potentially inappropriate for older patients. It is thought that the medications on this list cause adverse effects more commonly and should be avoided in older adult patients unless treatment with other medicines has failed. It is recommended that practitioners be aware of the medications on this list and educate clients regarding prescription and nonprescription medications. As the senior population continues to increase, there is a need to focus on reducing medication errors in this group.

As a rule, the elderly client will require smaller dosages of medications (as dosage size increases, the number of adverse effects and their severity increase), and the dosages should be given farther apart to prevent accumulation of medications and toxic effects. With aging, visual and hearing problems may develop. Special attention must be given when teaching clients about their medications to help prevent medication errors. Develop a relationship with the client; building rapport and trust is important for the elderly. Take time and talk to the elderly, listen to what they say, and never assume they do not know how much or what medications they are taking. Ascertain that all instructions are written as clearly as possible, choosing fonts that are friendly to older eyes. Make sure the client has appropriate measuring devices to facilitate ease and accuracy when measuring (e.g., a dropper or measuring cup with calibrated lines to indicate small dosages [0.2 mg, 0.4 mg, etc.]). To lessen the chance of taking too much medication or forgetting a dosage, try to establish specific times compatible with the client's routine for taking medications.

Omission of medications is a common cause of error for the elderly at home. This may be due to the cost of medication or forgetfulness. Establishing medication times when possible to coincide with the client's routine and engaging a family member or friend if possible in the teaching process may help in preventing omission of medications. Help the

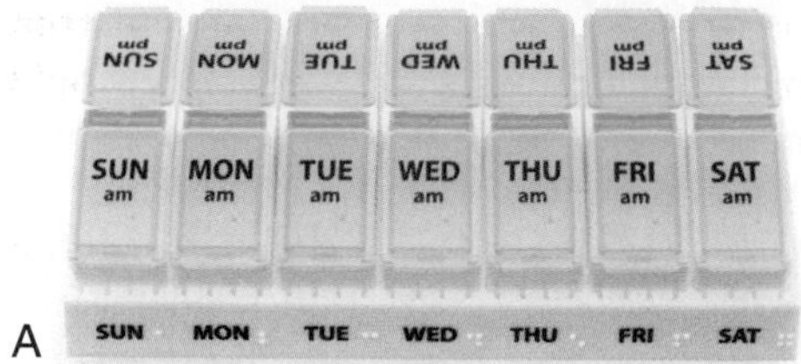

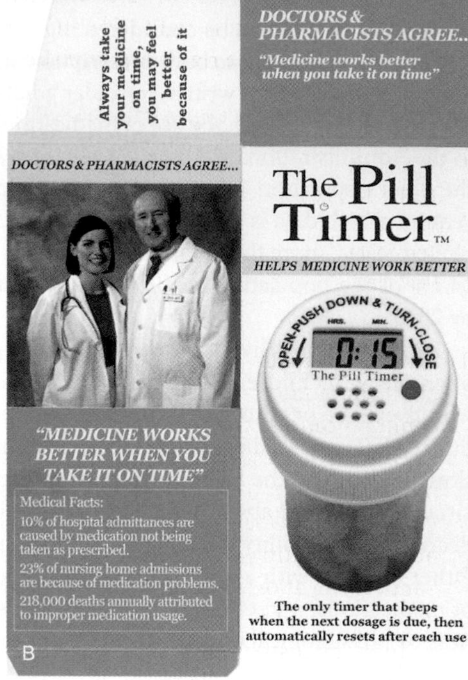

Figure 10-1 **A,** Container that holds a week's medications. **B,** The Pill Timer beeps, flashes, and automatically resets every time it is closed. (**A,** From Perry AG, Potter PA, Elkin MK, Ostendorf WR: *Nursing interventions and clinical skills,* ed 6, St Louis, 2016, Mosby.)

client recognize tablets by the name on the bottle, not by color. If the print on medications is too small for the client to read, encourage the use of a magnifying glass. Other measures might include providing a simple chart that outlines the medications to be taken, times they are to be taken, and special instructions if needed. Such a chart should be geared to the client's visual ability and comprehension level. Encourage the elderly client to request that childproof containers not be used; some older people will have difficulty opening child-resistant containers. Recommend medication aids for the client, such as special medication containers divided into separate compartments for storing daily or weekly medication dosages. (Figure 10-1 shows examples of medication containers.)

A careful and complete medication history, including illicit drugs, should be obtained from the elderly client. This should include over-the-counter medications, alternative medicines, and vitamins. The elderly client may think that these products are safe; however, they may cause dangerous interactions with prescribed medications. Encourage clients to check with their health care provider before taking over-the-counter medications.

When teaching the elderly, it is important to remember that they are mature adults who are capable of learning; they may need and deserve additional time for learning to take place. Be patient, use simple language, and maintain the independence of the elderly as much as possible. Always allow ample time for processing, individualize the teaching, and remember to always foster feelings of self-worth. Always have your clients demonstrate back to you what you have taught them. Correct teaching can decrease misunderstandings and errors in medication.

The Rights of Medication Administration

The "rights" of medication administration can be looked at as being standards. By definition, standards are actions that ensure safe nursing practice. The "rights" of medication administration are a set of safety checks that serve as guidelines for the practitioner to follow when administering medications to prevent errors and ensure client safety. The "rights" must be consistently followed when administering medications to a client. There have been many medication errors linked to inconsistency in following the "rights." Over the years there have been five, then six, and now in many places eight or more rights. There are six basic rights of medications administration that are required safety checks that must be performed with the administration of each and every medication to a client. The six basic rights include the right client, right medication, right dose, right route, right time, and right documentation. **A violation of any of the six basic rights constitutes a medication error.** Additional rights include right indication, right to know, and right to refuse. A new right being considered is the right response (Box 10-1).

BOX 10-1 The Rights of Medication Administration

1. Right client
2. Right medication
3. Right dose
4. Right route
5. Right time
6. Right documentation
7. Right indication
8. Right to know
9. Right to refuse
10. Right response

1. **The right client**—Always make sure you are administering medications to the right client. Failure to correctly identify the right client has been cited as one of the three most common causes of medication errors. Since 2003, TJC has required that clients be identified with at least two unique client identifiers (e.g., name, birth date, medical record number, but not the client's room number). This requirement was initiated as a National Patient Safety Goal; it has been a standard since 2004 and applies to both inpatient and outpatient settings. It is permissible to check the two identifiers with the client's armband, medication administration record, or chart and ask the client to state his or her name or parent to state the child's name.

   In many institutions, you may be required to scan the barcode on the client's identification bracelet as well as the medication being administered. In basic nursing education programs, emphasis is placed on establishing the correct identification of the client prior to medication administration. Students are required to compare two client-specific identifiers with the client's armband, medication administration record (MAR), or chart and by asking the client to state her or his name (as a third identifier). To avoid administering medications to the wrong client, the steps identified need to be consistently implemented regardless of how familiar the nurse is with the client. Always know and use the unique identifiers recognized and required by the facility. Advanced technology does not eliminate your responsibility to correctly identify a client. Misidentification can result in the wrong client receiving the wrong medication.

SAFETY ALERT!

Always verify your client's identity by using the two identifiers designated by your institution each time medications are administered. This will help ensure you have the right client and avoid an error.

2. **The right medication**—When medications are ordered, the nurse should compare the MAR (medication administration record) or computer record with the actual order. When administering medications, the nurse should check the label on the medication container against the order. Medications should be checked three times: before preparing, after preparing, and before replacing the container. With unit dosages (each medication dosage is prepared in the prescribed dosage, packaged, labeled, and ready to use), the label should still be checked three times. Remember, regardless of the medication distribution system, the medication label should be checked three times. Errors frequently occur because of similarity in medication names and similar packaging.

   Many medications have names that sound alike, or have names or packaging that is similar. TJC posts online an extensive list of look-alike/sound-alike (LASA) medications that pose a risk for error due to prescribing and administering one for the other. This list includes medications such as quinidine and quinine, Tegretol and Trental, OxyContin (controlled release) and oxycodone (immediate release). A complete listing can be found by going to the TJC website (www.JointCommission.org)

   ISMP and FDA also suggest the use of "Tall Man" lettering to alert health professionals to the potential for error with look-alike names. In the use of this method, the medication name is mixed-case or enlarged, bolded, or in italics to emphasize the differing portions of the two names. Tall Man lettering is being used at many institutions. See Appendix B, which shows a listing of the FDA and ISMP lists of look-alike drug names with recommended Tall Man lettering. The right medication also includes checking the expiration date on the medication label. If the medication has expired, contact the pharmacy for an updated supply and discard according to the institution policy.

Administer only medications that you have prepared and that are clearly labeled. Avoid distractions when preparing medications; do not multitask. Some institutions have instituted "no interruption zones" in areas such as the medication room to prevent distractions.

SAFETY ALERT!

If the medication name is not clear or the medication does not seem to be appropriate for the client, question the order. Always double-check that you have the correct medication. If you are unfamiliar with a medication, refer to a reference to ensure you have the correct medication and prevent errors.

3. **The right dose**—Always perform and check calculations carefully, without ignoring decimal points. If you misread a decimal point, the client could receive a dose significantly different from the one ordered. Risk of harm from dosage errors in the pediatric population is great. Caution should be taken when administering medications to children. Errors can occur because of the frequency of weight-based calculations, the need for decimal points, and fractional dosages (TJC, 2008). Many errors have occurred with infusion pumps and calculations involving administration of parenteral fluids and medications. Electronic infusion pumps have reduced medication errors. Although infusion pump technology has increased administration safety, the nurse cannot rely fully on these devices. It is a nursing responsibility to be trained in the use of infusion pumps and to be alert for potential problems.

   To ensure the right dose of medication, interpret abbreviations correctly. Factors such as illegible handwriting, miscalculation of the amount, and use of inappropriate abbreviations can result in administration of the wrong dose. Always have someone else check a dosage that causes concern. In some agencies, certain medication dosages are required to be checked by two nurses (e.g., insulin, heparin). These medications have been a common source of errors in administration. If a dosage or abbreviation in a written order is not clear, call the prescriber for verification; do not assume.

   Computer entry does not eliminate the use of incorrect dosing symbols. Nurses should always consult a reference to confirm the dosage when in doubt. After dosages are calculated, they should be administered using standard measuring devices, such as calibrated medicine droppers and cups. Always double check a dosage and confirm pump settings. Before administering medications, it is the responsibility of the nurse to question orders thought to be inappropriate. Examples of questionable orders include a single dose to be composed of more than two or three dosage units (e.g., tablets, capsules, vials) and orders for atypically high doses. In order to recognize unusual dosages, the nurse has the responsibility to become familiar with the usual medication dosages for the clients they care for. The same principle of questioning applies to the preparation of IV solutions. If more than two or three dosage units are needed to prepare the solution, this could signal an error.

   In later chapters you will learn to calculate the amount to administer to a client. Thinking what is reasonable and using a common sense approach when calculating dosages is imperative to prevent errors. Full attention to accurate dosage calculation ensures that you avoid error and harm to a client when administering medications.
4. **The right route**—Route refers to how a medication is administered (e.g. by mouth, injection). A medication intended for one route is unsafe if administered by another route. Oral medications (e.g. tablets, capsules, caplets) are administered by mouth. Nurses should always consult a reliable reference to confirm the correct route for a medication that is unfamiliar. Always check that the route, if listed on the medication label, matches the route ordered. If the route is not indicated, use a reference to identify the correct route. The route of the medication should be stated on the order. Do not assume which route is appropriate. Orders to administer medications by a feeding tube that should not

be crushed (e.g., enteric coated) require that the nurse seek clarification of the order or have the order changed by the prescriber to ensure safe medication administration.

5. **The right time**—Medications should be given at the correct time of day and interval (e.g., three times a day [t.i.d.] or every 6 hours [q6h]). Judgment should be used as to when medications should be given or not given. If several medications are ordered, set priorities and administer medications that must act at a certain time. For example, insulin should be given at an exact time before meals. The right time should also include the right time sequence! For example, a client may be receiving a diuretic b.i.d., and the institution may have b.i.d. as 9:00 AM and 9:00 PM. The nurse will need to know that the diuretic should not be given in the late evening, so that the individual is not going to the bathroom all night. This requires critical thinking. The nurse must know whether a time schedule can be altered or requires judgment in determining the proper time to be administered. Know the institutional policy concerning medication times.

   Factors such as the purpose of the medication, medication interactions, absorption of the medication, and side effects must be considered when medication times are scheduled. Administer medications at the right time. In most cases, this means the medication must be administered within 30 minutes of the scheduled time. (Up to 30 minutes before or after the scheduled time.) This is referred to as the "30 minute rule."

   The "30 minute rule" for medication administration, enacted by the Centers for Medicare & Medical Services (CMS), required that medications be given within 30 minutes before or 30 minutes after their scheduled time. According to the ISMP, who conducted a survey of nurses in response to the 30 minute rule, many nurses developed unsafe practices and workarounds that threatened client safety and increased the potential for medication errors. Some of the unsafe practices that resulted from time pressures included taking risky shortcuts including deception (e.g., medication documented as being given at a certain time when it was delayed or given beforehand); administering medications without performing assessments and/or checking vital signs, lab values, weight and allergy status; skipping barcode scanning; and skipping important double checks to save time.

   As a result of the survey findings, CMS provided hospitals the flexibility to establish policies and procedures for the timing of medication, which includes establishing policies for identification of medications that require exact or precise timing for administration and are not eligible for scheduled dosing times. CMS defines time-critical scheduled medications as those in which early or late administration longer than 30 minutes may cause harm or have a significant impact on the intended therapeutic or pharmacological effect. Non–time-critical scheduled medications are those in which a longer or shorter interval of time since the prior dose does not significantly alter the medication's therapeutic effect or otherwise cause harm and therefore the hospitals may establish, as appropriate, either a one- or two-hour window of administration.

   ISMP, in collaboration with a panel and organizations including TJC and American Nurses Association (ANA), developed Acute Care Guidelines for Timely Administration of Scheduled Medications. These guidelines can be reviewed on the ISMP website, www.ismp.org. **It is important that nurses are aware that hospitals will still be held accountable for the "30 minute rule" in the CMS Interpretive Guidelines.** Nurses must know the agency's policy regarding their medication administration policy.

   Before administering prn (when required, whenever necessary) medications, check to ascertain that adequate time has passed since the previous dose, or severe consequences may occur because the medication was administered to the client too soon.

   All medication orders should include the frequency that a medication is to be administered. Administration of a medication at the prescribed time or right time is important to maximize the therapeutic effect and maintain therapeutic blood levels. Errors have occurred in medication administration because of misinterpretation of time and frequency in medication orders. The Joint Commission has taken steps to prevent errors by prohibiting the use of certain abbreviations related to dosing frequency (e.g., qod and qd have been mistaken for each other; instead of qod, write "every other day" and instead of qd write "daily" or "every day").

6. **Right documentation**—Correct documentation is referred to as the sixth right of medication administration. Medications should be charted accurately as soon as they are given—on the right client's medication record, under the right date, and next to the right time. If a medication is refused, it should be documented as such with a notation on the medication record or in the nurse's notes. Never chart a medication as given before administering it or without documentation as to why it was not given. Follow the policy of the institution when documenting. All documentation should be legible. Unintentional overmedication of a client could result if a nurse fails to document a medication that was given and a nurse on a following shift also gives the medication to the client.

   Documentation of medications administered is done on the client's medication administration record (MAR), which is a paper form or electronic record that tracks the medications a client receives. A computerized record is used as a working document that records medications as they are administered and is referred to as an electronic medication administration record (eMAR). This system allows electronic tracking of medications administered to help reduce errors. With some of the electronic medication systems, the medication barcode and the client's identification band is scanned, and the information is documented into the client's eMAR. **Remember: "If it's not documented, it's not done."**

The six basic rights that have been discussed should always be consistently followed when administering medications. In addition to the six rights, the nurse should always view the client receiving medications as an important and valuable asset in the prevention of medication errors. Always listen to concerns verbalized by the client when administering medications regardless of the checks that you have performed before administration (e.g., "The other nurse just gave me medication," "I have never taken this medication before"). Statements such as these by a client should not be ignored. Always listen carefully and be attentive to the concerns of a client. Consider what the client verbalizes as correct and investigate concerns before administering the medication; this can be valuable in preventing medication errors.

SAFETY ALERT!

When a client questions a medication **STOP** and **LISTEN.** This may be the opportunity to identify an error before a client is harmed.

7. **The right indication**—This is also referred to as the right reason. The nurse has the responsibility for knowing the reason a medication is being administered to ensure it is being given for the right reason. If the nurse understands the reason for a medication that is ordered, it will help in the identification of when to hold or not give a medication that may cause harm if administered. Knowing why prevents errors. If in doubt about the reason for a medication that is ordered, verify the order with the prescriber before administering.
8. **The right to know—All clients have a right to be educated regarding the medication they are taking.** Clients are more likely to be compliant if they understand why they are taking a medication, and education allows them to make an informed decision. Information that clients should receive includes dose, reason, effect, and side effects of the medication.
9. **The right to refuse**—In addition to the six basic rights of medication administration, another right is a **client has the right to refuse medications.** When this occurs, the nurse needs to document the refusal correctly and make appropriate persons aware of the refusal. The right to refuse may be denied to the client who has a mental illness. A client deemed to be dangerous to self or others can be taken to court and mandated to take medication. Though the client has the right to refuse medication or treatment, the law referred to as Kendra's Law in New York state may provide some exception to a client's right to refuse treatment (e.g., medication). Kendra's Law is legislation designed to protect the public and individuals living with mental illness by ensuring that potentially dangerous mentally ill outpatients are safely and effectively treated.

Kendra's Law is court-ordered assisted outpatient treatment (AOT). It authorizes the courts to issue orders that would require mentally ill persons who are unlikely to survive safely in the community without supervision to accept medications and other needed mental health services. In other words, if a client is in the community and noncompliant with the treatment regimen (e.g., medication), the client can be petitioned to court by an individual (e.g., spouse, parent, adult roommate). The judge can then mandate the client to take medication if he or she is a danger to self or others. It is important to realize, however, that although there is a right to refuse, during an emergency situation, if danger is imminent, the client can be forcibly medicated by order of a judge.

Nurses should always be aware of the state laws, policies, and procedures for their jurisdiction relative to the administration of medications to refusing clients. It is extremely important for nurses to check frequently for side effects related to medications and to listen carefully to client complaints. The reason for the refusal of medications should be carefully analyzed and documented in all cases. Education of the client and a reassuring therapeutic relationship can assist in diminishing a client's refusal.

Another important right has to do with educating the client. **All clients have a right to be educated regarding the medication they are taking.** Clients are more likely to be compliant if they understand why they are taking a medication, and education allows them to make an informed decision.

Knowing the **right reason** for a medication being administered is an important right for the nurse to prevent medication errors. If the nurse understands the reason for a medication that is ordered, it will help in the identification of when to (hold) or not give a medication that may cause harm if administered.

10. **The right response**—This is a new right that is being considered by some facilities. This right applies to making certain the medication has the effect intended and includes monitoring the client and documenting. For example, if a sleep medication is ordered, is the client able to sleep?

According to *Fundamentals of Nursing* (Potter, Perry, Stockert, Hall, 2013), in accordance with The Patient Care Partnership (American Hospital Association, 2003) and because of the potential risks related to medication administration, a patient has the following rights: to refuse a medication regardless of the consequences; to not receive unnecessary medications; to have qualified nurses or physicians assess a medication history, including allergies and use of herbs; and to receive labeled medications safely without discomfort in accordance with the six rights of medication administration.

In addition to some specific mandates mentioned by The Joint Commission to ensure client safety and prevent the occurrence of medication errors, another National Patient Safety Goal focused on medications that clients may be taking, including herbals, vitamins, and nonprescription products. Patients and families may not accurately report all their medications and dosages, as well as home remedies. This can lead to errors in medication administration and adverse effects. Nurses need to get a thorough history of medications being taken by a client to prevent medication interactions that may be fatal to the client.

According to *Fundamentals of Nursing* (Potter, Perry, Stockert, Hall, 2013), there are six rights for safe medication administration, which include the right to a complete and clearly written order; the right to have access to information; and the right to stop, think, and be vigilant when administering medications.

Medication Reconciliation

According to Michael Cohen in the book titled *Medication Errors* (2010), "Poor communication about medications at transition points—admission, transfer, and discharge—is responsible for up to 50% of all medication errors and 20% of adverse drug events in the hospital." In response to this, TJC has focused on medication reconciliation as a National Patient Safety Goal to reduce the risk of errors during transition points. This National Patient Safety Goal requires hospitals to reconcile medications across the continuum of care. Medication reconciliation is a requirement for ambulatory care, assisted living, behavioral health, home care, and long-term organizations. Medication reconciliation is to be applied in any setting or service where medications are to be used or the client's response to treatment or service could be affected by medications that the client has been taking.

In the context of the goal, reconciliation is the process of comparing the medications that the client/patient/resident has been taking before the time of admission or entry into a new setting with the medications that the organization is about to provide. The purpose of the reconciliation is to avoid errors of transcription, omission, duplication of therapy, or drug-drug and drug-disease interactions.

Medication reconciliation is an important step in the prevention of medication errors and can assist in obtaining accurate medication histories and ensure continuity of appropriate therapy. This process should begin on admission; discharge orders should be compared and reconciled with the most recent inpatient medication orders and the original list of medications taken at home. Nurses can play a major role in the reconciliation process. This must become an important focus to prevent errors and misunderstanding regarding medications that a client may be taking, especially when discharged. Ensuring client knowledge regarding prehospital medications and posthospital medications may be a step in preventing errors and medication interactions. For additional information about medication reconciliation, refer to TJC's National Patient Safety Goals (http://www.jointcommission.org)

Client Education

One of the most important nursing functions is educating the client. Educating clients about their medications is imperative in preventing errors and improving the quality of health care. Educating clients regarding medications plays a role in preventing adverse reactions and achieving adherence to prescribed therapy; taking the correct dosage of the right medication at the right time helps prevent problems with medication administration. Remember that clients cannot be expected to follow a medication regimen—taking the correct dosage of the right medication at the right time—if they have not been taught. Not knowing what to do results in noncompliance, inaccurate dosages, and other problems. Nurses are in a unique position to teach clients, and this has been a traditional activity of nursing practice. Education should begin in the hospital and be a major part of discharge planning because, once discharged, clients need to have been educated about their medications to continue taking them safely and correctly at home. With today's emphasis on outpatient treatment and early discharge, thorough client education regarding medications is necessary.

When the nurse is teaching a client, it is important to thoroughly assess the needs of the client. Determine what the client knows about the medication prescribed; how to take the medication; and the frequency, time, and dosage. Identify the client's learning needs, including literacy level and language most easily and clearly understood. Identify relevant ethnic, cultural, and socioeconomic factors that may influence medication use; consider factors such as age and physical capabilities. A variety of teaching strategies may have to be used to facilitate and enhance learning. Return demonstrations on proper use of medication equipment and reading dosages, in addition to repeated instructions and directions, may be necessary, especially regarding management at home.

What a client needs to know about a medication varies with the medication. There may be numerous pieces of information clients should learn regarding their medications. The items discussed here relate particularly to dosage administration. To ensure that the client takes the right medication in the right dosage, by the right route at the right time, client education should include the following:

- Both the brand and generic names of the medication or medications being taken
- Clear explanation of the amount of the medication to be taken (e.g., one tablet or 1/2 tablet)
- Clear explanation of when to take the medication (Prepare a chart created with the client's lifestyle in mind. For example, if the medication is to be taken with meals, perhaps the chart can indicate the client's mealtime and the medication scheduled accordingly.)
- Clear demonstration of measuring oral dosages, such as liquids (encourage the use of appropriate measuring devices.)
- Clear explanation of the route of administration (e.g., place under tongue)

In addition to teaching clients about prescription medications they are taking, it is imperative that nurses question clients about any other over-the-counter medications they might be taking at home, including herbal medications. Some herbal medications might interact with medications they are taking (e.g., ephedra can accelerate heart rate, ginkgo and garlic may inhibit blood clotting). Nurses must be alert to any factors that may interfere with client safety.

Though nurses cannot ensure that clients will act on or retain everything they are taught, nurses are responsible for providing information to the client that will prevent error-prone situations and enable safe medication administration. Nurses evaluate retention by providing follow-up, and, if necessary, finding alternative ways of dealing with a client who has a "no way" attitude.

Home Care Considerations

Home health nursing has become a large part of the health care delivery system and continues to grow. This is due to factors such as the promotion of cost-effective health care and early discharge. Home care nursing may involve many activities, such as providing treatments, dressing changes, hospice care, client/family teaching, and medication administration. Medication administration involves administration of medications in various ways (e.g., IV, p.o., injection). The increased movement of nursing into the home of the client, which is not a controlled setting, has some important nursing implications. Home health nursing increases the autonomy of practice. The nurse must conduct a thorough assessment, communicate effectively, problem solve, and use expert critical thinking skills. Thinking must be rational, reasonable, and based on knowledge.

The principles regarding medication administration are the same as in a structured setting (e.g., hospital, acute care facility, nursing home). The six basic rights are still guidelines for the nurse to follow to ensure safe administration. It is imperative that the client be well educated about safe administration. Depending on the client's condition, home nursing services may be provided on a scheduled or intermittent basis to monitor the status of a client. Not all clients have a health aide, family member, or continuous nursing services in the home (around the clock). It is essential that the nurse calculate medication administration in a systematic, organized manner and adhere to the six rights of medication administration. The sixth right—documentation—is essential everywhere, including home health care. Documentation of medications is not just for legal purposes; it plays a significant role in cost reimbursement and payments. Correct interpretation of medication orders and validation are imperative. Proper education of the client concerning the medication, dosage, and route of administration is crucial in order for the client to manage in the home environment. Some may look at it as "the client being totally at your mercy." Clients depend on the nurse to provide direction for them to ensure safe home administration. The nurse must be able to teach the client to use appropriate measuring devices for measuring prescribed dosages and determining the accuracy of the dosage. When possible, encourage clients to use devices that are readily available in many pharmacies, such as calibrated oral syringes or plastic cups with measurements. Use of these devices can help prevent errors that often occur when clients measure their medication with household utensils. (As discussed in the chapters on systems of measure, the nurse must be able to convert dosages among the various systems.) The nurse providing services to the client in the home must be innovative and knowledgeable and demonstrate excellent critical thinking skills. Open communication with the client is essential. It is crucial to know what clients are taking and how. Remember that clients have to be taught. They may not know that they cannot resume previously taken medications or herbal remedies.

The Nurse's Role in Medication Error Prevention

In addition to the consistent use of the basic six rights of medication administration, nurses are essential to reducing medication errors and improving client outcomes. An effective way to reduce medication errors as identified in a report by the Institute of Medicine (IOM), *Preventing Medication Errors*, is a partnership between clients and their health care providers. Emphasis was placed on open communication between nurses and clients which not only included talking to clients but also listening. In response to this, TJC launched a Speak Up™ campaign that urged clients to take an active role in preventing errors by becoming more active in their care. When administering medications, client questions should be encouraged, and the nurse should be prepared to answer them. According to Cohen (2010),

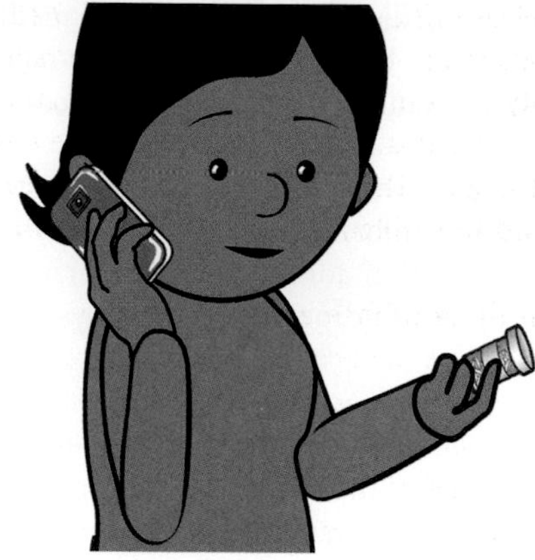
Julie says:
"Read the label on your medicine to make sure it's yours. If something doesn't seem right or if you don't understand, Speak Up!"
Watch the Speak Up™ videos online at www.jointcommission.org/speakup.
The Joint Commission

Figure 10-2 Sample of Speak Up Poster. (Copyright © The Joint Commission, 2013.)

"Patients should be encouraged to ask questions about their medications and seek satisfactory answers. Many errors have been prevented by observant and informed patients and their families." By way of brochures and posters displayed in health care facilities, clients are encouraged to use strategies to avoid medication mistakes. These include tips such as check your medications; ask questions; and make sure your doctors, nurses, and other caregivers check your wristband and ask your name before giving you medicine (Figure 10-2).

Nurses can reduce errors by making more use of information technologies when administering medications. Using reference information provided by a reliable source or downloaded content on personal digital assistants (PDAs), Smartphones, or iPads will enhance the nurse's ability to apply critical thinking when making judgments related to medication administration. With the increasing technology in health care, nurses must be able to identify safety risks and prevent adverse events when using it.

When medication errors occur, they should be reported following the organization's procedure for reporting. Nurses need to utilize information sources that provide vital information related to medication errors and preventing their occurrence (e.g., ISMP, TJC). Decreasing errors and preventing them requires the nurse to adhere to safety standards prescribed by organizations such as TJC and ISMP.

The prevention of medication errors, the use of technology in prevention, and the education of nurses with an emphasis on maintaining the safety of the client coincide with the Quality and Safe Education for Nurses (QSEN) goal to improve the quality and safety of client care. Medication administration and strategies to prevent errors (e.g., consistent use of the six basic rights, analyzing the causes of medication errors, discouraging the use of unsafe abbreviations, and the benefits of safety enhancing technologies such as barcoding) can be placed under competency 5, which is Safety.

Routes of Medication Administration

Route refers to how a medication is administered. Medications come in several forms for administration.

Oral (p.o.). Oral medication is administered by mouth (e.g., tablets, capsules, caplets, liquid solutions).

Sublingual (SL). Sublingual medications are placed under the tongue and designed to be readily absorbed through the blood vessels in this area. They should not be swallowed. Nitroglycerin is an example of a medication commonly administered by the sublingual route.

Sustained-release (SR), extended-release (XL), or delayed-release (DR) tablets or capsules release medication into the bloodstream over a period of time at specific intervals. Therefore, these forms of medication should not be opened, chewed or crushed.

Enteric-Coated Tablets/Capsules. Enteric-coated medications are covered with a special coating that does not dissolve in the stomach. The coating dissolves in the small intestine. This prevents gastrointestinal upset, and the tablet/capsule should be taken whole, never crushed.

Buccal. Buccal tablets are placed in the mouth against the mucous membranes of the cheek where the medication will dissolve. The medication is absorbed from the blood vessels of the cheek. Clients should be instructed not to chew or swallow the medication and not to take any liquids with it. Medications administered by the oral route will be discussed in more detail in Chapter 17, Calculation of Oral Medications.

Parenteral. Parenteral medications are administered by a route other than by mouth or gastrointestinal tract. Parenteral routes include intravenous (IV), intramuscular (IM), subcutaneous (subcut), and intradermal (ID). Parenteral routes will be discussed in more detail in Chapter 18, Parenteral Medications.

Insertion. Medication is placed into a body cavity, where the medication dissolves at body temperature (e.g., suppositories). Vaginal medications, creams, and tablets may also be inserted by using special applicators provided by the manufacturer.

Instillation. Medication is introduced in liquid form into a body cavity. It can also include placing an ointment into a body cavity, such as erythromycin eye ointment, which is placed in the conjunctiva of the eye. Nose drops and ear drops are also instillation medications.

Inhalation. Medication is administered into the respiratory tract, for example, through nebulizers used by clients for asthma. Bronchodilators and corticosteroids may be administered by inhalation through the mouth using an aerosolized, pressurized metered-dose inhaler (MDI). In some institutions, these medications are administered to the client with special equipment, such as positive pressure breathing equipment or the aerosol mask. Other medications in inhalation form include pentamidine, which is used to treat *Pneumocystis jiroveci*, a type of pneumonia found in clients with acquired immunodeficiency syndrome (AIDS). Devices such as "spacers" or "extenders" have been designed for use with inhalers to allow all of the metered dose to be inhaled, particularly in clients who have difficulty using inhalers.

Intranasal. A medicated solution is instilled into the nostrils. This method is used to administer corticosteroids, the antidiuretic hormone vasopressin, and a nasal mist influenza vaccine.

Topical. The medication is applied to the external surface of the skin. It can be in the form of lotion, ointment, or paste.

Percutaneous. Medications are applied to the skin or mucous membranes for absorption. This includes ointments, powders, and lotions for the skin; instillation of solutions onto the mucous membranes of the mouth, ear, nose, or vagina; and inhalation of aerosolized liquids for absorption through the lungs. The primary advantage is that the action of the drug, in general, is localized to the site of application.

Transdermal. Transdermal medication, which is becoming more popular, is contained in a patch or disk and applied topically. The medication is slowly released and absorbed through the skin and enters the systemic circulation. These topical applications may be applied for 24 hours or for as long as 7 days and have systemic effects. Examples include nitroglycerin for chest pain, nicotine transdermal (Nicoderm) for smoking cessation, clonidine for hypertension, fentanyl (Duragesic) for chronic pain, and birth control patches.

Forms of oral medications (tablets, capsules), oral solutions, and routes for parenteral medications are discussed in more detail in later chapters.

Some medications are supplied in multiple forms and therefore can be administered by a variety of routes. For example, Phenergan (promethazine hydrochloride) is supplied as a tablet, syrup, suppository, and solution for injection.

Equipment Used for Medication Administration

Medicine Cup. Equipment used for oral administration includes a 30-mL or 1-oz medication cup made of plastic, used to measure most liquid medications. The cup has measurements in all three systems of measure (Figure 10-3). By looking at the medicine cup, you can see that 30 mL = 1 oz, 5 mL = 1 tsp, and so forth. Remember that any volume less than 1 tsp (5 mL) should be measured with a more accurate device, such as an oral syringe, dropper, or calibrated spoon.

Although the medicine cup is commonly used for administering liquid medications, National Alert Network (NAN), in an article dated June 30, 2015, cited a fatal error reported to ISMP National Medication Errors Reporting Program in which there was confusion of two dosing scales on an oral liquid dosing cup. The cup had drams on it, and the nurse confused it with mL, resulting in a client receiving an overdose of morphine. According to the article, many facilities still use medicine cups that have measures such as drams, as well as household measures. To avoid dosing errors, the recommendations included that health care institutions purchase cups that have printed, rather than embossed, measurements so they are easier to read, and ideally the measuring cups should be printed with milliliters (mL) only. To avoid confusion with different measurement systems, organizations such as the American Academy of Pediatrics (AAP), the Institute for Safe Medication Practices (ISMP), and the Centers for Disease Control and Prevention (CDC) have called for adoption of the metric system (mL) as the standard for prescribing and measuring doses of liquid medications.

Soufflé Cup. A soufflé cup is a small paper or translucent plastic cup used for solid forms of medication, such as tablets and capsules (Figure 10-4).

Calibrated Dropper. A calibrated dropper may be used to administer small amounts of medication to an adult or child (Figure 10-5). The calibrations are usually in milliliters but can be in drops. Droppers are also used to dispense eye, nose, and ear medications in a squeeze drop bottle and designed for that purpose. The amount of the drop, abbreviated gtt, and size vary according to the diameter of the opening at the tip of the dropper. For this reason, it is important to remember that droppers should not be used as a medication measure unless they are calibrated. Also, because of variation, a properly calibrated dropper is often packaged with the medication (see Figure 10-5) and calibrated for the specified dose. Examples include children's vitamins; nystatin oral solution; furosemide oral solution; and OxyFast (oxycodone hydrochloride), a highly concentrated solution, which is a narcotic analgesic (Figure 10-6). The calibration allows for accurate dosing. Use the calibrated dropper only with the medicine for which it is designed or packaged with.

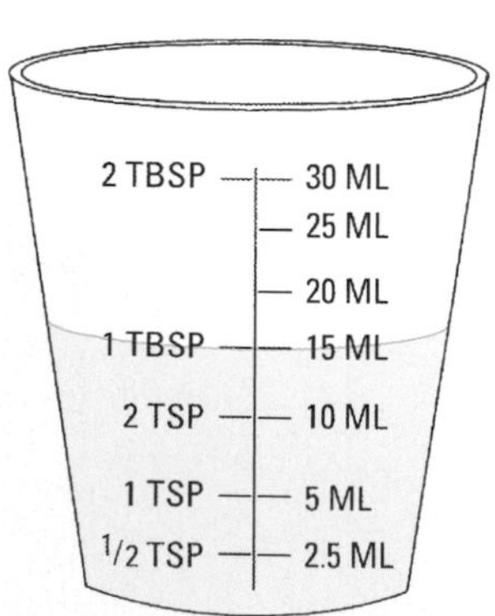

Figure 10-3 Medicine cup. (Modified from Mulholland JM and Turner SJ: *The nurse, the math, the meds: drug calculations using dimensional analysis,* ed 3, St Louis, 2015, Mosby.)

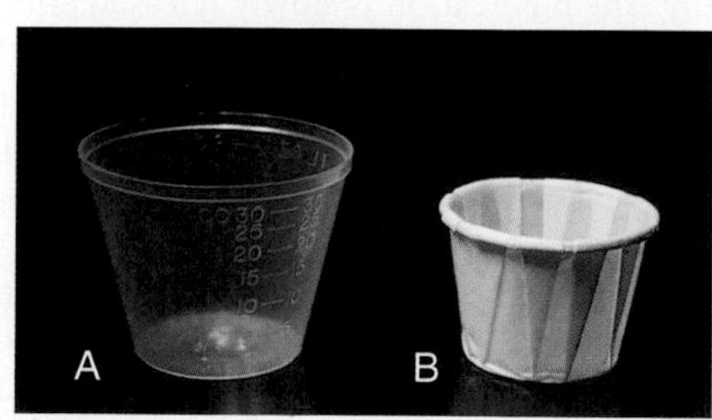

Figure 10-4 **A,** Plastic medicine cup. **B,** Soufflé cup. (Courtesy of Chuck Dresner. From Clayton BD, Willihnganz M: *Basic pharmacology for nurses,* ed 17, St Louis, 2017, Mosby.)

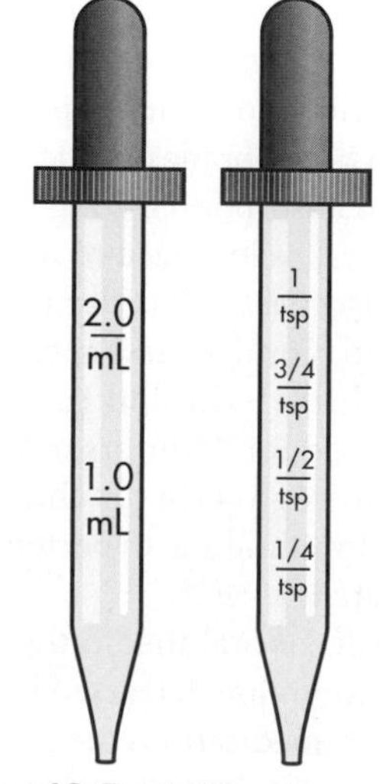

Figure 10-5 Medicine droppers.

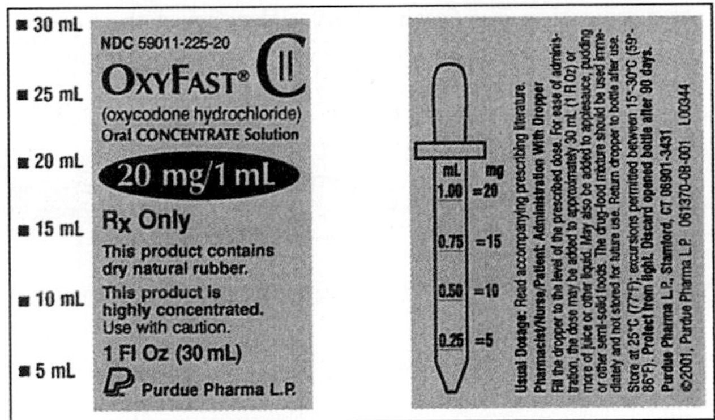

Figure 10-6 OxyFast label.

CRITICAL THINKING

BE SAFE. THINK: Drops from a dropper with a large opening provide more medication than drops from a smaller opening.

SAFETY ALERT!

Droppers are accurate when used to measure the specific medication they are calibrated to, not for measuring other medications. Do not interchange droppers that are packaged with medications. Using a dropper for the wrong medication could result in a serious medication error.

Nipple. An infant feeding nipple with additional holes may be used for administering oral medications to infants (Figure 10-7).

Oral Syringe. An oral syringe may be used to administer liquid medications orally to adults and children. No needle is attached (Figure 10-8).

Parenteral Syringe. A parenteral syringe is used for IM, subcut, ID, and IV medications. These syringes come in various sizes and are marked in milliliters or units. The specific types of syringes are discussed in more detail in Chapter 18. The barrel of the syringe holds the medication and has calibrations on it. The needle is attached to the tip. The

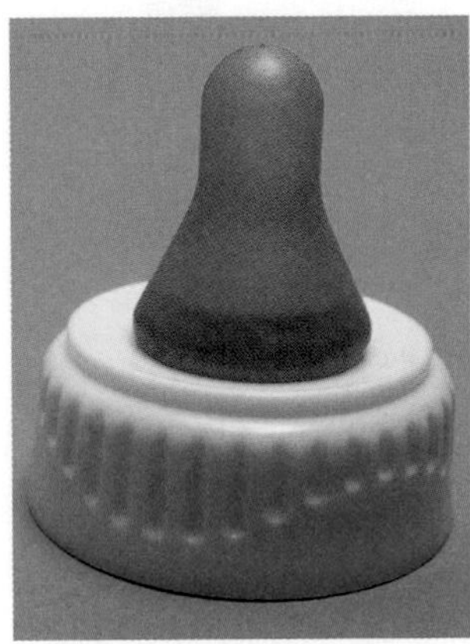

Figure 10-7 Nipple. (Modified from Clayton BD, Willihnganz M: *Basic pharmacology for nurses,* ed 17, St Louis, 2017, Mosby.)

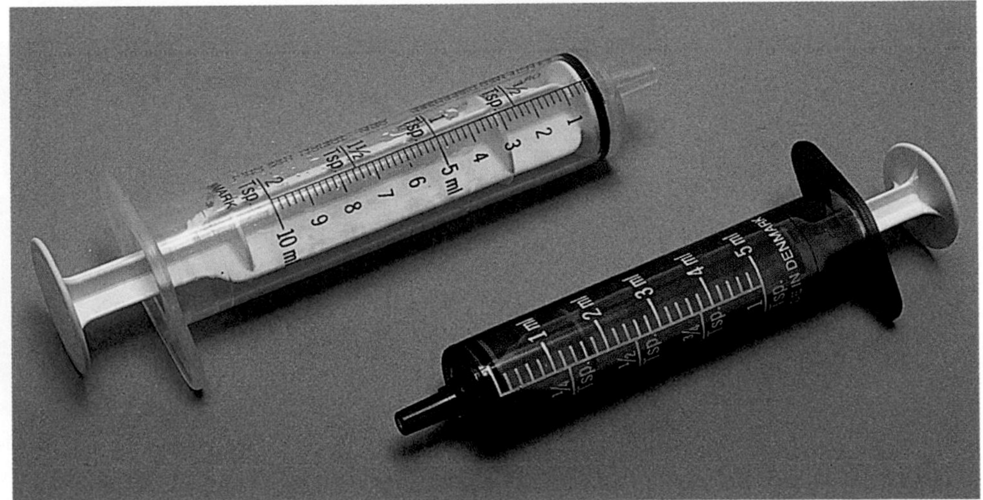

Figure 10-8 Oral syringes. (Courtesy of Chuck Dresner. From Clayton BD, Willihnganz M: *Basic pharmacology for nurses,* ed 17, St Louis, 2017, Mosby.)

plunger pushes the medication out (Figure 10-9). The size of the needle depends on how the medication is given (e.g., subcut or IM), the viscosity of the medication, and the size of the client. See Figure 10-10 for samples of the types of syringes.

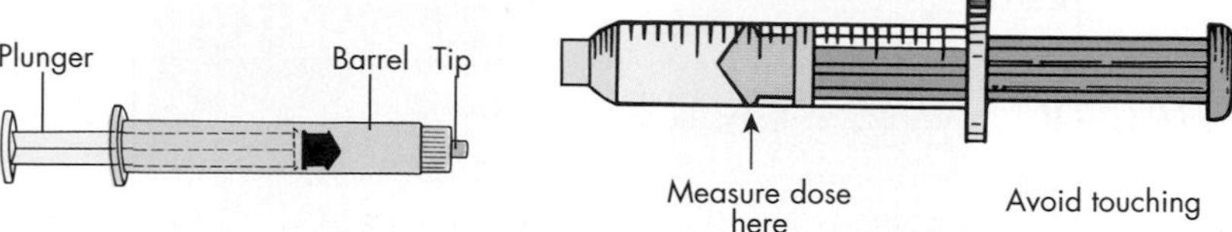

Figure 10-9 Parts of a syringe. (From Potter PA, Perry AG, Stockert P, Hall A: *Fundamentals of nursing,* ed 9, St Louis, 2016, Mosby.)

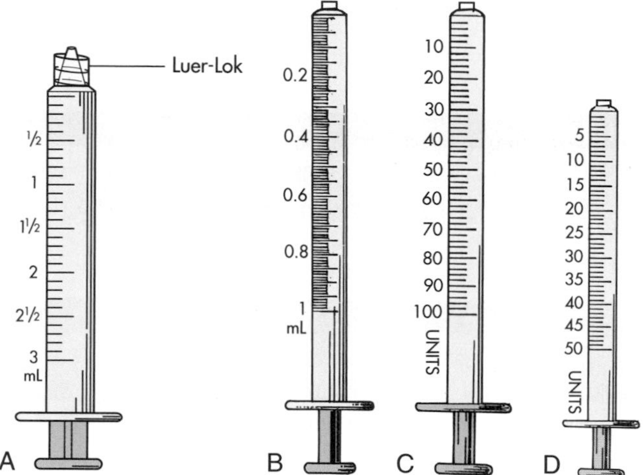

Figure 10-10 Types of syringes. **A,** Luer-Lok syringe marked in 0.1 (tenths). **B,** Tuberculin syringe marked in 0.01 (hundredths) for dosages of less than 1 mL. **C,** Insulin syringe marked in units (100). **D,** Lo-Dose Insulin syringe marked in units (50). (From Potter PA, Perry AG, Stockert P, Hall A: *Fundamentals of nursing,* ed 9, St Louis, 2016, Mosby.)

Equipment for Administering Oral Medications to a Child

Various types of calibrated equipment are on the market for administering medications to children. Most of the available equipment is for oral use. Caregivers should be instructed to always use calibrated measuring devices that are appropriate for measuring prescribed dosages when administering medications to a child. Household spoons vary in size and are not reliable devices for accurate dosing. Figure 10-11 presents samples of equipment used to administer oral medications to a child.

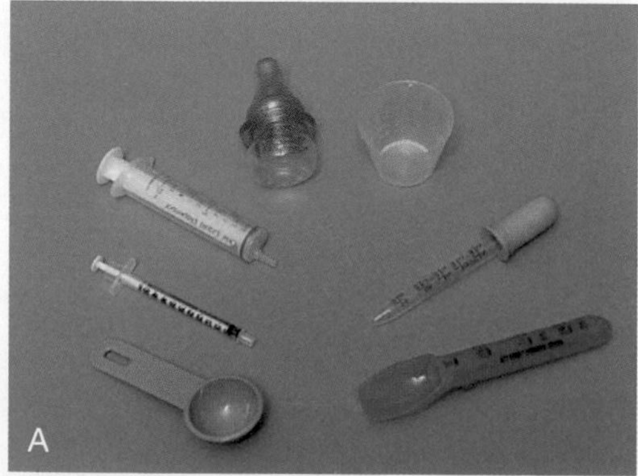

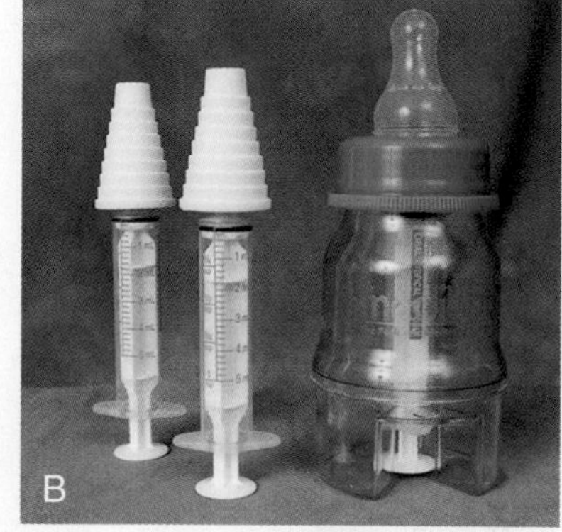

Figure 10-11 **A,** Acceptable devices for measuring and administering oral medication to children *(clockwise)*: measuring spoon, plastic syringes, calibrated nipple, plastic medicine cup, calibrated dropper, hollow-handled medicine spoon. **B,** Medibottle used to deliver oral medication via a syringe. (**A,** From Hockenberry MJ, Wilson D: *Wong's nursing care of infants and children,* ed 9, St Louis, 2011, Mosby. **B,** Courtesy Paul Vincent Kuntz, Texas Children's Hospital, Houston.)

SAFETY ALERT!

Remember, to prevent errors in medication administration, the device or equipment you use must be calibrated for the dose you need to administer in order to accurately measure the dose.

PRACTICE PROBLEMS

Answer the following questions by filling in the correct word or words to complete the sentence.

1. A dose for oral use that is less than 5 mL should not be measured in a

 ______________________.

2. The ______________________ and ______________________ need special considerations regarding medication dosages.

3. ______________________ refers to the way in which a medication is administered.

4. Children and the elderly usually require ______________________ dosages.

5. A ______________________ cup is used for dispensing solid forms of medication.

6. Application of medication to the external surface of the skin is referred to as the

 ______________________ route.

7. Medication administration is a process that requires critical thinking and the nursing process, which includes:

 a. ______________________ d. ______________________

 b. ______________________ e. ______________________

 c. ______________________

8. Being an autonomous thinker is an example of ______________________.

9. ______________________ droppers should be used for medication administration.

10. When medications are placed next to the cheek, they are administered by the

 ______________________ route.

Answers on p. 148

POINTS TO REMEMBER

- The basic six rights of medication administration serve as guidelines for nurses when administering medications (the right client, the right medication, the right dose, the right route, the right time, and the right documentation). Additional rights include the right indication, the right to know, the right to refuse, and the right response.
- Medication administration includes using critical thinking and the nursing process.
- There are numerous reasons for medication errors.
- Medication errors can harm clients physically and economically and can be fatal.
- Nurses are accountable for medications administered regardless of the reason for the error.

(continued)

- Nurses are responsible for ensuring the client's safety when administering medications. This includes ensuring that clients receive the right medication, the right dosage, by the right route, at the right time, with the right documentation.
- Nurses can play a major role in the medication reconciliation process.
- Nurses play a critical role in the prevention of medication errors.
- Talking to clients and listening to them can prevent errors. Encourage client questions.
- Know the policy of the institution regarding timely administration of medications.
- QSEN (The Quality and Safety Education for Nurses) goal is to improve the quality and safety of client care.
- Technology to prevent errors and medication safety is relevant to the QSEN safety competency and informatics.
- The elderly and children require special considerations with medication administration.
- Home health nursing increases the autonomy of nursing practice.
- A calibrated dropper should be used when administering medications with a dropper.
- Dosages less than 1 teaspoon should be measured with a device such as an oral syringe, dropper, or calibrated spoon.
- A medication cup has the capacity of 30 mL. A soufflé cup is used to dispense solid forms of medications.
- Medications are administered by various routes.

CHAPTER REVIEW

1. Name the six basic rights of medication administration

   Right ____________ Right ____________

   Right ____________ Right ____________

   Right ____________ Right ____________

2. The Joint Commission requires that clients be identified using ____________ client identifiers, neither of which can be the ____________.

3. A medication label should be read ____________ times.

4. Medications should be charted ____________ you have administered them.

5. Name three routes of medication administration. ____________

   ____

6. The medicine cup has a (an) ____________ capacity.

7. Droppers are calibrated to administer standardized drops regardless of what type of dropper is used. True or False? ____________

8. The syringe used to administer a dosage by mouth is referred to as a (an) ____________.

9. Volume on a syringe is indicated in ____________.

10. The medicine cup indicates that 2 tablespoons are approximately ____________ mL.

11. The ______________________ ______________________ lists medications that should be avoided in elderly clients.

12. ISMP is an abbreviation for ____.

13. TJC is an abbreviation for ____.

14. The route by which medicated solutions are instilled into the nostrils is __________.

15. Examples of medications that have been identified as high-alert medications are

    potassium chloride, ________________________, ________________________,

    and ________________________.

16. QSEN is an abbreviation for ________________________.

17. True or False. Medication calculations that are incorrect are an example of a

    medication error. ________________________.

18. True or False. Safe medication administration is the responsibility of only the nurse.

    ____

19. True or False. A nurse does not have to establish the identity of a client they know well. ________________________

20. True or False. Clients do not have the right to refuse medications. ______________

For questions 21-25, read the statements carefully and indicate which right of medication administration has been violated.

21. The medication label indicated for optic use, and the medication was instilled into

    the client's ears. The right ________________________.

22. The prescriber ordered Glipizide and the client received Glyburide. The right

    ________________________.

23. The nurse charted all her medications on the medication record before she

    administered them. The right ________________________.

24. The nurse administers a medication at 10 PM that was scheduled for 10 AM. The

    right ________________________.

25. The dosage to be administered was $1\frac{1}{2}$ tsp. The client received 15 mL. The right

    ________________________.

For questions 26-27: Identify the right that is violated.

26. A client asks why she is receiving a medication. The nurse knows why, does not tell the client, and administers the medication. The right ________________________

27. A client with a history of low blood pressure (hypotension) has an order for an antihypertensive medication. The right ____________________

28. According to the report, *Preventing Medication Errors*, by the Institute of Medicine, a strategy to effectively reduce errors is a partnership between ______________.

29. When a nurse is unfamiliar with a medication that has been ordered, the nurse should consult a ____________________.

30. SREs is an abbreviation for____________________________, which are endorsed by NQF. NQF is an abbreviation for__________________________.

Answers below

ANSWERS

Chapter 10

Answers to Practice Problems

1. medicine cup
2. elderly and children
3. route
4. smaller
5. souffle
6. topical
7. assessment, nursing diagnosis/nursing problem, planning, implementation, evaluation
8. critical thinking
9. calibrated
10. buccal

Answers to Chapter Review

1. medication, dosage, client, route, time, documentation
2. two unique, client's (patient's) room number
3. three
4. after
5. parenteral, oral, inhalation, insertion, topical, percutaneous, intranasal, instillation, sublingual, buccal, transdermal
6. 30 mL or 1 oz
7. False
8. oral syringe
9. milliliters (mL)
10. 30 mL
11. Beers criteria
12. Institute for Safe Medication Practices
13. The Joint Commission
14. intranasal
15. heparin, insulin, morphine, neuromuscular medications, chemotherapy medications
16. Quality and Safety Education for Nurses
17. True
18. False
19. False
20. False
21. Route
22. Medication
23. Documentation
24. Time
25. Dosage
26. Right to know
27. Right indication or right reason
28. Client/patient and health care provider
29. Reputable drug reference
30. Serious Reportable Events, National Quality Forum

CHAPTER 11
Understanding and Interpreting Medication Orders

Objectives

After reviewing this chapter, you should be able to:

1. Identify the components of a medication order
2. Identify the meanings of standard abbreviations used in medication administration
3. Interpret a given medication order
4. Identify abbreviations, acronyms, and symbols recommended by TJC's "Do Not Use" List and ISMP's List of Error-Prone Abbreviations, Symbols, and Dose Designations
5. Read and write correct medical notations

Before a nurse can administer any medication, there must be a written legal order for it. Medication orders can be written by physicians, dentists, physician's assistants, nurse midwives, or nurse practitioners, depending on state law. Health care providers use medication orders to convey the therapeutic plan for a client, which includes medications.

In the acute care setting, there are different types of medication orders that can be written:

- **Standing order.** Sometimes referred to as a routine order, a standing order may be written to indicate a medication is to be given for a specified number of doses. For example, ampicillin 1 g IV q6h for 4 doses. A standing order can also indicate that a medication should be administered until it is discontinued or is replaced by another order. For example, Colace 100 mg po tid. Most health care facilities have policies relating to automatic cancellation of an order after a certain time period. For example, 72 hours for narcotics; 30 days for standing orders.
- **prn order.** This order is administered as needed. This type of order allows for the nurse to exercise her judgment on when a medication should be administered based on the client's needs. For example, Tylenol 650 mg po q4h prn for temperature greater than 101° F.
- **Stat order.** This means a medication is to be given immediately but only once unless it is re-ordered. For example, Ativan 2 mg IM stat.
- **Single (one-time) order.** This order specifies a medication to be given only once at a specified time. For example, Demerol 50 mg IM and atropine 0.4 mg IM on call to the operating room.

Medication orders are written as prescriptions in private practice or in clinics. The medication the health care provider is ordering in these settings is written on a prescription form that usually comes as a pad and is filled by a pharmacist at a drug store (pharmacy) or the hospital. Medication orders are used by health care providers to communicate to the nurse or designated health care worker which medication or medications to administer to a client. Medication orders can be oral or written.

Regardless of the mechanism used for a medication order, the nurse has responsibilities relating to the order to ensure safe administration. The nursing responsibilities include interpreting the order, selecting the correct medication and dosage, administering the medication by the correct route at the right time to the right client, educating the client regarding the medication, monitoring the client's response to the medication, and documenting the medication administered. **Although the nurse is not the originator of the**

medication order, it is important to remember the nurse is the point person before the client receives the medication ordered. If a calculation or double check of an order is not done, the nurse who administers the medication shares the liability for the injury, even if the order was incorrect, and is responsible for the medication error.

Verbal Orders

Usually, medication orders must be written and signed by the prescribing practitioner or directly entered into the computer by the prescriber. Verbal orders are discouraged as a routine policy. However, certain situations or emergencies may require a verbal order that is stated directly in person or by telephone from a licensed physician or another qualified practitioner who is licensed to prescribe. In most health care institutions, the nurse or other authorized personnel can receive a verbal order. Such orders, however, are usually received by the nurse. Verbal orders can be particularly error prone for several reasons, including: the order being misheard, poor phone reception, sound-alike drug names, and the nurse assuming the intended order when the order given is incomplete.

Recognizing the errors that can occur with verbal orders and wanting to decrease the potential errors when an oral or telephone order is taken, The Joint Commission (TJC) requires that only "designated qualified staff" may accept verbal or telephone orders. TJC, which is the accrediting body for health care organizations and agencies, developed the National Patient Safety Goals (NPSGs), which are published annually, to address specific areas of concern in regards to client safety. NSPG 2 is designed to improve the effectiveness of communication among caregivers. TJC requires that the authorized individual receiving a verbal or telephone order first **write it down** in the patient's chart or enter it into the computer record; second, **read it back** to the prescriber; and then third, **receive confirmation** from the prescriber who gave the order that it is correct. For the nurse to only repeat back the order is not sufficient to prevent errors and is not allowed by TJC. Any questions or concerns relating to the order should be clarified with the prescriber during the conversation. A verbal order must contain the same elements as a written order and be accurate: the date of the order, name and dosage of the medication, route, frequency, any special instructions, and the name of the individual giving the order. TJC advises that in emergency situations, such as a code, doing a formal "read-back" is not feasible, and a "repeat-back" is acceptable to avoid compromising client safety.

It must be noted that it was a verbal or telephone order, and the signature of the nurse taking the order is required. Many institutions require that the order must be signed by the prescriber within 24 hours. Some institutions may require that medication orders written by a person other than a physician be countersigned by designated personnel.

TIPS FOR CLINICAL PRACTICE

It is important to be familiar with specific policies regarding verbal or telephone medication orders and responsibilities in this regard because they vary according to the institution or health care facility.

SAFETY ALERT!

Acceptance of a verbal order is a major responsibility and can lead to medication errors. Accept a verbal order only in an emergency situation. If you accept a verbal order, follow the policy of TJC. Always clarify questions about the order during the conversation. If you are unsure of the medication or the spelling, spell it back to the prescriber and get confirmation. NEVER ASSUME.

The medication order indicates the treatment plan or medication the health care provider has ordered for a client. Depending on the institution, the medication order may be written on a sheet labeled "physician's order sheet" or "order sheet." After the medication order has been written, the nurse or, in some institutions, a trained unit clerk transcribes the order. This means the order is written on the medication administration record (MAR). In an instance in which the nurse does not transcribe the order, the nurse is accountable for what is written and for verifying the order, initialing it, and checking it before administering.

At some institutions, computers are used for processing medication orders. Medication orders are either electronically transmitted or manually entered directly into the computer from an order form. The use of the computer allows immediate transmission of the order to the pharmacy. The computerized medication record can be seen directly on the computer screen or on a printed copy. Medication orders done by computer entry allow the prescriber to make changes if indicated, and the orders are signed by the prescriber with an assigned electronic code. Once the medication is received on the unit, the medication order is implemented and the client receives the medication.

Computerized physician order entry (CPOE), according to Cohen (2010), "could prevent many problems that occur with written orders as well as clearly communicating medication orders, and avoiding dosing mistakes; it would also help in preventing serious drug interactions and monitoring and documenting adverse events and therapeutic outcomes." In addition, the authors of the 2006 Institute of Medicine (IOM) report *Preventing Medication Errors* call for all health care providers to have plans in place for CPOE by 2008, and by 2010, IOM recommends that all prescribers be using electronic prescribing and all pharmacies be capable of accepting electronic prescriptions (Cohen, 2010).

In some institutions fax (facsimile) transmission may be used to avoid telephone orders. Faxed orders, however, may not be clearly legible and can also cause errors in interpretation. Cohen (2010) recommends that faxed orders be reviewed carefully and that the pharmacy verify the order before dispensing the medication or wait for the original.

Despite the advent of technology, there are institutions that still have handwritten orders and nurses must be familiar with transcription of orders.

Transcription of Medication Orders

Incorrect transcription of medication orders is one of the main causes of medication errors. According to Cohen (2010), illegible handwriting is a widely recognized cause of errors.

Before transcribing an order or preparing a dosage, the nurse must be familiar with reading and interpreting an order. To interpret a medication order, the nurse must know the components of a medication order, and the standard abbreviations and symbols used in writing a medication order, as well as those abbreviations and symbols that should not be used. Knowledge of error-prone abbreviations, symbols, and dose designations and abbreviations that should not be used will prevent misinterpretation and errors with medication orders which can be fatal to the client (QSEN Competency 5—Safety). The nurse therefore must memorize the abbreviations and symbols commonly used in medication orders. The abbreviations include units of measure, route, and frequency for the medication ordered. The common abbreviations and symbols used in medication administration are listed in Tables 11-1 and 11-2 and must be committed to memory, along with abbreviations related to systems of measure. TJC's "Do Not Use" List is shown in Appendix C, and the Institute for Safe Medication Practices' (ISMP's) List of Error-Prone Abbreviations, Symbols, and Dose Designations are in Appendix D.

Cohen (2010) recommended that the arrows ↑,↓ (up and down) to indicate increase and decrease should not be used. These symbols can be confused for numbers and letters.

TIPS FOR CLINICAL PRACTICE

The use of abbreviations, acronyms, and symbols in the writing of medication orders can have safety implications, and certain abbreviations can mean more than one thing. Care must be taken to use only abbreviations, acronyms, and symbols that have been approved.

TABLE 11-1 Symbols and Abbreviations for Units of Measure Used in Medication Administration

Abbreviation/Symbol	Meaning	Abbreviation/Symbol	Meaning
c, C	cup	mg	milligram
g	gram	mL	milliliter
gtt	drop	oz	ounce
kg	kilogram	pt	pint
L	liter	qt	quart
mcg	microgram	T, tbs	tablespoon
mEq*	milliequivalent	t, tsp	teaspoon

*mEq (milliequivalent) is a drug measure in which electrolytes are measured; it expresses the ionic activity of a medication.

TABLE 11-2 Commonly Used Medication Abbreviations

Abbreviation	Meaning	Abbreviation	Meaning
$\bar{a}$	before	$\bar{p}$	after
aa, $\overline{aa}$	of each	p.c., pc	after meals
a.c., ac	before meals	per	through or by
ad lib.	as desired, freely	pm, PM	evening, before midnight
am, AM	morning before noon	p.o.	by mouth, oral
amp	ampule	p.r.	by rectum
aq	aqueous, water	p.r.n., prn	when necessary/ required, as needed
b.i.d., bid	twice a day	q.	every
b.i.w.	twice a week	q.a.m.	every morning
$\bar{c}$	with	q.h., qh	every hour
c, C	cup	q2h, q4h, q6h, q8h, q12h	every 2 hours, every 4 hours, every 6 hours, every 8 hours, every 12 hours
cap, caps	capsule	q.i.d., qid	four times a day
CD	controlled dose	q.s.	a sufficient amount/ as much as needed
CR	controlled release	rect	rectum
dil.	dilute	$\bar{s}$	without
DS	double strength	sl, SL	sublingual
EC	enteric coated	sol, soln	solution
elix.	elixir	s.o.s., SOS	may be repeated once if necessary
fl, fld.	fluid	SR	sustained release
GT	gastrostomy tube	S&S	swish and swallow
gtt	drop	stat, STAT	immediately, at once
h, hr	hour	subcut	subcutaneous
ID	intradermal	supp	suppository
IM	intramuscular	susp	suspension
IV	intravenous	syp, syr	syrup
IVPB	intravenous piggyback	tab	tablet
IVSS	intravenous Soluset	t.i.d., tid	three times a day
KVO	keep vein open (a very slow infusion rate)	tr., tinct	tincture
LA	long acting	ung., oint	ointment
LOS	length of stay	vag, v	vaginally
min	minute	XL	long acting
mix	mixture	XR	extended release
NAS	intranasal		
NG, NGT	nasogastric tube		
noc, noct	at night		
n.p.o., NPO	nothing by mouth		
NS, N/S	normal saline		

Note: Abbreviations may be written with or without the use of periods; this does not alter the meaning.

CLINICAL **REASONING**

It is important for you to concentrate on understanding what abbreviations or symbols mean in the context of the order.

Writing a Medication Order

The health care provider writes a medication order on a form called the *physician's order sheet.* Order sheets vary from institution to institution. The order sheet should have the client's name on it. A prescription blank is used to write medication orders for clients who are being discharged from the hospital or are seeing the health care provider in an outpatient facility. Nurses often have to explain these orders to clients so they understand the dosages and other relevant information relating to their medications to ensure safety.

Components of a Medication Order

When a medication order is written, it must contain the following seven important parts or it is considered invalid or incomplete: (1) client's full name, (2) date and time the order was written, (3) name of the medication, (4) dosage of the medication, (5) route of administration, (6) frequency of administration, and (7) signature of the person writing the order. These parts of the medication order are discussed in detail in the following sections.

SAFETY ALERT!

If any of the components of a medication order are missing, the order is not complete and not a legal medication order. When in doubt, clarify the order with the prescriber.

Client's Full Name. Using the client's full name helps prevent confusion between one client and another, thereby preventing administration of the wrong medication to a client. Many institutions use a nameplate to imprint the client's name and record number on the order sheet; in addition, there is usually a place to indicate allergies. In institutions that use computers, the computer screen may also show identifying information for the client, such as age and known medication allergies.

Date and Time the Order Was Written. The date and time of the order include the month, day, year, and the time the order was written. This will help in determining the start and stop of the medication order. A record of the time the order was written is preferred in many institutions, but omission does not invalidate the order. This same information is required in computer entry of medication orders. In many institutions, the health care provider (or person legally authorized to write a medication order) is required to include the length of time the medication is to be given (e.g., 7 days); or he or she may use the abbreviation LOS (length of stay), which means the client is to receive the medication during the entire stay in the hospital. Even when not written as part of the order, LOS is implied unless stated otherwise. The policy of indicating the length of time a medication is to be given varies from institution to institution. At some institutions, if there is no specified time period for particular medications, it is assumed to be continued until otherwise stopped by the health care provider or a protocol in place for certain medications, such as controlled substances (narcotics). Some medications have automatic stop times according to the facility (e.g., narcotics, certain antibiotics).

Name of the Medication. The medication may be ordered by the generic or brand name (Figures 11-1 and 11-2). To avoid confusion with another medication, the name of the medication should be written clearly and spelled correctly.

Trade name—The brand name or proprietary name is the name under which a manufacturer markets the medication. The brand or trade name is followed by the registration symbol, ®. The name either starts with a capital letter or is all in capital letters on the label. It is generally the largest printed information on the label. A medication may have several trade names, according to the manufacturer. It is important to note that some medications may not have trade names.

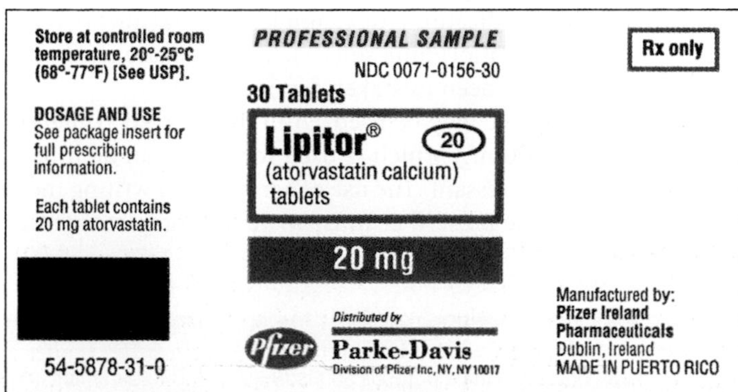

Figure 11-1 Lipitor label. Notice the two names. The first, *Lipitor,* is the trade name, identified by the registration symbol ®. The name in smaller and different print is *atorvastatin calcium,* the generic or official name.

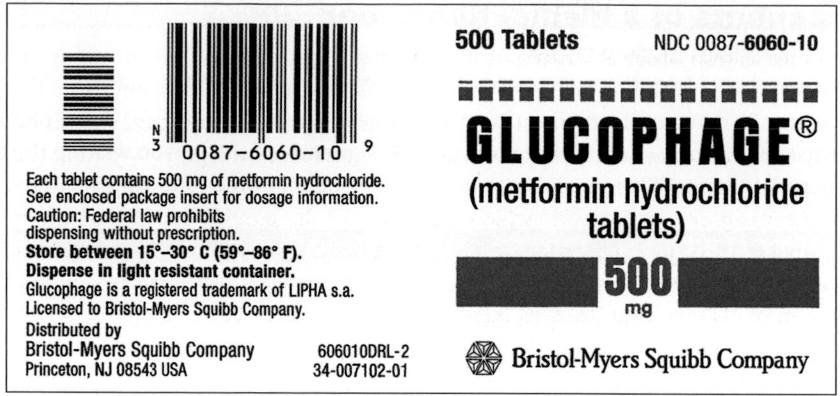

Figure 11-2 Glucophage label. Notice the two names. The first, *Glucophage,* is the trade name, identified by the registration symbol ®. The name in smaller and different print is *metformin hydrochloride*, the generic or official name.

Generic name—The proper name, chemical name, or nonproprietary name of the medication. It is a name given by the manufacturer that first created the medication. It is usually designated in lowercase letters or a different typeface. Sometimes the generic name is also placed in parentheses. The generic name is usually found under the brand or trade name. Occasionally, only the generic name will appear on the label. Each medication has only one generic name. A medication is licensed under its generic name. **By law, the generic name must appear on all medication labels.** The generic name is also registered with a national listing of medications: The United States Pharmacopeia (USP) and National Formulary (NF). This name is not specific to the manufacturer. Therefore, a medication label must indicate the generic name, and some labels may include a trade name. The prescriber may order medications using the generic name.

TIPS FOR CLINICAL PRACTICE

Nurses must be familiar with both the generic name and the trade name for a medication. To ensure correct medication identification, nurses should crosscheck trade and generic names as needed with a medication reference.

Checking the names of medications even when they are generic is essential in preventing errors. Some very different medications have similar generic names, such as pyridostigmine bromide (Mestinon), which is used to treat myasthenia gravis, and pyrimethamine (Daraprim), which is used to treat parasitic disorders, such as toxoplasmosis.

To ensure correct medication information, nurses should crosscheck trade and generic names as needed. When reading the name of a medication, never assume. Sometimes orders may be written with abbreviated medication names. This has been discouraged unless the abbreviation is common and approved. Some abbreviations used for medications can cause confusion with another medication; for example, $MgSO_4$ (intended use: magnesium sulfate) and MSO_4 (intended use: morphine sulfate). These two are cited on TJC's "Do Not Use" List because they have often been mistaken for each other.

For example, the acronym AZT may be used. "AZT 100 mg p.o." (intended medication order zidovudine [Retrovir], 100 mg, which is used for HIV) can be misread as azathioprine (Imuran), an immunosuppressant. The use of acronyms in writing medication orders is not recommended by TJC; the prescriber must write the complete medication name to avoid misinterpretation.

TIPS FOR CLINICAL PRACTICE

Nurses must be familiar with the names of medications (generic and trade). Many medications on the market have similar names and pronunciations but very different actions. Examples: Glyburide and Glipizide, Procardia and Procardia XL, Percocet and Percodan, quinine and quinidine.

SAFETY ALERT!

A case of mistaken identity with medications can have tragic results.

Dosage of the Medication. The amount and strength of the medication should be written clearly to avoid confusion. Dosage indicates the amount or weight provided in the form (e.g., per tablet, per milliliter).

To avoid misinterpretation, "U," which stands for units, should not be used when insulin, heparin, or any other medication order that uses units is written. The word *units* should be written out. This would also include "mU" (milliunits). Errors have occurred as a result of confusion of "U" with an "O" in a handwritten order. The abbreviation "U" for units is on TJC's Official "Do Not Use" List and on ISMP's List of Error-Prone Abbreviations, Symbols, and Dose Designations.

Example: 6U subcut stat of Humulin Regular Insulin. The U is almost completely closed and could be misread as 60 units. The *word units* should be written out. The handwritten letters "q.d.," when used in prescription writing, can be misinterpreted as "q.i.d." if the period is raised and the tail of the "q" interferes. Example: Lasix 40 mg qid.

Route of Administration. The route of administration is a very important part of a medication order because medications can be administered by several routes. Never assume that you know which route is appropriate. Standard and acceptable abbreviations should be used to indicate the route.

Examples: p.o. (oral, by mouth) IM (intramuscular)

ID (intradermal) IV (intravenous)

SAFETY ALERT!

Administering a medication by a route other than what the form indicates constitutes a medication error. Regardless of the source of an error, if you administer the wrong dosage, or give a medication by a route other than what it is intended for, you have made a medication error and are legally responsible for it.

Time and Frequency of Administration. Standard abbreviations should be used to indicate when and what times a medication is to be administered.

Examples: q.i.d. (four times a day), stat (immediately)

The time intervals at which a medication is administered are determined by the institution, and most health care facilities have routine times for administering medications.

Example: t.i.d. (three times a day) may be 9 AM, 1 PM, and 5 PM, or 10 AM, 2 PM, and 6 PM.

Factors such as the purpose of the medication, medication interactions, absorption of the medication, and side effects should be considered when medication times are scheduled. It is important to realize that when abbreviations such as b.i.d. and t.i.d. are used, the amount you calculate is for one dosage and not for the day's total. The frequency indicates the dosage (amount) of medication given at a single time.

Signature of the Person Writing the Order. For a medication order to be legal, it must be signed by the health care provider. The health care provider writing the order must include his or her signature on the order, and it should be legible. At some institutions, in addition to the signature of the physician or other person licensed to write orders, to ensure legibility the prescriber must stamp the order with a rubber stamp that has his or her name clearly printed on it after an order has been written. Orders that are done by computer entry require a signature created by using an assigned electronic code or electronic signature. In some institutions, depending on the rank of the physician or the person writing the order, an order may have to be co-signed by a senior physician.

Example: Residents or interns and persons other than a physician writing an order must secure the signature of an attending physician.

In addition to the seven required components of a medication order already discussed, any special instructions or parameters for certain medications need to be clearly written.

Examples:
1. Hold if blood pressure (BP) is below 100 systolic.
2. Administer a half-hour before meals ($\frac{1}{2}$ hour a.c.).

Medications ordered as needed or whenever necessary (p.r.n.) should indicate the purpose of administration as well. In addition, a frequency must be written to state the minimum time allowed between dosages. example q4h prn.

Examples:
1. For chest pain
2. Temperature above 101° F
3. For blood pressure (BP) greater than 140 systolic and 90 diastolic

In instances in which specific instructions are not stated, nursing judgment must be used to determine whether it is appropriate to administer a medication.

For dosage calculations, the nurse is usually concerned with the medication name, dosage of the medication, route, and time or frequency of administration. This information is necessary in determining a safe and reasonable dosage for a client.

SAFETY ALERT!

Never assume what an order states! Clarify an order when in doubt. If an order is not clear, or if essential components are omitted, it is not a legal order and should not be implemented. The nurse is accountable!

Interpreting a Medication Order

Medication orders should be written following a specific sequence:
1. Name of the medication
2. The dosage, expressed in standard abbreviations or symbols
3. Route
4. Frequency

Example:

Colace	100 mg	p.o.	t.i.d.
↓	↓	↓	↓
name of medication	dosage	route	frequency

This order means the prescriber wants the client to receive Colace (name of medication), which is a stool softener, 100 milligrams (dosage) by mouth (route), three times a day (frequency). The use of abbreviations in a medication order is a form of shorthand. For the purpose of interpreting orders, it is important for nurses to commit to memory common medical abbreviations as well as abbreviations related to the systems of measure. Refer to Tables 11-1 and 11-2 for medical abbreviations and symbols used in medication administration. Be systematic when interpreting the order to avoid an error. The medication order follows a specific sequence when it is written correctly (the name of the medication first, followed by the dosage, route, and frequency); interpret the order in this manner as well; avoid "scrambling the order."

Let's look at some medication orders for practice reading and interpreting.

Example 1: Buspar 15 mg po b.i.d.

This order means: Give Buspar 15 milligrams orally (by mouth) two times a day.

Example 2: Procaine Penicillin G 250,000 units IV q6h.

This order means: Give Procaine Penicillin G 250,000 units by intravenous injection every 6 hours.

Example 3: Motrin 400 mg po q6h prn for pain.

This order means: Give Motrin 400 milligrams orally (by mouth) every 6 hours whenever necessary (as required) for pain.

SAFETY ALERT!

p.r.n. must have a frequency that designates the minimum time allowed between doses.

Orders are transcribed in some institutions where unit dose (a system that uses single-unit packages of medications that are dispersed to fill each dose requirement) is used. In some institutions, more transcribing may be necessary because the MAR may have the capacity to be used for only a limited period (e.g., 3 days, 5 days). It is therefore necessary to transcribe orders again at the end of the designated period.

In facilities in which computers are used, the medication order is entered into the computer, and a printout lists the currently ordered medications. The computer is able to scan for information such as medication incompatibilities, safe dosage ranges, recommended administration times, and allergies; it can also indicate when a new order for a medication is required.

Computerized order entry and charting do not eliminate the nurse's responsibility for double-checking medication orders before administering. Nurses need to be aware of some of the problems that the use of certain abbreviations and acronyms has created. Use of certain abbreviations has created situations that can be harmful to clients and result in the potential for or actual error in medication administration. Recognize that use of certain abbreviations and symbols in medication orders can be misinterpreted and cause significant harm to clients.

As a result of increasing numbers of medication errors made due to misinterpretation of medical abbreviations, various organizations have identified a list of abbreviations, acronyms, and symbols to avoid because they are a common source of errors and can be easily misinterpreted. See TJC's official Do Not Use list in Appendix C. ISMP also published a list of error-prone abbreviations, symbols, and dose designations that includes TJC's "Do Not Use" List (Appendix D). ISMP has recommended that these abbreviations, symbols, and dose designations be strictly prohibited when communicating medical information, including medication orders.

For the safety of clients and to prevent errors in misinterpretation, prescribers responsible for writing medication orders ***must*** pay attention to what they write; it could save a life. In addition to knowing correct medication notations, those who administer medications must know the safe dosage and be able to recognize discrepancies in a dosage that can sometimes be caused by misinterpretation of an order.

SAFETY ALERT!

Acceptable abbreviations and medical notations are subject to change. Stay abreast of the guidelines and recommendations of TJC, ISMP, and your health care institution regarding acceptable abbreviations and medical notations.

When writing orders, prescribers should avoid nonstandard abbreviations and avoid abbreviations and symbols that have been identified as error prone. It is important to note that CPOE can still result in errors in medication orders. Therefore, all forms of communicating medical information, whether a written order or CPOE according to organizations which include ISMP, TJC, and the National Coordinating Council for Medication Error Reporting and Prevention (NCCMERP), should avoid the use of error prone abbreviations, symbols, and dose designations that have led to medication errors.

SAFETY ALERT!

The consequences of misinterpreting abbreviations, symbols, and dosages may be fatal.

POINTS TO REMEMBER

- A primary responsibility of the nurse is the safe administration of medications to a client.
- Interpret medication orders systematically, the way in which it is written (the name of the medication, the dosage, the route, and frequency).
- The seven components of a medication order are as follows:
  1. The full name of the client
  2. Date and time the order was written
  3. Name of the medication to be administered
  4. Dosage of the medication
  5. Route of administration
  6. Time or frequency of administration
  7. Signature of the person writing the order
- All medication orders must be legible, and standard abbreviations and symbols must be used.
- Memorize the meaning of common abbreviations and symbols.
- The nurse needs to be aware of acronyms, symbols, and abbreviations that should not be used. Their use can increase the potential for errors in medication administration.
- Oral (verbal) orders must be written down, read back to the prescriber, and confirmed with the prescriber that the order is correct.
- If any of the seven components of a medication order are missing or seem incorrect, the medication order is not legal. Do not assume—clarify the order!
- If you are in doubt as to the meaning of an order, clarify it with the prescriber before administering.
- Always crosscheck medications; misidentification can result in a medication error.

PRACTICE **PROBLEMS**

Interpret the following abbreviations.

1. p.c. ______________________
2. h ______________________
3. q12h ______________________
4. b.i.d. ______________________
5. p.r.n. ______________________

Interpret the following orders. Use either *administer* or *give* at the beginning of the sentence.

6. Zidovudine 200 mg p.o. q4h. ______________________

   ____

7. Procaine penicillin G 400,000 units IV q8h. ______________________

   ____

8. Gentamicin sulfate 45 mg IVPB q12h. ______________________

   ____

9. Regular Humulin insulin 5 units subcut, a.c. at 7:30 AM and at bedtime. __________

   ____

10. Vitamin B_{12} 1,000 mcg IM, every other day. ______________________

____

11. Prilosec 20 mg p.o. bid. ______________________

____

12. Tofranil 75 mg p.o. at bedtime. ______________________

____

13. Restoril 30 mg p.o. at bedtime. ______________________

____

14. Mylanta 30 mL p.o. q4h p.r.n. ______________________

____

15. Synthroid 200 mcg p.o. daily. ______________________

____

Answers on p. 162

CHAPTER REVIEW

List the seven components of a medication order.

1. ______________________
2. ______________________
3. ______________________
4. ______________________
5. ______________________
6. ______________________
7. ______________________

Write the meaning of the following abbreviations.

8. NAS ______________________
9. ad. lib. ______________________
10. subcut ______________________
11. c̄ ______________________
12. a.c. ______________________
13. q.i.d. ______________________
14. b.i.w. ______________________
15. elix. ______________________
16. syr ______________________
17. n.p.o. ______________________
18. sl ______________________

Give the abbreviations for the following:

19. after meals ______________________
20. three times a day ______________________
21. intramuscular ______________________
22. every eight hours ______________________

23. suppository ____________________

24. intravenous ____________________

25. may be repeated once if necessary ____

26. without ____________________

27. immediately ____________________

28. ointment ____________________

29. milliequivalent ____________________

30. by rectum ____________________

Interpret the following orders. Use either *administer* or *give* at the beginning of the sentence.

31. Methergine 0.2 mg p.o. q4h for 6 doses. ____________________

32. Digoxin 0.125 mg p.o. once a day. ____________________

33. Regular Humulin insulin 14 units subcut daily at 7:30 AM. ____________________

34. Demerol 50 mg IM and atropine 0.4 mg IM on call to the operating room.

35. Ampicillin 500 mg p.o. stat, and then 250 mg p.o. q.i.d. thereafter. ____________________

36. Lasix 40 mg IM stat. ____________________

37. Librium 50 mg p.o. q4h p.r.n. for agitation. ____________________

38. Tylenol 650 mg p.o. q4h p.r.n. for pain. ____________________

39. Mylicon 80 mg p.o. p.c. and bedtime. ____________________

40. Folic acid 1 mg p.o. every day. ____________________

41. Nembutal 100 mg p.o. at bedtime p.r.n. ____________________

42. Aspirin 600 mg p.o. q4h p.r.n. for temperature greater than 101° F. ____________________

43. Dilantin 100 mg p.o. t.i.d. ______________________________

44. Minipress 2 mg p.o. b.i.d.; hold for systolic BP less than 120. ______________________________

45. Compazine 10 mg IM q4h p.r.n. for nausea and vomiting. ______________________________

46. Ampicillin 1 g IVPB q6h for 4 doses. ______________________________

47. Heparin 5,000 units subcut q12h. ______________________________

48. Dilantin susp 200 mg by NGT q AM and 300 mg by NGT at bedtime. ______________________________

49. Benadryl 50 mg p.o. stat. ______________________________

50. Epogen 3,500 units subcut three times a week. ______________________________

51. Milk of magnesia 30 mL p.o. at bedtime p.r.n. for constipation. ______________________________

52. Septra DS 1 tab p.o. daily. ______________________________

53. Neomycin ophthalmic ointment 1% in the right eye t.i.d. ______________________________

54. Carafate 1 g via NGT q.i.d. ______________________________

55. Morphine sulfate 15 mg subcut stat and 10 mg subcut q4h p.r.n. for pain. ______________________________

56. Ampicillin 120 mg IVSS q6h for 7 days. ______________________________

57. Prednisone 10 mg p.o. at 10 a.m. every other day. ______________________________

Identify the missing part from the following medication orders. Assume that the date, time, and signature are included on the orders.

58. Dicloxacillin 250 mg q.i.d. ______

59. Synthroid 0.05 mg p.o. ______

60. Nitrofurantoin p.o. q6h for 10 days. ______

61. 25 mg p.o. q12h, hold if BP less than 100 systolic. ______

62. Solu-Cortef 100 q6h. ______

63. Describe what your action would be if the following order was written:

    Prilosec 20 mg daily. ______

Using the discussion on medication abbreviations, symbols, and acronyms that should not be used, identify the mistake in the following orders and correct each order.

64. Inderal20mg p.o. daily. ______

65. Lasix 10.0 mg p.o. b.i.d. ______

66. Humulin Regular insulin 4U IV stat. ______

67. Haldol .5 mg p.o. t.i.d. ______

Answers below and on p. 163

ANSWERS

Chapter 11

Answers to Practice Problems

1. after meals
2. hour
3. every 12 hours
4. twice daily, twice a day
5. when necessary/required, as needed
6. Give or administer zidovudine 200 milligrams orally (by mouth) every 4 hours.
7. Give or administer procaine penicillin G 400,000 units by intravenous injection every 8 hours.
8. Give or administer gentamicin sulfate 45 milligrams by intravenous piggyback injection every 12 hours.
9. Give or administer regular Humulin insulin 5 units by subcutaneous injection before the morning meal at 7:30 AM and at bedtime.
10. Give or administer vitamin B_{12} 1,000 micrograms by intramuscular injection every other day.
11. Give or administer Prilosec 20 milligrams orally (by mouth) twice a day (two times a day).
12. Give or administer Tofranil 75 milligrams orally (by mouth) at bedtime.
13. Give or administer Restoril 30 milligrams orally (by mouth) at bedtime.
14. Give or administer Mylanta 30 milliliters orally (by mouth) every 4 hours when necessary (when required).
15. Give or administer Synthroid 200 micrograms orally (by mouth) daily.

Answers to Chapter Review

1. name of the client
2. date and time the order was written
3. name of the medication
4. dosage of medication
5. route by which medication is to be administered
6. time and/or frequency of administration
7. signature of the person writing the order
8. intranasal
9. as desired
10. subcutaneous
11. with
12. before meals

13. four times a day
14. twice a week
15. elixir
16. syrup
17. nothing by mouth
18. sublingual
19. p.c. *or* pc
20. t.i.d. *or* tid
21. I.M. *or* IM
22. q.8.h. *or* q8h
23. supp
24. I.V. *or* IV
25. s.o.s. *or* sos
26. $\bar{s}$
27. stat *or* STAT
28. ung *or* oint
29. mEq
30. p.r. *or* pr
31. Give or administer Methergine 0.2 milligrams orally (by mouth) every 4 hours for 6 doses.
32. Give or administer digoxin 0.125 milligrams orally (by mouth) once a day.
33. Give or administer regular Humulin insulin 14 units by subcutaneous injection daily at 7:30 AM.
34. Give or administer Demerol 50 milligrams by intramuscular injection and atropine 0.4 milligrams by intramuscular injection on call to the operating room.
35. Give or administer ampicillin 500 milligrams orally (by mouth) immediately and then 250 milligrams orally (by mouth) four times a day thereafter.
36. Give or administer Lasix 40 milligrams by intramuscular injection immediately (at once).
37. Give or administer Librium 50 milligrams orally (by mouth) every 4 hours when necessary (when required) for agitation.
38. Give or administer Tylenol 650 milligrams orally (by mouth) every 4 hours when necessary (when required) for pain.
39. Give or administer Mylicon 80 milligrams orally (by mouth) after meals and at bedtime.
40. Give or administer folic acid 1 milligram orally (by mouth) every day.
41. Give or administer Nembutal 100 milligrams orally (by mouth) at bedtime when necessary (when required).
42. Give or administer aspirin 600 milligrams orally (by mouth) every 4 hours when necessary (when required) for temperature greater than 101° F.
43. Give or administer Dilantin 100 milligrams orally (by mouth) three times a day.
44. Give or administer Minipress 2 milligrams orally (by mouth) two times a day. Hold for systolic blood pressure less than 120.
45. Give or administer Compazine 10 milligrams by intramuscular injection every 4 hours when necessary (when required) for nausea and vomiting.
46. Give or administer ampicillin 1 gram by intravenous piggyback injection every 6 hours for 4 doses.
47. Give or administer heparin 5,000 units by subcutaneous injection every 12 hours.
48. Give or administer Dilantin suspension 200 milligrams by nasogastric tube every morning and 300 milligrams by nasogastric tube at bedtime.
49. Give or administer Benadryl 50 milligrams orally (by mouth) immediately (at once).
50. Give or administer Epogen 3,500 units by subcutaneous injection three times a week.
51. Give or administer milk of magnesia 30 milliliters orally (by mouth) at bedtime when necessary (when required) for constipation.
52. Give or administer Septra double-strength 1 tablet orally (by mouth) daily.
53. Give or administer neomycin ophthalmic ointment 1% to the right eye three times a day.
54. Give or administer Carafate 1 gram by nasogastric tube four times a day.
55. Give or administer morphine sulfate 15 milligrams by subcutaneous injection immediately (at once) and 10 milligrams by subcutaneous injection every 4 hours when necessary (when required) for pain.
56. Give or administer ampicillin 120 milligrams by intravenous Soluset injection every 6 hours for 7 days.
57. Give or administer prednisone 10 milligrams orally (by mouth) at 10 a.m. every other day.
58. route of administration
59. frequency of administration
60. dosage of medication (drug)
61. name of medication (drug)
62. dosage of medication (drug) and route of administration
63. Notify the prescriber that the order is incomplete; route is missing from the order; do not administer, order not legal. Never assume.
64. Inderal 20 mg p.o. daily. There should be adequate spacing between the medication name, dosage, and unit of measure. Could be misread as 120 mg, which is 6 times the dosage ordered.
65. Lasix 10 mg p.o. bid. Trailing zeros could cause dosage to be interpreted as 100 mg, which is 10 times the intended dose.
66. Humulin Regular Insulin 4 units IV stat. The abbreviation for units here could be misread as a zero, which could result in 10 times the dose being administered. Write out units.
67. Haldol 0.5 mg p.o. tid. Omission of the leading zero before the decimal point could result in the dosage being read as 5 mg, which would be 10 times the dosage ordered.

CHAPTER 12
Medication Administration Records and Medication Distribution Systems

Objectives

After reviewing the chapter, you should be able to:

1. State the components of a medication order
2. Identify the necessary components of a medication administration record (MAR)
3. Read an MAR and identify medications that are to be administered on a routine basis, including the name of the medication, the dosage, the route of administration, and the time of administration
4. Read an MAR and identify medications that are administered, including the name of the medication, the dosage, the route of administration, and the time of administration
5. Identify the various medication distribution systems used

Medication Orders

As already discussed, before any medication can be administered or transcribed, there must be an order. Hospitals usually have a special form for recording medication orders. The terms *medication orders* and *doctor's orders* are used interchangeably, and the forms vary from institution to institution. As more and more hospitals transition to the electronic medical record, handwritten medication order forms are gradually being replaced by computerized prescriber order entry. This should be computerized physician/prescriber order entry (CPOE). According to an article in the *American Journal of Nursing* titled "Health Information Technology and Nursing" (McBride et al., 2012), CPOE can improve quality of care and patient safety by preventing common prescribing errors and eliminate nurses' frustration in the face of illegible written orders, which can, for instance, require a nurse to make extra phone calls to clarify what's written." A medication order, whether handwritten or done by computer entry, must have the following components:

- Client's name
- Name of the medication
- Dosage
- Route frequency and any special instructions for medications if needed; for example, for moderate pain, hold for pulse less than 60.
- Signature of the prescriber

In institutions in which handwritten records are still used, after the medication order has been verified, the order is transcribed to a medication administration record (MAR).

Medication Administration Record

The medication administration record (MAR) is a form used to document medications a client has received and is currently receiving. MARs are legal documents that may be handwritten (Figure 12-1) or electronic (Figure 12-2). Electronic medication administration records (eMARs) are viewed and charted on the computer. There is no standard form for MARs; the form varies from institution to institution. The various MAR forms used at different institutions represent differences in form only; the essential information is common to all (the name of each medication, the dosage, route and frequency). Whether the MAR is electronic or handwritten, they contain the same information indicated on a medication order and specify the actual time to administer the medication or the actual time of administration. Regardless of the format used to document administration of medications, the documentation must be accurate, and legally all medications administered must be documented. Documentation is the sixth "right of medication administration." Documentation should follow the administration of medication and include not only medications administered but also documentation regarding refusals, delays in administration, and responses to medication administration (including adverse effects). Different forms may be used in the home care setting for the charting of medications that are administered.

DEPARTMENT OF NURSING
MEDICATION ADMINISTRATION RECORD

Identifying Client Information (Name, Room Number, Date of Birth, Medical Record Number)

Diagnosis:	
ALLERGIES: NKDA	Date: 4/2/2017

Order Date	Exp. Date	RN Initial	Medication-Dosage, Frequency, Route	Date 2017	4/2	4/3	4/4	4/5	4/6	4/7	4/8
				Time	Initial	Initial	Initial	Initial	Initial	Initial	Initial
4/2/17	5/2/17	DG	Colace 100 mg po bid	0900	DG	JN					
				1700	NN	NN					
4/2/17	5/2/17	DG	Furosemide 40 mg po daily	0900	DG						
4/2/17	5/2/17	DG	K-Dur 10 mEq po bid	0900	DG	JN					
				1700	NN	NN					
4/2/17	5/2/17	DG	Digoxin 0.125 mg po daily	0900	DG	JN					
			Check apical pulse (AP)	AP	76	80					
			Hold if less than 60 or above 100 beats per minute (bpm)								

	Initial	Print Name/Title		Initial	Print Name/Title		Initial	Print Name/Title
1	DG	Deborah Gray RN	5				9	
2	NN	Nancy Nurse RN	6				10	
3	JN	Jane Nightingale RN	7				11	
4			8				12	

Figure 12-1 Handwritten medication administration record (MAR). Note: This MAR is intended to show the basic information that would be included on a MAR.

FRIDAY 10/12/12 - 0700 thru SATURDAY 10/13/12 - 0659 Meyer, Lois M. WESOF W303-2 Age: 78 Sex: F Primary Dx: CP	Unit#: Admitted: 10/12/12 Ht: 152.40 cm Wt: kg	ST ANNE HOSPITAL MEDICATION ADMINISTRATION RECORD Acct#: Page: 1 Attending Dr: Thomas Smith, MD Run Date/Time: 10/12/12 - 2237 DOB: 06/23/1934		
ALLERGIES:	Drug: PCN. ERYTHROMYCIN. IV DYE Other: NO ALLERGIES RECORDED Pharmacy: IODINE (INCLUDES RADIOPAQUE AGENTS W/IODINE). MACROLIDE ANTIBIOTICS, PENICILLINS			

Init	IV Flushes: Routine	0700-1459	1500-2259	2300-0659
	Sodium Chloride 0.9% **IV** Flush peripheral IV lines with 5 mls 0.9 NS q 8 hours and central lines per protocol.	Time _____ Init _____ # Flushed_____	Time _____ Init _____ # Flushed_____	Time _____ Init _____ # Flushed_____

Init	SCHED MEDS	DOSE		0700-1459	1500-2259	2300-0659
	DOCUSATE SODIUM (DOCUSATE SODIUM) START: 10/12 D/C: 11/11/12 AT 2244	**100 MG**	PO Q12 RX 002306792			
	PRAVACHOL (PRAVASTATIN SODIUM) Give at: BEDTIME START: 10/12 D/C: 11/11/12 AT 2244	**80 MG**	PO RX 002306793			
	METOPROLOL TARTRATE (METOPROLOL TARTRATE) HOLD FOR SBP<110 OR HR<55 Check apical rate and BP before drug admin. START: 10/12 D/C: 11/11/12 AT 2244	**50 MG**	PO Q12 RX 002306794			
	ACCUPRIL (QUINAPRIL HCL) HOLD FOR SBP<120 START: 10/12 D/C: 11/11/12 AT 2244	**40 MG**	PO Q12 RX 002306795			
	NITROGLYCERIN 2% (NITROGLYCERIN 2%) HOLD FOR SBP<100 START: 10/12 D/C: 11/11/12 AT 2244	**1 INCH**	TP Q6 RX 002306796			0000 0600
	ALPRAZOLAM (ALPRAZOLAM) START: 10/12 D/C: 10/14/12 AT 1601	**0.25 MG**	PO Q8 RX 002306791			0000

Init	PRN MEDS	DOSE		0700-1459	1500-2259	2300-0659
	NITROSTAT 25 TABS/BOTTLE (NITROGLYCERIN) Chest discomfort. May repeat q 5 min x 3. If no relief after 3 doses. Stat ECG & call Physician. START: 10/12 D/C: 11/11/12 at 1833	**0.4 MG**	SL STAT RX 002306718 PRN			

Figure 12-2 Electronic medication administration record (eMAR). From Kee JL, Marshall SM: *Clinical calculations: with applications to general and specialty areas,* ed 8, St Louis, 2016, Saunders.

SAFETY ALERT!

Document properly and accurately any medications administered to prevent medication errors caused by over-medication or under-medication.

At some institutions, a complete schedule is written out for all the administration times for medications given on a continual or routine basis. In some institutions, the method of charting medications varies (e.g., some sign for the day and just put in times given). The charting for computerized records also varies. Each time a dosage is given, the nurse initials the record next to the time. Some institutions maintain separate records for routine, intravenous (IV), and as-needed (prn) medications (Figure 12-3) and for medications administered on a one-time basis, whereas in other institutions these are kept on the same record in a designated area.

TIPS FOR CLINICAL PRACTICE

Regardless of whether the MAR is handwritten or electronic, the nurse or other health care provider uses the record to check the medication order, prepare the correct dosage, and record the medication administered to a client.

DEPARTMENT OF NURSING
MEDICATION RECORD

Identifying Client Information (Name, Room Number, Date of Birth, Medical Record Number)

Diagnosis:	
ALLERGIES: NKDA	Date: 4/9/2017

Order Date	Exp. Date	Initials	PRN MEDICATIONS Med=Dose-Freq-Route								
4/10/17	4/13/17	DG	Percocet 2 tabs po q4h prn	Date	4/10/17	4/10/17					
			for pain for 3 days	Time	1800	2200					
				Initial	DG	DG					
4/10/17	4/17/17	NN	Tylenol 650 mg po q4h prn	Date	4/10/17						
			for temp greater than 101 F	Time	1400						
				Initial	NN						
4/10/17	4/17/17	JN	Robitussin DM 10 mL po	Date	4/11/17						
			q12 prn	Time	2200						
				Initial	JN						

	Initial	Print Name/Title		Initial	Print Name/Title		Initial	Print Name/Title
1	DG	Deborah Gray RN	5			9		
2	NN	Nancy Nurse RN	6			10		
3	JN	Jane Nightingale RN	7			11		
4			8			12		

Figure 12-3 Medication administration record (MAR) showing PRN medications.

Essential Components on a Medication Record

If a handwritten MAR is used, the information on the medication record must be legible and transcribed carefully to avoid errors. In addition to client information (name, date of birth, medical record number, allergies), the following information is necessary on all MARs regardless of the format:

1. **Dates.** This information usually includes the date the order was written, the date the medication is to be started (if different from the order date), and when to discontinue it.
2. **Medication information.** This includes the medication's full name, the dosage, the route, and the frequency. Abbreviations used on the medication record should be standard abbreviations and follow the guidelines and restrictions of The Joint Commission (TJC), ISMP, and the health care institution.
3. **Time of administration.** This will be based on the desired administration schedule stated on the order, such as t.i.d. The desired administration time is placed on the medication record and converted to time periods based on the institution's time intervals for scheduled or routine medications. (Thus t.i.d. may mean 9 AM, 1 PM, and 5 PM at one institution and 10 AM, 2 PM, and 6 PM at another.) A nurse

should always become familiar with the hours for medication administration designated by a specific institution. Medication times for p.r.n. and one-time dosages are recorded at the time they are administered. Abbreviations for time and frequency should adhere to TJC and ISMP guidelines.

4. **Initials.** Most medication records have a place for the initials of the person transcribing the medication to the MAR and the person administering the medication. The initials are then written under the signature section to identify who gave the medication. Some forms may request the title as well as the signature of the nurse. The policy regarding initialing after each administration varies by institution and by charting system used. See Figures 12-1 and 12-3 for examples.
5. **Special instructions (parameters).** Any special instructions relating to a medication should be indicated on the medication record. For example, "Hold if blood pressure less than 100 systolic" or "p.r.n. for pain." Refer to the Percocet and Tylenol order shown on the MAR in Figure 12-3.

In addition to the information listed above, some medication records may include legends, as well as an area for charting to indicate when a medication is omitted or a dosage is not given. Other medication records may have an area where the nurse can document the reason for omission of a medication directly on the medication record. Other information may include injection codes so the nurse may indicate the injection site for parenteral medications. In cases in which no injection codes are indicated, the nurse is still expected to indicate the injection site. Space may also be allotted for charting information such as pulse and blood pressure if this information is relevant to the medication.

TIPS FOR CLINICAL PRACTICE

The nurse must stay alert to the guidelines of TJC and ISMP regarding abbreviations and medical notations.

Documentation of Medications Administered

Handwritten MARs include an area for documenting medications administered. After administering the medication, the nurse or other qualified staff member must record his or her initials next to the time the medication was administered. For scheduled medications, a complete schedule is written out, and the initials are recorded next to each given time. As previously mentioned, this practice can vary by institution. With one-time dosages and p.r.n. medication, *the time of administration* is written and again initialed by the person administering it. The medication form has a place for the full name of each person administering medications, along with the identifying initials. This allows for immediate identification of the person's initials if necessary. When medications are not administered, some records have notations, such as an asterisk (*), a circle, or a number corresponding to a legend on the MAR, to indicate this, or there may be an area on the back or at the bottom of the MAR for charting medications not given. The type of notation used will depend on the institution. In addition to notations made on the MAR, most institutions require documentation in the proper section of the client's chart. (Some institutions have a section designated "nurse's notes." At other institutions, nurses may be charting on a progress note and indicate a notation as "nurse's notes."

In institutions in which the eMAR is used, the documentation of medications administered is done in the computer. The computerized MAR also allows the nurse to document comments regarding the medication administration at the computer terminal. Like CPOEs, the eMAR is gradually replacing the transcription tasks that were frequently done by nurses and identified as a major contributor to medication errors.

Regardless of whether the handwritten MAR or eMAR is used, documentation should be done immediately after medications are given. Remember, this practice will prevent forgetting to document, which can result in the administration of the medication by another nurse or health care provider who thought the medication was not administered. No documentation can be interpreted as not being administered.

Explanation of Medication Administration Records

Many types of MARs are used, and these forms vary among institutions. However, despite the variety of forms, MARs contain essential information that is common to all and to their purpose. The MAR is used to determine what medications are ordered and the dosage, route, and time at which each is to be given. The MAR is also verified with the prescriber's orders. Any MAR requiring transcription of orders should always be checked against the prescriber's orders. In institutions where personnel other than the nurse transcribe orders, the nurse must double-check the transcription to make sure there are no discrepancies. Regardless of the variation in format for MARs, the information common to all is as follows:

1. The name of the client and pertinent data related to the client
2. Medication (dosage, route)
3. Time/frequency desired for administration
4. A place to indicate allergies
5. A place for date, the initials of the person who administers the medication, and a section to identify the name of the person administering the medication

Sample MARs are included in this chapter. As you look at the sample records, it is important to locate and identify the information common to all MARs, with focus on medications that are given on a continual basis.

Use of Computers in Medication Administration

As in other businesses, the use of computers in health care facilities is increasing. As a result of the reported rise in medication errors, many health care facilities have instituted some form of computer-based medication administration.

To improve quality in health care and client safety, the Health Information Technology for Economic and Clinical Health Act (HITECH Act) of 2009 encourages the use of health care informatics systems and services such as electronic health records (EHRs). According to the article, "Health Information Technology and Nursing" (2012) in the *American Journal of Nursing*, "the Obama administration, convinced like its predecessor of the potential benefits of this technology, has pushed ahead, appropriating billions of dollars in the Health Information Technology for Economic and Clinical Health (HITECH) Act—passed as part of the American Recovery and Reinvestment Act of 2009—to promote and accelerate the implementation and adoption of EHRs in hospitals and ambulatory care clinics by 2015." The legislation also authorizes the offering of monetary incentives to eligible health care providers in order to offset the related costs of such technology and to encourage the adoption of the EHR system. In addition, this health information technology expands current Federal privacy and security protections for health information. As a result of this legislation, the Congressional Budget Office estimates that approximately 90% of doctors and 70% of hospitals will be using comprehensive electronic health records within the next decade.

The literature supports the fact that one of the main causes of medication errors is the incorrect transcription of the original prescriber's order. According to Michael Cohen in the book *Medication Errors* (2010), "In transcribed orders, stray marks as well as marks intended as initials, letters, check marks, and so forth can also obscure or change the appearance of a medication order. Handwritten MARs can contribute to errors if they are crowded or illegible or present drug information in an inconsistent manner." Typically, according to Cohen, "orders are transcribed onto the MAR exactly as written; the presentation of information may not be consistent, and error-prone abbreviations and dose expressions may be carried forth from the order."

Many health care facilities have moved away from the written medication order and transcription of orders to the MAR to a computer prescriber order entry (CPOE). This system was designed to eliminate the problem of unclear and ambiguous orders, which was identified as a common reason for medication errors. Medication orders of the prescriber are either electronically transmitted or manually entered into the system. The CPOE system accepts orders in a standard format conforming to strict criteria. Once the order has been entered into the system, it is transmitted to the pharmacy to be processed. Depending on the institution and the sophistication of the software, information such as medication incompatibilities, medication allergies, range of dosages, and recommended medication times may be part of the system. This shows the importance of computers to the safe administration of medication. With the computer used to process medication orders, orders can be viewed on the computer screen or on a printout. A corresponding MAR is available at some institutions based on the computerized order entry. The computerized MAR allows the nurse to enter the charting of medications into the computer, as well as any other essential information relating to medication administration. Each institution generates its own medication record, following a specific format.

At some institutions, after the entry of orders into the system, the computer automatically generates a list of all the medications to be given to clients on a unit and the times they are to be given. The computer has become an essential tool for medication administration at some institutions. It is important to note that the use of computers in reference to medication administration times varies from one institution to the next, and the sophistication of the computer system depends on the facility and the software purchased.

The use of computerized systems as a means of reducing errors in medication administration speaks to two QSEN competencies: safety to reduce risk of harm to clients, and the use of technology to mitigate errors.

Medication Distribution Systems

The medication distribution system varies from one institution to the next. The various distribution systems are discussed in the following sections.

Unit-Dose System

Many institutions use a system of medication administration referred to as a *unit dose drug dispensing system* (UDDS). This system has decreased medication preparation time because the medications are prepared daily in the pharmacy and sent to the unit. Medications are dispensed by the pharmacy in individual dosages as prescribed. Packages provide a single dosage of medication. The package is labeled with generic and trade names (and sometimes manufacturer, lot number, and expiration date). Depending on the distribution system, the individual packages may be labeled with the client's name and barcode. The medications are placed in a client-identified drawer in a large unit-dose cabinet at the nurse's station. "The value of unit dose dispensing in preventing errors should not be underestimated. TJC standards require medications to be dispensed in the most ready-to-administer form possible to minimize opportunities for error" (Cohen, 2010). Cohen points out that although unit-dose may be used, the system does not extend to all products. (For example, in many institutions, nurses are responsible for reconstituting or preparing IV doses from floor stock medications, and no policy exists for double-checking accuracy of calculation, preparation, and labeling.) Errors therefore occur that a fully implemented unit-dose system could have prevented.

Unit dose is also used as part of another medication system in some institutions (e.g., a computerized unit dose medication cart). In the computerized unit-dose system, each dosage for the client is released individually and recorded automatically. This system is used for monitoring controlled substances and other items used in the unit (e.g., medications used by the unit in large volumes). The type of medication form used for this system varies from one institution to another. In some instances, this system has decreased the amount of time spent transcribing orders or eliminated the need for transcription. In some institutions, however, transcription of medication orders to the MAR is still required. The prescriber's orders are therefore written on a separate order sheet and sent to the pharmacy. Figure 12-1 illustrates the transcription of orders to the MAR.

At some institutions the prescriber's order is done by computer entry, eliminating the need for transcription. Figure 12-4 shows a unit-dose cabinet.

Computer-Controlled Dispensing System

The use of automated dispensing cabinets (ADCs) is on the rise in health care facilities. This system is gaining increased popularity in many institutions and health care facilities. The computer-controlled dispensing system is supplied by the pharmacy daily with

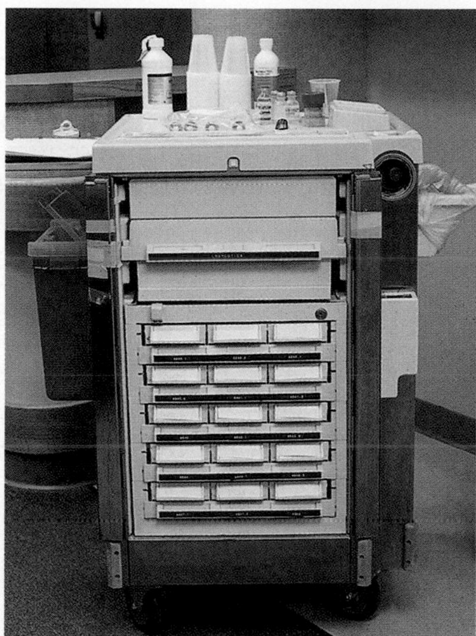

Figure 12-4 Unit dose cabinet. (From Clayton BD, Willihnganz M: *Basic pharmacology for nurses,* ed 17, St Louis, 2017, Mosby.)

stock medications. Controlled substances are also kept in the cart, and the system provides a detailed record indicating which controlled substances were used and by whom. The medication order is received by the pharmacy for the client and then entered into the system. To access medications in this system, the nurse uses a security code and password or biometric fingerprint scan.

The three most common dispensing systems are the Pyxis Med Station system (Figure 12-5), the Omnicell Omni Rx, and the AcuDose Rx.

The Omnicell system shown in Figure 12-6 is a mobile medication system that assists in providing for the safe and secure transportation of medications from the automated dispensing cabinets(ADC) to the client's bedside. This system allows for the nurse to retrieve medications that are scheduled and as needed medications. Medications administered as well as those wasted can now be recorded remotely using this system. This system allows nurses to retrieve all medications that are needed by the client without making trips to an ADC. A controlled substance management system is also part of this mobile unit that allows for an inventory of controlled substances that are used.

These systems allow storage of items such as vials and premixed IVs and allow nurses to obtain any medications stored in the device for any client and even to override the system in an emergency. However, overrides eliminate verification of medications by the pharmacy, which could result in an error. Currently, almost 90% of all automated dispensing cabinets are linked to pharmacy information systems, thereby decreasing errors by ensuring that the nurse can only access medications for a specific client.

Some institutions have added barcoding to this process during the administration phase of the medication process. At the client's bedside, the nurse uses a handheld scanner that records the barcode on the client's wristband and the unit-dose medication packet, linking this information to the client database. If there is an error, the administration process is halted; if the information is correct, the medication is administered and documentation in the MAR occurs automatically. Literature supports that use of ADCs has reduced medication errors by dispensing the correct medication.

Recognizing the need to guide health care organizations in the safest use of ADCs, ISMP has developed and posted guidelines that include 12 interdisciplinary core processes for safe use of ADCs (ISMP, 2008). These can be viewed on the ISMP website (www.ismp.org). The health care provider must still remember the importance of client safety and follow the "Six Rights of Medication Administration" when using technology.

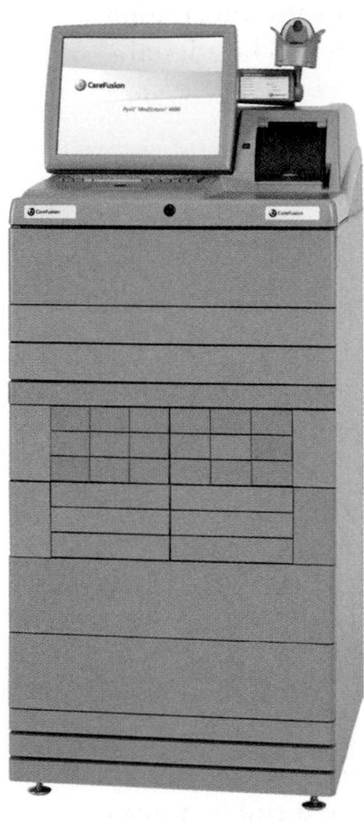

Figure 12-5 Pyxis Med Station. (Courtesy and © Becton, Dickinson and Company, Franklin Lakes, NJ.)

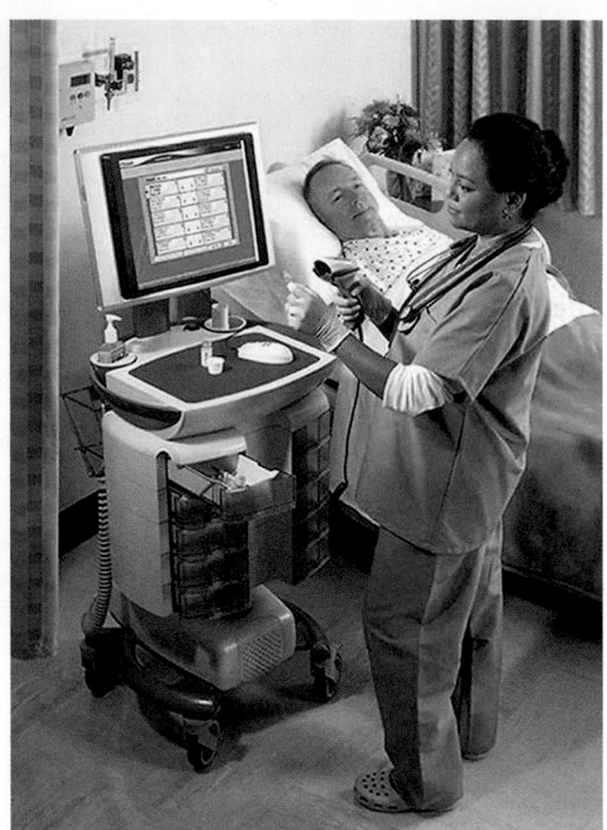

Figure 12-6 A nurse using the Omnicell Savvy Mobile Medication System at the patient's bedside. (Used with permission of Omnicell.)

Barcode Medication Delivery

Barcode medication delivery is increasing in some health care facilities. Studies have shown that barcode medication administration can reduce medication errors by 65% to 86% (Cohen, 2010). It was pioneered by the Veterans Affairs facilities. The basic system of barcoding verifies that a client receives the right dosage of the right medication by the right route at the right time. This system requires that each client wear an ID with a unique barcode to identify the individual. Each medication must therefore have a barcode. Computers installed at the client's bedside and/or handheld devices enable the nurse to scan the barcode on the client's identification band and the medication to be administered. Once the information has been validated to the client and the client's medication profile, the medication given is documented on an online MAR (see Figure 12-7 showing a barcode for unit medication dose, and Figure 12-8 showing a barcode

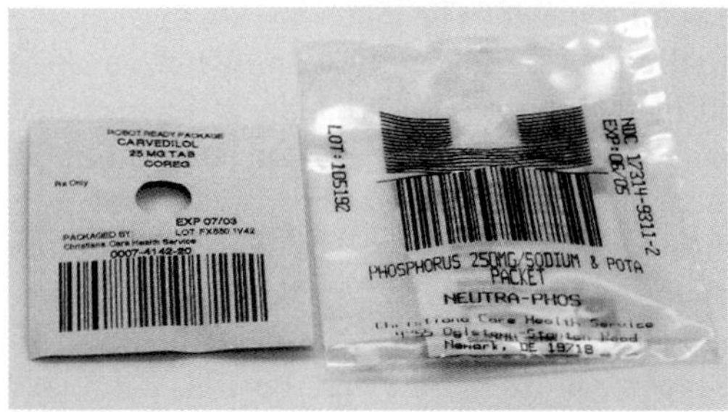

Figure 12-7 Barcode for unit drug dose. (From Kee JL, Marshall SM: *Clinical calculations: with applications to general and specialty areas,* ed 8, St Louis, 2016, Saunders.)

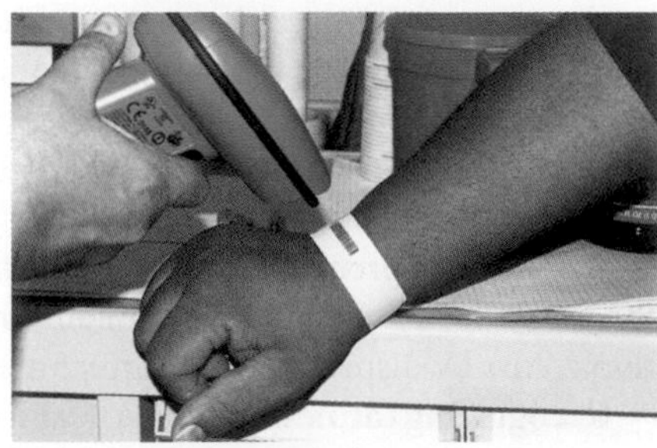

Figure 12-8 Barcode reader. (From Kee JL, Marshall SM: *Clinical calculations: with applications to general and specialty areas,* ed 8, St Louis, 2016, Saunders.)

reader). Barcoding is being added to some medication distribution systems as mentioned in the discussions of automated dispensing systems and unit-dose systems. Many pharmacists are using the barcode system to prepare unit-dose medications. Like other systems, barcode systems with additional features are also available. The complexity or simplicity of the barcode system depends on the institution. The barcode medication administration system allows overrides in cases where medications need to be administered in an emergency. However, literature points out that an override bypasses the important step of order verification by the pharmacist.

Additional Technology in Medication Administration

Additional technology designed to prevent medication errors includes computer-based drug administration (CBDA), a technological software system. The purpose of the software is to automate the medication administration process and improve accuracy and efficiency in documentation. The system comprises the computerized prescriber order system, the barcode administration system and the electronic medication administration record (eMAR), and the pharmacy information systems.

eMAR is a counterpart to the barcode medication system that acts as a stringent safeguard to ensure that the right client receives the right medication, the right dose, by the right route, and at the right time. eMAR uses the barcode on the client's arm band and the barcode on the medications supplied by the pharmacy. Before administering medications, barcodes on the client's arm band and the medication are scanned using the barcode scanner. The computer then checks the medications against the client's history (allergies, medication history) and lab results. The computer verifies and confirms that the nurse is administering the right medications to the right client in the right dosage, by the right route, and at the right time. The computer also alerts the nurse to any conditions that should be checked before administering the medication. The pharmacist and health care provider can access the computerized record to confirm medication delivery.

Advantages and Disadvantages of Technology

The nursing literature supports the belief that technology has decreased the number of medication errors; however, the risks of medication errors with technology have also been discussed. Even though the use of technology in the health care system has increased, it has been emphasized that technology as well as medication administration systems are not a total safeguard.

The use of technology cannot eliminate all medication errors, but it can provide safeguards that are not possible with the use of manual processes. According to Cohen (2010), "The implementation of any new technology requires adequate planning and preparation of the staff to properly use the safety features and not devise workarounds." Any technology implemented in a health care setting should not substitute for knowledge of the practitioner or eliminate the taking of basic safety precautions. Literature relating to the use of technology in the health care system reinforces the need for proper education of nurses and other health care providers to its use to avoid compromising client safety. The article, "Health Information Technology and Nursing" cited earlier indicates that the introduction of EHRs will present nurses with specific challenges, and nurses must be aware of the new types of errors EHRs can introduce, which may differ from those encountered in a paper chart system.

Basic safety precautions such as the rights of medication administration cannot be eliminated and can help in the reduction of medication errors even with the use of technology.

Some of the problems that can result in medication errors have been discussed in this chapter. It is important to remember that technology "can't improve safety unless system design and uses are carefully planned and properly implemented" (Cohen, 2010).

In addition to aspects such as being able to override systems, entry errors can occur with computer prescribed order entry when orders are entered by the health care provider. Safeguards on CPOE do not prevent a prescriber from entering an order into the wrong client record or selecting the wrong medication (Cohen, 2010). Barcoding, like automated dispensing cabinets, allows overrides in cases where medications need to be administered in an emergency. According to Cohen (2010), "All caregivers administering medications must understand that using an override bypasses the important step of order verification by a pharmacist." Cohen recommends that before a health care facility decides to use barcoding medication administration, facilities must anticipate failures and develop contingency plans for unexpected results. Newer systems of administration will have identified their own safety precautions to prevent errors.

It is important to be aware of the technological advances that have been instituted to decrease the occurrence of medication errors and to recognize that although their use has been shown to reduce errors, no system is completely without fault. Regardless of the medication system used, the nurse must recognize the importance of safety first and realize that no system eliminates the need for the nurse to follow the standard administration procedures for medication administration, such as verifying all aspects of the medication order—the right client, right medication, right dosage, right time, right route, and right documentation. In addition, the institution of technology into medication administration requires a collaborative approach and commitment by all health care providers who will be affected in the process. With the influx of new medications and technology in the health care system, nurses must be knowledgable and prepared to meet their responsibilities remembering client safety is the main focus.

Scheduling Medication Times

Many health care facilities have routine schedules for administering medications, which vary from one institution to another. Common abbreviations are used for scheduling and prescribing medications. As previously mentioned in this chapter, the nurse must become familiar with the administration schedule used at a specific institution. Table 12-1 shows some examples of commonly used abbreviations in scheduling of medications. The nurse must be knowledgeable about abbreviations prohibited for use by TJC and ISMP related to dosing frequency (QSEN Competency 5, Safety).

Military Time

Many hospitals and health care agencies use military time (international time). Medication orders may include the time of administration in military time when documenting the administration of medications on the MAR. The FDA recommends the use of military time. The nurse therefore needs to be familiar with how to convert traditional time to military time. Clinical facilities may use traditional or military (international) time for documentation. As a review, in military (international) time, the day begins after 0000, the first minute of the day is 0001, and day ends at 2400 (which is 12 midnight). (0000 is commonly used by the military.) To convert AM, omit the colon and AM and ensure that a 4-digit number is written, adding a zero in the beginning as needed. For each hour beginning with 1 PM standard time, add 12 hours to convert to military.

TABLE 12-1 Commonly Used Abbreviations for Scheduling Medications

Abbreviation	Meaning
a.c.*	before meals
b.i.d	twice a day
p.c.*	after meals
p.r.n.	as needed (when necessary/required)
q	every
q.h.	every hour
q2h, q3h, q4h	every 2 hours, 3 hours, 4 hours
q6h, q8h, q12h, q24h	every 6 hours, 8 hours, 12 hours, 24 hours
q.i.d.	four times a day
stat	immediately (at once), now
t.i.d.	three times a day

*Based on mealtimes.

Example: b.i.d. (twice a day) at a facility could be in standard time, for example, 9 (AM) and 5 (PM) or, in military time, 0900 and 1700.

Review content relating to converting time between traditional and military in Chapter 9 if necessary.

POINTS TO REMEMBER

- The system used for medication administration plays a role in determining the type of medication record used and whether transcription of orders is necessary.
- Regardless of the type of medication record used at an institution, the nurse should know the data that are essential for the medication record and understand the importance of accuracy and clarity on medication orders.
- Persons transcribing orders should transcribe them in ink and write legibly to avoid medication errors. All essential notations or instructions should be clearly written on the medication record. Notations used should follow TJC and ISMP regulations.
- Documentation of medications administered should be done promptly, accurately, and only by the person administering them.
- To avoid errors in administration, always check transcribed orders against the prescriber's orders.
- The use of technology has reduced medication errors.
- Nurses need to be aware of the different distribution systems in use.
- Regardless of the system used, safety is the priority, and the nurse must still use the process in medication administration of verifying the order, administering the medication to the right client, right dosage, right route, right time, and right documentation.
- A facility may use traditional or military (international) time to designate administration times. The FDA recommends the use of military time.

PRACTICE **PROBLEMS**

1. True or False? Illegible prescribers' handwriting is the most common reason for medication errors on handwritten MARs (medication administration records).

   ____

2. True or False? The use of technology is a foolproof method to prevent medication errors. ________________

3. True or False? Medication administration forms have information that is common to all, regardless of the form used. ________________

4. "The right ________________ must receive the right ________________ in the right ________________ by the right ________________ at the right ________________ followed by the right ________________."

5. The ________________ is responsible for the medication administered, regardless of the reason for the error.

6. The Pyxis is an example of ________________.

7. The ability to ________________ a system eliminates ________________ by the pharmacy, which increases the likelihood of a medication error.

8. True or False? All health care institutions document medications using traditional time. ________________

9. What is the last step in medication administration? ________________

10. CPOE is an abbreviation for ________________.

Refer to the handwritten MAR (Figure 12-1) to answer the following questions.

11. How many times a day is furosemide ordered? ________________

12. Identify the medications and their doses administered at 0900 ________________

13. K-Dur 10 mEq is ordered. What does mEq mean? ________________

14. What action must you take before administering Digoxin? ________________

15. What is the equivalent of the scheduled administration time for K-Dur in traditional time? ________________

Refer to the eMAR (Figure 12-2) to answer the following questions.

16. What medication is ordered to be administered at bedtime? ________________

17. Five (5) of the meds ordered have a discontinuation (D/C) date of 11/11/12 at 2244. What time is this in traditional time? ________________

Answers on p. 178

CHAPTER **REVIEW**

1. Who determines the medication administration times? ________________

2. Do b.i.d. and q2h have the same meaning? ________________ Explain: ________

____

____

3. What is the purpose of barcoding? ________________

4. The abbreviation *eMAR* stands for ________________.

5. Times for medication administration can be indicated in ________ or ________.

Refer to the eMAR in Figure 12-2 to answer the following questions.

6. Which medication is indicated as being prn? ________________

7. What is the route indicated for the prn medication? ________________

8. Which medication is ordered q8h? (include dosage and route) ________________

Refer to the MAR in Figure 12-3 to answer the following questions.

9. What would be the next time the client could receive Percocet if needed? (Give date and state time in traditional and international time.)

 ____

10. When could the client receive another dose of Robitussin DM if needed? (Give date and state time in traditional and international time.) ________________

Refer to the portion of the transcribed MAR provided to answer questions 11-15

11. What dosage of Neurontin should be administered? ________________

12. Are any of the medication orders incomplete? If so, which medication and what information is missing? ________________

		Time	5/2/17	5/3/17	5/4/17	5/5/17	5/6/17	5/7/17	5/8/17
5/2/17	Vasotec po qd	1000							
	Hold for SBP less than 100	B/P							
5/2/17	Neurontin 400 mg po tid	1000							
		1400							
		1800							
5/2/17	Heparin 5,000 U daily	1000							
5/2/17	Benadryl 50 mg po q6h prn for itching								

13. Indicate the time of day in traditional time that each medication should be given.

____

14. Which order(s) contain(s) error-prone abbreviations? How should the order be corrected? _______________

15. Why are no times listed for Benadryl? _______________

Answers below

ANSWERS

Chapter 12

Answers to Practice Problems

1. True
2. False
3. True
4. client, medication (drug), dosage (dose), route, time, documentation
5. nurse
6. automated dispensing cabinet (ADC). Sometimes referred to as computer-controlled dispensing system
7. override, verification
8. False
9. documentation
10. computer prescriber order entry
11. Once a day
12. Colace 100 mg, furosemide 40 mg, K-Dur 10 mEq, Digoxin 0.125 mg
13. Milliequivalent
14. Check the client's apical pulse
15. 9:00 AM, 5:00 PM
16. Pravachol (pravastatin sodium)
17. 10:44 PM

Answers to Chapter Review

1. hospital, institution, or health care facility
2. No, b.i.d. means the order will be given two times in 24 hours, whereas a q2h order would be given 12 times in 24 hours.
3. to ensure dispensing and administration of the correct medication to the right client
4. electronic medication administration record
5. traditional time, military time (international time)
6. Nitrostat (nitroglycerin)
7. sublingual (sl)
8. Alprazolam 0.25 mg (milligram) po (by mouth)
9. 4/11/17 2:00 AM, 0200
10. 4/12/17 10 AM, 1000
11. 400 mg
12. Yes. For Vasotec, the dosage is missing; for heparin, the route is missing.
13. Vasotec, 10:00 AM; Neurontin 10:00 AM, 2:00 PM, 6:00 PM; Heparin 10:00 AM.
14. Vasotec frequency should be stated as every day or daily. Heparin units should not be abbreviated.
15. Benadryl is ordered whenever necessary or required (prn). It is not given on a routine schedule and is charted each time it is given, spaced at 6-hour intervals.

CHAPTER 13
Reading Medication Labels

Objectives

After reviewing this chapter, you should be able to identify:

1. The trade and generic names of medications
2. The dosage strength of medications
3. The form in which a medication is supplied
4. The total volume of a medication container where indicated
5. Directions for mixing or preparing a medication where necessary
6. Information on combined-medication labels

Administering medications safely to a client begins with the nurse accurately reading and interpreting the information on a medication label. The medication label indicates the information you need to perform dosage calculations. Medication labels indicate the dosage contained in the package. Other pertinent information includes: the medication name, form, total volume, total amount in container (for solid forms of medication) route of administration, warnings, storage requirements, and manufacturing information. In addition, information regarding expiration dates and a National Drug Code (NDC) number is identifiable on a medication label. It is important to read the label carefully and recognize essential information.

SAFETY ALERT!

Always read the label carefully. Reading the label three (3) times will prevent an error in administration of the wrong medication.

Reading Medication Labels

The nurse should be able to recognize the following pertinent information on a medication label.

Generic Name

Every medication has an official name, referred to as the generic name. Medications have one generic name. By law, the generic name must be identified on all medication labels. If there is only one name on the medication, it is the generic name. The generic name is given by the manufacturer that first develops the medication, but the name is not specific to the manufacturer. It is also recorded with a national listing of medications: the United States Pharmacopeia (USP) and the National Formulary (NF). Medications have only one generic name. Prescribers are ordering medications more often by generic name. In many institutions, pharmacists are dispensing medications by generic name to decrease costs. Nurses therefore need to know the generic name as well as the trade name for medications, and crosscheck medications to prevent inaccurate medication identification.

On a medication label the generic name appears directly under the brand name and sometimes is placed inside parentheses. Sometimes only the generic name may appear on a medication label or package. This is common for medications that have been used for

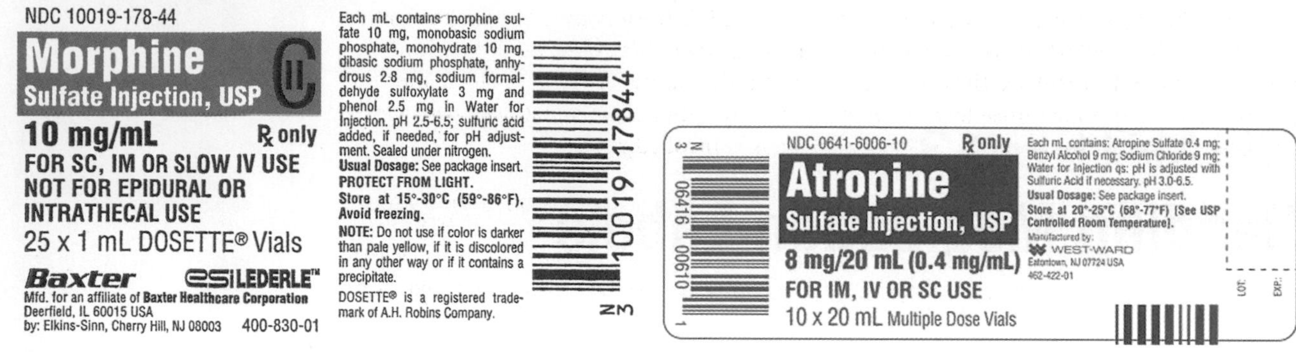

A B

Figure 13-1 **A,** Morphine label: 10 mg per mL. **B,** Atropine label: 8 mg per 20 mL (0.4 mg per mL).

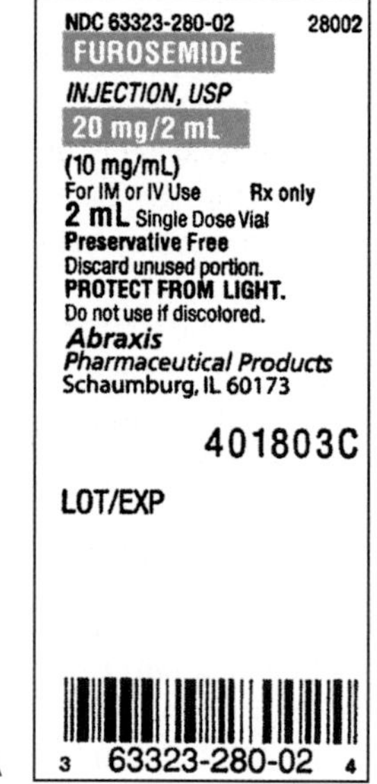

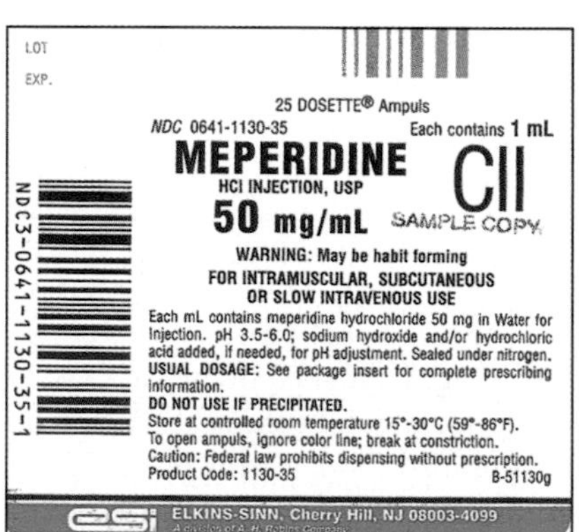

LOT
EXP.
25 DOSETTE® Ampuls
NDC 0641-1130-35
Each contains 1 mL
MEPERIDINE
CII
HCl INJECTION, USP
50 mg/mL
SAMPLE COPY
WARNING: May be habit forming
FOR INTRAMUSCULAR, SUBCUTANEOUS
OR SLOW INTRAVENOUS USE
Each mL contains meperidine hydrochloride 50 mg in Water for Injection. pH 3.5-6.0; sodium hydroxide and/or hydrochloric acid added, if needed, for pH adjustment. Sealed under nitrogen.
USUAL DOSAGE: See package insert for complete prescribing information.
DO NOT USE IF PRECIPITATED.
Store at controlled room temperature 15°-30°C (59°-86°F).
To open ampuls, ignore color line; break at constriction.
Caution: Federal law prohibits dispensing without prescription.
Product Code: 1130-35
B-51130g
NDC3-0641-1130-35-1
ELKINS-SINN, Cherry Hill, NJ 08003-4099

A B

Figure 13-2 **A,** Furosemide label: 20 mg per 2 mL (10 mg per mL). **B,** Meperidine label: 50 mg per mL.

many years, are well established, and do not require marketing under a different trade name. Examples include atropine and morphine (Figure 13-1, *A* and *B*). Other examples of medications commonly used in the clinical setting and often seen with only the generic name on the label are Lasix and Demerol. Lasix is the trade or brand name; however, it is often seen with the generic name only, furosemide, Figure 13-2, *A*. Figure 13-2, *B*, shows a Demerol label. Note that only meperidine is indicated on the label.

SAFETY ALERT!

It is important for the nurse to crosscheck all medications, whether just the generic name or both the trade and generic names are indicated on the label, to accurately identify a medication. Failure to crosscheck medications could lead to choosing the wrong medication, a violation of the rights of medication administration (the "right" medication).

Remember that even medications with similar names may have markedly different chemical structures and actions: for example, buspirone (BuSpar), which is an antianxiety medication, and bupropion (Welbutrin), which is used to treat major depressive disorder. Although the generic names are similar, the action, composition of the medications, and their use are different.

The Food and Drug Administration (FDA) now requires the "tall-man" letters be used in generic name pairs that are associated with errors. "Tall-man" uses mixed-case or enlarged letters to emphasize differing portions of the name. For example the two medications discussed using Tall-Man Letters are shown as: bus**PIR**one and bu**PROP**ion. Notice the letters are bolded and capitalized to indicate the differing portions of the name.

Notice that on all labels shown in Figures 13-1 and 13-2, the acronym USP appears after the name of the medication. As stated, this is one of the two official listings of medications. The other is NF. You will see these initials on medication labels. They are placed after the generic name. Do not confuse these abbreviations with other initials that designate a special form of a medication, such as CR, which means controlled release.

SAFETY ALERT!

It is important to avoid confusing these official listings with other initials or abbreviations on a medication label, which may serve to identify additional medications or specific actions or reactions to a medication. Use caution with medications that have similar spellings.

Trade Name

The trade name is also referred to as the *brand name* or *proprietary name;* it is the manufacturer's name for the medication. Notice that the brand name is very prominent on the label and is capitalized to market the medication. Medications can have multiple trade names.

In Figures 13-3 and 13-4, note that the trade name is listed before the generic name. A trade name is for the sole use of the company that manufacturers the medication. The trade name is identified by the ®, which is the registration symbol. The registered mark ® means the name has been legally registered with the U.S. Patent and Trademark Office.

Figure 13-3 shows the label for TriCor. TriCor is the trade name identified by the ® registration symbol. The name underneath in smaller print, fenofibrate, is the generic or official name of the medication. It is important to remember that a medication may be manufactured by different manufacturers but market it using different trade names.

Notice the ™ after the name Isentress. The trade name is the name given to the medication by the manufacturer and therefore cannot be used by another company. The medication name is a trademark for that company. Once the Patent and Trademark Office formally registers the trademark, the symbol ® then appears on the medication label. Figure 13-4 shows the label for Isentress. Isentress is the trade name identified by the ™ trademark symbol. The name underneath in smaller print and enclosed in parentheses, raltegravir, is the generic or official name.

Dosage Strength

Dosage strength refers to the weight or amount of the medication provided in a specific unit of measure (the weight per tablet, capsule, milliliter, etc.). For solid forms of medications, the dosage strength is the amount of medication per tablet, capsule, or other form. For liquid medications, the dosage strength is the amount of medication present in a certain amount of solution.

Examples:

- The dosage strength of the Tricor tablets shown in Figure 13-3 is 48 mg per tablet (the weight and specific unit of measurement).
- The dosage strength of the Isentress tablets shown in Figure 13-4 is 400 mg per tablet (the weight and specific unit of measurement).

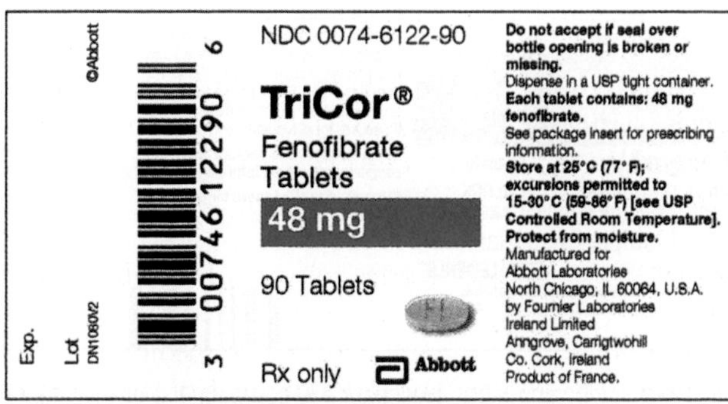

Figure 13-3 TriCor label.

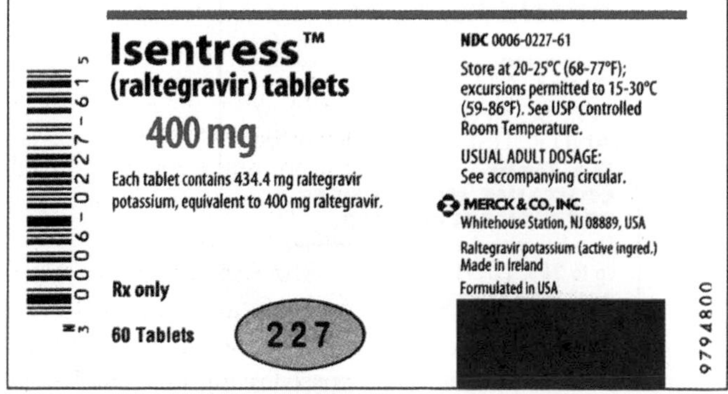

Figure 13-4 Isentress label.

- Namenda (oral solution), shown in Figure 13-5; the dosage strength is 2 mg per mL.
- Veetids (oral solution), shown in Figure 13-6, has two different but equivalent dosage strengths shown on the label: 125 mg (per 5 mL) or 200,000 units (per 5 mL). The prescriber therefore could order the medication in either unit of measurement.

Dosage strength can be expressed in different systems of measure. Some labels may state the dosage strength in apothecary and metric measures (e.g., nitroglycerin). Some oral liquids may state household measures (e.g., each 15 mL [one tablespoon] contains 80 mg).

Dosage Expressed as Ratio or Percent

Sometimes you may see solutions expressed (dosage) as a ratio or percentage. Refer to the labels in Figures 13-7 and 13-8. Notice that the labels also express the dosage strength in milligrams per milliliters.

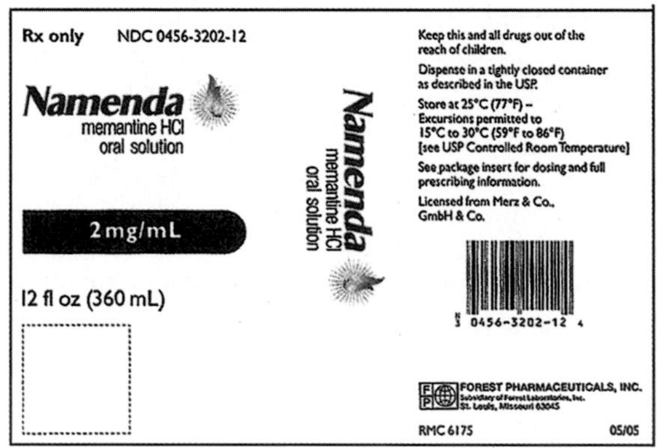

Figure 13-5 Namenda label.

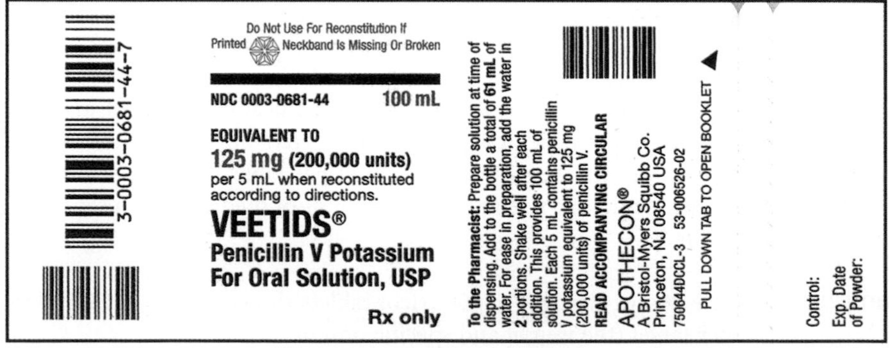

Figure 13-6 Veetids label.

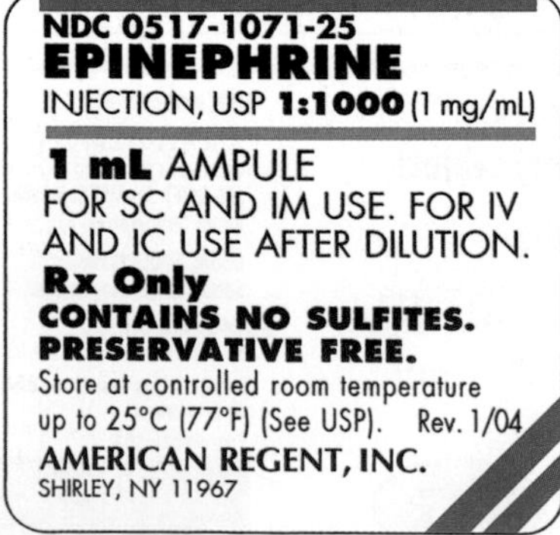

Figure 13-7 Epinephrine label. Epinephrine contains 1 g of medication per 1,000 mL solution (1:1,000) and 1 mg per mL.

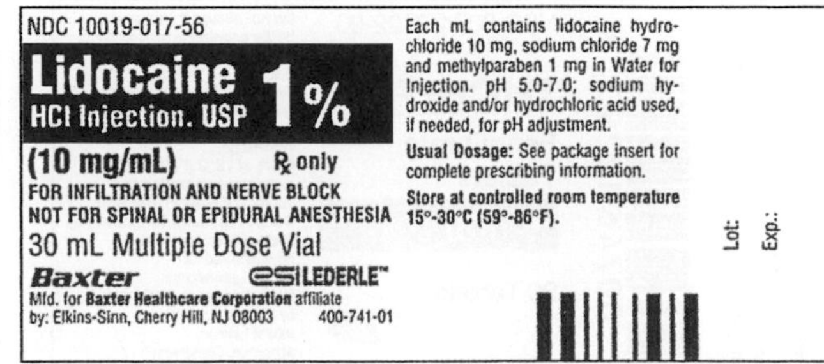

Figure 13-8 Lidocaine label. Lidocaine 1% contains 1 g of medication per 100 mL solution and 10 mg per mL.

> **SAFETY ALERT!**
>
> The Institute for Safe Medication Practices (ISMP) recommends that the slash mark (/) not be used to separate two doses to indicate *per* because it can be misread and mistaken as the number *1*. Use *per* rather than the slash mark. Example: Use 10 mg per 5 mL rather than 10 mg/5 mL, which could be misread as 10 mg and 15 mL. This will be followed in this text.

> **SAFETY ALERT!**
>
> Always read a medication label carefully to avoid errors. Medication names can be deceptively similar. Similarity in name does not mean similarity in action. For example, *Inderal* and *Inderide* are similar names, but the action and the contents of the medications are different. Inderal delivers a certain dose of propranolol hydrochloride; Inderide combines two antihypertensive agents (propranolol hydrochloride and hydrochlorothiazide, a diuretic-antihypertensive).

Form

The form specifies the type of preparation available in the package.

- Examples of forms include tablets, capsules, liquids, suppositories, and ointments. Solutions may be indicated by milliliters (mL) and described as oral suspension or aqueous solution. Some medications are available in powder or granular form or as patches.
- Labels may also indicate abbreviations or words that describe the form of the medication. Examples include CR (controlled release), LA (long acting), DS (double strength), SR (sustained release), XL (long acting), and ES (extra strength). Some labels may use abbreviations such as EC (enteric coated) or just indicate enteric coated. These medications should not be crushed. See label 13-9, *D*, for Ery tablets.
- Abbreviations that describe the form of a medication indicate whether the medication has been prepared in a way that allows extended action, or slow release, of the active ingredient. Often, these medications are given less frequently. Examples

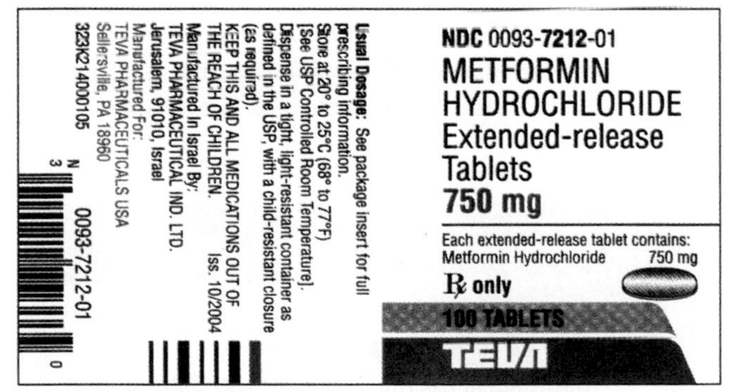

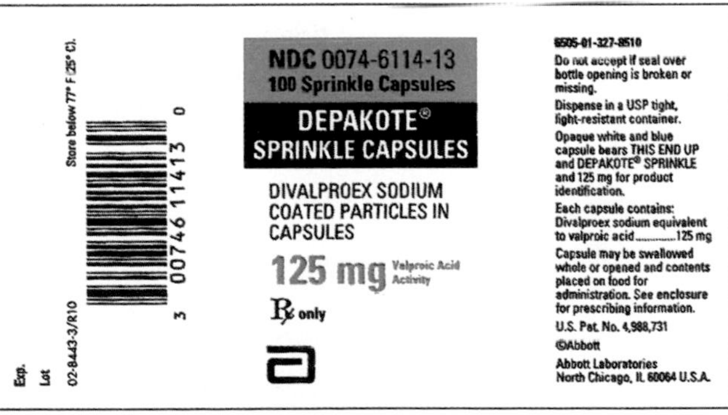

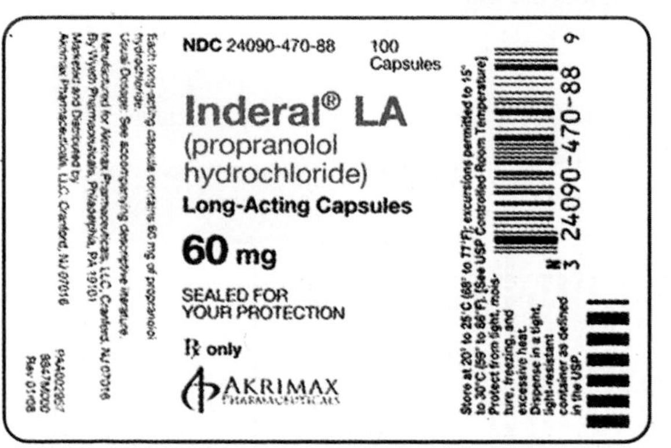

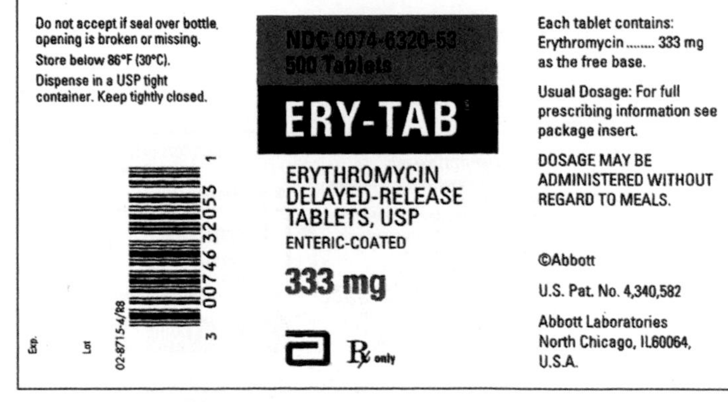

Figure 13-9 **A,** Metformin Hydrochloride Extended Release Tablets. **B,** Depakote Sprinkle Capsules. **C,** Inderal LA Long Acting Capsules. **D,** Ery Tab Delayed Release Tab and Enteric Coated.

include: Procardia XL, Inderal LA, Calan SR, and Metformin extended release. These special forms should be swallowed whole and never crushed. Always read labels carefully. Refer to labels in Figure 13-9, *A-D,* for samples of medication labels indicating special forms. Notice Figure 13-9, *B*. Note the label for Depakote Sprinkle states, "May be swallowed whole or opened and contents placed on food." Also notice label for Ery Tab; the tablets are enteric coated as well as delayed release.

SAFETY ALERT!

Administering the incorrect form of a medication is a medication error!

SAFETY ALERT!

Certain forms should not be crushed or dissolved for use through a nasogastric, gastrostomy, or jejunostomy tube without first consulting a pharmacist or medication guide for information regarding whether a medication can be crushed or altered. Altering oral medications by crushing may result in an alteration of the medication's action and cause unintended outcomes.

Barcoding Symbols

Notice that barcode symbols appear on some medication labels as thin and heavy lines arranged in a group. Barcodes are particularly important at institutions where barcoding is used as part of the medication distribution system. Refer to the barcodes indicated on the labels in Figures 13-1 to 13-6 and 13-8 to 13-9, *A-D*. Barcodes can also be used for stock reorder.

Route of Administration

The route of administration describes how the medication is to be administered.

Examples of routes of administration include oral, enteral (into the gastrointestinal tract through a tube), sublingual, injection (IV, IM, subcut), optical, topical, and others. The route of administration may not be stated directly for oral medications (see Figures 13-3, 13-4, and 13-9, *A*, *C*, and *D*). However, if a tablet or capsule is not to be swallowed, additional information will be given. For example, the label for Nitrostat® indicates it is administered sublingually (under the tongue) (Figure 13-10*A*). Another form for sublingual use is sublingual film. For example, Suboxone, which is used to treat opioid dependence, is a sublingual film.

Store at Controlled Room Temperature 20°-25°C (68°-77°F) [see USP].
Dispense in original, unopened container.
DOSAGE AND USE
See accompanying prescribing information.
Each tablet contains 0.3 mg nitroglycerin.
Keep this and all drugs out of the reach of children.
Warning–To prevent loss of potency, keep these tablets in the original container or in a supplemental Nitroglycerin container specifically labeled as being suitable for Nitroglycerin Tablets. Close tightly immediately after each use.
Manufactured by: Pfizer Pharmaceuticals LLC Vega Baja, PR 00694
8210
NDC 0071-0417-24
Rx only
100 Sublingual Tablets
Nitrostat®
(Nitroglycerin Tablets, USP)
0.3
0.3 mg (1/200 gr)
05-5930-32-2
Distributed by Pfizer Parke-Davis Division of Pfizer Inc, NY, NY 10017

A

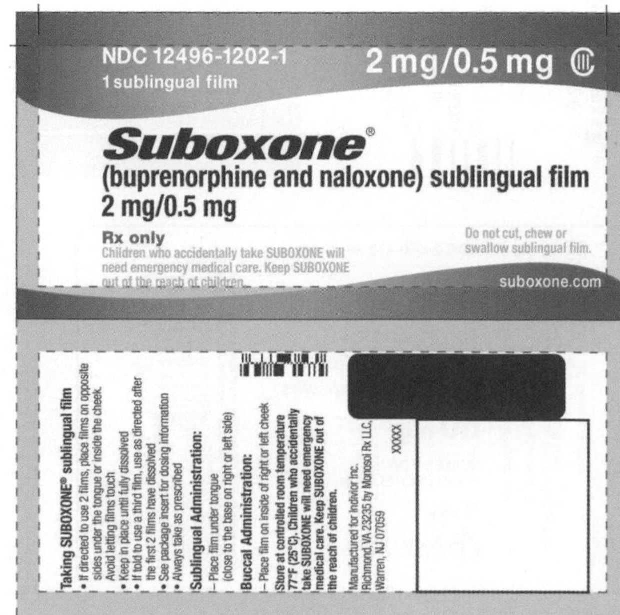

B

Figure 13-10 **A,** Nitrostat label (sublingual). **B,** Suboxone sublingual film.

The form allows for rapid absorption of medication, which is desired in the treatment of these clients. See Figure 13-10, *B*. However, unless specified otherwise, tablets, capsules, and caplets are always intended for oral use. Any form intended for oral use should be administered orally.

Because all tablets, capsules, and liquids are not always given orally, read the label carefully because any variation from oral administration is indicated on the label. Examples: sublingual tablets, otic suspension for use in ears; some capsules are placed in an inhaler and not swallowed.

Liquid medications may be administered orally or by injection. Labels for liquid medications will indicate the route, such as intravenous (IV), intramuscular (IM), or subcutaneous (subcut). See Figures 13-11 to 13-13. Labels will indicate routes for others as well.

Total Volume

On labels of solutions for injections or oral liquids, total volume, as well as dosage strength, is stated. Total volume refers to the quantity contained in a bottle, vial, or ampule. For liquids, total volume refers to the total fluid volume.

There have been documented medication errors caused by misinterpretation of dosage strength and total volume. Since 2009, the Food and Drug Administration (FDA) has required that the dosage strength per total volume be the prominent expression on single and multidose injectable product labels, followed in close proximity by the dosage strength per mL enclosed in parentheses (Cohen, 2010). Notice the clindamycin label shown in Figure 13-14

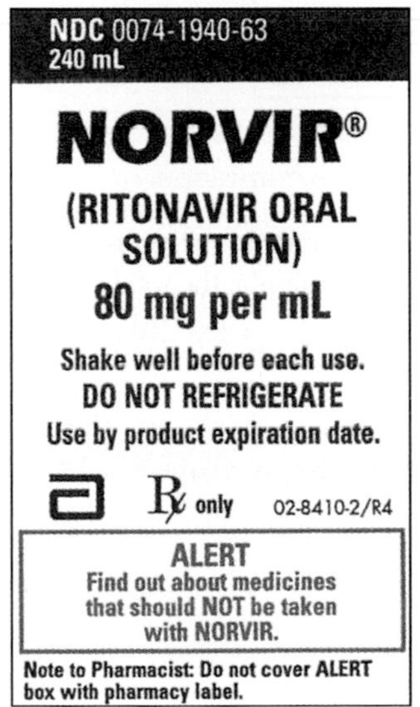

Figure 13-11 Norvir label (oral).

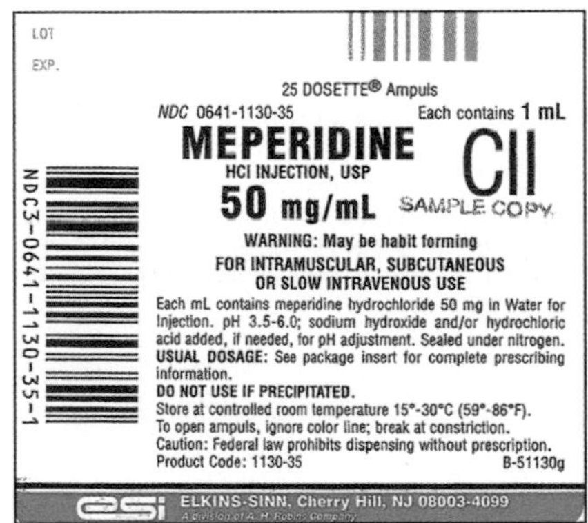

Figure 13-12 Meperidine label (IM, subcut, IV).

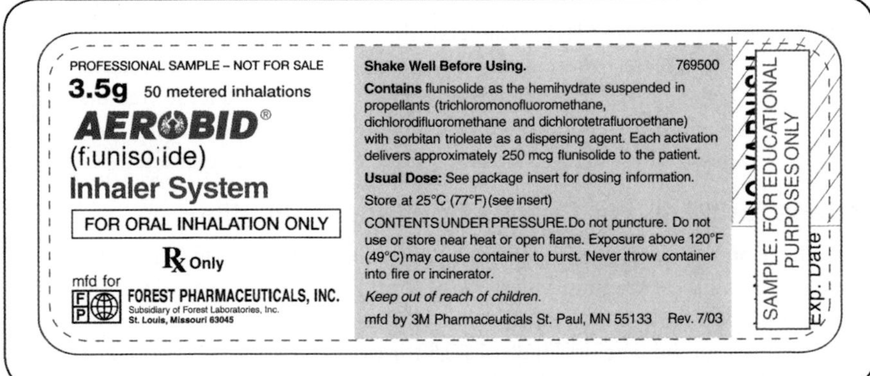

Figure 13-13 Aerobid label (oral inhalation).

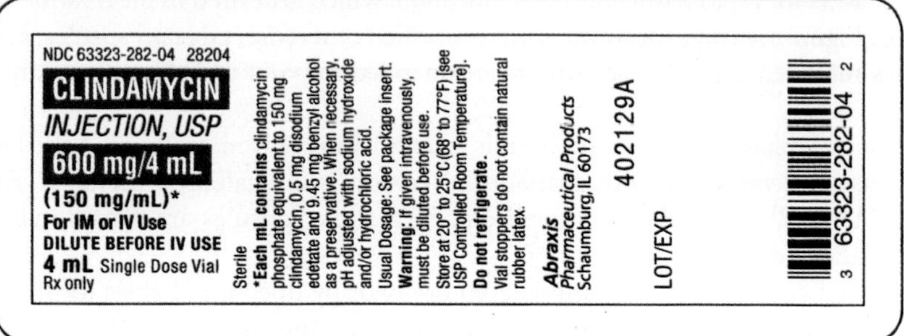

Figure 13-14 Clindamycin Injectable label.

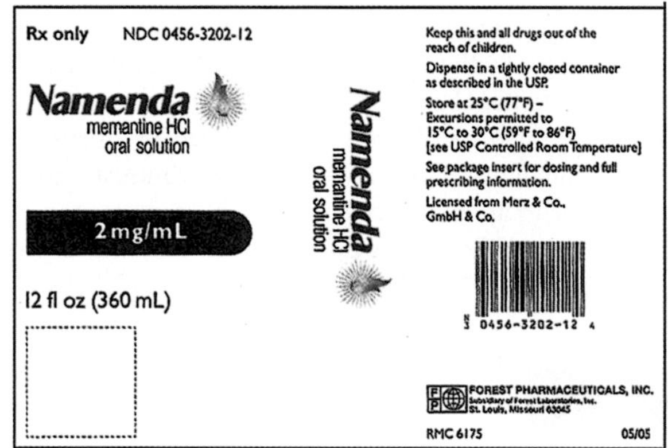

Figure 13-15 Namenda Oral Solution label, 360 mL (12 fluid ounces).

indicates 4 mL is the vial size (total volume). The dosage strength is stated for the entire vial (600 mg per 4 mL) and per mL (150 mg per mL). In Figure 13-15, Namenda, the total volume is 12 fluid ounces (360 mL), and the solution or liquid contains 2 mg per mL (dosage strength).

SAFETY ALERT!

It is important to recognize the difference between the amount per milliliter and the total volume to avoid confusion and errors. Do not confuse total volume, total amount in container with dosage strength. Confusing volume with dosage strength can cause a serious medication error.

Total Amount in Container

For solid forms of medication, such as tablets or capsules, the total amount is the total number of tablets or capsules in the container. The dosage strength, as well as the total amount in the container, is included on labels of solid forms of medication, such as tablets or capsules.

Examples: In Figure 13-3 (TriCor tablets), the total amount of tablets in the container is 90 tablets, whereas the dosage strength is 48 mg per tablet. In Figure 13-9, *A* (Metformin Hydrochloride Extended Release Tablets), the total amount of extended-release tablets in the container is 100 extended-release tablets, whereas the dosage strength is 750 mg per extended-release tablet.

Directions for Mixing or Reconstituting a Medication

When medication comes in a powdered form, the directions for how to mix or reconstitute it and with what solution are found on the label or package insert. The directions for reconstitution should be followed exactly as stated on the label for accuracy in administration. See the directions on the label in Figure 13-16 for cytarabine. In Figure 13-17 (amoxicillin label), the directions for mixing amoxicillin are shown on the side of the label. Reconstitution is discussed further in Chapter 19.

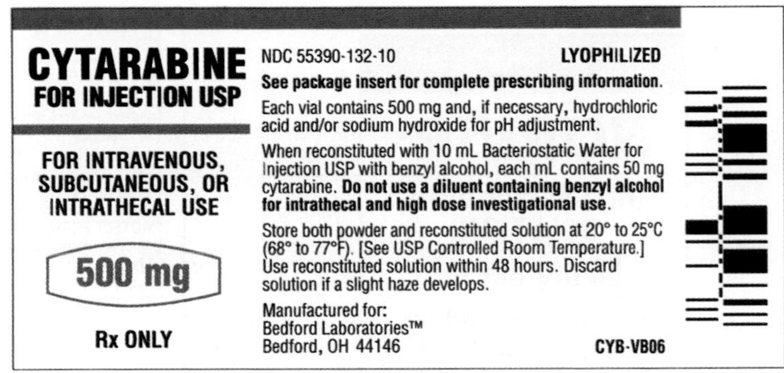

Figure 13-16 Cytarabine label (see directions).

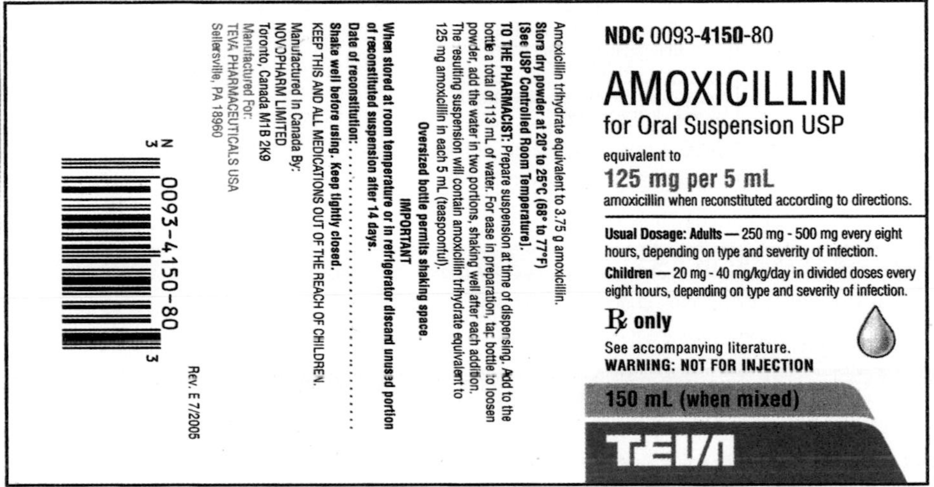

Figure 13-17 Amoxicillin label (see directions).

Precautions

Medications may come with warnings, alerts, or precautions that are related to safety, effectiveness, or administration considerations and need to be followed. Storage alerts might also be on the label. These precautions, warnings, and alerts may be printed on the label by the manufacturer or added by the pharmacy that dispenses the medication. Always read precautions or special alerts carefully, and follow the instructions given precisely. Examples of precautions, warnings, or alerts on a label may include the following: shake well, protect from light, may be habit forming. For example, refer to the lower left side of the Amoxicillin label in Figure 13-17 (Shake well before using. Keep tightly closed.). Notice the warning on the label for Demerol in Figure 13-18: "May be habit forming." Also notice the warning on the Amoxicillin label that states, "Not for Injection." Labels may also carry warnings for specific groups of clients. For example, a label may caution that you should find out which other medications may not be taken with the medication (refer to Norvir label, Figure 13-19).

Expiration Date

Medication labels contain information such as the expiration date (which may be indicated with the abbreviation *Exp*). Expiration dates indicate the last date on which a medication should be used. Typically, the date appears as the month/year. This information can be found on the back or side of a label. Medications requiring reconstitution provide specific expiration instructions. Refer to the Amoxicillin label in Figure 13-17: "Discard unused portion of reconstituted suspension after 14 days." In the hospital setting, medications that have expired should be returned to the pharmacy. Note the expiration date on the furosemide label (8/2012) in Figure 13-20. *Note:* Expiration dates must always be checked on medications, and expiration dates are always present on actual prescriptions. The labels shown in this text may not all have expiration dates because they are used solely for educational purposes.

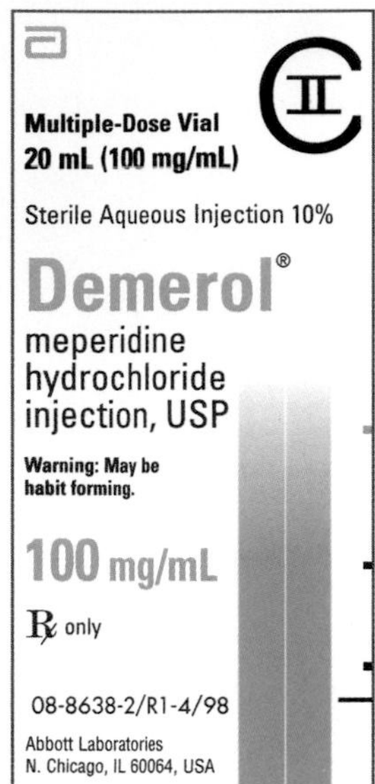

Figure 13-18 Demerol label. (Demerol may be habit forming.)

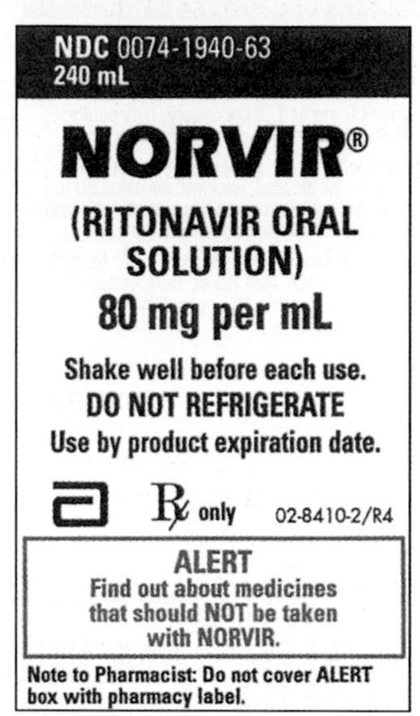

Figure 13-19 Norvir label. (Find out about medicines that should not be taken with Norvir).

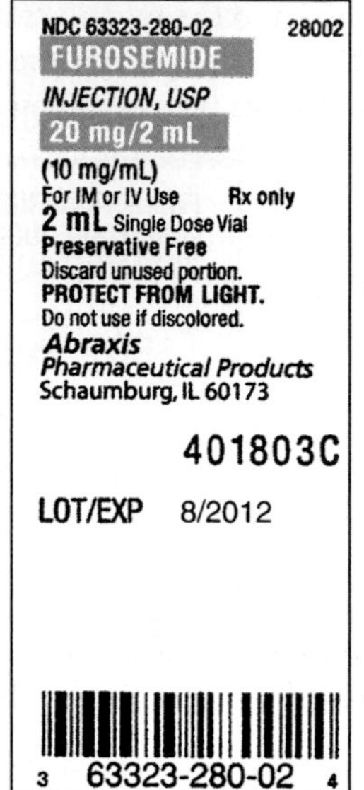

Figure 13-20 Furosemide label.

TIPS FOR CLINICAL PRACTICE

It is imperative that nurses check the expiration dates on medications as a routine habit.

SAFETY ALERT!

Remember to always read the expiration date. After the expiration date, the medication may lose its potency or cause adverse or different effects from the intended. Discard expired medications according to agency policy. For some medications, such as narcotics, disposal must be witnessed. Never give expired medications to a client! Clients must be educated in *all* aspects of medication administration, so teach them to check medications for expiration dates, and discard medications that have expired properly. Teach clients about community medication disposal days or days in some communities when they can take unused or expired medications to the police department. Encourage clients not to flush medications down the drainage system.

Storage Directions—This section of the medication label provides information as to how a medication should be stored to prevent the medication from losing its potency or effectiveness. Usually, information is given on the label relating to temperature for storing the medication. Refer to meperidine label 50 mg per mL (see Figure 13-2, *B*), and Tricor label (see Figure 13-3). When medications come in a powdered form and must be reconstituted, storage information is usually indicated on the label telling how long the medication is effective once it has been reconstituted. Refer to cytarabine label (see Figure 13-16) and Amoxicillin label (see Figure 13-17).

Lot/Control Numbers—Federal law requires that all medication packages be identified by a lot/control number. This number is important in the event that medications have to be recalled. Refer to furosemide label (see Figure 13-20), lot number 401803C.

National Drug Code (NDC) Number—This is a number required by federal law to be given to all medications. Each medication has a unique NDC number. The NDC number consists of NDC followed by three discrete groups of numbers (example: NDC 55390-132-10 for cytarabine).

Manufacturer's Name—All medication labels contain the name of the company that manufactured the medication (examples: Pharmacia & Upjohn, Lilly, or SmithKline Beecham). Abraxis is the manufacturer's name on the furosemide label in Figure 13-20. This information can be valuable; if you have questions about the medication, refer to the medication labels.

Abbreviations such as USP (United States Pharmacopoeia), NF (National Formulary)—USP and NF are the two official national lists of approved medications. Special guidelines are given to the manufacturer related to use and placement of these initials on medication labels. On the epinephrine label in Figure 13-7, notice that USP follows Epinephrine Injection. Notice the placement of USP on the lidocaine label (see Figure 13-8).

Some medication labels may indicate the usual medication dosage on the label, or the label may say to read the package insert for complete information. The usual dosage tells how much medication is given in a single dose or in a 24-hour period. See Figure 13-2, *B* (meperidine), which refers to the package insert, and Figure 13-17 (Amoxicillin), which states the usual adult and child dose.

Controlled Medication Labeling

Medications considered controlled substances are classified into schedules that rank them according to their abuse potential and physical and psychological dependence. They are ranked from Schedule I to Schedule V. Medications that have the highest abuse potential are Schedule I, and medications with the lowest or limited abuse potential are Schedule V medications. Refer to the label for meperidine in Figure 13-2, *B*, which states meperidine is Schedule II (notice the "C" with II).

Medication Labels for Combined Medications

Some medication labels may indicate that a medication contains two or more medications. Combination medications are sometimes ordered by the number of tablets, capsules, or milliliters to be given rather than by the dosage strength. Combined medications such as Sinemet, which comes in several strengths, cannot be ordered without a specific dosage; the number of tablets alone is insufficient to fill the order. **It must include the dosage!** Example: Sinemet 25 mg/100 mg, 1 tab po tid.

Example 1: The label for Sinemet, which is the trade name for an antiparkinsonian drug, indicates that the medication contains carbidopa and levodopa. The first number specifies the amount of carbidopa, and the second number represents the amount of levodopa. This is further indicated in fine print on the label. See sample labels in Figures 13-21, 13-22, and 13-23.

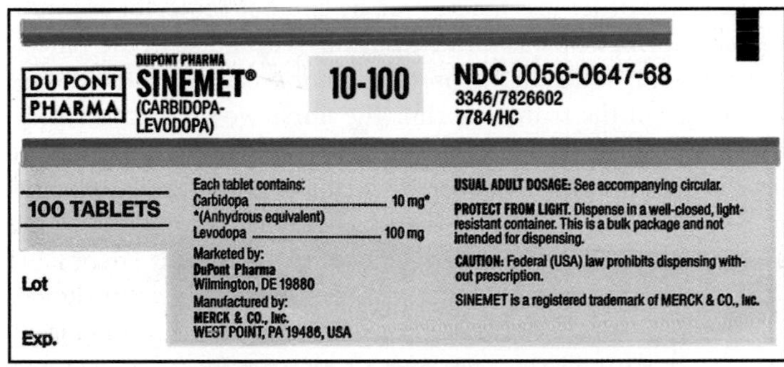

Figure 13-21 Sinemet 10-100 label. This label indicates the dosage strength of carbidopa as 10 mg and that of levodopa as 100 mg.

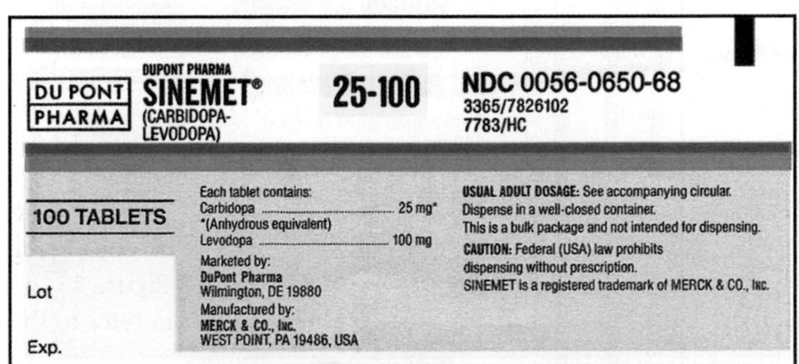

Figure 13-22 Sinemet 25-100 label. The dosage strength of carbidopa is 25 mg, and that of levodopa is 100 mg.

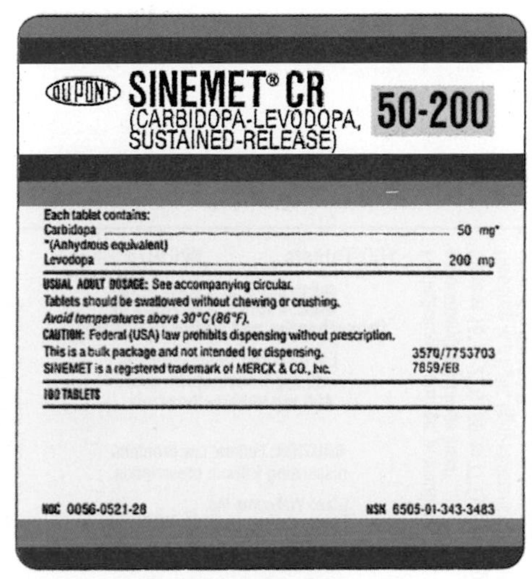

Figure 13-23 Sinemet® CR 50-200. CR indicates controlled release or sustained release tablet. The dosage strength of carbidopa is 50 mg, and that of levodopa is 200 mg.

Example 2: Percocet, which is used to treat moderate to severe pain, is a combination of oxycodone (narcotic pain reliever) and acetaminophen (non-narcotic pain reliever). The medication contains varying strengths of oxycodone (2.5 mg to 10 mg) and acetaminophen (325 mg to 650 mg). Orders for this medication must specify the dosage strength. Example: Percocet 2.5 mg/325 mg, 1-2 tabs p.o. q6h prn for pain.

Example 3: Septra, an antibacterial that is also manufactured under the trade name Bactrim, is a combination of trimethoprim and sulfamethoxazole. For example, a Septra tablet contains 80 mg of trimethoprim and 400 mg of sulfamethoxazole. A Septra DS (double-strength) tablet contains 160 mg of trimethoprim and 800 mg of sulfamethoxazole. See the labels for Septra in Figures 13-24 and 13-25.

Example 4: Tarka label. Note the different substances that are combined in each tablet and the ER (extended release following verapamil HCl) (Figure 13-27).

It is important to remember that some medications may not indicate their strength but are ordered by the number of tablets (e.g., multivitamin tablet 1 p.o. every day, Bactrim DS 1 tablet p.o. b.i.d.). This is because these medications are available in one strength only. This is also common with some medications that contain a combination of medications.

SAFETY ALERT!

The numbers following a medication name may be used to identify the dosage strengths of more than one medication in a preparation, and initials may be used to identify a special medication action. Read labels carefully to validate that you have the correct medication and dosage for combined medications.

Although tablets and capsules that contain more than one medication are often ordered by the brand name and number of tablets to be given (e.g., Septra DS 1 tab p.o. b.i.d.), the health care provider may order this medication by another route, for example, intravenous (IV). The injectable form, which is for IV infusion, is available in the generic name (see IV label in Figure 13-26). With the IV order, the nurse calculates the dosage to be given based on the strength of the trimethoprim. The nurse would learn such information described by using appropriate resources, such as a reference medication book (*Physician's Desk Reference [PDR]*), pharmacist, hospital formulary, and available information technology.

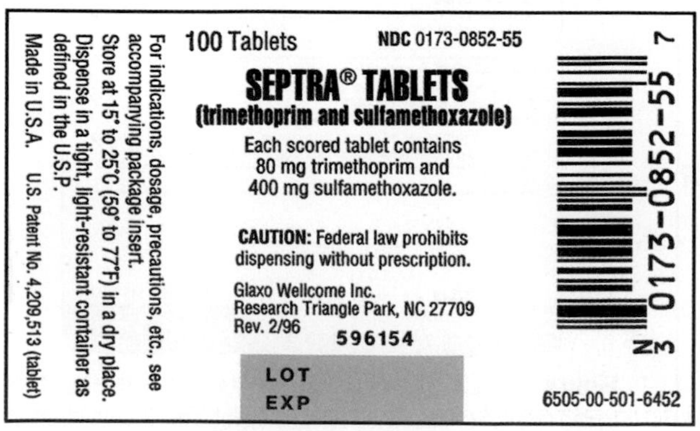

Figure 13-24 Septra label.

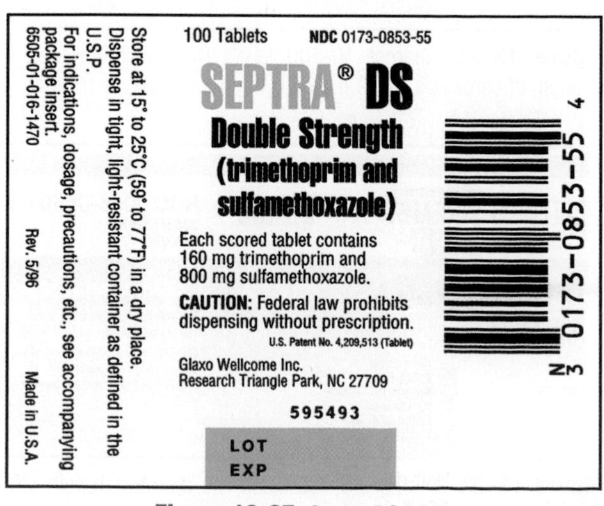

Figure 13-25 Septra DS label.

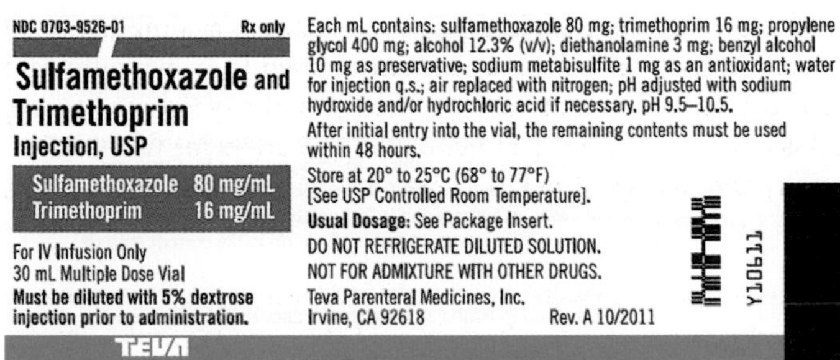

Figure 13-26 IV label for Sulfamethoxazole and Trimethoprim.

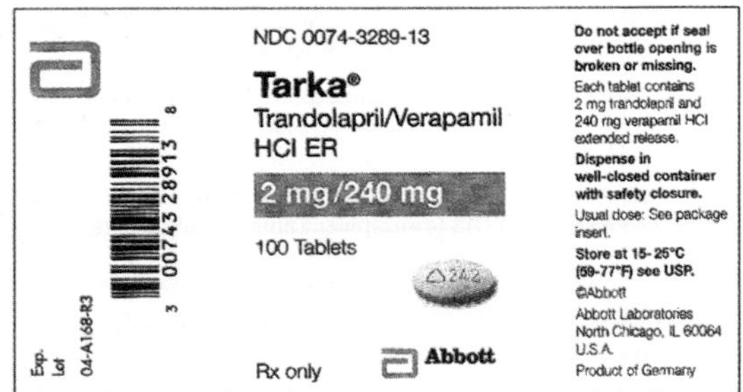

Figure 13-27 Tarka® label 2 mg/240 mg. The dosage strength of trandolapril is 2 mg, with 240 mg of verapamil HCl extended release.

Unit-Dose Packaging

Most medications administered in the hospital setting are available in unit dose. The pharmacy provides a 24-hour supply of each medication for the client. In unit dose, the medications will come to the unit in individually wrapped packets that are labeled for an individualized dosage for a specific client. The label on the package includes generic and trade names, manufacturer, lot number, and expiration date. Sometimes the package may only contain the generic name. The strength is indicated on the medication label. The nurse must read the label on unit-dose packages and note that sometimes, even with this method, calculation may be necessary. The pharmacy in some institutions provides the unit with a supply of medications available in multidose containers. These medications may be in unit-dose packaging but are used a great deal by the clients on the unit. Examples include Tylenol and aspirin. Some medications may also be dispensed in bottles—for example, 100 tablets of aspirin 325 mg.

Most hospital units have a combination of unit dose and multidose. However, multidose is rarely seen. Multidose packaging is the packaging of medications in containers that have more than one dose of the medication. The medications may be part of the floor stock. Tablets, capsules, powders, and liquid medications may be supplied in stock bottles for dispensing. Parenteral medications in liquid form or in powder that requires reconstitution may come in multidose vials. Figure 13-28 shows examples of unit-dose packaging.

Medication Information

To decrease errors and manage the risks of medications and adverse medication effects, the U.S. Food and Drug Administration (FDA) mandates the format in which medication information is provided on Prescription Medication Package Inserts. Since 2016, the FDA has mandated the new format for package inserts, which includes categories such as the highlights of prescribing information, boxed warning, recent major changes, indications and usage, and adverse reactions, which includes the following statement under the section, "To report SUSPECTED ADVERSE REACTIONS, Contact (Manufacturer) at (phone # and Web address) or FDA at 1-800-FDA-1088 or WWW.fda.gov/medwatch." See Figure 13-29, of an excerpt from the prescribing information for the medication Zyprexa (olanzapine).

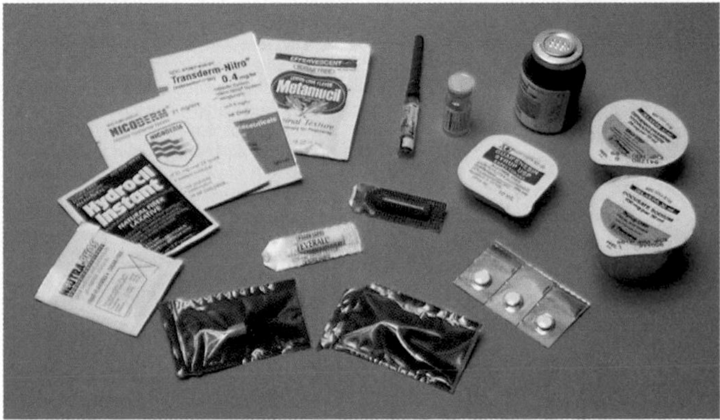

Figure 13-28 Unit-dose packages. (From Clayton BD and Willihnganz, M: *Basic pharmacology for nurses*, ed. 17, St Louis, 2017, Mosby.)

HIGHLIGHTS OF PRESCRIBING INFORMATION

These highlights do not include all the information needed to use ZYPREXA safely and effectively. See full prescribing information for ZYPREXA.

ZYPREXA (olanzapine) Tablet for Oral use
ZYPREXA ZYDIS (olanzapine) Tablet, Orally Disintegrating for Oral use
ZYPREXA IntraMuscular (olanzapine) Injection, Powder, For Solution for Intramuscular use

Initial U.S. Approval: 1996

WARNING: INCREASED MORTALITY IN ELDERLY PATIENTS WITH DEMENTIA-RELATED PSYCHOSIS

See full prescribing information for complete boxed warning.

- **Elderly patients with dementia-related psychosis treated with antipsychotic drugs are at an increased risk of death. ZYPREXA is not approved for the treatment of patients with dementia-related psychosis. (5.1, 5.14, 17.2)**
  When using ZYPREXA and fluoxetine in combination, also refer to the Boxed Warning section of the package insert for Symbyax.

RECENT MAJOR CHANGES

Indications and Usage:	
Schizophrenia (1.1)	12/2009
Bipolar I Disorder (Manic or Mixed Episodes) (1.2)	12/2009
Special Considerations in Treating Pediatric Schizophrenia and Bipolar I Disorder (1.3)	12/2009
ZYPREXA IntraMuscular: Agitation Associated with Schizophrenia and Bipolar I Mania (1.4)	12/2009
Dosage and Administration:	
Schizophrenia (2.1)	12/2009
Bipolar I Disorder (Manic or Mixed Episodes) (2.2)	12/2009
Warnings and Precautions:	
Orthostatic Hypotension (5.8)	05/2010
Leukopenia, Neutropenia, and Agranulocytosis (5.9)	08/2009
Hyperprolactinemia (5.15)	01/2010

INDICATIONS AND USAGE

ZYPREXA® (olanzapine) is an atypical antipsychotic indicated:

As oral formulation for the:

- Treatment of schizophrenia. (1.1)
  - Adults: Efficacy was established in three clinical trials in patients with schizophrenia: two 6-week trials and one maintenance trial. (14.1)
  - Adolescents (ages 13-17): Efficacy was established in one 6-week trial in patients with schizophrenia (14.1). The increased potential (in adolescents compared with adults) for weight gain and hyperlipidemia may lead clinicians to consider prescribing other drugs first in adolescents. (1.1)
- Acute treatment of manic or mixed episodes associated with bipolar I disorder and maintenance treatment of bipolar I disorder. (1.2)
  - Adults: Efficacy was established in three clinical trials in patients with manic or mixed episodes of bipolar I disorder: two 3- to 4-week trials and one maintenance trial. (14.2)
  - Adolescents (ages 13-17): Efficacy was established in one 3-week trial in patients with manic or mixed episodes associated with bipolar I disorder (14.2). The increased potential (in adolescents compared with adults) for weight gain and hyperlipidemia may lead clinicians to consider prescribing other drugs first in adolescents. (1.2)
- Medication therapy for pediatric patients with schizophrenia or bipolar I disorder should be undertaken only after a thorough diagnostic evaluation and with careful consideration of the potential risks. (1.3)
- Adjunct to valproate or lithium in the treatment of manic or mixed episodes associated with bipolar I disorder. (1.2)
  - Efficacy was established in two 6-week clinical trials in adults (14.2). Maintenance efficacy has not been systematically evaluated.

As ZYPREXA IntraMuscular for the:

- Treatment of acute agitation associated with schizophrenia and bipolar I mania. (1.4)
  - Efficacy was established in three 1-day trials in adults. (14.3)

As ZYPREXA and Fluoxetine in Combination for the:

- Treatment of depressive episodes associated with bipolar I disorder. (1.5)
  - Efficacy was established with Symbyax (olanzapine and fluoxetine in combination) in adults; refer to the product label for Symbyax.
- Treatment of treatment resistant depression (major depressive disorder in patients who do not respond to 2 separate trials of different antidepressants of adequate dose and duration in the current episode). (1.6)
  - Efficacy was established with Symbyax (olanzapine and fluoxetine in combination) in adults; refer to the product label for Symbyax.

DOSAGE AND ADMINISTRATION

Schizophrenia in adults (2.1)	Oral: Start at 5-10 mg once daily; Target: 10 mg/day within several days
Schizophrenia in adolescents (2.1)	Oral: Start at 2.5-5 mg once daily; Target: 10 mg/day
Bipolar I Disorder (manic or mixed episodes) in adults (2.2)	Oral: Start at 10 or 15 mg once daily
Bipolar I Disorder (manic or mixed episodes) in adolescents (2.2)	Oral: Start at 2.5-5 mg once daily; Target: 10 mg/day
Bipolar I Disorder (manic or mixed episodes) with lithium or valproate in adults (2.2)	Oral: Start at 10 mg once daily
Agitation associated with Schizophrenia and Bipolar I Mania in adults (2.4)	IM: 10 mg (5 mg or 7.5 mg when clinically warranted) Assess for orthostatic hypotension prior to subsequent dosing (max. 3 doses 2-4 hrs apart)
Depressive Episodes associated with Bipolar I Disorder in adults (2.5)	Oral in combination with fluoxetine: Start at 5 mg of oral olanzapine and 20 mg of fluoxetine once daily
Treatment Resistant Depression in adults (2.6)	Oral in combination with fluoxetine: Start at 5 mg of oral olanzapine and 20 mg of fluoxetine once daily

- Lower starting dose recommended in debilitated or pharmacodynamically sensitive patients or patients with predisposition to hypotensive reactions, or with potential for slowed metabolism. (2.1)
- Olanzapine may be given without regard to meals. (2.1)

ZYPREXA and Fluoxetine in Combination:

- Dosage adjustments, if indicated, should be made with the individual components according to efficacy and tolerability. (2.5, 2.6)
- Olanzapine monotherapy is not indicated for the treatment of depressive episodes associated with bipolar I disorder or treatment resistant depression. (2.5, 2.6)
- Safety of co-administration of doses above 18 mg olanzapine with 75 mg fluoxetine has not been evaluated. (2.5, 2.6)

DOSAGE FORMS AND STRENGTHS

- Tablets (not scored): 2.5, 5, 7.5, 10, 15, 20 mg (3)
- Orally Disintegrating Tablets (not scored): 5, 10, 15, 20 mg (3)
- Intramuscular Injection: 10 mg vial (3)

CONTRAINDICATIONS

- None with ZYPREXA monotherapy.
- When using ZYPREXA and fluoxetine in combination, also refer to the Contraindications section of the package insert for Symbyax®. (4)
- When using ZYPREXA in combination with lithium or valproate, refer to the Contraindications section of the package inserts for those products. (4)

WARNINGS AND PRECAUTIONS

- *Elderly Patients with Dementia-Related Psychosis:* Increased risk of death and increased incidence of cerebrovascular adverse events (e.g., stroke, transient ischemic attack). (5.1)
- *Suicide:* The possibility of a suicide attempt is inherent in schizophrenia and in bipolar I disorder, and close supervision of high-risk patients should accompany drug therapy; when using in combination with fluoxetine, also refer to the Boxed Warning and Warnings and Precautions sections of the package insert for Symbyax. (5.2)
- *Neuroleptic Malignant Syndrome:* Manage with immediate discontinuation and close monitoring. (5.3)

Figure 13-29 Prescribing information for Zyprexa.

- *Hyperglycemia:* In some cases extreme and associated with ketoacidosis or hyperosmolar coma or death, has been reported in patients taking olanzapine. Patients taking olanzapine should be monitored for symptoms of hyperglycemia and undergo fasting blood glucose testing at the beginning of, and periodically during, treatment. (5.4)
- *Hyperlipidemia:* Undesirable alterations in lipids have been observed. Appropriate clinical monitoring is recommended, including fasting blood lipid testing at the beginning of, and periodically during, treatment. (5.5)
- *Weight Gain:* Potential consequences of weight gain should be considered. Patients should receive regular monitoring of weight. (5.6)
- *Tardive Dyskinesia:* Discontinue if clinically appropriate. (5.7)
- *Orthostatic Hypotension:* Orthostatic hypotension associated with dizziness, tachycardia, bradycardia and, in some patients, syncope, may occur especially during initial dose titration. Use caution in patients with cardiovascular disease, cerebrovascular disease, and those conditions that could affect hemodynamic responses. (5.8)
- *Leukopenia, Neutropenia, and Agranulocytosis:* Has been reported with antipsychotics, including ZYPREXA. Patients with a history of a clinically significant low white blood cell count (WBC) or drug induced leukopenia/neutropenia should have their complete blood count (CBC) monitored frequently during the first few months of therapy and discontinuation of ZYPREXA should be considered at the first sign of a clinically significant decline in WBC in the absence of other causative factors. (5.9)
- *Seizures:* Use cautiously in patients with a history of seizures or with conditions that potentially lower the seizure threshold. (5.11)
- *Potential for Cognitive and Motor Impairment:* Has potential to impair judgment, thinking, and motor skills. Use caution when operating machinery. (5.12)
- *Hyperprolactinemia:* May elevate prolactin levels. (5.15)
- *Use in Combination with Fluoxetine, Lithium or Valproate:* Also refer to the package inserts for Symbyax, lithium, or valproate. (5.16)
- *Laboratory Tests:* Monitor fasting blood glucose and lipid profiles at the beginning of, and periodically during, treatment. (5.17)

---------------------------- ADVERSE REACTIONS ----------------------------

Most common adverse reactions (≥5% and at least twice that for placebo) associated with:

Oral Olanzapine Monotherapy:

- Schizophrenia (Adults) – postural hypotension, constipation, weight gain, dizziness, personality disorder, akathisia (6.1)
- Schizophrenia (Adolescents) – sedation, weight increased, headache, increased appetite, dizziness, abdominal pain, pain in extremity, fatigue, dry mouth (6.1)
- Manic or Mixed Episodes, Bipolar I Disorder (Adults) – asthenia, dry mouth, constipation, increased appetite, somnolence, dizziness, tremor (6.1)
- Manic or Mixed Episodes, Bipolar I Disorder (Adolescents) – sedation, weight increased, increased appetite, headache, fatigue, dizziness, dry mouth, abdominal pain, pain in extremity (6.1)

Combination of ZYPREXA and Lithium or Valproate:

- Manic or Mixed Episodes, Bipolar I Disorder (Adults) – dry mouth, weight gain, increased appetite, dizziness, back pain, constipation, speech disorder, increased salivation, amnesia, paresthesia (6.1)

ZYPREXA and Fluoxetine in Combination: Also refer to the Adverse Reactions section of the package insert for Symbyax. (6)

ZYPREXA IntraMuscular for Injection:

- Agitation with Schizophrenia and Bipolar I Mania (Adults) – somnolence (6.1)

To report SUSPECTED ADVERSE REACTIONS, contact Eli Lilly and Company at 1-800-LillyRx (1-800-545-5979) or FDA at 1-800-FDA-1088 or www.fda.gov/medwatch

---------------------------- DRUG INTERACTIONS ----------------------------

- *Diazepam:* May potentiate orthostatic hypotension. (7.1, 7.2)
- *Alcohol:* May potentiate orthostatic hypotension. (7.1)
- *Carbamazepine:* Increased clearance of olanzapine. (7.1)
- *Fluvoxamine:* May increase olanzapine levels. (7.1)
- *ZYPREXA and Fluoxetine in Combination:* Also refer to the Drug Interactions section of the package insert for Symbyax. (7.1)
- *CNS Acting Drugs:* Caution should be used when taken in combination with other centrally acting drugs and alcohol. (7.2)
- *Antihypertensive Agents:* Enhanced antihypertensive effect. (7.2)
- *Levodopa and Dopamine Agonists:* May antagonize levodopa/dopamine agonists. (7.2)
- *Lorazepam (IM):* Increased somnolence with IM olanzapine. (7.2)
- *Other Concomitant Drug Therapy:* When using olanzapine in combination with lithium or valproate, refer to the Drug Interactions sections of the package insert for those products. (7.2)

---------------------- USE IN SPECIFIC POPULATIONS ----------------------

- *Pregnancy:* ZYPREXA should be used during pregnancy only if the potential benefit justifies the potential risk to the fetus. (8.1)
- *Nursing Mothers:* Breast-feeding is not recommended. (8.3)
- *Pediatric Use:* Safety and effectiveness of ZYPREXA in children <13 years of age have not been established. (8.4)

See 17 for PATIENT COUNSELING INFORMATION and FDA-approved Medication Guide

Revised: 05/2010

Figure 13-29, cont'd

Over-the-Counter (OTC) Labels

Over-the-Counter (OTC) medicines are medications that a client can purchase without a prescription. The FDA requirements regarding the format for OTC include Medication Facts (the name of the medication and its purpose), uses of the medication, warnings, and directions of how to take the medication. The information is found on the packaging itself (see Figure 13-30, OTC label for Aleve). The OTC label is presented in a simpler format than the format for prescription medications.

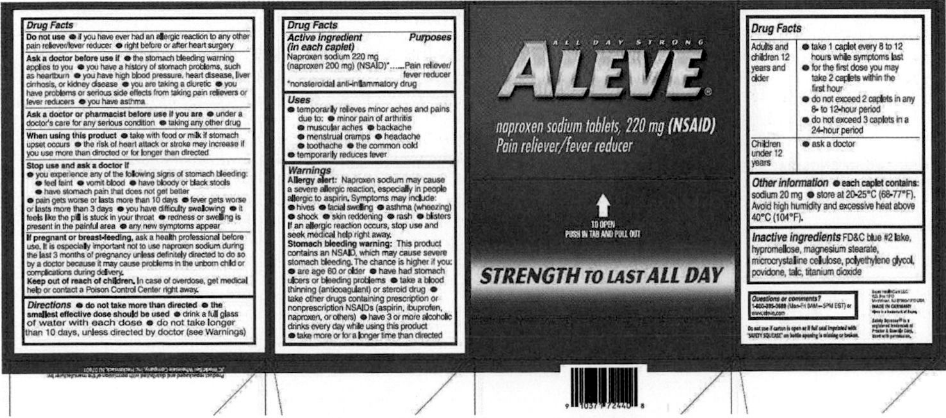

Figure 13-30 OTC label for Aleve.

The amount of information found on a medication label varies; however, some information is consistent on all labels and includes name of medication, dosage, amount in the package, manufacturer's name, expiration date, and lot/control number.

Clients should be encouraged to carefully read the information relating to medications they are taking. Prescription drug information is accessible on DailyMed, an interagency online health information clearinghouse created cooperatively by the FDA and the National Library of Medicine (NLM), available at http://dailymed.nlm.nih.gov. Clients should be made aware of this resource.

Let's examine some sample medication labels for review and identify some of the important information on labels.

1. In Figure 13-31, note the following:

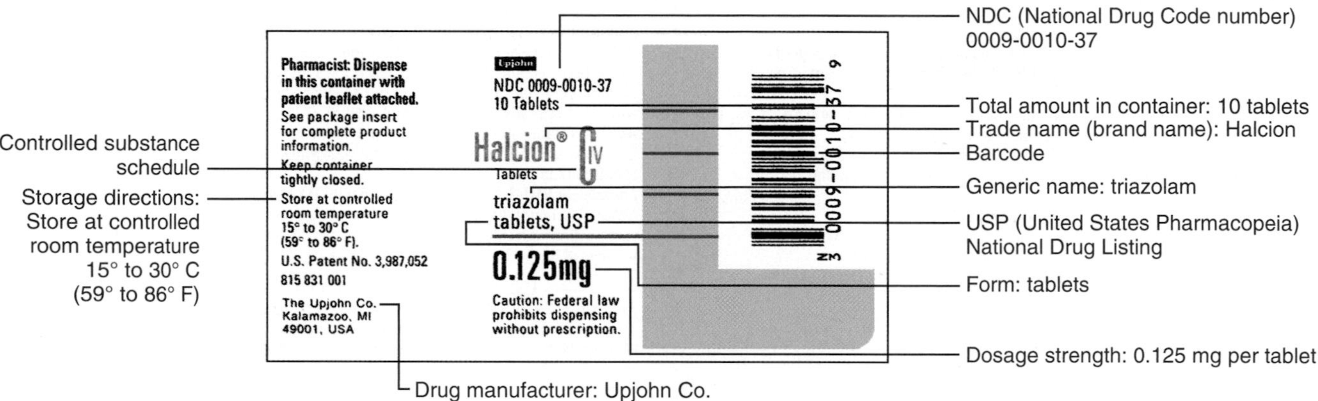

Figure 13-31 Halcion label.

2. In Figure 13-32, note the following:

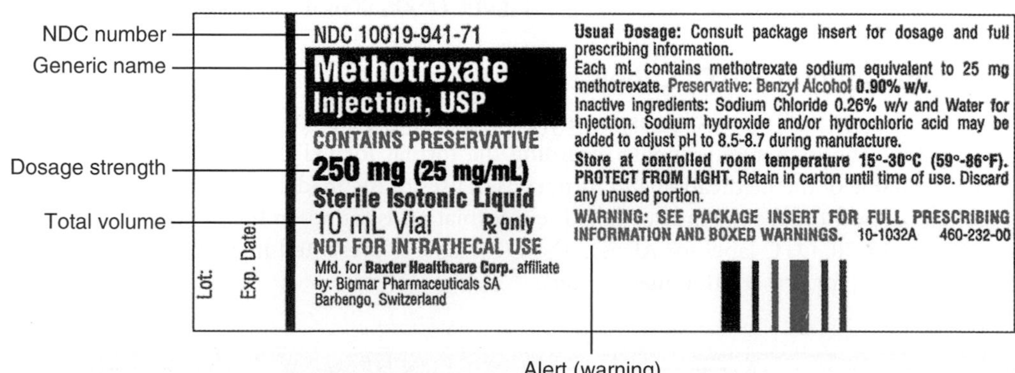

Figure 13-32 Methotrexate label. Injection is the route; injectable liquid is the form.

3. In Figure 13-33, note the following:

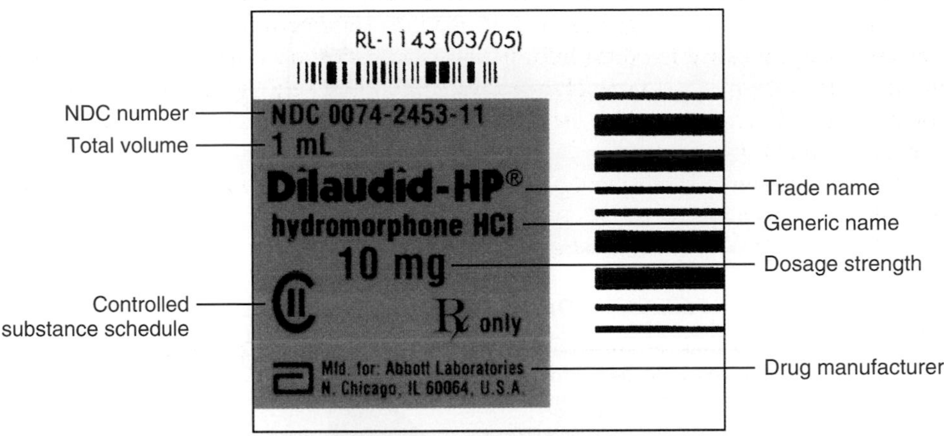

Figure 13-33 Dilaudid-HP (Dilaudid High Potency)

4. In Figure 13-34 note the following:

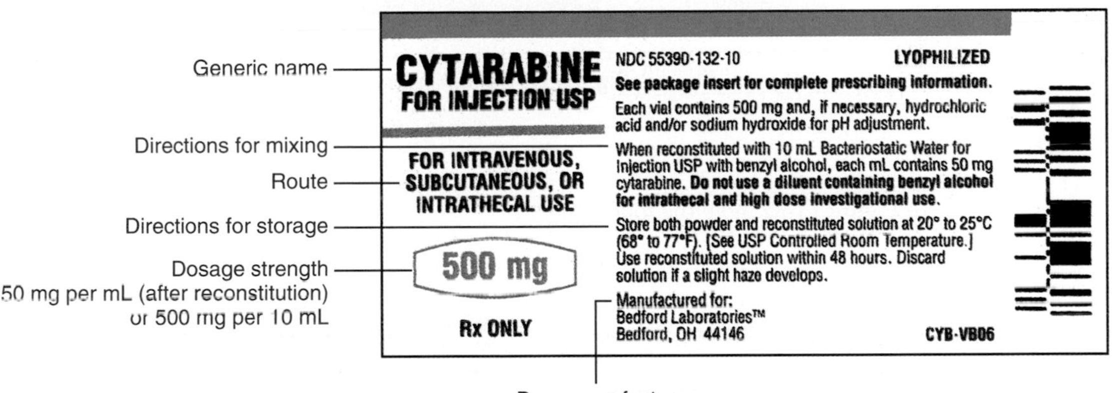

Figure 13-34 Cytarabine label. Form is powder; it must be diluted for use.

5. In Figure 13-35, note the following:

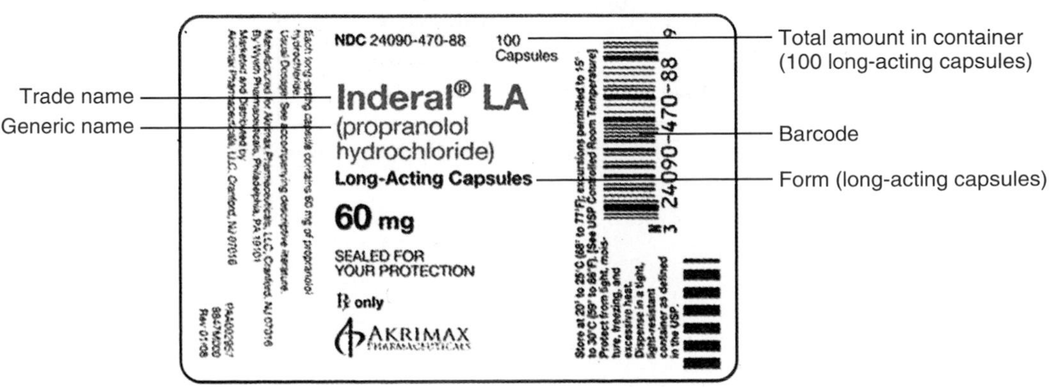

Figure 13-35 Inderal® LA label.

6. In Figure 13-36, note the following:

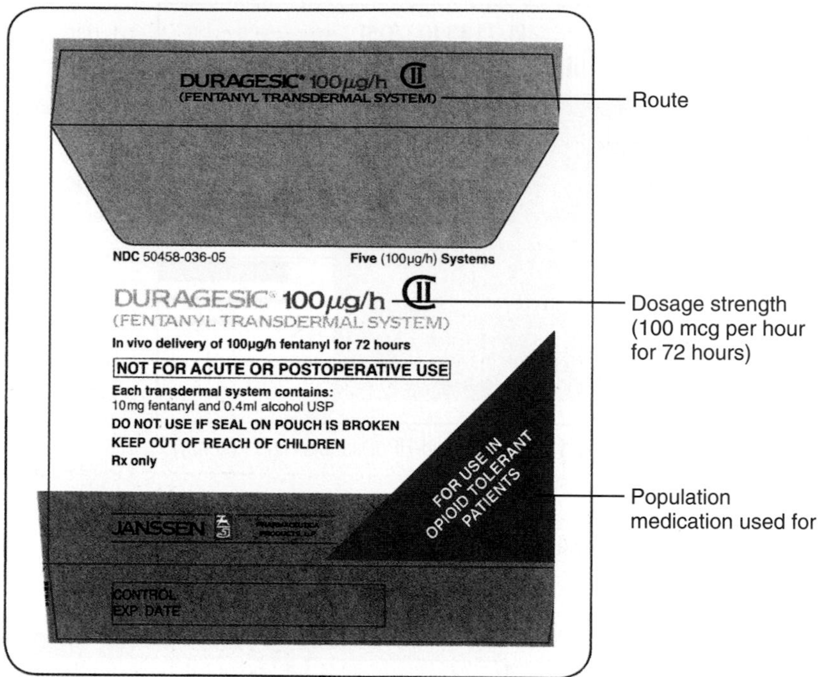

Figure 13-36 Duragesic label.

7. In Figure 13-37, note the following:

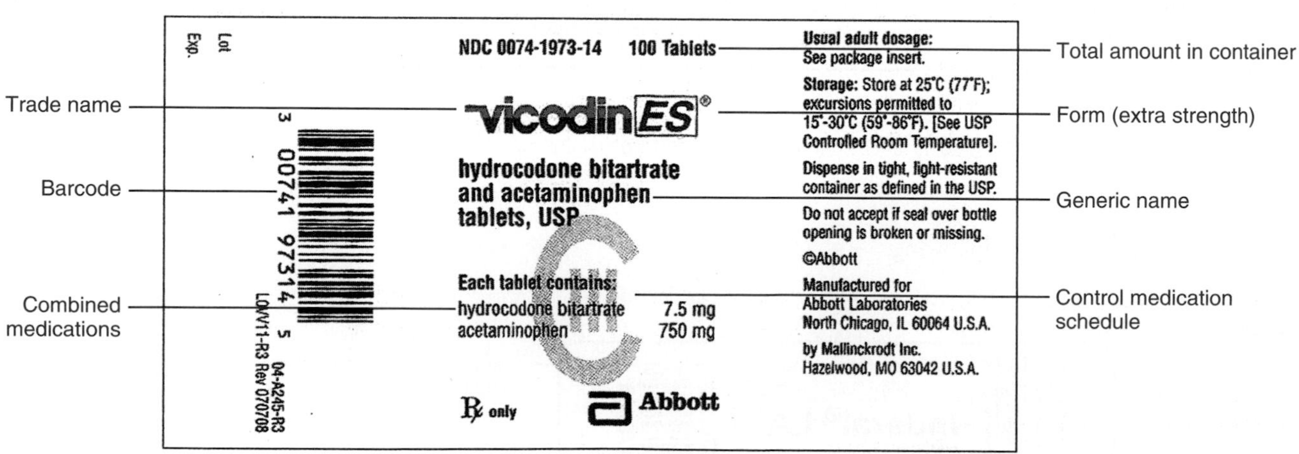

Figure 13-37 VicodinES. (Notice the initials ES next to the trade name to indicate a special form.)

8. In Figure 13-38, note the following:

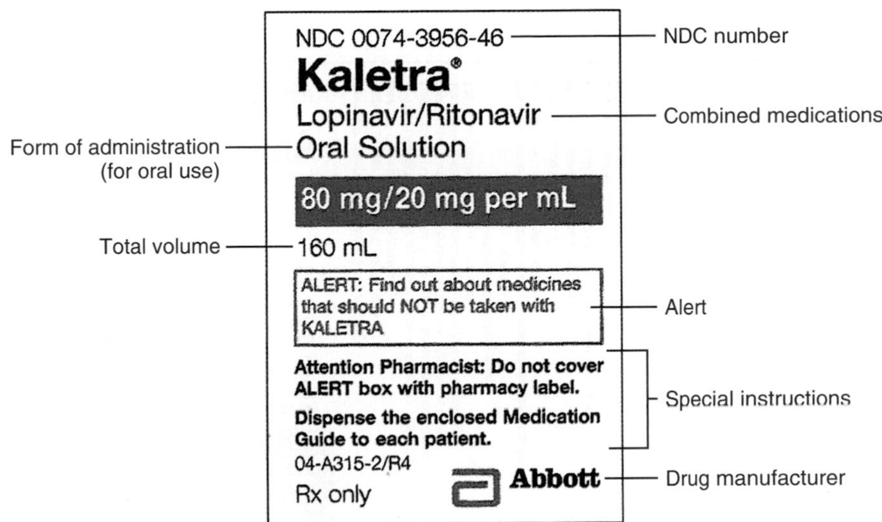

Figure 13-38 Kaletra label (combination medication: lopinavir 80 mg, ritonavir 20 mg).

POINTS TO REMEMBER

- Read medication labels three times.
- Identify directions for mixing when indicated.
- Read labels carefully, and do not confuse medication names; they are often deceptively similar. When in doubt, check appropriate resources, such as a reference book or the hospital pharmacist. Always cross-reference medication names to avoid administering the wrong medication.
- Read the label on combined medications carefully to ascertain whether you are administering the correct medication dosage.
- Extra abbreviations or initials after a medication name may identify additional medications in the preparation or a special action.
- Read labels carefully to identify trade and generic names, dosage strength, form, total amount in container, total volume, and route of administration.
- Do not confuse special forms such as SR (sustained release) and XL (extended release) with USP and NF official listing for medications.
- Read directions relating to storage.
- Carefully read alerts on medication labels.
- Do not administer expired medications.
- Controlled medication labels indicate the potential for abuse and are ranked Schedule I to Schedule V.
- When writing dosages, ISMP recommends using *per* instead of a slash (/) because of misinterpretation and being mistaken as the number *1*.
- Administering the incorrect form of a medication is a medication error.
- Be certain that you administer the right medication.

PRACTICE **PROBLEMS**

Use the labels to identify the information requested.

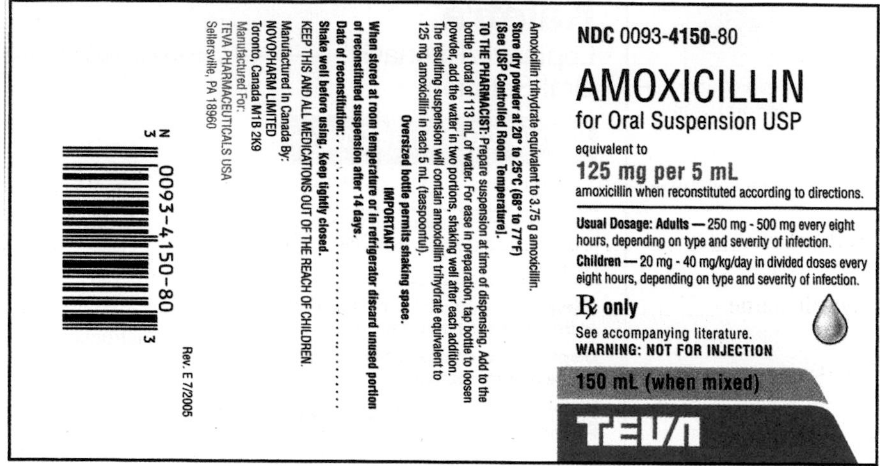

1. Trade name ____________________ Dosage strength when reconstituted ____________________

   Generic name ____________________

   Form ____________________ Total volume when mixed ____________________

   Warning ____________________

RANBAXY
CIV
NDC 63304-553-30
CLORAZEPATE DIPOTASSIUM
Tablets, USP
7.5 mg
PHARMACIST: Dispense the accompanying Medication Guide to each patient*
Rx only 30 Tablets

Each tablet contains 7.5 mg clorazepate dipotassium, USP.
USUAL DOSAGE: See package insert for full prescribing information.
Store at 20 - 25° C (68 - 77° F) [See USP Controlled Room Temperature].
Protect from moisture.
Keep bottle tightly closed.
Dispense in a USP tight, light-resistant container.
Do not accept if seal over bottle opening is broken or missing.
*To obtain the Medication Guide online please visit www.ranbaxyusa.com.

Manufactured for:
Ranbaxy Pharmaceuticals Inc.
Jacksonville, FL 32257 USA
by: Ohm Laboratories Inc.
North Brunswick, NJ 08902 USA

non varnish area
LOT:
EXP:

2. Trade name ____________________ Total amount in container __________

   Generic name ____________________ Controlled substance schedule ______

   Form ____________________ Pharmacist directions ______________

   Dosage strength ____________________

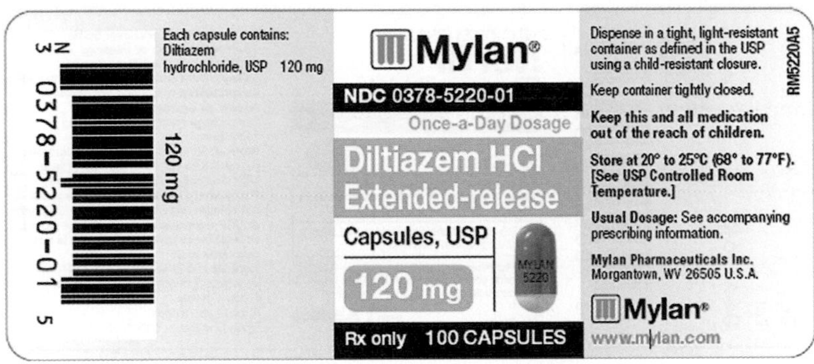

Each capsule contains:
Diltiazem hydrochloride, USP 120 mg
120 mg
N 3 0378-5220-01 5
Mylan®
NDC 0378-5220-01
Once-a-Day Dosage
Diltiazem HCl
Extended-release
Capsules, USP
120 mg
MYLAN 5220
Rx only 100 CAPSULES
Dispense in a tight, light-resistant container as defined in the USP using a child-resistant closure.
Keep container tightly closed.
Keep this and all medication out of the reach of children.
Store at 20° to 25°C (68° to 77°F). [See USP Controlled Room Temperature.]
Usual Dosage: See accompanying prescribing information.
Mylan Pharmaceuticals Inc. Morgantown, WV 26505 U.S.A.
Mylan®
www.mylan.com
RM5220A5

3. Trade name ____________ Dosage strength ____________

Generic name ____________ Total amount in container ________

Form ____________

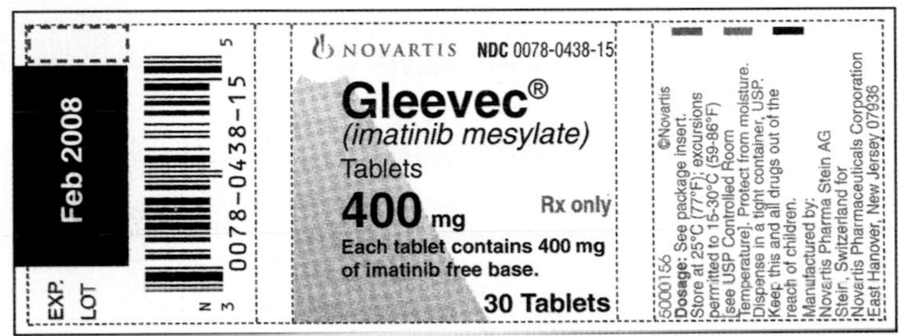

4. Trade name ____________ Dosage strength ____________

Generic name ____________ Total amount in container ________

Storage ____________

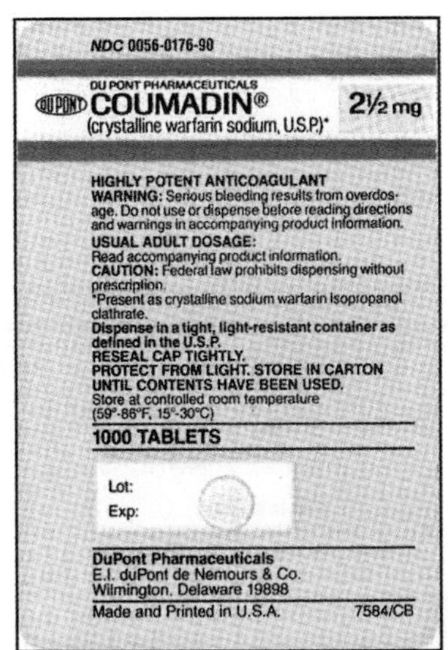

5. Trade name ____________ Form ____________

Dosage strength ____________ NDC number ____________

Total amount in container ________

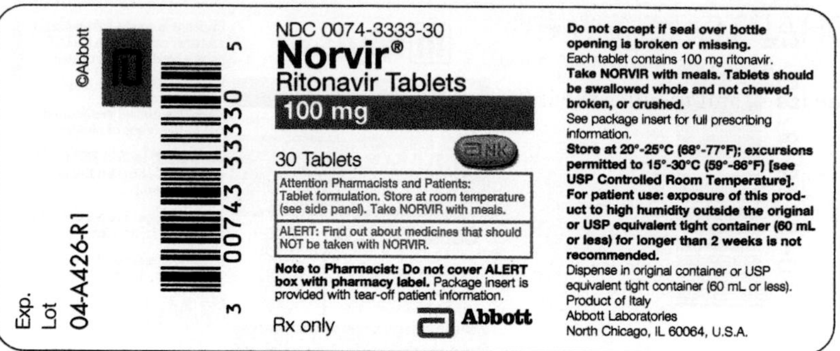

6. Trade name ____________ Total amount in container ________

Generic name ____________ Can this medication be crushed? ____

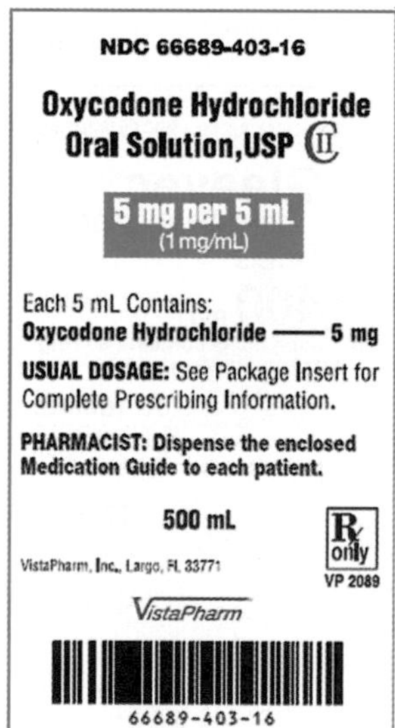

7. Generic name ____________ Total volume ____________

Form ____________ Usual dosage ____________

Dosage strength ____________

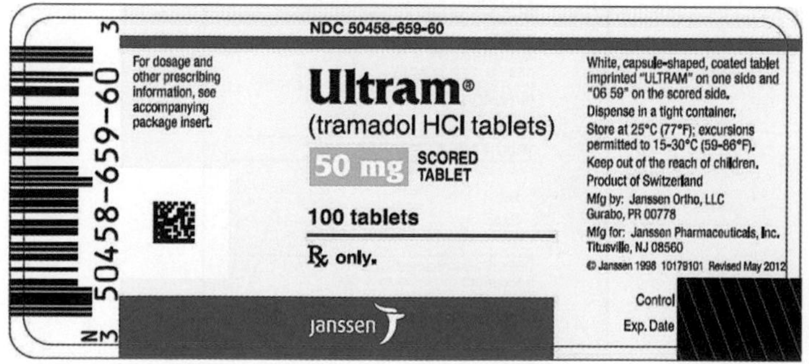

8. Trade name ____________ Dosage strength ____________

Generic name ____________ Total amount in container ________

Answers on pp. 215-216

CHAPTER REVIEW

Read the label, and identify the information requested.

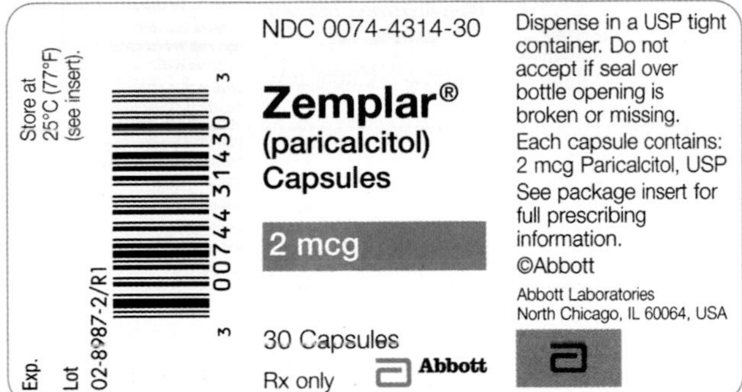

1. Trade name ______________ Form ______________

   Generic name ______________ Dosage strength ______________

   Total amount in container ______________

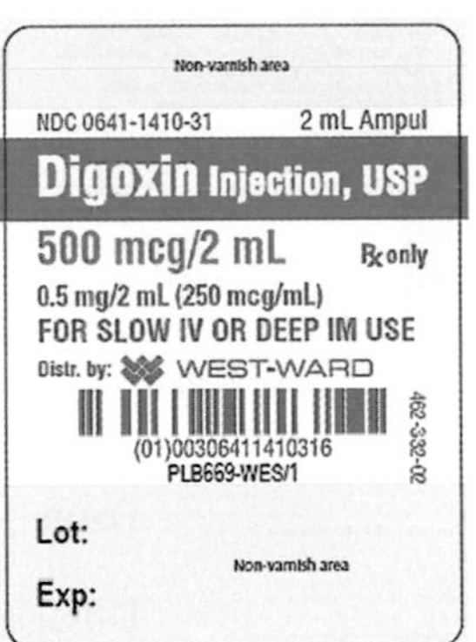

2. Trade name ______________ Form ______________

   Generic name ______________ Dosage strength ______________

   NDC number ______________

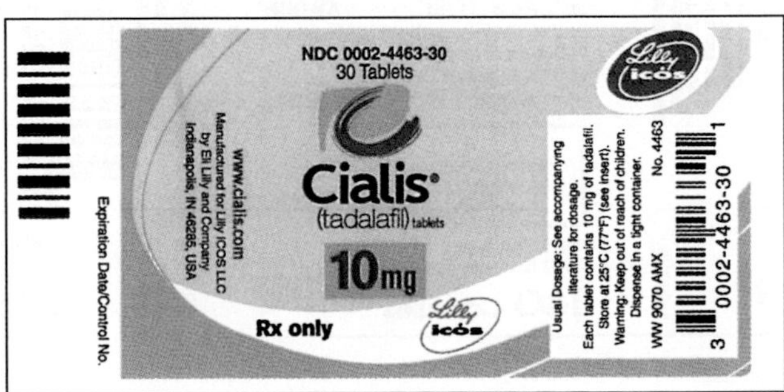

3. Trade name ______________ Form ______________

   Generic name ______________ Dosage strength ______________

   Storage ______________ Total amount in container ______________

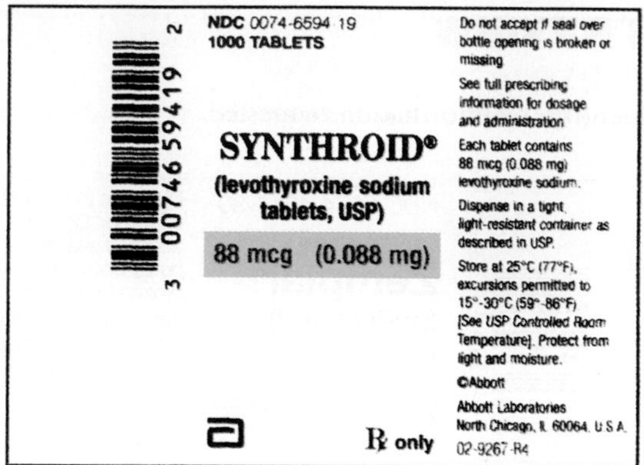

4. Trade name ____________ Form ____________

Generic name ____________ Dosage strength ____________

Total amount in container ________

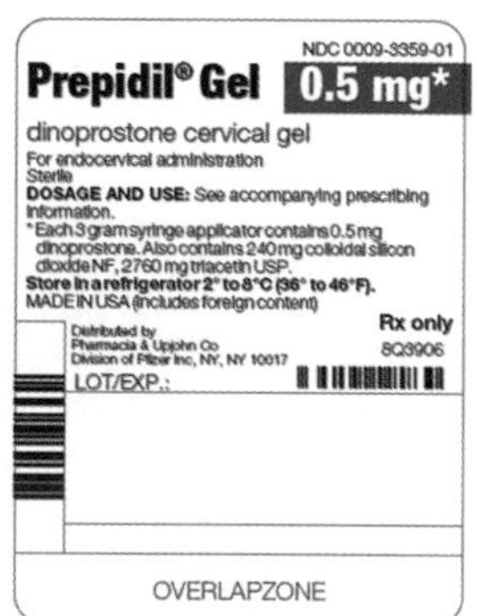

5. Trade name ____________ Form ____________

Generic name ____________ Dosage strength ____________

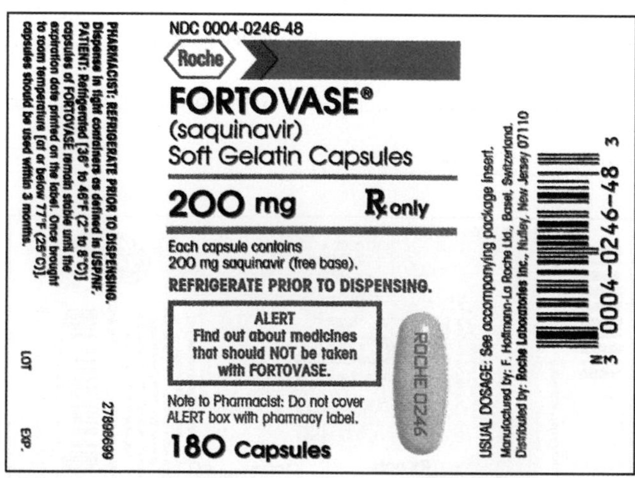

6. Trade name ____________ Form ____________

Generic name ____________ Dosage strength ____________

Usual dosage ____________ Total amount in container ________

Alert ____________

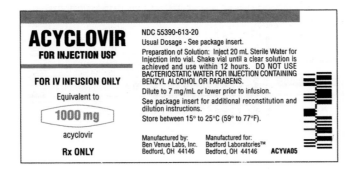

7. Trade name ____________________ Dosage strength after reconstitution

   Generic name ____________________ ____________________

   Form ____________________ Directions for use ____________________

   Directions for mixing ____________________

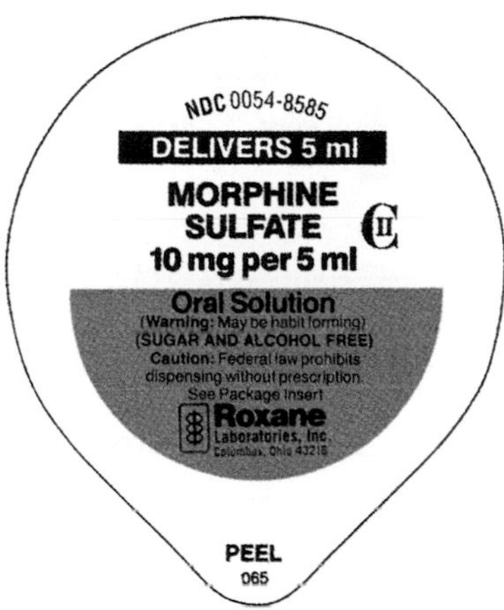

8. Generic name ____________________ Form ____________________

   NDC number ____________________ Dosage strength ____________________

   Total volume ____________________ Warning ____________________

   Controlled substance schedule ______

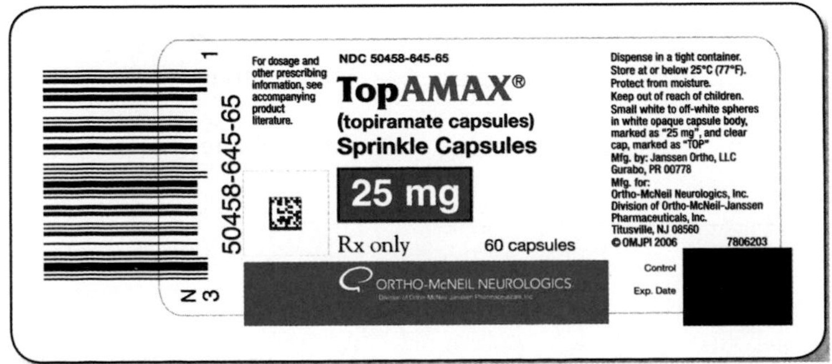

9. Trade name ____________________ Form ____________________

   Generic name ____________________ Dosage strength ____________________

   Total amount in container __________

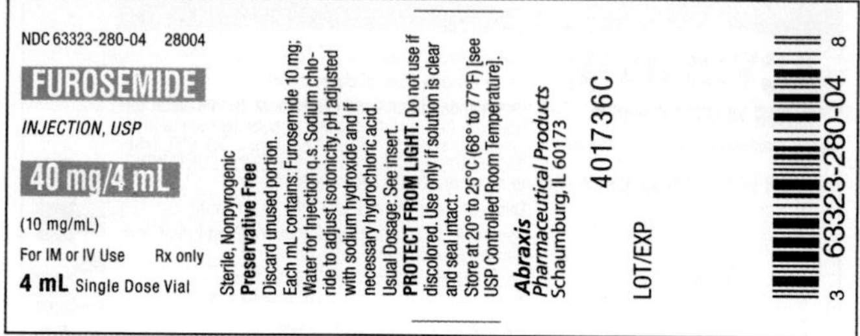

10. Generic name ____________ Form ____________

Dosage strength ____________ Total volume ____________

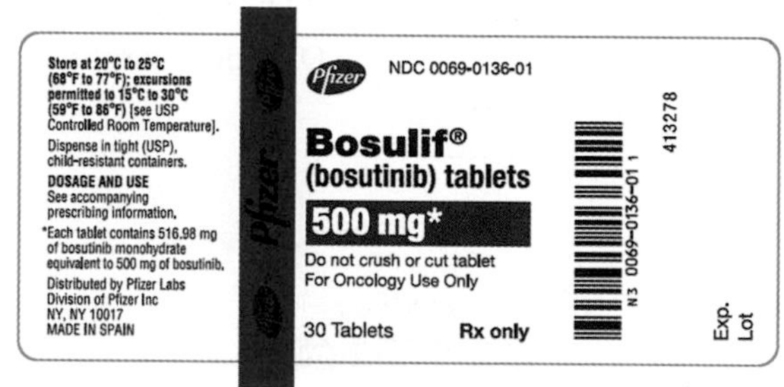

11. Trade name ____________ Form ____________

Generic name ____________ Dosage strength ____________

Total amount in container ____________ Directions for use ____________

Administration directions ____________

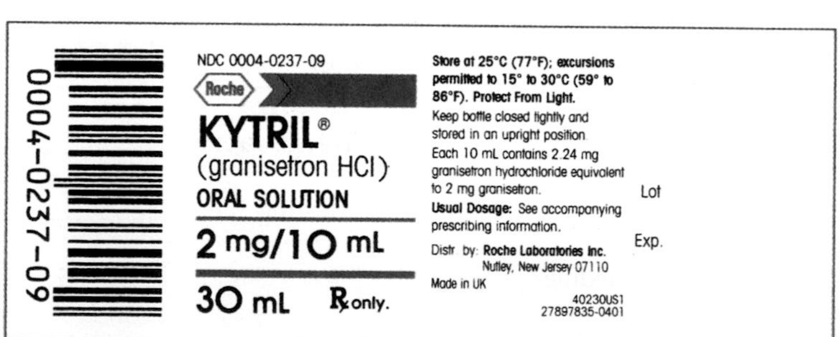

12. Trade name ____________ Dosage strength ____________

Generic name ____________ Total volume ____________

Form ____________

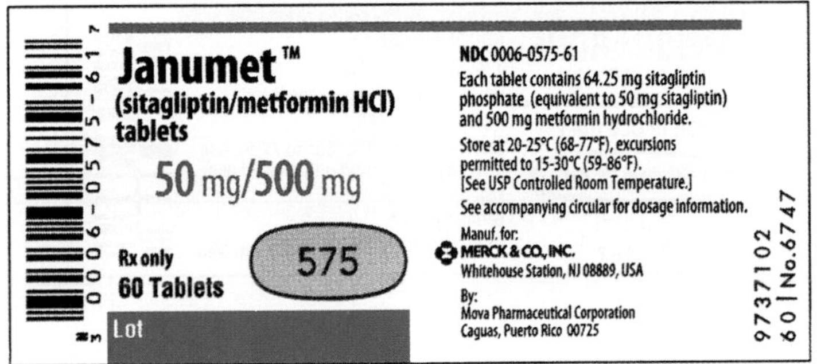

13. Trade name ____________________ Dosage strength ____________________

Generic name ____________________ NDC number ____________________

Form ____________________

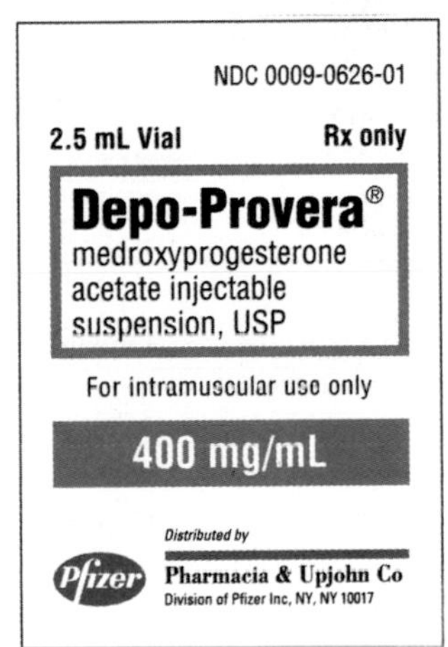

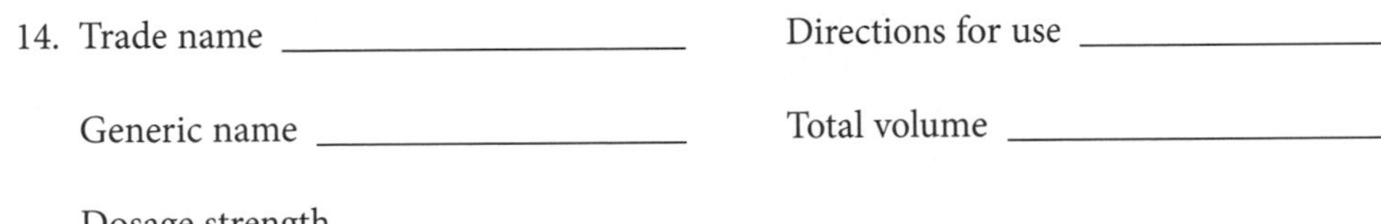

14. Trade name ____________________ Directions for use ____________________

Generic name ____________________ Total volume ____________________

Dosage strength ____________________

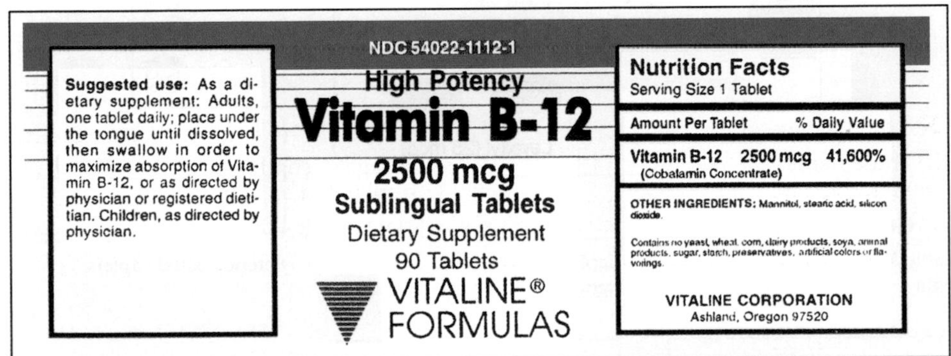

15. Total amount in container ____________ Dosage strength ____________________

Form ____________________ Suggested use ____________________

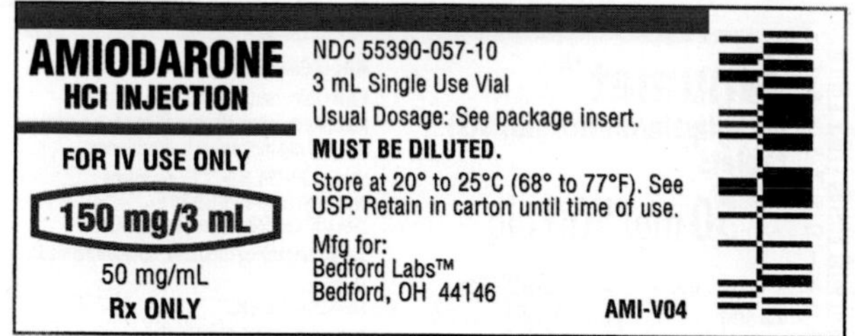

16. Generic name ____________ Usual dosage ____________

Form ____________ Dosage strength ____________

Directions for use ____________ Total volume ____________

Hydromorphone Hydrochloride Injection, USP 2 mg/mL

Warning: May be habit forming.

For IM, SC, or Slow IV Use.

Caution: Federal law prohibits dispensing without prescription.

ASTRA®
Astra Pharmaceutical Products, Inc.
Westborough, MA 01581

NDC 0186-1309-01
20 mL Multiple Dose Vial
Each mL contains: 2 mg hydromorphone hydrochloride (Warning: May be habit forming), 0.5 mg edetate disodium, 1.8 mg methylparaben, 0.2 mg propylparaben, and sodium hydroxide or hydrochloric acid to adjust pH. Filled under nitrogen. See package insert for prescribing information. Store at 15°–30°C (59°–86°F). **Protect from light.** Store in carton until time of use.
071212R01

APPROXIMATE VOLUME (mL) 20 15 10 5

17. Trade name ____________ Dosage strength ____________

Generic name ____________ Total volume ____________

Directions for use ____________ Warning ____________

Form ____________

Zocor® 40 mg
(Simvastatin)

Manuf. for:
MERCK & CO., INC.
Whitehouse Station, NJ 08889, USA
By: MERCK SHARP & DOHME LTD.
Cramlington, Northumberland, UK NE23 3JU
Formulated in UK

Each tablet contains 40 mg of simvastatin.

MSD 749

90 Tablets

Lot

N 3 0006-0749-54 4

NDC 0006-0749-54

USUAL ADULT DOSAGE:
See accompanying circular.

Store between 5-30°C (41-86°F).

Rx only

9782900
90| No.8148

18. Trade name ____________ Dosage strength ____________

Generic name ____________ NDC number ____________

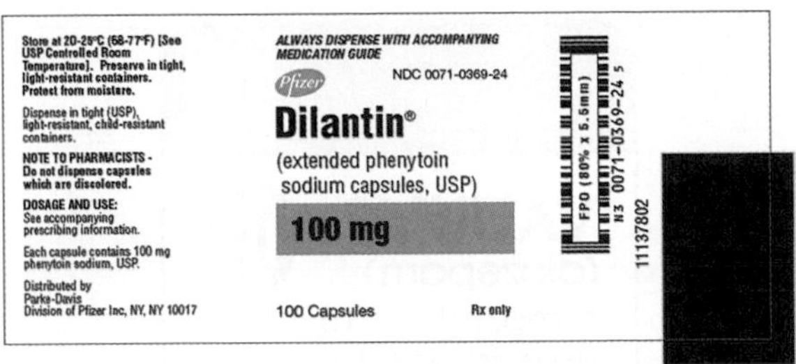

19. Generic name ____________ Dosage strength ____________

Form ____________ Total amount in container ____________

NDC number ____________ Dosage and use ____________

Instructions for dispensing ____________

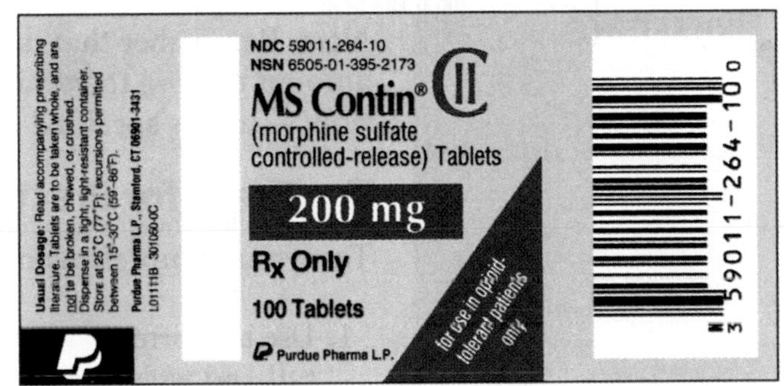

20. Trade name ____________ Total amount in container ____________

Generic name ____________ Controlled substance schedule ____________

Form ____________ Directions for use ____________

Dosage strength ____________

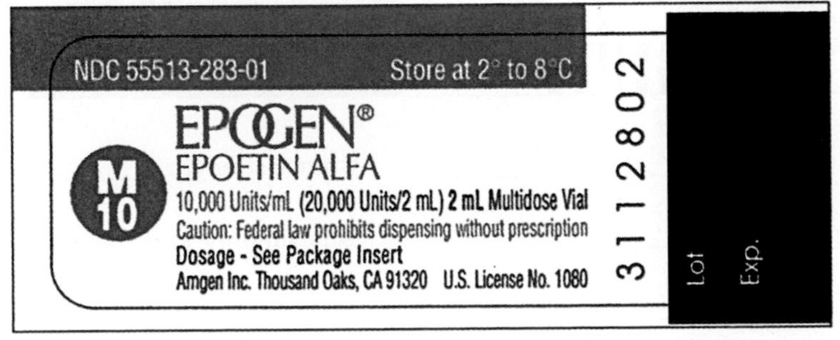

21. Trade name ____________ Total volume ____________

Generic name ____________ Dosage strength ____________

Storage information ____________

Roche Laboratories Inc.
Nutley, New Jersey 07110

VALIUM® CIV
(diazepam)
5 mg/mL 10 mL Vial
Sterile. For I.M. or I.V. Use.
Each mL contains 5 mg diazepam compounded with 40% propylene glycol, 10% ethyl alcohol; 5% sodium benzoate and benzoic acid as buffers; and 1.5% benzyl alcohol as preservative.
NOTE: Solution may appear colorless to light yellow.
℞ only.
STORE AT 59° TO 86° F (15° TO 30° C).
EXPIRES
25402082-0199

22. Trade name ____________________ Total volume ____________________

Generic name ____________________ Controlled substance schedule ______

Dosage strength ____________________

NDC 0093-7212-01
METFORMIN HYDROCHLORIDE Extended-release Tablets
750 mg
Each extended-release tablet contains:
Metformin Hydrochloride 750 mg
℞ only
100 TABLETS
TEVA

Usual Dosage: See package insert for full prescribing information.
Store at 20° to 25°C (68° to 77°F) [See USP Controlled Room Temperature].
Dispense in a tight, light-resistant container as defined in the USP, with a child-resistant closure (as required).
KEEP THIS AND ALL MEDICATIONS OUT OF THE REACH OF CHILDREN. Iss. 10/2004
Manufactured In Israel By:
TEVA PHARMACEUTICAL IND. LTD.
Jerusalem, 91010, Israel
Manufactured For:
TEVA PHARMACEUTICALS USA
Sellersville, PA 18960
323K214000105
N 3 0093-7212-01 0

23. Trade name ____________________ Dosage strength ____________________

Generic name ____________________ Total amount in container __________

Form ____________________

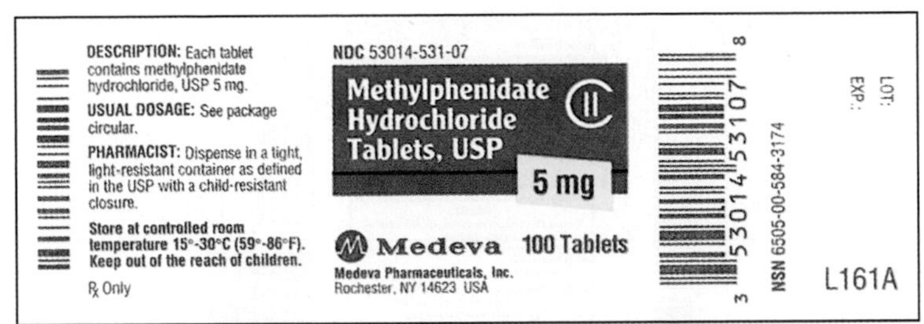

24. Generic name ______________ Dosage strength ______________

Instructions to pharmacist ______________

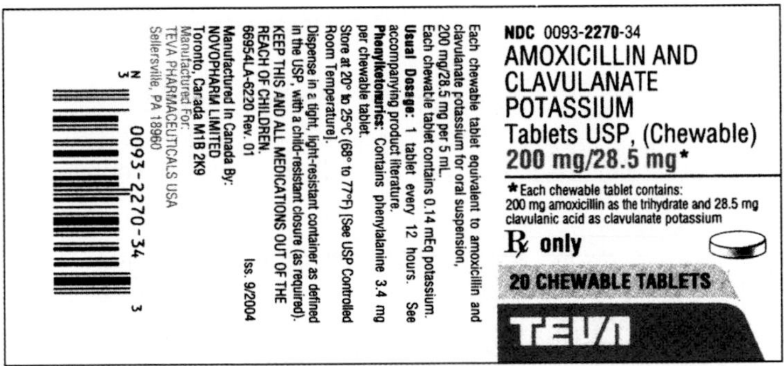

25. Generic name ______________ Form ______________

Dosage strength ______________ Total amount in container ______________

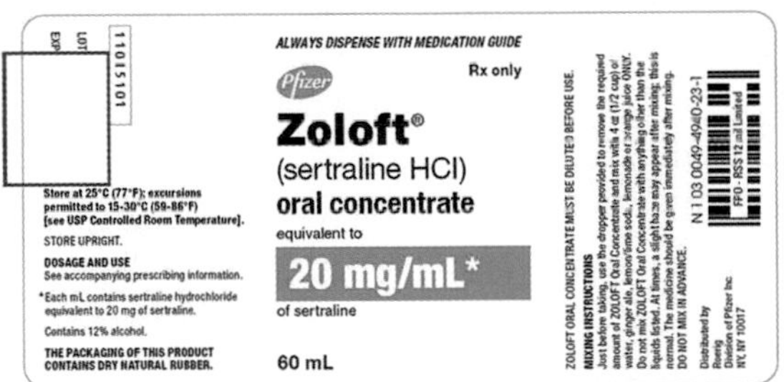

26. Generic name ______________ Directions for dispensing ______________

Form ______________ Total volume ______________

Dosage strength ______________

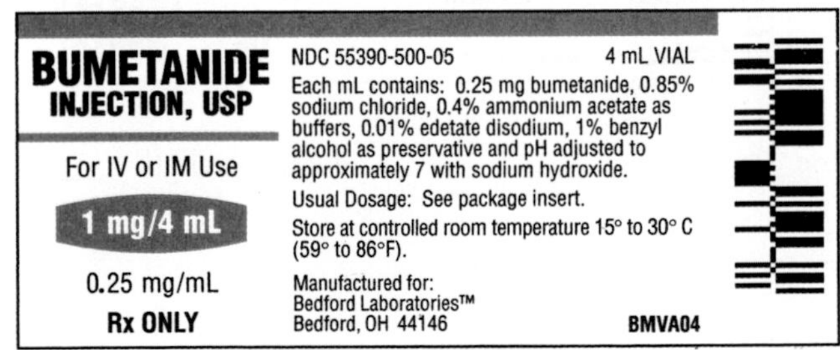

27. Generic name ______________ Dosage strength ______________

Form ______________ Directions for use ______________

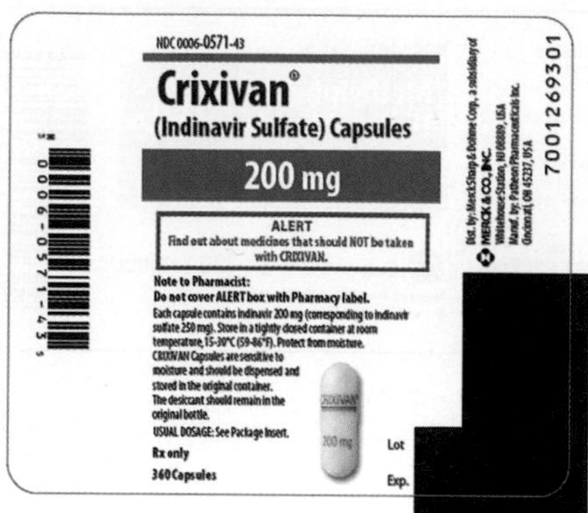

28. Trade name ____________ Dosage strength ____________

Generic name ____________ Alert ____________

Form ____________ Total amount in container ________

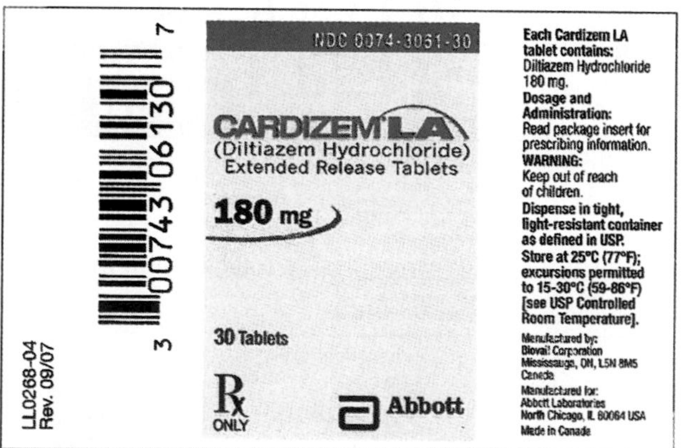

29. Trade name ____________ Dosage strength ____________

Generic name ____________ Total amount in container ________

Form ____________

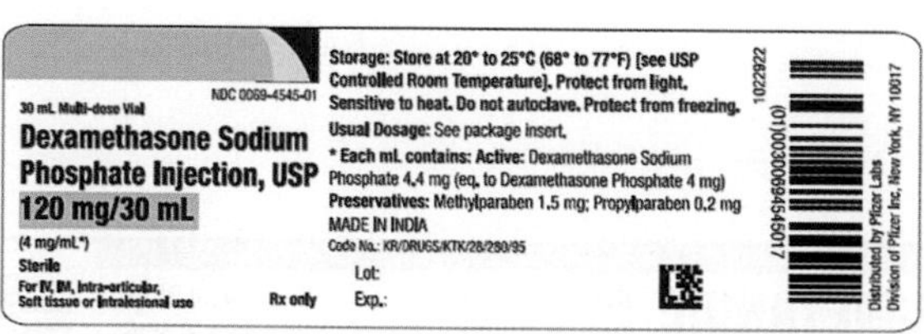

30. Generic name ____________ Dosage strength ____________

Form ____________

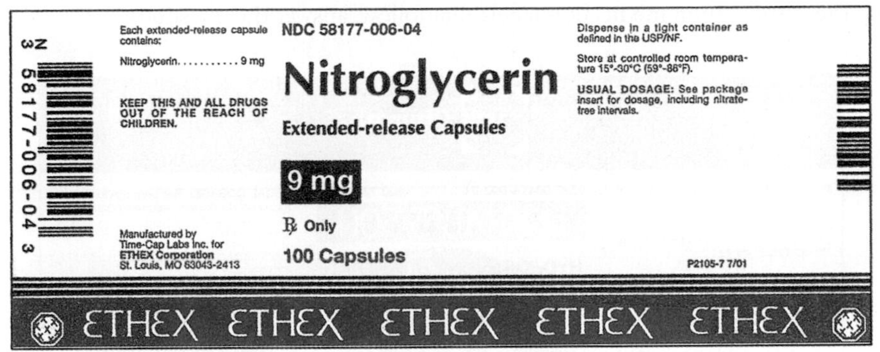

31. Trade name ____________________ Form ____________________

Generic name ____________________ Dosage strength ____________________

Storage information ____

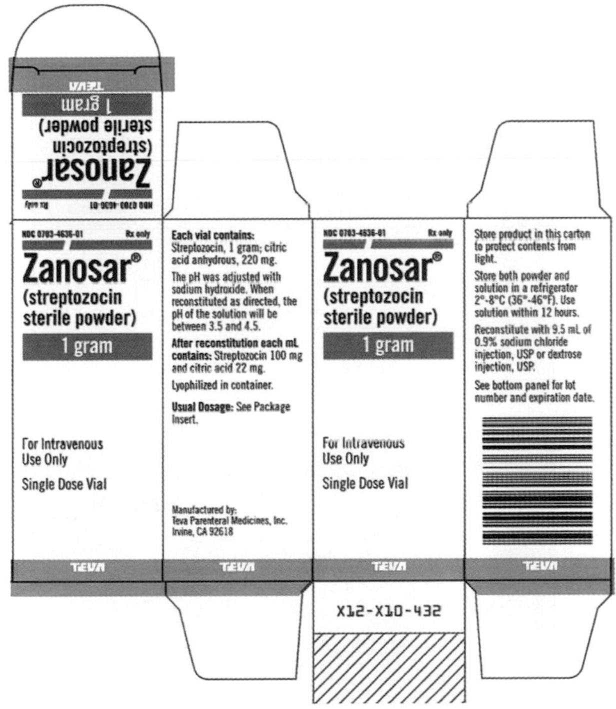

32. Trade name ____________________ Form ____________________

Generic name ____________________ Direction for use ____________________

Using the combination medication labels that follow, answer the questions:

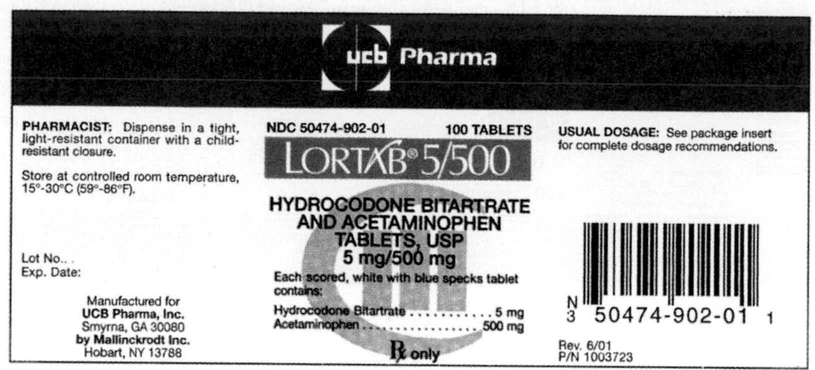

33. The route of administration for this medication would be ______________________.

34. This medication contains ________ mg of hydrocodone bitartrate and ________ mg of acetaminophen.

35. The total amount in the container is ______________________________.

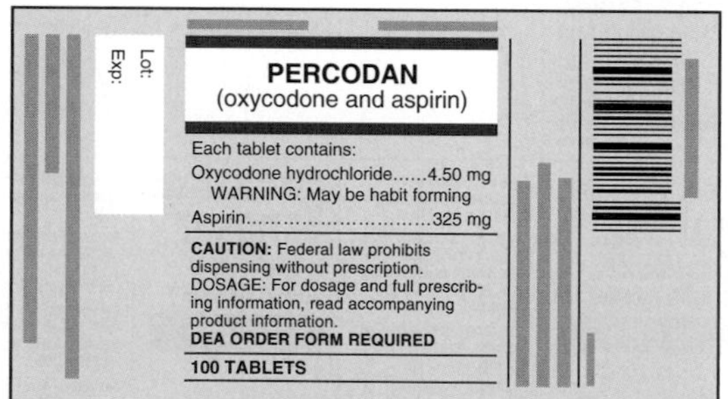

A

Lot:
Exp:
PERCOCET
(oxycodone and acetaminophen)
Each tablet contains:
Oxycodone hydrochloride.........5 mg
WARNING: May be habit forming
Acetaminophen.................325 mg
CAUTION: Federal law prohibits dispensing without prescription.
DOSAGE: For dosage and full prescribing information, read accompanying product information.
DEA ORDER FORM REQUIRED
100 TABLETS

B

36. The prescriber ordered Percocet 1 tab p.o. q4h p.r.n. for pain. The nurse would use which of the medications above to administer the dosage? ________________

37. The difference between the medications Percodan and Percocet is that Percodan contains ________ mg of oxycodone hydrochloride and ________ mg of aspirin. Percocet contains ________mg of oxycodone hydrochloride and ________ mg of acetaminophen.

38. If a client is allergic to aspirin, which medication should the client not be given?

____

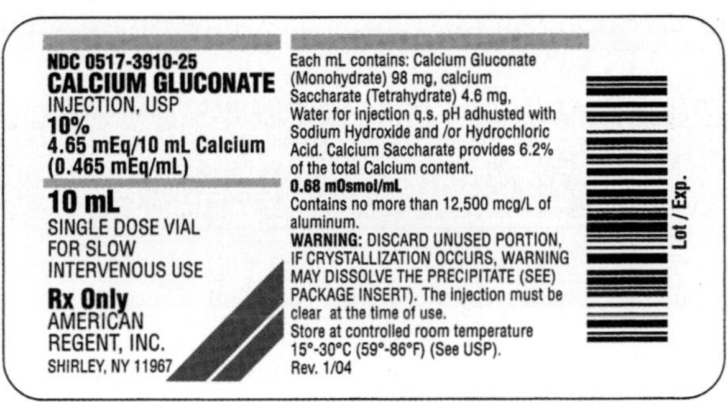

39. The dosage strength of this medication expressed as a percentage is _____________.

40. The dosage strength of this medication in milliequivalents per milliliter is ________.

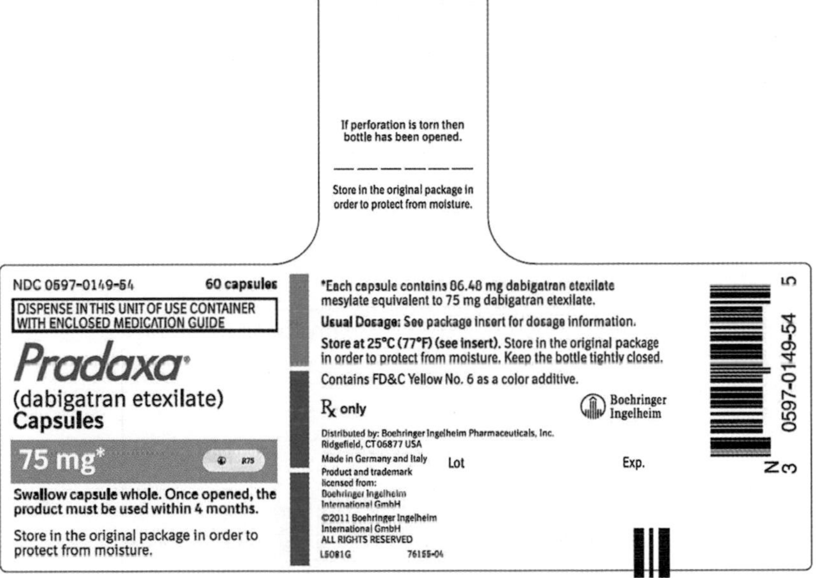

If perforation is torn then bottle has been opened.
Store in the original package in order to protect from moisture.
NDC 0597-0149-54
60 capsules
DISPENSE IN THIS UNIT OF USE CONTAINER WITH ENCLOSED MEDICATION GUIDE
Pradaxa®
(dabigatran etexilate)
Capsules
75 mg*
Swallow capsule whole. Once opened, the product must be used within 4 months.
Store in the original package in order to protect from moisture.
*Each capsule contains 86.48 mg dabigatran etexilate mesylate equivalent to 75 mg dabigatran etexilate.
Usual Dosage: See package insert for dosage information.
Store at 25°C (77°F) (see insert). Store in the original package in order to protect from moisture. Keep the bottle tightly closed.
Contains FD&C Yellow No. 6 as a color additive.
℞ only
Boehringer Ingelheim
Distributed by: Boehringer Ingelheim Pharmaceuticals, Inc. Ridgefield, CT 06877 USA
Made in Germany and Italy
Product and trademark licensed from: Boehringer Ingelheim International GmbH
©2011 Boehringer Ingelheim International GmbH
ALL RIGHTS RESERVED
Lot
Exp.
N 3 0597-0149-54 5

41. Trade name ____________________ Form _________________________

Generic name ____________________

How long can the medication be stored after opening? ____________________

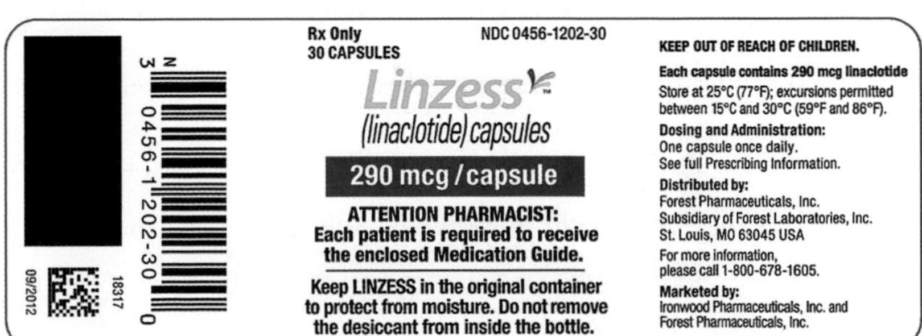

42. Trade name ____________________ Form _________________________

Generic name ____________________ Dosage strength __________________

Can the capsules be placed in another container? ____________________

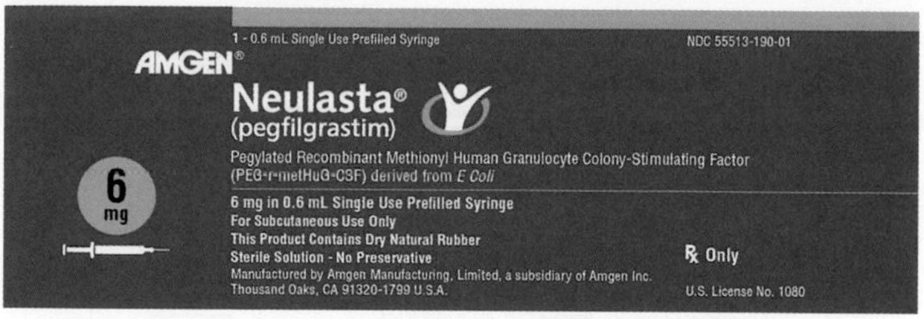

43. Trade name ____________ Dosage strength ____________

Generic name ____________ Directions for use ____________

Does this medication require you to draw it up in a syringe to administer? ________

Each tablet contains 300 mg canagliflozin.
NDC 50458-141-30 30 tablets
Invokana®
(canagliflozin)
Tablets 300 mg
Dispense with Medication Guide
300
© Janssen Pharmaceuticals, Inc. 2013
janssen
Rx only
Dosing: See package insert for full prescribing information.
Store at 25 °C (77 °F); with excursions permitted to 15 to 30 °C (59 to 86 °F).
Keep out of reach of children.
Active ingredient made in Belgium
Finished product manufactured by: Janssen Ortho, LLC Gurabo, PR 00778
Manufactured for: Janssen Pharmaceuticals, Inc. Titusville, NJ 08560
Licensed from Mitsubishi Tanabe Pharma Corporation
10280701
LOT:
EXP:

44. Generic name ____________ Drug manufacturer ____________

NDC number ____________ Directions for storage ____________

Dosage strength ____________

Dosage: take one capsule by mouth twice a day.
Store at 15°C to 30°C (59°F to 86°F). Protect from light. Store in original container.
Once the bottle is opened, use within 90 days.
Manufactured by: Biogen Idec Inc Cambridge, MA 02142
Tecfidera.com
NDC 64406-006-02 60 capsules
Tecfidera.
(dimethyl fumarate) delayed-release capsules
240 mg
Swallow capsule whole.
Rx only
Each capsule contains 240 mg dimethyl fumarate
LOT XXXXXX
EXP MM/YYYY

45. Generic name ____________ Dosage strength ____________

Form ____________

How long can the medication be stored after opening? ____________

Directions for administration ____________

NDC 0004-0800-85
Tamiflu®
(oseltamivir phosphate) Capsules
75 mg
Each capsule contains oseltamivir phosphate equivalent to 75 mg oseltamivir (free base).
℞ only
10 Capsules
Genentech

46. Trade name ____________ Form ____________

Generic name ____________ Dosage strength ____________

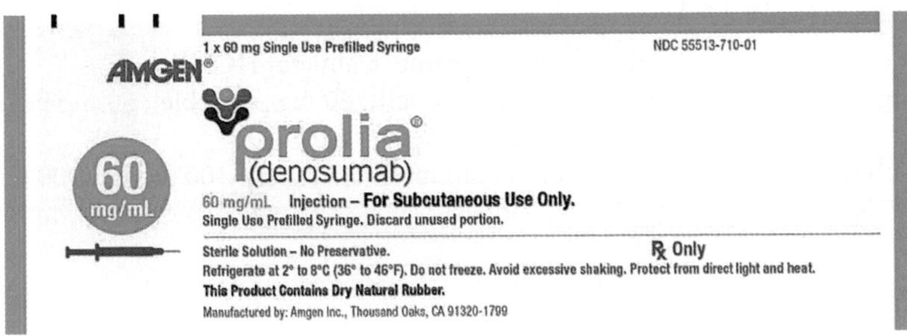

1 x 60 mg Single Use Prefilled Syringe
NDC 55513-710-01
AMGEN®
prolia®
(denosumab)
60 mg/mL
60 mg/mL Injection – For Subcutaneous Use Only.
Single Use Prefilled Syringe. Discard unused portion.
Sterile Solution – No Preservative.
℞ Only
Refrigerate at 2° to 8°C (36° to 46°F). Do not freeze. Avoid excessive shaking. Protect from direct light and heat.
This Product Contains Dry Natural Rubber.
Manufactured by: Amgen Inc., Thousand Oaks, CA 91320-1799

47. Generic name ____________ Directions for use ____________

Dosage strength ____________ Storage ____________

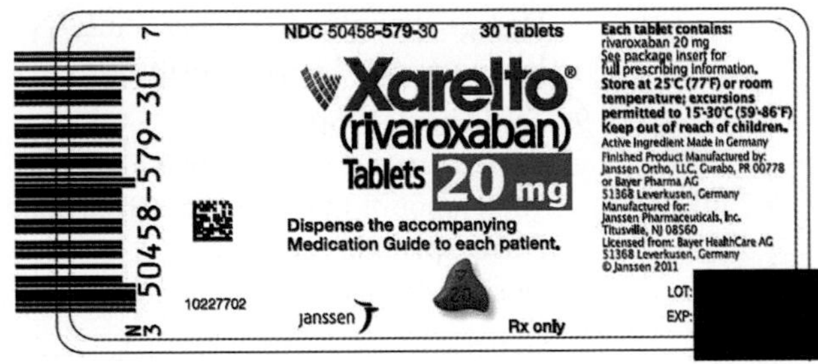

48. Trade name ____________ Dispensing directions ____________

NDC number ____________ Total amount in container ____________

Dosage strength ____________

Answers on pp. 216-218

ANSWERS

Chapter 13

Answers to Practice Problems

1. Trade name: no trade name stated
   Generic name: amoxicillin
   Form: powder; oral suspension when reconstituted
   Dosage strength (when reconstituted): 125 mg per 5 mL
   Total volume when mixed: 150 mL
   Warning: not for injection
2. Trade name: none stated
   Generic name: clorazepate dipotassium
   Form: tablets
   Dosage strength: 7.5 mg per tablet
   Total amount in container: 30 tablets
   Controlled substance schedule: 4, IV
   Pharmacist instructions: Dispense the accompanying medication guide to each patient.
3. Trade name: none stated
   Generic name: Diltiazem HCl
   Form: extended-release capsules
   Dosage strength: 120 mg per extended-release capsule
   Total amount in container: 100 extended-release capsules
4. Trade name: Gleevec
   Generic name: imatinib mesylate
   Dosage strength: 400 mg per tab
   Total amount in container: 30 tablets (tabs)
   Storage: See package insert. Store at 25° C (77° F); excursions permitted to 15° to 30° C.
5. Trade name: Coumadin
   Dosage strength: 2.5 mg per tablet
   Total amount in container: 1,000 tablets (tabs)
   Form: tablets
   NDC number: 0056-0176-90
6. Trade name: Norvir
   Generic name: ritonavir
   Total amount in container: 30 tablets
   Can this medication be crushed? No, label indicates tablets should be swallowed whole and not chewed, broken, or crushed.

7. Generic name: oxycodone hydrochloride
   Form: oral solution
   Dosage strength: 5 mg per 5 mL; 1 mg per mL
   Total volume: 500 mL
   Usual dosage: See package insert for complete prescribing information

8. Trade name: Ultram
   Generic name: tramadol HCl
   Dosage strength: 50 mg per tablet; 50 mg per scored tablet
   Total amount in container: 100 tablets; 100 scored tablets

Answers to Chapter Review

1. Trade name: Zemplar
   Generic name: paricalcitol
   Total amount in container: 30 capsules
   Form: capsules
   Dosage strength: 2 mcg per capsule
2. Trade name: no trade name stated
   Generic name: digoxin
   NDC number: 0641-1410-31
   Form: Injectable liquid
   Dosage strength: 500 mcg per 2 mL, 0.5 mg per 2 mL, 250 mcg per mL
3. Trade name: Cialis
   Generic name: tadalafil
   Storage: Store at 25° C (77° F).
   Form: tablets (tabs)
   Dosage strength: 10 mg per tablet (tab)
   Total amount in container: 30 tablets (tabs)
4. Trade name: Synthroid
   Generic name: levothyroxine sodium
   Total amount in container: 1,000 tablets
   Form: tablets
   Dosage strength: 88 mcg per tablet; 0.088 mg per tablet
5. Trade name: Prepidil Gel
   Generic name: dinoprostone
   Form: topical gel (cervical)
   Dosage strength: 0.5 mg
6. Trade name: Fortovase
   Generic name: saquinavir
   Usual dosage: See accompanying package insert.
   Alert: Find out about medicines that should not be taken with Fortovase.
   Form: capsules; soft gelatin capsules
   Dosage strength: 200 mg per soft gelatin capsule (caps)
   Total amount in container: 180 soft gelatin capsules (caps)
7. Trade name: no trade name stated
   Generic name: acyclovir
   Form: powder (injectable liquid once reconstituted)
   Directions for mixing: Inject 20 mL sterile water for injection into vial, shake vial until a clear solution is achieved, and use within 12 hours. Do not use bacteriostatic water for injection containing benzyl alcohol or parabens.
   Dosage strength after reconstitution: 1,000 mg per 20 mL
   Directions for use: For IV infusion only; dilute to 7 mg per mL or lower prior to infusion
8. Generic name: morphine sulfate
   NDC number: 0054-8585
   Total volume: 5 mL
   Controlled substance schedule: 2, II
   Form: oral solution
   Dosage strength: 10 mg per 5 mL
   Warning: may be habit forming
9. Trade name: Topamax
   Generic name: topiramate
   Total amount in container: 60 sprinkle capsules
   Form: sprinkle capsules
   Dosage strength: 25 mg per sprinkle capsule
10. Generic name: furosemide
    Dosage strength: 40 mg per 4 mL, 10 mg per mL
    Form: injectable liquid
    Total volume: 4 mL
11. Trade name: Bosulif
    Generic name: bosutinib
    Total amount in container: 30 tablets
    Administration directions: Do not crush or cut tablet.
    Form: tablet
    Dosage strength: 500 mg per tablet
    Directions for use: For oncology use only
12. Trade name: Kytril
    Generic name: granisetron HCl
    Form: oral solution
    Dosage strength: 2 mg per 10 mL
    Total volume: 30 mL
13. Trade name: Janumet
    Generic name: sitagliptin/metformin HCl
    Form: tablets
    Dosage strength: 64.25 mg sitagliptin phosphate (equivalent to 50 mg sitagliptin) and 500 mg per tablet of metformin HCl
    NDC number: 0006-0575-61
14. Trade name: Depo-Provera
    Generic name: medroxyprogesterone acetate
    Dosage strength: 400 mg per mL
    Directions for use: For intramuscular use only
    Total volume: 2.5 mL
15. Total amount in container: 90 sublingual tablets (tabs)
    Form: sublingual tablets (tabs)
    Dosage strength: 2,500 mcg per sublingual tablet (tab)
    Suggested use: As a dietary supplement

16. Generic name: amiodarone HCl
    Form: injectable liquid
    Directions for use: For IV use only; must be diluted
    Usual dosage: See package insert
    Dosage strength: 150 mg per 3 mL; 50 mg per mL
    Total volume: 3 mL
17. Trade name: no trade name stated
    Generic name: hydromorphone hydrochloride
    Directions for use: IM, SC (subcut), or slow IV use
    Form: injectable liquid
    Dosage strength: 2 mg per mL
    Total volume: 20 mL
    Warning: may be habit forming
18. Trade name: Zocor
    Generic name: simvastatin
    Dosage strength: 40 mg per tablet (tab)
    NDC number: 0006-0749-54
19. Generic name: extended phenytoin sodium
    Form: extended release capsules
    NDC number: 0071-0369-24
    Instructions for dispensing: Do not dispense capsules that are discolored.
    Dosage strength: 100 mg per extended capsule
    Total amount in container: 100 extended capsules
    Dosage and use: See accompanying information.
20. Trade name: MS Contin
    Generic name: morphine sulfate
    Form: controlled release tablets
    Dosage strength: 200 mg per controlled release tablet
    Total amount in container: 100 controlled release tablets.
    Controlled substance schedule: 2, II
    Directions for use: For use in opioid tolerant patients only
21. Trade name: Epogen
    Generic name: epoetin alfa
    Storage: Store at 2° to 8° C.
    Total volume: 2 mL
    Dosage strength: 10,000 units per mL, 20,000 units per 2 mL
22. Trade name: Valium
    Generic name: diazepam
    Dosage strength: 5 mg per mL
    Total volume: 10 mL
    Controlled substance schedule: 4, IV
23. Trade name: no trade name stated
    Generic name: metformin hydrochloride
    Form: extended-release tablets
    Dosage strength: 750 mg per extended-release tablet
    Total amount in container: 100 extended-release tablets
24. Generic name: methylphenidate hydrochloride
    Instructions to pharmacist: Dispense in a tight, light-resistant container as defined in the USP with a child-resistant closure.
    Dosage strength: 5 mg per tablet (tab)
25. Generic name: amoxicillin and clavulanate potassium
    Dosage strength: 200 mg amoxicillin per chewable tablet and 28.5 mg clavulanate potassium per chewable tablet
    Form: chewable tablets (tabs)
    Total amount in container: 20 chewable tablets
26. Generic name: sertraline HCl
    Form: oral concentrate
    Dosage strength: 20 mg per mL
    Total volume: 60 mL
27. Generic name: bumetanide
    Form: injectable liquid
    Dosage strength: 1 mg per 4 mL; 0.25 mg per mL
    Directions for use: for IM or IV use
28. Trade name: Crixivan
    Generic name: indinavir sulfate
    Form: capsules
    Dosage strength: 200 mg per capsule
    Alert: Find out about medications that should not be taken with Crixivan
    Total amount in container: 360 capsules
29. Trade name: Cardizem LA
    Generic name: diltiazem hydrochloride
    Form: extended-release tablets (tabs)
    Dosage strength: 180 mg per extended-release tablet (tab)
    Total amount in container: 30 extended-release tablets (tabs)
30. Generic name: dexamethasone sodium phosphate
    Form: injectable liquid
    Dosage strength: 120 mg per 30 mL; 4 mg per mL
31. Trade name: no trade name stated
    Generic name: nitroglycerin
    Storage information: Store at controlled room temperature: 15° to 30° C (59° to 86° F).
    Form: extended-release capsules
    Dosage strength: 9 mg per extended-release capsule (cap)
32. Trade name: Zanosar
    Generic name: streptozocin
    Form: sterile powder (injectable liquid once reconstituted)
    Directions for use: For intravenous use only.
33. by mouth, p.o.
34. 5 mg of hydrocodone bitartrate and 500 mg of acetaminophen
35. 100 tablets
36. B (Percocet)
37. 4.5 mg of oxycodone hydrochloride and 325 mg of aspirin. Percocet contains 5 mg of oxycodone hydrochloride and 325 mg of acetaminophen.
38. Percodan (it contains aspirin)
39. 10%

40. 0.465 mEq per mL
41. Trade name: Pradaxa
    Generic name: dabigatran etexilate
    Form: capsules
    How long can this medication be stored after opening? 4 months
42. Trade name: Linzess
    Generic name: linaclotide
    Can the capsules be placed in another container? NO
    Directions say to keep in original container to protect from moisture. Do not remove desiccant from inside bottle.
    Form: capsules
    Dosage strength: 290 mcg per capsule
43. Trade name: Neulasta
    Generic name: pegfilgrastim
    Does the medication require you to draw it up in a syringe to administer? No. The medication is available in prefilled syringe for single use.
    Dosage strength: 6 mg in 0.6 mL
    Directions for use: For subcutaneous use only.
44. Generic name: canagliflozin
    NDC number: 50458-141-30
    Dosage strength: 300 mg per tablet
    Drug manufacturer: Janssen Pharmaceuticals, Inc.
    Directions for storage: Store at 25° C (77° F) with excursions permitted to 15 to 30° C (59-86° F)
45. Generic name: dimethyl fumarate
    Form: delayed-release capsules
    How long can the medication be stored after opening? 90 days
    Directions for administration: Swallow capsule whole.
    Dosage strength: 240 mg per delayed release capsule.
46. Trade name: Tamiflu
    Generic name: oseltamivir phosphate
    Form: capsules
    Dosage strength: 75 mg per capsule
47. Generic name: denosumab
    Dosage strength: 60 mg per mL
    Directions for use: For subcutaneous use only.
    Storage: refrigerate at 2° to 8° C (36° to 46° F)
    Do not freeze. Avoid excessive shaking. Protect from direct light and heat.
48. Trade name: Xarelto
    NDC number: 50458-579-30
    Dosage strength: 20 mg per tablet
    Dispensing directions: Dispense the accompanying medication guide to each patient.
    Total amount in container: 30 tablets

CHAPTER 14
Dosage Calculation Using the Ratio and Proportion Method

Objectives

After reviewing this chapter, you should be able to:

1. State a ratio and proportion to solve a given dosage calculation problem
2. Solve simple calculation problems using the ratio and proportion method

Several methods are used for calculating dosages. The most common methods are *ratio and proportion* and *use of a formula.* After presentation of the various methods, students can choose the method they find easiest and most logical to use. First, let's discuss calculating by using ratio and proportion. If necessary, review Chapter 4 on ratio and proportion.

Use of Ratio and Proportion in Dosage Calculation

When you know three of the four values of a proportion, you can solve the proportion to determine the unknown quantity. In dosage calculation, it is often necessary to find only one unknown quantity. As you recall from Chapter 4 (ratio and proportion), the proportion can be set up stating the terms using colons (ratio format) or as a fraction. Recall that a proportion is a relationship comparing two ratios. Remember, in addition to solving for the unknown quantity, it is essential to also be competent in setting up the proportion correctly.

SAFETY ALERT!

If you set up the proportion incorrectly, you could calculate the dose incorrectly and administer the wrong dose, which could have serious consequences for the client.

For example, suppose you had a medication with a dosage strength of 50 mg per 1 mL, and the prescriber orders a dosage of 25 mg. A ratio and proportion may be used to determine how many milliliters to administer. Remember to include units when writing a ratio and proportion to avoid errors.

When setting up the ratio and proportion using the fraction format to calculate dosages, the known ratio is what you have available, or the information on the medication label, and is stated first (placed on the left side of the proportion). The desired, or what is ordered to be administered, is the unknown (placed on the right side). Therefore, using the example, the ratio and proportion would be stated as follows:

Example 1:

$$\underset{\text{(known)}}{\frac{50\text{ mg}}{1\text{ mL}}} = \underset{\text{(unknown)}}{\frac{25\text{ mg}}{x\text{ mL}}}$$

When writing the ratio and proportion using the colons (ratio format), the known ratio, what you have available or the information on the medication label, is stated first, and the unknown ratio is stated second.

Example 1:

$$\underset{\text{(known)}}{50\text{ mg}:1\text{ mL}} = \underset{\text{(unknown)}}{25\text{ mg}:x\text{ mL}}$$

Solution: To solve for x, use the principles presented in Chapter 4 on ratio and proportion.

$$\underset{\text{(known)}}{\frac{50\text{ mg}}{1\text{ mL}}} = \underset{\text{(unknown)}}{\frac{25\text{ mg}}{x\text{ mL}}}$$

$$\frac{50x}{50} = \frac{25}{50}$$

$$x = 0.5\text{ mL}$$

Remember that, as shown, the known is stated as the first fraction, and the unknown as the second. When stated in fraction format, solve by cross multiplication.

or

$$\underset{\text{(known)}}{50\text{ mg}:1\text{ mL}} = \underset{\text{(unknown)}}{25\text{ mg}:x\text{ mL}}$$

$$50x = \text{product of extremes}$$

$$25 = \text{product of means}$$

$$50x = 25 \text{ is the equation}$$

$$\frac{50x}{50} = \frac{25}{50} \quad \text{(Divide both sides by 50, the number in front of } x.\text{)}$$

$$x = 0.5\text{ mL}$$

SAFETY ALERT!

It is important to remember when stating ratios that the units of measure should be stated in the same sequence (in the examples, $\frac{\text{mg}}{\text{mL}} = \frac{\text{mg}}{\text{mL}}$ or mg : mL = mg : mL). Labeling the terms in the ratios, including x, is also essential. These pointers are crucial to preventing calculation errors.

Example 2: Order: 40 mg p.o. of a medication.

Available: 20 mg tablets (tab, tabs). How many tabs will you administer?

Solution:

$$\underset{\text{(known)}}{\frac{20\text{ mg}}{1\text{ tab}}} = \underset{\text{(unknown)}}{\frac{40\text{ mg}}{x\text{ tab}}}$$

$$\frac{20x}{20} = \frac{40}{20}$$

$$x = 2\text{ tabs}$$

or

$$\underset{\text{(known)}}{20\text{ mg}:1\text{ tab}} = \underset{\text{(unknown)}}{40\text{ mg}:x\text{ tab}}$$

$$\frac{20x}{20} = \frac{40}{20}$$

$$x = 2\text{ tabs}$$

Example 3: Order: 1 g p.o. of an antibiotic

Available: 500 mg capsules (cap, caps). How many caps will you administer?

Solution: Notice that the dosage ordered is in a different unit from what is available. Proceed first by changing the units of measure so they are the same. As shown in Chapter 8, ratio and proportion can be used for conversion.

After making the conversion, set up the problem and calculate the dosage to be given. In this example, the conversion required is within the same system (metric).

In this example, grams are converted to milligrams by using the equivalent 1,000 mg = 1 g. After making the conversion of 1 g to 1,000 mg, the ratio is stated as follows:

$$\underset{\text{(known)}}{\frac{500\text{ mg}}{1\text{ cap}}} = \underset{\text{(unknown)}}{\frac{1{,}000\text{ mg}}{x\text{ caps}}} \quad \textit{or} \quad \underset{\text{(known)}}{500\text{ mg}:1\text{ cap}} = \underset{\text{(unknown)}}{1{,}000\text{ mg}:x\text{ caps}}$$

$$x = 2\text{ caps} \qquad\qquad x = 2\text{ caps}$$

An alternate method of solving might be to convert milligrams to grams. In doing this, 500 mg would be converted to grams by using the same equivalent: 1,000 mg = 1 g. However, decimals are common when measures are changed from smaller to larger in the metric system: 500 mg = 0.5 g. Even though converting the milligrams to grams would net the same final answer, *conversions that net decimals are often the source of calculation errors.* Therefore, if possible, avoid conversions that require their use. As a rule, it is best to convert to the measure stated on the medication label. Doing this consistently can prevent confusion. As with the other examples, this proportion could be stated as a fraction as well.

For the purpose of learning to calculate dosages by using ratio and proportion, this chapter emphasizes the mathematics used to calculate the answer. Determining whether an answer is logical is essential and necessary in the calculation of medication. An answer *must make sense.* Determining whether an answer is logical will be discussed further in later chapters covering the calculation of dosages by various routes.

POINTS TO REMEMBER

Important Points When Calculating Dosages Using Ratio and Proportion

- Make sure all terms are in the same unit and system of measure before calculating. If they are not, a conversion will be necessary before calculating the dosage.
- When conversion of units is required, conversions can be made by converting what is ordered to the units in which the medication is available or by changing what is available to the units in which the medication is ordered. Be consistent as to how you make conversions. It is usual to convert what is ordered to the same unit and system of measure you have the medication available in.
- When stating ratios, the known is stated first. The known ratio is what is available or on hand or the information obtained from the medication label.
- The unknown ratio is stated second. The unknown ratio is the dosage desired, or what the prescriber has ordered.
- The terms of the ratios in a proportion must be written in the same sequence.

  Example: mg : mL = mg : mL *or* $\frac{\text{mg}}{\text{mL}} = \frac{\text{mg}}{\text{mL}}$.
- Label all terms of the ratios in the proportion, including *x*.
- Before calculating the dosage, make a mental estimate of the approximate and reasonable answer.
- Label the value you obtain for *x* (e.g., mL, tabs). Double-check the label for *x* by referring back to the label of *x* in the original ratio and proportion; it should be the same.
- A proportion can be stated in a horizontal fashion using colons (ratio format) or as a fraction.
- Double-check all work.
- Be consistent in how ratios are stated and conversions are done.
- An error in the setup of the ratio and proportion can cause an error in calculation.

PRACTICE **PROBLEMS**

Answer the following questions by indicating whether you need less than 1 tab or more than 1 tab. Refer to Chapter 4 if you have difficulty in answering the questions in this area.

1. A client is to receive 0.2 mg of a medication. The tablets available are 0.4 mg.

   How many tablets do you need? ______________________

2. A client is to receive 1.25 mg of a medication. The tablets available are 0.625 mg.

   How many tablets do you need? ______________________

3. A client is to receive 7.5 mg of a medication. The tablets available are 15 mg.

   How many tablets do you need? ______________________

4. A client is to receive 10 mg of a medication. The tablets available are 20 mg.

   How many tablets do you need? ______________________

5. A client is to receive 100 mg of a medication. The tablets available are 50 mg.

   How many tablets do you need? ______________________

Solve the following problems using ratio and proportion. Express your answer in mL to the nearest tenth where indicated, and include the label on the answer.

6. Order: 7.5 mg p.o. of a medication.

   Available: Tablets labeled 5 mg ______________________

7. Order: 45 mg p.o. of a medication.

   Available: Tablets labeled 30 mg ______________________

8. Order: 90 mg p.o. of a medication.

   Available: Capsules labeled 100 mg ______________________

9. Order: 0.25 mg IM of a medication.

   Available: 0.5 mg per mL ______________________

10. Order: 100 mg p.o. of a liquid medication.

    Available: 125 mg per 5 mL ______________________

11. Order: 20 mEq IV of a medication.

    Available: 40 mEq per 10 mL ______________________

12. Order: 5,000 units subcut of a medication.

    Available: 10,000 units per mL ______________________

13. Order: 50 mg IM of a medication.

    Available: 80 mg per 2 mL ____________________

14. Order: 0.5 g p.o. of an antibiotic.

    Available: Capsules labeled 250 mg ____________________

15. Order: 400 mg p.o. of a liquid medication.

    Available: 125 mg per 5 mL ____________________

16. Order: 50 mg IM of a medication.

    Available: 80 mg per mL ____________________

17. Order: 60 mg IM of a medication.

    Available: 30 mg per mL ____________________

18. Order: 15 mg of a medication.

    Available: Tablets labeled 5 mg. ____________________

19. Order: 0.24 g p.o. of a liquid medication.

    Available: 80 mg per 7.5 mL ____________________

20. Order: 20 g p.o. of a liquid medication.

    Available: 10 g per 15 mL ____________________

21. Order: 0.125 mg IM of a medication.

    Available: 0.5 mg per 2 mL ____________________

22. Order: 0.75 mg IM of a medication.

    Available: 0.25 mg per mL ____________________

23. Order: 375 mg p.o. of a liquid medication.

    Available: 125 mg per 5 mL ____________________

24. Order: 10,000 units subcut of a medication.

    Available: 7,500 units per mL ____________________

25. Order: 0.45 mg p.o. of a medication.

    Available: Tablets labeled 0.3 mg ____________________

26. Order: 20 mg IM of a medication.

    Available: 25 mg per 1.5 mL ____________________

27. Order: 150 mg IV of a medication.

    Available: 80 mg per mL ______________________

28. Order: 2 mg IM of a medication.

    Available: 1.5 mg per 0.5 mL ______________________

29. Order: 500 mcg IV of a medication.

    Available: 750 mcg per 3 mL ______________________

30. Order: 0.15 mg IM of a medication.

    Available: 0.2 mg per 1.5 mL ______________________

31. Order: 1,100 units subcut of a medication.

    Available: 1,000 units per 1.5 mL ______________________

32. Order: 0.6 g IV of a medication.

    Available: 1 g per 3.6 mL ______________________

33. Order: 3 g IV of a medication.

    Available: 1.5 g per mL ______________________

34. Order: 35 mg IM of a medication.

    Available: 40 mg per 2.5 mL ______________________

35. Order: 0.3 mg subcut of a medication.

    Available: 1,000 mcg per 2 mL ______________________

36. Order: 200 mg IM of a medication.

    Available: 0.5 g per 2 mL ______________________

37. Order: 10 mEq IV of a medication.

    Available: 20 mEq per 10 mL ______________________

38. Order: 165 mg IV of a medication.

    Available: 55 mg per 1.1 mL ______________________

39. Order: 35 mg subcut of a medication.

    Available: 45 mg per 1.2 mL ______________________

40. Order: 700 mg IM of a medication.

    Available: 1,000 mg per 2.3 mL ______________________

Write a proportion and solve for the following unknown quantity.

41. If 15 mL of solution contains 75 mg of medication, how many mg of medication are in 60 mL of solution?

42. A client must take three tablets per day for 28 days. How many tablets should the pharmacy supply to fill this order?

43. A health care provider is instructed to administer 700 mL of a solution every 8 hours. How many hours will be needed to administer 2,100 mL?

44. Two tablets contain a total of 6.25 mg of a medication. How many milligrams of medication are in 10 tablets?

45. If 80 mg of medication is in 480 mL of solution, how many milliliters of solution contain 60 milligrams?

Answers on pp. 243-246

CHAPTER **REVIEW**

Part I

Read the medication labels where available, and calculate the number of tablets or capsules necessary to provide the dosage ordered. Include the label on your answer.

1. Order: Phenobarbital 15 mg p.o. t.i.d.

   Available: Phenobarbital tablets labeled 15 mg ____________________

2. Order: Erythromycin (delayed release capsules) 0.5 g p.o. q12h for 10 days.

   Available:

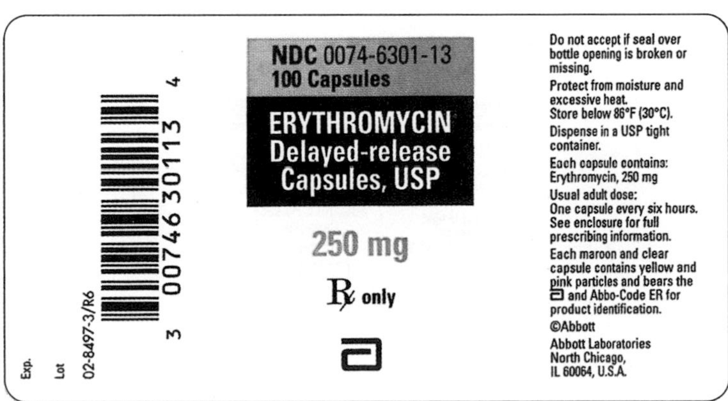

____

3. Order: Persantine 50 mg p.o. q.i.d.

   Available:

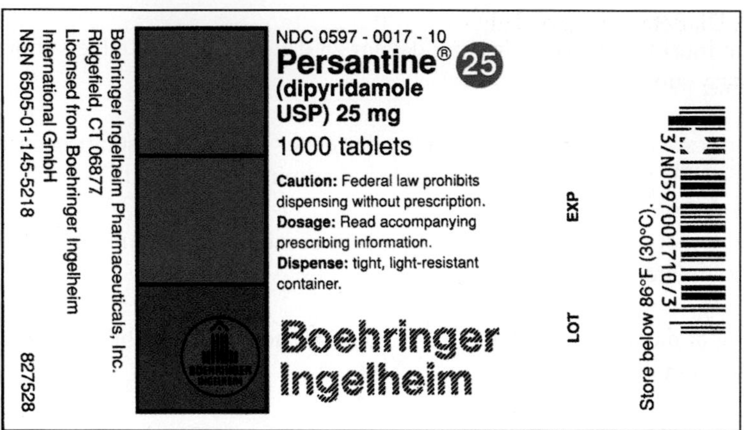

____

4. Order: Phenobarbital 60 mg p.o. at bedtime.

   Available: Scored phenobarbital tablets (can be broken in half) labeled 30 mg

____

5. Order: Baclofen 20 mg p.o. t.i.d.

   Available: Scored baclofen tablets (can be broken in half) labeled 10 mg.

____

6. Order: Dilatrate-SR 80 mg p.o. q12h.

   Available:

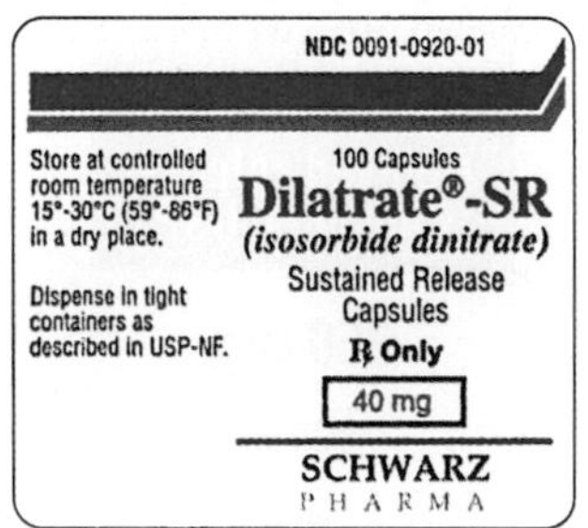

____

7. Order: Dexamethasone 4 mg p.o. q6h.

   Available: Dexamethasone tablets labeled 2 mg ____________________

8. Order: DiaBeta 5 mg p.o. daily.

   Available:

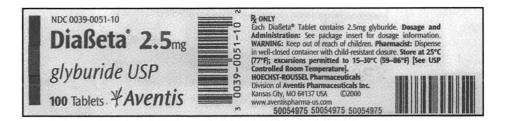

____

9. Order: Digoxin 125 mcg p.o. daily.

   Available: Scored digoxin tablets (can be broken in half).

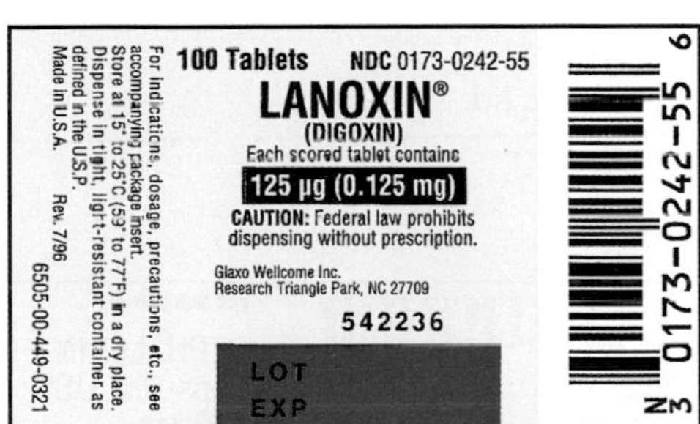

____

10. Order: Synthroid 0.05 mg p.o. daily.

    Available: Synthroid tablets labeled 50 mcg (0.05 mg)

____

11. Order: Tranxene 30 mg p.o. at bedtime.

    Available:

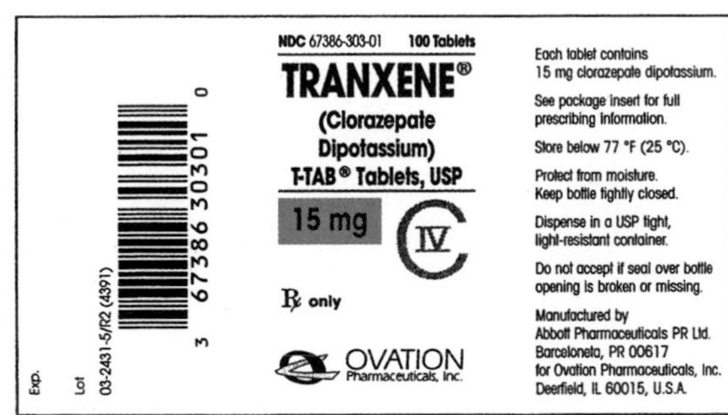

____

12. Order: Phenobarbital 60 mg p.o. at bedtime.

    Available: Phenobarbital tablets labeled 60 mg

    ____

13. Order: Tigan 200 mg p.o. t.i.d. p.r.n. for nausea.

    Available:

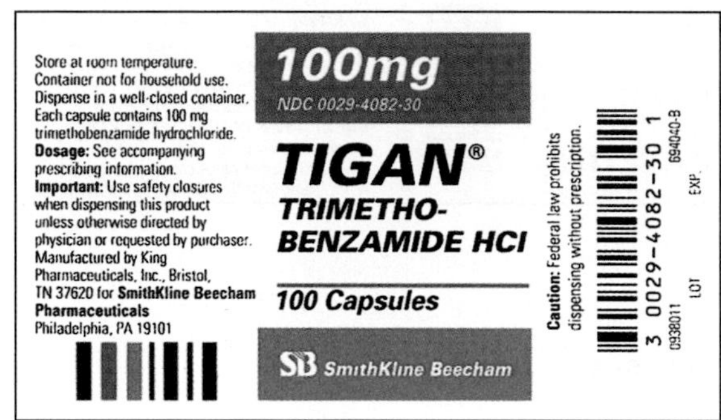

____

14. Order: Cephalexin 0.5 g p.o. q.i.d.

    Available:

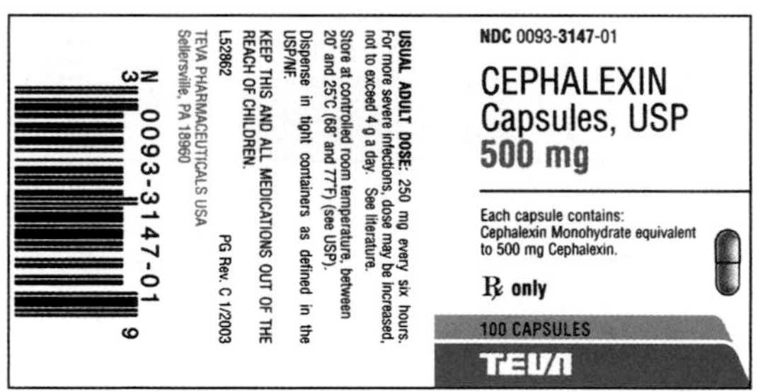

____

15. Order: Cogentin 2 mg p.o. b.i.d.

    Available: Cogentin tablets labeled 1 mg ______________________

16. Order: Amoxicillin and clavulanate potassium 400 mg/57 mg p.o. q8h.

    Available:

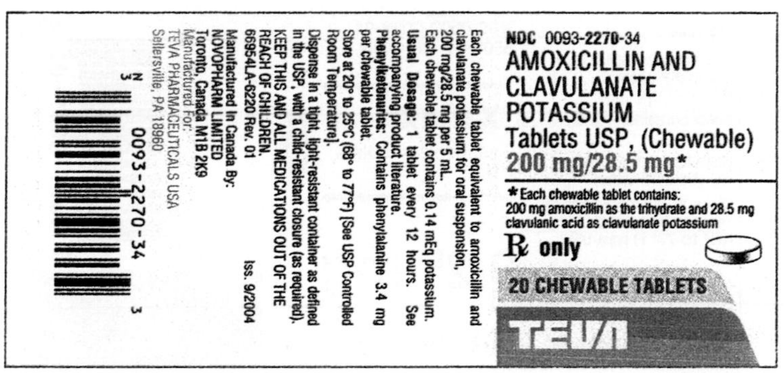

17. Order: Zovirax 400 mg p.o. b.i.d. for 7 days.

    Available: Zovirax capsules labeled 200 mg

18. Order: Rifampin 0.6 g p.o. daily.

    Available:

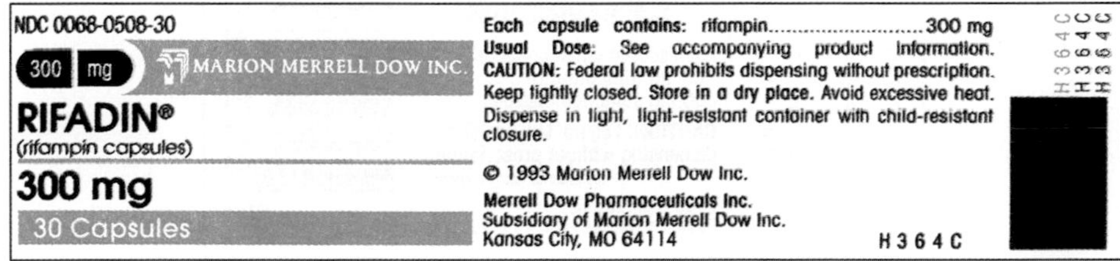

19. Order: Carafate 1,000 mg p.o. b.i.d.

    Available: Carafate tablets labeled 1 g

20. Order: Cardizem 240 mg p.o. daily.

    Available: Cardizem tablets labeled 120 mg

21. Order: Xanax 0.5 mg p.o. b.i.d.

    Available: Scored tablets (can be broken in half)

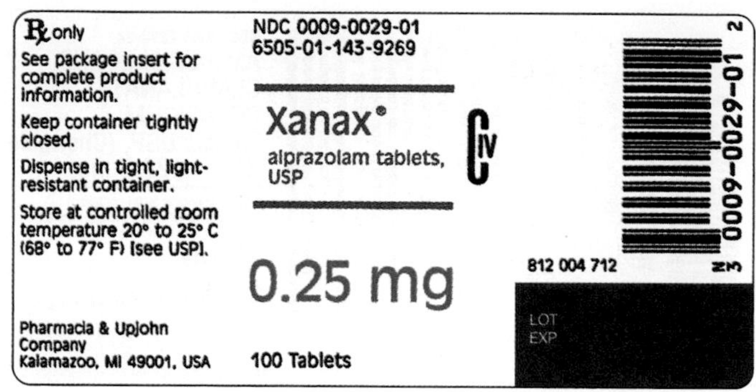

____

22. Order: Septra DS 1 tab p.o. daily 3 times per week (Mon, Wed, Fri).

    Available:

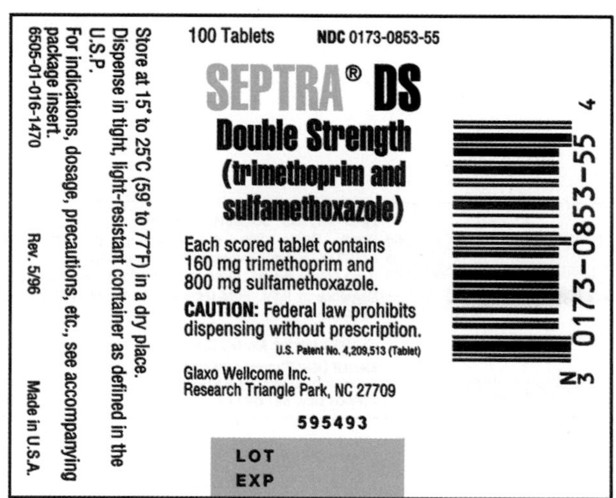

____

23. Order: Lotrel 2.5/10 2 caps p.o. daily.

    Available:

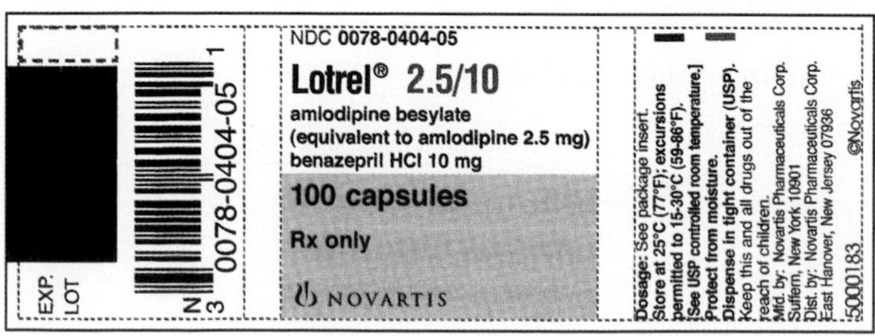

____

24. Order: Retrovir 0.2 g p.o. t.i.d.

    Available: Retrovir capsules labeled 100 mg

    ____

25. Order: Prandin 1 mg p.o. b.i.d.

    Available:

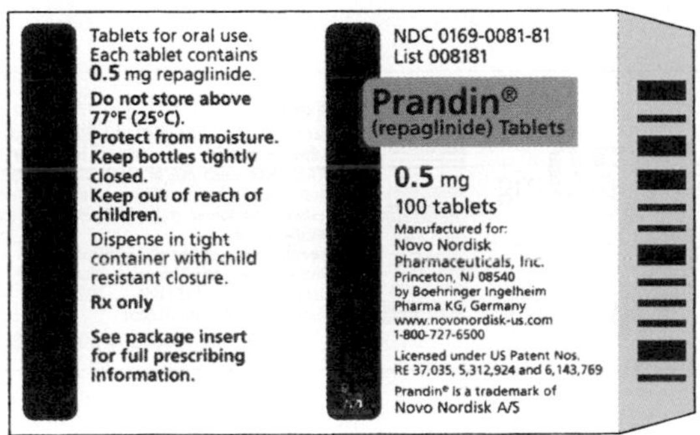

    ____

26. Order: Risperdal 1 mg p.o. b.i.d.

    Available:

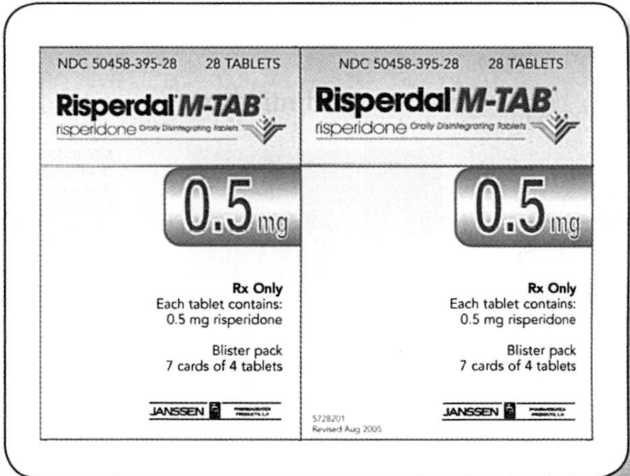

    ____

27. Order: Flagyl 0.5 g p.o. q8h.

    Available:

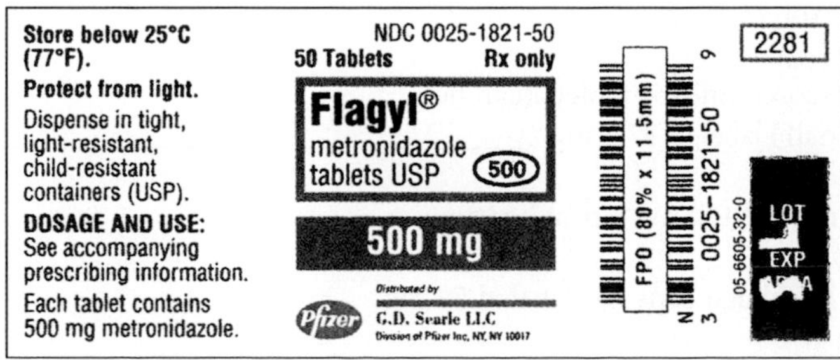

    ____

28. Order: Lopressor 100 mg p.o. b.i.d.

    Available: Lopressor tablets labeled 50 mg ______________________

29. Order: Lasix 60 mg p.o. daily.

    Available:

____

30. Order: Motrin 0.6 g p.o. q6h p.r.n. for pain.

    Available: Motrin tablets labeled 300 mg ______________________

31. Order: Potassium chloride extended release 30 mEq p.o. daily.

    Available:

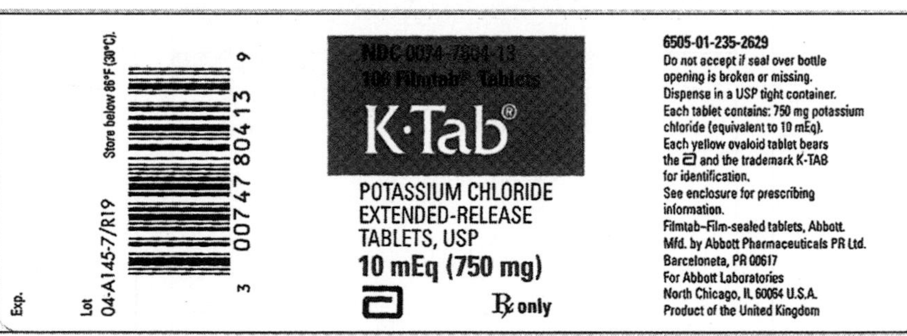

____

32. Order: Mevacor 20 mg p.o. daily at 6 PM.

    Available: Mevacor tablets labeled 10 mg ______________________

33. Order: Effexor 75 mg p.o. b.i.d.

    Available: Scored Effexor tablets (can be broken in half) labeled 37.5 mg ______________________

34. Order: Nembutal 100 mg p.o. at bedtime.

    Available: Nembutal capsules labeled 50 mg

____

35. Order: Geodon 40 mg p.o. b.i.d.

Available:

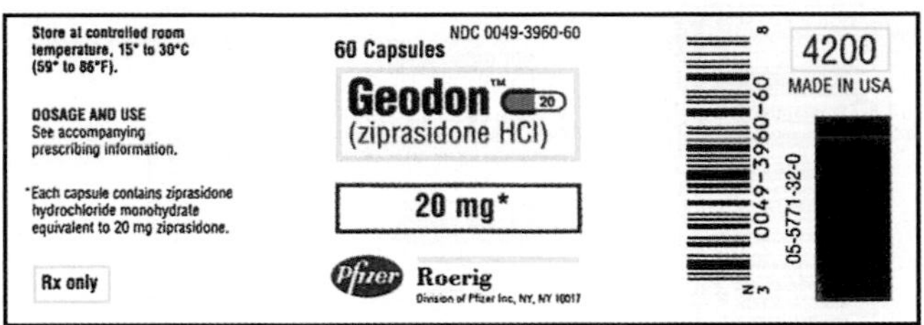

____

36. Order: Zarontin 750 mg p.o. b.i.d.

Available:

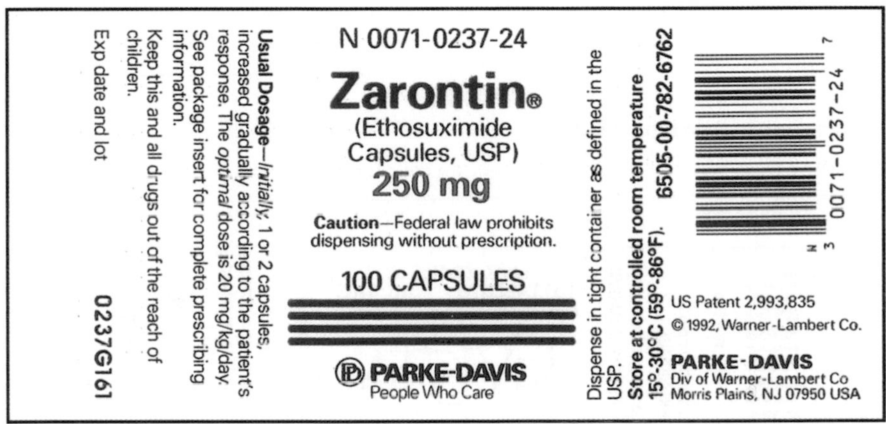

____

37. Order: Effient 10 mg p.o. daily.

Available:

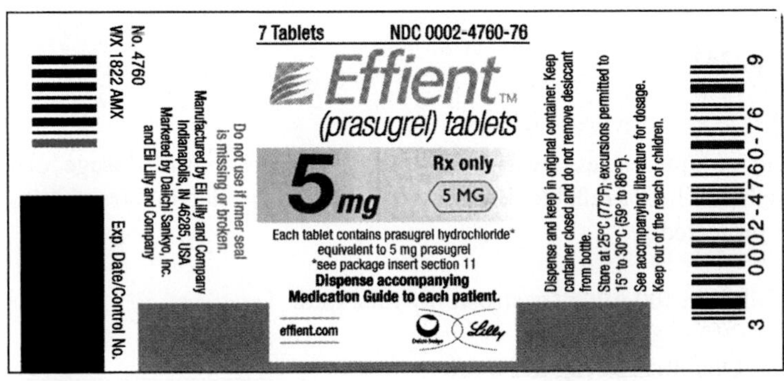

____

38. Order: Levothroid 0.112 mg p.o. every day.

    Available: Scored tablets (can be broken in half)

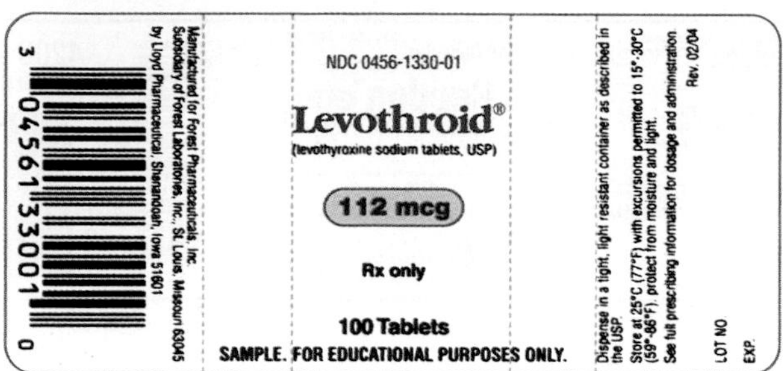

____

39. Order: Lanoxin 0.125 mg p.o. every day.

    Available: Lanoxin scored tablets (can be broken in half) labeled 250 mcg (0.25 mg)

____

40. Order: Evista 0.06 g p.o. daily.

    Available:

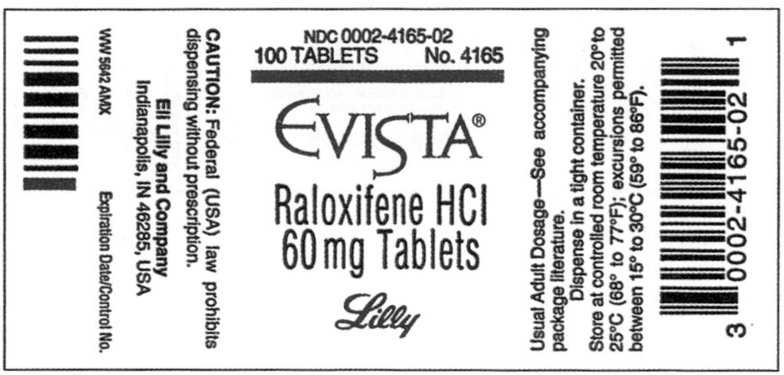

____

Answers on p. 247

Part II

Calculate the volume necessary (in milliliters) to provide the dosage ordered, using medication labels where available. Express your answer as a decimal fraction to the nearest tenth where indicated.

41. Order: Dilantin 100 mg by gastrostomy tube t.i.d.

    Available: Dilantin 125 mg per 5 mL _______________

42. Order: Benadryl 50 mg p.o. at bedtime.

    Available: Benadryl elixir 12.5 mg per 5 mL _______________

43. Order: Gentamicin 50 mg IM q8h.

 Available:

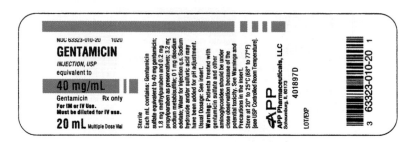

____

44. Order: Vibramycin 100 mg p.o. q12h.

 Available:

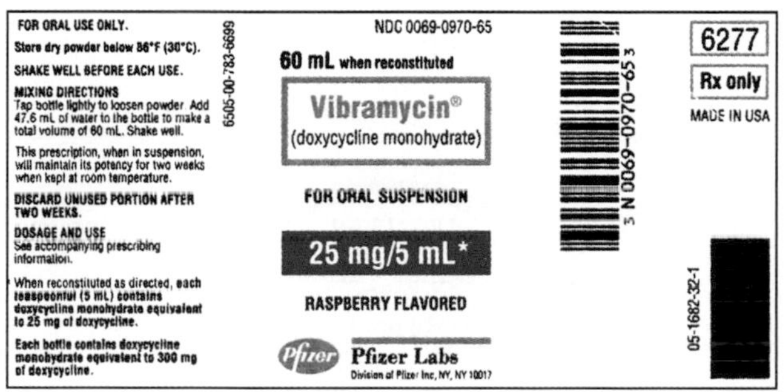

____

45. Order: Meperidine hydrochloride 50 mg IM q4h p.r.n. for pain.

 Available: Meperidine 75 mg per mL ________________

46. Order: Gentamicin 90 mg IV q8h.

 Available: Gentamicin 40 mg per mL ________________

47. Order: Morphine 15 mg subcut q4h p.r.n. for pain.

 Available: Morphine labeled 15 mg per mL

____

48. Order: Vitamin B_{12} (Cyanocobalamin) 1,000 mcg IM once monthly.

    Available:

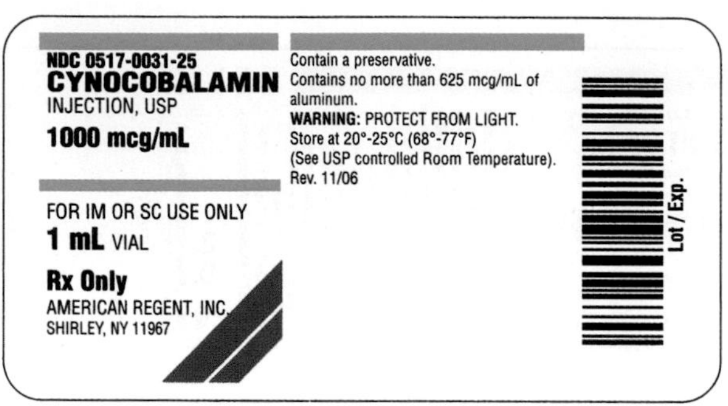

____

49. Order: Morphine 10 mg subcut stat. (Express answer in hundredths.)

    Available: Morphine 15 mg per mL. _______________

50. Order: Potassium chloride 20 mEq p.o. daily.

    Available:

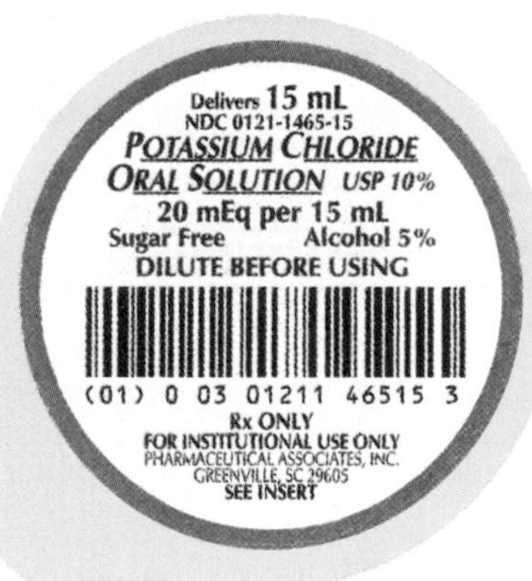

____

51. Order: Nystatin oral suspension 100,000 units swish and swallow q6h.

    Available: Nystatin oral suspension labeled 100,000 units per mL

____

52. Order: Heparin 5,000 units subcut daily.

    Available:

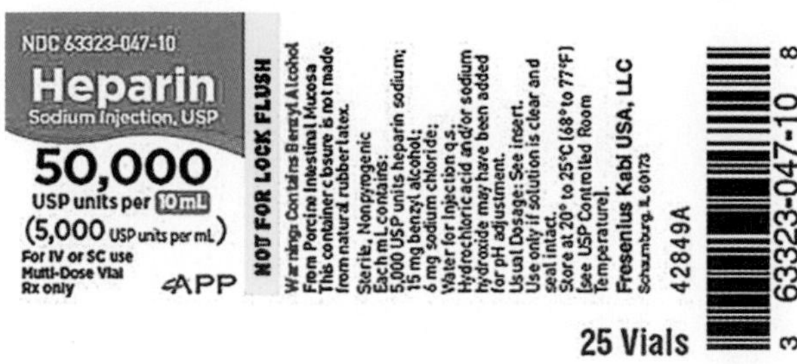

____

53. Order: Atropine 0.2 mg subcut stat.

    Available:

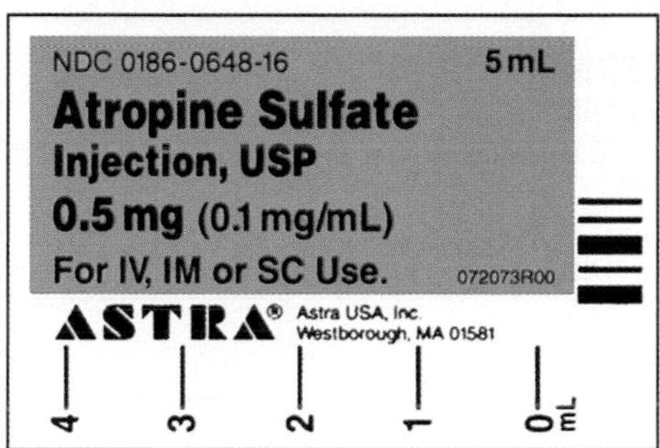

____

54. Order: Amoxicillin 500 mg p.o. q6h for 7 days.

    Available:

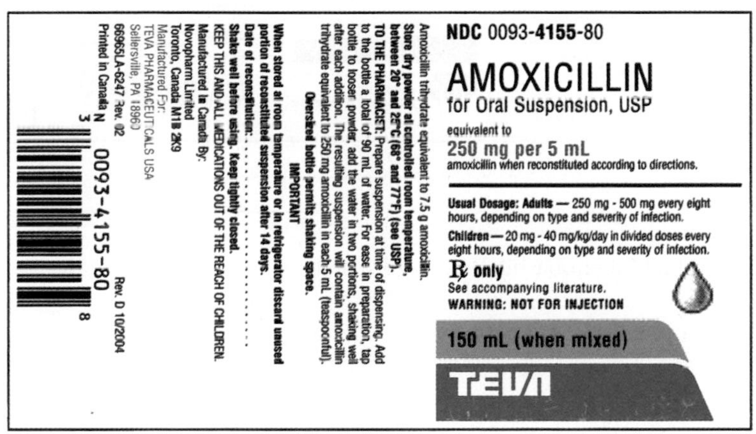

____

55. Order: Heparin 7,500 units subcut daily. Express answer in hundredths.

    Available: Heparin 10,000 units per mL ____________________

56. Order: Methylprednisolone 70 mg IV daily.

    Available: Methylprednisolone labeled 40 mg per mL

____

57. Order: Lorazepam 2 mg IM q4h p.r.n. for agitation.

 Available:

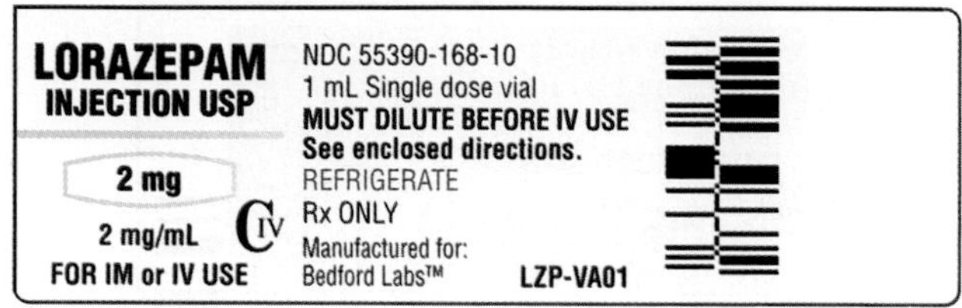

____

58. Order: Vistaril 25 mg IM on call to operating room (OR).

 Available:

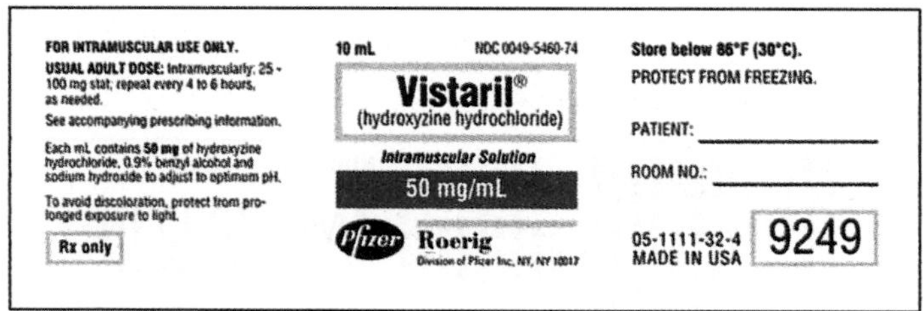

____

59. Order: Luminal (phenobarbital) 90 mg IM stat.

 Available: Luminal 130 mg per ml

____

60. Order: Sandostatin 200 mcg subcut q12h.

 Available:

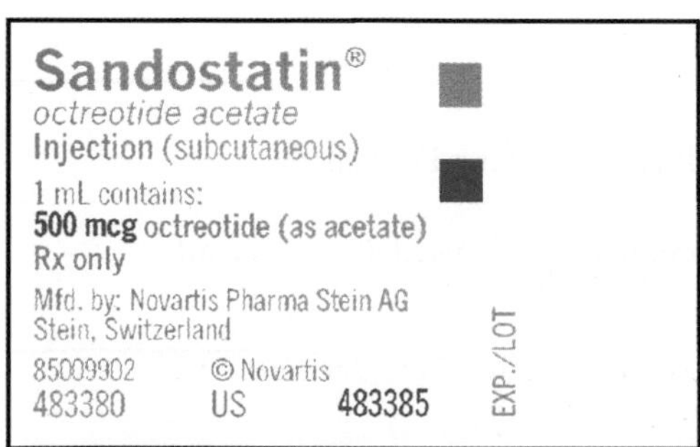

____

61. Order: Ranitidine 150 mg IV daily.

Available:

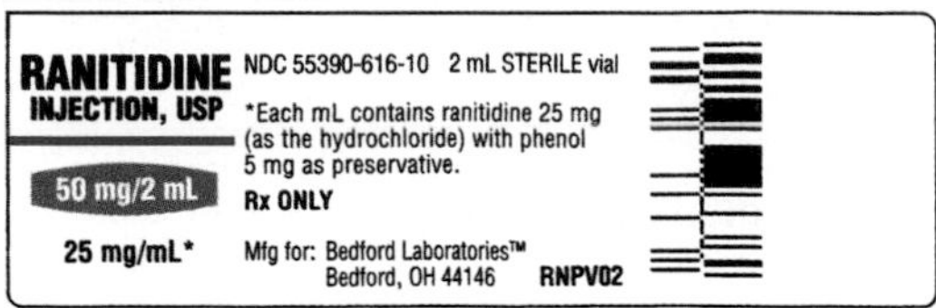

____

62. Order: Amoxicillin 0.5 g p.o. q8h.

Available: Amoxicillin Oral Suspension labeled 400 mg per 5 mL

____

63. Order: Thorazine concentrate 75 mg p.o. daily.

Available: Thorazine concentrate labeled 100 mg per mL

____

64. Order: Trileptal 300 mg p.o. b.i.d.

Available:

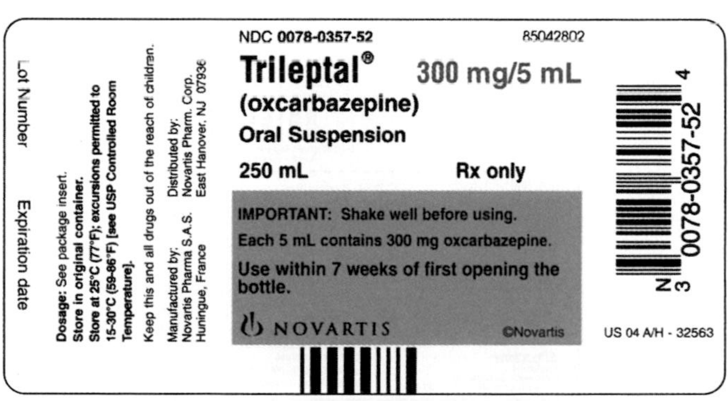

____

65. Order: Epivir 0.3 g p.o. b.i.d.

Available: Epivir oral solution labeled 10 mg per mL

____

66. Order: Cipro 0.4 g IV q12h.

    Available: Cipro (IV) labeled 400 mg per 40 mL

    ____

67. Order: Prozac 40 mg p.o. daily.

    Available: Prozac oral solution labeled 20 mg per 5 mL

    ____

68. Order: Depo-Provera 0.4 g IM at bedtime once a week on Thursday.

    Available:

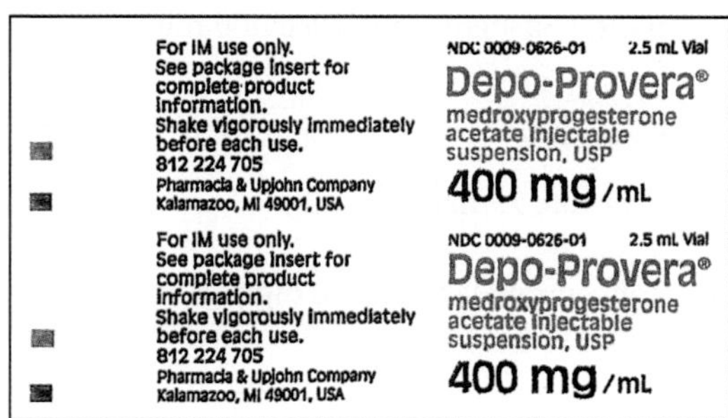

    ____

69. Order: Diphenhydramine 35 mg IM q6h p.r.n. for itching.

    Available:

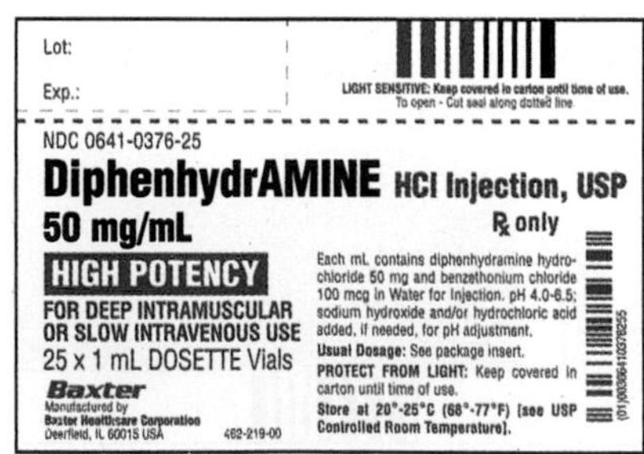

    ____

70. Order: Lactulose 30 g p.o. t.i.d.

    Available: Lactulose oral solution labeled 10 g per 15 mL

    ____

71. Order: Mellaril 40 mg p.o. b.i.d.

    Available: Mellaril concentrate 30 mg per mL ______________

72. Order: Compazine 7 mg IM q4h p.r.n. for vomiting.

    Available:

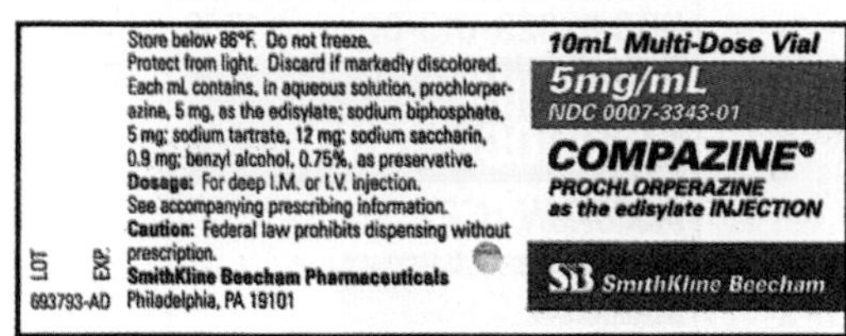
Store below 86°F. Do not freeze.
Protect from light. Discard if markedly discolored.
Each mL contains, in aqueous solution, prochlorperazine, 5 mg, as the edisylate; sodium biphosphate, 5 mg; sodium tartrate, 12 mg; sodium saccharin, 0.9 mg; benzyl alcohol, 0.75%, as preservative.
Dosage: For deep I.M. or I.V. injection.
See accompanying prescribing information.
Caution: Federal law prohibits dispensing without prescription.
SmithKline Beecham Pharmaceuticals
Philadelphia, PA 19101
LOT
EXP.
693793-AD
10mL Multi-Dose Vial
5mg/mL
NDC 0007-3343-01
COMPAZINE®
PROCHLORPERAZINE
as the edisylate INJECTION
SB SmithKline Beecham

____

73. Order: Cefaclor 0.5 g p.o. q8h.

    Available:

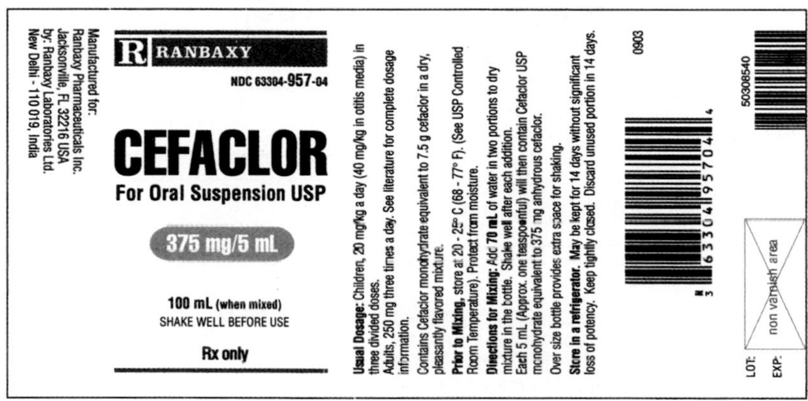

____

74. Order: Dilantin suspension 200 mg per nasogastric tube every day.

    Available:

Dilantin-125®
(Phenytoin Oral Suspension, USP)
125 mg per 5 mL potency
Important—Another strength available; verify unspecified prescriptions.
Caution—Federal law prohibits dispensing without prescription.

____

75. Order: Celestone 7 mg IM stat.

    Available: Celestone labeled 6 mg per mL

____

76. Order: Thiamine hydrochloride 75 mg IM every day.

Available:

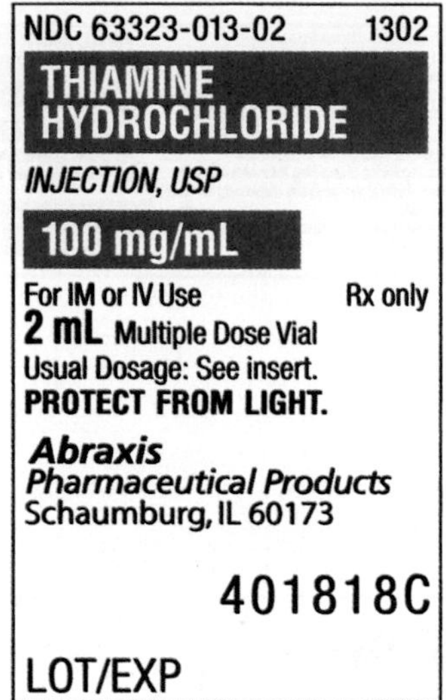

____

77. Order: Epinephrine 0.25 mg IV stat.

Available:

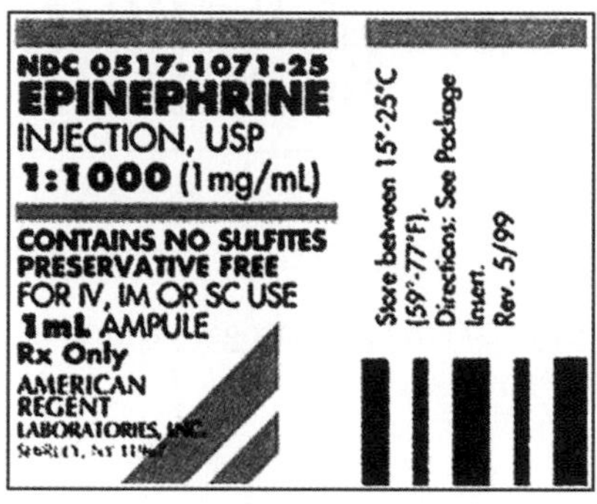

____

78. Order: Alprazolam 0.25 mg p.o. b.i.d. (Express answer in hundredths.)

Available:

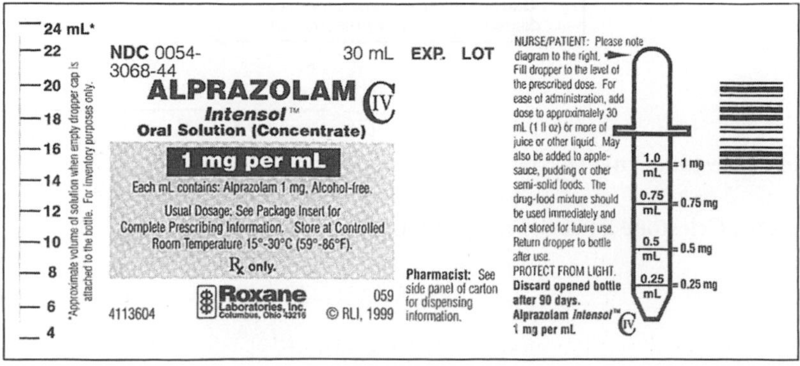

____

79. Order: Vantin 100 mg p.o. q12h for 10 days.

    Available: Vantin Oral Suspension labeled 50 mg per 5 mL

    ____

80. Order: Zithromax oral suspension 500 mg p.o. for 1 dose stat then 250 mg daily for 3 days. Determine the amount to administer for the stat dose.

    Available:

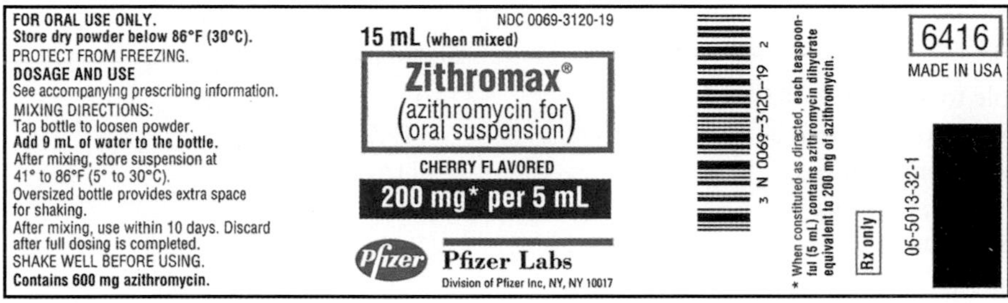

____

Answers on p. 247

ANSWERS

Chapter 14

Answers to Practice Problems

1. Less than 1 tab
2. More than 1 tab
3. Less than 1 tab
4. Less than 1 tab
5. More than 1 tab
6. $$\frac{5\text{ mg}}{1\text{ tab}} = \frac{7.5\text{ mg}}{x\text{ tab}}$$
   $$\frac{5x}{5} = \frac{7.5}{5}$$
   or
   $$5\text{ mg} : 1\text{ tab} = 7.5\text{ mg} : x\text{ tab}$$
   $$\frac{5x}{5} = \frac{7.5}{5}$$
   $$x = \frac{7.5}{5}$$
   $x = 1.5$ tabs or $1\frac{1}{2}$ tabs. 5 mg is less than 7.5 mg; therefore you will need more than 1 tab to administer the dosage.
7. $$\frac{30\text{ mg}}{1\text{ tab}} = \frac{45\text{ mg}}{x\text{ tab}}$$
   $$\frac{30x}{30} = \frac{45}{30}$$
   $$x = \frac{45}{30}$$
   or
   $$30\text{ mg} : 1\text{ tab} = 45\text{ mg} : x\text{ tab}$$
   $$\frac{30x}{30} = \frac{45}{30}$$
   $$x = \frac{45}{30}$$
   $x = 1.5$ tabs or $1\frac{1}{2}$ tabs. 45 mg is more than 30 mg; therefore you need more than 1 tab to administer the dosage.

8. $$\frac{100\text{ mg}}{1\text{ cap}} = \frac{90\text{ mg}}{x\text{ cap}}$$
$$\frac{100x}{100} = \frac{90}{100}$$
$$x = \frac{90}{100}$$

or

$$100\text{ mg}:1\text{ cap} = 90\text{ mg}:x\text{ cap}$$
$$\frac{100x}{100} = \frac{90}{100}$$
$$x = \frac{90}{100}$$

$x = 1$ cap. It would be impossible to administer 0.9 of a capsule. A 10% margin of difference is allowed between what is ordered and what is administered. When this 10% safety margin is used, no more than 110 mg and no less than 90 mg may be given.

The prescriber ordered (90 mg). The capsules available are 100 mg. Capsules are not divisible. Administering 1 cap is within the 10% margin of difference allowed.

9. $$\frac{0.5\text{ mg}}{1\text{ mL}} = \frac{0.25\text{ mg}}{x\text{ mL}}$$
$$\frac{0.5x}{0.5} = \frac{0.25}{0.5}$$
$$x = \frac{0.25}{0.5}$$

or

$$0.5\text{ mg}:1\text{ mL} = 0.25\text{ mg}:x\text{ mL}$$
$$\frac{0.5x}{0.5} = \frac{0.25}{0.5}$$
$$x = \frac{0.25}{0.5}$$

$x = 0.5$ mL, 0.25 mg is less than 0.5 mg; you will need less than 1 mL to administer the dosage.

10. $$\frac{125\text{ mg}}{5\text{ mL}} = \frac{100\text{ mg}}{x\text{ mL}}$$
$$\frac{125x}{125} = \frac{500}{125}$$
$$x = \frac{500}{125}$$

or

$$125\text{ mg}:5\text{ mL} = 100\text{ mg}:x\text{ mL}$$
$$\frac{125x}{125} = \frac{500}{125}$$
$$x = \frac{500}{125}$$

$x = 4$ mL. 100 mg is less than 125 mg; therefore you will need less than 5 mL to administer the dosage.

11. $$\frac{40\text{ mEq}}{10\text{ mL}} = \frac{20\text{ mEq}}{x\text{ mL}}$$
$$\frac{40x}{40} = \frac{200}{40}$$
$$40\text{ mEq}:10\text{ mL} = 20\text{ mEq}:x\text{ mL}$$
$$\frac{40x}{40} = \frac{200}{40}$$
$$x = \frac{200}{40}$$

$x = 5$ mL. 20 mEq is less than 40 mEq; you will need less than 10 mL to administer the dosage.

12. $$\frac{10{,}000\text{ units}}{1\text{ mL}} = \frac{5{,}000\text{ units}}{x\text{ mL}}$$
$$\frac{10{,}000x}{10{,}000} = \frac{5{,}000}{10{,}000}$$
$$x = \frac{5{,}000}{10{,}000}$$

or

$$10{,}000\text{ units}:1\text{ mL} = 5{,}000\text{ units}:x\text{ mL}$$
$$\frac{10{,}000x}{10{,}000} = \frac{5{,}000}{10{,}000}$$
$$x = \frac{5{,}000}{10{,}000}$$

$x = 0.5$ mL, 10,000 units is more than 5,000 units; therefore you will need less than 1 mL to administer the dosage.

13. $$\frac{80\text{ mg}}{2\text{ mL}} = \frac{50\text{ mg}}{x\text{ mL}}$$
$$\frac{80x}{80} = \frac{100}{80}$$
$$x = \frac{100}{80}$$

or

$$80\text{ mg}:2\text{ mL} = 50\text{ mg}:x\text{ mL}$$
$$\frac{80x}{80} = \frac{100}{80}$$
$$x = \frac{100}{80}$$

$x = 1.25 = 1.3$ mL. 50 mg is less than 80 mg; therefore you will need less than 2 mL to administer the dosage.

14. Equivalent: 1,000 mg = 1 g (0.5 g = 500 mg)

$$\frac{250 \text{ mg}}{1 \text{ cap}} = \frac{500 \text{ mg}}{x \text{ cap}}$$
$$\frac{250x}{250} = \frac{500}{250}$$

or

$$250 \text{ mg} : 1 \text{ cap} = 500 \text{ mg} : x \text{ cap}$$
$$\frac{250x}{250} = \frac{500}{250}$$
$$x = \frac{500}{250}$$

$x = 2$ caps. 500 mg is more than 250 mg; therefore you will need more than 1 cap to administer the dosage.

15.
$$\frac{125 \text{ mg}}{5 \text{ mL}} = \frac{400 \text{ mg}}{x \text{ mL}}$$
$$\frac{125x}{125} = \frac{2{,}000}{125}$$
$$x = \frac{2{,}000}{125}$$

or

$$125 \text{ mg} : 5 \text{ mL} = 400 \text{ mg} : x \text{ mL}$$
$$\frac{125x}{125} = \frac{2{,}000}{125}$$
$$x = \frac{2{,}000}{125}$$

$x = 16$ mL. 400 mg is larger than 125 mg; therefore you will need more than 5 mL to administer the dosage.

16.
$$\frac{80 \text{ mg}}{1 \text{ mL}} = \frac{50 \text{ mg}}{x \text{ mL}}$$
$$\frac{80x}{80} = \frac{50}{80}$$
$$x = \frac{50}{80}$$

or

$$80 \text{ mg} : 1 \text{ mL} = 50 \text{ mg} : x \text{ mL}$$
$$\frac{80x}{80} = \frac{50}{80}$$
$$x = \frac{50}{80}$$

$x = 0.62 = 0.6$ mL. 50 mg is less than 80 mg; therefore you will need less than 1 mL to administer the dosage.

17.
$$\frac{30 \text{ mg}}{1 \text{ mL}} = \frac{60 \text{ mg}}{x \text{ mL}}$$
$$\frac{30x}{30} = \frac{60}{30}$$
$$x = \frac{60}{30}$$

or

$$30 \text{ mg} : 1 \text{ mL} = 60 \text{ mg} : x \text{ mL}$$
$$\frac{30x}{30} = \frac{60}{30}$$
$$x = \frac{60}{30}$$

$x = 2$ mL. 60 mg is more than 30 mg; therefore you will need more than 1 mL to administer the dosage.

18.
$$\frac{5 \text{ mg}}{1 \text{ tab}} = \frac{15 \text{ mg}}{x \text{ tab}}$$
$$\frac{5x}{5} = \frac{15}{5}$$

or

$$5 \text{ mg} : 1 \text{ tab} = 15 \text{ mg} : x \text{ tab}$$
$$\frac{5x}{5} = \frac{15}{5}$$
$$x = \frac{15}{5}$$

$x = 3$ tabs. 15 mg is more than 5 mg; therefore you will need more than 1 tab to administer the dosage.

19. Equivalent: 1,000 mg = 1 g (0.24 g = 240 mg)

$$\frac{80 \text{ mg}}{7.5 \text{ mL}} = \frac{240 \text{ mg}}{x \text{ mL}}$$
$$\frac{80x}{80} = \frac{1{,}800}{80}$$
$$x = \frac{1{,}800}{80}$$

or

$$80 \text{ mg} : 7.5 \text{ mL} = 240 \text{ mg} : x \text{ mL}$$
$$\frac{80x}{80} = \frac{1{,}800}{80}$$
$$x = \frac{1{,}800}{80}$$

$x = 22.5$ mL. 240 mg is more than 80 mg; therefore you would need more than 7.5 mL to administer the dosage.

20. $$\frac{10\text{ g}}{15\text{ mL}} = \frac{20\text{ g}}{x\text{ mL}}$$
$$\frac{10\,x}{10} = \frac{300}{10}$$
$$x = \frac{300}{10}$$

or

$$10\text{ g}:15\text{ mL} = 20\text{ g}:x\text{ mL}$$
$$\frac{10x}{10} = \frac{300}{10}$$
$$x = \frac{300}{10}$$

$x = 30$ mL. 20 g is more than 10 g; therefore you would need more than 15 mL to administer the dosage.

21. $$\frac{0.5\text{ mg}}{2\text{ mL}} = \frac{0.125\text{ mg}}{x\text{ mL}}$$
$$\frac{0.5\,x}{0.5} = \frac{0.25}{0.5}$$

or

$$0.5\text{ mg}:2\text{ mL} = 0.125\text{ mg}:x\text{ mL}$$
$$\frac{0.5x}{0.5} = \frac{0.25}{0.5}$$
$$x = \frac{0.25}{0.5}$$

$x = 0.5$ mL, 0.125 mg is less than 0.5 mg; therefore you will need less than 2 mL to administer the dosage.

22. $$\frac{0.25\text{ mg}}{1\text{ mL}} = \frac{0.75\text{ mg}}{x\text{ mL}}$$
$$\frac{0.25\,x}{0.25} = \frac{0.75}{0.25}$$

or

$$0.25\text{ mg}:1\text{ mL} = 0.75\text{ mg}:x\text{ mL}$$
$$\frac{0.25x}{0.25} = \frac{0.75}{0.25}$$
$$x = \frac{0.75}{0.25}$$

$x = 3$ mL. 0.75 mg is more than 0.25 mg; therefore you will need more than 1 mL to administer the dosage.

23. $$\frac{125\text{ mg}}{5\text{ mL}} = \frac{375\text{ mg}}{x\text{ mL}}$$
$$\frac{125x}{125} = \frac{1{,}875}{125}$$

or

$$125\text{ mg}:5\text{ mL} = 375\text{ mg}:x\text{ mL}$$
$$\frac{125x}{125} = \frac{1{,}875}{125}$$
$$x = \frac{1{,}875}{125}$$

$x = 15$ mL. 375 mg is more than 125 mg; therefore you will need more than 5 mL to administer the dosage.

24. $$\frac{7{,}500\text{ units}}{1\text{ mL}} = \frac{10{,}000\text{ units}}{x\text{ mL}}$$
$$\frac{7{,}500x}{7{,}500} = \frac{10{,}000}{7{,}500}$$

or

$$7{,}500\text{ units}:1\text{ mL} = 10{,}000\text{ units}:x\text{ mL}$$
$$\frac{7{,}500x}{7{,}500} = \frac{10{,}000}{7{,}500}$$
$$x = \frac{10{,}000}{7{,}500}$$

$x = 1.33 = 1.3$ mL. 10,000 units is more than 7,500 units; therefore you will need more than 1 mL to administer the dosage.

25. $$\frac{0.3\text{ mg}}{1\text{ tab}} = \frac{0.45\text{ mg}}{x\text{ tab}}$$
$$\frac{0.3x}{0.3} = \frac{0.45}{0.3}$$

or

$$0.3\text{ mg}:1\text{ tab} = 0.45\text{ mg}:x\text{ tab}$$
$$\frac{0.3x}{0.3} = \frac{0.45}{0.3}$$
$$x = \frac{0.45}{0.3}$$

$x = 1.5$ tabs or $1\frac{1}{2}$ tabs. 0.45 mg is more than 0.3 mg; therefore you will need more than 1 tab to administer the dosage.

NOTE

For questions 26-45 and Chapter Review Parts I and II, answers only are provided. Refer to setup for problems 1-25 if needed.

26. 1.2 mL
27. 1.9 mL
28. 0.7 mL
29. 2 mL
30. 1.1 mL
31. 1.7 mL
32. 2.2 mL
33. 2 mL
34. 2.2 mL
35. 0.6 mL
36. 0.8 mL
37. 5 mL
38. 3.3 mL
39. 0.9 mL
40. 1.6 mL
41. 300 mg
42. 84 tablets
43. 24 hours
44. 31.25 mg
45. 360 mL

Answers to Chapter Review Part I

1. 1 tab
2. 2 delayed release caps
3. 2 tabs
4. 2 tabs
5. 2 tabs
6. 2 sustained release (SR) caps
7. 2 tabs
8. 2 tabs
9. 1 tab
10. 1 tab
11. 2 tabs
12. 1 tab
13. 2 caps
14. 1 cap
15. 2 tabs
16. 2 tabs (chewable)
17. 2 caps
18. 2 caps
19. 1 tab
20. 2 tabs
21. 2 tabs
22. 1 tab (DS)
23. 2 caps
24. 2 caps
25. 2 tabs
26. 2 tabs
27. 1 tab
28. 2 tabs
29. 3 tabs
30. 2 tabs
31. 3 tabs
32. 2 tabs
33. 2 tabs
34. 2 caps
35. 2 caps
36. 3 caps
37. 2 tabs
38. 1 tab
39. $\frac{1}{2}$ tab *or* 0.5 tab
40. 1 tab

Answers to Chapter Review Part II

41. 4 mL
42. 20 mL
43. 1.3 mL
44. 20 mL
45. 0.7 mL
46. 2.3 mL
47. 1 mL
48. 1 mL
49. 0.67 mL
50. 15 mL
51. 1 mL
52. 1 mL
53. 2 mL
54. 10 mL
55. 0.75 mL
56. 1.8 mL
57. 1 mL
58. 0.5 mL
59. 0.7 mL
60. 0.4 mL
61. 6 mL
62. 6.3 mL
63. 0.8 mL
64. 5 mL
65. 30 mL
66. 40 mL
67. 10 mL
68. 1 mL
69. 0.7 mL
70. 45 mL
71. 1.3 mL
72. 1.4 mL
73. 6.7 mL
74. 8 mL
75. 1.2 mL
76. 0.8 mL
77. 0.3 mL
78. 0.25 mL
79. 10 mL
80. 12.5 mL

CHAPTER 15
Dosage Calculation Using the Formula Method

Objectives

After reviewing this chapter, you should be able to:

1. Identify the information from a calculation problem to place into the formula given
2. Calculate medication dosages using the formula $\frac{D}{H} \times Q = x$
3. Calculate the number of tablets or capsules to administer
4. Calculate the volume to administer for medications in solution

This chapter shows how to use a commonly used *formula method* to calculate the amount to administer. Using a *formula method* to calculate requires determining the components of the formula from the problem and substituting the information from the problem into the formula.

Total reliance on a formula without thinking and asking yourself whether an answer is reasonable can result in errors in calculation and an administration error.

When using a formula, always use it consistently and in its entirety to avoid calculation errors. Always ask, "Is the answer obtained reasonable?"

You will learn, for example, that the maximum number of tablets or capsules for a single dosage is usually three. Anything exceeding that should be a red flag to you, even if the answer is obtained from the use of a formula. Use formulas to validate the dosage you think is reasonable, not the reverse. **Think** before you calculate. Always estimate **before** applying a formula. Thinking first will allow you to detect errors and alert you to try again and question the results you obtained.

SAFETY ALERT!

Avoid Dosage Calculation Errors

Do not rely solely on formulas when calculating dosages to be administered. Use critical thinking skills such as considering what the answer should be, reasoning, problem solving, and finding rational justification for your answer. Formulas should be used as tools for validating the dosage you THINK should be given.

Formula for Calculating Dosages

The formula presented in this chapter can be used when calculating dosages in the same system of measurement. When the dosage desired and the dosage on hand are in different systems, convert them to the same system before using the formula, using one of the methods learned for conversion. It is important to learn and memorize the following formula and its components:

$$\frac{D}{H} \times Q = x$$

Let's examine the terms in the formula before using it.

D = The dosage desired, or what the prescriber has ordered, including the units of measurement. Examples: mg, g, etc.
H = The dosage strength available, what is on hand, or the weight of the medication on the label, including the unit of measurement. Examples: mg, g, etc.
Q = The quantity or the unit of measure that contains the dosage that is available, in other words, the number of tablets, capsules, milliliters, etc. that contains the available dosage. "Q" is labeled accordingly as tablet, capsule, milliliter, etc.
x = The unknown, the dosage you are looking for, the dosage you are going to administer, how many milliliters, tablets, etc. you will give.

Note: The unknown "x" and "Q" are always labeled the same (e.g., tabs, mL).

Always get into the habit of inserting the quantity value for **"Q"** into the formula, even though when solving problems that involve solid forms of medication (tabs, caps), **"Q"** is always 1. This will prevent errors when calculating dosages for medications in solution (oral liquids or injectables) in which the solution quantity can be more or less than 1. (such as per 10 mL). When solving problems for medications in solution, the amount for **"Q"** varies and must always be included.

The available dosage on the label for medications in solution may indicate the quantity of medication per 1 milliliter or per multiple milliliters of solution, such as 80 mg per 2 mL, 125 mg per 5 mL. Some liquid medications may also express the quantity in amounts less than a milliliter, such as 2 mg per 0.5 mL.

When setting up the formula, notice that **"D,"** which is the dosage desired, is in the numerator, and **"H."** which is the dosage strength available, is placed in the denominator of the fraction.

All terms of the formula, including "x," must be labeled to ensure accuracy.

SAFETY ALERT!

Omission of the amount for **"Q"** can render an error in dosage calculation. Labeling of all terms of the formula, including "x," is a safeguard to prevent errors in calculation. Always think first, what is a reasonable amount to administer, and calculate the dosage using the formula.

Using the Formula Method

Let's review the steps for using the formula (Box 15-1) before beginning to calculate dosages.

BOX 15-1 Steps for Using the Formula

1. Memorize the formula, or verify the formula from a resource.
2. Place the information from the problem into the formula in the correct position, with all terms in the formula labeled correctly, including "*x*."
3. Make sure that all measures are in the same units and system of measure; if not, a conversion must be done *before* calculating the dosage.
4. Think logically, and consider what a reasonable amount to administer would be.
5. Calculate your answer, using the formula $\frac{D}{H} \times Q = x$.
6. Label all answers—tabs, caps, mL, etc.

Now we will look at sample problems illustrating the use of the formula.

Example 1: Order: 0.375 mg p.o. of a medication.

Available: Tablets labeled 0.25 mg

Solution: The dosage 0.375 mg is desired; the dosage strength available is 0.25 mg per tablet. No conversion is necessary. What is desired is in the same system and unit of measure as what you have on hand.

✓ FORMULA SETUP

$$\frac{D}{H} \times Q = x$$

The desired (D) is 0.375 mg. You have on hand (H) 0.25 mg per (Q) 1 tablet. The label on x is tablet. Notice that the label on x is always the same as Q.

$$\frac{\text{(D) 0.375 mg}}{\text{(H) 0.25 mg}} \times \text{(Q) 1 tab} = x \text{ tab}$$

$$x = \frac{0.375}{0.25} \times 1$$

$$x = \frac{0.375}{0.25}$$

$$x = 1.5 = 1\tfrac{1}{2} \text{ tabs}$$

Therefore $x = 1.5$ tabs, or $1\frac{1}{2}$ tabs. (Because 0.375 mg is larger than 0.25 mg, you will need more than 1 tab to administer 0.375 mg.) *Note:* Although 1.5 tabs is the same as $1\frac{1}{2}$ tabs, for administration purposes, it would be best to state it as $1\frac{1}{2}$ tabs.

Example 2: Order: 7,000 units IM of a medication.

Available: 10,000 units in 2 mL

Solution:

$$\frac{\text{(D) 7,000 units}}{\text{(H) 10,000 units}} \times \text{(Q) 2 mL} = x \text{ mL}$$

$$x = \frac{7{,}0\cancel{00}}{10{,}0\cancel{00}} \times 2$$

$$x = \frac{14}{10}$$

$$x = 1.4 \text{ mL}$$

SAFETY ALERT!

Omitting Q here could result in an error. A liquid form of medication is involved; Q must be included because the amount varies and is not always per 1 mL.

RULE

Rule for Different Units or Systems of Measure

Whenever the desired amount and the dosage on hand are in different units or systems of measure, follow these steps:

1. Choose the identified equivalent (the conversion factor needed to make the conversion).
2. Convert what is ordered to the same units or system of measure as what is available by using one of the methods presented in the chapter on converting.
3. Use the formula $\frac{D}{H} \times Q = x$ to calculate the dosage to administer.

Remember that despite The Joint Commission (TJC) recommendation to discontinue the use of the apothecary system, you may still see these measures indicated on medication labels. A common medication seen with apothecary measures is Nitrostat (Nitroglycerine); however, the metric equivalent is also indicated on the label. Always look carefully for the metric dosage strength and use it to calculate dosages.

TIPS FOR CLINICAL PRACTICE

The metric system is the principal system used for medications. When converting is required before calculating a dosage, convert measures to their metric equivalent when possible to decrease the chance of error in calculation.

Example 3: Order: 0.1 mg p.o. of a medication daily

Available: Tablets labeled 50 mcg

Solution: Convert 0.1 mg to mcg. The equivalent to use is 1 mg = 1,000 mcg. Therefore, 0.1 mg = 100 mcg

Now that you have everything in the same system and units of measure, use the formula presented to calculate the dosage to be administered.

Solution:

$$\frac{\text{(D) 100 mcg}}{\text{(H) 50 mcg}} \times \text{(Q) 1 tab} = x \text{ tab}$$

$$x = \frac{100}{50} \times 1$$

$$x = \frac{100}{50}$$

$$x = 2 \text{ tabs}$$

Therefore, $x = 2$ tabs. (Because 100 mcg is a larger dosage than 50 mcg, it will take more than 1 tab to administer the desired dosage.)

Example 4: Order: 0.2 g p.o. of a liquid medication.

Available: 125 mg per 5 mL.

Solution: Convert 0.2 g to mg. The equivalent to use is 1,000 mg = 1 g. Therefore, 0.2 g = 200 mg.

Now that everything is in the same system and units of measure, use the formula presented to calculate the dosage to be administered.

$$\frac{\text{(D) 200 mg}}{\text{(H) 125 mg}} \times \text{(Q) 5 mL} = x \text{ mL}$$

$$x = \frac{200 \times 5}{125}$$

$$x = \frac{1{,}000}{125}$$

$$x = 8 \text{ mL}$$

Therefore, $x = 8$ mL (Because 200 mg is a larger dose than 125 mg, it will take more than 5 mL to administer the desired dosage.)

Example 5: Order: 10 mg subcutaneous of a medication.

Available: 30 mg per mL (Express the answer to the nearest tenth.)

Solution: No conversion is required; the dosage ordered is in the same system and unit of measurement as the available.

$$\frac{(D)\ 10\ \text{mg}}{(H)\ 30\ \text{mg}} \times (Q)\ 1\ \text{mL} = x\ \text{mL}$$

$$x = \frac{10}{30} \times 1$$

$$x = \frac{10}{30}$$

$$x = \frac{1}{3} = 3\overline{)1.00}^{\,0.33} = 0.33 = 0.3\ \text{mL}$$

Therefore, $x = 0.33 = 0.3$ mL rounded to the nearest tenth. (Because 30 mg is larger than 10 mg, it will take less than 1 mL to administer the required dosage.) Milliliter is a metric measure expressed as a decimal number.

CRITICAL THINKING

Use critical thinking before and after formulaic calculating. It is an essential step in estimating what is reasonable and logical in terms of a dosage. This will help prevent errors in calculation caused by setting up the problem incorrectly or careless math and will remind you to double-check your calculation and identify any error.

Remember to memorize the formula presented and follow the steps sequentially.

- Check **first** to see if a conversion is required; if so, **convert** so that everything is in the same units and system of measure.
- **Think** critically as to a reasonable answer.
- Set up terms in the formula and **calculate** to validate the dosage you anticipated was reasonable using the formula.

SAFETY ALERT!

Always double-check your math. Errors can be made in simple calculations because of lack of caution. Always ask yourself whether the answer you have obtained is reasonable and correct.

POINTS TO REMEMBER

- The formula $\frac{D}{H} \times Q = x$ can be used to calculate the dosage to be administered.
- The Q is always 1 for solid forms of medications (tabs, caps, etc.) but varies when medications are in liquid form. Do not omit "Q" even when 1.
- Before the dosage to be given is calculated, the dosage desired must be in the same units and system of measure as the dosage available or a conversion is necessary.
- Set up the terms in the formula labeled with the units of measure, including "*x*."
- Think about what a reasonable answer would be.
- Calculate the dosage to administer using the formula to validate your answer as to what was reasonable.
- Double-check all your math, and think logically about the answer obtained.
- Label all answers obtained (e.g., tabs, caps, mL).
- The use of a formula does not eliminate the need to think critically.
- Always systematically follow these steps: **Convert** if necessary, **THINK** about what would be a reasonable answer, set up the terms in the formula, **Calculate** the dosage to administer using the formula.

PRACTICE PROBLEMS

Calculate the following problems using the formula presented in this chapter. Label answers correctly: tabs, caps.

1. Order: 0.4 mg p.o.

   Available: Tablets labeled 0.2 mg ______________________

2. Order: 0.75 g p.o.

   Available: Capsules labeled 250 mg ______________________

3. Order: 90 mg p.o.

   Available: Tablets labeled 60 mg ______________________

4. Order: 7.5 mg p.o.

   Available: Tablets labeled 2.5 mg ______________________

5. Order: 0.05 mg p.o.

   Available: Tablets labeled 25 mcg ______________________

6. Order: 0.4 mg p.o.

   Available: Tablets labeled 200 mcg ______________________

7. Order: 1,000 mg p.o.

   Available: Tablets labeled 500 mg ______________________

8. Order: 0.6 g p.o.

   Available: Capsules labeled 600 mg ______________________

9. Order: 1.25 mg p.o.

   Available: Tablets labeled 625 mcg ______________________

Calculate the following in milliliters; round to the nearest tenth where indicated. Label answers in mL.

10. Order: 10 mg subcut.

    Available: 15 mg per mL ______________________

11. Order: 400 mg p.o.

    Available: Oral solution labeled 200 mg per 5 mL ______________________

12. Order: 15 mEq p.o.

    Available: Oral solution labeled 20 mEq per10 mL ______________________

13. Order: 125 mg p.o.

    Available: Oral solution labeled 250 mg per 5 mL ______________

14. Order: 0.025 mg p.o.

    Available: Oral solution labeled 0.05 mg per 5 mL ______________

15. Order: 375 mg p.o.

    Available: Oral solution labeled 125 mg per 5 mL ______________

Answers on pp. 268-269

CHAPTER **REVIEW**

Calculate the following dosages using the medication label or information provided. Label answers correctly: tabs, caps, mL. Answers expressed in milliliters should be rounded to the nearest tenth where indicated.

1. Order: Phenobarbital 30 mg p.o. t.i.d.

   Available: Phenobarbital tablets labeled 30 mg ______________

2. Order: Crixivan 0.8 g p.o. q8h

   Available: Crixivan capsules labeled 400 mg ______________

3. Order: Feldene 20 mg p.o. daily.

   Available:

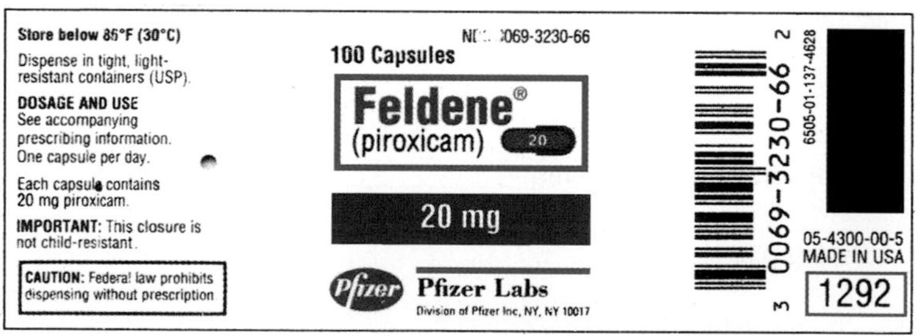

____

4. Order: Hydrodiuril 50 mg p.o. b.i.d.

   Available:

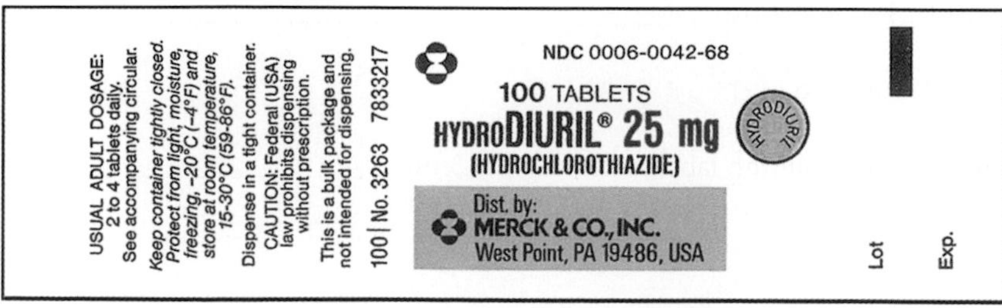

____

5. Order: Tylenol 650 mg p.o. q4h p.r.n. for pain.

   Available:

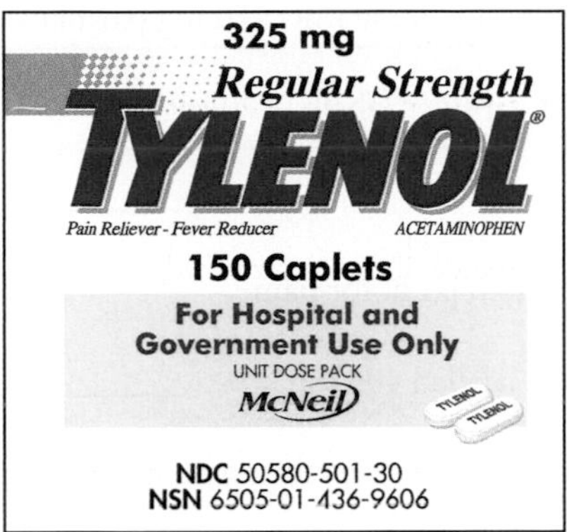

____

6. Order: Digoxin 0.375 mg p.o. daily.

   Available:

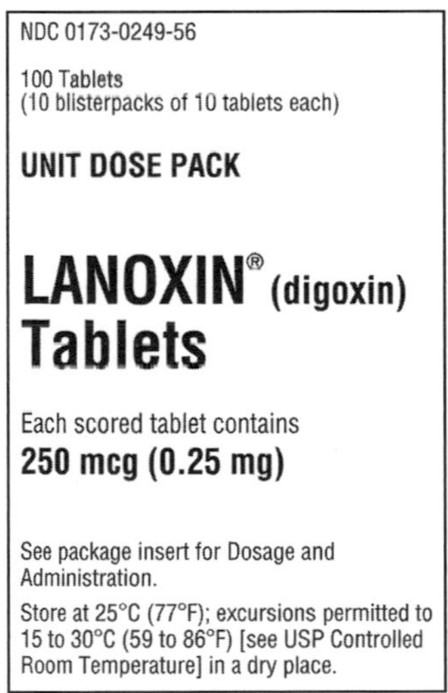

____

7. Order: Flagyl 0.5 g p.o. b.i.d. for 1 week.

   Available:

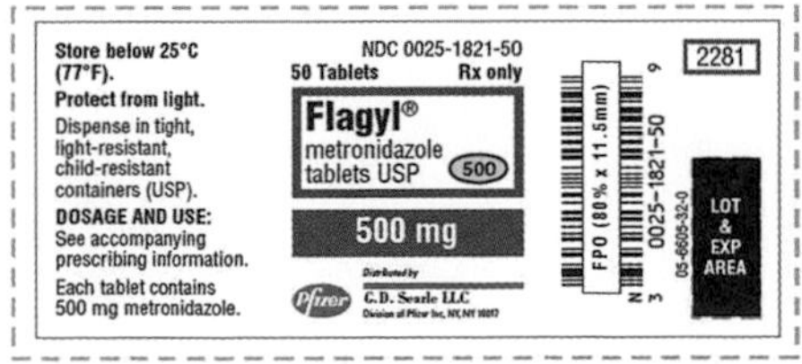

____

8. Order: Seconal 100 mg p.o. at bedtime.

   Available: Seconal capsules labeled 100 mg ______________

9. Order: Verapamil Sustained Release (SR) 240 mg p.o. daily.

   Available: Verapamil SR capsules labeled 120 mg

   ____

10. Order: Motrin 0.8 g p.o. q8h p.r.n. for pain.

    Available: Motrin tablets labeled 400 mg ______________

11. Order: Morphine (immediate release tablets) 30 mg p.o. q4h p.r.n. for pain.

    Available: Scored tablets (can be broken in half).

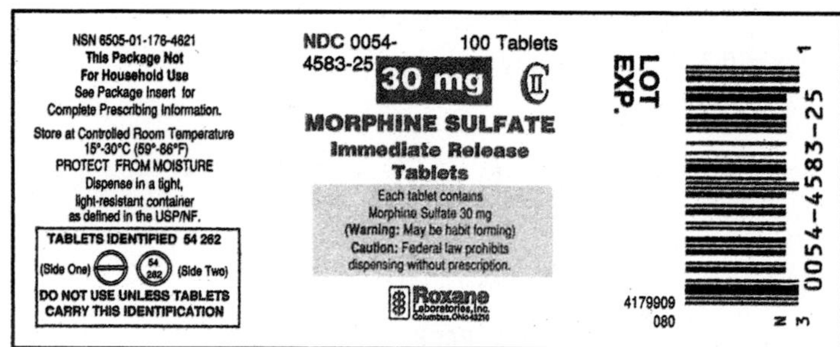

    ____

12. Order: Cephradine 0.5 g p.o. q6h.

    Available: Cephradine 250 mg caps. ______________

13. Order: Cogentin 0.5 mg p.o. at bedtime.

    Available:

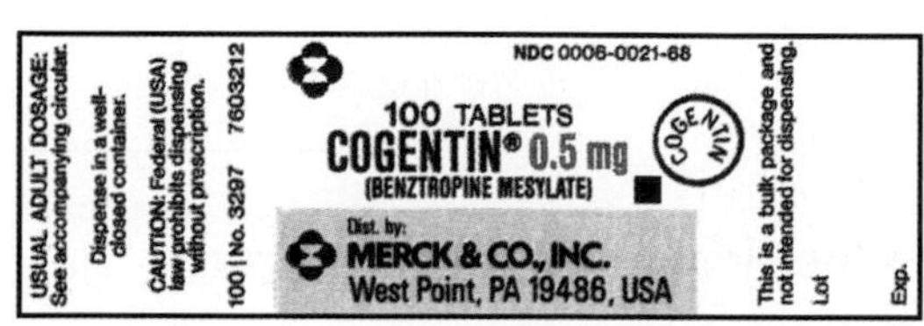

    ____

14. Order: Librium 50 mg p.o. q4h p.r.n. for 24 hours for acute alcohol withdrawal.

    Available:

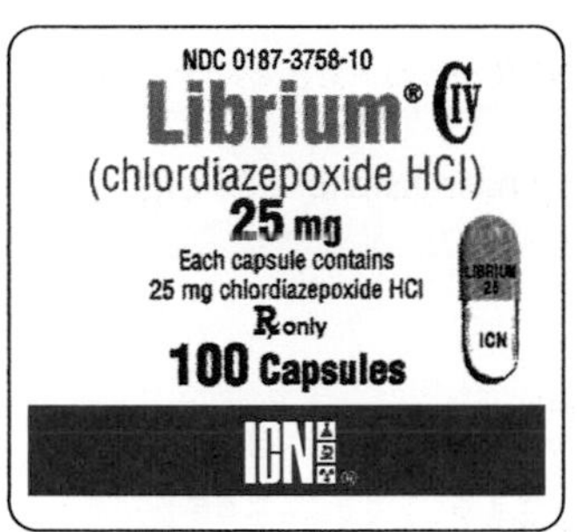

____

15. Order: Dilantin (extended capsules) 60 mg p.o. b.i.d.

    Available: Dilantin (extended capsules) labeled 30 mg

____

16. Order: Meperidine hydrochloride 50 mg I.M. q4h p.r.n. for pain.

    Available: Meperidine hydrochloride 75 mg per mL

____

17. Order: Methylprednisolone sodium succinate 60 mg IV daily.

    Available: Methylprednisolone sodium succinate labeled 40 mg per mL

____

18. Order: Diltiazem 20 mg IV stat.

    Available:

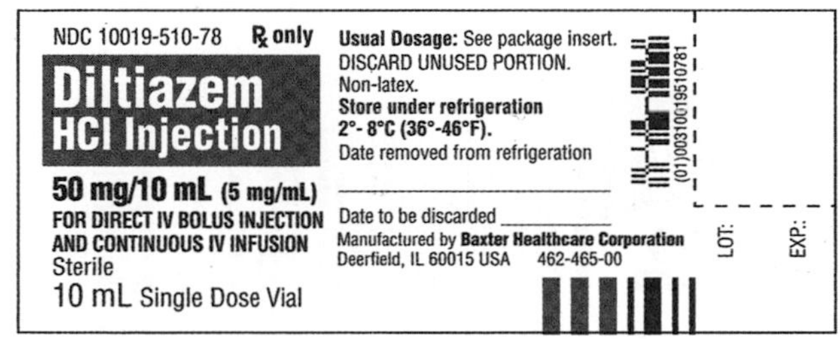

____

19. Order: Amoxicillin 300 mg p.o. q8h.

    Available: Amoxicillin oral suspension labeled 125 mg per 5 mL

    ____

20. Order: Amoxicillin 0.5 g by nasogastric tube q6h.

    Available:

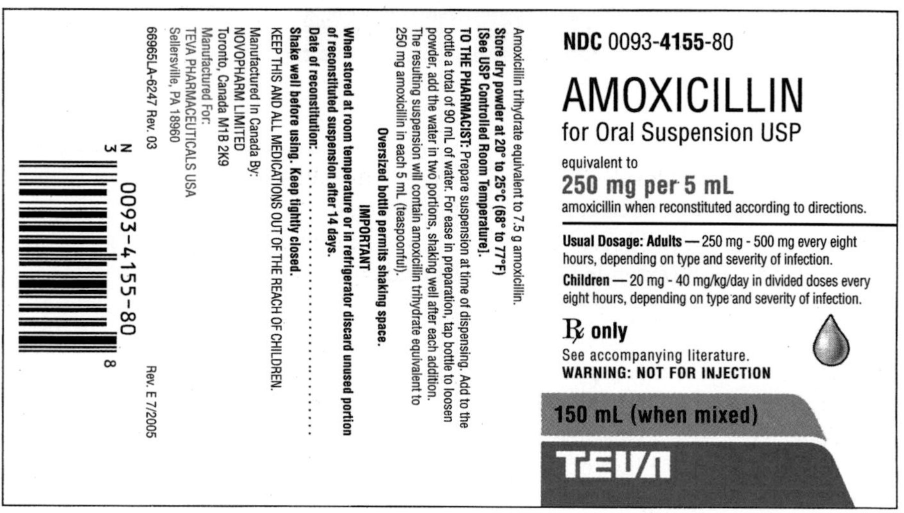

    ____

21. Order: Phenobarbital elixir 45 mg p.o. b.i.d.

    Available: Phenobarbital elixir 20 mg per 5 mL

    ____

22. Order: Heparin 3,000 units subcut b.i.d.

    Available:

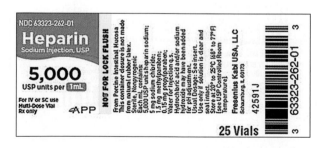

    ____

23. Order: Procaine Penicillin G 600,000 units IM q12h.

    Available: Procaine Penicillin G 300,000 units per mL

    ____

24. Order: Gentamicin 70 mg IV q8h.

    Available:

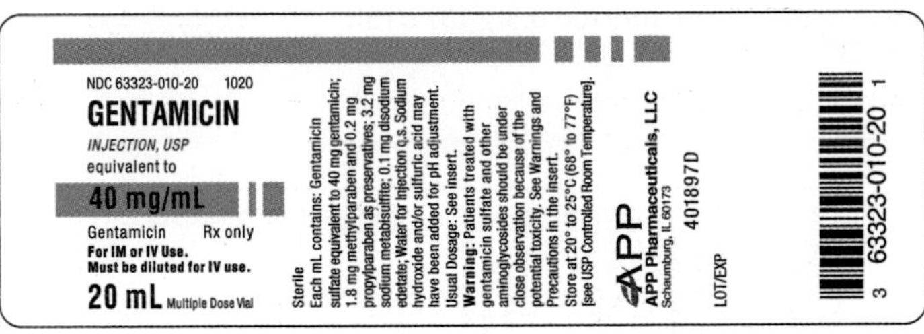
NDC 63323-010-20 1020
GENTAMICIN
INJECTION, USP
equivalent to
40 mg/mL
Gentamicin Rx only
For IM or IV Use.
Must be diluted for IV use.
20 mL Multiple Dose Vial
Sterile
Each mL contains: Gentamicin sulfate equivalent to 40 mg gentamicin; 1.8 mg methylparaben and 0.2 mg propylparaben as preservatives; 3.2 mg sodium metabisulfite; 0.1 mg disodium edetate; Water for Injection q.s. Sodium hydroxide and/or sulfuric acid may have been added for pH adjustment.
Usual Dosage: See insert.
Warning: Patients treated with gentamicin sulfate and other aminoglycosides should be under close observation because of the potential toxicity. See Warnings and Precautions in the insert.
Store at 20° to 25°C (68° to 77°F) [see USP Controlled Room Temperature].
APP
APP Pharmaceuticals, LLC
Schaumburg, IL 60173
401897D
LOT/EXP
3 63323-010-20 1

____

25. Order: Potassium chloride 20 mEq IV in 1,000 mL 0.9% normal saline.

    Available: Potassium chloride 20 mL vial labeled 40 mEq (2 mEq per mL)

____

26. Order: Folic acid 1,000 mcg IM daily for 10 days.

    Available: Folic acid 5,000 mcg per mL ____________________

27. Order: Vistaril 100 mg IM stat.

    Available: Vistaril 50 mg per mL ____________________

28. Order: Morphine sulfate 6 mg subcut q4h p.r.n. for pain.

    Available:

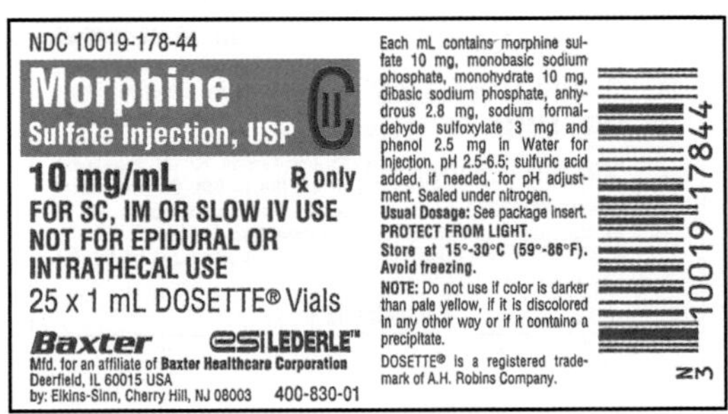
NDC 10019-178-44
Morphine
Sulfate Injection, USP
CII
10 mg/mL
℞ only
FOR SC, IM OR SLOW IV USE
NOT FOR EPIDURAL OR INTRATHECAL USE
25 x 1 mL DOSETTE® Vials
Baxter
ESI LEDERLE
Mfd. for an affiliate of Baxter Healthcare Corporation
Deerfield, IL 60015 USA
by: Elkins-Sinn, Cherry Hill, NJ 08003
400-830-01
Each mL contains morphine sulfate 10 mg, monobasic sodium phosphate, monohydrate 10 mg, dibasic sodium phosphate, anhydrous 2.8 mg, sodium formaldehyde sulfoxylate 3 mg and phenol 2.5 mg in Water for Injection. pH 2.5-6.5; sulfuric acid added, if needed, for pH adjustment. Sealed under nitrogen.
Usual Dosage: See package insert.
PROTECT FROM LIGHT.
Store at 15°-30°C (59°-86°F). Avoid freezing.
NOTE: Do not use if color is darker than pale yellow, if it is discolored in any other way or if it contains a precipitate.
DOSETTE® is a registered trademark of A.H. Robins Company.
N 3 10019 17844

____

29. Order: Atropine 0.3 mg IM stat.

    Available: Atropine 0.4 mg per mL ____________________

30. Order: Stadol 1 mg IM q4h p.r.n. for pain.

    Available: Stadol labeled 2 mg per mL ____________________

31. Order: Ativan 1 mg IM stat.

    Available: Ativan 4 mg per mL ______________________

32. Order: Lincomycin hydrochloride 0.5 g IM q12h.

    Available:

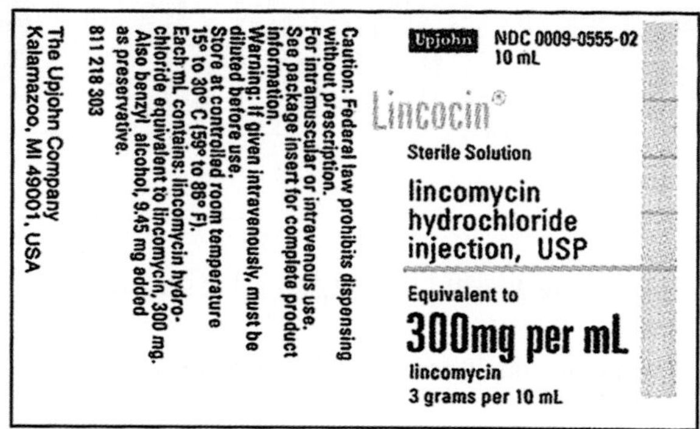

____

33. Order: Robinul 0.4 mg IM stat on call to OR.

    Available: Robinul labeled 0.2 mg per mL

____

34. Order: Aminophylline 80 mg IV q6h.

    Available:

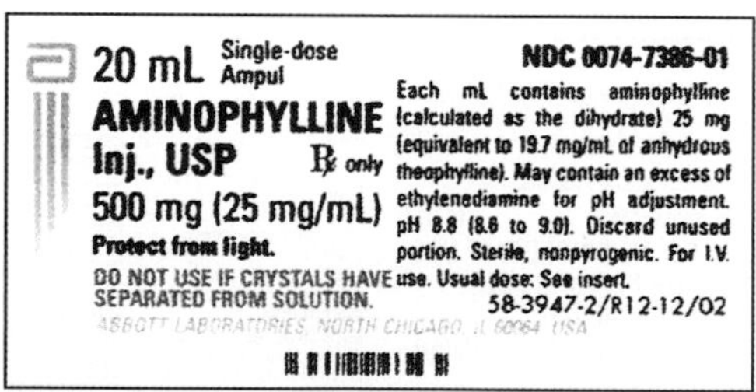

____

35. Order: Lithium citrate oral solution 300 mg p.o. t.i.d.

    Available: Lithium citrate 300 mg per 5 mL

____

36. Order: Sinemet 25-100 p.o. q.i.d.

Available:

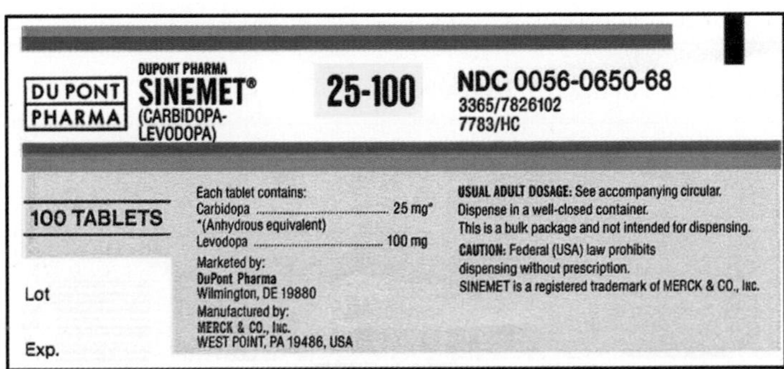

____

37. Order: Lopid 0.6 g p.o. b.i.d. 30 minutes before meals.

Available:

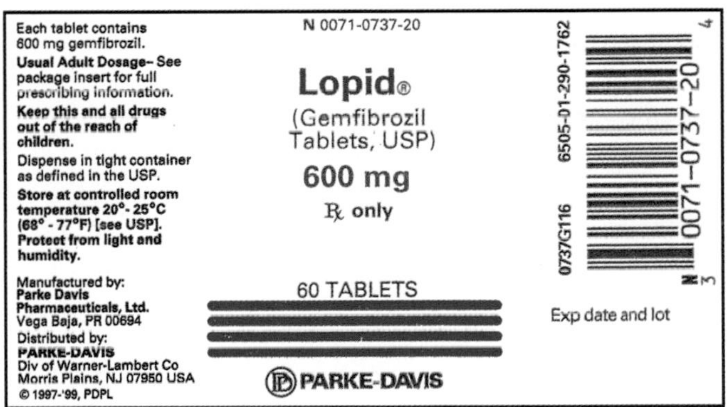

____

38. Order: Tricor 108 mg p.o. daily.

Available:

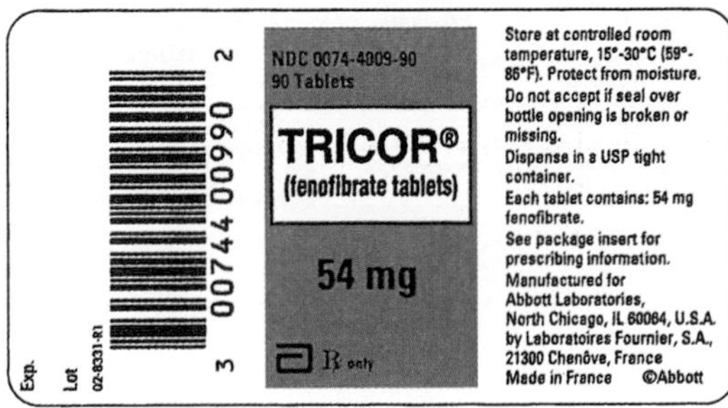

____

39. Order: Potassium chloride 10 mEq IV in 1,000 mL D5W.

    Available: Potassium chloride 20 mL vial labeled 40 mEq (2 mEq per mL)

    ____

40. Order: Prednisone 7.5 mg p.o. b.i.d.

    Available:

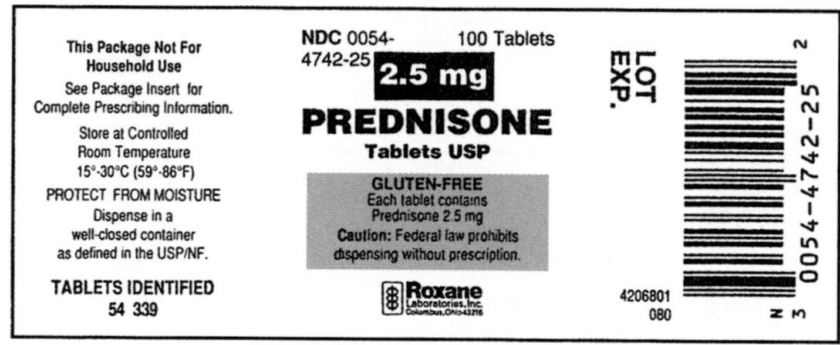

    ____

41. Order: Tagamet 800 mg p.o. at bedtime.

    Available: Tagamet tablets labeled 400 mg

    ____

42. Order: Depo-Provera 650 mg IM once a week (on Mondays).

    Available: Depo-Provera labeled 400 mg per mL

    ____

43. Order: Tagamet 0.4 g IV b.i.d.

    Available:

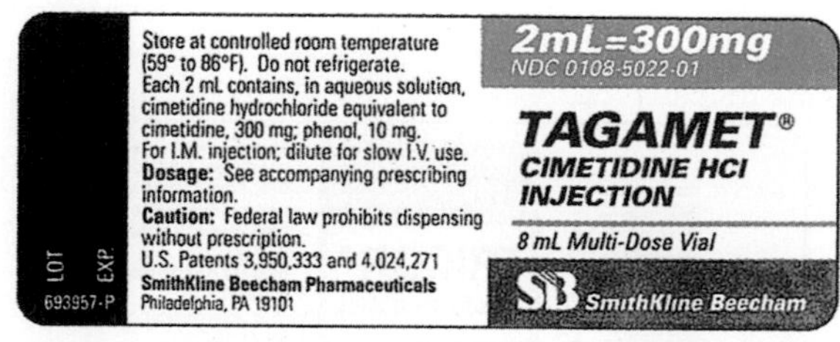
Store at controlled room temperature (59° to 86°F). Do not refrigerate.
Each 2 mL contains, in aqueous solution, cimetidine hydrochloride equivalent to cimetidine, 300 mg; phenol, 10 mg.
For I.M. injection; dilute for slow I.V. use.
Dosage: See accompanying prescribing information.
Caution: Federal law prohibits dispensing without prescription.
U.S. Patents 3,950,333 and 4,024,271
SmithKline Beecham Pharmaceuticals
Philadelphia, PA 19101
LOT
EXP
693957-P
2mL=300mg
NDC 0108-5022-01
TAGAMET®
CIMETIDINE HCl INJECTION
8 mL Multi-Dose Vial
SB SmithKline Beecham

    ____

44. Order: Doxycycline 0.1 g IVPB q12h.

Available:

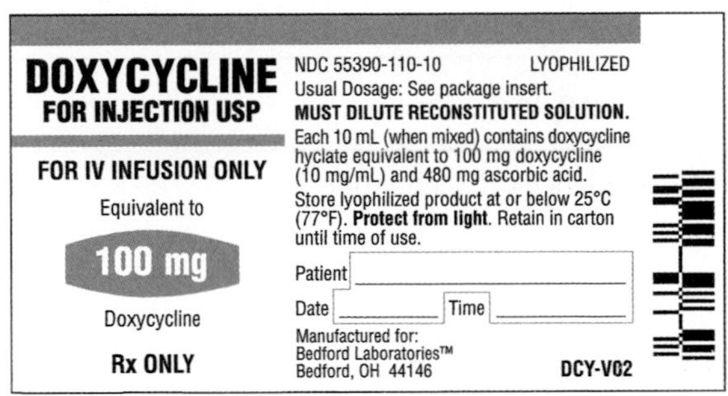

____

45. Order: Cipro 1.5 g p.o. q12h.

Available: Cipro tablets labeled 750 mg _______________

46. Order: Vasotec 5 mg p.o. daily.

Available:

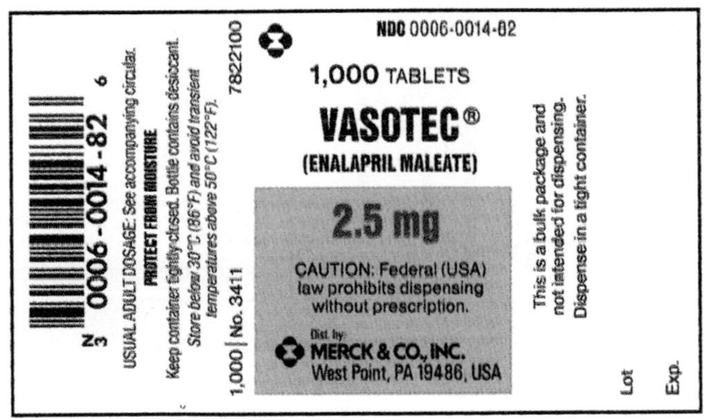

____

47. Order: Clozaril 50 mg p.o. b.i.d.

Available:

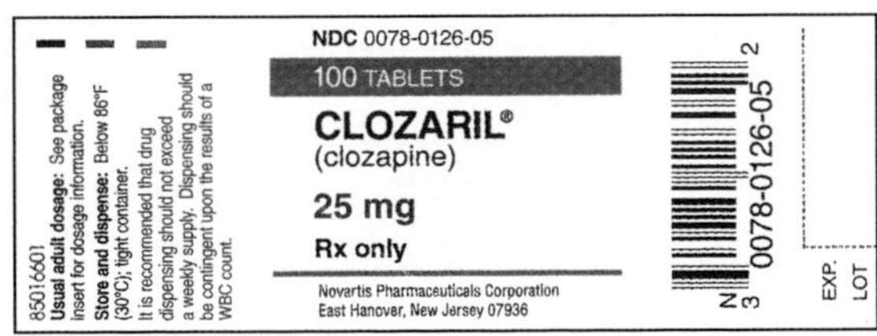

____

48. Order: Clindamycin 450 mg p.o. q.i.d. for 5 days.

    Available: Clindamycin oral solution labeled 75 mg per 5 mL

    ____

49. Order: Benadryl 30 mg p.o. t.i.d.

    Available: Oral solution labeled 12.5 mg per 5 mL

    ____

50. Order: Primidone 125 mg p.o. daily.

    Available: Oral solution labeled 250 mg per 5 mL

    ____

51. Order: Metformin hydrochloride (extended release) 750 mg p.o. b.i.d. with meals.

    Available:

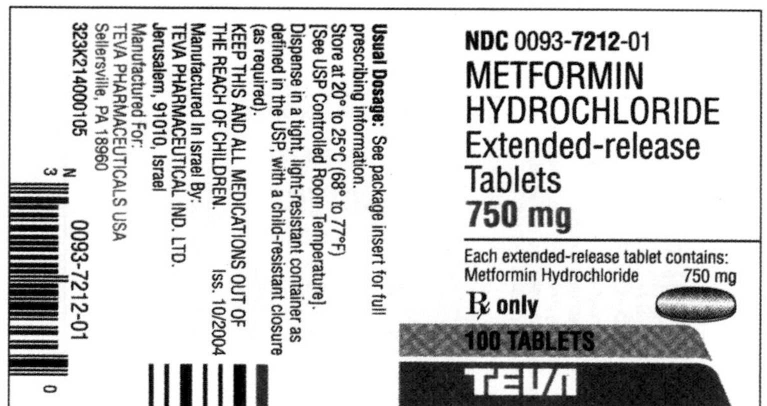

    ____

52. Order: Inderal 40 mg p.o. b.i.d.

    Available:

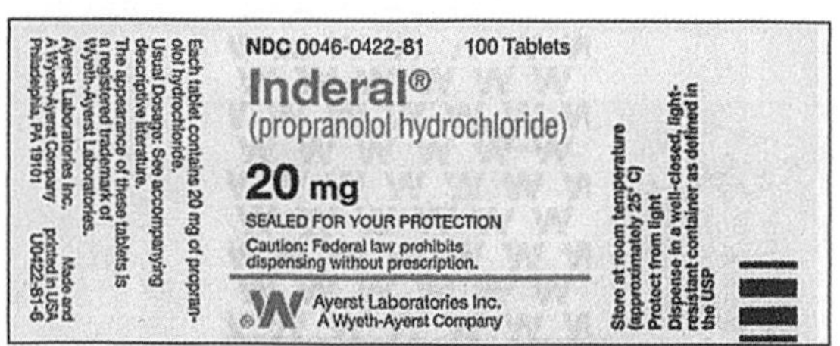

    ____

53. Order: Lasix 30 mg p.o. every day at 9 AM.

Available: Scored tablets (can be broken in half)

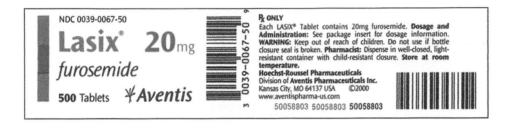

____

54. Order: Janumet 50 mg/1,000 mg p.o. b.i.d.

Available:

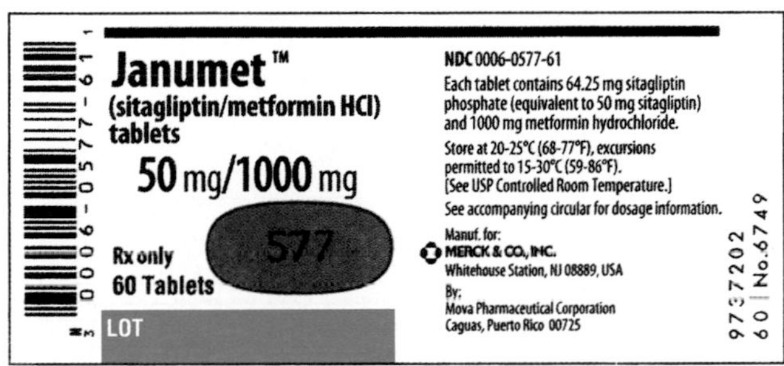

____

55. Order: Targretin 150 mg p.o. daily ac.

Available:

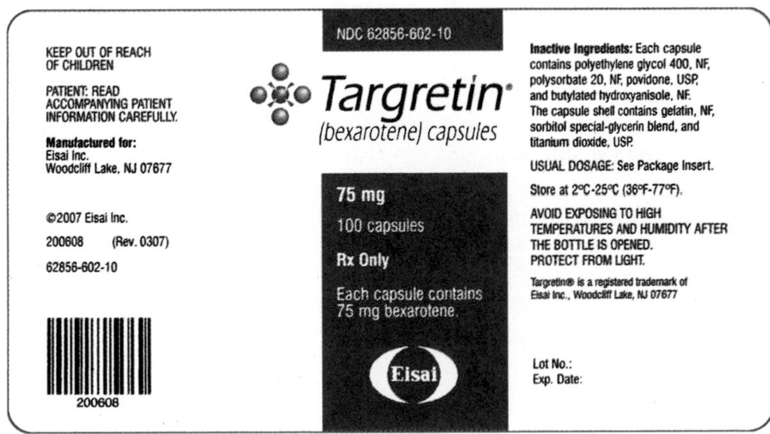

____

56. Order: Glyburide 7.5 mg p.o. daily with breakfast.

    Available: Glyburide tablets labeled 2.5 mg

    ____

57. Order: Biaxin 0.5 g p.o. q12h for 10 days.

    Available:

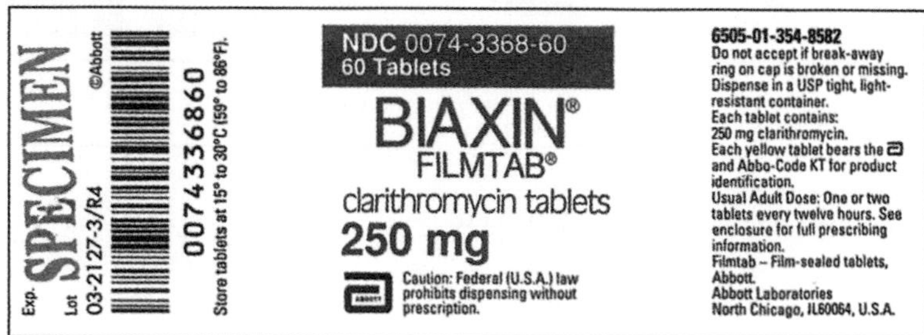

    ____

58. Order: Aricept 5 mg p.o. every day at bedtime.

    Available:

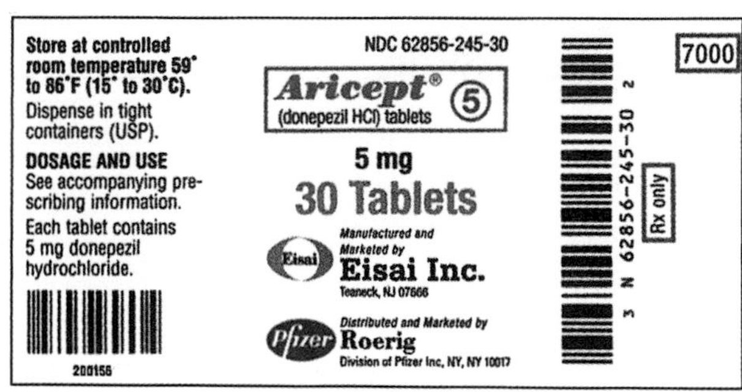

    ____

59. Order: Lasix 8 mg IM stat.

    Available: Lasix labeled 20 mg per 2 mL ______________________

60. Order: Toprol-XL 0.2 g p.o. every day.

Available:

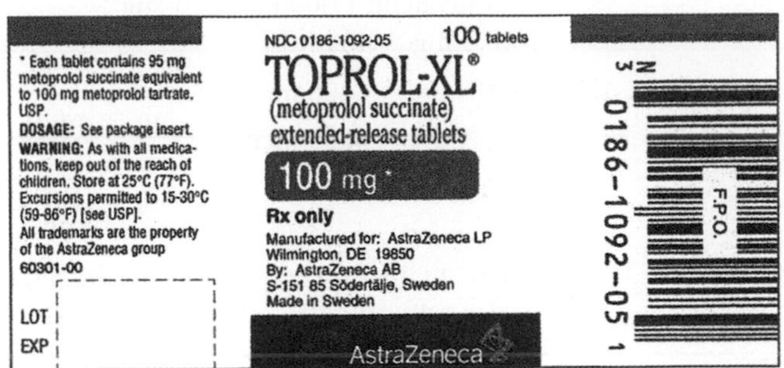

____

Answers on p. 269

ANSWERS

Chapter 15

Answers to Practice Problems

1. $\frac{0.4\text{ mg}}{0.2\text{ mg}} \times 1\text{ tab} = x\text{ tab}$

$$x = \frac{0.4}{0.2}$$

$x = 2$ tabs. 0.4 mg is greater than 0.2 mg; therefore you will need more than 1 tab to administer the dosage.

2. Equivalent: 1,000 mg = 1 g (0.75 g = 750 mg)

$$\frac{750\text{ mg}}{250\text{ mg}} \times 1\text{ cap} = x\text{ cap}$$

$$x = \frac{750}{250}$$

$x = 3$ caps. 750 mg is larger than 250 mg; therefore you will need more than 1 cap to administer the dosage.

3. $\frac{90\text{ mg}}{60\text{ mg}} \times 1\text{ tab} = x\text{ tab}$

$$x = \frac{90}{60}$$

$x = 1.5$ or $1\frac{1}{2}$ tabs. 90 mg is larger than 60 mg; therefore you will need more than 1 tab to administer the dosage.

4. $\frac{7.5\text{ mg}}{2.5\text{ mg}} \times 1\text{ tab} = x\text{ tab}$

$$x = \frac{7.5}{2.5}$$

$x = 3$ tabs. 7.5 mg is larger than 2.5 mg; therefore you will need more than 1 tab to administer the dosage.

5. Equivalent: 1,000 mcg = 1 mg (0.05 mg = 50 mcg)

$$\frac{50\text{ mcg}}{25\text{ mcg}} \times 1\text{ tab} = x\text{ tab}$$

$$x = \frac{50}{25}$$

$x = 2$ tabs. 50 mcg is larger than 25 mcg; therefore you will need more than 1 tab to administer the dosage.

6. Equivalent: 1,000 mcg = 1 mg (0.4 mg = 400 mcg)

$$\frac{400\text{ mcg}}{200\text{ mcg}} \times 1\text{ tab} = x\text{ tab}$$

$$x = \frac{400}{200}$$

$x = 2$ tabs. 400 mcg is larger than 200 mcg; therefore you will need more than 1 tab to administer the dosage.

7. $\frac{1{,}000\text{ mg}}{500\text{ mg}} \times 1\text{ tab} = x\text{ tab}$

$$x = \frac{1{,}000}{500}$$

$x = 2$ tabs. 1,000 mg is more than 500 mg; therefore you will need more than 1 tab to administer the dosage.

8. Equivalent: 1,000 mg = 1 g (0.6 g = 600 mg)

$$\frac{600\text{ mg}}{600\text{ mg}} \times 1\text{ cap} = x\text{ cap}$$

$$x = \frac{600}{600}$$

$x = 1$ cap. 0.6 g = 600 mg. 600-mg caps are available; therefore give 1 cap to administer the dosage.

9. Equivalent: 1,000 mcg = 1 mg (1.25 mg = 1,250 mcg)

$$\frac{1{,}250\text{ mcg}}{625\text{ mcg}} \times 1\text{ tab} = x\text{ tab}$$

$$x = \frac{1{,}250}{625}$$

$x = 2$ tabs. 1,250 mcg is more than 625 mcg; therefore you will need more than one tab to administer the dosage.

10. $\frac{10\text{ mg}}{15\text{ mg}} \times 1\text{ mL} = x\text{ mL}$

$$x = \frac{10}{15}$$

$x = 0.66 = 0.7$ mL. 10 mg is less than 15 mg; therefore you will need less than 1 mL to administer the dosage.

11. $\frac{400\text{ mg}}{200\text{ mg}} \times 5\text{ mL} = x\text{ mL}$

$$x = \frac{2{,}000}{200}$$

$x = 10$ mL. 400 mg is more than 200 mg; therefore you will need more than 5 mL to administer the dosage.

12. $\frac{15 \text{ mEq}}{20 \text{ mEq}} \times 10 \text{ mL} = x \text{ mL}$

$$x = \frac{150}{20}$$

$x = 7.5$ mL. 15 mEq is less than 20 mEq; therefore you will need less than 10 mL to administer the dosage.

13. $\frac{125 \text{ mg}}{250 \text{ mg}} \times 5 \text{ mL} = x \text{ mL}$

$$x = \frac{625}{250}$$

$x = 2.5$ mL. 125 mg is less than 250 mg; therefore you will need less than 5 mL to administer the dosage.

14. $\frac{0.025 \text{ mg}}{0.05 \text{ mg}} \times 5 \text{ mL} = x \text{ mL}$

$$x = \frac{0.125}{0.05}$$

$x = 2.5$ mL. 0.025 mg is less than 0.05 mg; therefore you will need less than 5 mL to administer the dosage.

15. $\frac{375 \text{ mg}}{125 \text{ mg}} \times 5 \text{ mL} = x \text{ mL}$

$$x = \frac{1{,}875}{125}$$

$x = 15$ mL. 375 mg is more than 125 mg; therefore you will need more than 5 mL to administer the dosage.

Answers to Chapter Review

NOTE

For Chapter Review Problems, only answers are shown. If needed, review setup of problems in Practice Problems 1-15.

1. 1 tab
2. 2 caps
3. 1 cap
4. 2 tabs
5. 2 caplets
6. $1\frac{1}{2}$ tabs *or* 1.5 tabs
7. 1 tab
8. 1 cap
9. 2 caps (SR)
10. 2 tabs
11. 1 tab
12. 2 caps
13. 1 tab
14. 2 caps
15. 2 caps (extended)
16. 0.7 mL
17. 1.5 mL
18. 4 mL
19. 12 mL
20. 10 mL
21. 11.3 mL
22. 0.6 mL
23. 2 mL
24. 1.8 mL
25. 10 mL
26. 0.2 mL
27. 2 mL
28. 0.6 mL
29. 0.8 mL
30. 0.5 mL
31. 0.3 mL
32. 1.7 mL
33. 2 mL
34. 3.2 mL
35. 5 mL
36. 1 tab
37. 1 tab
38. 2 tabs
39. 5 mL
40. 3 tabs
41. 2 tabs
42. 1.6 mL
43. 2.7 mL
44. 10 mL
45. 2 tabs
46. 2 tabs
47. 2 tabs
48. 30 mL
49. 12 mL
50. 2.5 mL
51. 1 tab (extended release)
52. 2 tabs
53. $1\frac{1}{2}$ tabs *or* 1.5 tabs
54. 1 tab
55. 2 caps
56. 3 tabs
57. 2 tabs *or* 2 film tabs
58. 1 tab
59. 0.8 mL
60. 2 tabs (extended release)

CHAPTER 16
Dosage Calculation Using the Dimensional Analysis Method

Objectives

After reviewing this chapter, you should be able to:

1. Define dimensional analysis
2. Implement unit cancellation in dimensional analysis
3. Perform conversions using dimensional analysis
4. Use dimensional analysis to calculate dosages

In this chapter, you will learn how to use *dimensional analysis* as a method for calculating dosages. It was introduced as a conversion method in Chapter 8. You may prefer *dimensional analysis* to *ratio and proportion* or *formula method.* When using *dimensional analysis,* there is no memorization of a formula required, and one equation may be used even if a conversion is required. However, memorization of the common equivalents is still a **must**.

Dimensional analysis is the use of a simple technique with a fancy name for the process of manipulating units. By manipulating units, you are able to eliminate or cancel unwanted units. It is considered a commonsense approach and, as already stated, it eliminates the need to memorize a formula and only one equation is needed. Once the concepts related to dimensional analysis are mastered, it can be used to calculate dosages.

Dimensional analysis is also referred to as the *factor-label method* or the *unit factor method.* Dimensional analysis can be viewed as a problem-solving method. Dimensional analysis can be used for all calculations you may encounter once you become comfortable with the process. This chapter will discuss dimensional analysis and provide examples of how it might be used in calculating dosages. Although some may find the formalism of the term *dimensional analysis* intimidating at first, you will find it is quite simple once you have worked a few problems. This method can be used for all calculations. Dimensional analysis will be demonstrated as we proceed through the chapters. *Note:* Remember, as stated in the discussion of calculation methods, it is important that you understand that you as the learner must choose a method of calculation you are comfortable with and use it consistently.

Understanding the Basics of Dimensional Analysis

Let's begin by looking at how the process works in making conversions before we look at its use in calculating dosages. As you recall from previous chapters, you learned what were referred to as *equivalents* or *conversion factors:* for example, 1 g = 1,000 mg, 1 kg = 1,000 g. When we begin using this process for dosage calculations, you will quickly see how dimensional analysis allows multiple factors to be entered in one equation. This method is particularly useful when you have a medication ordered in one unit, and it is available in another unit. Although multiple factors can be placed in a dimensional analysis equation, you can decide to do the conversion before you set up the equation using one of the methods learned in earlier chapters, or you can use dimensional analysis to perform the conversion before calculating the dosage.

Performing Conversions Using Dimensional Analysis

The equivalents (or conversion factors) you learned can be written in a fraction format without changing the value of the unit. This is important to understand when using dimensional analysis. Let's look at the equivalent 1 kg = 1,000 g.

This can be written as:

$$\frac{1\text{ kg}}{1{,}000\text{ g}} \quad or \quad \frac{1{,}000\text{ g}}{1\text{ kg}}$$

Now let's look at the basics in using dimensional analysis for converting units of measure. It is necessary to state the equivalent (conversion factor) in fraction format, maintaining the desired unit in the numerator. In dimensional analysis, how the fraction is written is important. How the fraction is written is based on the unit you want to cancel (or eliminate) to get the unit desired. An equivalent (conversion factor) will give you two fractions:

Examples:

$$2.2\text{ lb} = 1\text{ kg} = \frac{2.2\text{ lb}}{1\text{ kg}} \quad or \quad \frac{1\text{ kg}}{2.2\text{ lb}}$$

$$1{,}000\text{ mcg} = 1\text{ mg} = \frac{1{,}000\text{ mcg}}{1\text{ mg}} \quad or \quad \frac{1\text{ mg}}{1{,}000\text{ mcg}}$$

To Make Conversions Using Dimensional Analysis

1. Identify the desired unit.
2. Identify the equivalent (conversion factor) needed.
3. Write the equivalent (conversion factor) in fraction format, keeping the desired unit in the numerator of the fraction. This is written first in the equation. (Notice the unit in the numerator is the same as the unit you desire.)
4. Label all factors in the equation, and label what you desire *x* (unit desired).
5. Identify unwanted or undesired units, and cancel them. Reduce to lowest terms if possible.
6. If all the labels except the answer label (unit desired) are not eliminated, recheck the equation.
7. Perform the mathematical process indicated.

SAFETY ALERT!

Stating the equivalent incorrectly will not allow you to eliminate desired units. Knowing when the equation is set up correctly is an important part of the concept of dimensional analysis.

Let's look at examples to demonstrate the dimensional analysis process.

Example 1: 1.5 g = ________ mg

1. The desired unit is mg.
2. Equivalent (conversion factor): 1,000 mg = 1 g
3. Write the equivalent (conversion factor), keeping mg in the numerator to allow you to cancel the unwanted unit, g. (Notice the unit in the numerator of the first fraction is the same as the unit you are looking for.)
4. Write the equivalent (conversion factor) first stated as a fraction, followed by a multiplication sign (×).
5. Perform the indicated mathematical operations.

Setup:

$$x\text{ mg} = \frac{1{,}000\text{ mg}}{1\text{ }\cancel{g}} \times 1.5\text{ }\cancel{g}$$

or

$$x\text{ mg} = \frac{1{,}000\text{ mg}}{1\text{ }\cancel{g}} \times \frac{1.5\text{ }\cancel{g}}{1}$$

$$1{,}000 \times 1.5 = 1{,}500\text{ mg}$$

$$x = 1{,}500\text{ mg}$$

The problem in Example 1 could be done by decimal movement. It is shown in this format to illustrate dimensional analysis.

Example 2: 110 lb = ________ kg

1. The desired unit is kg.
2. Equivalent (conversion factor): 2.2 lb = 1 kg
3. Proceed to set up the problem as outlined.

RULE

Placing a 1 under a value does not alter the value of the number. What you desire or are looking for is labeled *x*.

Setup:

$$x\text{ kg} = \frac{1\text{ kg}}{2.2\text{ }\cancel{\text{lb}}} \times 110\text{ }\cancel{\text{lb}}$$

or

$$x\text{ kg} = \frac{1\text{ kg}}{2.2\text{ }\cancel{\text{lb}}} \times \frac{110\text{ }\cancel{\text{lb}}}{1}$$

$$x = \frac{110}{2.2}$$

$$x = 50\text{ kg}$$

RULE

All factors entered in the equation must always include the quantity and unit of measure. State all answers following the rules of the system. When there is more than one equivalent (conversion factor) for a unit of measure, use the equivalent (conversion factor) used most often.

PRACTICE **PROBLEMS**

Set up the following problems using the dimensional analysis format; cancel the units. Do not solve.

1. $8\frac{1}{2}$ tsp = ____________________ mL
2. 15 mg = ____________________ g
3. 400 mcg = ____________________ mg
4. 2 tbs = ____________________ mL
5. 0.007 g = ____________________ mg
6. 0.5 L = ____________________ mL
7. 529 mg = ____________________ g
8. 1,600 mL = ____________________ L
9. 46.4 kg = ____________________ lb
10. 5 cm = ____________________ in

Answers on p. 286

POINTS TO REMEMBER

- Identify the desired unit, and label it *x*.
- State the equivalent (conversion factor) in fraction format with the desired unit in the numerator.
- Label all factors in the equation, including "*x*."
- State the equivalent first in the equation, followed by a multiplication sign (×).
- Remember the rules relating to conversions.
- Cancel the undesired units.

Dosage Calculation Using Dimensional Analysis

As stated, dimensional analysis can be used to calculate dosages with the use of a single equation. A single equation can also be used to calculate the dosage when the dosage desired is in units that differ from what is available. When using dimensional analysis to calculate dosages, it is important to extract the essential information needed from the problem.

In earlier chapters relating to calculating dosages, you learned how to read medication labels. Remember, dosages are always expressed in relation to the form or unit of measure (e.g., milliliters) that contains them.

Examples: 100 mg per tab, 500 mg per cap, 40 mg per 2 mL.

When dimensional analysis is used to calculate dosages, the above examples become crucial factors in the equation and are entered as a fraction with a numerator and denominator.

Steps in Calculating Dosages Using Dimensional Analysis

1. Identify the unit of measure desired in the calculation. With solid forms, the unit will be tab or cap. For parenteral and oral liquids, the unit is milliliter.
2. On the left side of the equation, place the name or appropriate abbreviation for x, what you desire or are looking for (e.g., tab, cap, mL).
3. On the right side of the equation, place the available information from the problem in a fraction format. The abbreviation or unit matching the desired unit must be placed in the numerator.
4. Enter the additional factors from the problem, usually what is ordered. Set up the numerator so that it matches the unit in the previous denominator.
5. Cancel out the like units of measurement on the right side of the equation. The remaining unit should match the unit on the left side of the equation and be the unit desired. Reduce to lowest terms if possible.
6. Solve for the unknown x.

Let's look at an example using these steps.

Example 1: Order: Lasix 40 mg p.o. daily

Available: Tablets labeled 20 mg

1. Place the unit of measure desired in the calculation on the left side of the equation, and label it x.

$$x \text{ tab} =$$

2. Place the information from the problem on the right side of the equation in a fraction format with the unit matching the desired unit in the numerator. (In this problem each tab contains 20 mg.) You must always think about what is a reasonable answer.

$$x \text{ tab} = \frac{1 \text{ tab}}{20 \text{ mg}}$$

3. Enter the additional factors from the problem, what is ordered, matching the numerator in the previous denominator (in the problem the order is 40 mg). Placing a 1 under it does not change the value.

$$\underset{\substack{\text{Amount to}\\\text{administer}\\\downarrow}}{x \text{ tab}} = \underset{\substack{\text{Available}\\\text{dosage}\\\downarrow}}{\frac{1 \text{ tab}}{20 \text{ mg}}} \times \underset{\substack{\text{Ordered}\\\text{dosage}\\\downarrow}}{\frac{40 \text{ mg}}{1}}$$

4. Cancel the like units of measurement on the right side of the equation. The remaining unit of measurement should be what is desired. Match the unit of measurement on the left side. Proceed with the mathematical process. Notice that after cancellation of units (mg), the desired unit of measure to be administered remains (e.g., tabs in this problem).

$$x \text{ tab} = \frac{1 \text{ tab}}{20 \cancel{\text{mg}}} \times \frac{40 \cancel{\text{mg}}}{1}$$

$$x = \frac{1 \times 40}{20}$$

$$x = \frac{40}{20}$$

$$x = 2 \text{ tabs}$$

Now let's look at an example with parenteral medications. You would follow the same steps illustrated in Example 1.

Example 2: Order: Gentamicin 55 mg IM q8h

Available: Gentamicin 80 mg per 2 mL (round answer to the nearest tenth)

1. On the left side of the equation, place the unit desired in this problem (mL).

$$x \text{ mL} =$$

2. On the right side, place the available information from the problem in fraction format, placing the unit matching the unit desired in the numerator. Think what is reasonable to administer.

$$x \text{ mL} = \frac{2 \text{ mL}}{80 \text{ mg}}$$

3. Enter the additional factors from the problem, what is ordered matching the numerator in the previous denominator (in this problem, the order is 55 mg).

Amount to administer ↓ Available dosage ↓ Ordered dosage ↓

$$x \text{ mL} = \frac{2 \text{ mL}}{80 \text{ mg}} \times \frac{55 \text{ mg}}{1}$$

4. Cancel out the like units of measurement on the right side of the equation. The remaining unit of measurement should match the unit on the left side of the equation and be the unit desired.

$$x \text{ mL} = \frac{2 \text{ mL}}{80 \cancel{\text{mg}}} \times \frac{55 \cancel{\text{mg}}}{1}$$

$$x = \frac{2 \times 55}{80}$$

$$x = \frac{110}{80} = 1.37$$

$$x = 1.4 \text{ mL}$$

As already mentioned, dimensional analysis can be used when a medication is ordered in one unit of measurement and available in another, thereby necessitating a conversion. However, the same steps are followed as previously shown.

- An additional fraction is entered into the equation as the second fraction. This fraction is the equivalent (or conversion factor) needed. The numerator must match the unit of the previous denominator.
- The last fraction is the medication ordered. This is written so that the numerator of the fraction matches the unit in the denominator of the fraction immediately before.

Let's look at an example:

Example 3: Order: Ampicillin 0.5 g IM q6h

Available: Ampicillin labeled 250 mg per mL

1. On the left side of the equation, place the unit of measure desired in the calculation, and label it *x*.

$$x \text{ mL} =$$

2. Place the information from the problem on the right side of the equation in a fraction format, placing the unit matching the unit desired in the numerator. Think about what is a reasonable amount to administer.

$$x \text{ mL} = \frac{1 \text{ mL}}{250 \text{ mg}}$$

3. The order is for 0.5 g, and the medication is available in 250 mg; a conversion is therefore needed.
   From previous chapters, we know 1 g = 1,000 mg; this fraction is placed next in the form of a fraction (the numerator of the fraction must match the denominator of the immediately previous fraction).

$$x \text{ mL} = \frac{1 \text{ mL}}{250 \text{ mg}} \times \frac{1{,}000 \text{ mg}}{1 \text{ g}}$$

4. Next, place the amount of medication ordered in the equation. This will match the denominator of the fraction immediately before. In this problem, it is 0.5 g.

$$x \text{ mL} = \underset{\substack{\text{Available}\\\text{dosage}\\\downarrow}}{\frac{1 \text{ mL}}{250 \text{ mg}}} \times \underset{\substack{\text{Conversion}\\\text{factor}\\\downarrow}}{\frac{1{,}000 \text{ mg}}{1 \text{ g}}} \times \underset{\substack{\text{Dose}\\\text{ordered}\\\downarrow}}{\frac{0.5 \text{ g}}{1}}$$

5. Cancel out like units of measurement on the right side of the equation; the remaining unit of measurement should match the unit on the left side of equation and be the desired unit. Notice that mg and g cancel, leaving the desired unit, mL.

$$x \text{ mL} = \frac{1 \text{ mL}}{250 \cancel{\text{mg}}} \times \frac{1{,}000 \cancel{\text{mg}}}{1 \cancel{\text{g}}} \times \frac{0.5 \cancel{\text{g}}}{1}$$

$$x = \frac{1{,}000 \times 0.5}{250}$$

$$x = \frac{500}{250}$$

$$x = 2 \text{ mL}$$

SAFETY ALERT!

Incorrect placement of units of measure into the equation will not allow cancellation of units and can result in an error in calculation. Dimensional analysis does not eliminate thinking about what a reasonable answer should be.

POINTS TO REMEMBER

When using dimensional analysis to calculate dosages:

- First determine units of the medication you want to administer; for example, tabs, caps, mL, and so on. The unit desired is written **FIRST** to the left of the equation followed by an equal sign (=).
- The units in the numerator on the left of the equal sign are the same units placed in the numerator of the **first fraction** on the right side of the equation.
- If a conversion is necessary, the conversion factor is also entered into the right side of the equation, as the second fraction.
- The ordered dosage is added at the end as the final fraction.
- Cancel the like units. When all the cancellations have been made, only the units desired remain (e.g., tab, caps, mL).
- Always determine the units and **THINK** about what a reasonable answer is, set up the equation, and cancel the units.
- All factors entered into the equation must include the quantity and unit of measure.
- Incorrect placement of units of measurement will not allow you to cancel units and can result in an incorrect answer.
- Thinking and reasoning are essential even with dimensional analysis.

PRACTICE **PROBLEMS**

Set up the following problems using dimensional analysis. Do not solve.

11. A dose strength of 0.3 g has been ordered.

    Available: 0.4 g per 1.5 mL ______________________

12. A dose strength of 15 mg is ordered.

    Available: 15 mg per mL ______________________

13. Order: Ampicillin 1 g p.o. stat.

    Available: Ampicillin capsules labeled 500 mg ______________________

14. Order: Cefaclor 250 mg p.o. t.i.d.

    Available: Cefaclor oral suspension labeled 125 mg per 5 mL

    ____

15. Order: Ranitidine 150 mg I.V. daily.

Available:

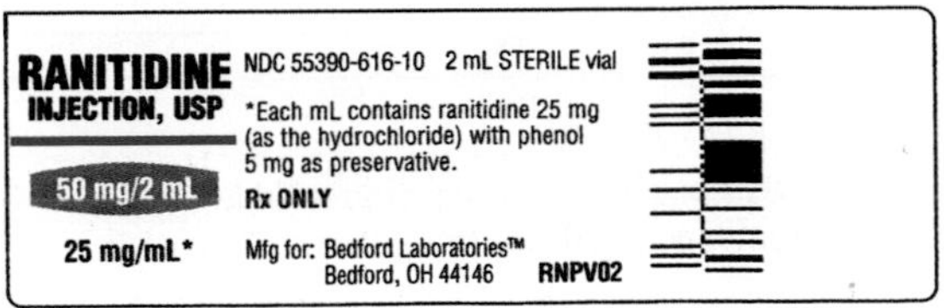

____

16. Order: Aldomet 0.5 g p.o. daily.

Available: Aldomet tablets labeled 250 mg

____

17. Order: Digoxin 0.125 mg p.o. daily.

Available: Scored tablets (can be broken in half)

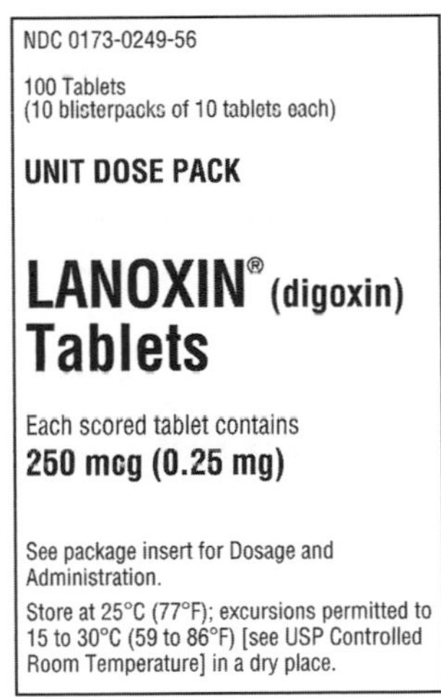

____

18. Order: Dilantin 300 mg p.o. t.i.d.

Available: Dilantin oral suspension labeled 125 mg per 5 mL

____

19. Order: Cipro 0.5 g p.o. q12h

    Available: Cipro tablets labeled 250 mg

    ____

20. Order: Clindamycin 0.3 g IV q6h.

    Available: Clindamycin labeled 150 mg per mL

    ____

Answers on p. 286

CHAPTER REVIEW

Calculate the following medication dosages using the dimensional analysis method. Use medication labels or information provided. Label answers correctly: tab, caps, mL. Answers expressed in milliliters should be expressed to the nearest tenth, except where indicated.

1. Order: Antivert 50 mg p.o. daily.

   Available:

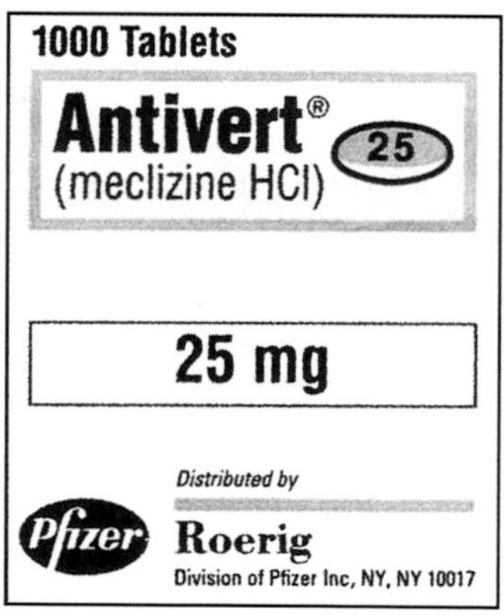

____

2. Order: Potassium chloride 20 mEq in 1 L of D5W.

   Available:

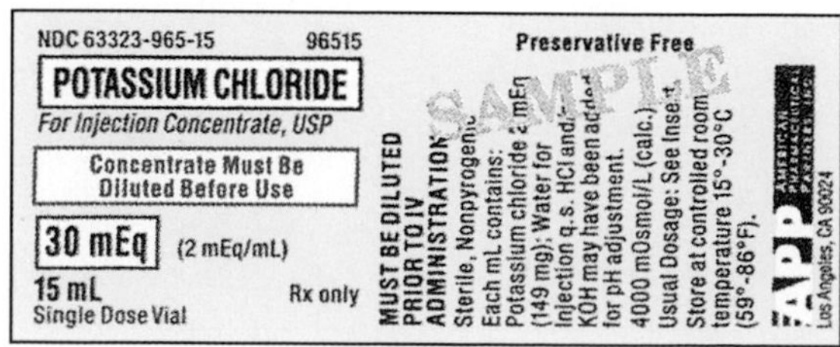

____

3. Order: Morphine sulfate 20 mg IM stat.

   Available:

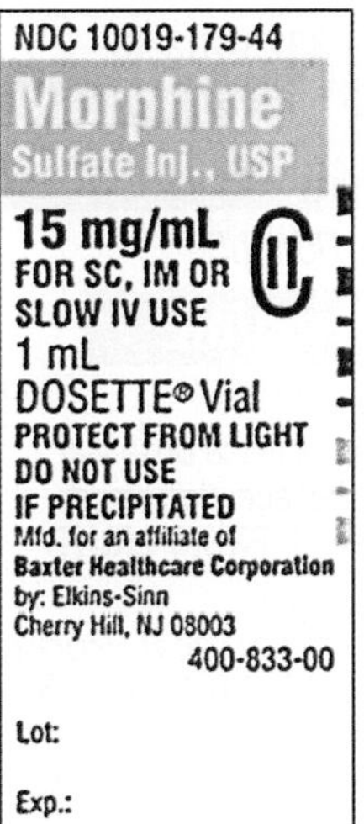

____

4. Order: Lexapro 20 mg p.o. daily

   Available:

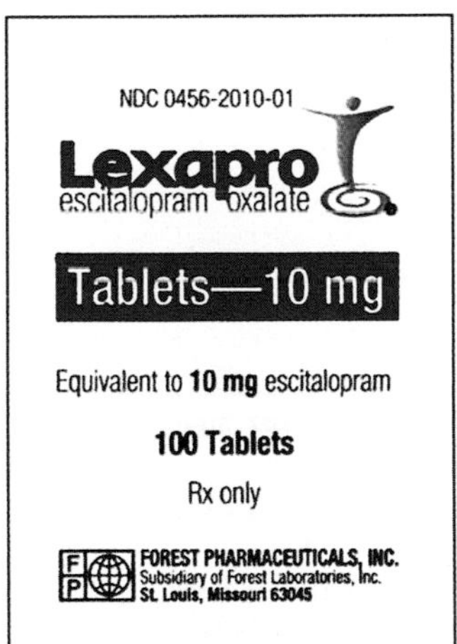

____

5. Order: Capoten 25 mg p.o. daily.

   Available: Capoten tablets labeled 12.5 mg

____

6. Order: Thiamine 80 mg IM stat.

   Available:

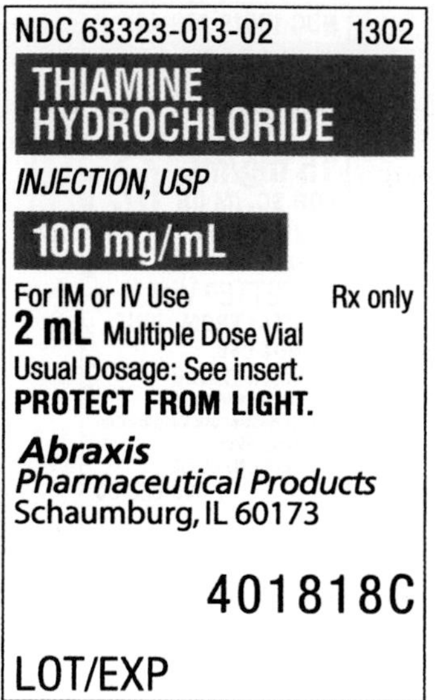

____

7. Order: Heparin 6,500 units subcut q12h.

   Available: Heparin labeled 10,000 units per mL (Express answer in hundredths.)

____

8. Order: Terbutaline 5 mg p.o. t.i.d.

   Available:

USUAL DOSAGE:
See package insert for prescribing information.
Dispense in a tight, light-resistant container as defined in the USP with a child-resistant closure.
Store at 20°-25°C (68°-77°F) [See USP Controlled Room Temperature]. Excursion permitted 15°-30°C (59°-86°F)
Rev. 03/05
N 3 0527-1318-01 5

NDC 0527-1318-01
LANNETT
TERBUTALINE SULFATE TABLETS, USP
2.5 mg
Rx Only
100 TABLETS

Each tablet contains:
Terbutaline, USP ...... 2.5 mg
Inactive Ingredients:
Anhydrous lactose, magnesium stearate, microcrystalline cellulose, povidone, and pregelatinized starch.
Manufactured by:
Lannett Company, Inc.
Philadelphia, PA 19136
Exp. Date:
Lot No.:

____

9. Order: Trandate 200 mg p.o. b.i.d.

   Available: Trandate tablets labeled 100 mg

____

10. Order: Solu-Medrol 175 mg IV daily.

Available: Solu-Medrol labeled 500 mg per 8 mL

____

11. Order: Trental (ER) 0.4 g p.o. t.i.d.

Available: Trental ER tablets labeled 400 mg

____

12. Order: Biaxin 0.5 g p.o. q12h for 7 days.

Available:

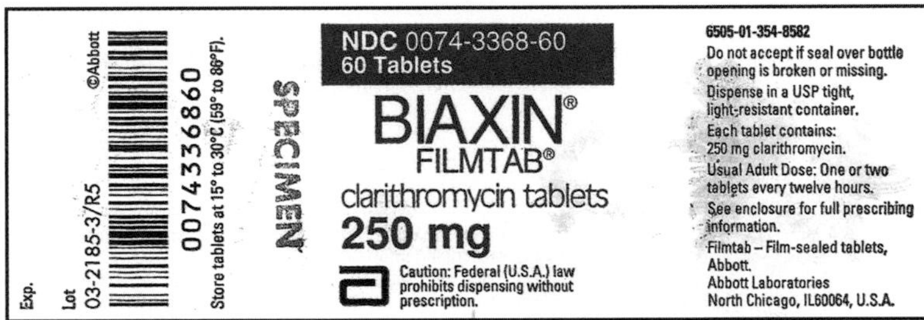

____

13. Order: Clonazepam 0.5 mg p.o. b.i.d.

Available:

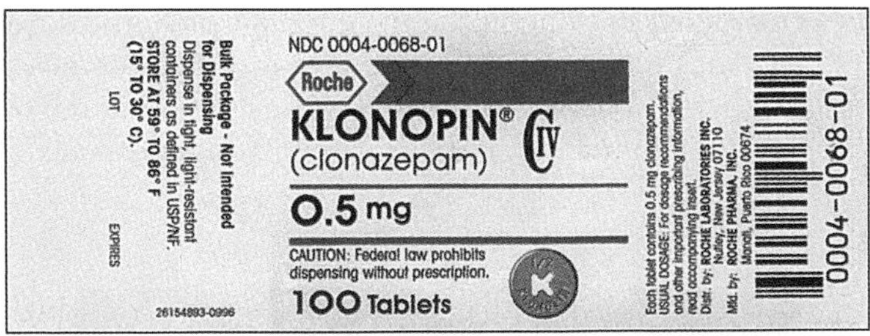

____

14. Order: Quinidine gluconate 200 mg IM q8h.

Available: Quinidine gluconate labeled 80 mg per mL

____

15. Order: Protamine sulfate 25 mg IV stat.

    Available:

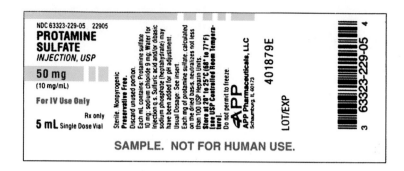

____

16. Order: Methotrexate 15 mg IM every week (on Monday).

    Available:

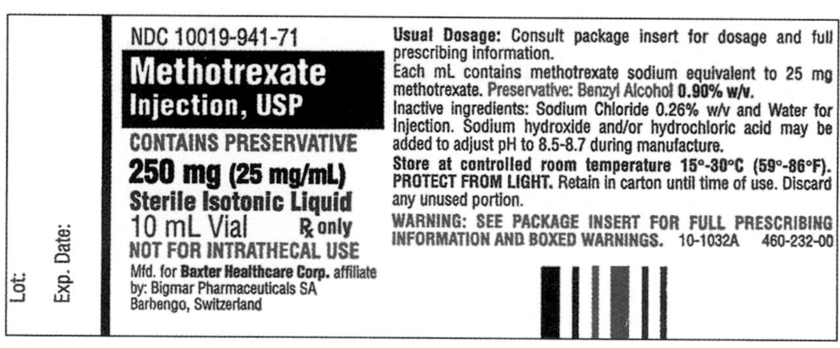

____

17. Order: Uniphyl 0.4 g p.o. b.i.d.

    Available:

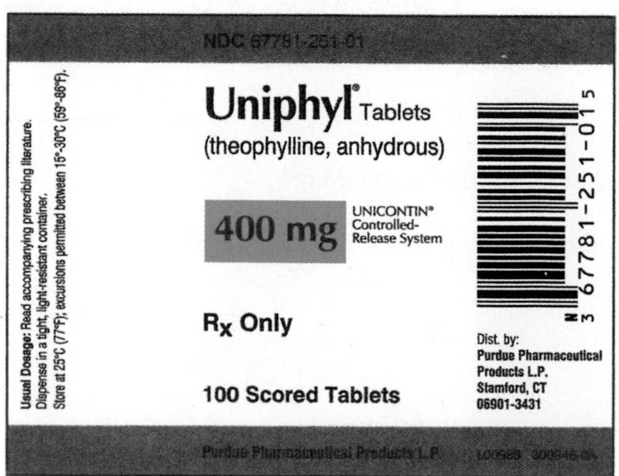

____

18. Order: Diphenhydramine 60 mg IM stat.

    Available: Diphenhydramine labeled 50 mg per mL

    ____

19. Order: Cefaclor 0.4 g p.o. q8h.

    Available:

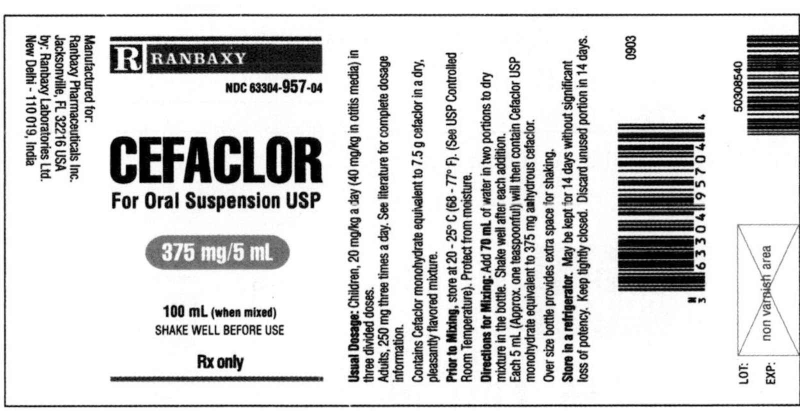

____

20. Order: Synthroid 0.075 mg p.o. daily.

    Available: Scored tablets (can be broken in half) labeled 50 mcg (0.05 mg)

    ____

21. Order: Haloperidol decanoate 0.05 g IM every 2 weeks.

    Available:

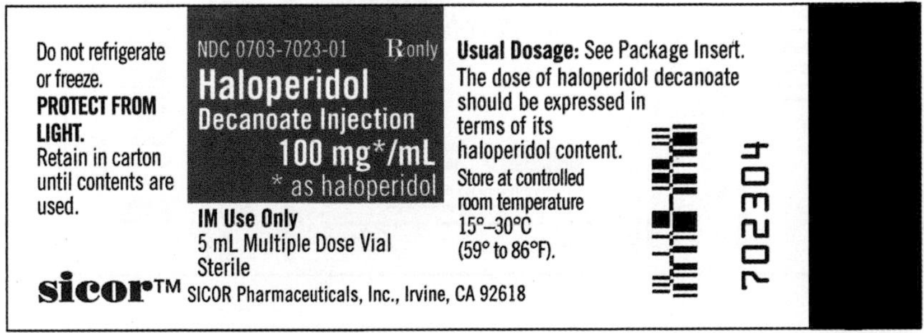

____

22. Order: Dexamethasone 1.5 mg IV stat.

    Available:

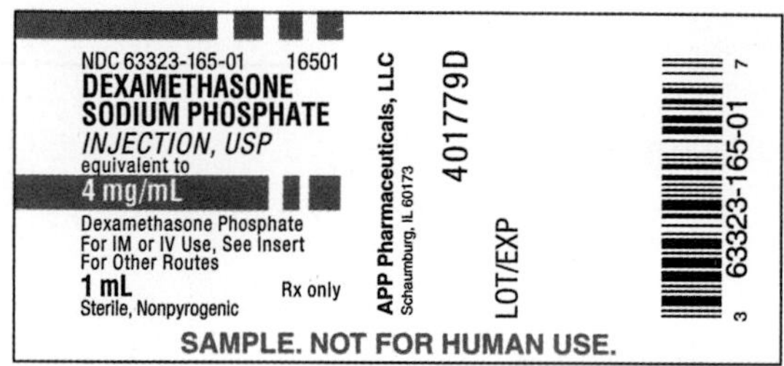

____

23. Order: Heparin 5,000 units subcut stat.

    Available:

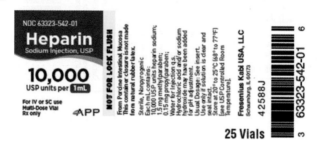

____

24. Order: Strattera 0.1 g p.o. daily.

    Available:

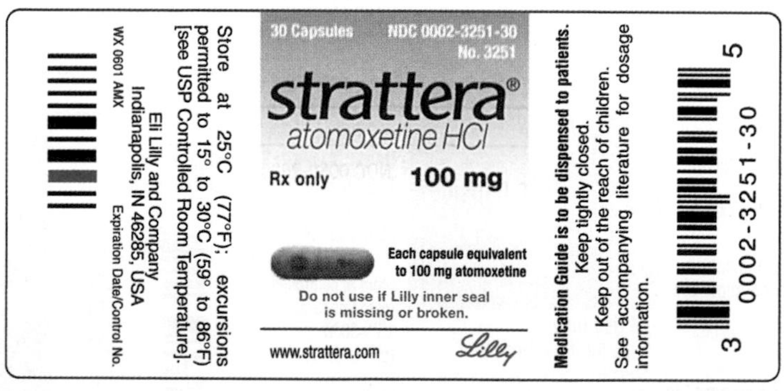

____

25. Order: Erythromycin oral suspension 150 mg p.o. b.i.d.

    Available: Erythromycin oral suspension labeled 200 mg per 5 mL

____

26. Order: Aranesp 0.02 mg subcut once weekly.

Available:

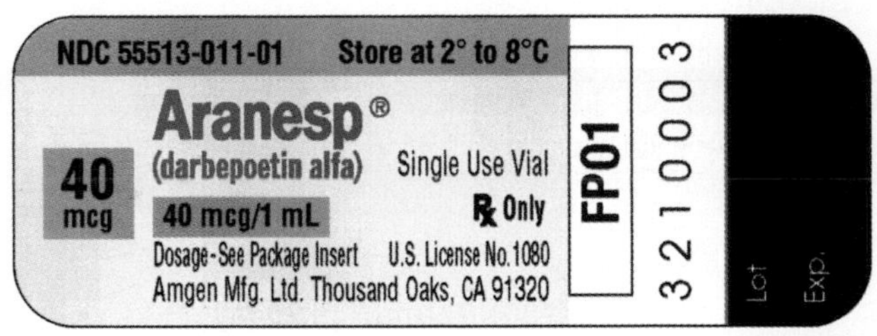

____

For questions 27 through 35, set up the problem using dimensional analysis and make the conversion as indicated.

27. 3 qt = ______________________________ mL

28. 79 lb = ______________________________ kg (round to nearest tenth)

29. 5 mcg = ______________________________ mg

30. 2,400 mL = ______________________________ L

31. 8 in = ______________________________ cm

32. 1.25 mcg = ______________________________ mg

33. 240 mL = ______________________________ oz

34. 1.75 mg − ______________________________ mcg

35. 125 mL = ______________________________ L

Answers on pp. 286-289

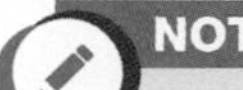

ANSWERS

Chapter 16

Answers to Practice Problems

> **NOTE**
>
> The following problems could be set up without placing 1 under a value; placing a 1 under the value as shown in the setup for problems 1-20 does not alter the value of the number.

1. $x \text{ mL} = \dfrac{5 \text{ mL}}{1 \cancel{\text{tsp}}} \times \dfrac{8\frac{1}{2} \cancel{\text{tsp}}}{1}$

2. $x \text{ g} = \dfrac{1 \text{ g}}{1{,}000 \cancel{\text{mg}}} \times \dfrac{15 \cancel{\text{mg}}}{1}$

3. $x \text{ mg} = \dfrac{1 \text{ mg}}{1{,}000 \cancel{\text{mcg}}} \times \dfrac{400 \cancel{\text{mcg}}}{1}$

4. $x \text{ mL} = \dfrac{15 \text{ mL}}{1 \cancel{\text{tbs}}} \times \dfrac{2 \cancel{\text{tbs}}}{1}$

5. $x \text{ mg} = \dfrac{1{,}000 \text{ mg}}{1 \cancel{\text{g}}} \times \dfrac{0.007 \cancel{\text{g}}}{1}$

6. $x \text{ mL} = \dfrac{1{,}000 \text{ mL}}{1 \cancel{\text{L}}} \times \dfrac{0.5 \cancel{\text{L}}}{1}$

7. $x \text{ g} = \dfrac{1 \text{ g}}{1{,}000 \cancel{\text{mg}}} \times \dfrac{529 \cancel{\text{mg}}}{1}$

8. $x \text{ L} = \dfrac{1 \text{ L}}{1{,}000 \cancel{\text{mL}}} \times \dfrac{1{,}600 \cancel{\text{mL}}}{1}$

9. $x \text{ lb} = \dfrac{2.2 \text{ lb}}{1 \cancel{\text{kg}}} \times \dfrac{46.4 \cancel{\text{kg}}}{1}$

10. $x \text{ inch} = \dfrac{1 \text{ inch}}{2.5 \cancel{\text{cm}}} \times \dfrac{5 \cancel{\text{cm}}}{1}$

11. $x \text{ mL} = \dfrac{1.5 \text{ mL}}{0.4 \cancel{\text{g}}} \times \dfrac{0.3 \cancel{\text{g}}}{1}$

12. $x \text{ mL} = \dfrac{1 \text{ mL}}{15 \cancel{\text{mg}}} \times \dfrac{15 \cancel{\text{mg}}}{1}$

13. $x \text{ cap} = \dfrac{1 \text{ cap}}{500 \cancel{\text{mg}}} \times \dfrac{1{,}000 \cancel{\text{mg}}}{1 \cancel{\text{g}}} \times \dfrac{1 \cancel{\text{g}}}{1}$

14. $x \text{ mL} = \dfrac{5 \text{ mL}}{125 \cancel{\text{mg}}} \times \dfrac{250 \cancel{\text{mg}}}{1}$

15. $x \text{ mL} = \dfrac{1 \text{ mL}}{25 \cancel{\text{mg}}} \times \dfrac{150 \cancel{\text{mg}}}{1}$

    or

    $x \text{ mL} = \dfrac{2 \text{ mL}}{50 \cancel{\text{mg}}} \times \dfrac{150 \cancel{\text{mg}}}{1}$

16. $x \text{ tab} = \dfrac{1 \text{ tab}}{250 \cancel{\text{mg}}} \times \dfrac{1{,}000 \cancel{\text{mg}}}{1 \cancel{\text{g}}} \times \dfrac{0.5 \cancel{\text{g}}}{1}$

17. $x \text{ tab} = \dfrac{1 \text{ tab}}{0.25 \cancel{\text{mg}}} \times \dfrac{0.125 \cancel{\text{mg}}}{1}$

18. $x \text{ mL} = \dfrac{5 \text{ mL}}{125 \cancel{\text{mg}}} \times \dfrac{300 \cancel{\text{mg}}}{1}$

19. $x \text{ tabs} = \dfrac{1 \text{ tab}}{250 \cancel{\text{mg}}} \times \dfrac{1{,}000 \cancel{\text{mg}}}{1 \cancel{\text{g}}} \times \dfrac{0.5 \cancel{\text{g}}}{1}$

20. $x \text{ mL} = \dfrac{1 \text{ mL}}{150 \cancel{\text{mg}}} \times \dfrac{1{,}000 \cancel{\text{mg}}}{1 \cancel{\text{g}}} \times \dfrac{0.3 \cancel{\text{g}}}{1}$

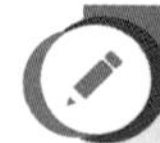

> **NOTE**
>
> Placing a 1 under the value does not alter the value of the number.

Answers to Chapter Review

1. $x \text{ tab} = \dfrac{1 \text{ tab}}{25 \cancel{\text{mg}}} \times \dfrac{50 \cancel{\text{mg}}}{1}$

   $x = \dfrac{50}{25}$

   $x = 2 \text{ tabs}$

2. $x \text{ mL} = \dfrac{15 \text{ mL}}{\underset{3}{\cancel{30}} \cancel{\text{mEq}}} \times \dfrac{\overset{2}{\cancel{20}} \cancel{\text{mEq}}}{1}$

   $x = \dfrac{15 \times 2}{3}$

   $x = \dfrac{30}{3}$

   $x = 10 \text{ mL}$

3. $x \text{ mL} = \dfrac{1 \text{ mL}}{15 \cancel{\text{mg}}} \times \dfrac{20 \cancel{\text{mg}}}{1}$

   $x = \dfrac{20}{15}$

   $x = 1.3 \text{ mL}$

4. $x \text{ tabs} = \dfrac{1 \text{ tab}}{10 \cancel{\text{mg}}} \times \dfrac{20 \cancel{\text{mg}}}{1}$

   $x = \dfrac{20}{10}$

   $x = 2 \text{ tabs}$

5. $x \text{ tab} = \frac{1 \text{ tab}}{12.5 \cancel{\text{mg}}} \times \frac{25 \cancel{\text{mg}}}{1}$

$x = \frac{25}{12.5}$

$x = 2 \text{ tabs}$

6. $x \text{ mL} = \frac{1 \text{ mL}}{100 \cancel{\text{mg}}} \times \frac{80 \cancel{\text{mg}}}{1}$

$x = \frac{80}{100}$

$x = 0.8 \text{ mL}$

7. $x \text{ mL} = \frac{1 \text{ mL}}{10{,}000 \cancel{\text{units}}} \times \frac{6{,}500 \cancel{\text{units}}}{1}$

$x = \frac{6{,}500}{10{,}000}$

$x = 0.65 \text{ mL}$

8. $x \text{ tabs} = \frac{1 \text{ tab}}{2.5 \cancel{\text{mg}}} \times \frac{5 \cancel{\text{mg}}}{1}$

$x = \frac{5}{2.5}$

$x = 2 \text{ tabs}$

9. $x \text{ tabs} = \frac{1 \text{ tab}}{100 \cancel{\text{mg}}} \times \frac{200 \cancel{\text{mg}}}{1}$

$x = \frac{200}{100}$

$x = 2 \text{ tabs}$

10. $x \text{ mL} = \frac{8 \text{ mL}}{500 \cancel{\text{mg}}} \times \frac{175 \cancel{\text{mg}}}{1}$

$x = \frac{8 \times 175}{500}$

$x = \frac{1{,}400}{500}$

$x = 2.8 \text{ mL}$

11. $x \text{ tab} = \frac{1 \text{ tab}}{400 \cancel{\text{mg}}} \times \frac{1{,}000 \cancel{\text{mg}}}{1 \cancel{\text{g}}} \times \frac{0.4 \cancel{\text{g}}}{1}$

$x = \frac{1{,}000 \times 0.4}{400}$

$x = \frac{400}{400}$

$x = 1 \text{ tab (ER)}$

12. $x \text{ tab} = \frac{1 \text{ tab}}{\overset{}{\underset{1}{\cancel{250}}} \cancel{\text{mg}}} \times \frac{\overset{4}{\cancel{1{,}000}} \cancel{\text{mg}}}{1 \cancel{\text{g}}} \times \frac{0.5 \cancel{\text{g}}}{1}$

$x = \frac{4 \times 0.5}{1}$

$x = \frac{2}{1}$

$x = 2 \text{ tab (film tab)}$

13. $x \text{ tab} = \frac{1 \text{ tab}}{0.5 \cancel{\text{mg}}} \times \frac{0.5 \cancel{\text{mg}}}{1}$

$x = \frac{0.5}{0.5}$

$x = 1 \text{ tab}$

14. $x \text{ mL} = \frac{1 \text{ mL}}{80 \cancel{\text{mg}}} \times \frac{200 \cancel{\text{mg}}}{1}$

$x = \frac{200}{80}$

$x = 2.5 \text{ mL}$

15. $x \text{ mL} = \frac{1 \text{ mL}}{10 \cancel{\text{mg}}} \times \frac{25 \cancel{\text{mg}}}{1}$

$x = \frac{25}{10}$

$x = 2.5 \text{ mL}$

or

$x \text{ mL} = \frac{5 \text{ mL}}{50 \cancel{\text{mg}}} \times \frac{25 \cancel{\text{mg}}}{1}$

$x = \frac{5 \times 25}{50}$

$x = \frac{125}{50}$

$x = 2.5 \text{ mL}$

16. $x \text{ mL} = \frac{1 \text{ mL}}{25 \cancel{\text{mg}}} \times \frac{15 \cancel{\text{mg}}}{1}$

$x = \frac{15}{25}$

$x = 0.6 \text{ mL}$

or

$x \text{ mL} = \frac{10 \text{ mL}}{250 \cancel{\text{mg}}} \times \frac{15 \cancel{\text{mg}}}{1}$

$x = \frac{10 \times 15}{250}$

$x = \frac{150}{250}$

$x = 0.6 \text{ mL}$

17. $x \text{ tabs} = \frac{1 \text{ tab}}{400 \cancel{\text{mg}}} \times \frac{1{,}000 \cancel{\text{mg}}}{1 \cancel{\text{g}}} \times \frac{0.4 \cancel{\text{g}}}{1}$

$x = \frac{1{,}000 \times 0.4}{400}$

$x = \frac{400}{400}$

$x = 1 \text{ tab}$

18. $x \text{ mL} = \frac{1 \text{ mL}}{50 \cancel{\text{mg}}} \times \frac{60 \cancel{\text{mg}}}{1}$

$x = \frac{60}{50}$

$x = 1.2 \text{ mL}$

19. $x \text{ mL} = \frac{5 \text{ mL}}{375 \cancel{\text{mg}}} \times \frac{1{,}000 \cancel{\text{mg}}}{1 \cancel{\text{g}}} \times \frac{0.4 \cancel{\text{g}}}{1}$

$x = \frac{5{,}000 \times 0.4}{375}$

$x = \frac{2{,}000}{375}$

$x = 5.33 \text{ mL} = 5.3 \text{ mL}$ (to the nearest tenth)

20. $x \text{ tab} = \frac{1 \text{ tab}}{0.05 \cancel{\text{mg}}} \times \frac{0.075 \cancel{\text{mg}}}{1}$

$x = \frac{0.075}{0.05}$

$x = 1.5$ tabs or $1\frac{1}{2}$ tabs ($1\frac{1}{2}$ tabs preferred for administration purposes)

21. $x \text{ mL} = \frac{1 \text{ mL}}{100 \cancel{\text{mg}}} \times \frac{1{,}000 \cancel{\text{mg}}}{1 \cancel{\text{g}}} \times \frac{0.05 \cancel{\text{g}}}{1}$

$x = \frac{1{,}000 \times 0.05}{100}$

$x = \frac{50}{100}$

$x = 0.5 \text{ mL}$

22. $x \text{ mL} = \frac{1 \text{ mL}}{4 \cancel{\text{mg}}} \times \frac{1.5 \cancel{\text{mg}}}{1}$

$x = \frac{1.5}{4}$

$x = 0.37 \text{ mL} = 0.4 \text{ mL}$ (to the nearest tenth)

23. $x \text{ mL} = \frac{1 \text{ mL}}{10{,}000 \cancel{\text{units}}} \times \frac{5{,}000 \cancel{\text{units}}}{1}$

$x = \frac{5{,}000}{10{,}000}$

$x = 0.5 \text{ mL}$

24. $x \text{ caps} = \frac{1 \text{ caps}}{100 \cancel{\text{mg}}} \times \frac{1{,}000 \cancel{\text{mg}}}{1 \cancel{\text{g}}} \times \frac{0.1 \cancel{\text{g}}}{1}$

$x = \frac{1{,}000 \times 0.1}{100}$

$x = \frac{100}{100}$

$x = 1 \text{ caps}$

25. $x \text{ mL} = \frac{5 \text{ mL}}{200 \cancel{\text{mg}}} \times \frac{150 \cancel{\text{mg}}}{1}$

$x = \frac{5 \times 150}{200}$

$x = \frac{750}{200}$

$x = 3.75 \text{ mL} = 3.8 \text{ mL}$ (to the nearest tenth)

26. $x \text{ mL} = \frac{1 \text{ mL}}{40 \cancel{\text{mcg}}} \times \frac{1{,}000 \cancel{\text{mcg}}}{1} \times \frac{0.02 \cancel{\text{mg}}}{1}$

$x = \frac{1{,}000 \times 0.02}{40}$

$x = \frac{20}{40}$

$x = 0.5 \text{ mL}$

27. $x \text{ mL} = \frac{1{,}000 \text{ mL}}{1 \cancel{\text{qt}}} \times \frac{3 \cancel{\text{qt}}}{1}$

$x = \frac{1{,}000 \times 3}{1}$

$x = \frac{3{,}000}{1}$

$x = 3{,}000 \text{ mL}$

28. $x \text{ kg} = \frac{1 \text{ kg}}{2.2 \cancel{\text{lb}}} \times \frac{79 \cancel{\text{lb}}}{1}$

$x = \frac{79}{2.2}$

$x = 35.9 \text{ kg}$ (to the nearest tenth)

29. $x \text{ mg} = \frac{1 \text{ mg}}{1{,}000 \cancel{\text{mcg}}} \times \frac{5 \cancel{\text{mcg}}}{1}$

$x = \frac{5}{1{,}000}$

$x = 0.005 \text{ mg}$

30. $x \text{ L} = \frac{1 \text{ L}}{1{,}000 \cancel{\text{mL}}} \times \frac{2{,}400 \cancel{\text{mL}}}{1}$

$x = \frac{2{,}400}{1{,}000}$

$x = 2.4 \text{ L}$

31. $x \text{ cm} = \frac{2.5 \text{ cm}}{1 \cancel{\text{in}}} \times \frac{8 \cancel{\text{in}}}{1}$

$x = \frac{2.5 \times 8}{1}$

$x = 20 \text{ cm}$

32. $x \text{ mg} = \frac{1 \text{ mg}}{1{,}000 \cancel{\text{mcg}}} \times \frac{1.25 \cancel{\text{mcg}}}{1}$

$x = \frac{1.25}{1{,}000}$

$x = 0.00125 \text{ mg}$

33. $x \text{ oz} = \frac{1 \text{ oz}}{30 \cancel{\text{mL}}} \times \frac{240 \cancel{\text{mL}}}{1}$

$x = \frac{240}{30}$

$x = 8 \text{ oz}$

34. $x \text{ mcg} = \frac{1{,}000 \text{ mcg}}{1 \cancel{\text{mg}}} \times \frac{1.75 \cancel{\text{mg}}}{1}$

$x = \frac{1{,}000 \times 1.75}{1}$

$x = 1{,}750 \text{ mcg}$

35. $x \text{ L} = \frac{1 \text{ L}}{1{,}000 \cancel{\text{mL}}} \times \frac{125 \cancel{\text{mL}}}{1}$

$x = \frac{125}{1{,}000}$

$x = 0.125 \text{ L}$

UNIT FOUR

Oral and Parenteral Dosage Forms and Insulin

Oral medications are the easiest, most economical, and most frequently used medications, but sometimes parenteral (nongastrointestinal tract) dosage routes are necessary. Both oral and parenteral medications are available in liquid or powder form. Medications that are available in powdered form must be reconstituted and administered in liquid form. In addition to oral and parenteral dosage forms, this unit examines the varying types of insulin.

Chapter 17 Oral Medications

Chapter 18 Parenteral Medications

Chapter 19 Reconstitution of Solutions

Chapter 20 Insulin

CHAPTER 17
Oral Medications

Objectives

After reviewing this chapter, you should be able to:

1. Identify the forms of oral medication
2. Identify the terms on the medication label to be used in calculation of dosages
3. Calculate dosages for oral and liquid medications using ratio and proportion, the formula method, or dimensional analysis
4. Apply principles learned concerning tablet and liquid preparations to obtain a rational answer

The term *enteral* is used to describe medications that are administered directly into the gastrointestinal tract. With the enteral route, medications can be administered orally, rectally, or, when the oral route is unavailable, through a tube (e.g., nasogastric tube [NGT] or percutaneous endoscopic gastrostomy [PEG]).

Enteral medications are most commonly administered by the oral route (by mouth, or p.o., an abbreviation for the Latin phrase *per os*). Medications that are administered orally come in several forms, including tablets (tab/tabs), capsules (cap/caps), caplets, and liquid preparations. The administration of medications orally is considered to be the easiest, most convenient, and relatively most economical.

In an effort to increase medication safety and reduce errors, safety organizations have recommended that all medications be available in unit-dose packaging. Many health care institutions use a combination of unit-dose and bulk packaging. The Joint Commission (TJC) standards require "medications to be dispensed in the most ready-to-administer forms possible to minimize opportunities for error."

Practice problems provided in this chapter will require careful reading of labels in order to safely and accurately calculate a dose to administer. To calculate dosages appropriately, the nurse needs to understand the principles that apply to administration of medications by the oral route. Calculations involving tablets and capsules and their preparation for administration are usually simple. Let's discuss the various forms of solid medications, beginning with tablets.

Forms of Solid Medications

Tablets

Tablets are the most common form of solid oral medications. Tablets are preparations of powdered medications that have been molded into various sizes, shapes, and are available in many colors. Dosage strength of tablets can be expressed in metric or apothecary units (e.g., milligrams and grains). When the apothecary measure is indicated on the label of tablets, the apothecary measure is usually in parentheses with the metric conversion beside it. Many of the newer labels include only metric measures on the label.

There are some tablets designed for chewing, and some are made to be dissolved in water resulting in a liquid that the client drinks. Always check the medication label or a reliable drug reference to determine how a tablet is meant to be administered.

Let's begin with a discussion of the various types of tablets.

Caplets. A caplet is a tablet that has an elongated shape (oval) and is coated for ease of swallowing. Tylenol is available in caplet form.

Scored Tablets Scored tablets are designed to administer a dosage that is less than what is available in a single tablet. In other words, scored tablets have indentations, grooves, or markings that allow for ease in breaking the tablet. Most often, scored tablets divide into halves, but some are scored to divide into thirds or quarters. The medication in scored tablets is evenly distributed throughout the tablet and allows the dose to be divided evenly when a tablet is scored. Tablets may be broken only if they are scored. The groove or indentation on the tablet serves as a guide for breaking the tablet into fractional pieces. Hands should be washed and gloves worn when breaking tablets.

Figure 17-1 shows an example of a scored tablet.

Breaking scored tablets to administer an ordered dosage is allowed but not optimal. Always check to see if the tablet is available in another dosage strength before breaking a scored tablet. **Safety is always first.** Use practices that promote client safety (Quality and Safety Education for Nurses [QSEN]).

ISMP (2006) states to "verify suitability before prescribing, dispensing or administering half tablets, check drug references to ensure that it is safe. If unsure, contact the manufacturer. Ensure that patients have the required level of understanding, ability, and motivation to split the tablets. If a patient cannot be expected to split his or her own tablets, enlist the aid of a qualified family member."

It is safest and most accurate to administer the least number of whole, undivided tablets possible. Breaking tablets should be done only if tablets are scored and no other option exists to administer the dosage. Research (Verrue et al, 2011) has shown that splitting tablets that are not scored may result in uneven parts and inaccurate dosage.

Splitting tablets in half, even if they are scored with a line down the middle, leads to medication errors. Medications need to be provided in the correct dose whenever possible.

SAFETY ALERT!

Breaking an unscored tablet is risky and dangerous and can lead to administration of an unintended dosage. Question and/or verify any order as well as any calculation you perform that indicates administering a portion of a tablet that is not scored.

In order to break tablets evenly, a tablet cutter should be used. Clients breaking tablets at home should be told to use a pill or tablet cutter, which is readily available in most pharmacies. In addition, ensure that the client fully understands how to use the device and has a clear understanding regarding splitting the tablet. For the client who cannot split the tablet, the help of a qualified family member might be needed. Pill or tablet cutters should be washed following use to remove powder or particles.

Figure 17-2 shows a pill/tablet cutter. Always consult an appropriate medication reference before cutting a tablet.

Many tablets come in a form that allows slow and steady release of the active drug. These forms cannot be cut, crushed, or chewed. Capsules and enteric-coated, timed-release, sustained-release, and controlled-release tablets should be swallowed whole. Consult a drug reference or pharmacist when in doubt about the safety of cutting or crushing tablets or capsules.

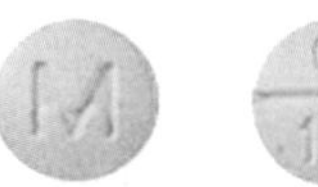

Figure 17-1 Clonazepam tablet scored.

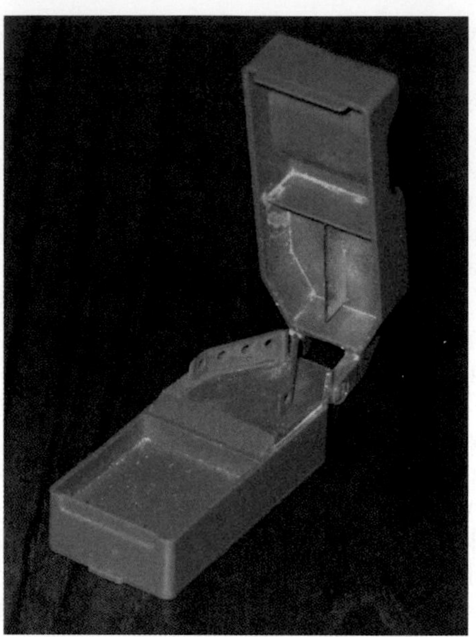

Figure 17-2 Pill/tablet cutter. (From Kee JL, Marshall SM: *Clinical calculations: with applications to general and specialty areas,* ed 8, St Louis, 2016, Saunders.)

TIPS FOR CLINICAL PRACTICE

If the calculation of a medication dosage requires that a tablet be cut in half, divide the tablet along the scoring created by the manufacturer. Use a pill or tablet cutter to divide a tablet in half to help ensure acccuracy of a dose.

Enteric-Coated Tablets. Enteric-coated tablets have a special coating that protects them from the effects of gastric secretions and prevents them from dissolving in the stomach. They are dissolved and absorbed in the small intestines. Enseal is also used to indicate enteric coated.

The enteric coating also prevents the medication from becoming a source of irritation to the gastric mucosa, thereby preventing gastrointestinal upset. Examples include enteric-coated aspirin and iron tablets, such as ferrous gluconate. Enteric-coated tablets should never be crushed, broken or chewed, because crushing, breaking and chewing them destroys the special coating and defeats its purpose. They must be swallowed whole with their coating intact.

Sublingual Tablets. Sublingual tablets are designed to be placed under the tongue for rapid absorption into the bloodstream by the network of blood vessels in this area. Sublingual tablets should never be swallowed, because this will prevent them from achieving their desired effect. Nitroglycerin, which is used for the relief of acute chest pain, is usually administered sublingually. Figure 17-3, *A,* shows placement of sublingual tablets.

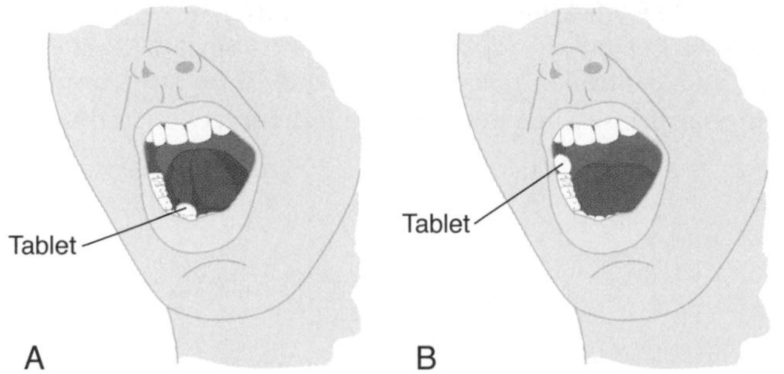

Figure 17-3 Sublingual **(A)** and buccal **(B)** tablets. (From Potter PA, Perry AG, Stockert P, Hall A: *Fundamentals of nursing,* ed 9, St Louis, 2016, Mosby.)

Buccal Tablets. Buccal tablets are placed between the gums and cheek for absorption from the blood vessels of the cheek. Clients should be instructed not to chew, swallow, or take liquids. Buccal tablets are designed to be absorbed through the mucous membranes of the mouth. Figure 17-3, *B,* shows placement of buccal tablets.

Layered Tablets. Some tablets contain different layers or have cores that separate different medications that may be incompatible with one another; thus incompatible ingredients may be separated and released at different times as the tablet passes through the gastrointestinal tract (Figure 17-4).

Medications in a layered form have become available in which one or more medications can be released immediately from the coating, whereas the same or other medications can be released on a sustained basis from the tablet core. An example of this is Ambien CR. Ambien CR is formulated in a two-layer tablet. The first layer of the tablet dissolves quickly to help in falling asleep, and the second layer dissolves slowly over the night to help the person stay asleep.

Film Tab. A film tab is a tablet sealed with a film. The special coating helps protect the stomach. Some medications that come as film tabs include Biaxin (clarithromycin) and E.E.S. 400 (erythromycin).

Orally Disintegrating Tablets. Orally disintegrating tablets dissolve rapidly, usually within seconds of being placed on the tongue. They are used for their rapid onset of action. Examples of use include treatment of migraine headaches, for clients who have difficulty swallowing, and in clients in whom administration must be ensured because the client often attempts to avoid taking their medications (e.g., the mentally ill). Klonopin (clonazepam), an anticonvulsant, is an example of an orally disintegrating tablet.

A **sublingual film** is now available. The film is placed under the tongue for rapid disintegration. Suboxone (used to manage opiate addiction) is an example of this form. The rapid action of the film is advantageous because the client is unable to retrieve the medication for possible sale on the street. Suboxone film can be abused in the same manner as other opioids.

Chewable Tablets. Chewable tablets are designed to be chewed, and must be chewed to be effective. Examples of medications that come in chewable form include: Amoxicillin and clavulanate potassium tablets, and calcium supplement tablets.

Timed-Release and Extended-Release Tablets. Look for abbreviations such as SA, LA, or XL. Medication from these types of tablets is not released immediately but released over a period of time at specific intervals. These types of preparations should not be crushed, chewed, or broken; they should be swallowed whole. If a timed-release or extended-release tablet is crushed, chewed, or broken, all of the medication will be administered at one time and absorbed rapidly. Examples include Procardia, Calan, and theophylline.

Capsules

A capsule is a form of medication that is oval-shaped or round and contains medication in powder, liquid, or oil enclosed in a hard or soft gelatin. Capsules are available in a variety of colors and sizes. Some capsules have special shapes and colorings to identify which company produced them. Capsules usually have a gelatin shell that has two pieces that fit together. Capsules are not divided or crushed but are administered whole to achieve the desired effect. There are some capsules that may be separated to remove the medication, which is then mixed with food for ease of administration for clients who have difficulty swallowing. Nurses should always check a drug reference to determine which capsules may be opened and mixed with food. Examples of medications that come in capsule form are ampicillin, tetracycline and Colace. In addition to capsules, some labels may include the term *Kapseals* (e.g., "Kapseals" is seen on the label for Dilantin extended capsules).

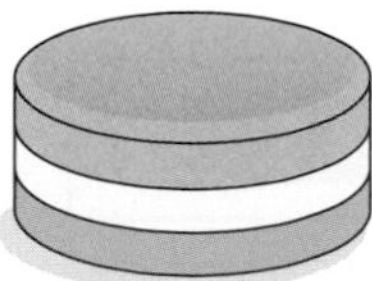

Figure 17-4 Layered tablet.

Spansules are special capsules that contain granules of medications. Spansules may be opened and mixed with food; however, the granules cannot be crushed or dissolved. The granules delay the release of the medication.

Gelcaps are gelatin shells that usually contain liquid medication. Gelcaps are not designed to be opened or crushed. Lanoxicaps are an example of a capsule that has liquid (digoxin solution) medication contained within a soft gelatin shell.

Sprinkle capsules are also available for oral administration. Sprinkle capsules can be swallowed whole or opened and sprinkled on a food such as apple sauce. Topamax and Depakote are examples of such a medication.

Crushing Tablets or Opening Capsules

Not all medications can be crushed or opened for administration to clients. The Institute for Safe Medication Practice (ISMP; http://www.ismp.org/tools/donotcrush) publishes a list of medications that are not safe for crushing. Medications may sometimes be ordered for administration enterally or into the gastrointestinal tract by a specially placed tube. For example, a nasogastric tube (NG/NGT) (a tube inserted through the nose into the gastric [stomach] region), a gastrostomy tube (GT) inserted directly through the abdomen into the stomach, percutaneous endoscopic gastrostomy (PEG). Medications administered by a tube will have to be crushed and dissolved in a small amount of warm water. Determine whether an alternative form of the medication exists if it cannot be crushed, such as oral liquid form.

To maintain safety of the client and prevent an incorrect dose or unintended effect, do not crush or open capsules or tablets that are labeled time-release, sustained-release, delayed-release, or extended-release. Tablets that are sublingual, buccal, or enteric-coated are never crushed. Capsules are not crushed or opened unless they are designed to be. Always consult a drug reference or pharmacist before crushing a tablet or opening a capsule to ensure that a medication can be safely administered to avoid harm to a client.

> **SAFETY ALERT!**
>
> Medications such as time-release, sustained-release, extended-release, and delayed-release tablets and capsules have special coatings to prevent the medication from being absorbed too quickly. Altering medications that should be administered whole may result in alteration of the medication action (e.g., increasing the rate of absorption or causing the medication to be inactivated) and cause unintended effects.

Although there are other forms of solid preparations for oral administration, such as lozenges and troches, tablets, capsules, and pulvules (proprietary capsules containing a dosage of a medication in powdered form) are the most common forms of solids requiring calculation encountered by the nurse. Figure 17-5 shows various forms of solid oral medications.

Calculating Dosages Involving Tablets and Capsules

When administering solid forms of oral medications (tablets and capsules), the nurse rarely performs complex calculations to determine the number of tablets or capsules needed to administer the dosage ordered. Accurate and safe dosage calculation includes requiring

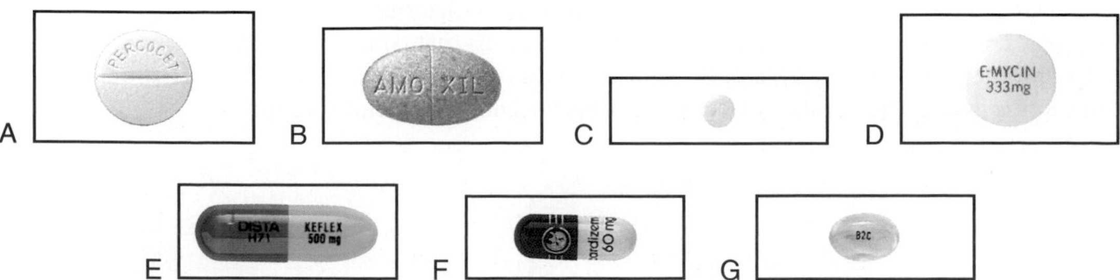

Figure 17-5 Types of oral medications. **A,** Scored tablet. **B,** Chewable tablet. **C,** Sublingual. **D,** Timed-release tablet. **E,** Capsule. **F,** Timed-release capsule. **G,** Gelatin capsule.

that the nurse understands the medication order, reads the medication label carefully to identify the dosage strength (also referred to as the dosage strength available, what is on hand or available), which is the amount of medication contained in each tablet or capsule, and accurately calculate the dose to administer. To foster clinical reasoning skills and help determine whether the calculated dosage is sensible, accurate, and safe to administer, and to avoid calculation errors, the nurse **must** integrate the following points as an integral part of calculation of dosages involving tablets and capsules.

POINTS TO REMEMBER

- Converting medication measures from one system to another and one unit to another to determine the dosage to be administered can result in discrepancies, depending on the conversion factor used.
- When the precise number of tablets or capsules is determined and you find that administering the amount calculated is unrealistic or impossible, always use the following rule to avoid an error in administration: *No more than 10% variation should exist between the dosage ordered and the dosage administered.* For example, you may determine that a client should receive 0.9 tablet or 0.9 capsule. Administration of such an amount accurately would be impossible. Following the stated rule, if you determined that 0.9 tablet or 0.9 capsule should be given, you could safely administer 1 tab or 1 cap. This variation usually occurs when conversions are made between apothecary and metric measurements because approximate equivalents are used. There should be no conversion to apothecary. If apothecary measure is indicated, the metric conversion will be beside the apothecary measure, which is often in parenthesis. The 10% variation rule is often applied with adults but not necessarily with the pediatric clients.
- Capsules are not scored and cannot be divided. They are administered in whole amounts only. If a client has difficulty swallowing a capsule, check to see if a liquid preparation of the same medication is available. Never crush or open a timed-release capsule or empty its contents into a liquid or food; this may cause release of all the medication at once.
- **Tablets and capsules** may be available in different strengths for administration, and you may have a choice when giving a dosage. For example, 75 mg of a medication may be ordered. When you check what is available, it may be in tablet or capsule form as 10, 25, or 50 mg. In deciding the best combination of tablets or capsules to give, the nurse should always choose the strength that would allow the least number of tablets or capsules to be administered without breaking a tablet, if possible, because breaking is found to result in variations in dosage. In the example given, the best combination for administering 75 mg is one 50 mg tablet or capsule and one 25 mg tablet or capsule.
- Only scored tablets are intended to be divided. It is safest and most accurate not to divide tablets, and give the fewest number of whole, undivided tablets possible.

RULE

Three (3) tablets or capsules are typically the maximum administered to achieve a single dose. Always **stop, think,** and **recheck** a calculation if a single dose requires more. Question the order before administering if it exceeds three (3).

- It is important to note that although the maximum number of tablets or capsules given to a client is usually three, there may be exceptions, including calcium tablets and some of the solid forms of HIV medications (e.g., tablets, capsules). Example: ritonavir 400 mg po q12h (available 100 mg per tab). Although many HIV medications are available in liquid form, many clients have a preference for tablets or capsules.
- **Remember:** Unless the medication is an exception, more than three (3) tablets or capsules to achieve a single dose is unusual and may indicate an error in interpretation of the order, transcription, or calculation. Think! Always question any order that exceeds this amount.
- When calculating dosages using ratio and proportion, the formula method, or dimensional analysis, remember that each tablet or capsule contains a certain amount of medication per tablet or capsule. Example: 325 mg per tablet, 500 mg per capsule. The dosage strength indicated on a label is per tablet or per capsule. This is particularly important when you are reading a medication label on a bottle or single unit-dose package.

continued

- In calculating oral dosages, you may encounter measures other than metric measures. For example, electrolytes such as potassium will indicate the number of milliequivalents (mEq) per tablet. Units is another measure you may see for oral antibiotics or vitamins. For example, a vitamin E capsule will indicate 400 units per capsule. Measurements of units and milliequivalents are specific to the medication they are being used for. There is no conversion between these and other systems of measure. (These are discussed in Chapter 18.)
- Always consult a medication reference or pharmacist when in doubt as to whether a capsule may be opened or whether a tablet can be crushed.

SAFETY ALERT!

Regardless of the source of an error, if you administer the wrong dose or give a medication by a route other than that intended, you have committed a medication error and are legally responsible for the error. Always think of the reasonableness of what you have calculated to administer and double-check the dose and route for a medication before administering.

Remembering the points mentioned will be helpful before starting to calculate dosages. Any of the methods presented in Chapters 14, 15, and 16 can be used to determine the dosage to be administered.

To compute dosages accurately, it is necessary to review a few reminders that were presented in previous chapters:

1. Read the order carefully and:
   a. Identify known factors.
   b. Identify unknown factors.
   c. Eliminate unnecessary information that is not relevant.
2. Make sure that what is ordered and what is available are in the same system of measurement and units, or a conversion will be necessary. When a conversion is necessary, it is usual to convert what is ordered into what you have available or what is indicated on the medication label. You can, however, convert the measure in which the medication is available into the same units and system of measure as the dosage ordered. The choice is usually based on whichever is easier to calculate. Use any of the methods presented in Chapters 8, 14, and 16 to make conversions consistent to avoid confusion. If necessary, go back and review these methods.
3. Consider what would be a reasonable answer based on what is ordered.
4. Set up the problem using ratio and proportion, the formula method, or dimensional analysis. Label each component in the setup, including *x*.
5. Label the final answer (tablet, capsule).
6. For administration purposes, for oral dosages that are given in fractional dosages (e.g., scored tablets), state answers to problems in fractions. Example: $\frac{1}{2}$ tab or $1\frac{1}{2}$ tabs, instead of 0.5 tabs or 1.5 tabs.

Here are some sample problems calculating the number of tablets or capsules to administer.

Example 1: Order: Digoxin 0.375 mg p.o. daily

Available: Digoxin (scored tablets) labeled 0.25 mg

✓ PROBLEM SETUP

1. No conversion is necessary; the units are in the same system of measure.
   Order: 0.375 mg
   Available: 0.25 mg
2. Think critically: Tablets are scored; 0.375 mg is larger than 0.25 mg; therefore, you will need more than 1 tab to administer the correct dosage.
3. Solve using ratio and proportion, the formula method, or dimensional analysis.

✓ Solution Using Ratio and Proportion

$$0.25 \text{ mg} : 1 \text{ tab} = 0.375 \text{ mg} : x \text{ tab}$$

(known) (unknown)

(what is available) (what is ordered)

$$\frac{0.25x}{0.25} = \frac{0.375}{0.25}$$

$$x = \frac{0.375}{0.25}$$

Therefore, $x = 1.5$ tabs or $1\frac{1}{2}$ tabs. (It is best to state it as $1\frac{1}{2}$ tabs for administration purposes.) You can administer $1\frac{1}{2}$ tabs because tablets are scored.

Note: Ratio and proportion could be stated in fraction format as well. If necessary, review Chapter 4 on ratio and proportion.

✓ Solution Using the Formula Method

$$\frac{\text{(D) } 0.375 \text{ mg}}{\text{(H) } 0.25 \text{ mg}} \times \text{(Q) } 1 \text{ tab} = x \text{ tab}$$

$$x = \frac{0.375}{0.25}$$

$$x = 1\frac{1}{2} \text{ tabs}$$

✓ Solution Using Dimensional Analysis

$$x \text{ tab} = \frac{1 \text{ tab}}{0.25 \cancel{\text{mg}}} \times \frac{0.375 \cancel{\text{mg}}}{1}$$

$$x = \frac{0.375}{0.25}$$

$$x = 1\frac{1}{2} \text{ tabs}$$

Example 2: Order: Ampicillin 0.5 g p.o. q6h

Available: Ampicillin capsules labeled 250 mg per capsule

1. Order: 0.5 g
   Available: 250 mg capsules
2. After making the necessary conversion, think about what is a reasonable amount to administer. (*Note:* Before calculating the dosage to be administered, the ordered dosage and the available dosage must be in the same unit of measure.)
3. Calculate the dosage to be administered using ratio and proportion, the formula method, or dimensional analysis.
4. Label your final answer (tablets, capsules).

PROBLEM SETUP

1. Convert grams to milligrams. Equivalent: 1,000 mg = 1 g

$$1{,}000 \text{ mg} : 1 \text{ g} = x \text{ mg} : 0.5 \text{ g}$$
$$x = 1{,}000 \times 0.5$$
$$x = 500 \text{ mg}$$

   Therefore, 0.5 g is equal to 500 mg. Converting the grams to milligrams eliminated a decimal, which is often the source of calculation errors. Converting milligrams to grams would necessitate a decimal. Whenever possible, conversions that result in a decimal should be avoided to decrease the chance of error in calculating. Remember, a ratio and proportion could also be stated as a fraction. If necessary, review Chapter 4 on ratio and proportion. Because the measures are metric in this problem (grams, milligrams), the other method that can be used is to move the decimal the desired number of places (0.5 g = 0.500 = 500 mg).
2. After making the conversion, you are now ready to calculate the dosage to be given, using ratio and proportion, the formula method, or dimensional analysis. In this problem we will use the answer obtained from converting what was ordered to what is available (0.5 g = 500 mg). Remember that if dimensional analysis is used, you need only one equation; even if conversion is required, you can choose to do conversion first and then set the problem up in dimensional analysis.

✓ Solution Using Ratio and Proportion

$$250 \text{ mg} : 1 \text{ cap} = 500 \text{ mg} : x \text{ cap}$$
$$\frac{250x}{250} = \frac{500}{250}$$
$$x = \frac{500}{250}$$
$$x = 2 \text{ caps}$$

✓ Solution Using the Formula Method

$$\frac{(D)\ 500 \text{ mg}}{(H)\ 250 \text{ mg}} \times (Q)\ 1 \text{ cap} = x \text{ cap}$$
$$x = \frac{500}{250}$$
$$x = 2 \text{ cap}$$

✓ Solution Using Dimensional Analysis

$$x \text{ caps} = \frac{1 \text{ cap}}{250 \cancel{\text{mg}}} \times \frac{1{,}000 \cancel{\text{mg}}}{1 \cancel{\text{g}}} \times \frac{0.5 \cancel{\text{g}}}{1}$$
$$x = \frac{1{,}000 \times 0.5}{250}$$
$$x = \frac{500}{250}$$
$$x = 2 \text{ caps}$$

Set up if conversion done first, then set up in dimensional analysis to calculate dosage:

$$x \text{ mg} = \frac{1{,}000 \text{ mg}}{1 \cancel{g}} \times 0.5 \cancel{g}$$

$$x = \frac{1{,}000 \times 0.5}{1}$$

$$x = \frac{500}{1}$$

$$x = 500 \text{ mg}$$

Set up in dimensional analysis after conversion made:

$$x \text{ caps} = \frac{1 \text{ cap}}{250 \cancel{mg}} \times \frac{500 \cancel{mg}}{1}$$

$$x = \frac{500}{250}$$

$$x = 2 \text{ caps}$$

Note: It is easier to set up the problem by using one equation that will allow you to convert and calculate the dosage required.

As discussed before, Nitroglycerin (anti-anginal) is administered sublingually, but it is also available in extended-release capsules. See Figure 17-6 with samples of labels.

Notice the label on Nitrostat (Nitroglycerin) sublingual tablets is in grains (gr) in parentheses and the metric equivalent in milligrams is also indicated. In performing calculations always look for and use the metric equivalent. In an emergency situation the sublingual form would be administered for immediate effect. Sublingual as well as extended-release must be administered whole.

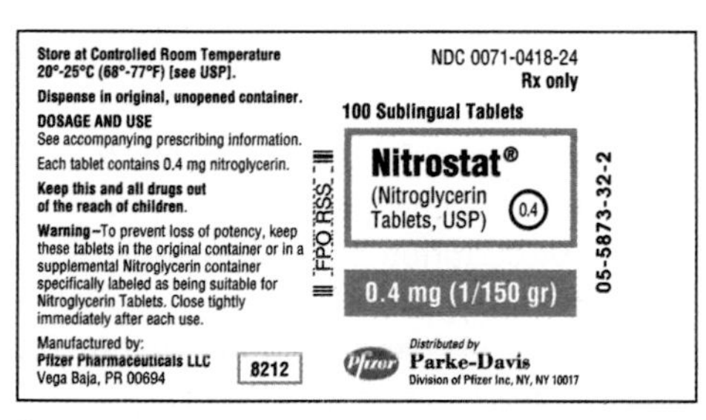

A

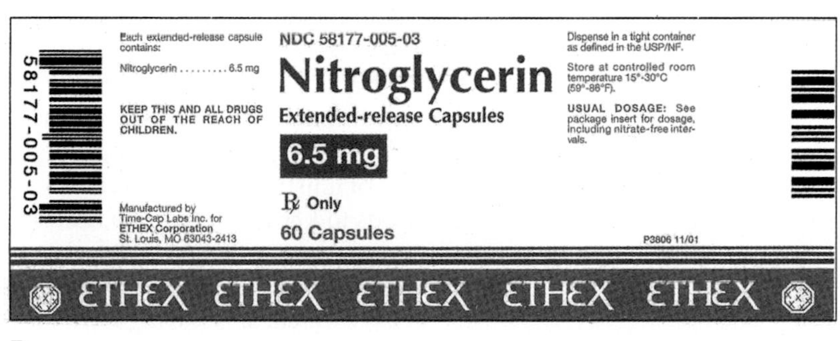

B

Figure 17-6 **A,** Nitrostat 0.4 mg sublingual tablets. **B,** Nitroglycerin 6.5 mg extended-release capsules.

Example 3: Order: Thorazine 100 mg p.o. t.i.d.

Available: Thorazine tablets labeled 25 mg and 50 mg

✓ PROBLEM SETUP

1. No conversion is necessary.
2. Thinking critically: 100 mg is larger than 25 or 50 mg. Therefore, more than 1 tab is needed to administer the dosage. The client should always be given the strength of tablets or capsules that would require the least number to be taken.
3. In this problem, selection of the 50-mg tablets would require the client to receive 2 tabs, whereas using 25 mg tablets would require 4 tabs to be administered.

✓ Solution Using Ratio and Proportion

$$50 \text{ mg} : 1 \text{ tab} = 100 \text{ mg} : x \text{ tab}$$

$$\frac{50x}{50} = \frac{100}{50}$$

$$x = 2 \text{ tabs } (50 \text{ mg each})$$

Note: The number of tablets is specified as well as the strength of the tablets.

✓ Solution Using the Formula Method

$$\frac{(\text{D})\ 100 \text{ mg}}{(\text{H})\ 50 \text{ mg}} \times (\text{Q})\ 1 \text{ tab} = x \text{ tab}$$

$$x = \frac{100}{50}$$

$$x = 2 \text{ tabs } (50 \text{ mg each})$$

✓ Solution Using Dimensional Analysis

$$x \text{ tab} = \frac{1 \text{ tab}}{50 \cancel{\text{mg}}} \times \frac{100 \cancel{\text{mg}}}{1}$$

$$x = \frac{100}{50}$$

$$x = 2 \text{ tabs } (50 \text{ mg each})$$

Example 3 could have been calculated without the use of ratio and proportion, dimensional analysis, or a formula. This is common when problems provide more than one dosage strength. In the case where a conversion is required, you would perform the conversion and choose the appropriate dosage strength to administer the least number of tablets or capsules. Add the dosage strengths chosen to ensure that it is equivalent to what is ordered.

Variation of Tablet and Capsule Problems

You will at times find it necessary to decide how many tablets or capsules are needed. This requires knowing the dosage and frequency. Numerous scenarios could arise, but for the purpose of illustration, let's look at two examples. A client is going out of town on vacation and needs to know whether it is necessary to refill the prescription before leaving.

Example 1: A client has an order for Valium 10 mg p.o. q.i.d. and has 5 mg tablets. The client is leaving town for 7 days and asks how many tablets to bring.

Solution: To obtain a dosage of 10 mg, the client requires two 5-mg tablets each time. Therefore, eight 5-mg tablets are necessary to administer the dosage q.i.d. (four times a day).

Number of tablets needed per day (8) × Number of days needed for (7) = Total number of tablets needed

$$8 \times 7 = 56$$

Answer: The total number of tablets needed for 7 days would be 56 tablets.

Example 2: A client is instructed to take 30 mg of a medication stat as an initial dose and 20 mg tid thereafter. The tablets available are 10 mg tablets. What is the total number of tablets the client will need for 3 days?

Solution: To obtain a dose of 30 mg, the client will require three 10-mg tablets for the stat dose, and six 10-mg tablets are needed to administer the dose t.i.d. (three times a day).

Number of tablets needed per day (6) × Number of days needed for (3) = Total number of tablets needed.

$6 \times 3 = 18 + 3 \text{ (stat dose)} = 21 \text{ tablets}$

Answer: The total number of tablets needed for 3 days is 21 tablets.

Determining the Dosage to Be Given Each Time

Example: A client is to receive 1 gram of a medication p.o. daily. The medication should be given in four equally divided doses.

How many milligrams should the client receive each time the medication is administered?

Solution: $\frac{\text{Total daily allowance}}{\text{Number of doses per day}} = \text{Dosage to be administered}$

Answer: $\frac{1 \text{ g (1,000 mg)}}{4} = 250 \text{ mg}$ each time the medication is administered.

POINTS TO REMEMBER

- The maximum number of tablets and capsules to administer to achieve a single desired dosage is usually three. Question any order for more than this before administering.
- Before calculating a dosage, make sure that the dosage ordered and what is available are in the same system and units of measurement. When a conversion is required, it is usually best to convert the dosage ordered to what is available.
- No more than a 10% variation should exist between the dosage ordered and the dosage administered for adults. Remember, this should only occur when you are converting between apothecary and metric systems because of using approximate equivalents. When possible, always convert to a metric measure or use the metric measure indicated on a label.
- Regardless of the method used to calculate a dosage, it is important to develop the ability to think critically about what is a reasonable amount. Think and question any dosage that seems unreasonable.
- State dosages as you are actually going to administer them. Example: 0.5 tab = $\frac{1}{2}$ tab.
- Tablets that are not scored should not be broken.
- It is safer to administer the least number of whole tablets possible without scoring.
- Read labels carefully and choose the correct medication to administer to match the order and dosage amount.
- When there is a choice of tablets or capsules in varying strengths, choose the strength that allows administration of the least number of tablets or capsules.
- Consult a medication reference or pharmacist when in doubt about a dosage to be administered and whether tablets can be crushed or capsules opened.

PRACTICE PROBLEMS

Calculate the correct number of tablets or capsules to be administered in the following problems using the labels or information provided. Use any of the methods presented to calculate the dosage. Remember to label your answers correctly: tabs, caps.

1. Order: Synthroid 0.025 mg p.o. every day.

   Available: Scored tablets

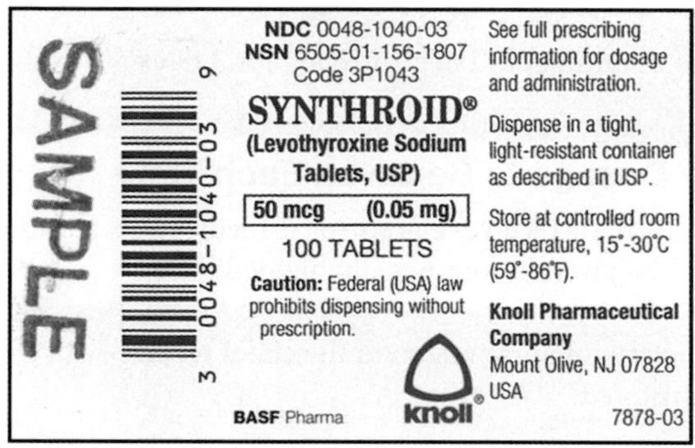

____

2. Order: Strattera 50 mg p.o. daily.

   Available:

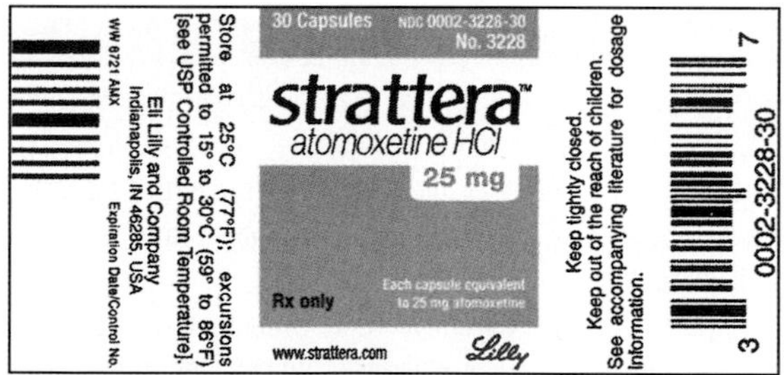

____

3. Order: Relafen 1 g p.o. daily.

   Available:

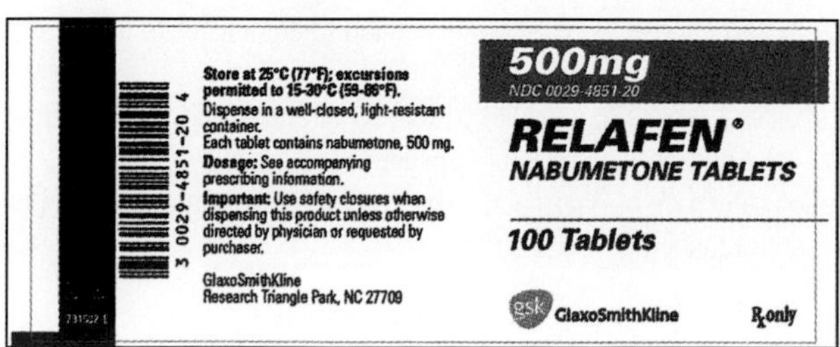

500mg
RELAFEN®
NABUMETONE TABLETS
100 Tablets
GlaxoSmithKline
℞only
Store at 25°C (77°F); excursions permitted to 15-30°C (59-86°F).
Dispense in a well-closed, light-resistant container.
Each tablet contains nabumetone, 500 mg.
Dosage: See accompanying prescribing information.
Important: Use safety closures when dispensing this product unless otherwise directed by physician or requested by purchaser.
GlaxoSmithKline
Research Triangle Park, NC 27709
3 0029-4851-20 4

____

4. Order: Coumadin 7.5 mg p.o. at bedtime.

   Available: Scored tablets

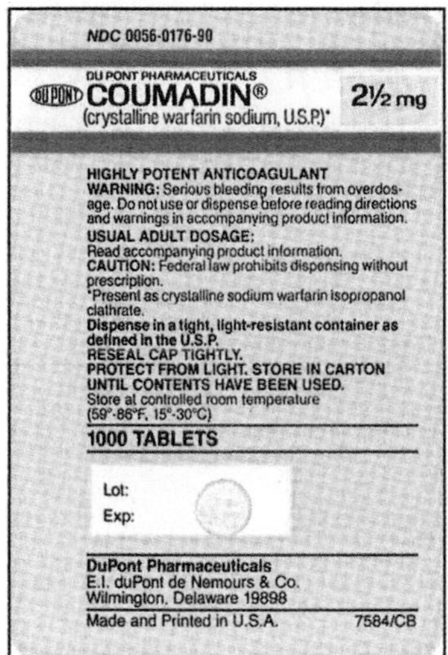

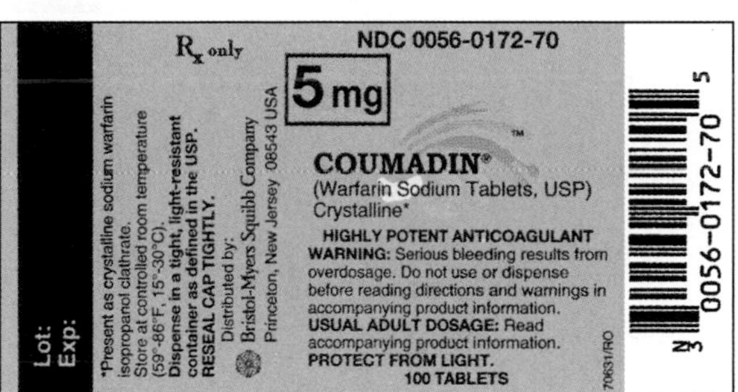

What is the appropriate strength tablet to use? ____________

5. Order: Lanoxin 0.125 mg p.o. daily.

   Available: Scored tablets

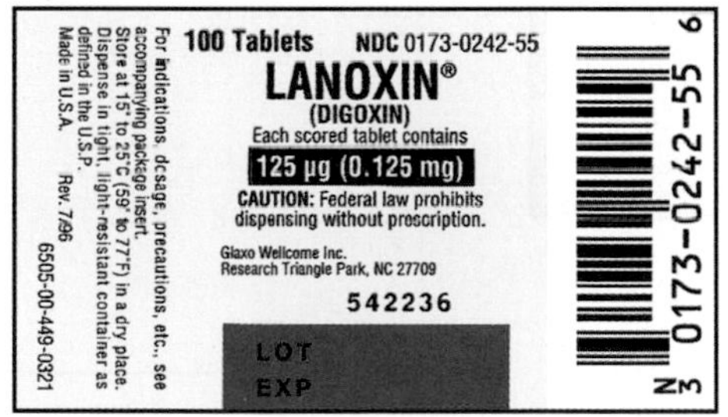

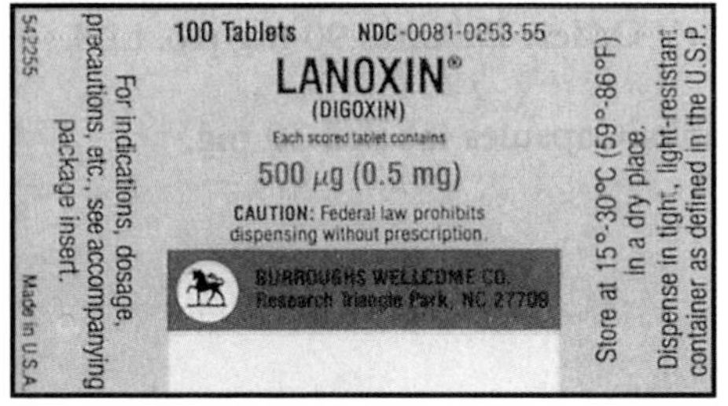

   a. What is the appropriate strength tablet to use? ____________

   b. What will you administer? ____________

6. Order: Ampicillin 1 g p.o. q6h.

   Available: Ampicillin capsules labeled 500 mg and 250 mg

   a. Which strength capsule is appropriate to use? ____________

   b. How many capsules are needed for one dosage? ____________

   c. What is the total number of capsules needed if the medication is ordered for 7 days? ____________

7. Order: Eliquis 10 mg p.o. b.i.d. for 7 days.

   Available:

   a. What is the appropriate strength tablet to use? ______________

   b. What will you administer? ______________

8. Order: Baclofen 15 mg p.o. t.i.d. for 3 days.

   Available: Scored tablets

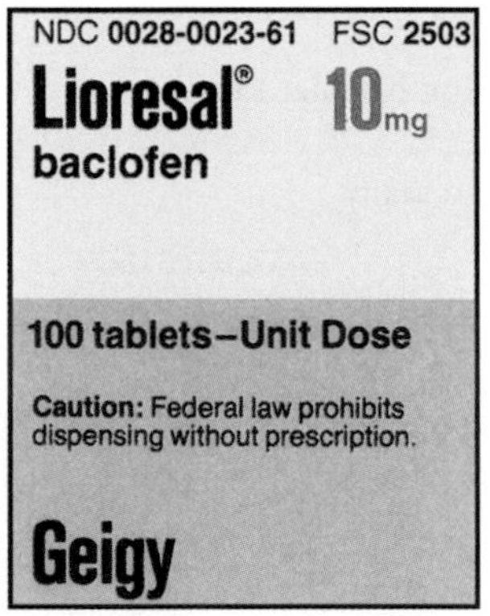

   a. How many tablets are needed for one dosage? ______________

   b. What is the total number of milligrams the client will receive in 3 days? ______________

9. Order: Dilaudid 4 mg p.o. q4h prn for moderate pain.

   Available: Dilaudid tablets labeled 2 mg

   ____

10. Order: Uniphyl 0.4 g p.o. daily.

Available:

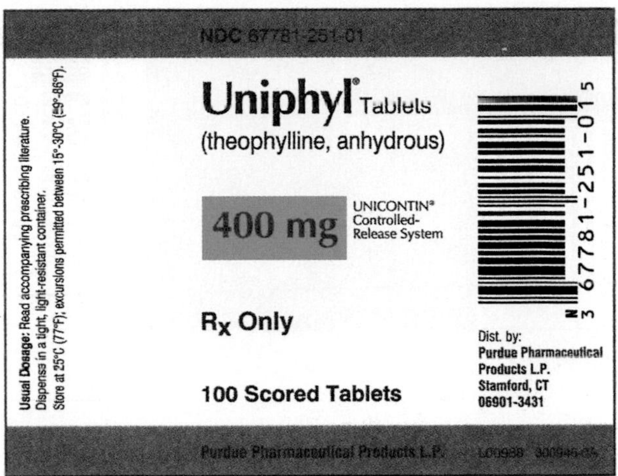

____

11. Order: Dilantin 90 mg (extended-release) p.o. t.i.d. ______________

Available: Dilantin capsules (extended-release) labeled 30 mg ______________

12. Order: Tegretol 200 mg p.o. t.i.d.

Available:

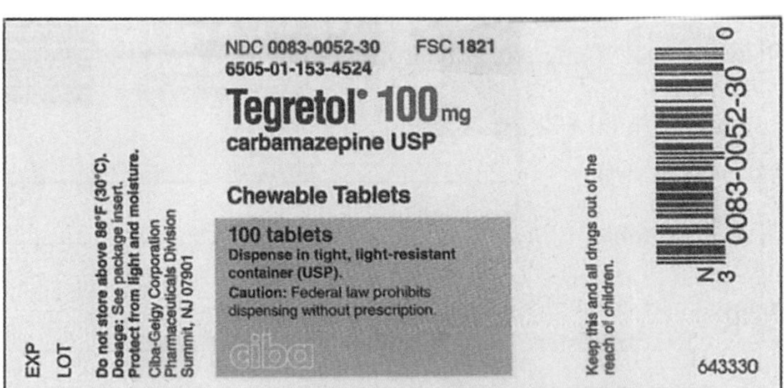

How many tablets will you administer for each dosage? ______________

13. Order: Clarinex 5 mg p.o. daily.

    Available:

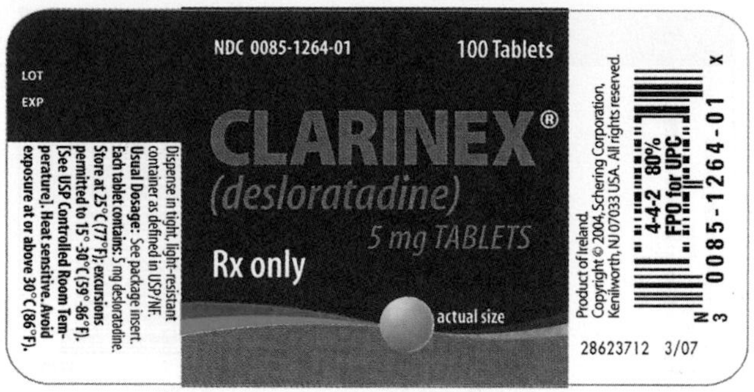

____

14. Order: Rexulti 1 mg p.o. daily for 4 days for a client with schizophrenia.

    Available:

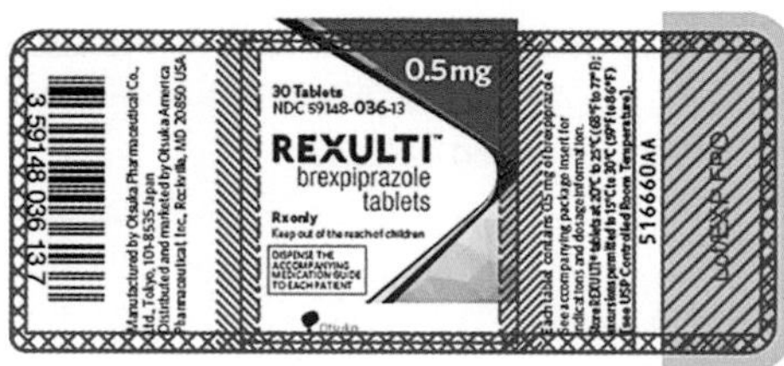

____

15. Order: Phenobarbital 90 mg p.o. at bedtime.

    Available: Phenobarbital 15 mg tabs and 30 mg tabs.

    a. Which strength tablet is best to administer? _______________

    b. How many tablets of which strength will you prepare to administer? _______________

16. Order: Ziagen 0.6 g p.o. daily.

    Available:

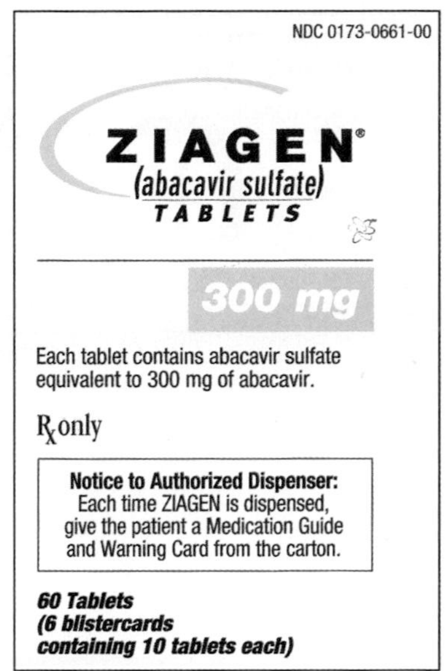

____

17. Order: Thorazine 100 mg p.o. t.i.d.

    Available:

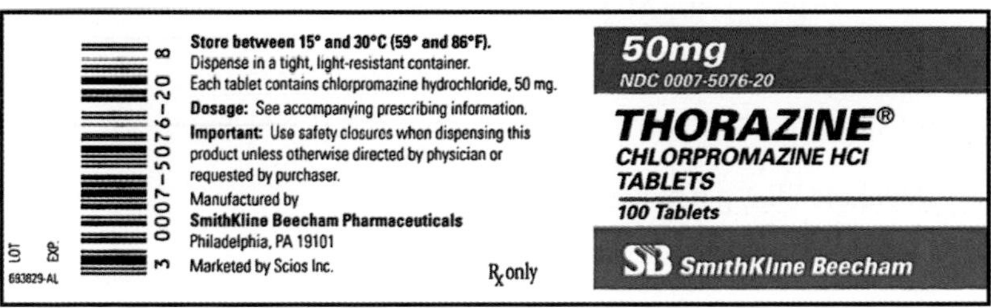

    How many tablets are needed for 3 days? ____________________

18. Order: Verapamil 120 mg p.o. t.i.d. Hold for systolic blood pressure less than 100, heart rate less than 55.

    Available: Verapamil scored tablets labeled 80 mg and 40 mg

    How many tablets of which strength will you administer? ____________________

19. Order: OxyContin (controlled-release) 20 mg p.o. q12h for pain management.

Available:

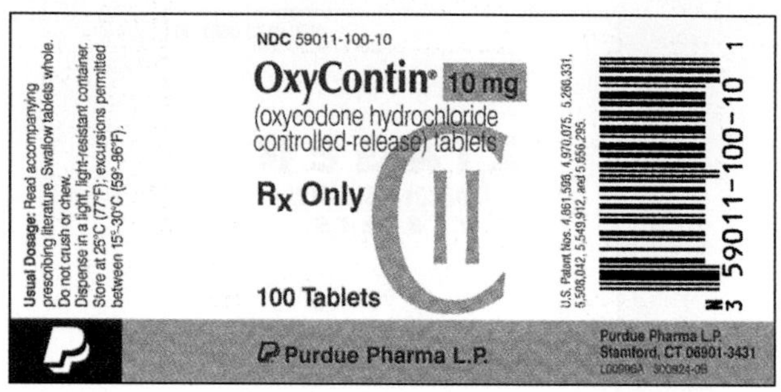

____

20. Order: Cogentin 1 mg p.o. t.i.d.

Available:

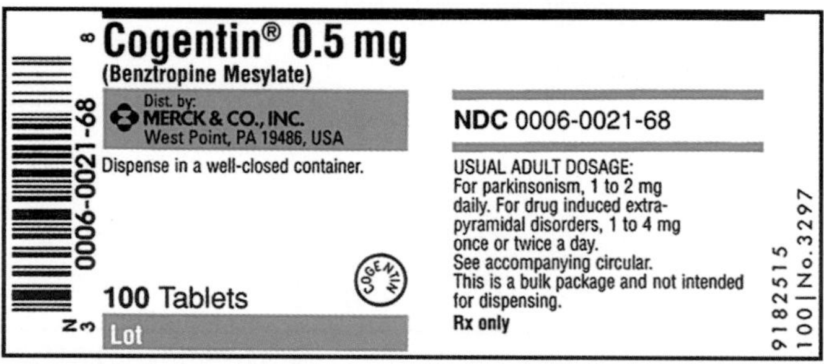

____

21. Order: Depakote ER 1 g p.o. daily.

Available:

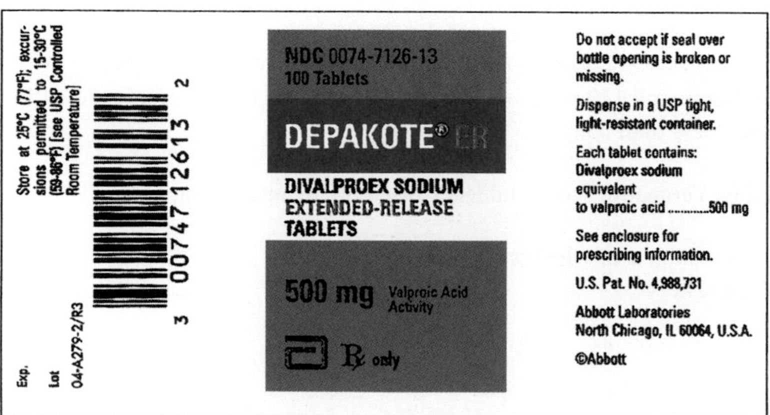

____

22. Order: Zyvox 0.6 g p.o. q12h for 10 days.

    Available:

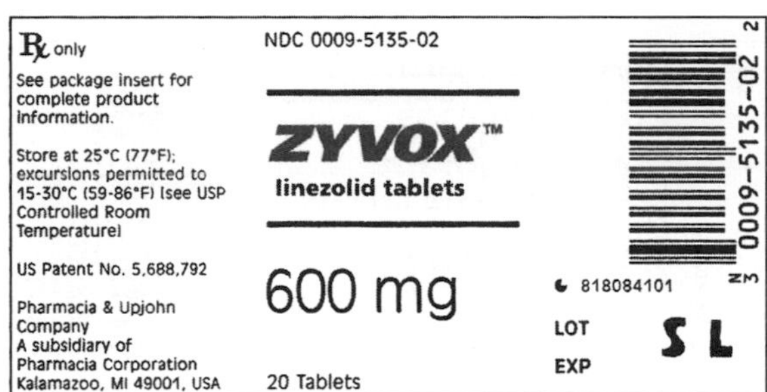

____

23. Order: Dexamethasone 6 mg p.o. daily.

    Available: Dexamethasone (scored tablets) labeled 0.5 mg, 4 mg, and 6 mg

    How many tablets of which strength will you administer? ____________________

24. Order: Pyridium 0.2 g p.o. q8h.

    Available:

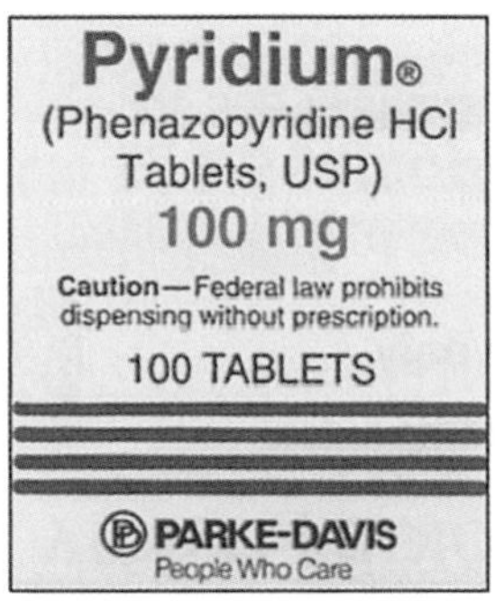

____

25. Order: Tecfidera DR 240 mg p.o. b.i.d. for a client with multiple sclerosis.

    Available:

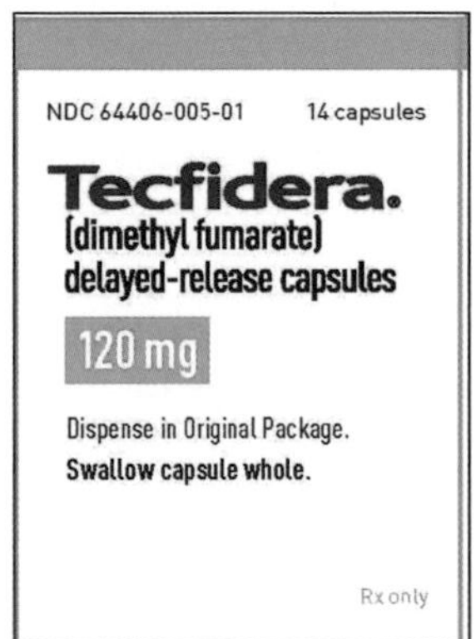

____

26. Order: Glyset 100 mg p.o. t.i.d. at the start of each meal.

Available:

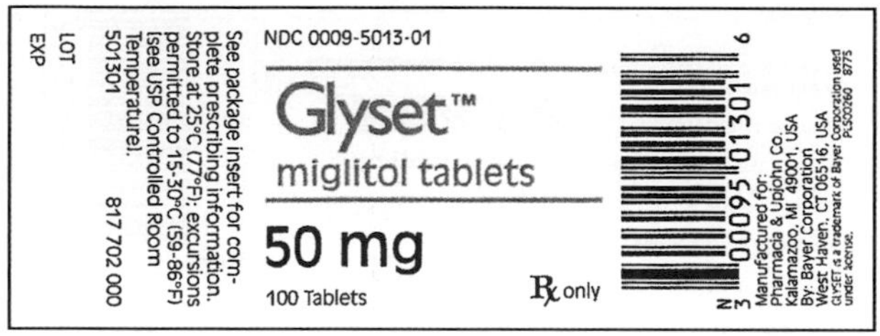

____

27. Order: Tagamet (cimetidine) 400 mg p.o. b.i.d.

Available: Tagamet (cimetidine) tablets labeled 200 mg

How many tablets will you administer for each dosage? ________________

28. Order: Indocin SR 150 mg p.o. b.i.d.

Available:

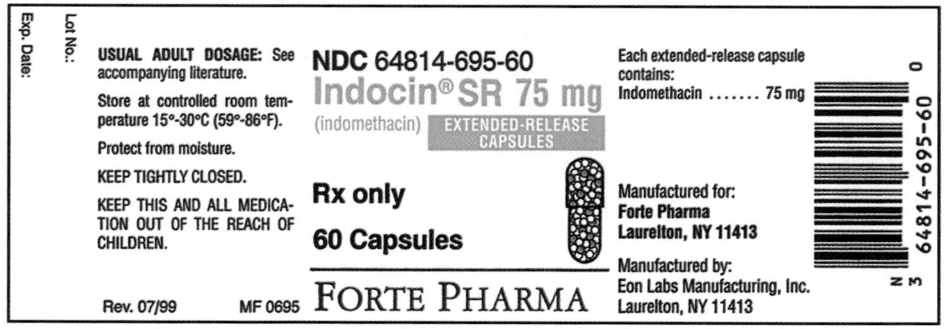

How many capsules will you administer for each dosage? ________________

29. Order: Azulfidine (sulfasalazine) 1 g p.o. q6h.

Available:

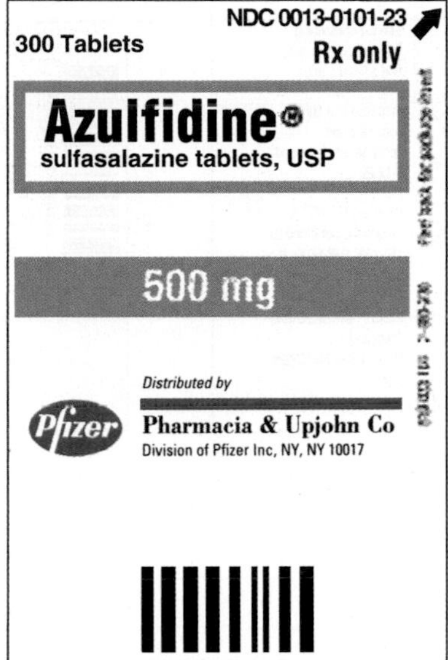

How many tablets will you administer for each dosage? ______________

30. Order: Cymbalta (delayed-release capsules) 60 mg p.o. daily.

Available:

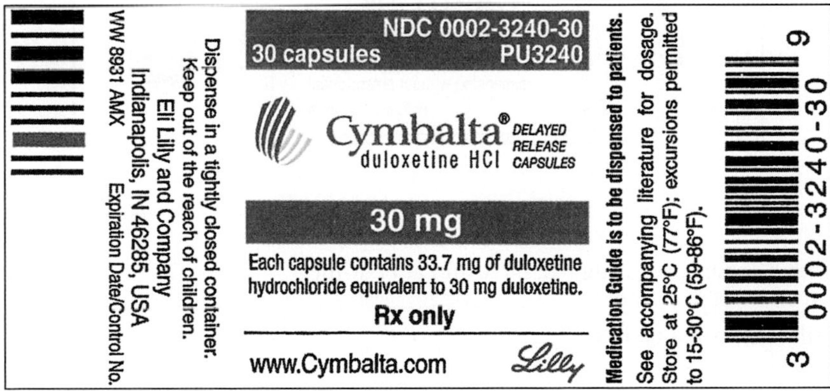

How many capsules will you administer for each dosage? ______________

31. Order: Synthroid 75 mcg p.o. daily.

    Available: Scored tablets

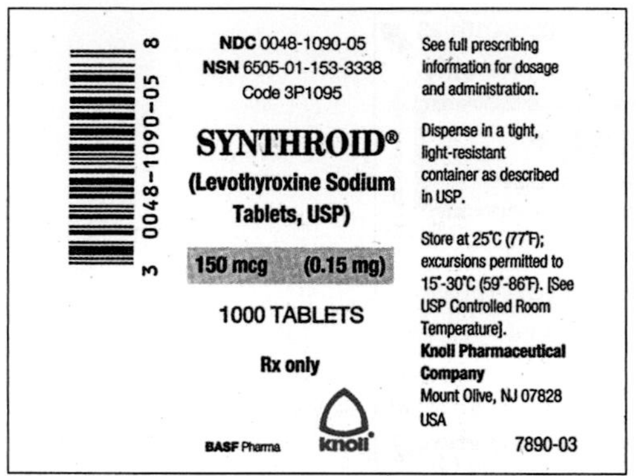

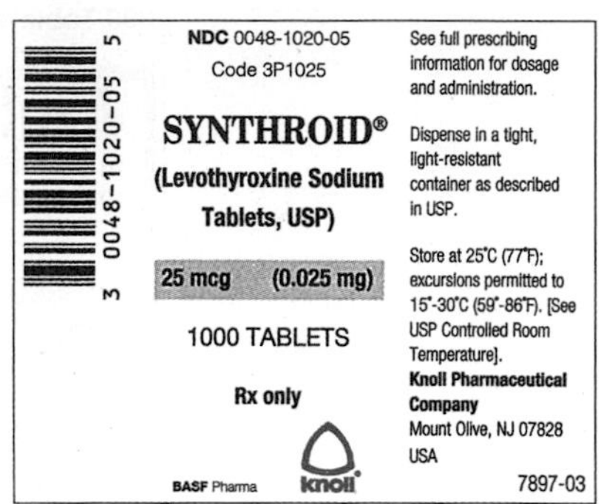

    How many tablets of which strength will you use to administer the dosage? __________

32. Order: Capoten 25 mg p.o. q8h.

    Available:

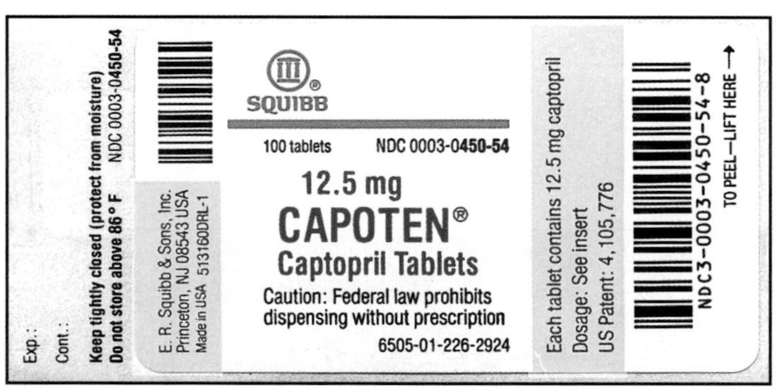

____

33. Order: Clonazepam 1 mg p.o. b.i.d. and at bedtime.

    Available: Scored tablets

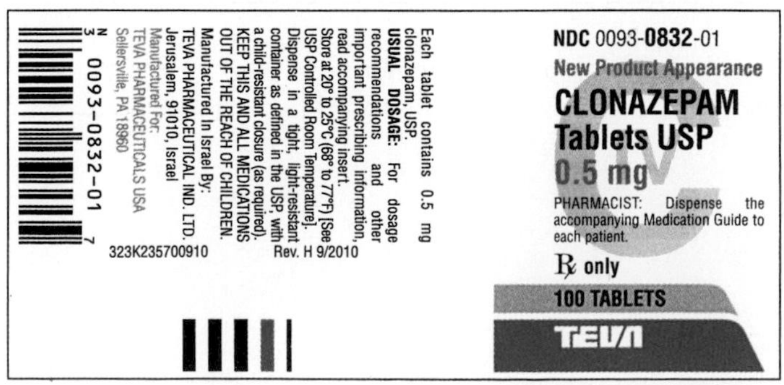

____

34. Order: Amoxicillin and Clavulanate Potassium 400 mg/57 mg p.o. q8h (dosage based on Amoxicillin).

Available:

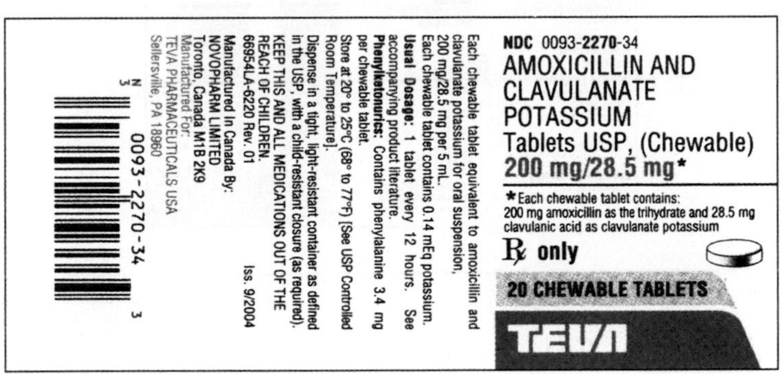

____

35. Order: Levothroid 0.137 mg p.o. daily.

Available: Levothroid tablets labeled 137 mcg

____

36. Order: Lyrica 50 mg p.o. t.i.d.

Available:

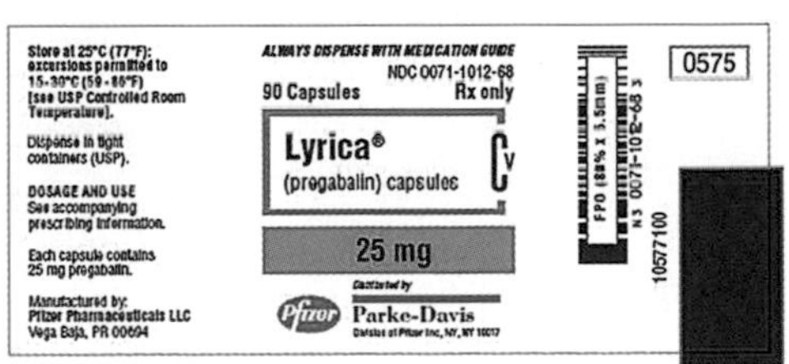

____

37. Order: Dilantin (extended-release capsules) 0.2 g p.o. t.i.d.

Available: Dilantin (extended-release capsules) labeled 100 mg

____

38. Order: Motrin 800 mg p.o. q6h p.r.n. for pain.

    Available:

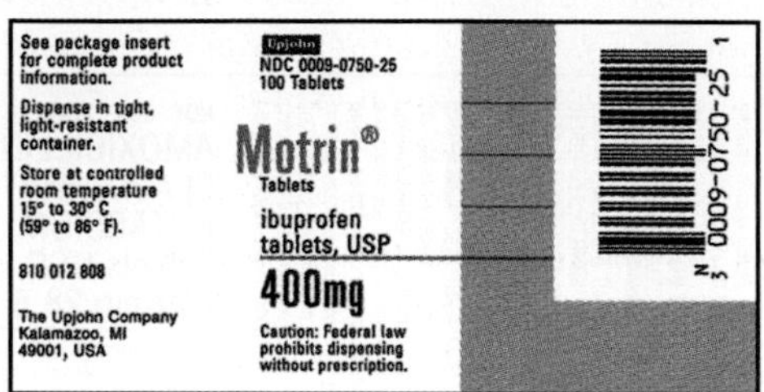

39. Order: Procardia XL 60 mg p.o. daily.

    Available: Procardia XL labeled 30 mg per tablet.

40. Order: Minoxidil 0.03 g p.o. daily.

    Available:

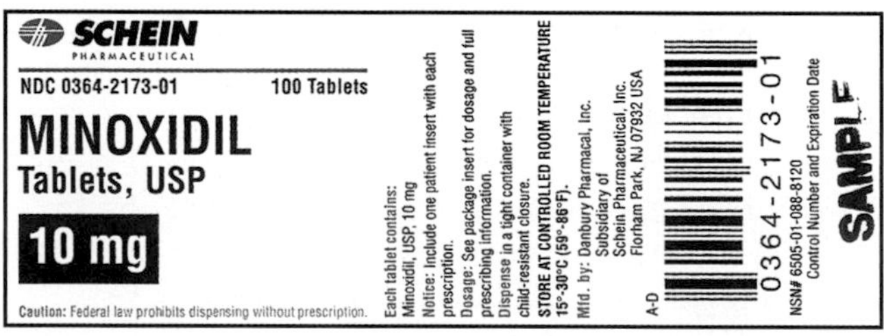

41. Order: Inderal LA 120 mg p.o. every day.

    Available:

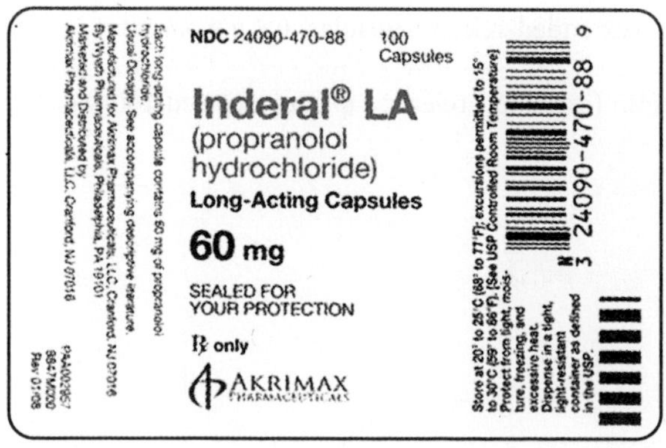

Answers on pp. 352-355

Calculating Oral Liquids

Enteral medications are also available in liquid form for administration orally or through various types of tubes placed into the stomach or intestines. Examples: nasogastric (tube in nose to stomach), gastrostomy (tube placed directly into the stomach), or jejunostomy (tube directly into intestines). Liquid medications are also desirable for use in:

- Clients who have dysphagia (difficulty swallowing)
- Young children, infants, and elderly clients
- Instances when medications that cannot be crushed for administration are ordered; then the availability of the medication in liquid form should be investigated.

Liquid medications are prepared in different forms, as follows:

1. ***Elixir***—Alcohol solution that is sweet and aromatic.
   Example: Phenobarbital elixir.
2. ***Suspension***—One or more medications finely divided into a liquid such as water.
   Example: Penicillin suspension.
3. ***Syrup***—Medication dissolved in concentrated solution of sugar and water.
   Example: Colace.

Liquid medications also come as tincture, emulsions, and extract preparations for oral use. Although oral liquids may be administered by means other than by mouth (e.g., nasogastric tube, gastrostomy), they should **never** be given by any other route, such as the intravenous (IV) route or by injection.

In the beginning of this chapter, you learned how to calculate medications that were in solid form (tablets, capsules). You calculated the number of tablets or capsules that contained the ordered dosage.

The labels on medications in liquid form indicate the specific amount or weight of a medication in a given amount of solution. You must calculate the volume or amount of liquid that contains the ordered dosage. The methods presented in Chapters 14 to 16 can be used to calculate the volume or amount to administer the ordered dosage. There are some oral liquid medications that do not require calculation because, when ordered, the specific amount to be administered is stated. Examples: Milk of Magnesia 1 ounce p.o. at bedtime; Robitussin 15 mL p.o. q4h prn; Fer-in-Sol 0.2 mL p.o. daily.

The medication label on oral liquids may indicate the amount of medication per milliliter, ounce, etc. For example, 25 mg per mL, 200 mg per mL (Figure 17-7, *A*). The amount may also be expressed in terms of multiple milliliters of solution, such as 80 mg per 2 mL, 250 mg per 5 mL (Figure 17-7, *B*).

Oral liquids can be measured in small amounts of volume, and a greater range of dosages can be ordered for administration. When calculating oral liquid medications, the stock, or what you have available, is in liquid form; therefore, the label (unit) on your answer will always be expressed in liquid measures such as milliliters.

According to Cohen (2010, Abridged edition), *Medication Errors,* "Many dosage errors occur with oral liquid medications. This dosage form may seem to have less potential for harm than injectable medications, but oral liquids are the least likely form to be dispensed in unit doses, and they are prescribed most often for pediatric and geriatric patients."

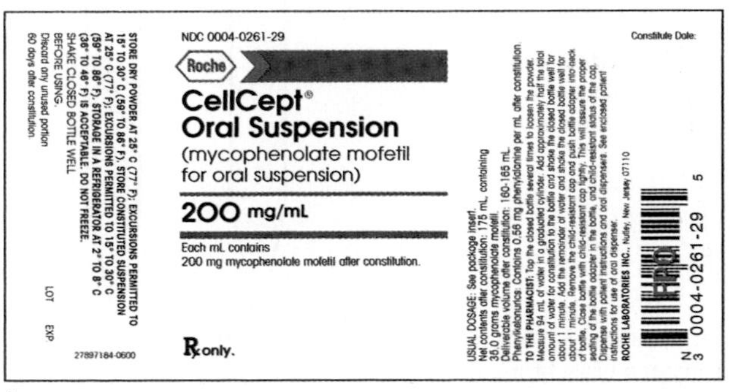

A

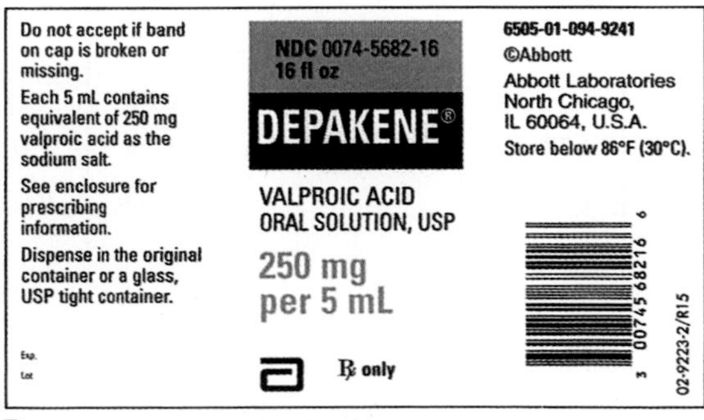

B

Figure 17-7 **A,** CellCept oral suspension 200 mg per mL. **B,** Depakene oral solution 250 mg per mL.

The reason for dosing errors include inaccurate measurements of oral liquids and the use of improper measuring devices. The use of calibrated measuring devices (droppers, calibrated spoons) should be used in the hospital, and clients educated on the importance of this at home as opposed to using household spoons. Let's discuss the measurement of oral liquids.

Measuring Oral Liquids

The administration of oral liquids requires careful measurement. There can be a greater range of dosages ordered and administered with oral liquids. Several types of equipment are used to administer enteral liquid medications. These include medicine cups, droppers, oral syringes, and calibrated spoons.

1. **The standard medicine cup** usually is plastic, has a capacity of 30 milliliters (1 fluid ounce), and is used to measure most liquid medications for oral administration. Most medication cups typically indicate metric, household, and apothecary systems of measurement on the cup. Therefore cups include units such as tablespoons (tbs), teaspoons (tsp), milliliters (mL), drams (dr), and ounces (oz). It is important to note that dram, a unit of measurement in the apothecary system, is no longer used but may still appear on medicine cups in some health care facilities. In some cases cubic centimeters (cc), formerly used interchangeably with milliliters (mL), may still appear on medicine cups. The correct unit is mL.

SAFETY ALERT!

To prevent medication errors, take care and do not confuse the **dosing scales on a medication cup when pouring medications.**

As a result of errors that have occurred with nurses confusing dosing scales on a plastic oral liquid dosing cup, there have been recommendations to move toward full use of metric dosing, including medicine cups that allow measurement in milliliters only. (National Alert Network, June 30, 2015-based on information from the National Medication Errors Reporting Program operated by the Institute for Safe Medication Practices.)

Figure 17-8 shows one view of a medication cup.

When measuring liquid medications, the medication cup should be placed on a flat surface, poured at eye level, and read at the bottom of the meniscus (a curvature made by the solution). See Figure 17-9. Always pour liquid medications with the label facing you to avoid covering the label with your hand or obscuring label information if the medication drips down the side of the container.

2. **Calibrated droppers** are used for measuring and administering small volumes of liquid medications (Figure 17-10). They may be used to administer certain liquid medications

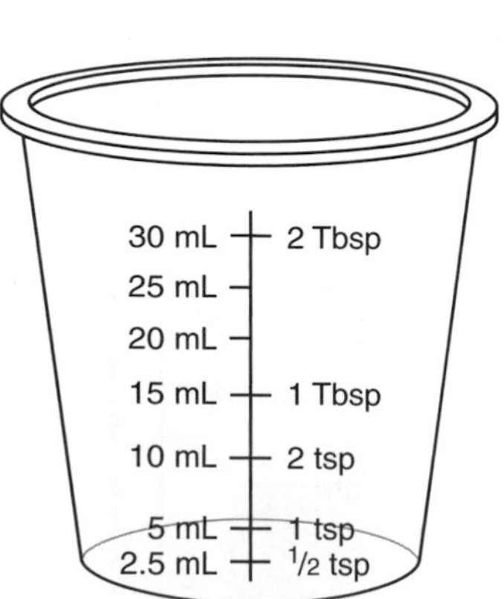

Figure 17-8 Medicine cup.

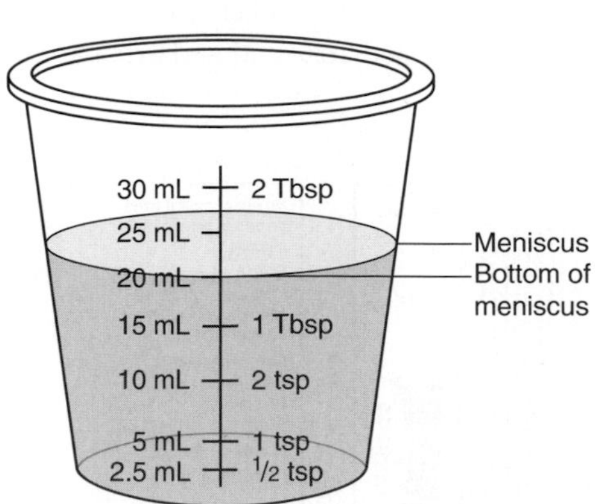

Figure 17-9 Reading meniscus. The meniscus is caused by the surface tension of the solution against the walls of the container. The surface tension causes the formation of a concave or hollowed curvature on the surface of the solution. Read the level at the lowest point of the concave.

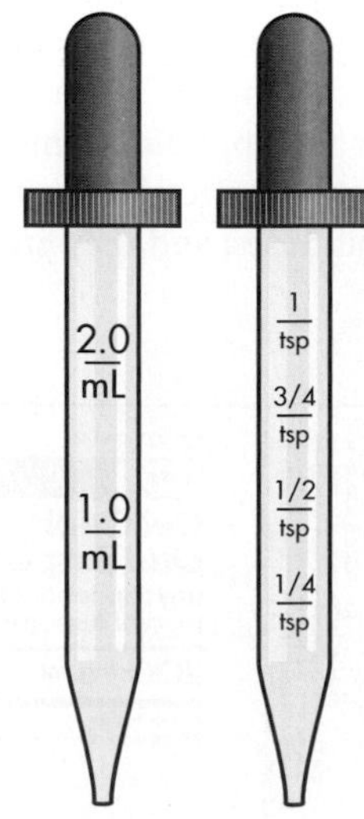

Figure 17-10 Medicine droppers.

to the eyes, ears, and nose. Another common use is for administration of oral pediatric doses such as vitamins. Droppers have different sized openings that produce different amounts of medication with each drop. Some medications come with a dropper that indicates the dropper is calibrated for the specified dose and can only be used for the medication it is packaged with, to ensure accurate dosing. Some medicine droppers are calibrated in milliliters, drops, teaspoons, or by actual dosage.

SAFETY ALERT!

A calibrated **dropper** should be used **ONLY** for the medication **for which it is intended; droppers are not interchangeable.** Drop size varies from one dropper to another.

Clients who are being discharged and taking oral medications at home should be instructed to use only the dropper or other measuring devices that come with the particular medication as opposed to a household spoon.

3. Syringes may also be used to measure medications. The medication is poured in a medication cup and drawn up in the syringe without the use of a needle. This is often done when the amount desired cannot be measured accurately in a cup. For example, 6.3 mL cannot be measured accurately in the standard medication cup; however, the medication may be drawn up in a syringe and then squirted into a cup or administered orally with the use of a hypodermic syringe without the needle. This practice is discouraged to prevent confusion with route of administration. Solutions for oral use should be measured by using a specially calibrated **oral syringe** (Figure 17-11). **Oral syringes** are used to measure and administer oral liquids to ensure accurate and safe dosages. Oral syringes have unique features that distinguish them from syringes used for injections. Oral syringes (often available in colors) are not sterile; some are labeled "For oral use only." An eccentric or off-center tip alerts the nurse that a needle should not be attached to this syringe. The tip of an oral syringe does not fit adapters and devices made for injectable syringes, such as IV tubing. This prevents medications for oral use from being injected IV or into tissue, which can cause injury or death. Oral syringes are calibrated in tenths of a milliliter and may have teaspoon and tablespoon markings.

SAFETY ALERT!

To prevent confusion with the route of administration, only use oral syringes to measure and administer oral medications. Oral medications are **never** injected.

Figure 17-12 shows how to fill a syringe from a medicine cup. Some oral liquid medications come in containers that allow the client to drink right out of the container, eliminating the need to transfer it to a medication cup.

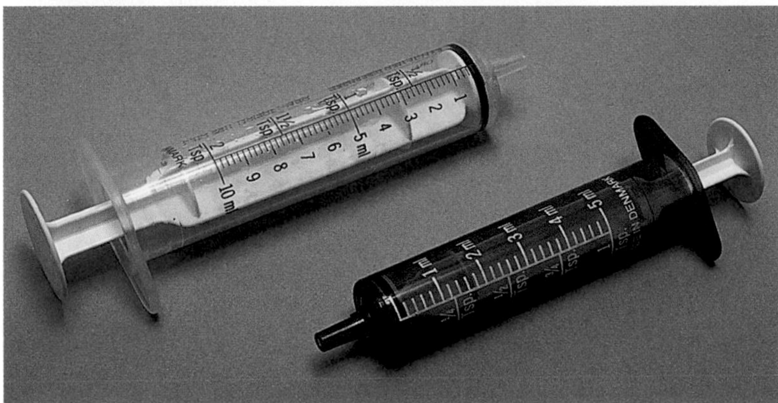

Figure 17-11 Oral syringes. (Courtesy Chuck Dresner. From Clayton BD, Willihnganz M: *Basic pharmacology for nurses,* ed 17, St Louis, 2017, Mosby.)

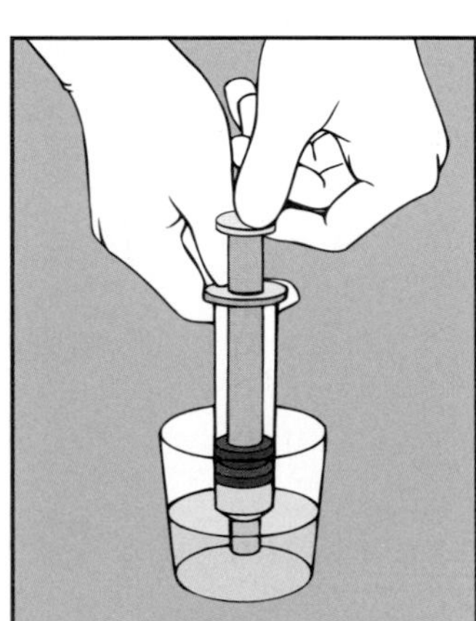

Figure 17-12 Filling a syringe directly from medicine cup. (Modified from Clayton BD, Willihnganz M: *Basic pharmacology for nurses,* ed 17, St Louis, 2017, Mosby.)

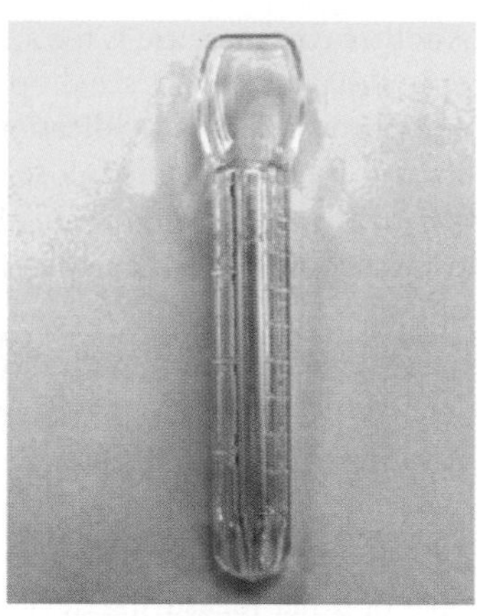

Figure 17-13 Calibrated spoons. (From Mulholland JM and Turner SJ: *The nurse, the math, the meds: drug calculations using dimensional analysis,* ed 3, St Louis, 2015, Mosby.)

4. Calibrated spoons are often used to administer oral liquids to children or elderly clients. Some spoons for children are shaped like animals. Household spoons vary in size and are not reliable for accurate dosing. Always encourage the use of calibrated spoons for medications that are measured by teaspoons, tablespoons, or milliliters (Figure 17-13).

Before we proceed to calculate liquid medications, let's review some helpful pointers.

1. The label on the medication container must be read carefully to determine the dosage strength in the volume of solution because it varies.

SAFETY ALERT!

Do not confuse dosage strength with total volume. Read labels carefully. Confusing dosage strength with total volume can result in errors when performing calculations and lead to the administration of an unintended dose.

For example, the label on a medication may indicate a total volume of 100 mL, but the dosage strength may be 125 mg per 5 mL. It must be noted that dosage strength can be written on solutions in several ways to indicate the same thing. For example, 125 mg per 5 mL may be written as 125 mg/5 mL or 125 mg = 5 mL. Other examples of dosage strength are 20 mg per mL, 20 mg/mL, 200 mg/5 mL, and 200 mg per 5 mL.

SAFETY ALERT!

Although dosage strengths may be written on solutions in several ways when dosages are written—for example, 40 mg per 2 mL or 40 mg/2 mL—ISMP (Institute for Safe Medication Practices; http://www.ismp.org/Tools/errorproneabbreviations) recommends that the "/" (slash mark) not be used to separate doses. The slash mark has been mistaken as the number 1. Use "per" rather than a slash mark to separate doses.

2. Answers are labeled using liquid measures. Example: mL.
3. Calculations can be done by using the same methods (ratio and proportion, the formula method, or dimensional analysis) and the same steps as for solid forms of oral medications.

Now let's look at some sample problems that involve the calculation of oral liquids.

Example 1: Order: Dilantin 200 mg p.o. t.i.d.

Available: Dilantin suspension labeled 125 mg per 5 mL

✓ PROBLEM SETUP

1. No conversion is required. Everything is in the same units of measure and the same system.
   Order: 200 mg
   Available: 125 mg per 5 mL

2. Think critically: What would be a logical answer? Looking at Example 1, you can assume the answer will be greater than 5 mL.
3. Set up the problem using ratio and proportion, the formula method, or dimensional analysis.
4. Label the final answer with the correct unit of measure. In this case the units will be milliliters. Remember: The answer has no meaning if written without the appropriate unit of measure.

✓ Solution Using Ratio and Proportion

$$125\text{ mg} : 5\text{ mL} = 200\text{ mg} : x\text{ mL}$$

$$\text{(known)} \qquad \text{(unknown)}$$

$$125x = 200 \times 5$$

$$\frac{125x}{125} = \frac{1{,}000}{125}$$

$$x = \frac{1{,}000}{125}$$

$$x = 8\text{ mL}$$

Note: Reduction of numbers can be done to make them smaller and easier to deal with.

✓ Solution Using the Formula Method

$$\frac{\text{(D) }200\text{ mg}}{\text{(H) }125\text{ mg}} \times \text{(Q) }5\text{ mL} = x\text{ mL}$$

$$x = \frac{200}{125} \times 5$$

$$x = \frac{1{,}000}{125}$$

$$x = 8\text{ mL}$$

✓ Solution Using Dimensional Analysis

$$x\text{ mL} = \frac{5\text{ mL}}{125\text{ }\cancel{\text{mg}}} \times \frac{200\text{ }\cancel{\text{mg}}}{1}$$

$$x = \frac{1{,}000}{125}$$

$$x = 8\text{ mL}$$

Example 2: Order: Lactulose 30 g p.o. b.i.d.

Available: Lactulose labeled 10 g per 15 mL

✓ Solution Using Ratio and Proportion

$$10\text{ g} : 15\text{ mL} = 30\text{ g} : x\text{ mL}$$

$$\frac{10x}{10} = \frac{450}{10}$$

$$x = \frac{450}{10}$$

$$x = 45\text{ mL}$$

✓ Solution Using the Formula Method

$$\frac{\text{(D) } 30 \text{ g}}{\text{(H) } 10 \text{ g}} \times \text{(Q) } 15 \text{ mL} = x \text{ mL}$$

$$x = \frac{30 \times 15}{10}$$

$$x = \frac{450}{10}$$

$$x = 45 \text{ mL}$$

✓ Solution Using Dimensional Analysis

$$x \text{ mL} = \frac{15 \text{ mL}}{10 \not{g}} \times \frac{30 \not{g}}{1}$$

$$x = \frac{450}{10}$$

$$x = 45 \text{ mL}$$

Example 3: Order: Omnicef 0.3 g p.o. q 12 h.

Available: Omnicef oral suspension labeled 125 mg per 5 mL

1. Convert grams to milligrams. 1,000 mg = 1 g.
   Any of the methods presented for converting can be used. Because the measures are metric in this problem (grams, milligrams), the other method that can be used is to move the decimal point the desired number of places. (Remember, a conversion is necessary before calculating the dose. What the prescriber ordered is in grams here, and the medication is available in milligrams.)

   (0.3 g = 0.300 = 300 mg)

✓ Solution Using Ratio and Proportion

$$125 \text{ mg} : 5 \text{ mL} = 300 \text{ mg} : x \text{ mL}$$

$$\frac{125x}{125} = \frac{300 \times 5}{125}$$

$$x = \frac{1{,}500}{125}$$

$$x = 12 \text{ mL}$$

✓ Solution Using the Formula Method

$$\frac{\text{(D) } 300 \text{ mg}}{\text{(H) } 125 \text{ mg}} \times \text{(Q) } 5 \text{ mL} = x \text{ mL}$$

$$x = \frac{300 \times 5}{125}$$

$$x = \frac{1{,}500}{125}$$

$$x = 12 \text{ mL}$$

✓ Solution Using Dimensional Analysis

$$x \text{ mL} = \frac{5 \text{ mL}}{125 \cancel{\text{mg}}} \times \frac{1{,}000 \cancel{\text{mg}}}{1 \cancel{\text{g}}} \times \frac{0.3 \cancel{\text{g}}}{1}$$

$$x = \frac{5{,}000 \times 0.3}{125}$$

$$x = \frac{1{,}500}{125}$$

$$x = 12 \text{ mL}$$

POINTS TO REMEMBER

- Liquid medications can be calculated using the same methods as those used for solid forms (tabs, caps).
- Read labels carefully on medications; identify the dosage strength of the medication contained in a certain amount (volume) of solution.
- Do not confuse dosage strength (amount of medication contained in a certain amount of solution) with total volume (the amount in the container).
- Administration of accurate dosages of liquid medications requires the use of calibrated devices (calibrated droppers, calibrated spoons, and oral syringes).
- Oral syringes are designed for oral use only. Use oral syringes to measure and administer oral liquids.
- When using a medication cup to administer oral liquid medications, pour the medication at eye level and read at eye level at bottom of meniscus on a flat surface.
- The use of ratio and proportion, the formula method, or dimensional analysis is a means of validating an answer; however, it still requires thinking in terms of the dosage you will administer and applying principles learned to calculate dosages that are sensible and safe.
- Use "per" to separate dosages when writing, not a slash mark. Example: 125 mg per 5 mL, not 125 mg/5 mL.
- Do not use the dropper packaged with a particular medication to administer other medications.

PRACTICE **PROBLEMS**

Calculate the following dosages for oral liquids in milliliters using the labels or information provided. Do not forget to label your answer. Round answers to the nearest tenth where indicated.

42. Order: Lyrica 50 mg p.o. t.i.d.

Available:

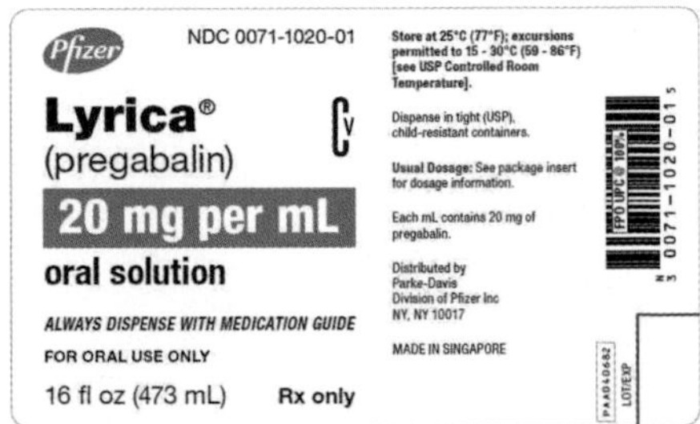

____

43. Order: Biaxin 100 mg p.o. q12h.

Available:

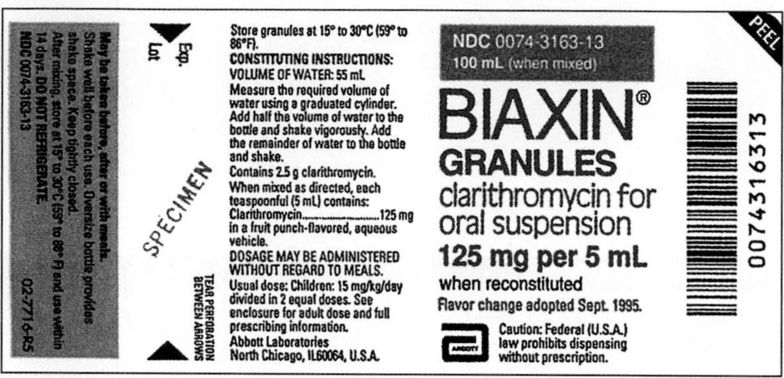

____

44. Order: Potassium chloride 40 mEq p.o. daily.

Available: Potassium chloride oral solution labeled 40 mEq per 15 mL

____

45. Order: Theophylline elixir 120 mg p.o. b.i.d.

Available: Theophylline elixir 80 mg per 15 mL ________________

46. Order: Erythromycin oral suspension 250 mg p.o. q6h.

Available: Erythromycin oral suspension labeled 200 mg per 5 mL

____

47. Order: Dilantin 100 mg p.o. t.i.d.

Available: Dilantin suspension 125 mg per 5 mL ________________

48. Order: Digoxin 125 mcg p.o. every day.

Available:

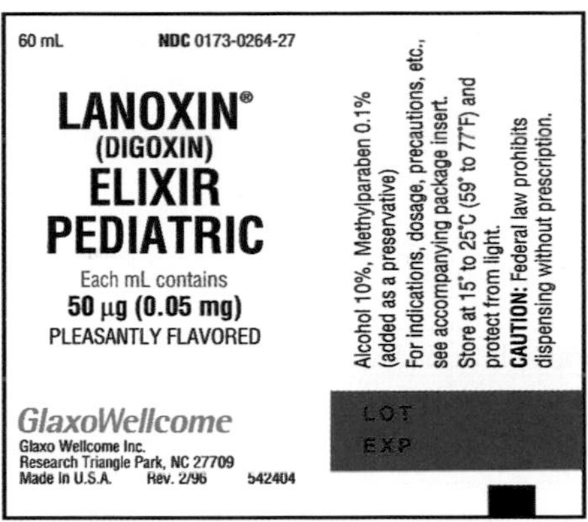

____

49. Order: Imodium (loperamide hydrochloride) 4 mg p.o. as initial dose and then 2 mg after each loose stool.

Available:

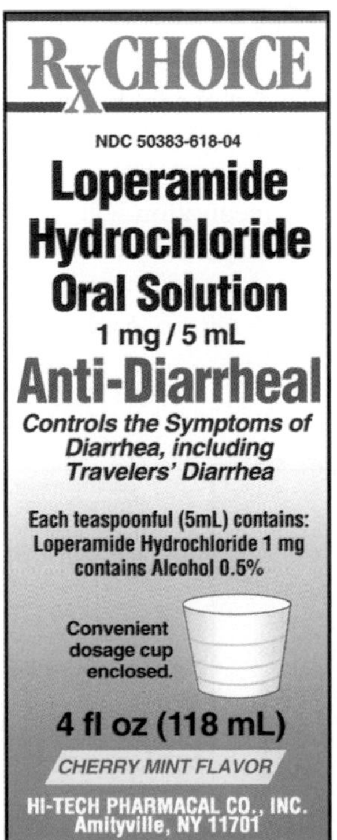

How many mL will you administer for the initial dose? ______________________

50. Order: Amoxicillin 0.5 g p.o. q6h.

    Available: Amoxicillin oral suspension labeled 125 mg per 5 mL

    ____

51. Order: Phenobarbital 60 mg p.o. at bedtime.

    Available: Phenobarbital elixir 20 mg per 5 mL ____________________

52. Order: Mellaril 150 mg p.o. b.i.d.

    Available: Mellaril oral solution labeled 30 mg per mL

    ____

53. Order: Diphenhydramine HCl 25 mg p.o. b.i.d. p.r.n. for agitation.

    Available: Diphenhydramine hydrochloride elixir 12.5 mg per 5 mL

    ____

54. Order: Lithium carbonate 600 mg p.o. at bedtime.

    Available: Lithium citrate syrup. Each 5 mL contains lithium carbonate 300 mg. Each unit-dose container contains 5 mL

    a. How many milliliters are needed to administer the required dosage? ____________________

    b. How many containers of the medication will you need to administer the dosage? ____________________

55. Promethazine Hydrochloride 12.5 mg p.o. q.i.d.

    Available:

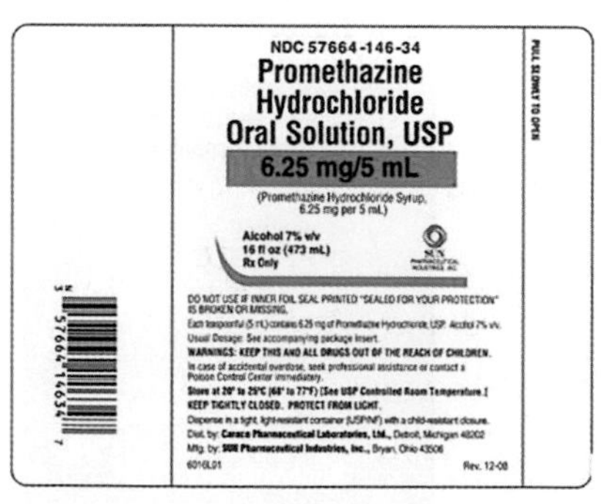

____

56. Order: E.E.S. 0.5 g by gastrostomy tube q6h.

Available:

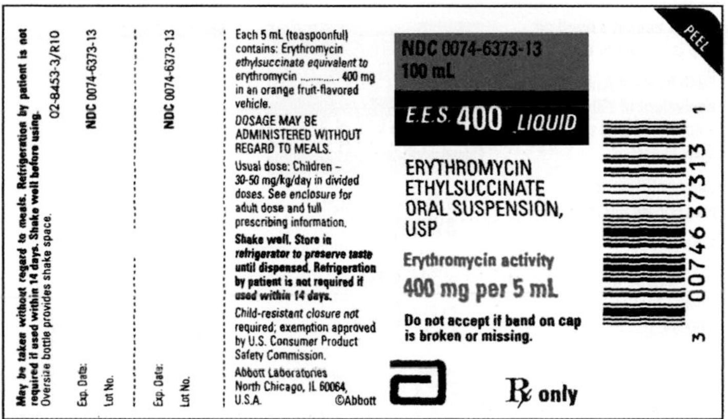

____

57. Order: Penicillin V Potassium 500,000 units p.o. q.i.d.

Available:

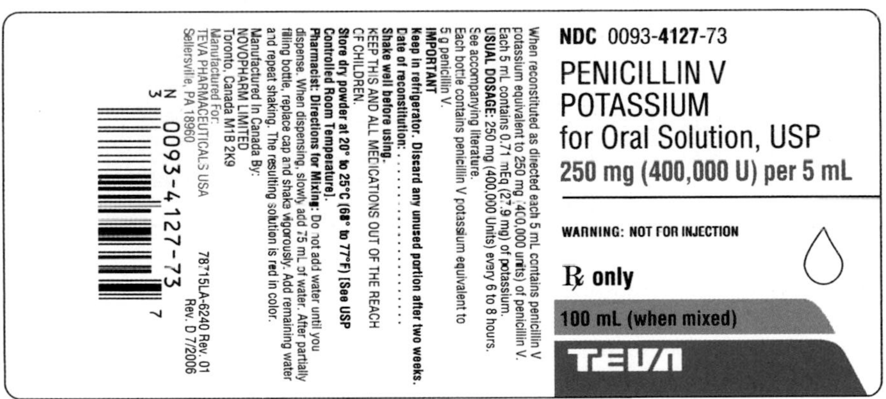

____

58. Order: Keflex 1 g by nasogastric tube q6h.

Available: Keflex oral suspension 125 mg per 5 mL ______________________

59. Order: Depakene 500 mg p.o. daily.

Available:

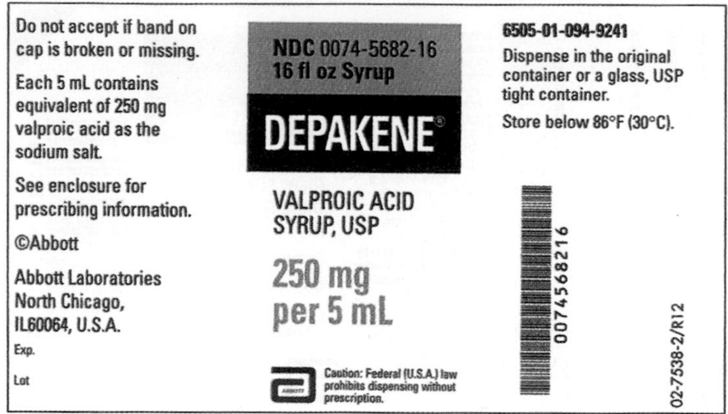

60. Order: Tamiflu 75 mg p.o. b.i.d. for 5 days.

Available:

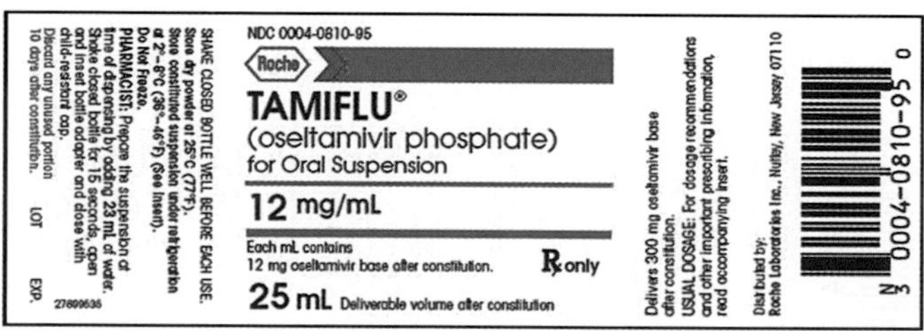

61. Order: Tagamet 400 mg p.o. q6h.

Available: Tagamet oral liquid labeled 300 mg per 5 mL

62. Order: Epivir 150 mg p.o. b.i.d.

Available:

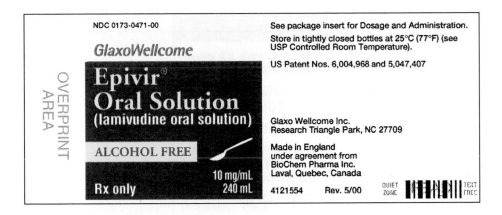

____

63. Order: Retrovir 0.3 g p.o. b.i.d.

Available: Retrovir (zidovudine) syrup labeled 50 mg per 5 mL

____

64. Order: Amoxicillin 375 mg p.o. q8h.

Available:

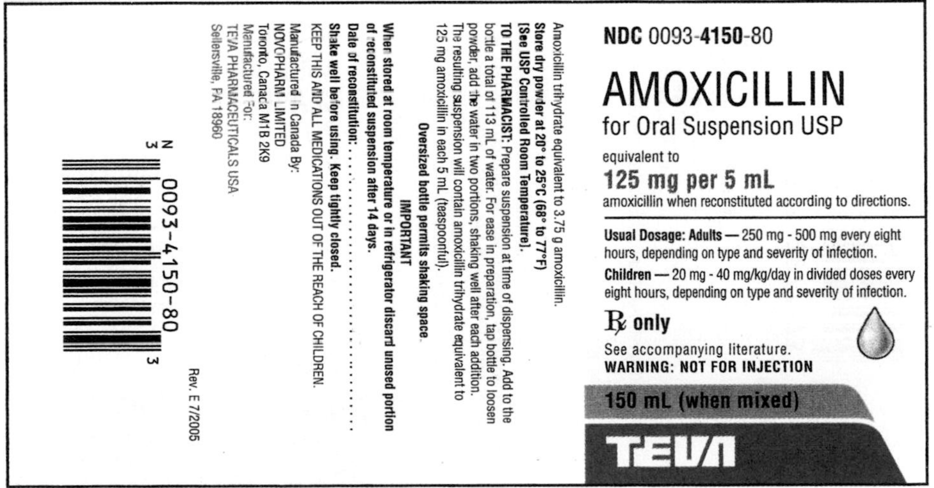

____

65. Order: Norvir 600 mg p.o. b.i.d.

Available:

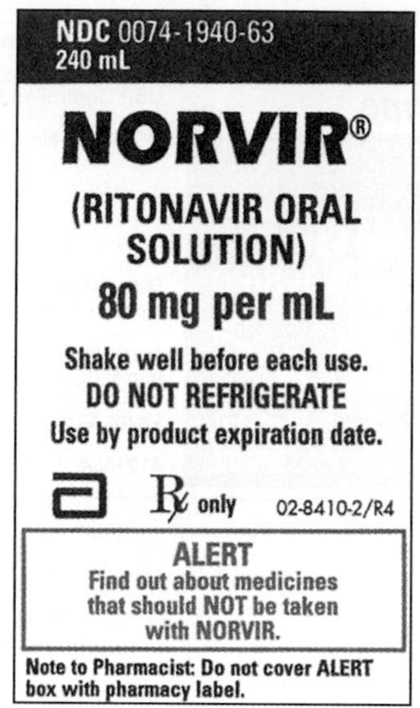

____

66. Order: Amoxicillin and Clavulanate Potassium 0.25 g p.o. q8h (ordered according to the dose of amoxicillin).

Available:

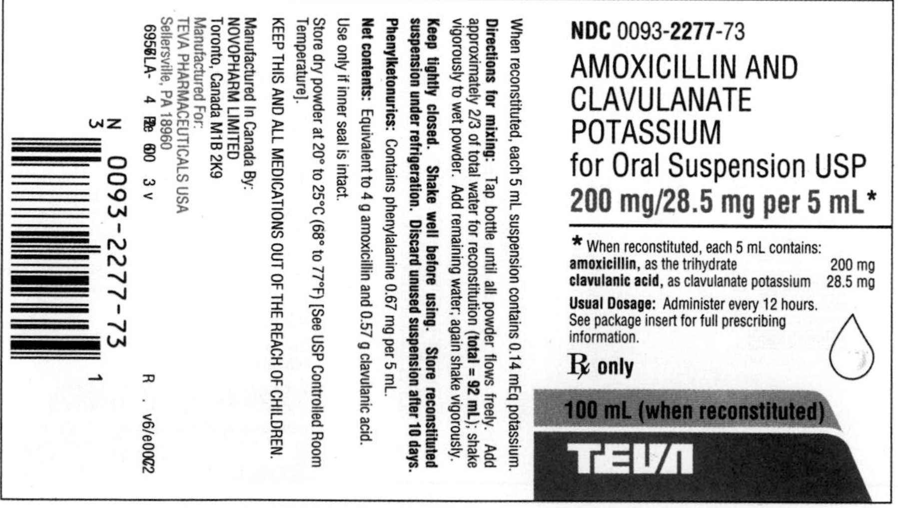

____

67. Order: Zovirax 200 mg p.o. q4h for 5 days.

Available:

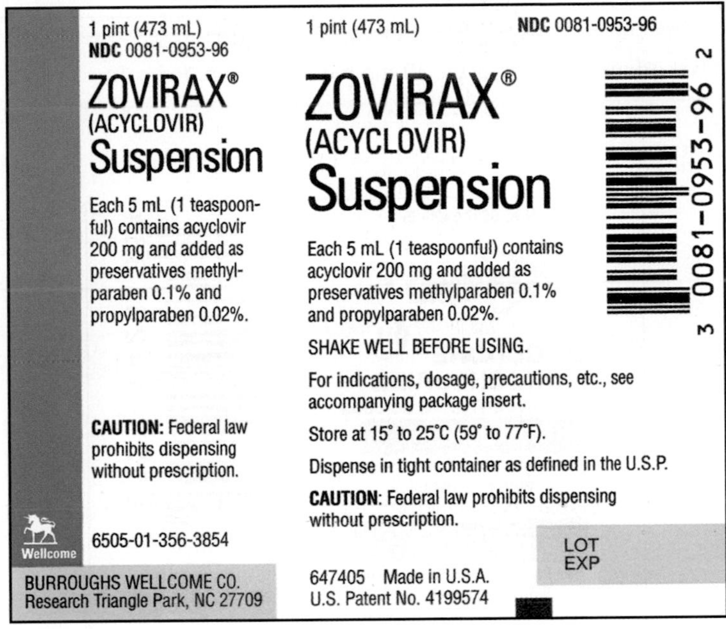

____

68. Order: Prozac 30 mg p.o. every day in AM.

Available:

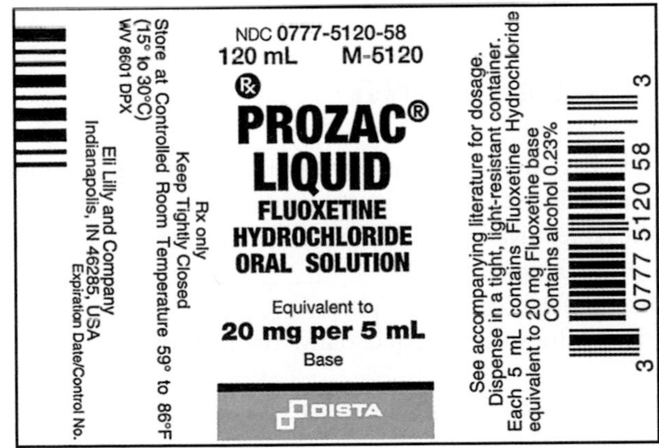

____

69. Order: Zantac 150 mg by nasogastric tube b.i.d.

    Available: Zantac syrup labeled 15 mg per mL

    ____

70. Order: Oxycodone Hydrochloride 30 mg p.o. q12h p.r.n. for pain.

    Available:

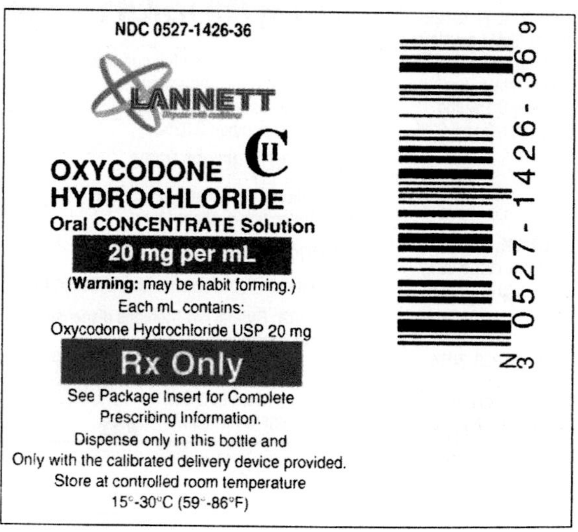

____

Answers on pp. 355-357

CLINICAL **REASONING**

1. **Scenario:** Order: Digoxin 0.75 mg p.o. daily. In preparing to administer medications, you find 0.125 mg tabs (scored) in the medication drawer for the client.
   a. Based on the tablets available, how many would you have to administer? ________
   b. What action should you take? ________
   c. What is the rationale for your action? ________
2. **Scenario:** Order: Diflucan 150 mg p.o. daily. The pharmacy sends two 100-mg unscored tabs.
   a. What action should you take to administer the dosage ordered? ________
   b. What is the rationale for your action? ________

3. **Scenario:** Order: Percocet 2 tabs p.o. q4h p.r.n. for pain for a client who is allergic to aspirin. The nurse administers Percodan 2 tabs.

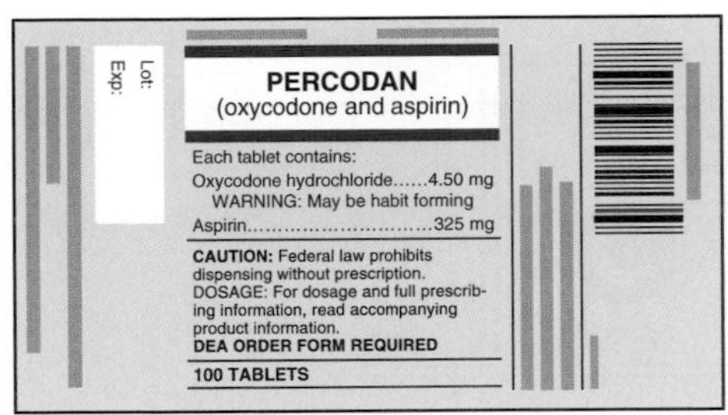

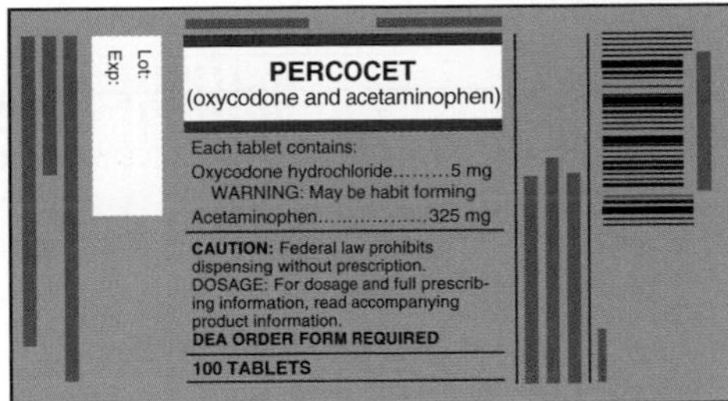

a. What client right was violated? ______________________
b. What contributed to the error? ______________________
c. What is the potential outcome of the error? ______________________
d. What preventive measures could have been taken to prevent the error? __________

Answers on p. 358

CHAPTER **REVIEW**

Calculate the following dosages using the medication label or information provided. Express volume answers in milliliters; round answers to the nearest tenth as indicated. Remember to label answers: tab, caps, mL.

1. Order: Tylenol 975 mg p.o. q6h p.r.n. for earache.

Available:

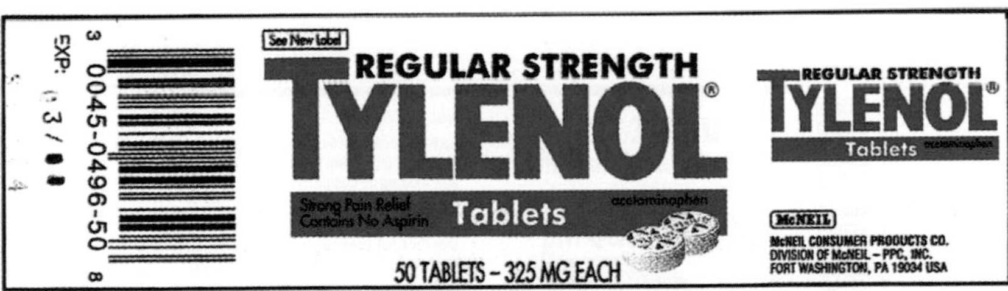

____

2. Order: Tamiflu 75 mg p.o. b.i.d. for a client with influenza.

Available:

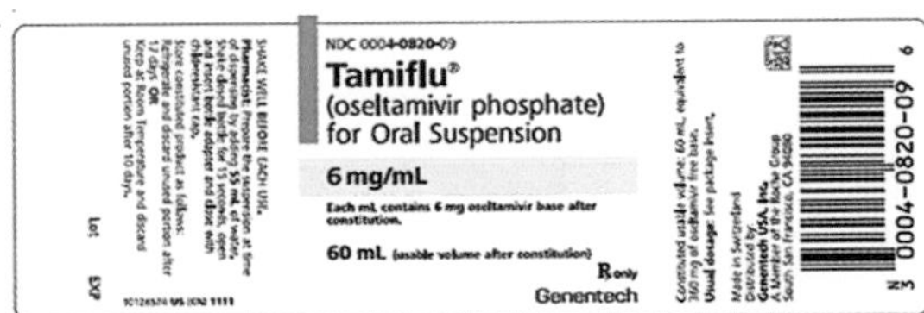

____

3. Order: Xifaxan 0.55 g p.o. t.i.d. for 14 days.

   Available:

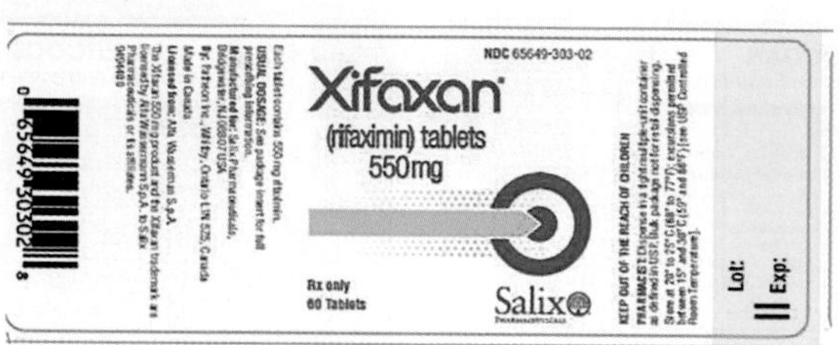

____

4. Order: Carvedilol 18.75 mg p.o. b.i.d.

   Available:

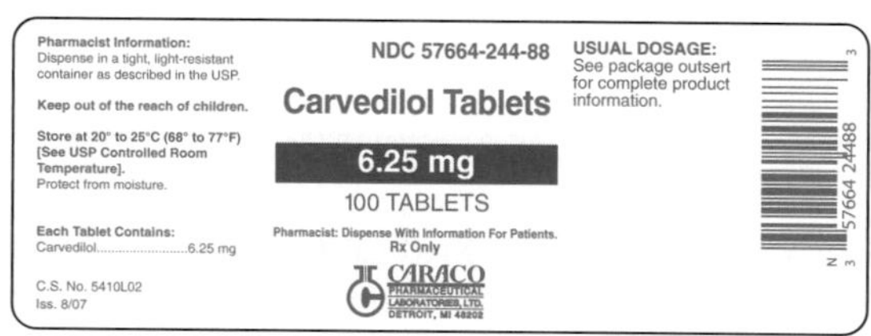

____

5. Order: Janumet 50 mg/1,000 mg p.o. b.i.d.

   Available:

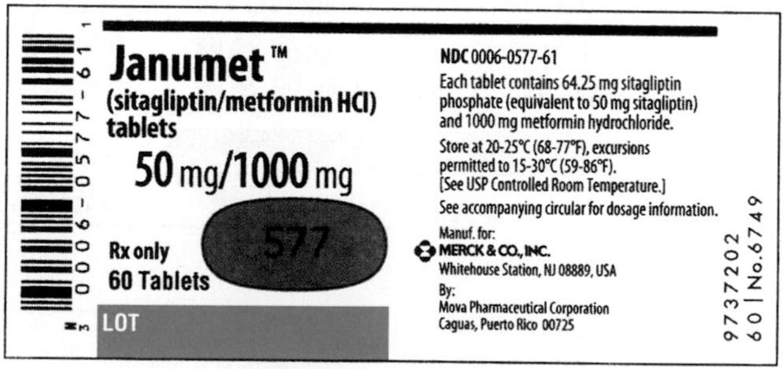

____

6. Order: Zithromax 250 mg p.o. daily for 3 days.

   Available:

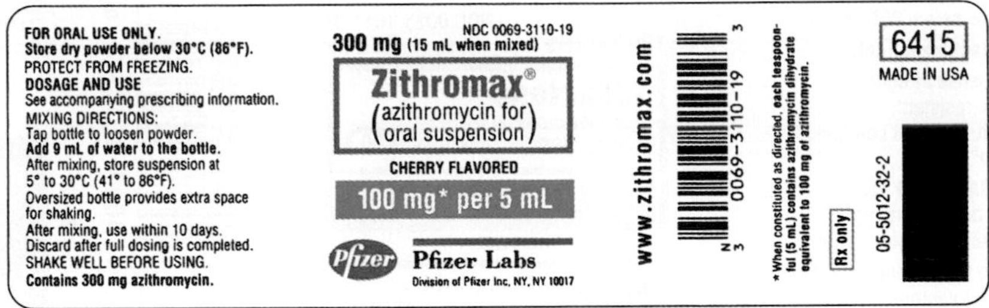

____

7. Order: Cialis 20 mg p.o. 1 hr before sexual activity for a client with erectile dysfunction.

   Available:

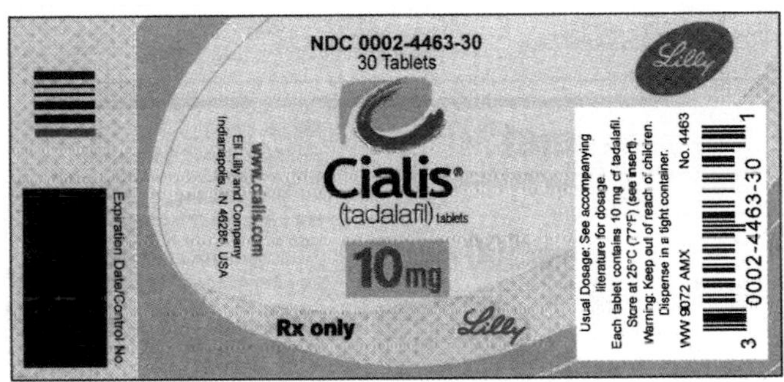

____

8. Order: Ativan 1 mg p.o. q4h p.r.n. for agitation.

   Available: Ativan tablets labeled 0.5 mg

____

9. Order: Lopressor 25 mg per nasogastric tube b.i.d.

   Available: Scored Lopressor tablets labeled 50 mg

____

10. Order: Aldactone 100 mg p.o. daily.

    Available:

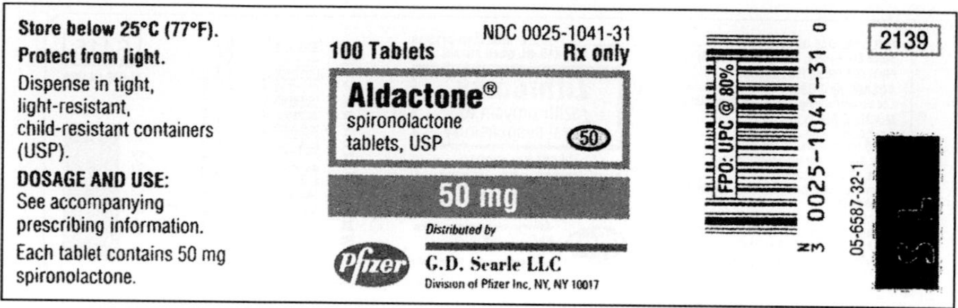

____

11. Order: Digoxin 0.1 mg p.o. daily.

    Available: Lanoxin (digoxin) elixir labeled 50 mcg (0.05 mg) per mL

____

12. Order: Amoxicillin 0.475 g p.o. q6h.

    Available:

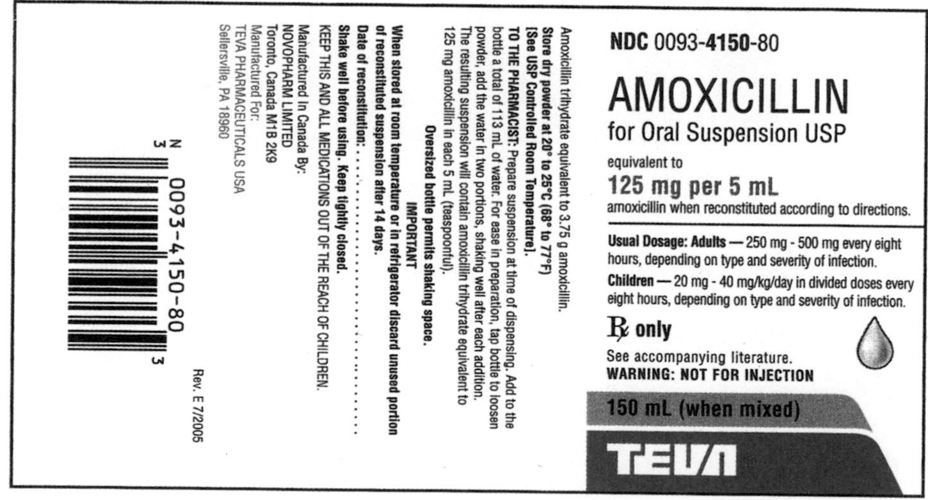

____

13. Order: Hydrochlorothiazide 12.5 mg p.o. daily. Hold for blood pressure less than 90/60.

    Available: Scored tablets

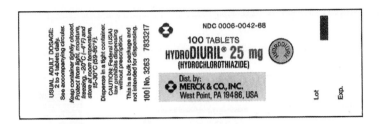

14. Order: Tylenol 500 mg by nasogastric tube q4h p.r.n. for temp greater than 101.4° F.

    Available:

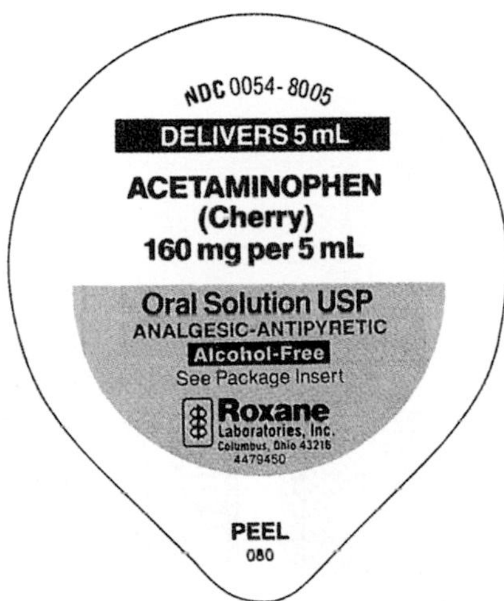

15. Order: Linzess 290 mcg p.o. daily for a client with irritable bowel syndrome with constipation (IBS-C).

    Available:

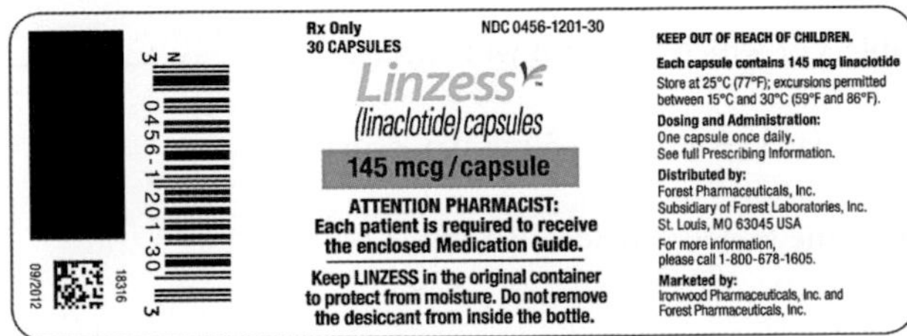

16. Order: Elixophyllin Elixir 300 mg by nasogastric tube b.i.d.

    Available: Elixophyllin liquid labeled 160 mg per 15 mL

    ____

17. Order: Xanax 0.75 mg p.o. t.i.d.

    Available:

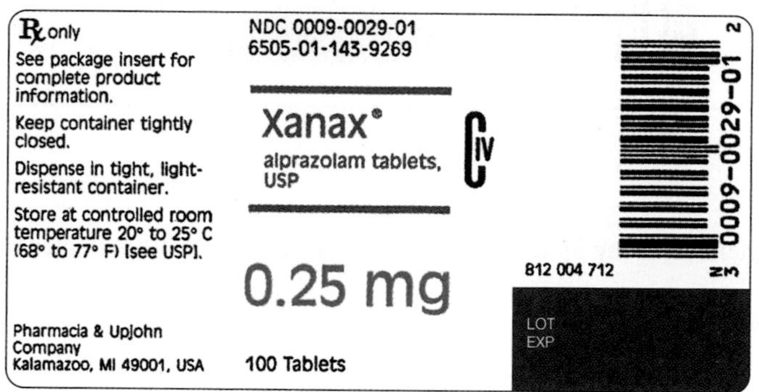

____

18. Order: Rexulti 3 mg p.o. daily.

    Available:

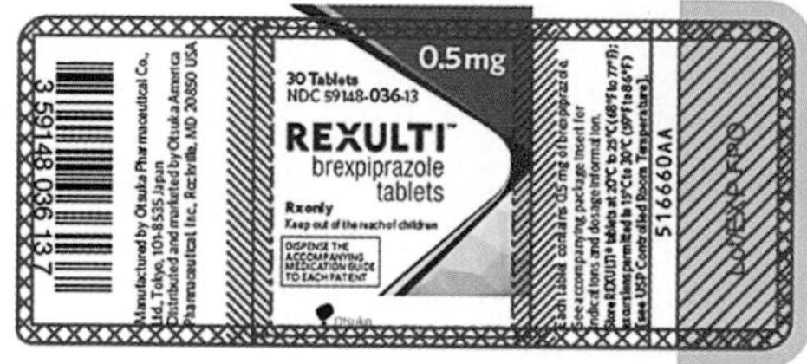

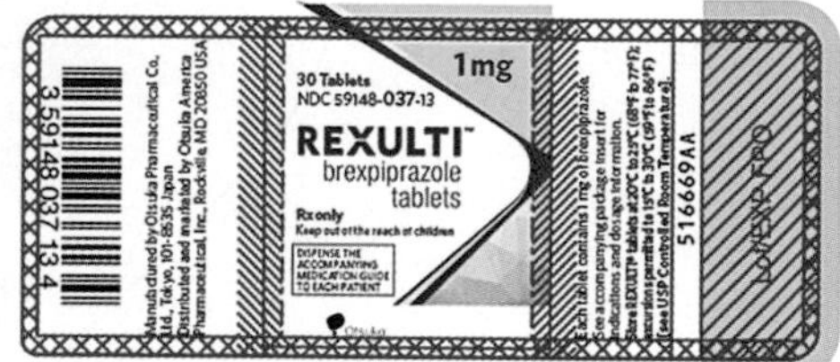

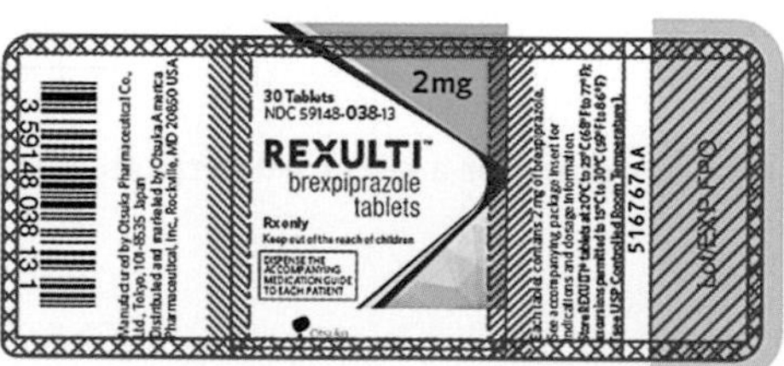

How many tablets of which strength will you use? ______________

19. Order: Meclizine HCl (Antivert) 25 mg p.o. every day.

    Available: Meclizine tablets labeled 12.5 mg

    ____

20. Order: Erythromycin (Delayed Release) 0.5 g p.o. b.i.d.

Available:

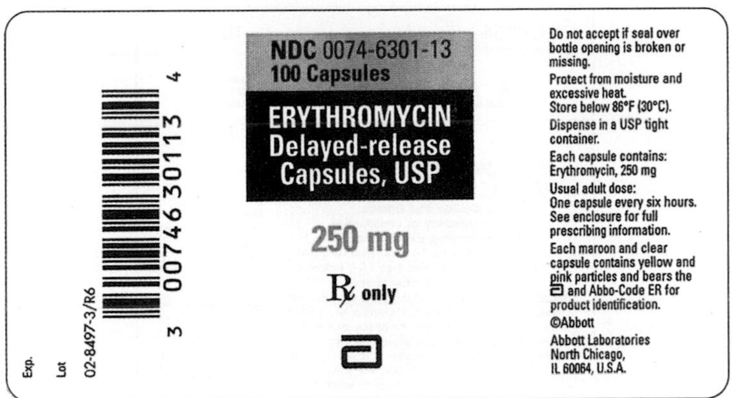

____

21. Order: Clonidine 0.5 mg p.o. t.i.d. Hold for blood pressure less than 100/60.

Available: Clonidine tablets labeled 0.1 mg, 0.2 mg, 0.3 mg

Which would be the best combination to administer to the client? ______________

22. Order: Invokana 0.3 g p.o. daily.

Available:

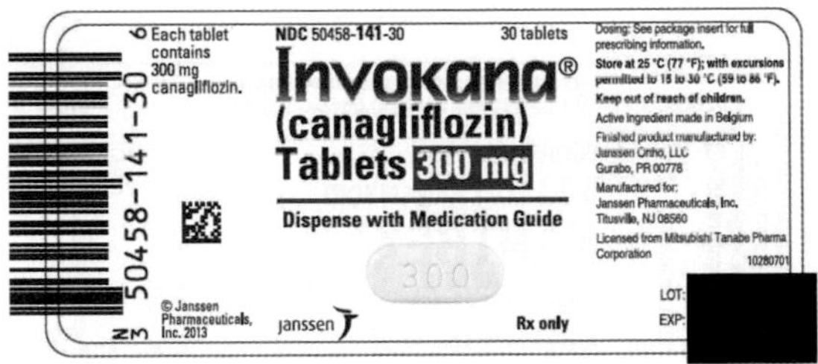

____

23. Order: Procanbid extended release 1 g p.o. q12h.

Available:

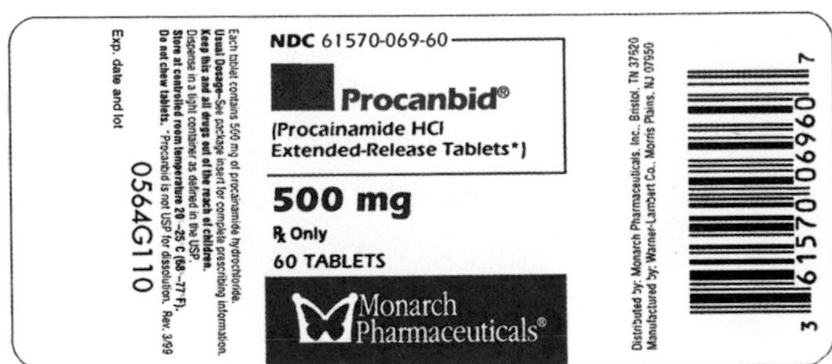

____

24. Order: Lactulose 20 g by gastrostomy tube b.i.d.

    Available:

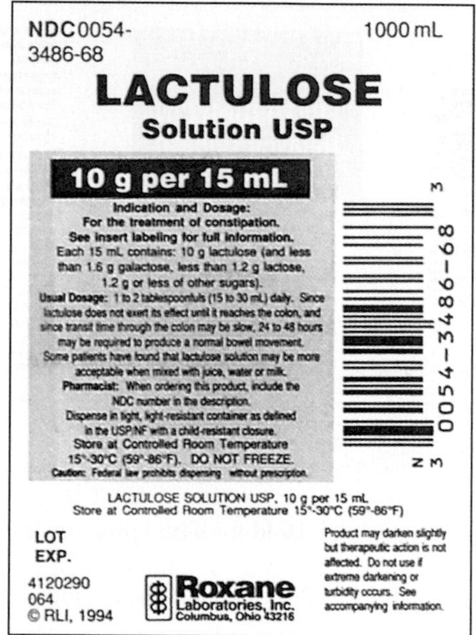
NDC 0054-3486-68
1000 mL
LACTULOSE
Solution USP
10 g per 15 mL
Indication and Dosage:
For the treatment of constipation.
See insert labeling for full information.
Each 15 mL contains: 10 g lactulose (and less than 1.6 g galactose, less than 1.2 g lactose, 1.2 g or less of other sugars).
Usual Dosage: 1 to 2 tablespoonfuls (15 to 30 mL) daily. Since lactulose does not exert its effect until it reaches the colon, and since transit time through the colon may be slow, 24 to 48 hours may be required to produce a normal bowel movement.
Some patients have found that lactulose solution may be more acceptable when mixed with juice, water or milk.
Pharmacist: When ordering this product, include the NDC number in the description.
Dispense in tight, light-resistant container as defined in the USP/NF with a child-resistant closure.
Store at Controlled Room Temperature 15°-30°C (59°-86°F). DO NOT FREEZE.
Caution: Federal law prohibits dispensing without prescription.
LACTULOSE SOLUTION USP, 10 g per 15 mL
Store at Controlled Room Temperature 15°-30°C (59°-86°F)
LOT
EXP.
4120290
064
© RLI, 1994
Roxane Laboratories, Inc.
Columbus, Ohio 43216
Product may darken slightly but therapeutic action is not affected. Do not use if extreme darkening or turbidity occurs. See accompanying information.
N 3 0054-3486-68 3

____

25. Order: Kanamycin (Kantrex) 1 g p.o. q6h for 5 days.

    Available:

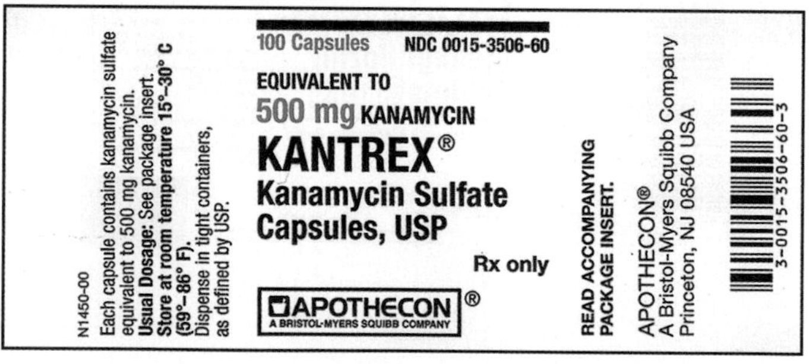

____

26. Order: Clozaril 50 mg p.o. daily.

Available:

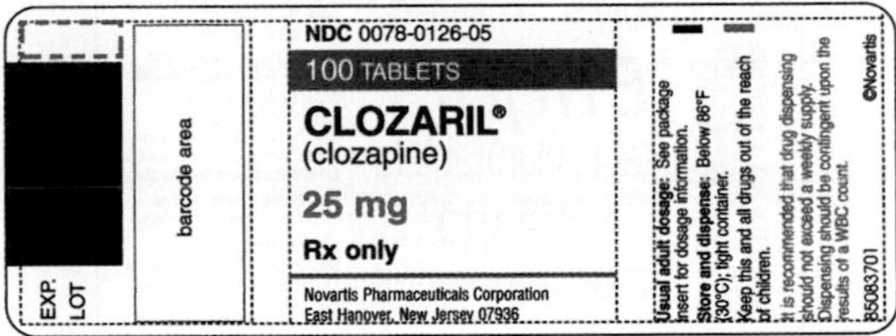

a. How many tabs will you administer for each dosage? ____________

b. How many tabs will be needed for 7 days? ____________

27. Order: Lipitor 30 mg p.o. every day.

Available:

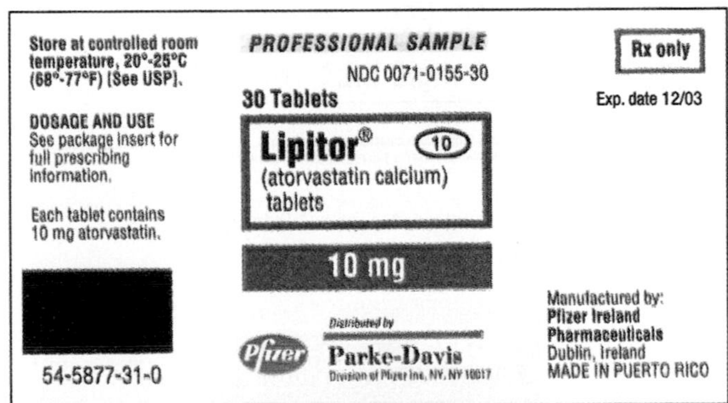

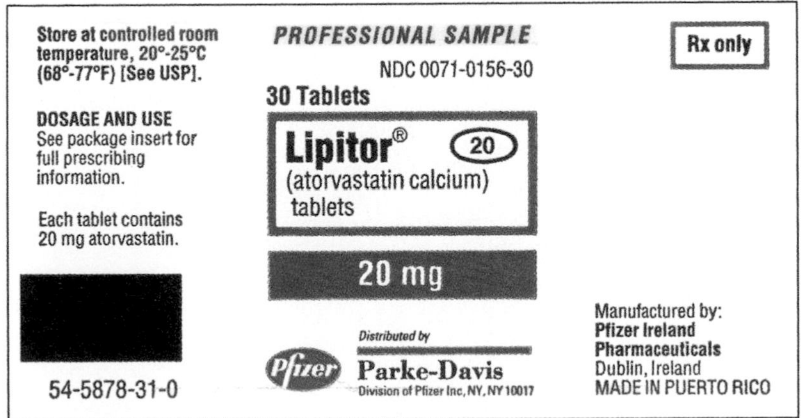

What will you administer to the client? ____________

28. Order: Eliquis 5 mg p.o. b.i.d.

    Available:

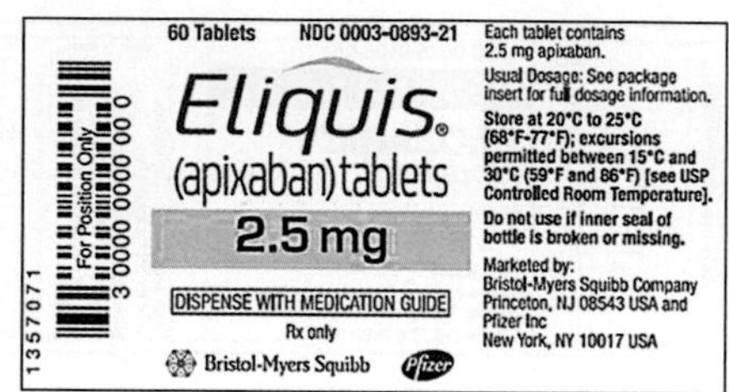

____

29. Order: Cefprozil 0.5 g p.o. q12h.

    Available:

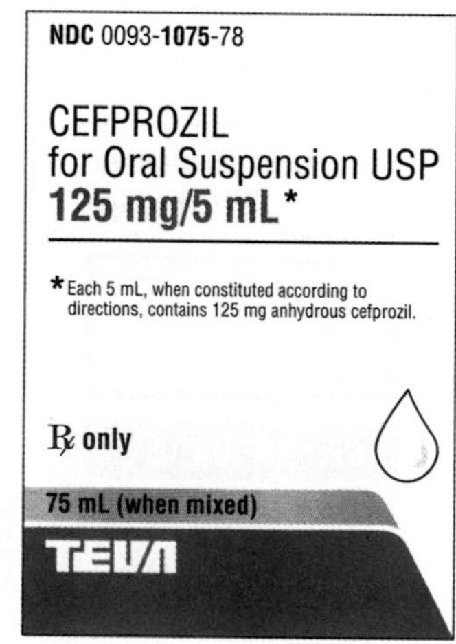

____

30. Order: Nexium (delayed release) 40 mg p.o. every day for 4 weeks.

Available:

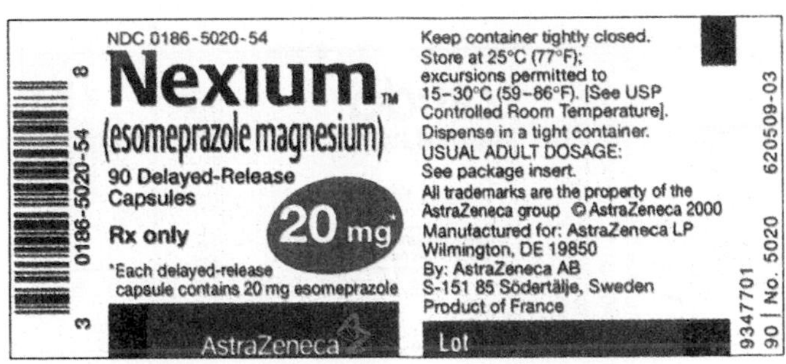

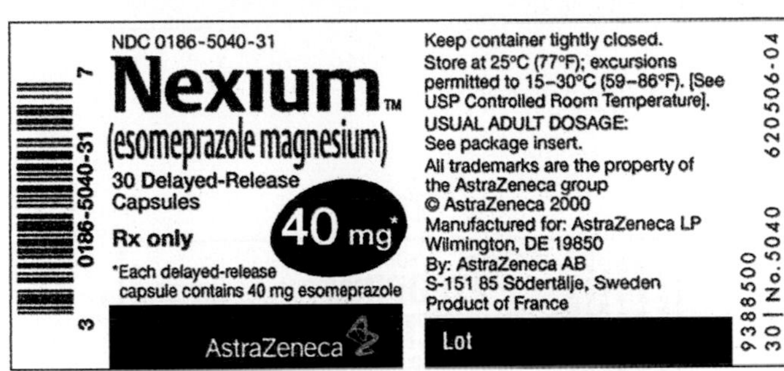

What will you administer to the client? ____________________

31. Order: Compazine 7.5 mg p.o. t.i.d.

Available:

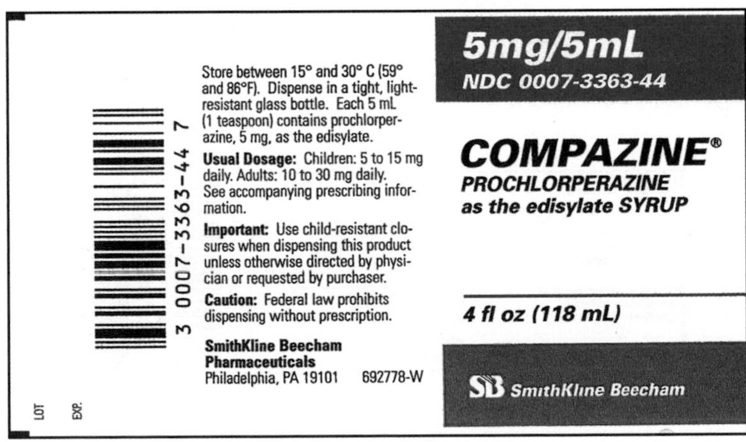
5mg/5mL
NDC 0007-3363-44
COMPAZINE®
PROCHLORPERAZINE as the edisylate SYRUP
4 fl oz (118 mL)
SB SmithKline Beecham
Store between 15° and 30° C (59° and 86°F). Dispense in a tight, light-resistant glass bottle. Each 5 mL (1 teaspoon) contains prochlorperazine, 5 mg, as the edisylate.
Usual Dosage: Children: 5 to 15 mg daily. Adults: 10 to 30 mg daily. See accompanying prescribing information.
Important: Use child-resistant closures when dispensing this product unless otherwise directed by physician or requested by purchaser.
Caution: Federal law prohibits dispensing without prescription.
SmithKline Beecham Pharmaceuticals Philadelphia, PA 19101 692778-W
3 0007-3363-44 7
LOT
EXP.

____

32. Order: Latuda 120 mg p.o. daily.

    Available:

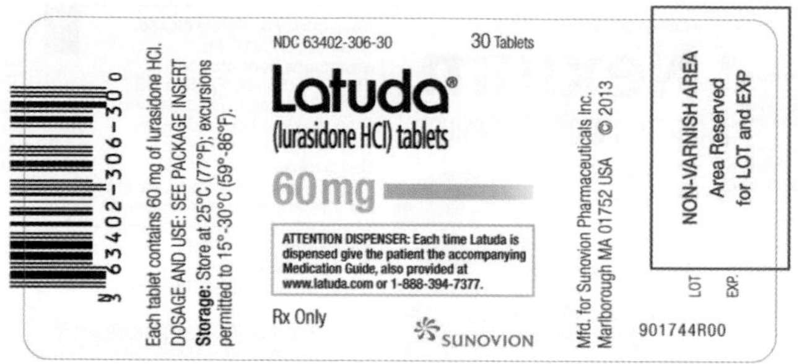

____

33. Order: Allopurinol 0.25 g p.o. every day.

    Available: Scored tablets

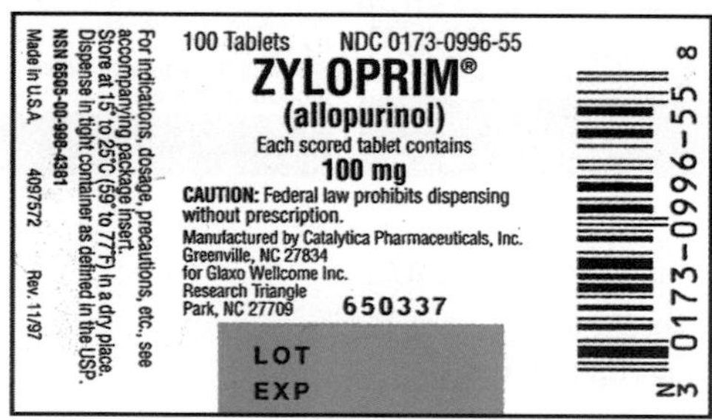

____

34. Order: Geodon 120 mg p.o. b.i.d.

    Available:

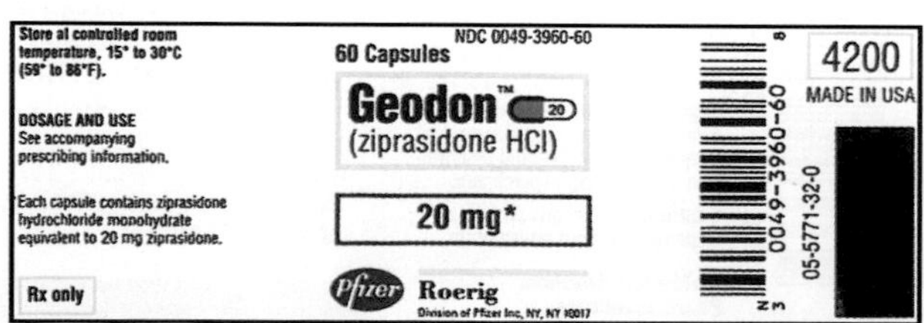

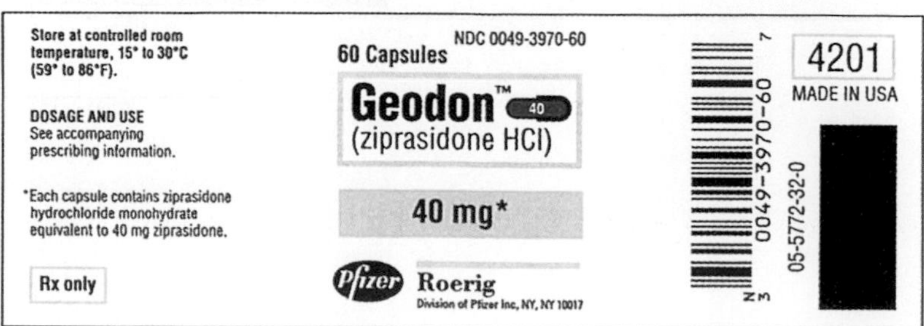

What will you administer to the client? ______________

35. Order: Lasix (furosemide) 100 mg by gastrostomy tube once a day.

Available:

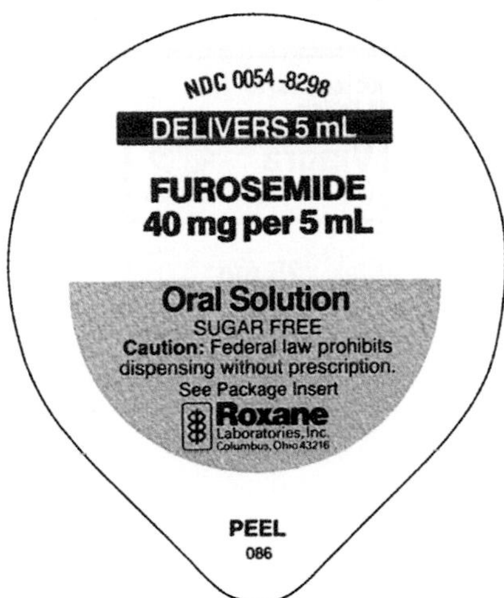

____

36. Order: Strattera 0.1 g p.o. daily.

Available:

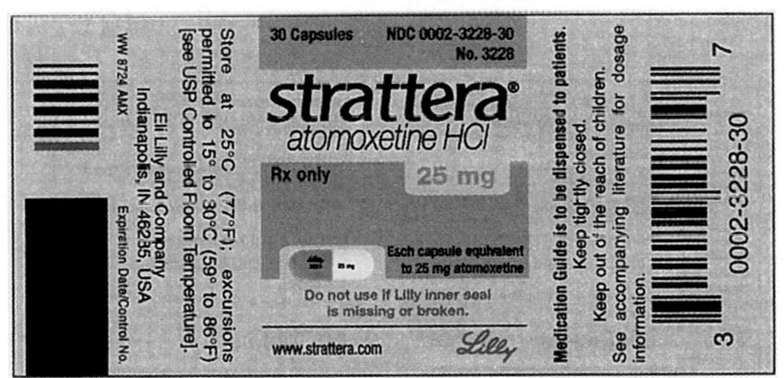

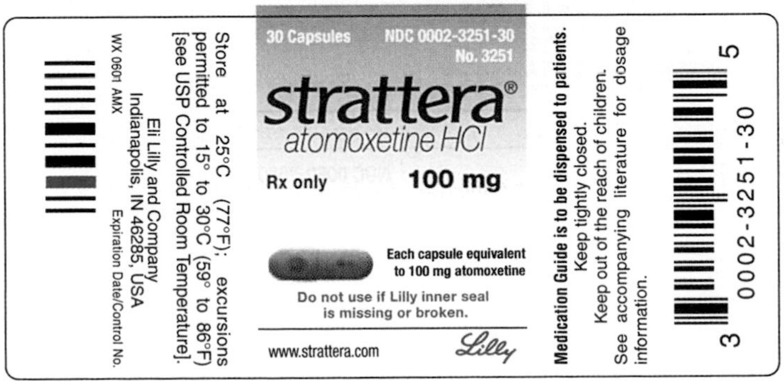

Which dosage strength will you administer? ______________________

37. Order: Viagra 50 mg p.o. ½ hour before sexual activity for a client with erectile dysfunction.

    Available:

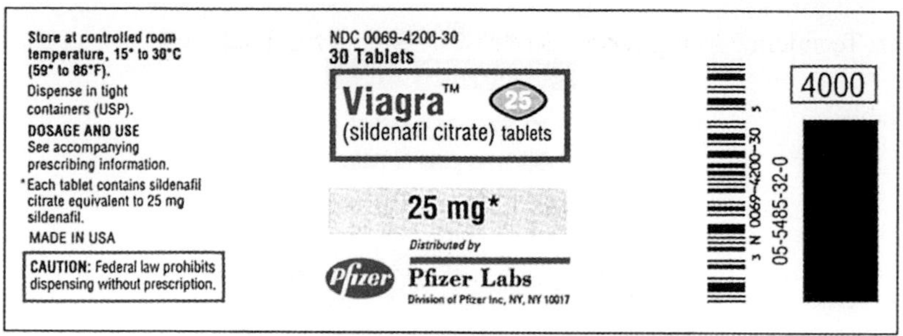

____

38. Order: Suboxone 16 mg/4 mg sublingual daily.

    Available:

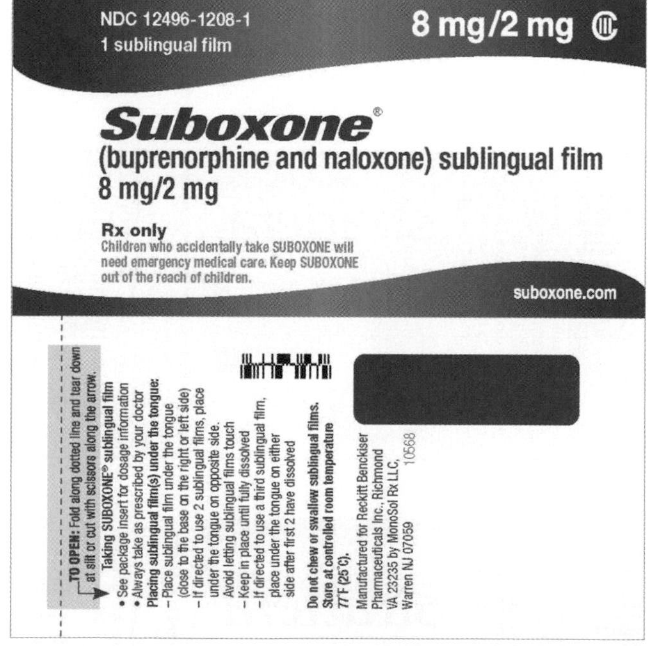

____

39. Order: Valproic acid (Depakene) 1 g p.o. every day.

Available: Depakene (valproic acid) syrup labeled 250 mg per 5 mL

____

40. Order: Tecfidera 240 mg (delayed-release capsules) p.o. b.i.d.

Available:

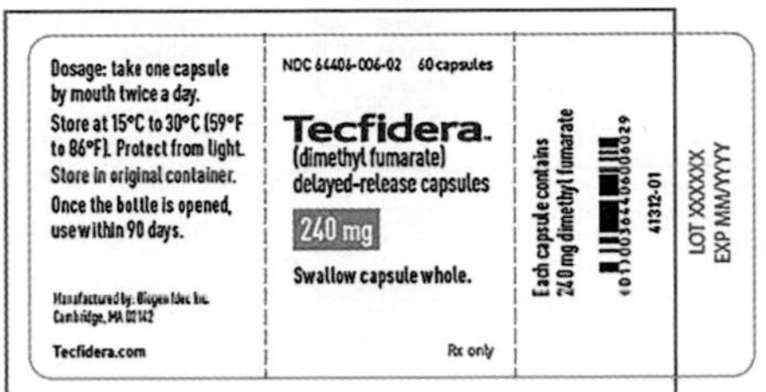

____

41. Order: Zyprexa 10 mg p.o. b.i.d.

Available:

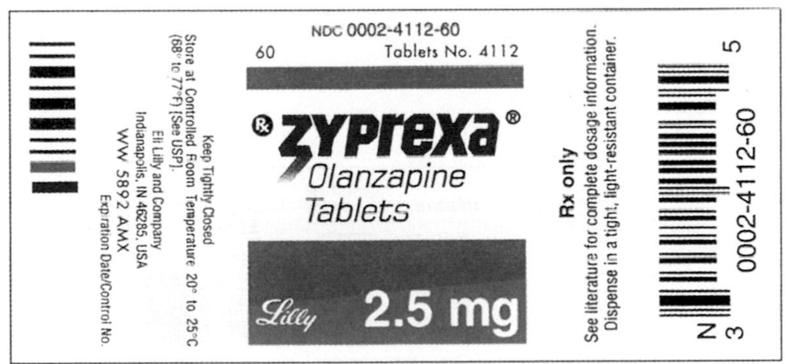

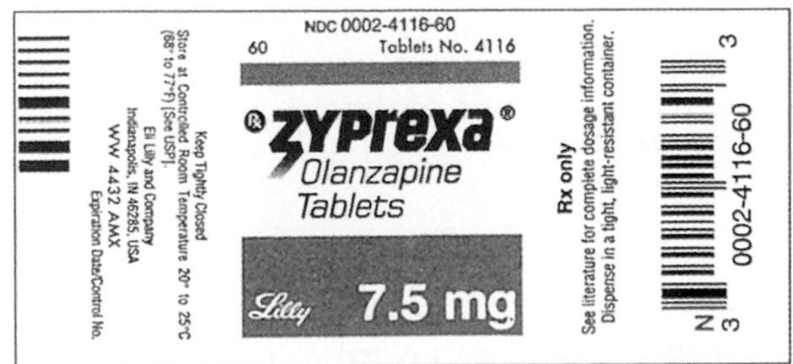

What will you administer to the client? ______________________

42. Order: Wellbutrin 150 mg p.o. b.i.d.

Available:

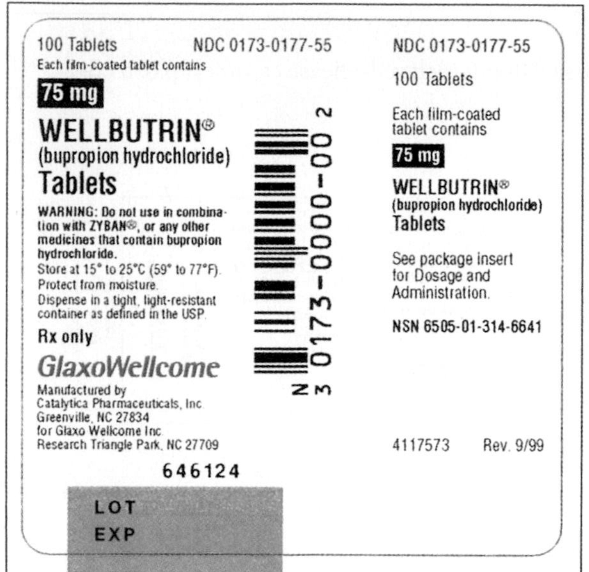

43. Order: Zoloft 150 mg p.o. daily

Available: Scored tablets

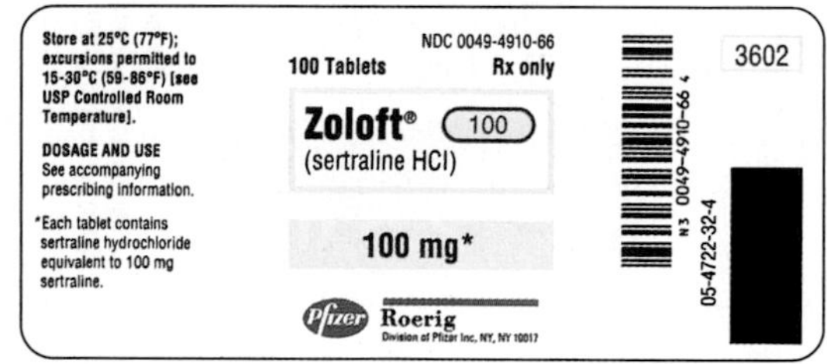

44. Order: Famvir 0.25 g p.o. t.i.d. for 5 days.

Available:

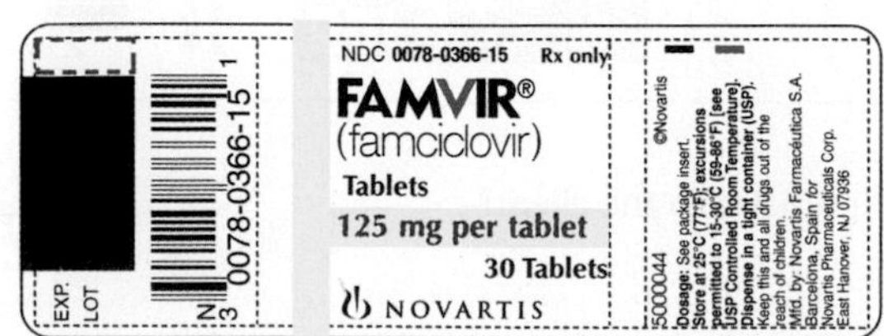

45. Order: Cytotec 200 mcg p.o. q.i.d.

Available:

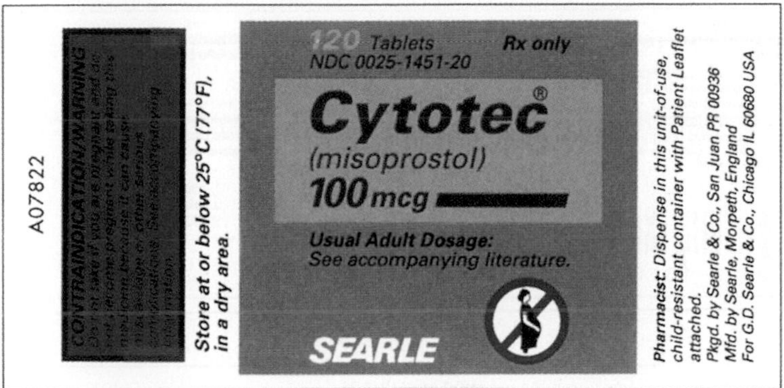

____

46. Order: Trileptal 0.6 g p.o. b.i.d.

Available:

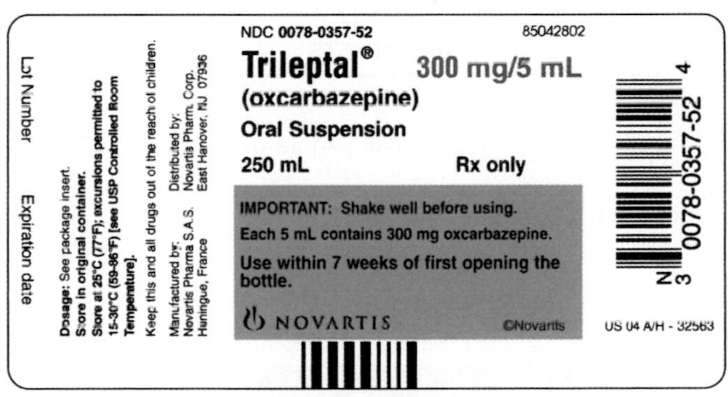

____

47. Order: Benadryl 100 mg p.o. at bedtime.

Available: Benadryl capsules labeled 50 mg

____

48. Order: Dexamethasone 1.5 mg p.o. b.i.d.

Available:

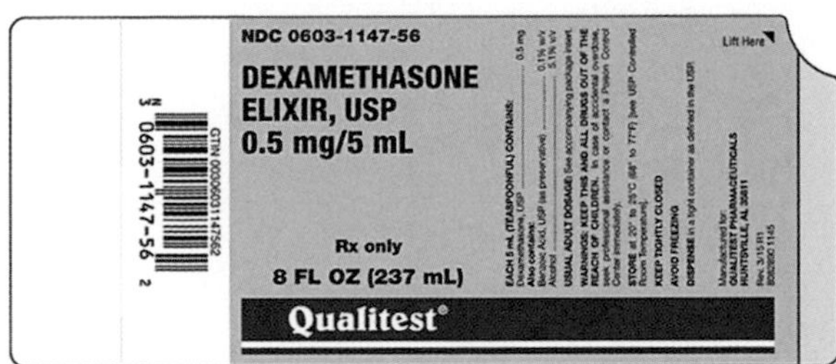

____

49. Order: Terbutaline 15 mg p.o. daily.

Available:

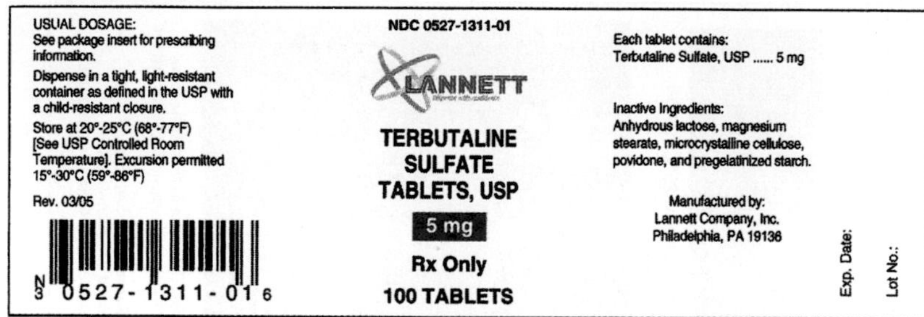

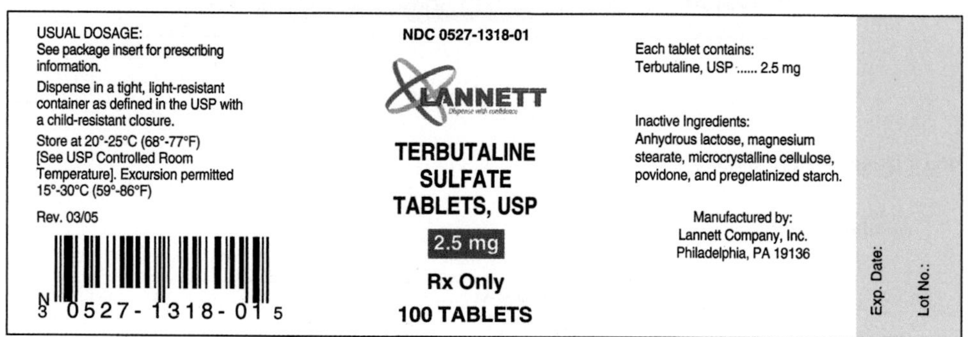

How many of which dosage strength will you administer? ______________________

50. Order: Ery-Tab 0.666 g p.o. q6h.

Available:

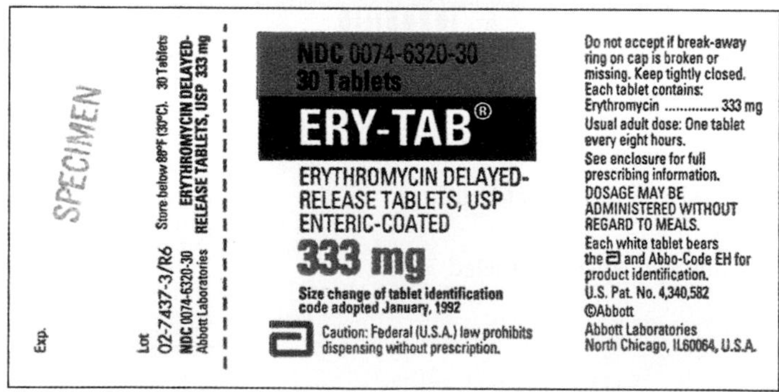

____

51. Order: Oxbutynin chloride 10 mg p.o. b.i.d.

Available:

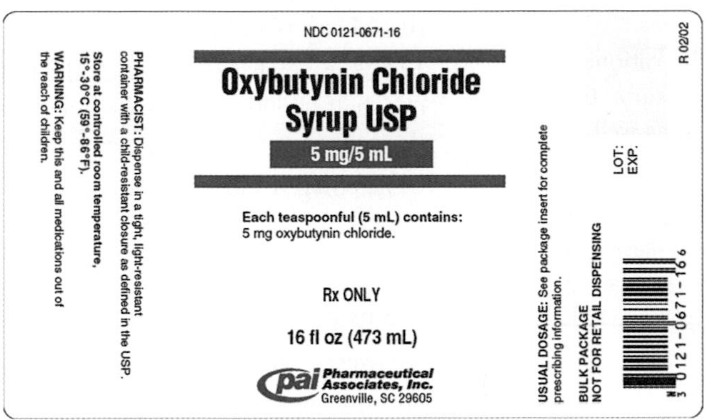

____

52. Order: Lyrica 75 mg p.o. b.i.d.

Available:

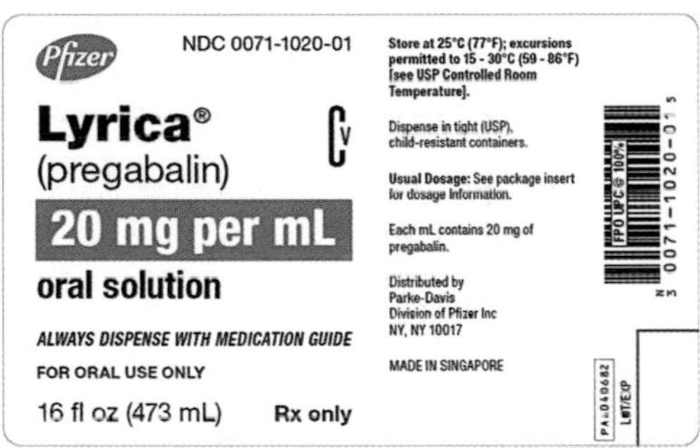

____

Answers on p. 358

evolve

For additional practice problems, refer to the Oral Dosages section of the Elsevier's Interactive Drug Calculation Application, Version 1 on Evolve.

ANSWERS

Chapter 17

Answers to Practice Problems

The answers to the practice problems include the rationale for the answer where indicated. Where necessary, the methods for calculation of the dosage are shown as well.

NOTE

Unless stated, no conversion is required to calculate dosage. In problems that required a conversion before calculating the dosage, the problem setup shown illustrates the problem after appropriate conversions have been made.

1. 0.025 mg = 25 mcg (1,000 mg = 1 mg)

   50 mcg : 1 tab = 25 mcg : x tab

   or

   $$\frac{25 \text{ mcg}}{50 \text{ mcg}} \times 1 \text{ tab} = x \text{ tab}$$

   Answer: 0.5 or $\frac{1}{2}$ tab. This is an acceptable answer, because the tabs are scored. (For administration purposes, state as $\frac{1}{2}$ tab.) Note that the problem could have been done without converting by using the dosage indicated on the label in mg. This would net the same answer.

   or

   0.05 mg : 1 tab = 0.025 mg : x tab

   $$\frac{0.025 \text{ mg}}{0.05 \text{ mg}} \times 1 \text{ tab} = x \text{ tab}$$

2. 25 mg : 1 cap = 50 mg : x cap

   or

   $$\frac{50 \text{ mg}}{25 \text{ mg}} \times 1 \text{ cap} = x \text{ cap}$$

   Answer: 2 caps. The dosage ordered is greater than what is available; therefore you will need more than 1 cap to administer the dosage.

3. Conversion is necessary: 1,000 mg = 1 g.

   Therefore 1 g = 1,000 mg.

   500 mg : 1 tab = 1,000 mg : x tab

   or

   $$\frac{1{,}000 \text{ mg}}{500 \text{ mg}} \times 1 \text{ tab} = x \text{ tab}$$

   Answer: 2 tabs. The dosage ordered is greater than what is available; therefore you will need more than 1 tab to administer the dosage.

4. It would be best to administer one of the 5-mg tablets and one of the 2.5 mg ($2\frac{1}{2}$ mg) tablets (5 mg + 2.5 mg = 7.5 mg).

5. a. 125-mcg tablet is the appropriate strength to use (0.125 mg = 125 mcg).

   b. 1- 125 mcg tab. Even though the tablets are scored, one-half of 500 mcg would still be twice the dosage desired.

   125 mcg : 1 tab = 125 mcg : x tab

   or

   $$\frac{125 \text{ mcg}}{125 \text{ mcg}} \times 1 \text{ tab} = x \text{ tab}$$

   Answer: 1 tab

6. a. 500-mg caps would be appropriate to use.

   b. 2 caps (500 mg each). 1,000 mg = 1 g; therefore 2 caps of 500 mg each would be the least number of capsules. Using the 250-mg strength capsules would require 4 caps.

   c. 2 caps q6h = 8 caps. Multiplying the number of caps needed by the number of days gives you the number of capsules required.

   8 (number of caps per day) × 7 (number of days) = 56 (total caps needed)

   500 mg : 1 cap = 1,000 mg : x cap

   $$\frac{1{,}000 \text{ mg}}{500 \text{ mg}} \times 1 \text{ cap} = x \text{ cap}$$

   $$x = 2 \text{ caps}$$

7. a. 5-mg tablets

   b. Two 5-mg tablets. This strength will allow the client to take two tablets to achieve the desired dosage, as opposed to four 2.5-mg tabs. This dosage is logical because the maximum number of tablets administered is generally three.

   5 mg : 1 tab = 10 mg : x tab

   or

   $$\frac{10 \text{ mg}}{5 \text{ mg}} \times 1 \text{ tab} = x \text{ tab}$$

   Answer: Two (2) 5 mg tabs

8. a. $1\frac{1}{2}$ tabs; the tablets are scored. (State as $1\frac{1}{2}$ tabs for administration purposes.)

   10 mg : 1 tab = 15 mg : x tab

   $$\frac{15 \text{ mg}}{10 \text{ mg}} \times 1 \text{ tab} = x \text{ tab}$$

   $$x = 1\frac{1}{2} \text{ tab}$$

   b. 15 mg × 3 (t.i.d.) = 45 mg/day. The total number of milligrams received for 3 days is 135 mg.

   45 mg × 3 = 135 mg

9. $2 \text{ mg} : 1 \text{ tab} = 4 \text{ mg} : x \text{ tab}$

$$\frac{4 \text{ mg}}{2 \text{ mg}} \times 1 \text{ tab} = x \text{ tab}$$

Answer: 2 tabs. The dosage ordered is greater than what is available; therefore, you will need more than 1 tab to administer the dosage.

10. $0.4 \text{ g} = 400 \text{ mg } (1 \text{ g} = 1{,}000 \text{ mg})$

$400 \text{ mg} : 1 \text{ tab} = 400 \text{ mg} : x \text{ tab}$

$$\frac{400 \text{ mg}}{400 \text{ mg}} \times 1 \text{ tab} = x \text{ tab}$$

Answer: 1 tab. 1 tab, 400 mg, is equal to 0.4 g; therefore, only 1 tab is needed to administer the dosage.

11. $30 \text{ mg} : 1 \text{ cap} = 90 \text{ mg} : x \text{ cap}$

or

$$\frac{90 \text{ mg}}{30 \text{ mg}} \times 1 \text{ cap} = x \text{ cap}$$

Answer: 3 caps. The dosage ordered is greater than what is available. You will need more than 1 cap to administer the dosage.

12. $100 \text{ mg} : 1 \text{ tab} = 200 \text{ mg} : x \text{ tab}$

or

$$\frac{200 \text{ mg}}{100 \text{ mg}} \times 1 \text{ tab} = x \text{ tab}$$

Answer: 2 tabs (chewable). The dosage ordered is greater than what is available; therefore you will need more than 1 tab to administer the dosage.

13. $5 \text{ mg} : 1 \text{ tab} = 5 \text{ mg} : x \text{ tab}$

$$\frac{5 \text{ mg}}{5 \text{ mg}} \times 1 \text{ tab} = x \text{ tab}$$

Answer: 1 tab. 1 tab, 5 mg, is equal to the available; therefore, only 1 tab is needed to administer the dosage.

14. $0.5 \text{ mg} : 1 \text{ tab} = 1 \text{ mg} : x \text{ tab}$

or

$$\frac{1 \text{ mg}}{0.5 \text{ mg}} \times 1 \text{ tab} = x \text{ tab}$$

Answer: 2 tabs. The dosage ordered is more than what is available; therefore you will need more than 1 tab to administer the dosage.

15. a. 30-mg tablets

b. Three 30-mg tablets. This strength will allow the client to take three tabs to achieve the desired dosage, as opposed to six 15 mg tabs. This dosage is logical because the maximum number of tablets administered is generally three.

$30 \text{ mg} : 1 \text{ tab} = 90 \text{ mg} : x \text{ tab}$

or

$$\frac{90 \text{ mg}}{30 \text{ mg}} \times 1 \text{ tab} = x \text{ tab}$$

Answer: three 30 mg tabs

16. $0.6 \text{ g} = 600 \text{ mg } (1 \text{ g} = 1{,}000 \text{ mg})$

$300 \text{ mg} : 1 \text{ tab} = 600 \text{ mg} : x \text{ tab}$

$$\frac{600 \text{ mg}}{300 \text{ mg}} \times 1 \text{ tab} = x \text{ tab}$$

Answer: 2 tabs. The dosage ordered is greater than what is available; therefore, you will need more than 1 tab to administer the dosage.

17. $50 \text{ mg} : 1 \text{ tab} = 100 \text{ mg} : x \text{ tab}$

or

$$\frac{100 \text{ mg}}{50 \text{ mg}} \times 1 \text{ tab} = x \text{ tab}$$

Answer: You need 2 tabs to administer 100 mg. 2 tabs t.i.d. (3 times a day) = 6 tabs × 3 days = 18 tabs.

18. It would be best to administer one 80-mg tablet and one 40-mg tablet (80 + 40 = 120 mg). This would be the least number of tablets.

19. $10 \text{ mg} : 1 \text{ tab} = 20 \text{ mg} : x \text{ tab}$

or

$$\frac{20 \text{ mg}}{10 \text{ mg}} \times 1 \text{ tab} = x \text{ tab}$$

Answer: 2 tabs (controlled release). The dosage ordered is larger than the available dosage; therefore more than 1 tab will be required.

20. $0.5 \text{ mg} : 1 \text{ tab} = 1 \text{ mg} : x \text{ tab}$

or

$$\frac{1 \text{ mg}}{0.5 \text{ mg}} \times 1 \text{ tab} = x \text{ tab}$$

$$x = 2 \text{ tabs}$$

Answer: 2 tabs. The dosage ordered is more than what is available; therefore you will need more than 1 tab to administer the dosage.

21. $1 \text{ g} = 1{,}000 \text{ mg}$

$500 \text{ mg} : 1 \text{ tab} = 1{,}000 \text{ mg} : x \text{ tab}$

$$\frac{1{,}000 \text{ mg}}{500 \text{ mg}} \times 1 \text{ tab} = x \text{ tab}$$

Answer: 2 tabs (extended release). The dosage ordered is greater than what is available; therefore, you will need more than 1 tab to administer the dosage.

22. Conversion is required. Equivalent: 1,000 mg = 1 g; therefore 0.6 g = 600 mg

$600 \text{ mg} : 1 \text{ tab} = 600 \text{ mg} : x \text{ tab}$

or

$$\frac{600 \text{ mg}}{600 \text{ mg}} \times 1 \text{ tab} = x \text{ tab}$$

Answer: 1 tab. 0.6 mg = 600 mg, which is equal to 1 tab.

23. Choose the 6-mg tab and give 1 tab, which allows the client to swallow the least number of tabs without dividing tabs.

$6 \text{ mg} : 1 \text{ tab} = 6 \text{ mg} : x \text{ tab}$

or

$$\frac{6 \text{ mg}}{6 \text{ mg}} \times 1 \text{ tab} = x \text{ tab}$$

Answer: one 6-mg tab

24. Conversion is required. Equivalent: 1,000 mg = 1 g; therefore 0.2 g = 200 mg.

$100 \text{ mg} : 1 \text{ tab} = 200 \text{ mg} : x \text{ tab}$

or

$$\frac{200 \text{ mg}}{100 \text{ mg}} \times 1 \text{ tab} = x \text{ tab}$$

Answer: 2 tabs. The dosage ordered is larger than what is available; therefore you will need more than 1 tab is needed to administer the dosage.

25. $120 \text{ mg} : 1 \text{ cap} = 240 \text{ mg} : x \text{ cap}$

or

$$\frac{240 \text{ mg}}{120 \text{ mg}} \times 1 \text{ cap} = x \text{ cap}$$

Answer: 2 delayed-release capsules. The dosage ordered is greater than what is available. You will need more than 1 cap to administer the dosage.

26. $50 \text{ mg} : 1 \text{ tab} = 100 \text{ mg} : x \text{ tab}$

or

$$\frac{100 \text{ mg}}{50 \text{ mg}} \times 1 \text{ tab} = x \text{ tab}$$

Answer: 2 tabs. The dosage ordered is more than what is available. You will need more than 1 tab to administer the dosage.

27. $200 \text{ mg} : 1 \text{ tab} = 400 \text{ mg} : x \text{ tab}$

or

$$\frac{400 \text{ mg}}{200 \text{ mg}} \times 1 \text{ tab} = x \text{ tab}$$

Answer: 2 tabs. The dosage ordered is more than what is available. You will need more than 1 tab to administer the dosage.

28. $75 \text{ mg} : 1 \text{ cap} = 150 \text{ mg} : x \text{ cap}$

or

$$\frac{150 \text{ mg}}{75 \text{ mg}} \times 1 \text{ cap} = x \text{ cap}$$

Answer: 2 caps (extended release). The dosage ordered is more than what is available. You will need more than 1 cap to administer the dosage.

29. Change 1 g to 1,000 mg (1,000 mg = 1 g)

$500 \text{ mg} : 1 \text{ tab} = 1{,}000 \text{ mg} : x \text{ tab}$

or

$$\frac{1{,}000 \text{ mg}}{500 \text{ mg}} \times 1 \text{ tab} = x \text{ tab}$$

Answer: 2 tabs. The dosage ordered is greater than what is available. You will need more than 1 tab to administer the dosage.

30. $30 \text{ mg} : 1 \text{ cap} = 60 \text{ mg} : x \text{ cap}$

or

$$\frac{60 \text{ mg}}{30 \text{ mg}} \times 1 \text{ cap} = x \text{ cap}$$

Answer: 2 caps (delayed release). The dosage ordered is more than what is available. You will need more than 1 cap to administer the dosage.

31. It would be best to administer 3–25 mcg tablets. Although the tabs are scored, it is best to administer tabs whole rather than breaking them. Variation in dosage can occur if tablets are broken.

32. $12.5 \text{ mg} : 1 \text{ tab} = 25 \text{ mg} : x \text{ tab}$

or

$$\frac{25 \text{ mg}}{12.5 \text{ mg}} \times 1 \text{ tab} = x \text{ tab}$$

Answer: 2 tabs. The dosage ordered is more than what is available. You will need more than 1 tab to administer the dosage.

33. $0.5 \text{ mg} : 1 \text{ tab} = 1 \text{ mg} : x \text{ tab}$

$$\frac{1 \text{ mg}}{0.5 \text{ mg}} \times 1 \text{ tab} = x \text{ tab}$$

Answer: 2 tabs. The dosage ordered is more than what is available; therefore, you will need more than 1 tab to administer the dosage.

34. $200 \text{ mg} : 1 \text{ tab} = 400 \text{ mg} : x \text{ tab}$

$$\frac{400 \text{ mg}}{200 \text{ mg}} \times 1 \text{ tab} = x \text{ tab}$$

Answer: 2 tabs (chewable). The dosage ordered is more than what is available; therefore, you will need more than 1 tab to administer the dosage.

35. $0.137 \text{ mg} = 137 \text{ mcg}.$

$137 \text{ mcg} : 1 \text{ tab} = 137 \text{ mcg} : x \text{ tab}$

$$\frac{137 \text{ mcg}}{137 \text{ mcg}} \times 1 \text{ tab} = x \text{ tab}$$

Answer: 1 tab. 0.137 mg = 137 mcg, which is equal to 1 tab and is the available dosage strength.

36. $25\text{ mg}:1\text{ cap} = 50\text{ mg}:x\text{ cap}$

or

$$\frac{50\text{ mg}}{25\text{ mg}} \times 1\text{ cap} = x\text{ cap}$$

Answer: 2 caps. The dosage ordered is greater than what is available. You will need more than 1 cap to administer the dosage.

37. Conversion is necessary. 1,000 mg = 1 g; therefore 0.2 g = 200 mg.

$100\text{ mg}:1\text{ cap} = 200\text{ mg}:x\text{ cap}$

or

$$\frac{200\text{ mg}}{100\text{ mg}} \times 1\text{ cap} = x\text{ cap}$$

Answer: 2 caps (extended release). The dosage ordered is greater than what is available. You will need more than 1 cap to administer the dosage.

38. $400\text{ mg}:1\text{ tab} = 800\text{ mg}:x\text{ tab}$

or

$$\frac{800\text{ mg}}{400\text{ mg}} \times 1\text{ tab} = x\text{ tab}$$

Answer: 2 tabs. The dosage ordered is greater than what is available. You will need more than 1 tab to administer the dosage.

39. $30\text{ mg}:1\text{ tab} = 60\text{ mg}:x\text{ tab}$

or

$$\frac{60\text{ mg}}{30\text{ mg}} \times 1\text{ tab} = x\text{ tab}$$

Answer: 2 tabs (XL). The dosage ordered is greater than what is available. You will need more than 1 tab to administer the dosage.

40. Conversion: 1,000 mg = 1 g. Therefore 0.03 g = 30 mg.

$10\text{ mg}:1\text{ tab} = 30\text{ mg}:x\text{ tab}$

or

$$\frac{30\text{ mg}}{10\text{ mg}} \times 1\text{ tab} = x\text{ tab}$$

Answer: 3 tabs. The dosage ordered is greater than what is available. You will need more than 1 tab to administer the dosage. Three is the maximum number of tablets that should generally be given.

41. $60\text{ mg}:1\text{ cap} = 120\text{ mg}:x\text{ cap}$

$$\frac{120\text{ mg}}{60\text{ mg}} \times 1\text{ cap} = x\text{ cap}$$

Answer: 2 caps (LA). The dosage ordered is greater than what is available. You will need more than 1 cap to administer the dosage.

NOTE

The setup shown for problems that required conversions reflects conversion of what the prescriber ordered to what is available. Unless stated in problems 42-70, no conversion is required to calculate the dosage.

42. $20\text{ mg}:1\text{ mL} = 50\text{ mg}:x\text{ mL}$

or

$$\frac{50\text{ mg}}{20\text{ mg}} \times 1\text{ mL} = x\text{ mL}$$

Answer: 2.5 mL. The dosage ordered is more than the available strength. You will need more than 1 mL to administer the dosage.

43. $125\text{ mg}:5\text{ mL} = 100\text{ mg}:x\text{ mL}$

or

$$\frac{100\text{ mg}}{125\text{ mg}} \times 5\text{ mL} = x\text{ mL}$$

Answer: 4 mL. The dosage ordered is less than the available strength; therefore less than 5 mL will be needed to administer the required dosage.

44. $40\text{ mEq}:15\text{ mL} = 40\text{ mEq}:x\text{ mL}$

or

$$\frac{40\text{ mEq}}{40\text{ mEq}} \times 15\text{ mL} = x\text{ mL}$$

Answer: 15 mL. The dosage ordered is contained in 15 mL of the medication.

45. $80\text{ mg}:15\text{ mL} = 120\text{ mg}:x\text{ mL}$

or

$$\frac{120\text{ mg}}{80\text{ mg}} \times 15\text{ mL} = x\text{ mL}$$

Answer: 22.5 mL. The dosage ordered is more than the available strength; therefore you will need more than 15 mL to administer the dosage.

46. $200\text{ mg}:5\text{ mL} = 250\text{ mg}:x\text{ mL}$

or

$$\frac{250\text{ mg}}{200\text{ mg}} \times 5\text{ mL} = x\text{ mL}$$

Answer: 6.3 mL. The dosage ordered is greater than the available strength; therefore more than 5 mL will be needed to administer the required dosage. The answer to the nearest tenth is 6.3 mL.

47. $125\text{ mg}:5\text{ mL} = 100\text{ mg}:x\text{ mL}$

or

$$\frac{100\text{ mg}}{125\text{ mg}} \times 5\text{ mL} = x\text{ mL}$$

Answer: 4 mL. The amount ordered is less than the available strength; therefore less than 5 mL will be needed to administer the required dosage.

48. Use the microgram equivalent to calculate the dosage.

$50 \text{ mcg} : 1 \text{ mL} = 125 \text{ mcg} : x \text{ mL}$

or

$$\frac{125 \text{ mcg}}{50 \text{ mcg}} \times 1 \text{ mL} = x \text{ mL}$$

Answer: 2.5 mL. (2.5 mL is metric and stated with decimal.) The dosage ordered is larger than the available strength; therefore you will need more than 1 mL to administer the dosage.

49. $1 \text{ mg} : 5 \text{ mL} = 4 \text{ mg} : x \text{ mL}$

or

$$\frac{4 \text{ mg}}{1 \text{ mg}} \times 5 \text{ mL} = x \text{ mL}$$

Answer: 20 mL. The dosage ordered is more than the available strength; therefore you will need more than 5 mL to administer the required dosage.

50. Conversion is required. Equivalent: 1,000 mg = 1 g. Therefore 0.5 g = 500 mg.

$125 \text{ mg} : 5 \text{ mL} = 500 \text{ mg} : x \text{ mL}$

or

$$\frac{500 \text{ mg}}{125 \text{ mg}} \times 5 \text{ mL} = x \text{ mL}$$

Answer: 20 mL. The dosage ordered is four times larger than the available strength; therefore more than 5 mL will be needed to administer the dosage.

51. $20 \text{ mg} : 5 \text{ mL} = 60 \text{ mg} : x \text{ mL}$

or

$$\frac{60 \text{ mg}}{20 \text{ mg}} \times 5 \text{ mL} = x \text{ mL}$$

Answer: 15 mL. The dosage ordered is more than the available strength. You will need more than 5 mL to administer the dosage.

52. $30 \text{ mg} : 1 \text{ mL} = 150 \text{ mg} : x \text{ mL}$

or

$$\frac{150 \text{ mg}}{30 \text{ mg}} \times 1 \text{ mL} = x \text{ mL}$$

Answer: 5 mL. The dosage ordered is five times larger than the available strength. You will need more than 1 mL to administer the required dosage.

53. $12.5 \text{ mg} : 5 \text{ mL} = 25 \text{ mg} : x \text{ mL}$

or

$$\frac{25 \text{ mg}}{12.5 \text{ mg}} \times 5 \text{ mL} = x \text{ mL}$$

Answer: 10 mL. The dosage needed is two times more than the available strength; therefore you will need more than 5 mL to administer the required dosage.

54. The label indicates that 5 mL = 300 mg of the medication.

$300 \text{ mg} : 5 \text{ mL} = 600 \text{ mg} : x \text{ mL}$

or

$$\frac{600 \text{ mg}}{300 \text{ mg}} \times 5 \text{ mL} = x \text{ mL}$$

a. 10 mL. The dosage ordered is two times more than the available strength. You will need more than 5 mL to administer the required dosage.
b. Two containers are needed. One container contains 300 mg.

55. $6.25 \text{ mg} : 5 \text{ mL} = 12.5 \text{ mg} : x \text{ mL}$

or

$$\frac{12.5 \text{ mg}}{6.25 \text{ mg}} \times 5 \text{ mL} = x \text{ mL}$$

Answer: 10 mL. The dosage ordered is more than the available strength. You will need more than 5 mL to administer the dosage.

56. Conversion is required. 1,000 mg = 1 g. Therefore 0.5 g = 500 mg.

$400 \text{ mg} : 5 \text{ mL} = 500 \text{ mg} : x \text{ mL}$

$$\frac{500 \text{ mg}}{400 \text{ mg}} \times 5 \text{ mL} = x \text{ mL}$$

Answer: 6.25 = 6.3 mL. The dosage ordered is larger than the available strength. You will need more than 5 mL to administer the dosage.

57. $400{,}000 \text{ units} : 5 \text{ mL} = 500{,}000 \text{ units} : x \text{ mL}$

$$\frac{500{,}000 \text{ units}}{400{,}000 \text{ units}} \times 5 \text{ mL} = x \text{ mL}$$

Answer: $x = 6.25 = 6.3$ mL. The dosage ordered is larger than the available strength. You will need more than 5 mL to administer the required dosage.

58. Conversion is required. Equivalent: 1 g = 1,000 mg.

$125 \text{ mg} : 5 \text{ mL} = 1{,}000 \text{ mg} : x \text{ mL}$

or

$$\frac{1{,}000 \text{ mg}}{125 \text{ mg}} \times 5 \text{ mL} = x \text{ mL}$$

Answer: 40 mL. The dosage ordered is more than the strength available. You will need more than 5 mL to administer the dosage.

59. $250 \text{ mg} : 5 \text{ mL} = 500 \text{ mg} : x \text{ mL}$

$$\frac{500 \text{ mg}}{250 \text{ mg}} \times 5 \text{ mL} = x \text{ mL}$$

Answer: 10 mL. The dosage ordered is larger than the available strength. You will need more than 5 mL to administer the dosage.

60. $12 \text{ mg} : 1 \text{ mL} = 75 \text{ mg} : x \text{ mL}$

or

$$\frac{75 \text{ mg}}{12 \text{ mg}} \times 1 \text{ mL} = x \text{ mL}$$

Answer: 6.25 = 6.3 mL. The dosage ordered is more than the available strength. You will need more than 1 mL to administer the dosage.

61. $300 \text{ mg} : 5 \text{ mL} = 400 \text{ mg} : x \text{ mL}$

or

$$\frac{400 \text{ mg}}{300 \text{ mg}} \times 5 \text{ mL} = x \text{ mL}$$

Answer: 6.66 = 6.7 mL to the nearest tenth. The dosage ordered is more than the available strength. You will need more than 5 mL to administer the dosage.

62. $10 \text{ mg} : 1 \text{ mL} = 150 \text{ mg} : x \text{ mL}$

or

$$\frac{150 \text{ mg}}{10 \text{ mg}} \times 1 \text{ mL} = x \text{ mL}$$

Answer: 15 mL. The dosage ordered is greater than the available strength; therefore you will need more than 1 mL to administer the required dosage.

63. Conversion is necessary. 1,000 mg = 1 g; therefore 0.3 g = 300 mg.

$50 \text{ mg} : 5 \text{ mL} = 300 \text{ mg} : x \text{ mL}$

or

$$\frac{300 \text{ mg}}{50 \text{ mg}} \times 5 \text{ mL} = x \text{ mL}$$

Answer: 30 mL. The dosage ordered is greater than the available strength; therefore you will need more than 5 mL to administer the required dosage.

64. $125 \text{ mg} : 5 \text{ mL} = 375 \text{ mg} : x \text{ mL}$

$$\frac{375 \text{ mg}}{125 \text{ mg}} \times 5 \text{ mL} = x \text{ mL}$$

Answer: 15 mL. The dosage ordered is three times more than the available strength. You will need more than 5 mL to administer the required dosage.

65. $80 \text{ mg} : 1 \text{ mL} = 600 \text{ mg} : x \text{ mL}$

or

$$\frac{600 \text{ mg}}{80 \text{ mg}} \times 1 \text{ mL} = x \text{ mL}$$

Answer: 7.5 mL. The dosage ordered is greater than the available strength; therefore you will need more than 1 mL to administer the required dosage.

66. Conversion necessary. 1,000 mg = 1 g; therefore, 0.25 g = 250 mg.

$200 \text{ mg} : 5 \text{ mL} = 250 \text{ mg} : x \text{ mL}$

or

$$\frac{250 \text{ mg}}{200 \text{ mg}} \times 5 \text{ mL} = x \text{ mL}$$

Answer: 6.25 = 6.3 mL. The dosage ordered is more than the available strength. You will need more than 5 mL to administer the dosage.

67. $200 \text{ mg} : 5 \text{ mL} = 200 \text{ mg} : x \text{ mL}$

or

$$\frac{200 \text{ mg}}{200 \text{ mg}} \times 5 \text{ mL} = x \text{ mL}$$

Answer: 5 mL. The dosage ordered is equivalent to the available strength. Label indicates 200 mg = 5 mL.

68. $20 \text{ mg} : 5 \text{ mL} = 30 \text{ mg} : x \text{ mL}$

or

$$\frac{30 \text{ mg}}{20 \text{ mg}} \times 5 \text{ mL} = x \text{ mL}$$

Answer: 7.5 mL. The dosage ordered is greater than the available strength; therefore you will need more than 5 mL to administer the required dosage.

69. $15 \text{ mg} : 1 \text{ mL} = 150 \text{ mg} : x \text{ mL}$

or

$$\frac{150 \text{ mg}}{15 \text{ mg}} \times 1 \text{ mL} = x \text{ mL}$$

Answer: 10 mL. The dosage ordered is 10 times more than the available strength; therefore you will need more than 1 mL to administer the required dosage.

70. $20 \text{ mg} : 1 \text{ mL} = 30 \text{ mg} : x \text{ mL}$

or

$$\frac{30 \text{ mg}}{20 \text{ mg}} \times 1 \text{ mL} = x \text{ mL}$$

Answer: 1.5 mL, the dosage ordered is greater than the available strength; therefore you will need more than 1 mL to administer the required dosage.

Answers to Clinical Reasoning Questions

1. a. 6 tablets
   b. Question the order before administering. Double-check your calculation with another nurse. If order is correct, check with the pharmacy regarding available dosage strengths for the medication. Check a reliable and reputable medication reference for the usual dosage and action of this medication.
   c. Any calculation that requires you to administer more than the maximum number of tablets or capsules, which is usually three (3), to achieve a single dose should be questioned and calculation rechecked. An unusual number of tablets or capsules should alert the nurse to a possible error in prescribing, transcribing, or calculation.
2. a. After checking a reliable and reputable drug resource for the usual dosage, contact the pharmacy regarding the available dosage strengths for the medication.
   b. The dosage ordered would require that the tablets be broken to administer the dosage. The tablets are unscored and should not be broken. Unscored tablets will not break evenly, and there is no way to determine the dosage being administered. Breaking an unscored tablet could lead to the administration of an unintended dosage.
3. a. The right medication
   b. In preparing the medication, the nurse did not read the label carefully and administered Percodan, the wrong medication, which has a similar spelling to Percocet. By not reading the label carefully, the nurse did not notice that combination medications contain more than one medication; in this case, Percodan contained aspirin. Percocet contained Tylenol.
   c. A medication error occurred because the wrong medication was administered. The client was allergic to aspirin and could have had a reaction from mild to a severe anaphylactic reaction (dyspnea, airway obstruction, shock, and in some cases death).
   d. The error could have been prevented by carefully reading the medication label three times while preparing the medication. The nurse must use caution when administering medications that look alike or that have similar spellings. Tablets or capsules that contain more than one medication must be read carefully. (Percocet contains acetaminophen [Tylenol] and Percodan contains aspirin.)

NOTE

Refer to problems 1-70 for setup of problems if needed.

Answers to Chapter Review

1. 3 tabs
2. 12.5 mL
3. 1 tab
4. 3 tabs
5. 1 tab
6. 12.5 mL
7. 2 tabs
8. 2 tabs
9. $\frac{1}{2}$ tab
10. 2 tabs
11. 2 mL
12. 19 mL
13. $\frac{1}{2}$ tab
14. 15.6 mL
15. 2 caps
16. 28.1 mL
17. 3 tabs
18. 1- 2 mg tab and 1- 1 mg tab
19. 2 tabs
20. 2 caps (delayed release)
21. 1- 0.3 mg tab and 1- 0.2 mg tab
22. 1 tab
23. 2 tabs (extended release)
24. 30 mL
25. 2 caps
26. a. 2 tabs
    b. 14 tabs
27. 1- 10 mg tab and 1- 20 mg tab
28. 2 tabs
29. 20 mL
30. 1- 40 mg tab
31. 7.5 mL
32. 2 tabs
33. $2\frac{1}{2}$ tabs
34. 3- 40 mg caps
35. 12.5 mL
36. 100 mg caps
37. 2 tabs
38. 2 sublingual tabs
39. 20 mL
40. 1 delayed release tab
41. 1- 7.5 mg tab and 1- 2.5 mg tab
42. 2 tabs
43. $1\frac{1}{2}$ tabs
44. 2 tabs
45. 2 tabs
46. 10 mL
47. 2 caps
48. 15 mL
49. 3-5 mg tabs
50. 2 tabs (delayed release; enteric coated)
51. 10 mL
52. 3.8 mL

CHAPTER 18
Parenteral Medications

Objectives

After reviewing this chapter, you should be able to:

1. Identify the various types of syringes used for parenteral administration
2. Read parenteral solution labels and identify dosage strengths
3. Read and measure dosages on a syringe
4. Calculate dosages of parenteral medications already in solution
5. Identify the appropriate syringe to administer the dosage based on the dosage calculation

The term *parenteral* is used to indicate medications by any route other than through the gastrointestinal (GI) system. Parenteral is commonly used to refer to medications administered by injection with the use of a needle and syringe. Common parenteral routes include intramuscular (IM), subcutaneous (subcut), and intravenous (IV). Of the three routes, the IV route produces the desired effect more rapidly, as the medication is injected directly into the bloodstream. Intradermal (ID) is a less common injection route and is mainly used for skin testing, such as for allergy test or tuberculin skin test.

Medications administered by the parenteral route generally act more quickly than oral medications because they are absorbed more rapidly into the bloodstream. This chapter will focus on calculation of medications administered IM, subcut, and IV.

- **IM**—Indicates an injection given into a muscle, such as Demerol for pain.
- **Subcut**—Injection into the subcutaneous tissue, below the skin, such as insulin used in the management of diabetes.
- **IV**—Injection given directly into the vein. This can be direct (IV push), or the medication can be diluted in a larger volume of intravenous fluid and infused over a period of time (IV infusion). Antibiotics and other medications may be administered IV.
- **ID**—Injection administered just under the skin is mainly used for diagnostic purposes. Example: used to administer purified protein derivative (PPD) skin test to test for exposure to tuberculosis.

When the rapid action of a medication is necessary or a client cannot take the medication orally, the parenteral route may be preferred. For example, a client is unable to take a medication orally because of emesis (vomiting) or a nonfunctioning gastrointestinal (GI) tract, or the client is unconscious.

Medications for parenteral use are available as a sterile solution or liquid that can be absorbed and distributed without causing irritation to the tissues. Parenteral medications are also available in powder form that must be diluted with a liquid or solvent (reconstituted) before they can be used. Reconstitution of medications in powder form will be covered in Chapter 19.

Parenteral Medication Packaging

Medications for parenteral use come packaged in a variety of forms, including ampules, vials, mix-o-vials, premeasured (pre-filled) syringes, and cartridges.

1. **Ampule**—Sealed glass container that contains a typical single dose of medication. It has a constricted neck that is designed to snap open. The neck of the ampule may be scored or have a darkened line or ring around it to indicate where it should be snapped (broken open) to withdraw the medication. The neck is snapped off by using a plastic protective sleeve, an alcohol wipe, or sterile gauze. A filter needle (a needle with a filter inside) should always be attached to the syringe to withdraw the medication from the ampule, the filter needle removed, and an appropriate needle used for administration. A filter needle prevents the withdrawal of glass or rubber particulate (Elkin et al., 2011).

   The medication is withdrawn into the syringe by gently pulling back on the plunger, which creates a negative pressure and allows the medication to be pulled into the syringe (Figure 18-1).
2. **Vial**—A vial is a plastic or glass container that has a rubber stopper or diaphragm on the top. The rubber stopper is covered with a metal lid or plastic cover to maintain sterility until the vial is used for the first time. Multi-dose vials contain more than one dosage of the medication. Single-dose vials contain the amount of medication for a typical single dose. Many medications are prepared as single-dose to reduce the chance of error. Even if medication is in a single-dosage vial, it should still be measured and not just drawn up. According to the Centers for Disease Control and Prevention (CDC; cdc.gov/injection safety/providers/provider_faqs_ singlevials.html), medication vials labeled "single dose" or "single use" should be used once and are meant for one patient use. The lack of antimicrobial preservatives in a single-dose vial places client at risk for life-threatening infections when used more than once. The practice of splitting single-dose/single-use medications vials into new doses for multiple clients is also a practice that places clients at risk for infection.

   When possible, the CDC also recommends multi-dose vials be used for a single client use and not opened or punctured in the immediate client area (example: client room). This practice will prevent contamination of vial (direct or indirect), which can lead to infections in subsequent clients. CDC recommends once a multi-dose vial is opened or punctured, it should be discarded within 28 days unless the manufacturer specifies a different expiration date for the opened vial. A vial that has not been opened or punctured with a needle should be discarded according to the manufacturer's expiration date. The medication in a vial may be in liquid (solution) form (Figure 18-2), or may contain a powder that must be reconstituted before administration (discussed in Chapter 19) (Figure 18-3).

   In contrast to the ampule, the vial is a closed system. Before a solution can be withdrawn from a vial, the same volume of air must be injected into the vial. For large

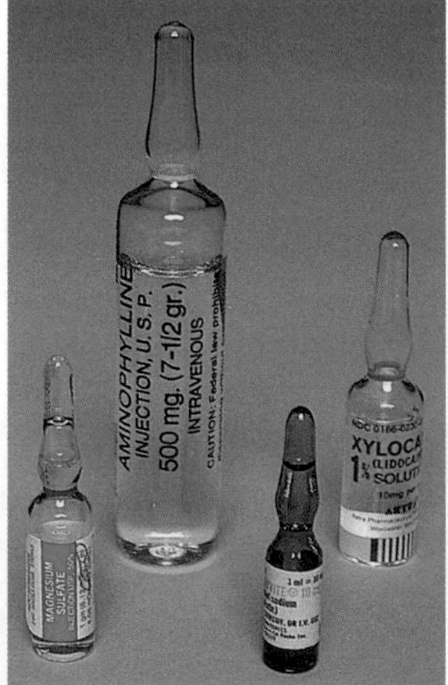

Figure 18-1 Medication in ampules. (From Perry AG, Potter PA, Elkin MK, Ostendorf WR: *Nursing interventions and clinical skills,* ed 6, St Louis, 2016, Mosby.)

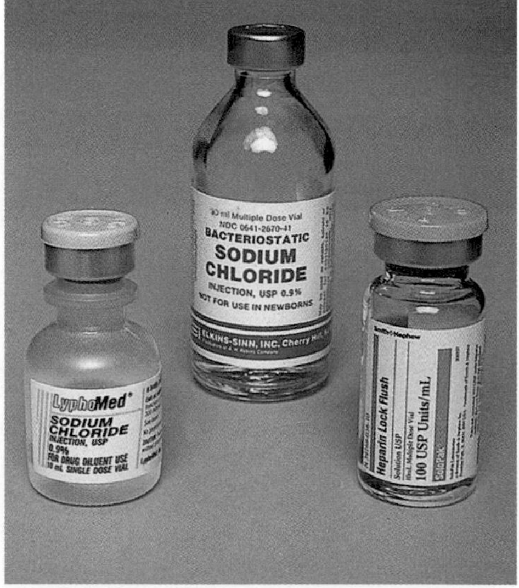

Figure 18-2 Medication in vials. (From Perry AG, Potter PA, Elkin MK, Ostendorf WR: *Nursing interventions and clinical skills,* ed 6, St Louis, 2016, Mosby.)

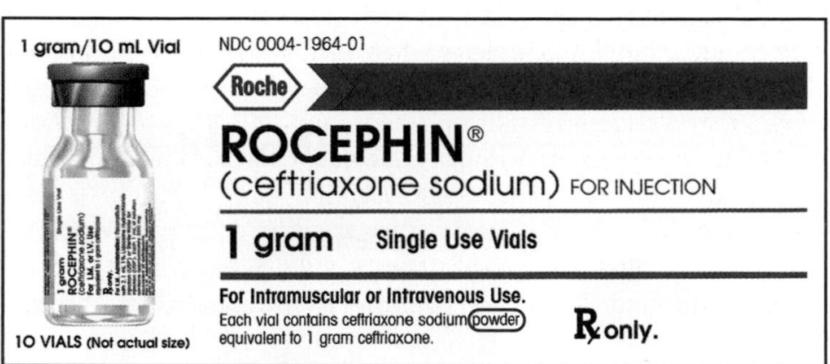
1 gram/10 mL Vial
NDC 0004-1964-01
Roche
ROCEPHIN®
(ceftriaxone sodium) FOR INJECTION
1 gram Single Use Vials
For Intramuscular or Intravenous Use.
Each vial contains ceftriaxone sodium (powder) equivalent to 1 gram ceftriaxone.
℞ only.
10 VIALS (Not actual size)

Figure 18-3 Medication in powder form.

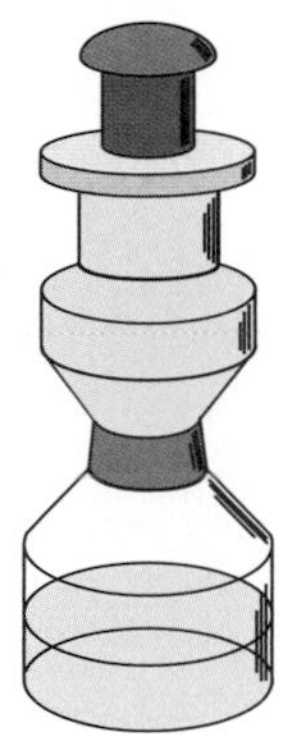

Figure 18-4 Mix-o-vial. (From Clayton BD, Willihnganz M: *Basic pharmacology for nurses,* ed 17, St Louis, 2017, Mosby.)

volumes of solution to be withdrawn, a small volume of air is required to initiate the flow of medication.

TIPS FOR CLINICAL PRACTICE

It is important to note that for both single-dose vials and ampules, there is a little extra medication present; it is most important to carefully measure the amount of medication to be withdrawn.

3. **Mix-o-vial**—Some medications come in mix-o-vials (Figure 18-4). The vial usually contains a single dosage of medication. The mix-o-vial has two compartments separated by a rubber stopper. The top compartment contains the sterile liquid (diluent), and the bottom compartment contains the powdered medication. When pressure is applied to the top of the vial, the rubber stopper that separates the medication and liquid is released. This allows the liquid and medication to be mixed, thereby dissolving the medication (Figure 18-5).
4. **Cartridge**—Some medications are packaged in a prefilled glass or plastic container. The cartridge is clearly marked, indicating the amount of medication in it. Certain cartridges require a special holder called a *Tubex* or *Carpuject* to release the medication from the cartridge. The cartridge contains a single dosage of medication. The white plastic portion on the end of the carpuject can also be removed, exposing a rubber stopper in which a needle can be inserted to remove calculated amounts.

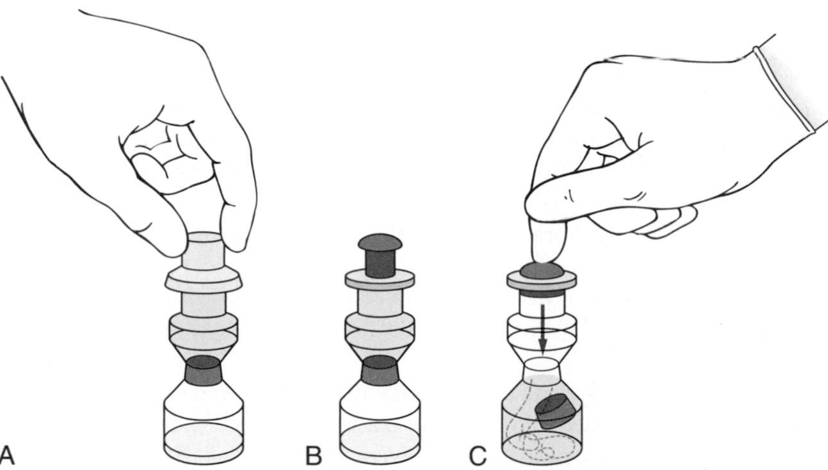

Figure 18-5 Mix-o-vial directions. **A,** Remove plastic lid protector. **B,** Powdered drug is in lower half; diluent is in upper half. **C,** Push firmly on the diaphragm-plunger. Downward pressure dislodges the divider between the two chambers. (Modified from Clayton BD, Willihnganz M: *Basic pharmacology for nurses,* ed 17, St Louis, 2017, Mosby.)

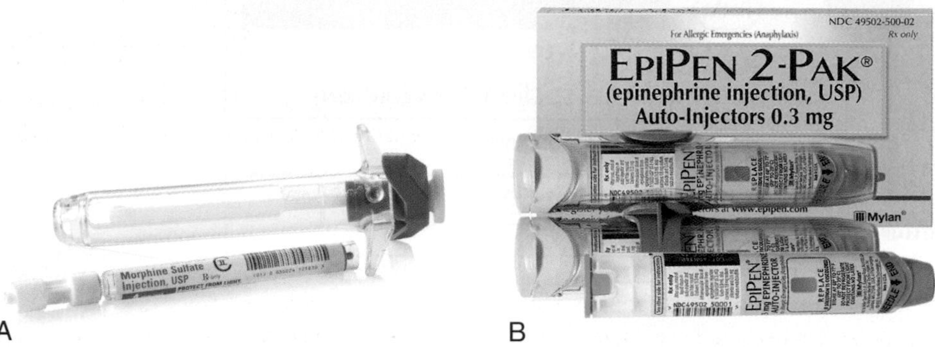

Figure 18-6 **A,** Carpuject syringe holder and needleless, prefilled sterile cartridge. **B,** EpiPen 2-Pak. (**A,** From Hospira, Inc., Lake Forest, IL. **B,** From Mylan Specialty L.P., Basking Ridge, NJ.)

If the dosage to be administered is less than the amount contained in the unit, discard the unneeded portion, if any (in the presence of another nurse when medication is a narcotic), and then administer the medication (Figure 18-6, *A*).

5. **Prefilled syringe (premeasured)**—The medication comes prepared for administration in a syringe, with the needle attached or without a needle attached. Prefilled syringes are single-dose syringes that come with a specific amount of medication contained in the syringe and are designed to be used only once. The amount desired is calculated, the excess disposed of (in the presence of another nurse when the medication is a narcotic), and the calculated dosage is administered. EpiPen, Hepatitis B vaccine, Lovenox, and emergency medications such as sodium bicarbonate and atropine are examples of medications that come in prefilled syringe (Figure 18-6, B). An insulin pen is also an example of a prefilled syringe. The insulin pen is used to administer insulin. The pen is loaded with an insulin cartridge, and the dial on the pen is adjusted to the ordered dose of insulin. A disposable needle is attached to the pen, and the insulin administered. Insulin pens are discussed in more detail in Chapter 20.

SAFETY ALERT!

To safely administer the prescribed amount from a cartridge and prefilled syringe, the amount of medication in excess of what is prescribed should be discarded before administration.

Syringes

Various-sized syringes are available for use. They have different capacities and specific calibrations. Syringes are made of plastic and glass, but plastic syringes are more commonly used. They are disposable and designed for one-time use only. Syringes have three parts (Figure 18-7):

1. **The barrel**—The outer calibrated portion that holds the medication. It has calibrations (markings) on the outer portion.
2. **The plunger**—The inner device that is moved backward to withdraw and measure the medication and is pushed to eject the medication from the syringe. The plunger fits into the barrel.
3. **The tip**—The end of the syringe that holds the needle. The needle slips on to the tip (non-Luer-Lok) or can be twisted and locked in place (Luer-Lok™). This design prevents the inadvertent removal of the needle (Potter, Perry, Stockert, Hall, 2013). See Figure 18-8.

Needles come in various lengths and diameters. The nurse chooses the needle according to the client's size, the type of tissue being injected into, and the viscosity of the medication to be injected. Some syringes also come with a needle attached that cannot be detached from the syringe.

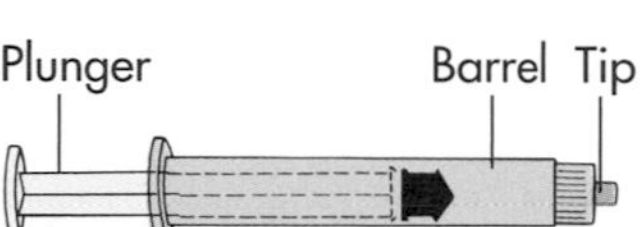

Figure 18-7 Parts of a syringe. (From Perry AG, Potter PA, Elkin MK, Ostendorf WR: *Nursing interventions and clinical skills,* ed 6, St Louis, 2016, Mosby.)

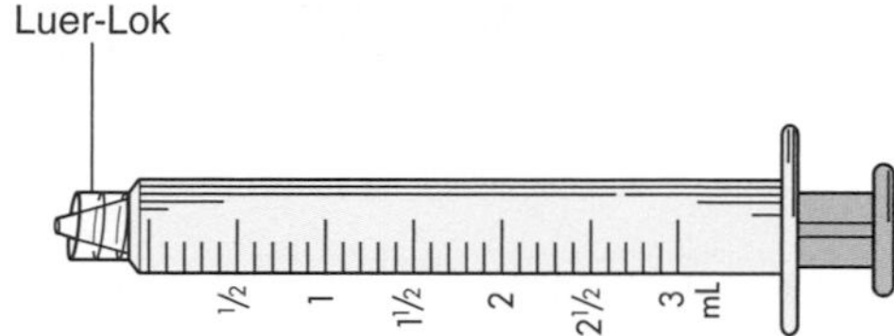

Figure 18-8 3-mL Luer-Lok syringe. (From Potter PA, Perry AG, Stockert P, Hall A: *Fundamentals of nursing,* ed 9, St Louis, 2016, Mosby.)

Safety Needles and Needleless Syringe

Needle-stick prevention is the **only** way to prevent transmission of blood-borne pathogens from contaminated needles. Consequently, this has resulted in special prevention techniques (e.g., no recapping of a needle after use) and development of special equipment, such as syringes with a sheath or guard that covers the needle after it is withdrawn from the skin, thereby decreasing the chance of needle-stick injury (Figure 18-9). Another advance in safety needle technology is the safety glide syringe, which contains a protective needle guard that can be activated by a single finger to cover and seal the needle after injection (Figure 18-10). Following the administration of an injection, the nurse should always activate the safety device. Safety syringes are available in various sizes and shapes. Needleless syringe systems have also been designed to prevent needle sticks. It may be used to withdraw medication from a vial, and to add medication to IV for medication administration (Figure 18-11).

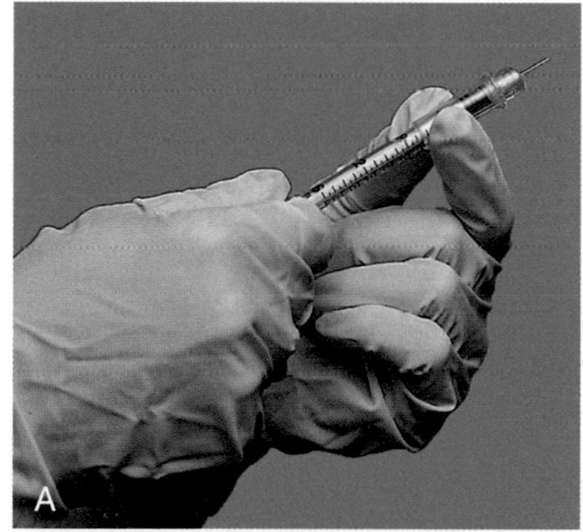

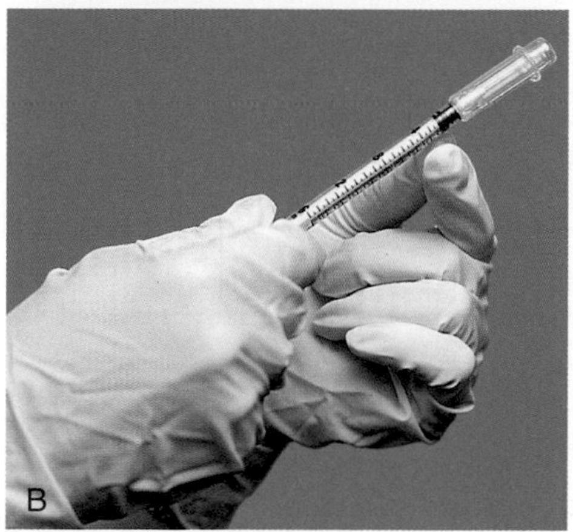

Figure 18-9 Needle with plastic guard to prevent needle sticks. **A,** Position of guard before injection. **B,** After injection the guard locks in place, covering the needle. (From Perry AG, Potter PA, Elkin MK, Ostendorf WR: *Nursing interventions and clinical skills,* ed 6, St Louis, 2016, Mosby.)

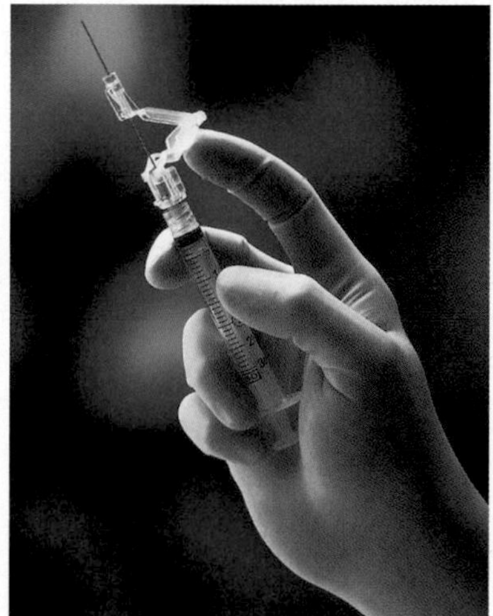

Figure 18-10 BD SafetyGlide™ needle. (From Becton, Dickinson, and Company, Franklin Lakes, NJ.)

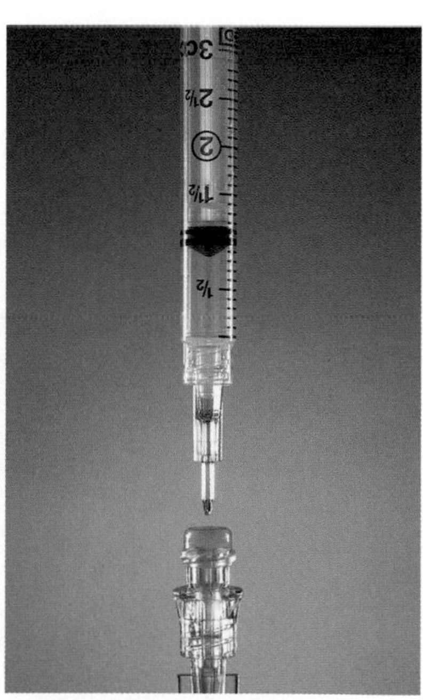

Figure 18-11 Needleless syringe system. (From Becton, Dickinson, and Company, Franklin Lakes, NJ.)

SAFETY ALERT!

Protection from needle-stick injuries requires that needles are never recapped and always correctly disposed of in special puncture resistant containers.

Types of Syringes

The three types of syringes are hypodermic, tuberculin, and insulin.

Hypodermic Syringes. **Hypodermic** syringes (a syringe with a needle) come in a variety of sizes, from 0.5 mL up to 60 mL and larger. Syringes are calibrated or marked in milliliters but hold varying capacities. Of the small-capacity syringes, the 3-mL syringe is used most often for the administration of medication that is more than 1 mL; however, hypodermic syringes are also available in larger sizes (10 mL 20 mL, 50 mL, and larger). Although many syringes are labeled in milliliters, a few syringes are still labeled with cubic centimeters (cc). Many manufacturers are now phasing in syringes labeled in milliliters. **It is important to note that milliliter (mL) is correct. The milliliter is a measure of volume, the cubic centimeter is a three-dimensional measure of space and represents the space that a milliliter occupies. The terms, although sometimes used interchangeably, are not the same.** This text shows mL on syringes, not cc (Figure 18-12).

SAFETY ALERT!

It is critical that the scale (calibrations) on small hypodermics be read carefully. Misreading the calibrations could lead to a medication error.

For small hypodermics, decimal numbers are used to express dosages (e.g., 1.2 mL, 0.3 mL). Notice that small hypodermics up to 3-mL size also have fractions on them (see Figure 18-12, *A*). There are, however, some syringes that indicate 0.5 mL, 1.5 mL, etc., instead of fractions. The use of decimals on the syringes correlates with the use of decimals in the metric system; therefore, a dosage should be stated in milliliters as a decimal.

Notice in Figure 18-12, *A* (3-mL syringe) the side that indicates mL. There are 10 spaces between the largest markings. This indicates that the syringe is marked in tenths of a milliliter. Each of the lines is 0.1 mL. The longer lines indicate half (0.5) and full milliliter measures.

In Figure 18-12, *B*, the 1-mL syringe is marked in hundredths (0.01) of a milliliter and tenths (0.1) of a milliliter. Each of the small lines is 0.01 mL, with the slightly longer lines equal to 0.05, 0.1, 0.15, 0.2, and so on.

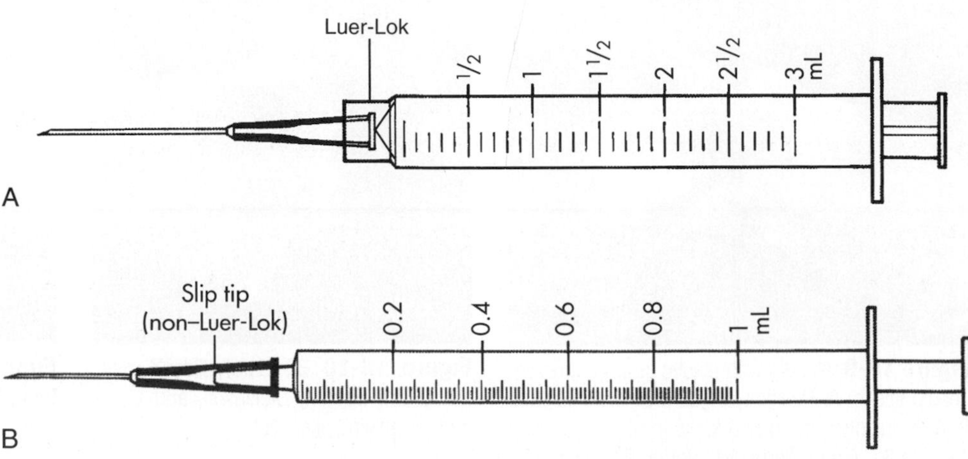

Figure 18-12 3-mL and 1-mL syringes.

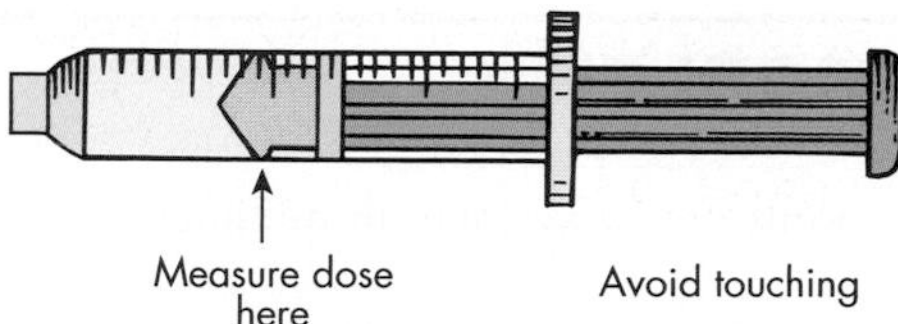

Figure 18-13 Reading measured amount of medication in a syringe. (From Potter PA, Perry AG, Stockert P, Hall A: *Fundamentals of nursing,* ed 9, St Louis, 2016, Mosby.)

When looking at the syringe shown in Figure 18-13, notice the rubber ring. When you are measuring medication and reading the medication withdrawn, the forward edge of the plunger head indicates the amount of medication withdrawn. Do not become confused by the second, bottom ring or by the raised section (middle) of the suction tip. The point where the rubber plunger edge makes contact with the barrel is the spot that should be lined up with the amount desired.

SAFETY ALERT!

Understanding the calibration marks on a syringe is critical to accurately measure a medication dosage. The volume of medication represented by the calibrations is different depending on the size of the syringe being used. Never assume what the calibrations on a syringe mean. Check the calibrations carefully. If medication is not accurately measured, an incorrect dosage can be administered, resulting in serious consequences to the client.

Let's examine the syringes below to illustrate specific amounts in a syringe. (Syringe **A** shows a volume of 0.7 mL filled in, and syringe **B,** 1.7 mL.)

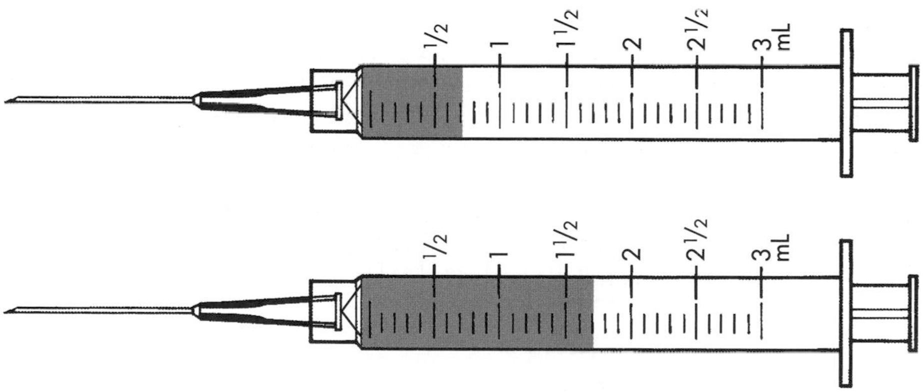

Because the small-capacity syringes are used most often to administer medications, it is very important to know how to read them to withdraw amounts accurately.

POINTS TO REMEMBER

- Small-capacity hypodermics are calibrated in milliliters; the 3-mL size syringe is used most often to administer dosages greater than 1 mL. Dosages administered with them must correlate to the calibration. Minims are no longer used.
- Syringes are labeled with the abbreviation mL. More and more syringes are being manufactured using just mL.
- The milliliter (mL) is the correct measure for volume. Although a few syringes may still indicate cubic centimeters (cc), technically this is incorrect.

PRACTICE PROBLEMS

Shade in the indicated amounts on the syringes in milliliters.

1. 0.8 mL

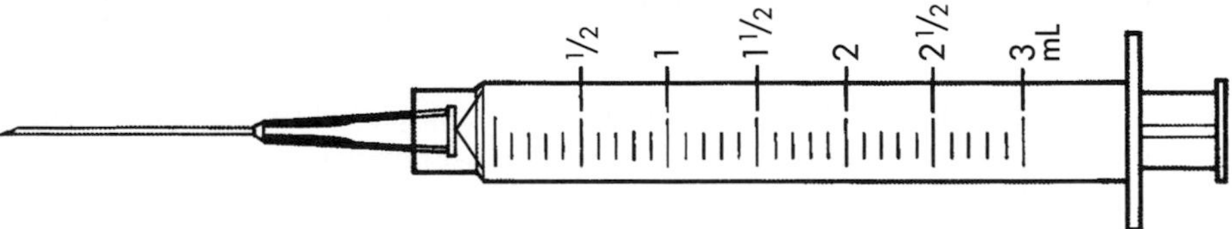

2. 1.2 mL

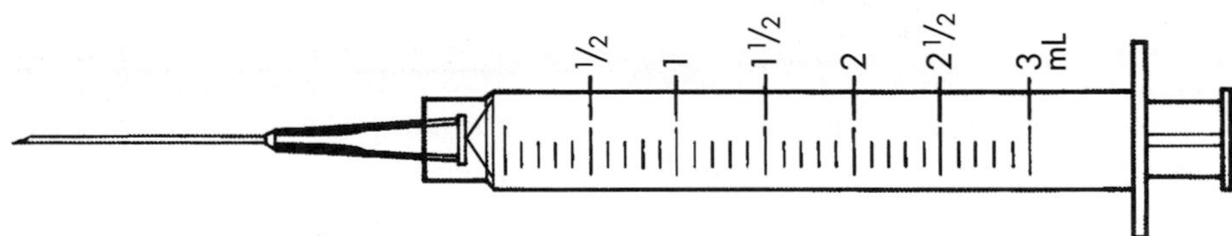

3. 1.5 mL

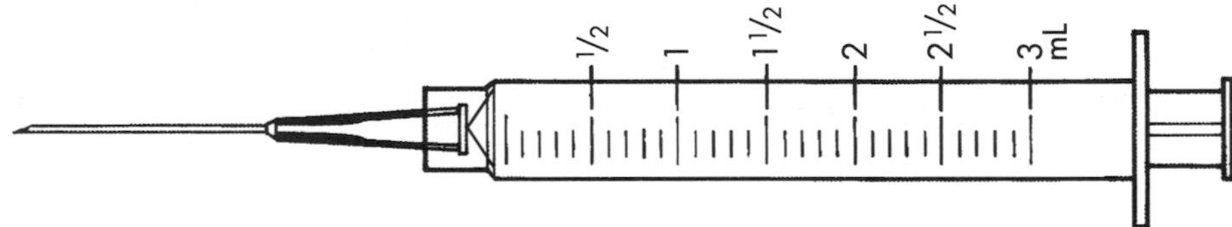

4. 2.4 mL

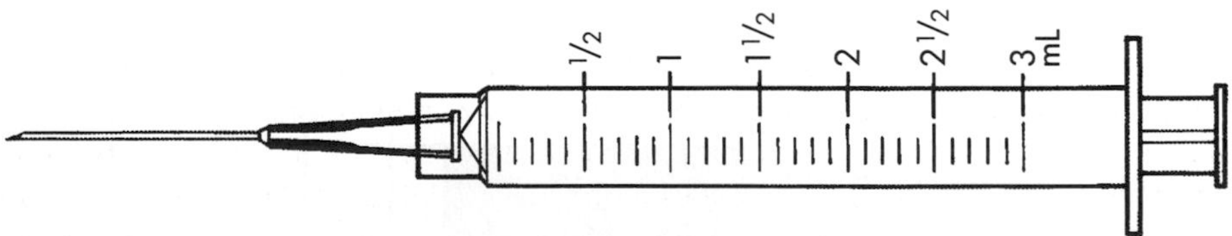

Indicate the number of milliliters shaded in on the following syringes.

5.

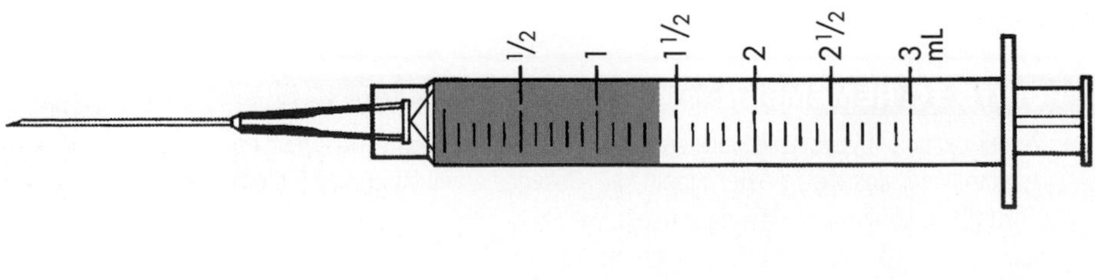

____

6.

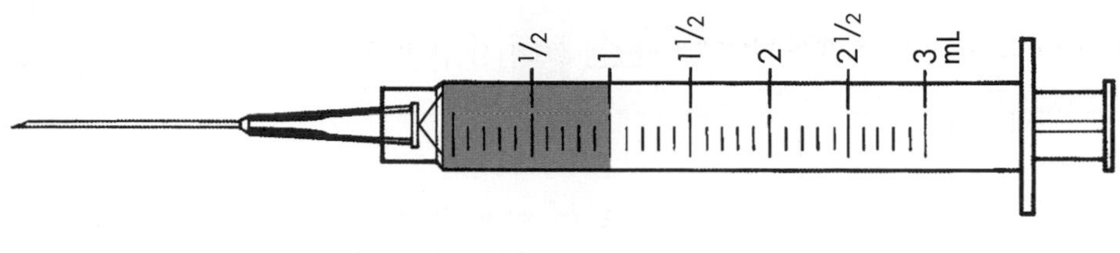

7.

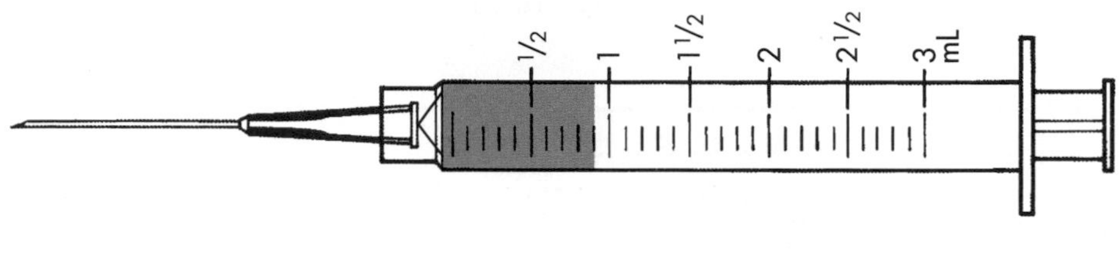

8.

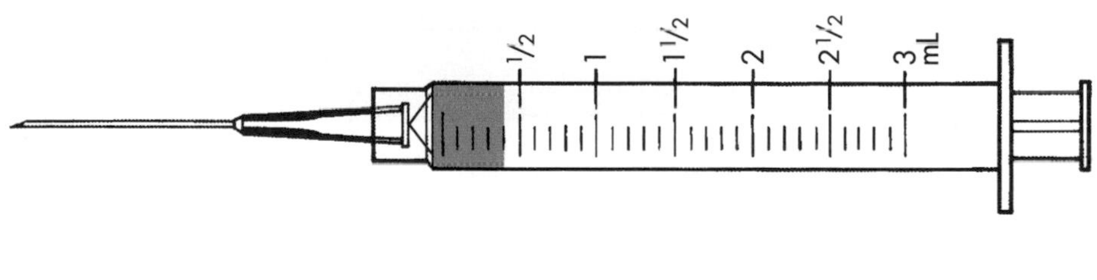

Answers on pp. 416-417

Large-Capacity Syringes. The larger hypodermics (5, 6, 10, and 12 mL) are used when volumes larger than 3 mL are desired. These syringes are used to measure whole numbers of milliliters as opposed to smaller units such as a tenth of a milliliter. Syringes 5, 6, 10, and 12 mL in size are calibrated in increments of fifths of a milliliter (0.2 mL), with the whole numbers indicated by the long lines. Figure 18-14, *A,* shows 0.8 mL of medication measured in a 5-mL syringe, and Figure 18-14, *B,* shows 7.8 mL measured in a 10-mL syringe. Syringes that are 20 mL and larger are calibrated in whole milliliter increments and can have other measures, such as ounces, on them.

The larger-size syringes (5, 6, 10, 12, and higher) are commonly used to prepare medications for intravenous administration. These syringes are sometimes referred to as *intravenous syringes.*

TIPS FOR CLINICAL PRACTICE

The larger the syringe, the larger the calibration. Example: In 5-mL and 10-mL syringes, each shorter calibration measures two tenths of a milliliter (0.2 mL). To be safe, always examine the calibration of the syringes and use the one best suited for the volume to be administered.

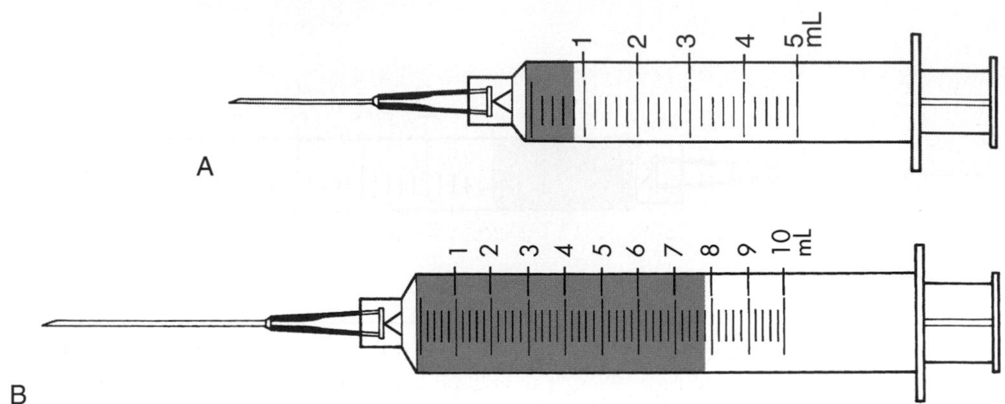

Figure 18-14 Large hypodermics. **A,** 5-mL syringe filled with 0.8 mL. **B,** 10-mL syringe filled with 7.8 mL.

PRACTICE PROBLEMS

Indicate the number of milliliters shaded in on the following syringes.

9.

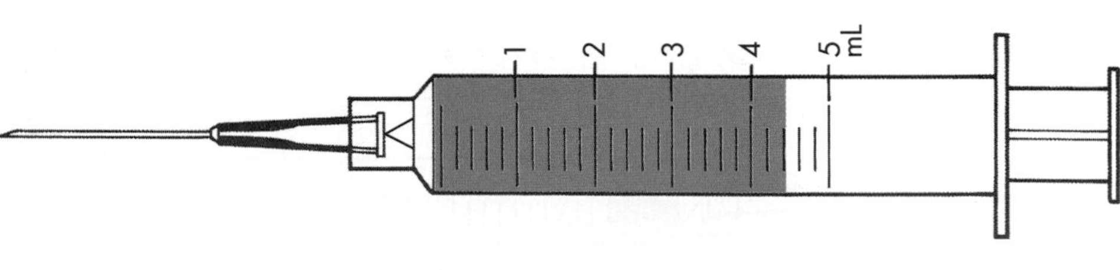

____

10.

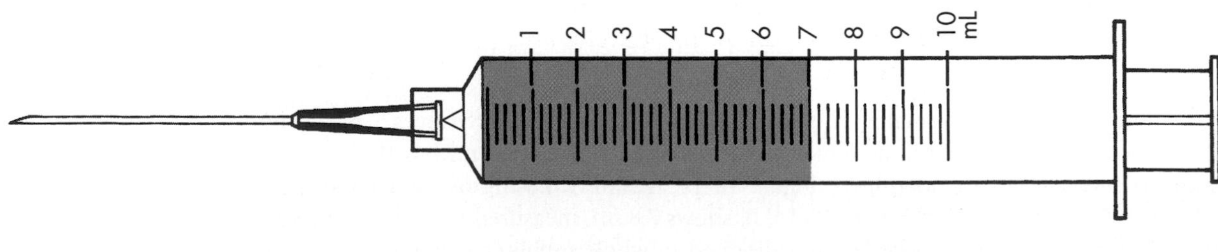

____

11.

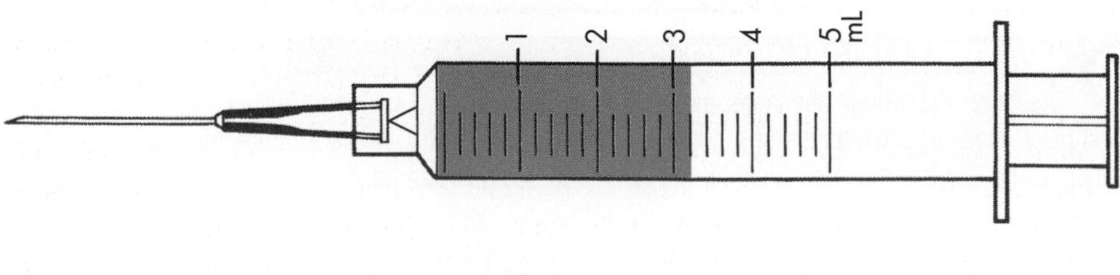

____

Answers on p. 417

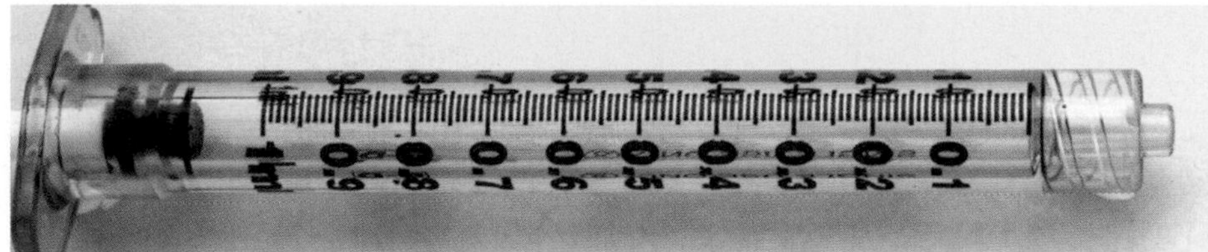

Figure 18-15 Tuberculin syringe.

Tuberculin Syringe. A tuberculin syringe is a narrow syringe that has a capacity of 0.5 mL or 1 mL. The 1-mL size is used most often. The volume of a tuberculin syringe can be measured on the milliliter scale. On the milliliter side of the syringe, the syringe is calibrated in hundredths (0.01 mL) and tenths (0.1 mL) of a milliliter. The markings on the syringe (lines) are closer together to indicate how small the calibrations are (Figure 18-15).

Tuberculin syringes are used to accurately measure medications given in very small volumes (e.g., heparin). This syringe is also often used in pediatrics and for diagnostic purposes (e.g., skin testing for tuberculosis). Vaccines are also administered using a tuberculin syringe. It is recommended that dosages less than 0.5 mL be measured with a tuberculin syringe to make certain that the correct dosage is administered to a client. Dosages such as 0.42 mL and 0.37 mL can be measured accurately with a tuberculin syringe. Measuring the correct dose with a tuberculin syringe requires extreme care. Read the markings carefully to avoid error.

SAFETY ALERT!

The calibrations on hypodermic syringes differ. Be careful when measuring medications in a syringe. Being off by even a small amount on the syringe scale can be critical. The syringe you use to administer medication must provide the calibration you need to accurately measure the dose.

Insulin syringes are used for the subcutaneous (subcut) injection of insulin and are calibrated in units rather than milliliters (mL). Insulin is measured in units and always ordered in units. Insulin syringes are calibrated for the administration of standard U-100 insulin only. The common strength of insulin is 100 units per milliliter, which is referred to as units 100 insulin and is abbreviated as "U-100." Insulin syringes should not be used for administration of nonstandard strengths of insulin (e.g., U-500 insulin). To avoid errors and ensure client safety, an order for nonstandard insulin should contain the number of units as well as the volume in milliliters. For example, if the order were "Humulin *Regular* U-500 insulin 140 units (*0.28 mL*) subcut stat," then 0.28 mL of U-500 insulin would be administered using a 1-mL tuberculin syringe. Calculation involving U-500 insulin will be discussed in Chapter 20.

SAFETY ALERT!

The insulin syringe marked U-100 is to be used for the administration of U-100 Insulin only. U-100 insulin indicates 100 units per milliliter. Never measure other medications measured in units in an insulin syringe, for example, heparin or U-500 insulin.

Insulin syringes are available in three sizes: 100 unit (1 mL), 50 unit (0.5 mL), and 30 unit (0.3 mL). The 100 unit (1 mL) is often referred to as the "standard" insulin syringe. The 50-unit (0.5 mL) and 30-unit (0.3 mL) insulin syringes are called Lo-Dose insulin syringes because they are designed to deliver low doses of insulin (50 units or less). Lo-Dose insulin syringes are designed to deliver low doses of insulin with greater accuracy, and should be used.

- **50 unit Lo-Dose** insulin syringe has a capacity of 50 units. It is calibrated in 1-unit increments up to 50 units per 0.5 mL. If available, a 50-unit (0.5 mL) insulin syringe should be used to administer doses of 50 units or less (Figure 18-16, *B*).
- **30 unit Lo-Dose** insulin syringe has a capacity of 30 units (0.3 mL). It is calibrated in 1-unit increments, or 30 units per 0.3 mL, and should be used to administer doses of 30 units or less. The 30-unit insulin syringe is commonly used in pediatrics for the administration of insulin (Figure 18-16, *C*).

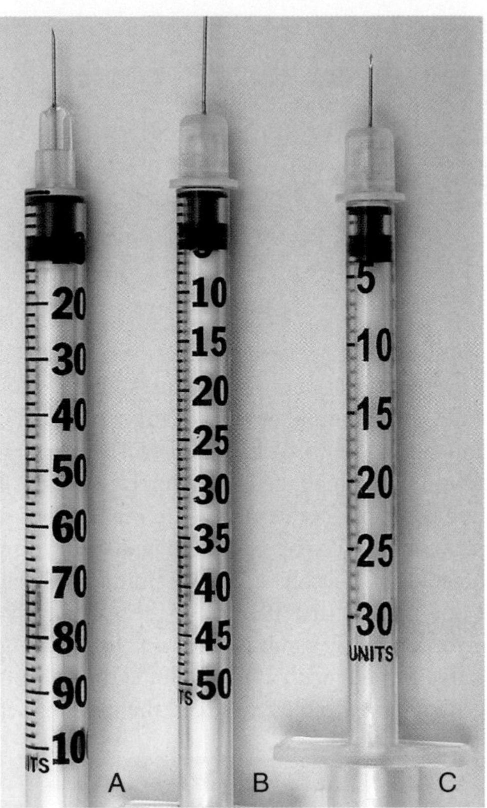

Figure 18-16 Insulin syringes. **A,** 1-mL size (100 units). **B,** Lo-Dose (50 units). **C,** Lo-Dose (30 units). (From Macklin D, Chernecky L, Infortuna H: *Math for clinical practice,* ed. 2, St. Louis, 2010, Mosby.)

Note that the Lo-Dose insulin syringe has an enlarged scale and is easy to read.

- **The standard U-100** syringe has a capacity of 100 units of insulin per milliliter. A single-scaled standard 100 unit insulin syringe is calibrated in 2-unit increments (see Figure 18-16, *A*). Odd number of units (e.g., 27 units) would have to be measured between the even calibrations.

Measurement of dosages that are approximate (in between lines) should be avoided.

The second type of 100-unit insulin syringe is the **dual-scale** version, which is calibrated in 2-unit increments. It has a scale with even-numbered 2-unit increments on one side (2, 4, etc.). It is calibrated on the opposite side in odd-numbered 2-unit increments (1, 3, etc.). The best method for using this type of syringe is the following. Measure odd dosages on the left and even dosages using the scale on the right (Figure 18-17). It is not necessary to use the various methods of calculation presented for insulin because the insulin syringe is designed to measure insulin dosages. Reading insulin syringes and being attentive to the calibrations is an essential skill for safety. Insulin dosages are discussed in more detail in Chapter 20.

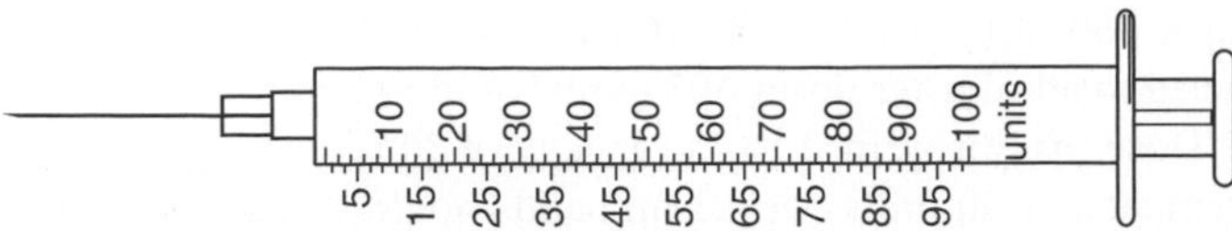

Figure 18-17 1-mL capacity insulin syringe (100 units) with dual scale odd and even calibrations. (From Becton, Dickinson, and Company, Franklin Lakes, NJ.)

SAFETY ALERT!

Insulin is a high-alert medication. All insulin dosages should be checked by another nurse before administration to a client.

TIPS FOR CLINICAL PRACTICE

It is important to note that insulin syringes do not have detachable needles. The needle, hub, and barrel are inseparable.

CLINICAL **REASONING**

- Dosages must be measurable and appropriate for the syringe used.
- The insulin syringe and the tuberculin syringe are different. Confusion of the two can cause a medication error.
- Measure insulin in an insulin syringe only.
- If the dosage cannot be accurately measured, do not administer.

POINTS TO REMEMBER

- When parenteral medications are prepared for administration, it is important to use the correct syringe for accurate administration of the dosage.
- Most medications are prepared and labeled with the dosage strength given per milliliter (mL). Remember that although you may see these terms used interchangeably and as equivalent measures (1 cc = 1 mL), technically they are not equivalents; milliliter should be used instead of cubic centimeter.
- Small-capacity hypodermic syringes are marked in tenths of a milliliter (0.1 mL). The 3-mL size is used most often to administer medication volumes greater than 1 mL.
- Hypodermic syringes—5, 6, 10, and 12 mL—are marked in increments of 0.2 mL and 1 mL.
- Hypodermic syringes—20 mL and larger—are marked in 1-mL increments and may have other markings, such as ounces.
- Tuberculin syringes or 1-mL syringes are small syringes marked in tenths and hundredths of a milliliter. They are used to administer small dosages and are recommended for use with a dosage less than 0.5 mL.
- Insulin syringes are marked U-100 for administration with U-100 insulin only. Insulin is measured in units and should be administered only with an insulin syringe.
- Dosages involving milliliters should be expressed as decimals even when the syringe is marked with fractions. The milliliter is a metric measure.

Before proceeding to discuss calculation of parenteral dosages, it is necessary to review some specifics in terms of reading labels. Reading the label and understanding what information is essential are important in determining the correct dosage to administer.

Reading Parenteral Labels

The information contained on the parenteral label is similar to the information on an oral liquid label. It contains the total volume of the container and the dosage strength (amount of medication in solution) expressed in milliliters (Table 18-1). It is important to read the label carefully to determine the dosage strength and volume. Let's examine some labels.

TABLE 18-1 Sample Dosage Strengths

Label	Interpretation
Diazepam 5 mg/mL	1 mL contains 5 mg of Diazepam
Inapsine 2.5 mg/mL	1 mL contains 2.5 mg of Inapsine
Digoxin 500 mcg/2 mL	2 mL contains 500 mcg of Digoxin

The slash (/) mark used here to illustrate expression of the dosage strength as written on label. When expressing dosage strengths do not use the slash mark. Use per. For example, per mL is recommended by ISMP and is on the list of Error-Prone Abbreviations, Symbols, and Dose Designation. The slash mark has been mistaken for the number (1).

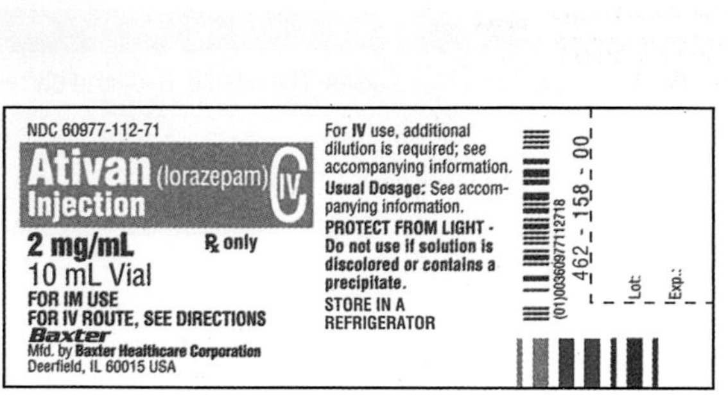

Figure 18-18 Ativan label.

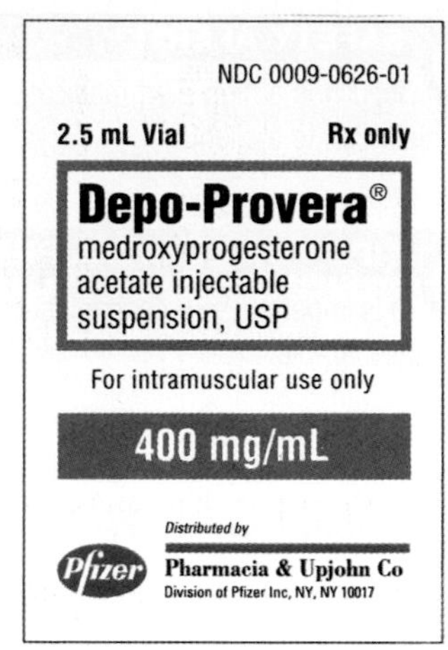

Figure 18-19 Depo-Provera label.

The Ativan label in Figure 18-18 tells us that the total size of the vial is 10 mL. The dosage strength is 2 mg per mL. The Depo-Provera label shown in Figure 18-19 indicates that the total vial size is 2.5 mL and that there are 400 mg per mL.

Dosage strengths for parenteral medications are commonly seen expressed as the amount of medication contained in a volume of solution and expressed in milliliters. Parenteral labels can also express the dosage strength for medications in percentage strengths, ratios, units, or milliequivalents. Read labels carefully to identify the unit of measure as well as the dosage strength.

PRACTICE PROBLEMS

Use the labels provided to answer the questions.

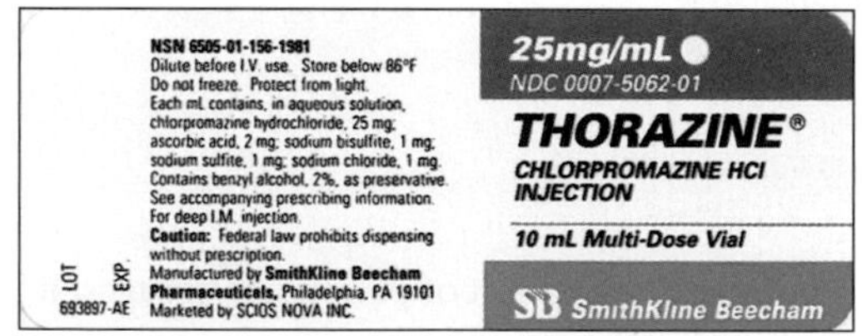

Using the Thorazine label above, answer the following questions:

12. a. What is the total volume of the vial? ____________

    b. What is the dosage strength? ____________

    c. If 50 mg was ordered, how many milliliters would this be? ____________

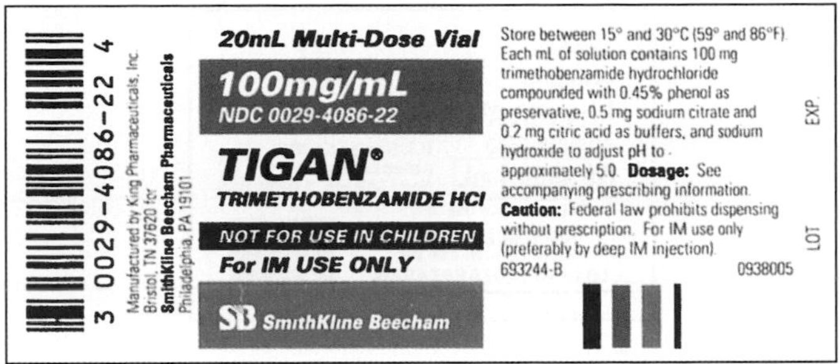

Using the Tigan label above, answer the following questions:

13. a. What is the total volume of the vial? ______________

b. What is the dosage strength? ______________

c. If 50 mg was ordered, how many milliliters would this be? ______________

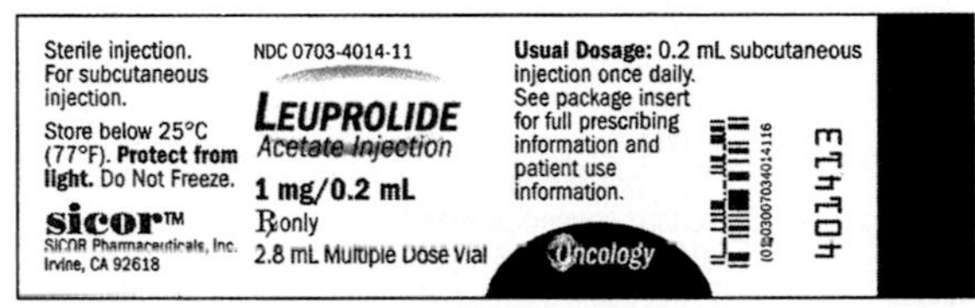

Using the leuprolide acetate label above, answer the following questions:

14. a. What is the total volume of the vial? ______________

b. What is the dosage strength? ______________

c. What is the route of administration? ______________

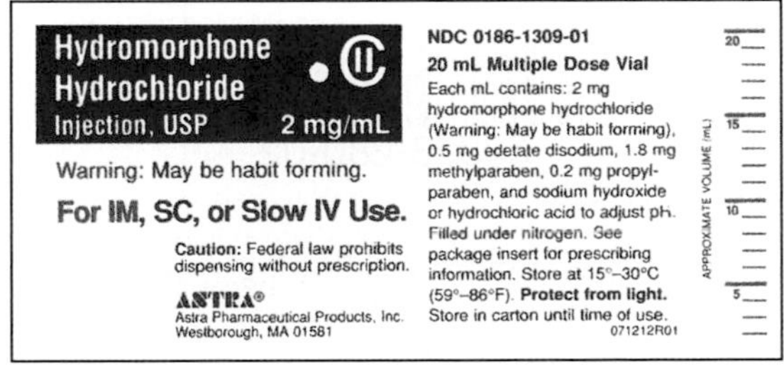

Using the hydromorphone label above, answer the following questions:

15. a. What is the total volume of the vial? ______________

b. What is the dosage strength? ______________

c. What is the controlled substance schedule? ______________

Exp./Lot
04-A132-R1
0.4 mL
HUMIRA®
adalimumab
20 mg/0.4 mL
NDC 0074-9374-02
U.S. License No. 0043 Rx only
Abbott Laboratories
North Chicago, IL 60064, USA
For Subcutaneous Use Only
(01)10300749374026

Using the Humira label above, answer the following questions:

16. a. What is the route of administration? ____________________

    b. What is the dosage strength? ____________________

NDC 63323-280-02 28002
FUROSEMIDE
INJECTION, USP
20 mg/2 mL
(10 mg/mL)
For IM or IV Use Rx only
2 mL Single Dose Vial
Preservative Free
Discard unused portion.
PROTECT FROM LIGHT.
Do not use if discolored.
Abraxis
Pharmaceutical Products
Schaumburg, IL 60173
401803C
LOT/EXP
3 63323-280-02 4

Using the furosemide label above, answer the following questions:

17. a. What is the total volume of the vial? ____________________

    b. What is the dosage strength? ____________________

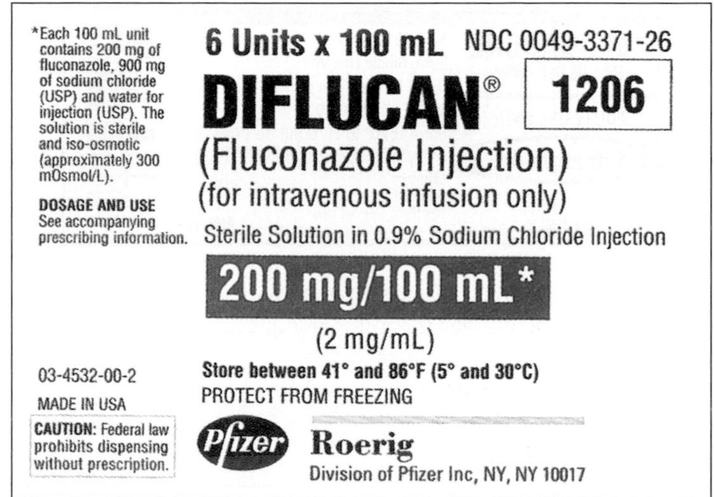

Using the Diflucan label above, answer the following questions:

18. a. What is the dosage strength? ____________________

    b. What is the route of administration? ____________________

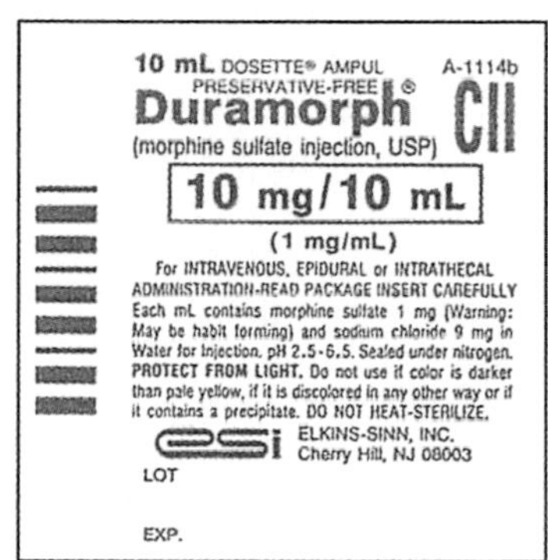

Using the Duramorph label above, answer the following questions:

19. a. What is the total volume of the ampule? ____________________

    b. What is the dosage strength? ____________________

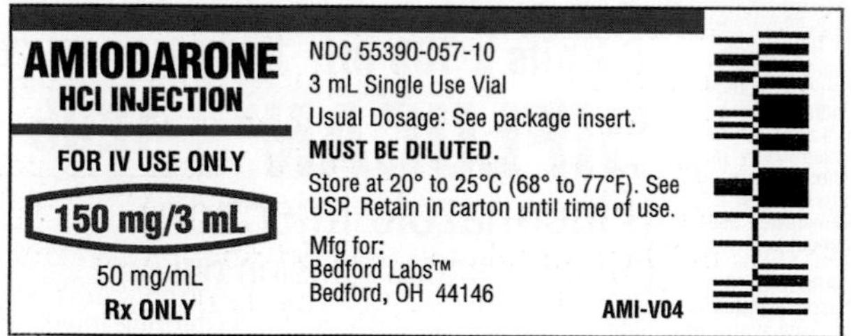

Using the Amiodarone label above, answer the following questions:

20. a. What is the total volume of the vial? ______________

b. What is the dosage strength? ______________

c. What is the route of administration? ______________

Answers on p. 417

Medications Labeled in Percentage Strengths

Medications that are labeled as percentage solutions give information such as the percentage of the solution and the total volume of the vial or ampule. Although percentage is used, metric measures are used as well. Example: In the figure below, which shows a label of lidocaine 1%, notice that there are 10 mg per mL. As discussed in Chapter 5, percentage solutions express the number of grams of the medication per 100 mL of solution. In the lidocaine label shown, lidocaine 1% contains 1 g of medication per 100 mL of solution, 1 g per 100 mL = 1,000 mg per 100 mL = 10 mg per mL.

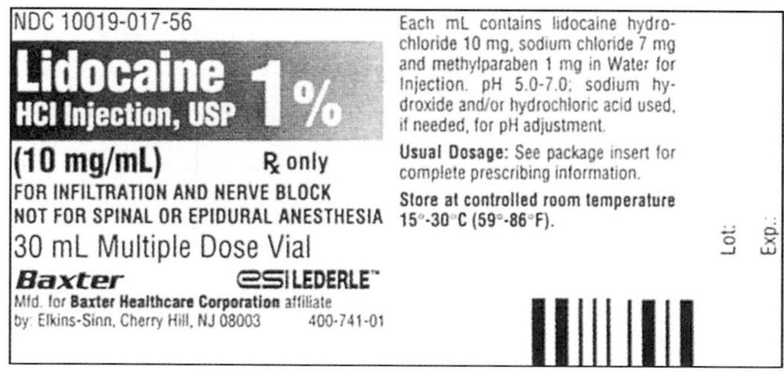

Often no calculation is necessary when medications expressed in percentage strength are given. The prescriber usually states the number of milliliters to prepare or may state it in the number of ampules or vials. Example: Calcium gluconate 10% may be ordered as "Administer one vial of 10% calcium gluconate or 10 mL of 10% calcium gluconate" (see label below).

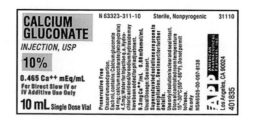

Solutions Expressed in Ratio Strength

A medication commonly expressed in terms of ratio strength is epinephrine. Medications expressed this way include metric measures as well and are often ordered by the number of milliliters. Example: Epinephrine may state 1 : 1,000 and indicate 1 mg per mL. Ratio solutions, as discussed in Chapter 4 on ratio and proportion, express the number of grams of the medication per total milliliters of solution. Epinephrine 1 : 1,000 contains 1 g medication per 1,000 mL solution, 1 g : 1,000 mL = 1,000 mg : 1,000 mL = 1 mg : 1 mL. (See the label below.)

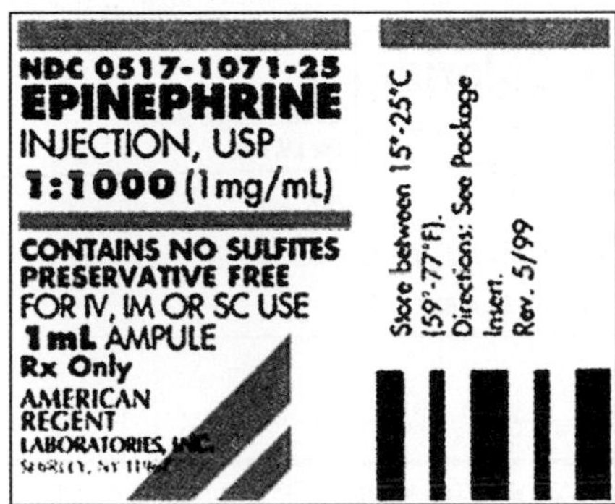

Parenteral Medications Measured in Units

Some medications measured in units for parenteral administration are heparin, Pitocin, insulin, and penicillin. Notice that the labels indicate how many units per milliliters. Examples: Insulin 100 units per mL, heparin 5,000 units per mL. Units express the amount of medication present in 1 mL of solution, and they are specific to the medication for which they are used. Units measure a medication in terms of its action (see heparin and insulin labels below).

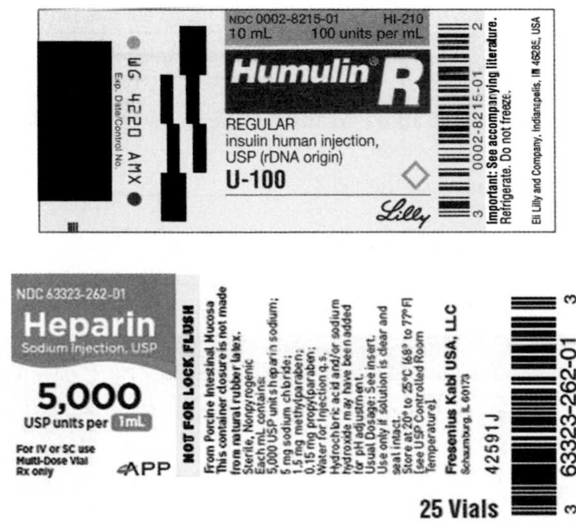

Parenteral Medications in Milliequivalents

Potassium and sodium bicarbonate are medications that are expressed in milliequivalents. Like units, milliequivalents are specific measurements that have no conversion to another system and are specific to the medication used. Milliequivalents (mEq) are used to measure electrolytes (e.g., potassium) and the ionic activity of a medication. Milliequivalents are also defined as an expression of the number of grams of a medication contained in 1 mL of a normal solution. This definition is often used by a chemist or pharmacist. (See Potassium label below.)

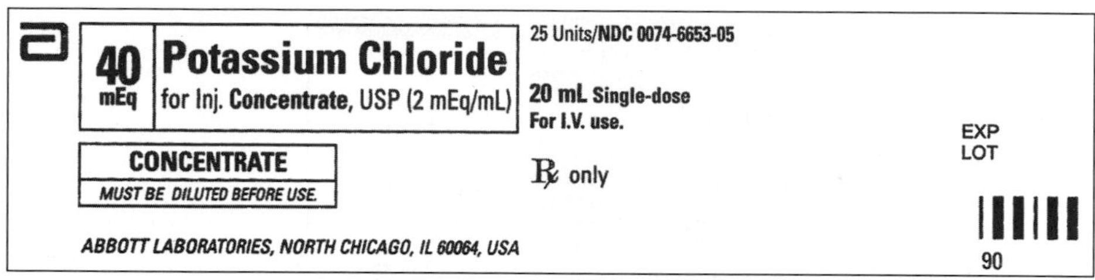

PRACTICE PROBLEMS

Use the labels provided to answer the questions.

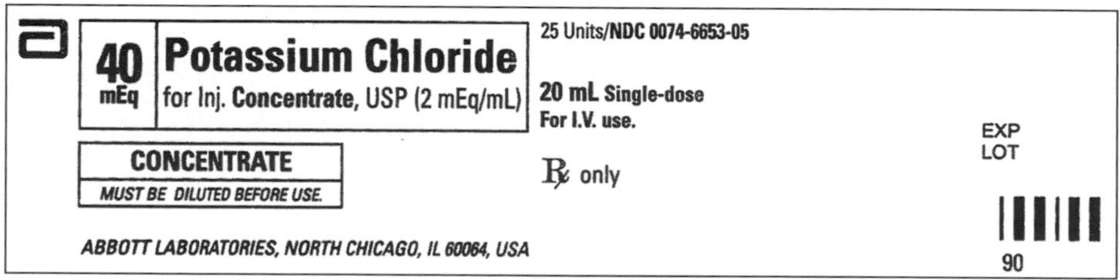

Use the potassium chloride label above to answer the following questions:

21. a. What is the total volume of the vial? __________

    b. What is the dosage in milliequivalents per milliliter? __________

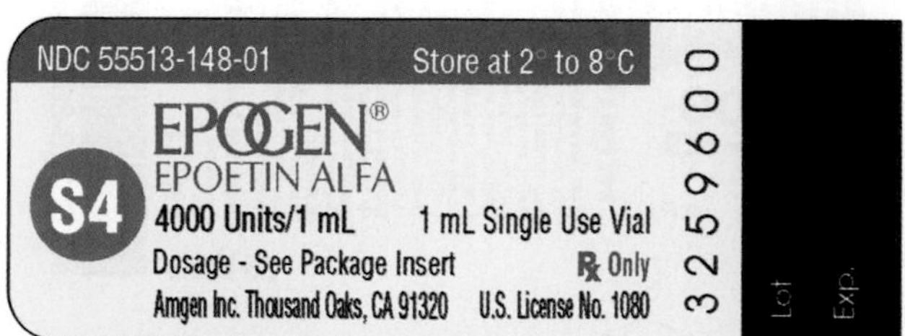

Use the Epogen label above to answer the following questions:

22. a. What is the total volume of the vial? __________

    b. What is the dosage strength? __________

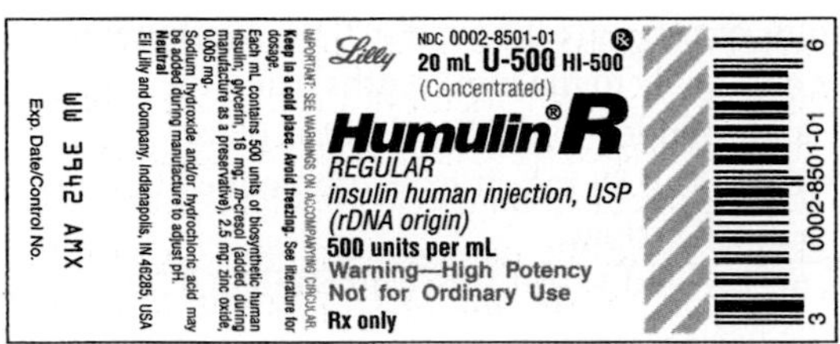

Use the insulin label above to answer the following questions:

23. a. What is the total volume of the vial? ______________________

    b. What is the dosage strength? ______________________

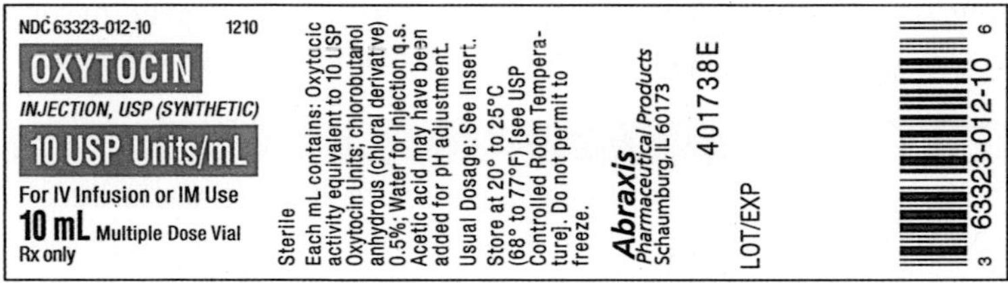
NDC 63323-012-10
1210
OXYTOCIN
INJECTION, USP (SYNTHETIC)
10 USP Units/mL
For IV Infusion or IM Use
10 mL Multiple Dose Vial
Rx only
Sterile
Each mL contains: Oxytocic activity equivalent to 10 USP Oxytocin Units; chlorobutanol anhydrous (chloral derivative) 0.5%; Water for Injection q.s. Acetic acid may have been added for pH adjustment.
Usual Dosage: See Insert.
Store at 20° to 25°C (68° to 77°F) [see USP Controlled Room Temperature]. Do not permit to freeze.
Abraxis
Pharmaceutical Products
Schaumburg, IL 60173
401738E
LOT/EXP
3 63323-012-10 6

Use the oxytocin label above to answer the following questions:

24. a. What is the total volume of the vial? ______________________

    b. What is the dosage strength? ______________________

Answers on pp. 417-418

TIPS FOR CLINICAL PRACTICE

It is important to read the labels on parenteral medications carefully. Labels on parenteral medications include a variety of units to express dosage strengths. To calculate dosages to administer, it is important to know the strength of the medication in solution per milliliter. Confusing dosage strength with total volume can lead to a medication error.

Calculating Parenteral Dosages

As previously stated, parenteral dosages can be calculated by using the same methods used to compute oral dosages. Ratio and proportion, the formula method, and dimensional analysis have been presented in earlier chapters. The following guidelines will help you calculate a dosage that is logical, reasonable, and accurate.

Guidelines for Calculating Parenteral Dosages

- To calculate parenteral dosages, convert if necessary, **THINK,** and calculate using one of the methods presented (ratio and proportion, the formula method, or dimensional analysis).

Calculate dosages and prepare injectable dosages using the following guidelines:

- The 3-mL syringe is calibrated in 0.1-mL increments. Round milliliters to the nearest tenth to measure in a 3-mL syringe; **never round to a whole unit.** If math calculation does not work out evenly to the tenths place, then carry division to the hundredths place (two decimal places) and round to the nearest tenth.

  Example: 1.75 mL = 1.8 mL

- The 1-mL (tuberculin syringe) is calibrated in 0.01-mL increments. If the math calculation does not work out evenly to the hundredths place, then the division is carried to the thousandths place and rounded to the hundredths place.
  Example: 0.876 mL = 0.88 mL. It is recommended that dosages less than 0.5 mL be measured with a 1-mL syringe.
- Large syringes (5-, 6-, 10-, and 12-mL) are calibrated in 0.2-mL increments. Dosages are also expressed to the nearest tenth.
- Dosages administered should be measured in milliliters, and the answer should be labeled accordingly.
- Standard U-100 insulin is administered and measured in units.

For injectable medications, there are guidelines as to the amount of medication that can be administered in a single site. It is recommended that when the amount exceeds the amount that can be administered in a single site, divide the amount into two injections. When administering medications by injection, the condition of the client, site selected, and absorption and consistency of the medication must be considered. Depending on his or her condition, a client may not be able to tolerate the maximum dosage volumes.

SAFETY ALERT!

When the dosage for parenteral administration exceeds the guidelines of volume that can be administered in a single injection site, the dosage should be questioned and calculation double-checked. Dosages larger than the maximum volume are rare and can cause harm to the client.

The maximum volume to administer in a single intramuscular site is as follows:

Intramuscular

- Average adult = 3 mL (for deltoid muscle, 1 mL)
- Children ages 6 to 12 years = 2 mL
- Children 0 to 5 years = 1 mL

It should be noted that IM injections are less common in the clinical setting than in the past.

Subcutaneous

The maximum for an adult is 1 mL.

Intravenous

Injectable solutions that are added to an IV solution may have a volume greater than 5 mL.

TIPS FOR CLINICAL PRACTICE

It is critical to choose the correct size syringe to ensure accurate measurement.

Calculating Injectable Medications According to the Syringe

Now that you have an understanding of syringes and guidelines, let's begin calculating dosages.

Now, with the guidelines in mind, let's look at some sample problems. Regardless of what method you use to calculate, the following steps are used:

1. Check to make sure everything is in the same system and unit of measure.
2. Think critically and estimate what the logical volume to administer should be.
3. Calculate: use ratio and proportion, the formula method, or dimensional analysis to calculate the dosage.
4. Consider the type of syringe being used. **The cardinal rule should always be that any dosage given must be able to be measured accurately in the syringe you are using.**

Let's look at some sample problems calculating parenteral dosages.

Example 1: Order: Gentamicin 75 mg IM q8h

Available: Gentamicin labeled 40 mg per mL

Note: No conversion is necessary here. Think—The dosage ordered is going to be more than 1 mL but less than 2 mL. Set up and solve.

✓ Solution Using Ratio and Proportion

$$40 \text{ mg} : 1 \text{ mL} = 75 \text{ mg} : x \text{ mL}$$

$$\frac{40x}{40} = \frac{75}{40}$$

$$x = 1.87 = 1.9 \text{ mL}$$

Answer: 1.9 mL

The answer here is rounded to the nearest tenth of a milliliter. Remember that you are using a small hypodermic syringe marked in tenths of a milliliter.

✓ Solution Using the Formula Method

$$\frac{\text{(D) } 75 \text{ mg}}{\text{(H) } 40 \text{ mg}} \times \text{(Q) } 1 \text{ mL} = x \text{ mL}$$

$$x = \frac{75}{40}$$

$$x = 1.87 = 1.9 \text{ mL}$$

Answer: 1.9 mL

✓ Solution Using Dimensional Analysis

$$x \text{ mL} = \frac{1 \text{ mL}}{40 \cancel{\text{mg}}} \times \frac{75 \cancel{\text{mg}}}{1}$$

$$x = \frac{75}{40}$$

$$x = 1.87 = 1.9 \text{ mL}$$

Answer: 1.9 mL

Refer to the syringe below illustrating 1.9 mL shaded in on the syringe.

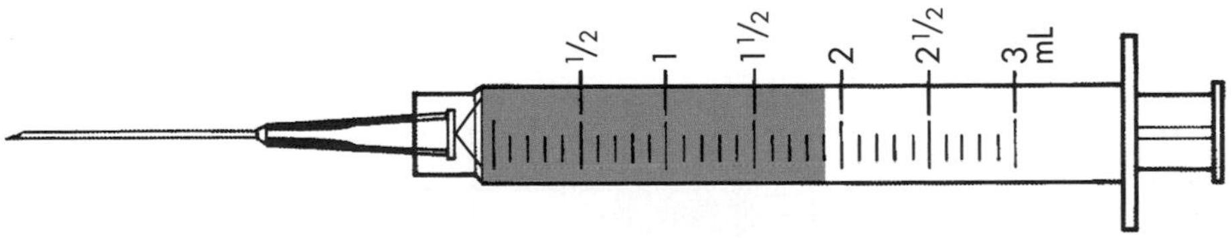

Example 2: Order: Ceftriaxone 0.25 g IM stat q12h

Available: Ceftriaxone labeled 350 mg per 1 mL

In this problem, a conversion is necessary. Equivalent: 1,000 mg = 1 g. Convert what is ordered to what is available: 0.25 g = 250 mg.

Think—The dosage you will need to give is less than 1 mL, and it is being given intramuscularly. The dosage therefore should fall within the range that is safe for IM administration. The solution, after making conversion, is as follows:

✓ Solution Using Ratio and Proportion

$$350 \text{ mg} : 1 \text{ mL} = 250 \text{ mg} : x \text{ mL}$$

$$\frac{350x}{350} = \frac{250}{350}$$

$$x = \frac{250}{350}$$

$$x = 0.71 = 0.7 \text{ mL}$$

Answer: 0.7 mL

✓ Solution Using the Formula Method

$$\frac{\text{(D) } 250 \text{ mg}}{\text{(H) } 350 \text{ mg}} \times \text{(Q) } 1 \text{ mL} = x \text{ mL}$$

$$x = \frac{250}{350}$$

$$x = 0.71 = 0.7 \text{ mL}$$

✓ Solution Using Dimensional Analysis

$$x \text{ mL} = \frac{1 \text{ mL}}{350 \cancel{\text{mg}}} \times \frac{1{,}000 \cancel{\text{mg}}}{1 \cancel{\text{g}}} \times \frac{0.25 \cancel{\text{g}}}{1}$$

$$x = \frac{1{,}000 \times 0.25}{350}$$

$$x = \frac{250}{350}$$

$$x = 0.71 = 0.7 \text{ mL}$$

Answer: 0.7 mL

Refer to the syringe below illustrating 0.7 mL drawn up.

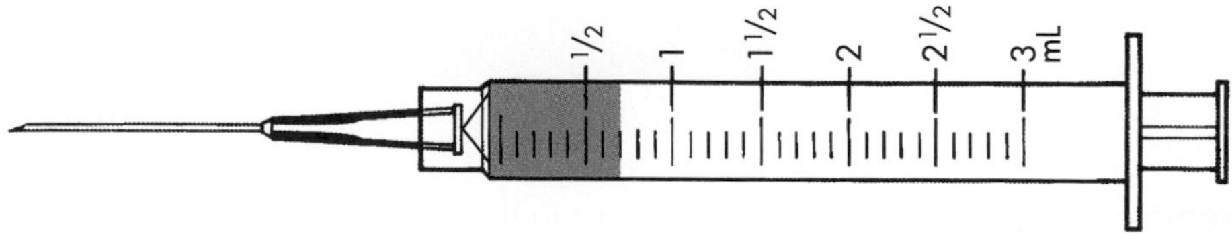

Example 3: Order: Atropine sulfate 0.6 mg IM stat

Available: Atropine sulfate in 20-mL vial labeled 0.4 mg per mL

PROBLEM SETUP

1. No conversion is necessary.
2. Think—You will need more than 1 mL to administer the required dosage.
3. Set up the problem, and calculate the dosage to be administered.

✓ Solution Using Ratio and Proportion

$$0.4\text{ mg} : 1\text{ mL} = 0.6\text{ mg} : x\text{ mL}$$

$$\frac{0.4x}{0.4} = \frac{0.6}{0.4}$$

$$x = \frac{0.6}{0.4}$$

$$x = 1.5\text{ mL}$$

Answer: 1.5 mL

Note that some small hypodermics have fraction markings; however, milliliter is metric and should be stated by using a decimal.

✓ Solution Using the Formula Method

$$\frac{\text{(D) } 0.6\text{ mg}}{\text{(H) } 0.4\text{ mg}} \times \text{(Q) } 1\text{ mL} = x\text{ mL}$$

$$x = \frac{0.6}{0.4}$$

$$x = 1.5\text{ mL}$$

Answer: 1.5 mL

✓ Solution Using Dimensional Analysis

$$x\text{ mL} = \frac{1\text{ mL}}{0.4\text{ }\cancel{\text{mg}}} \times \frac{0.6\text{ }\cancel{\text{mg}}}{1}$$

$$x = \frac{0.6}{0.4}$$

$$x = 1.5\text{ mL}$$

Answer: 1.5 mL

Refer to the illustration below showing 1.5 mL shaded in on the syringe.

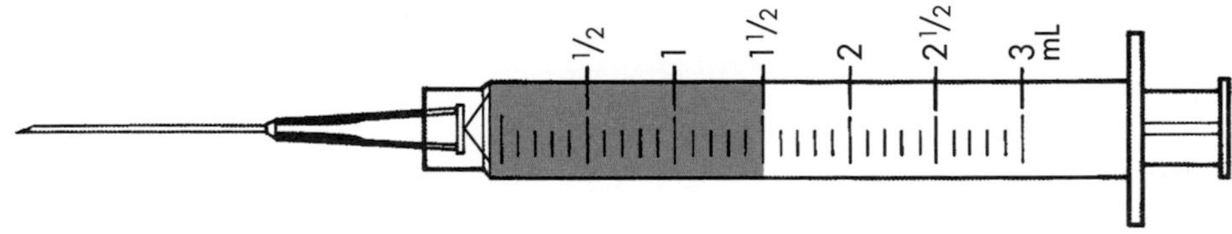

Calculating Dosages for Medications in Units

As previously mentioned, certain medications are measured in units. Some medications measured in units include vitamins, antibiotics, insulin, and heparin. The calculation of insulin will be discussed in Chapter 20. Insulin syringes are used for insulin only. In determining the dosage to administer when medications are measured in units, use the same steps as with other parenteral medications. Dosages of certain medications such as heparin are administered with a tuberculin syringe, as opposed to a hypodermic syringe (2, $2\frac{1}{2}$, 3 mL). Because of its effects, heparin is never rounded off; rather, exact dosages are given. Heparin will also be discussed in more detail in Chapter 23. Let's look at sample problems with units.

Example 1: Order: Heparin 750 units subcut daily

Available: Heparin 1,000 units per mL

Using a 1-mL (tuberculin) syringe, calculate the dosage to be administered.

✓ PROBLEM SETUP

1. No conversion is required. No conversion exists for units.
2. Think—The dosage to be given is less than 1 mL. This dosage can be accurately measured in a 1-mL tuberculin syringe. Heparin is administered in exact dosages.
3. Set up the problem, and calculate the dosage to be given.

SAFETY ALERT!

Because of the action of heparin, an exact dosage is crucial; the dosage should not be rounded off.

✓ Solution Using Ratio and Proportion

$$1{,}000 \text{ units} : 1 \text{ mL} = 750 \text{ units} : x \text{ mL}$$

$$\frac{1{,}000x}{1{,}000} = \frac{750}{1{,}000}$$

$$x = \frac{75}{1{,}000}$$

$$x = 0.75 \text{ mL}$$

Answer: 0.75 mL

✓ Solution Using the Formula Method

$$\frac{\text{(D) } 750 \text{ units}}{\text{(H) } 1{,}000 \text{ units}} \times \text{(Q) } 1 \text{ mL} = x \text{ mL}$$

$$x = \frac{750}{1{,}000}$$

$$x = 0.75 \text{ mL}$$

Answer: 0.75 mL

✓ Solution Using Dimensional Analysis

$$x \text{ mL} = \frac{1 \text{ mL}}{1{,}00\cancel{0} \cancel{\text{units}}} \times \frac{75\cancel{0} \cancel{\text{units}}}{1}$$

Note cancellation of zeros to make numbers smaller.)

$$x = \frac{75}{100}$$

$$x = 0.75 \text{ mL}$$

Answer: 0.75 mL

Refer to the syringe illustrating 0.75 mL shaded in.

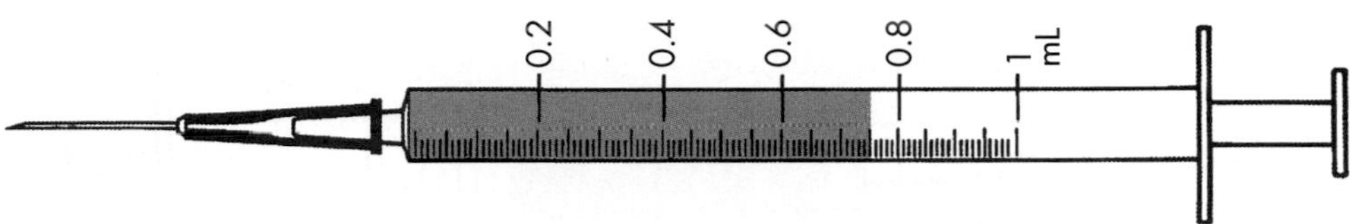

Example 2: Order: Penicillin G procaine, 500,000 units IM b.i.d.

Available: Penicillin G procaine labeled 300,000 units per mL

✓ PROBLEM SETUP

1. No conversion is required.
2. Think—The dosage ordered is more than the available strength. Therefore, more than 1 mL would be required to administer the dosage.
3. Set up the problem using ratio and proportion, the formula method, or dimensional analysis to calculate the dosage.

✓ Solution Using Ratio and Proportion

$$300{,}000 \text{ units} : 1 \text{ mL} = 500{,}000 \text{ units} : x \text{ mL}$$

$$\frac{300{,}000x}{300{,}000} = \frac{500{,}000}{300{,}000}$$

$$x = 1.66 \text{ mL} = 1.7 \text{ mL}$$

Answer: 1.7 mL

Note: Math was carried two decimal places to round to 1.7 mL. Small hypodermic marked in tenths of a mL.

✓ Solution Using the Formula Method

$$\frac{(D)\ 500{,}000 \text{ units}}{(H)\ 300{,}000 \text{ units}} \times (Q)\ 1 \text{ mL} = x \text{ mL}$$

$$x = \frac{5\cancel{00{,}000}}{3\cancel{00{,}000}}$$

$$x = 1.66 = 1.7 \text{ mL}$$

Answer: 1.7 mL

✓ Solution Using Dimensional Analysis

$$x \text{ mL} = \frac{1 \text{ mL}}{300{,}000 \cancel{\text{units}}} \times \frac{500{,}000 \cancel{\text{units}}}{1}$$

$$x = \frac{5\cancel{00{,}000}}{3\cancel{00{,}000}}$$

$$x = 1.66 = 1.7 \text{ mL}$$

Answer: 1.7 mL

Refer to the syringe illustrating 1.7 mL shaded in.

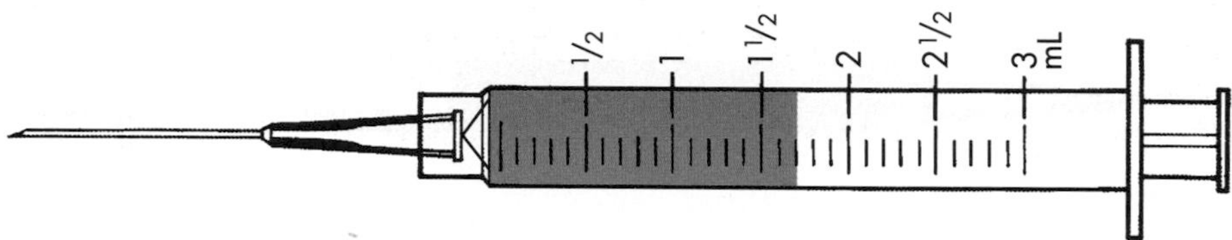

SAFETY ALERT!

Read orders carefully when they are expressed in units. Units should **NOT** be abbreviated in orders. To avoid confusion, The Joint Commission (TJC) has placed the abbreviations for units (U) on the "do not use" list. This abbreviation is also on ISMP's (Institute for Safe Medication Practices') Error Prone Abbreviations, Symbols, and Dose Designations. Prescribers are required to write out the word units to help prevent misinterpretation of an order—for example, "50 U" as "500 units." (Notice that the U is almost closed; it could be mistaken for a zero and misinterpreted as 500 units.) This error could be fatal.

Mixing Medications in the Same Syringe

Two medications may be mixed in one syringe if they are compatible with each other and the total amount does not exceed the amount that can be safely administered in a site. Always consult a reliable reference in regard to compatibility of medications before mixing medications.

When mixing two medications for administration in one syringe, calculate the dosage to be administered in milliliters to the nearest tenth for each of the medications ordered. Then add the results to find the total volume to be combined and administered.

Example: Order: Demerol 65 mg IM and Vistaril 25 mg IM q4h p.r.n. for pain

Available: Demerol 75 mg per mL and Vistaril 50 mg per mL

Solution: Demerol dosage 0.86 = 0.9 mL

Visatril dosage 0.5 mL

0.9 mL Demerol + 0.5 mL Vistaril = 1.4 mL (total volume)

Dosage shaded in one syringe:

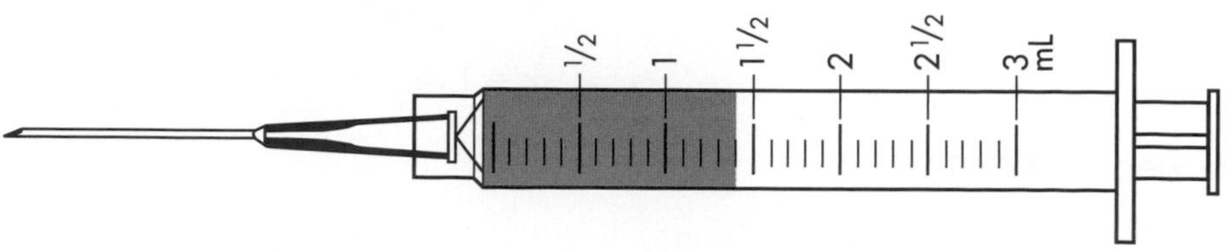

POINTS TO REMEMBER

- Read labels carefully. Do not confuse dosage strength with total volume.
- There is no conversion of units and milliequivalents.
- Do not exceed the dosage administration guidelines for parental administration. (IM—maximum 3 mL for an average-size adult, 1 mL per site for deltoid, 2 mL for children ages 6–12, 0–5 years 1 mL.)
- Subcut maximum 1 mL.
- Calculate parenteral dosage problems using any of the methods presented (ratio and proportion, formula method, or dimensional analysis).
- 3-mL syringe calibrated in 0.1 mL. Round mL to the nearest tenth.
- 1-mL syringe calibrated in 0.01-mL and 0.1 increments. Math that does not terminate evenly in hundredths is carried to thousandths and rounded to hundredths.
- 5-, 6-, and 12-mL syringes are calibrated in 0.2 mL. Dosages are expressed to the nearest tenth.
- Two medications can be administered in the same syringe if compatible. Calculate the dosage to be administered in mL to the nearest tenth for each of the medications. Add the result to get the total volume to administer.
- Choose the correct size syringe for the dosage to administer. Read the calibrations carefully.

PRACTICE **PROBLEMS**

Calculate the dosages for the problems below, and indicate the number of milliliters you will administer. Shade in the dosage on the syringe provided. Use medication labels or information provided to calculate the volume necessary to administer the dosage ordered. Express your answers in milliliters to the nearest tenth except where indicated.

25. Order: Compazine 10 mg IM q4h p.r.n.

    Available:

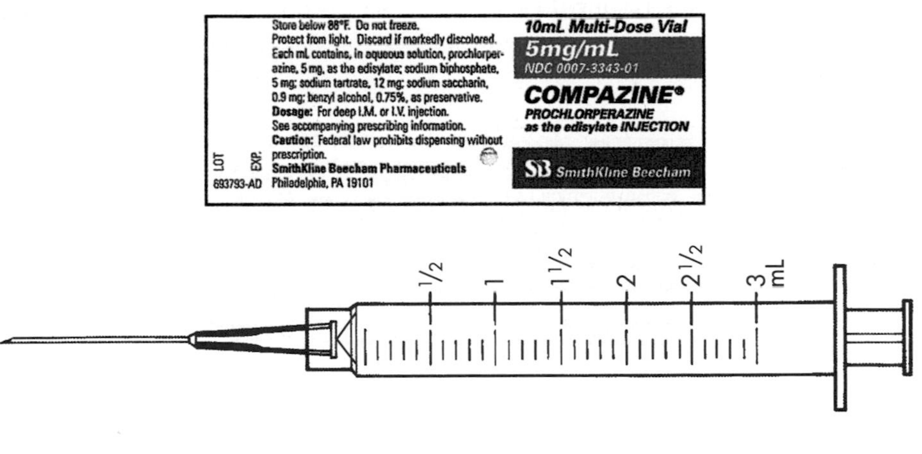

____

26. Order: Thiamine 75 mg IM daily.

Available:

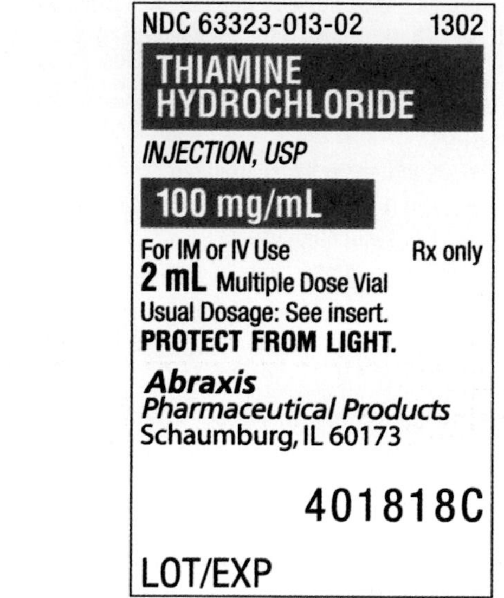

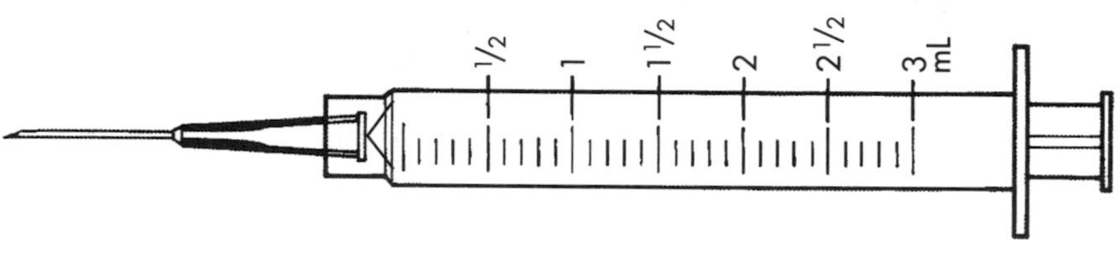

____

27. Order: Phenobarbital 120 mg IM at bedtime.

Available:

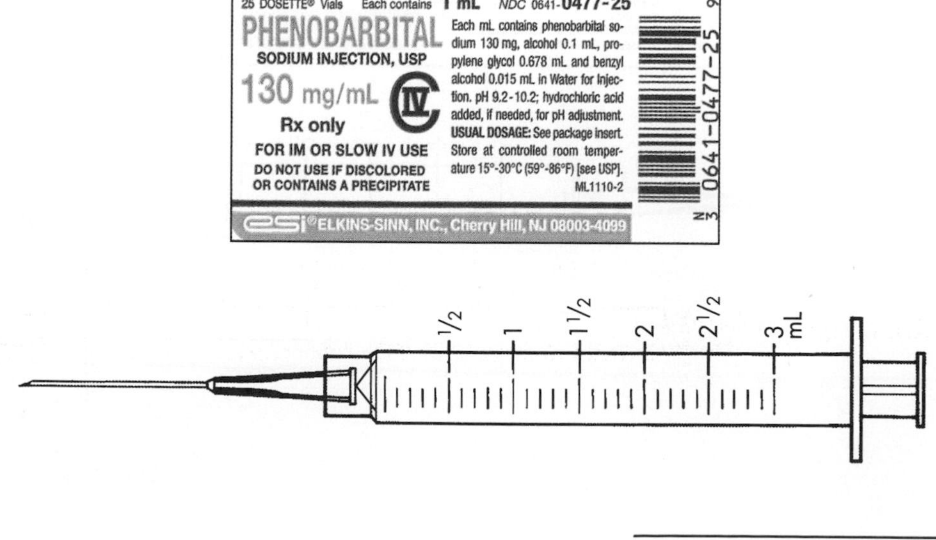

____

28. Order: Valium (diazepam) 8 mg IM q4h p.r.n. for agitation.

Available:

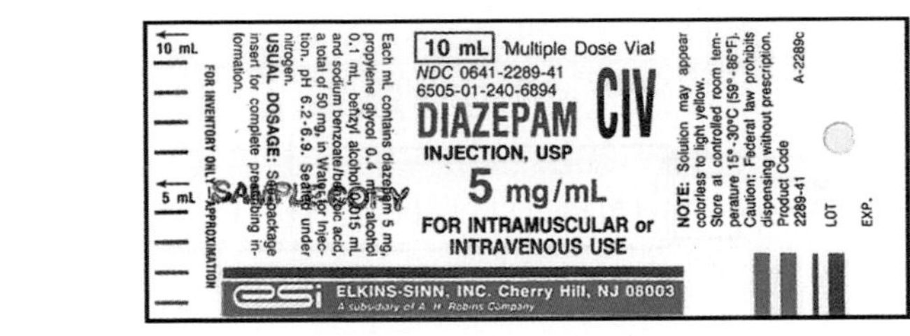

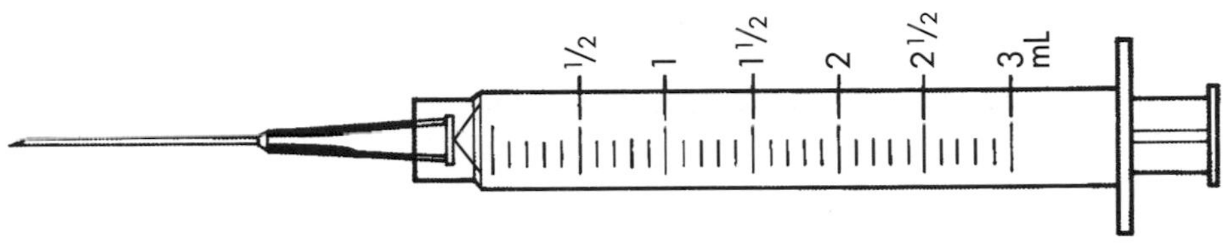

____

29. Order: Sandostatin 0.05 mg subcut daily.

Available:

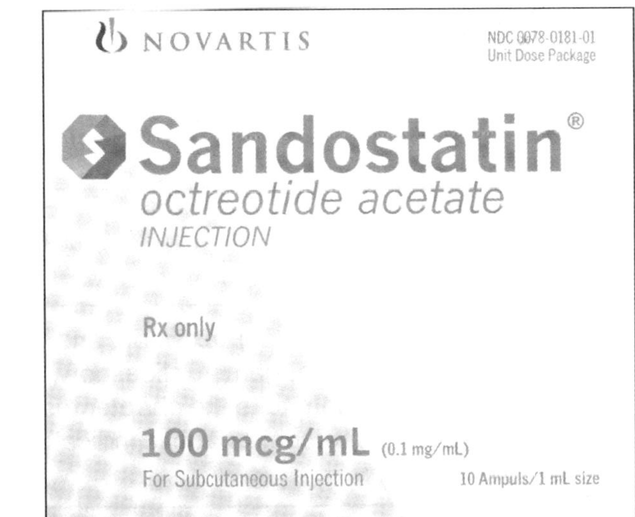

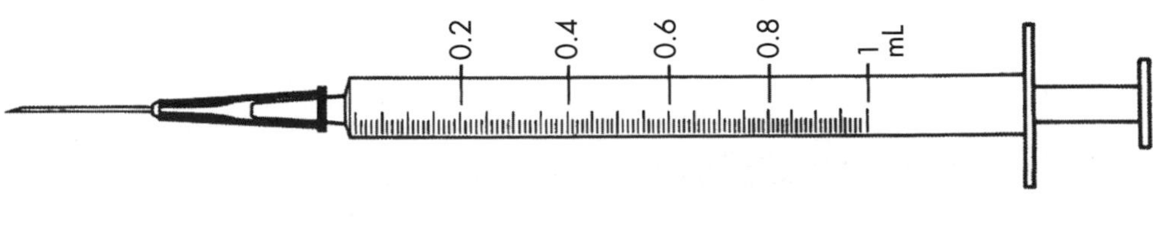

____

30. Order: Demerol 50 mg IM and Vistaril 25 mg IM q4h p.r.n. for pain.

    Available: Demerol labeled 75 mg per mL
    Vistaril labeled 50 mg per mL

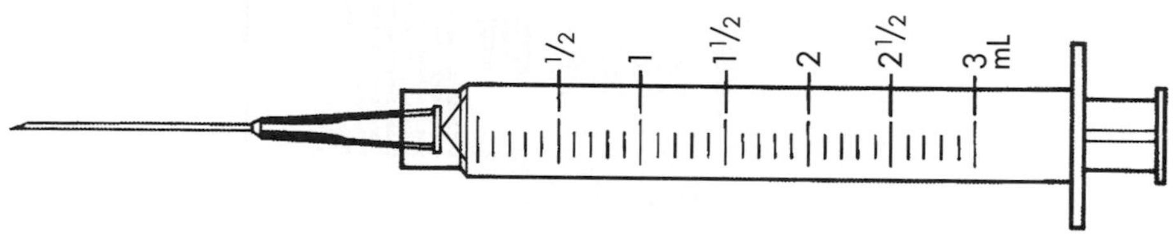

____

31. Order: Haloperidol decanoate 125 mg IM monthly.

    Available:

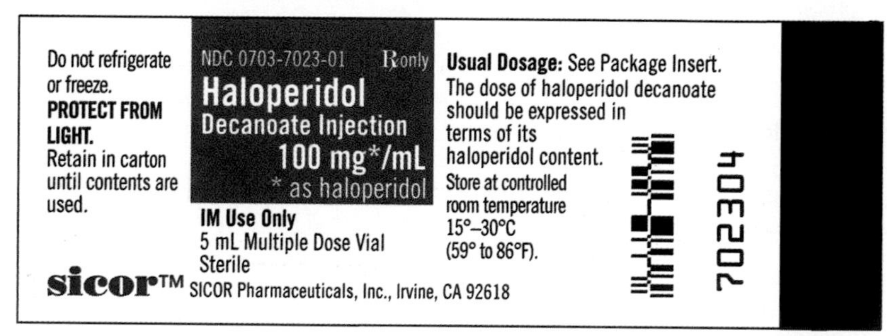

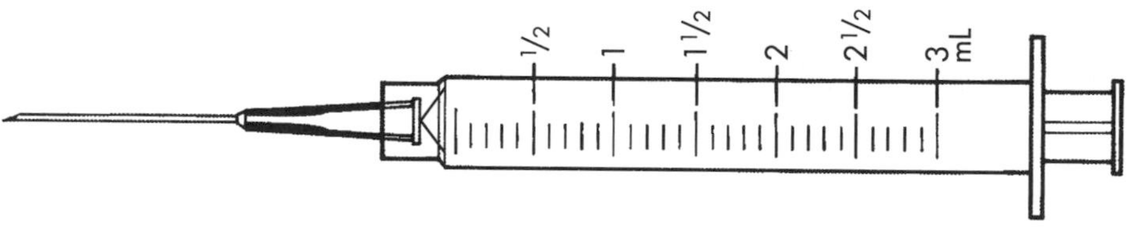

____

32. Order: Heparin 5,000 units subcut b.i.d.

    Available: Heparin 20,000 units per mL

    Express your answer in hundredths.

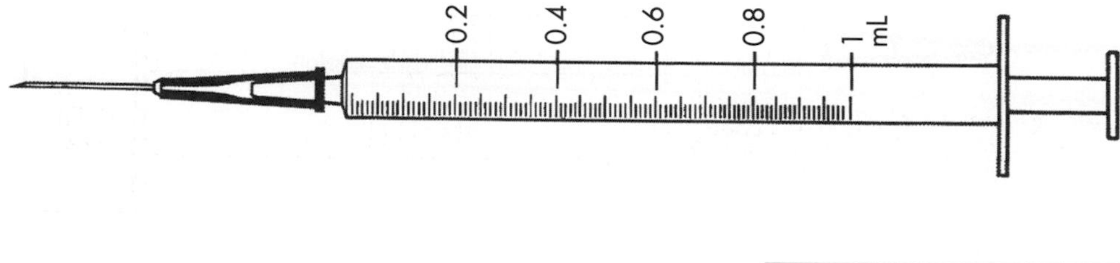

____

33. Order: Morphine sulfate 15 mg IM q4h p.r.n. for pain.

Available:

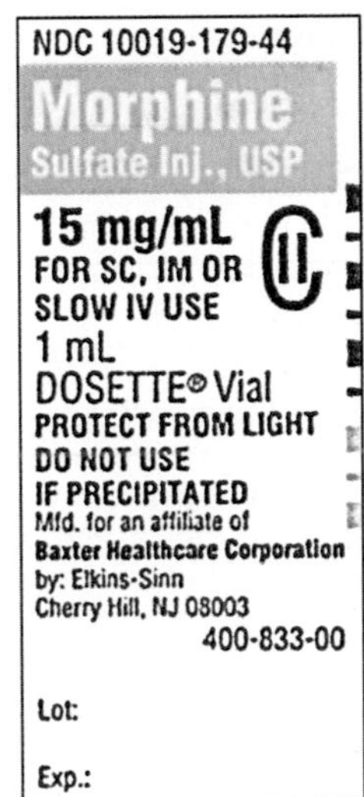

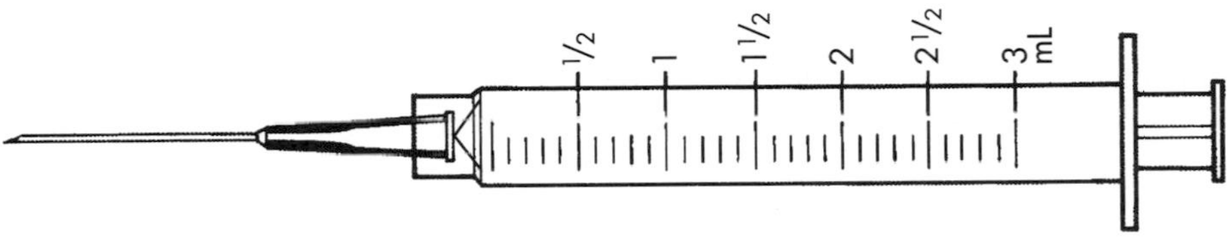

____

34. Order: Lasix (furosemide) 20 mg IM stat.

Available:

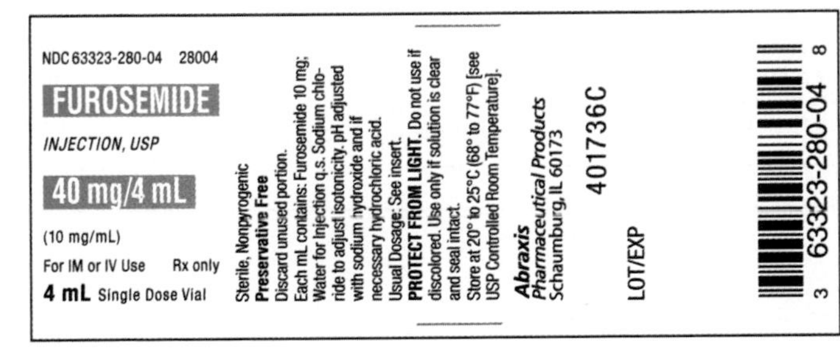

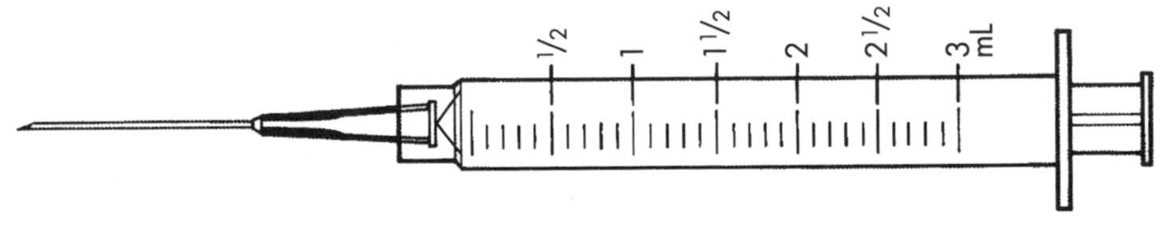

____

Answers on p. 417-418

CLINICAL REASONING

Scenario: Prescriber ordered the following:

Hydroxyzine 50 mg IM q4h p.r.n. for anxiety.

The nurse, in error, administered hydralazine 50 mg IM from a vial labeled 20 mg per mL and administered 2.5 mL.

a. What client right was violated? ______________________

b. What contributed to the error made? ______________________

c. What is the potential outcome from the error? ______________________

d. What measures could have been taken to prevent the error? ______________________

Answers on p. 419

CHAPTER REVIEW

Calculate the dosages for the problems that follow, and indicate the number of milliliters you will administer. Shade in the dosage on the syringe provided. Use medication labels or information provided to calculate the volume necessary to administer the dosage ordered. Express your answers to the nearest tenth except where indicated.

1. Order: Clindamycin 0.3 g IM q6h.

   Available:

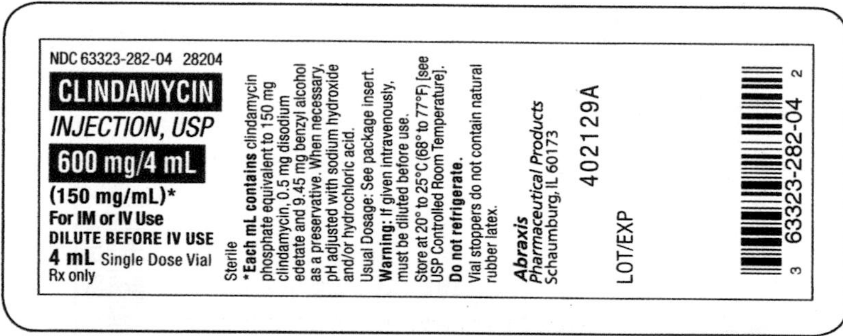

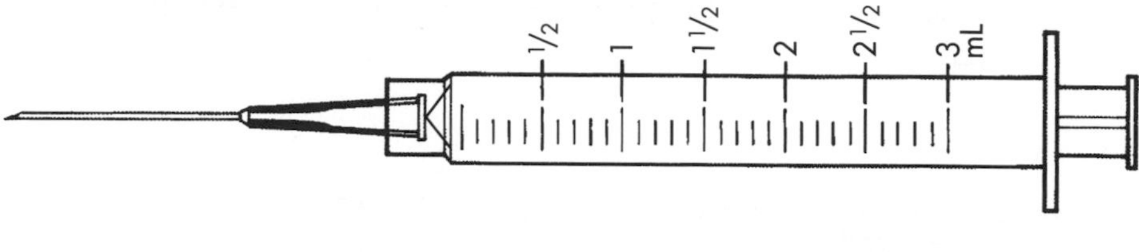

____

2. Order: Sandostatin 175 mcg subcut q12h. (Express your answer in hundredths.)

Available:

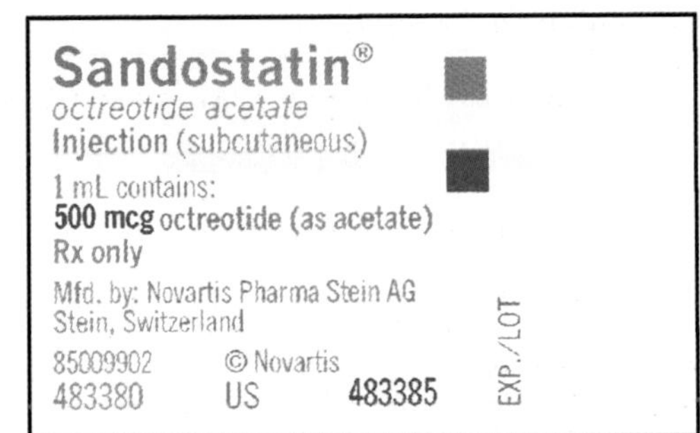

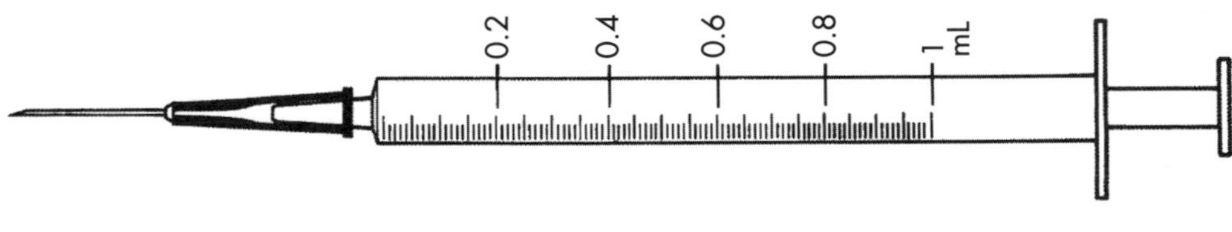

3. Order: Ketorolac 25 mg IM q6h p.r.n. for pain.

Available:

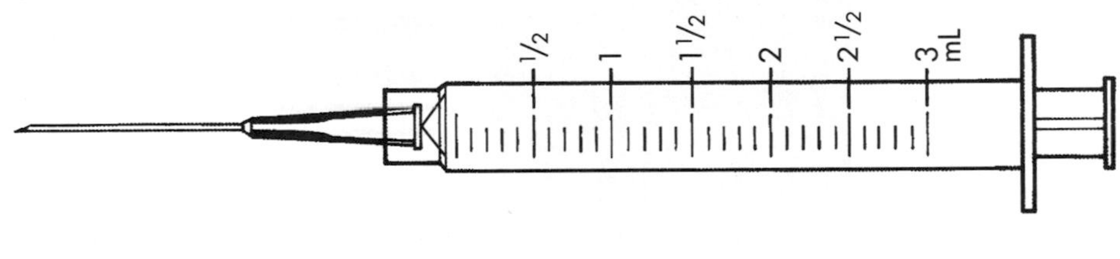

4. Order: Digoxin 100 mcg IM daily.

Available:

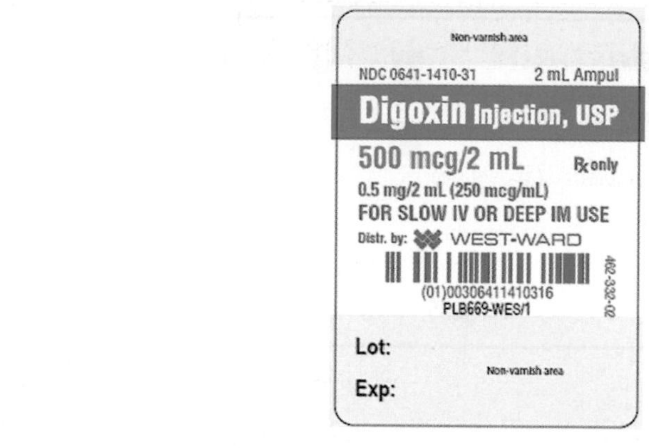

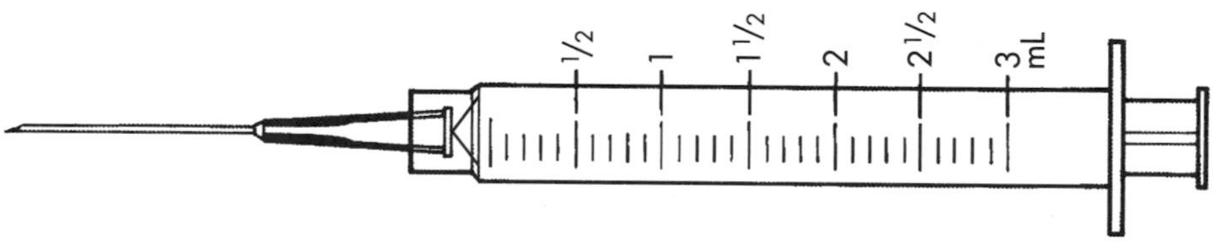

____

5. Order: Dilaudid HP 4 mg subcut q4h p.r.n. for pain.

Available:

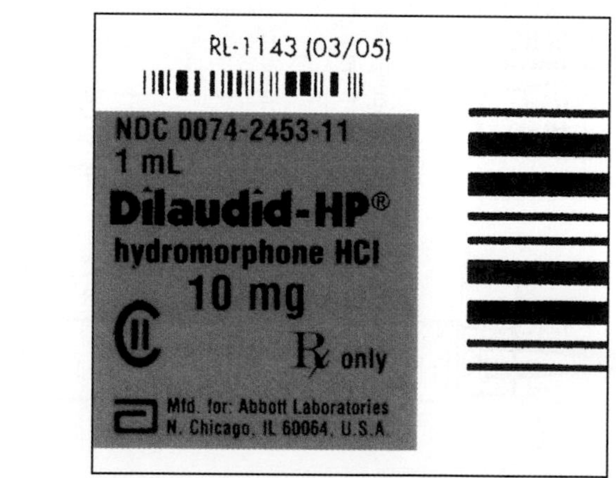

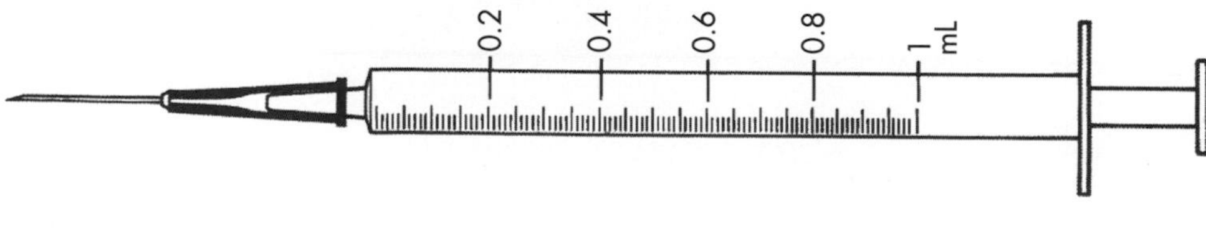

____

6. Order: Bicillin C-R (900/300) 1,200,000 units IM stat.

Available:

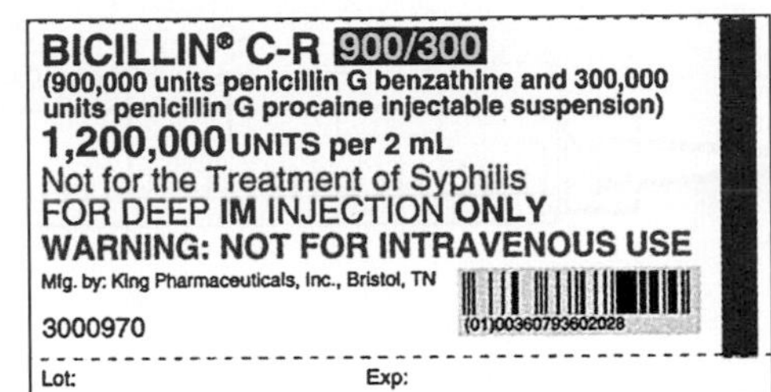

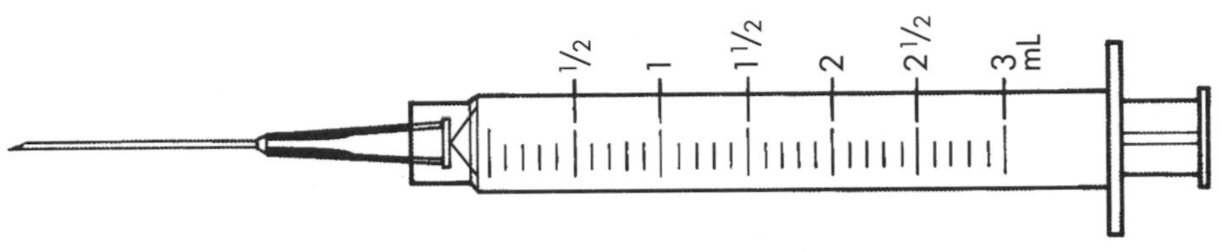

____

7. Order: Methylprednisolone 100 mg IV q8h for 2 doses.

Available:

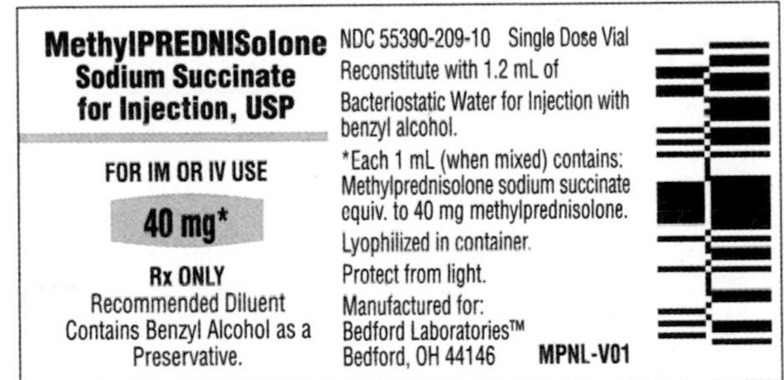

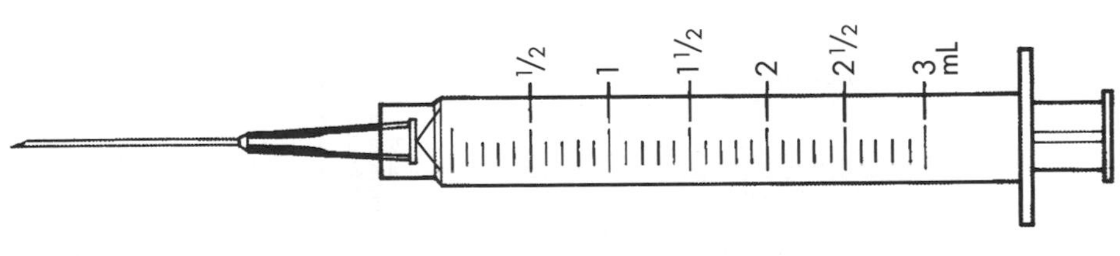

____

8. Order: Methergine 0.4 mg IM q4h for 3 doses.

   Available: Methergine labeled 0.2 mg per mL

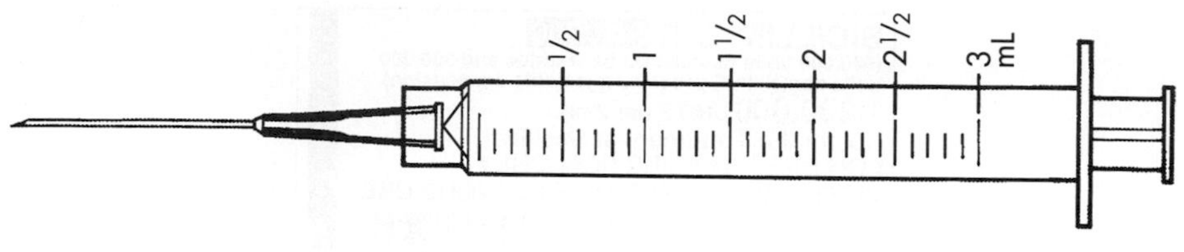

____

9. Order: Heparin 8,000 units subcut q12h.

   Available:

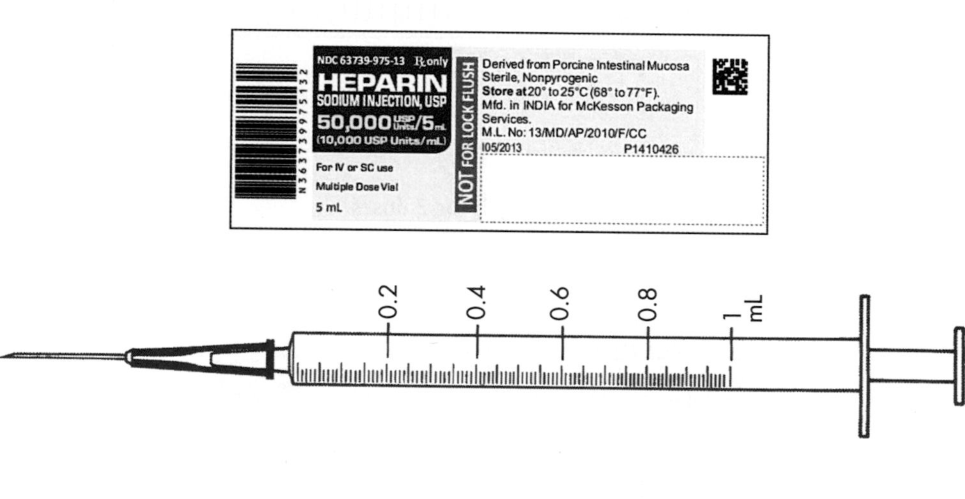

____

10. Order: Dilantin 200 mg IV stat.

    Available:

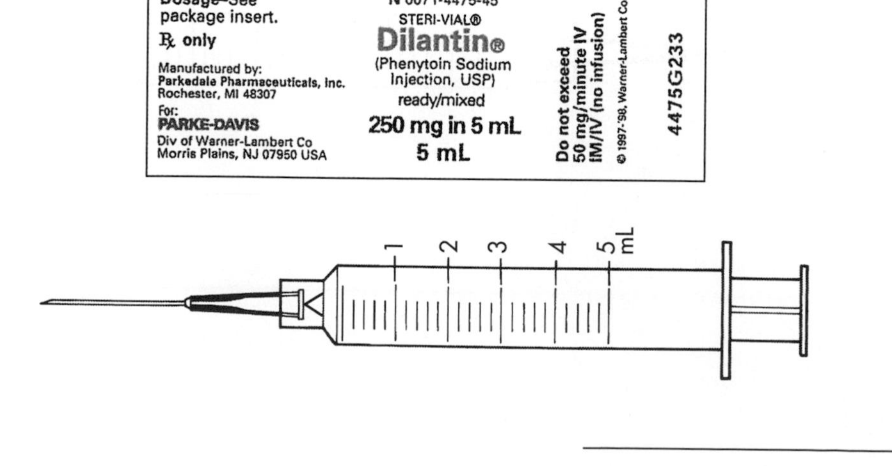

____

11. Order: Vitamin K (AquaMEPHYTON) 10 mg IM daily for 3 days.

Available:

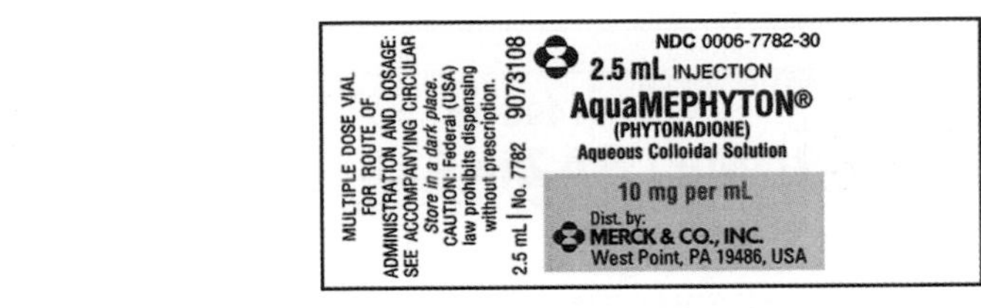

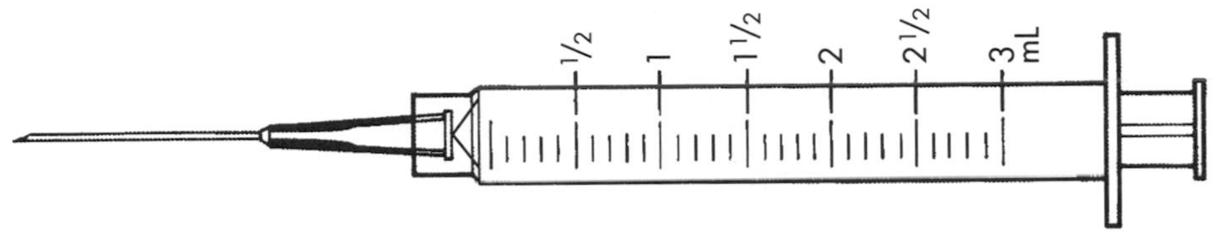

____

12. Order: Famotidine 40 mg IV at bedtime.

Available:

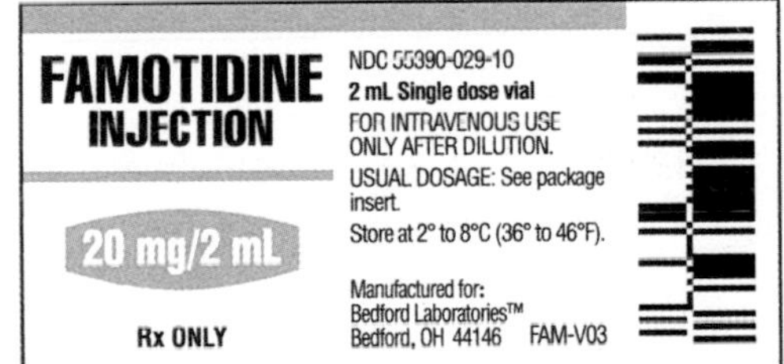

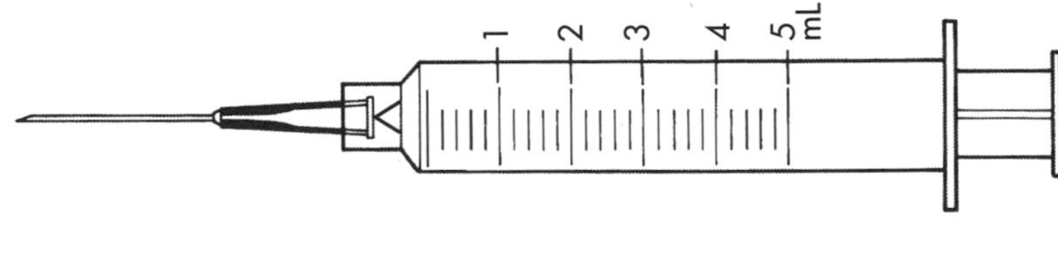

____

13. Order: Phenergan (promethazine HCl) 25 mg IM q4h p.r.n. for nausea.

 Available:

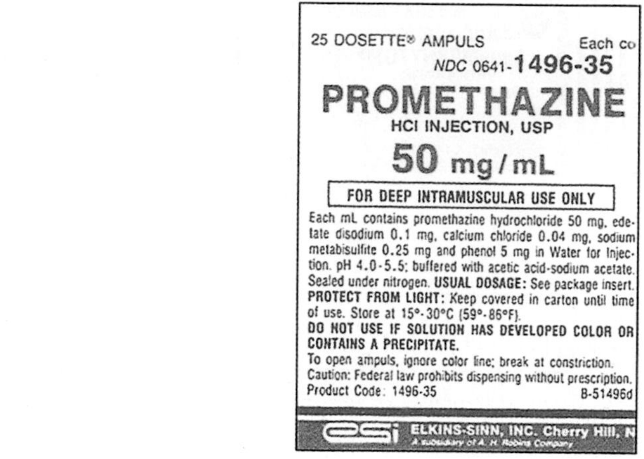

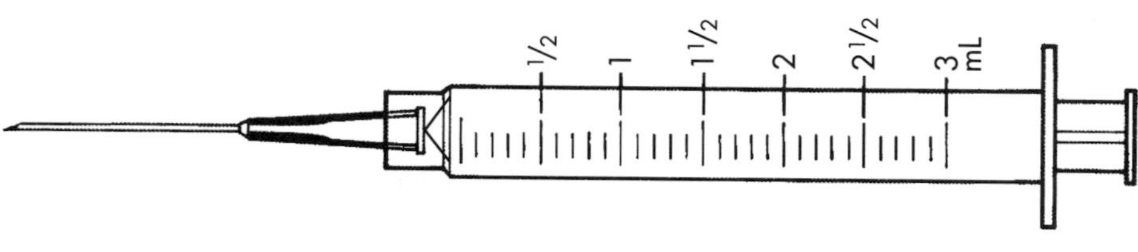

____

14. Order: Stadol 1.5 mg IM q4h p.r.n. for pain.

 Available: Stadol labeled 2 mg per mL

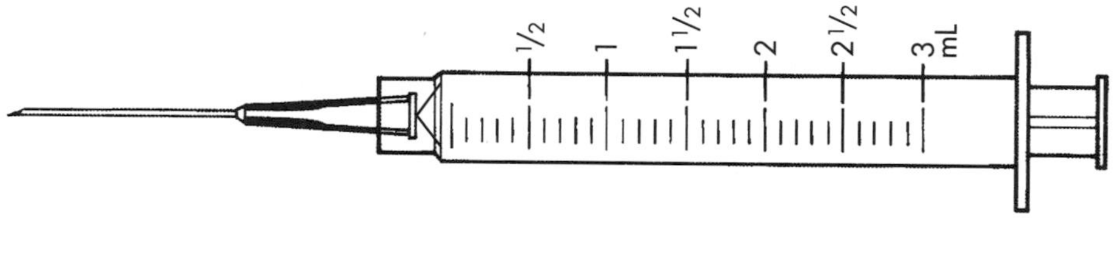

____

15. Order: Tobramycin 50 mg IM q8h.

Available:

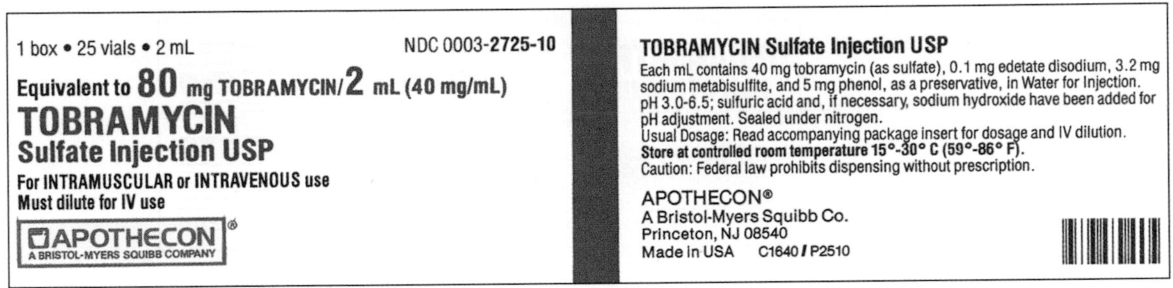

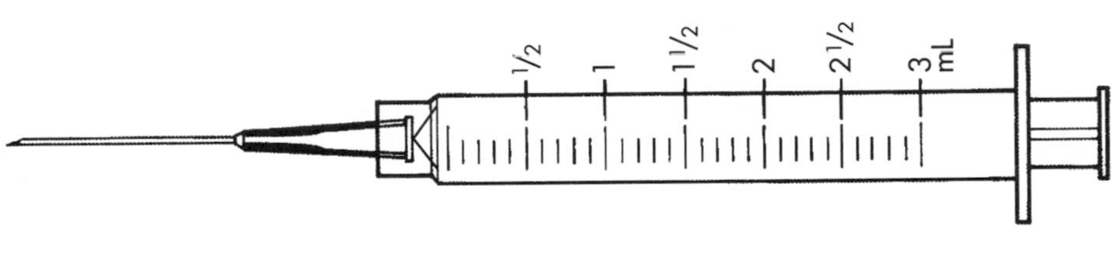

____

16. Order: Diphenhydramine 25 mg IM q6h p.r.n. for itching.

Available:

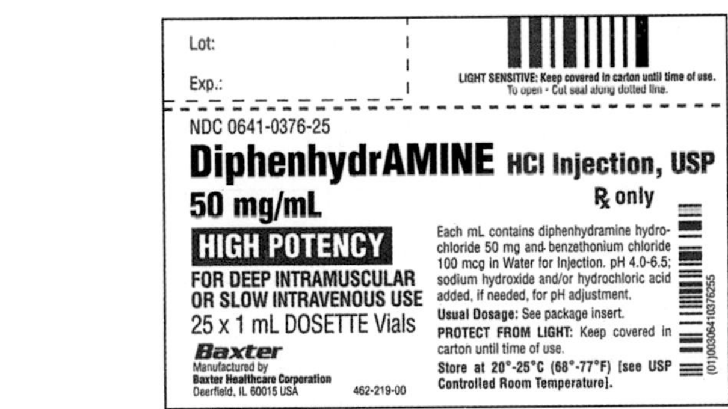

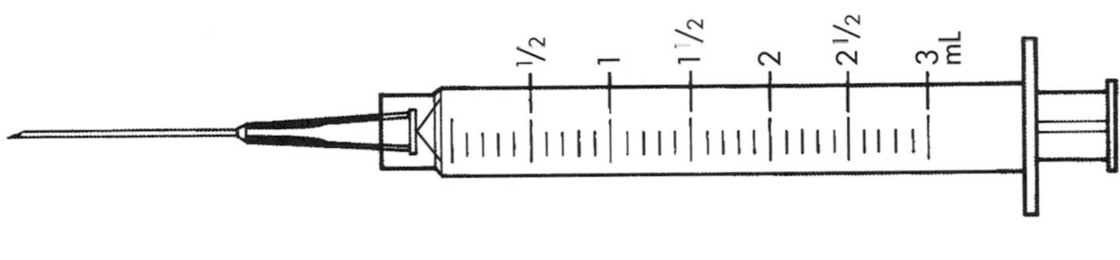

____

17. Order: Ondansetron 3 mg IV stat.

Available:

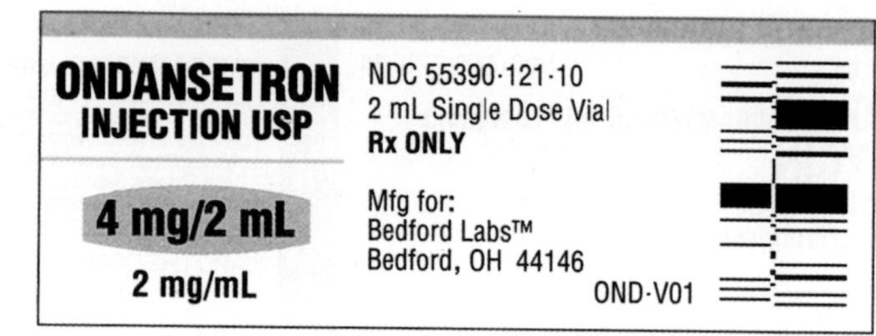

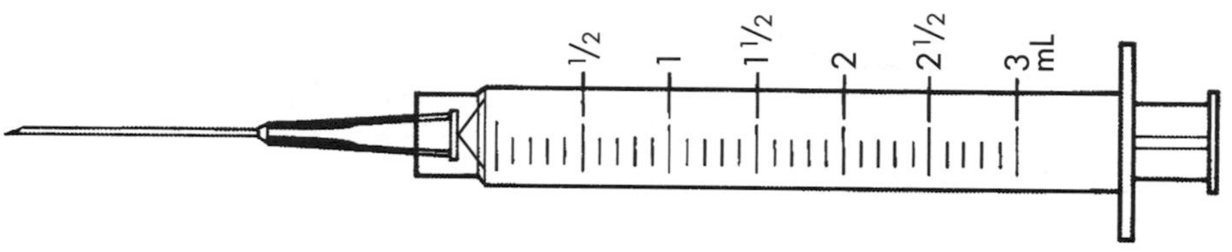

____

18. Order: Solu-Cortef 400 mg IV every day for a severe inflammation for 5 days.

Available:

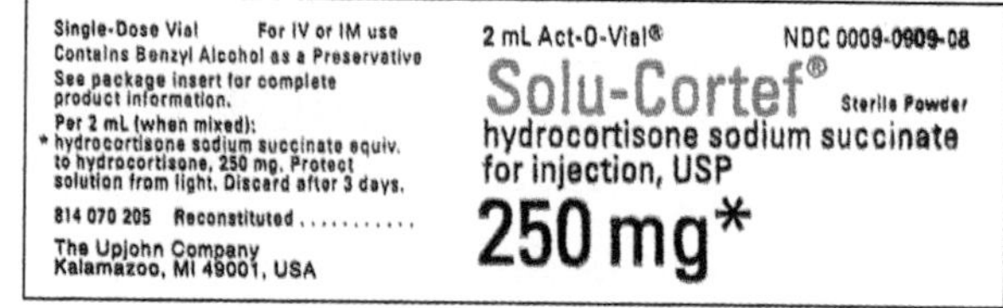

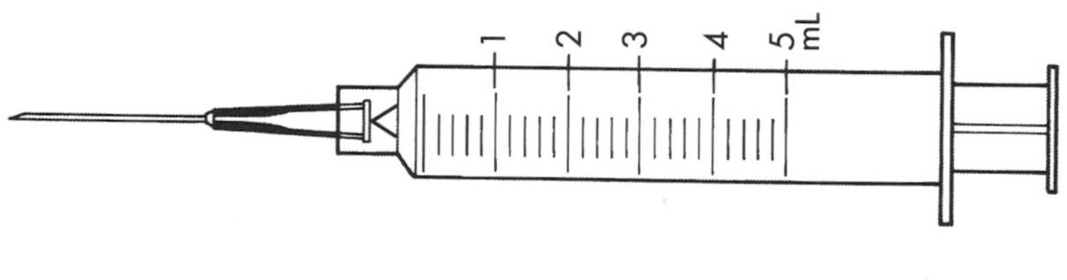

____

19. Order: Naloxone 0.2 mg IM stat.

Available:

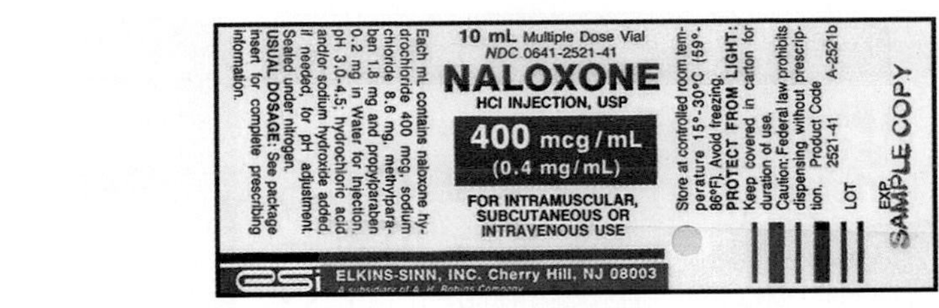

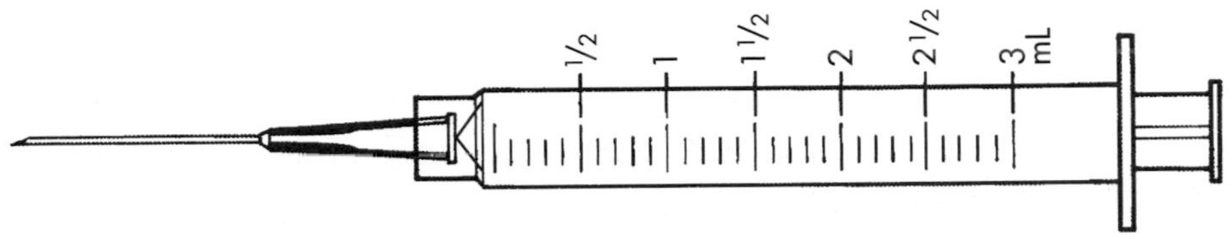

____

20. Order: Robinul (glycopyrrolate) 200 mcg IM on call to the O.R.

Available:

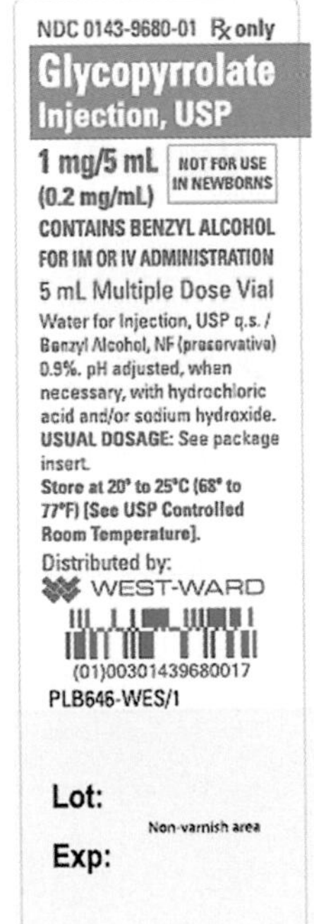

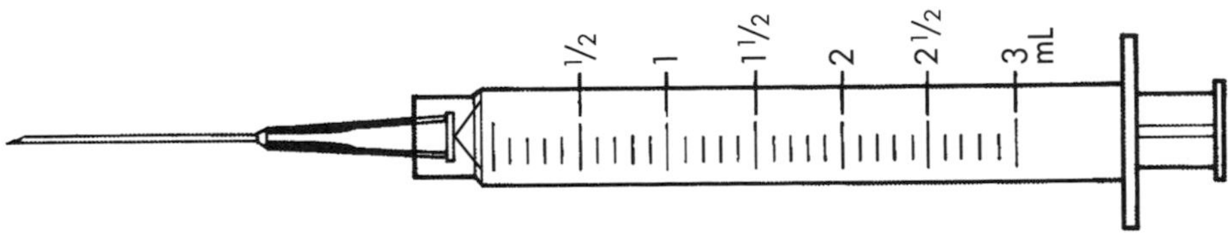

____

21. Order: Aranesp 30 mcg subcut stat. (Express your answer in hundredths.)

Available:

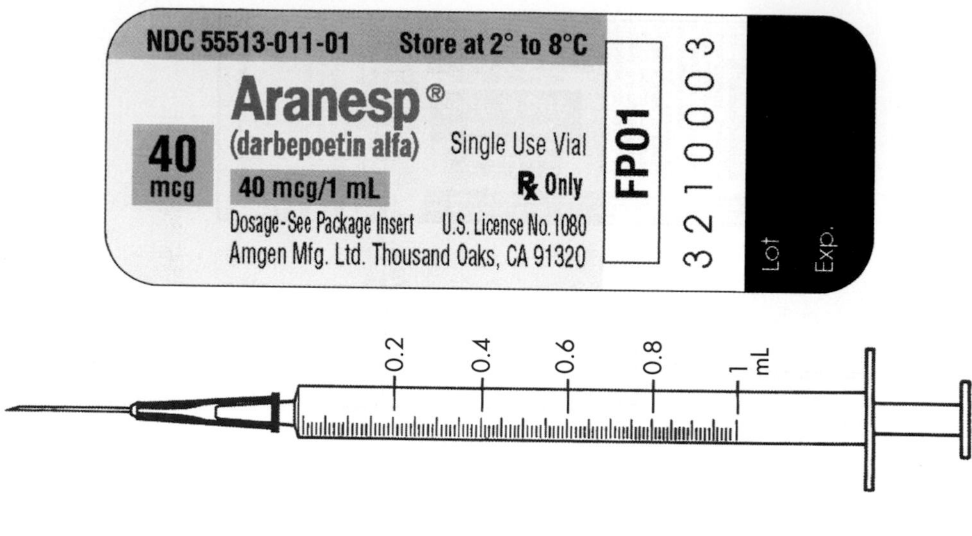

____

22. Order: Vistaril 35 mg IM stat.

Available:

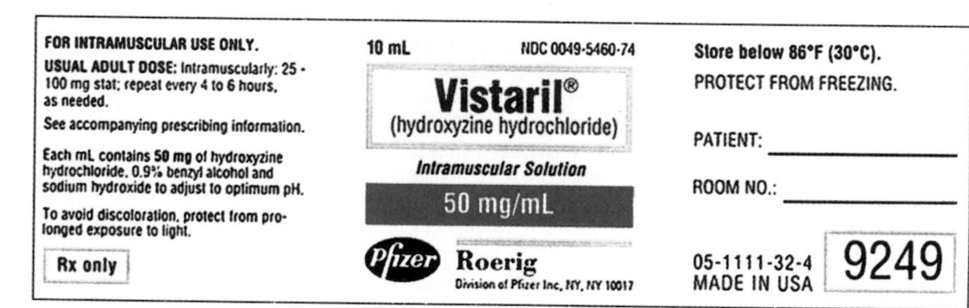

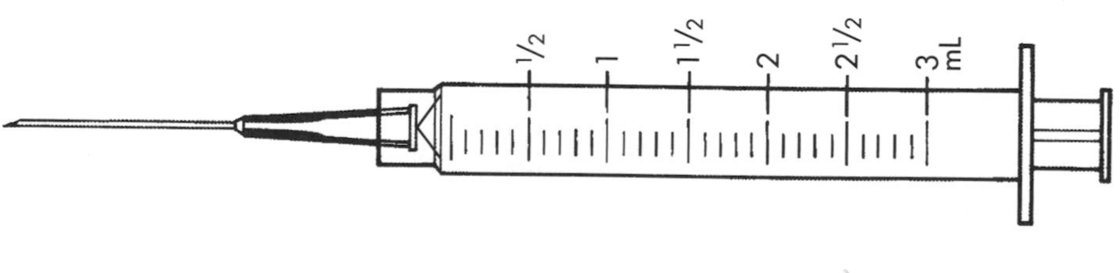

____

23. Order: Meperidine (Demerol) 60 mg IM q4h p.r.n. for pain.

Available:

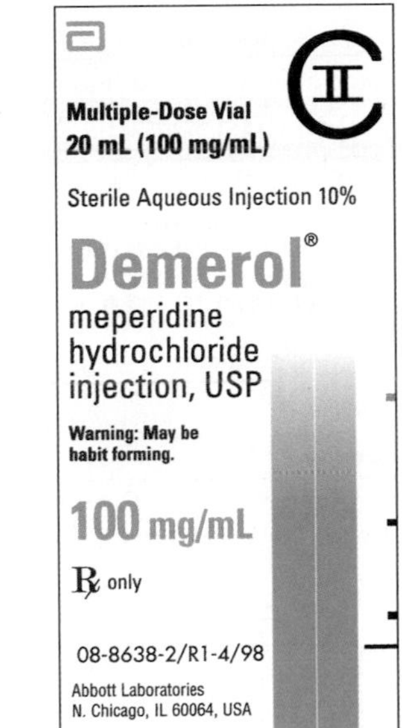

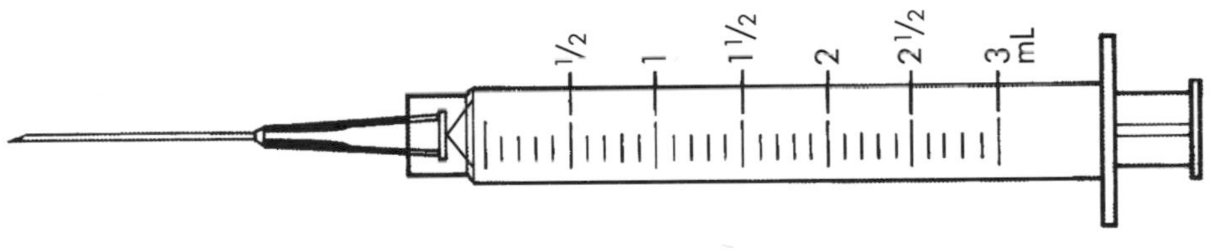

____

24. Order: Ranitidine 50 mg IV q6h.

Available:

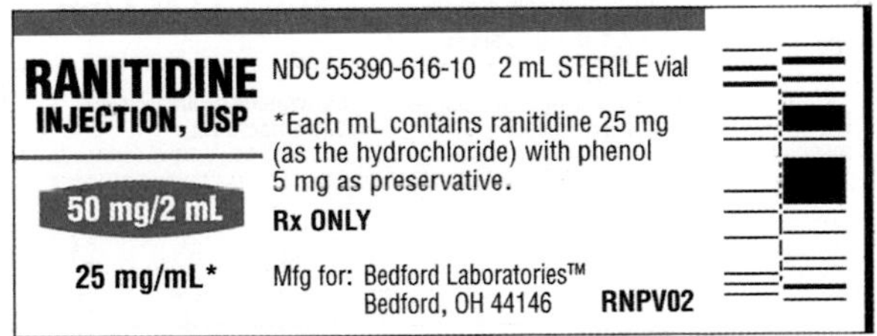

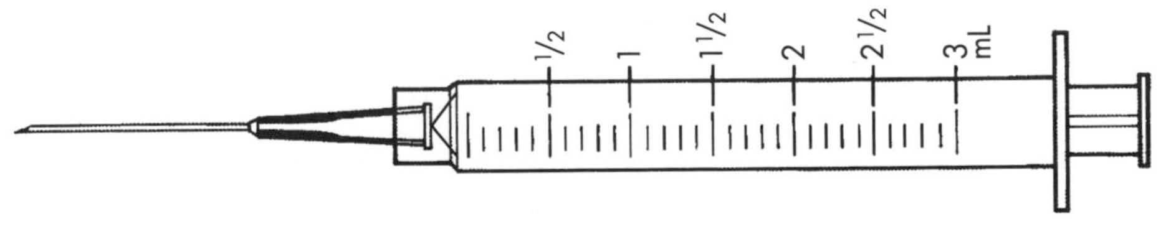

____

25. Order: Digoxin 0.4 mg IM stat.

Available:

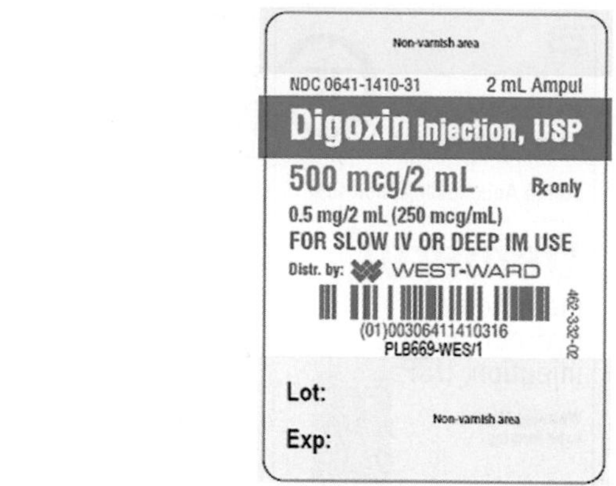

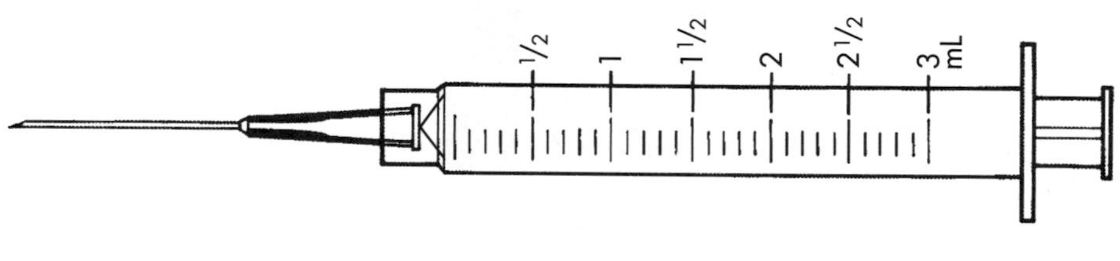

26. Order: Lincocin 500 mg IV q8h.

Available:

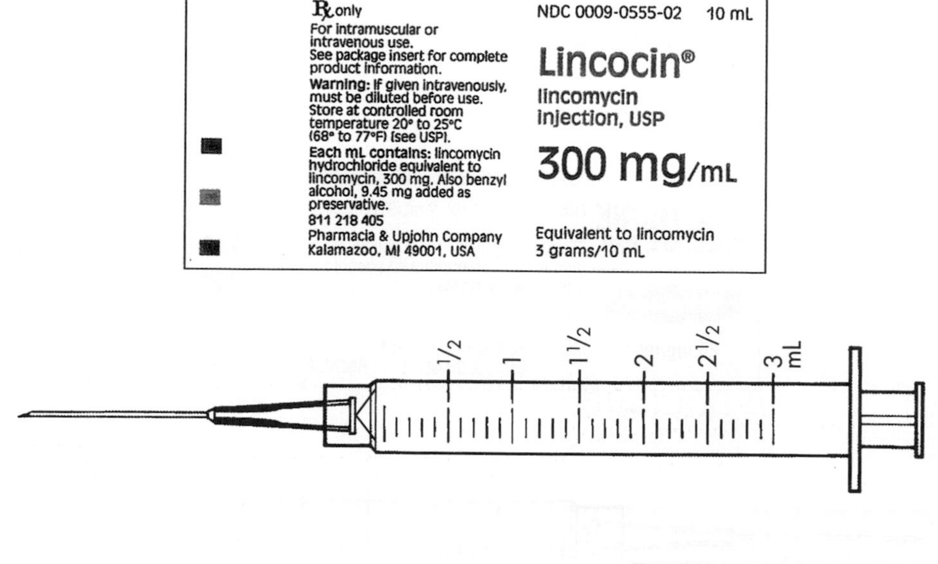

27. Order: Ativan 1.5 mg IM b.i.d. p.r.n. for agitation.

Available:

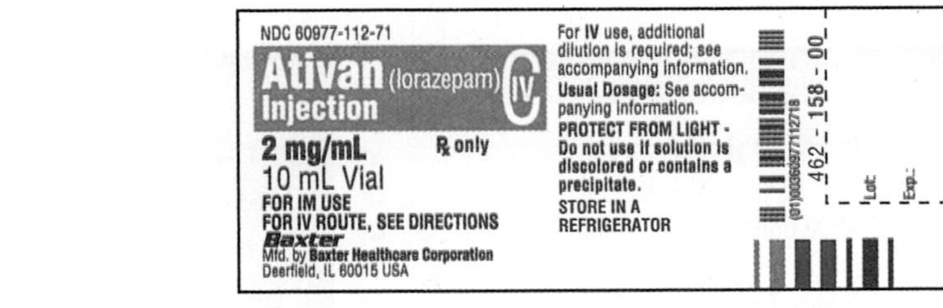

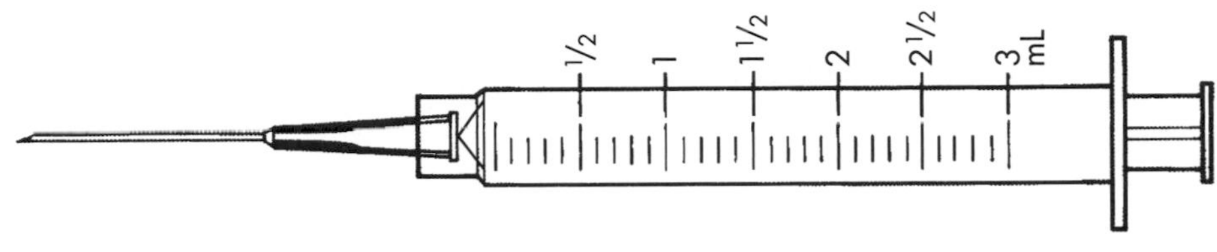

28. Order: Depo-Provera 0.65 g IM once a week (on Thursdays).

Available:

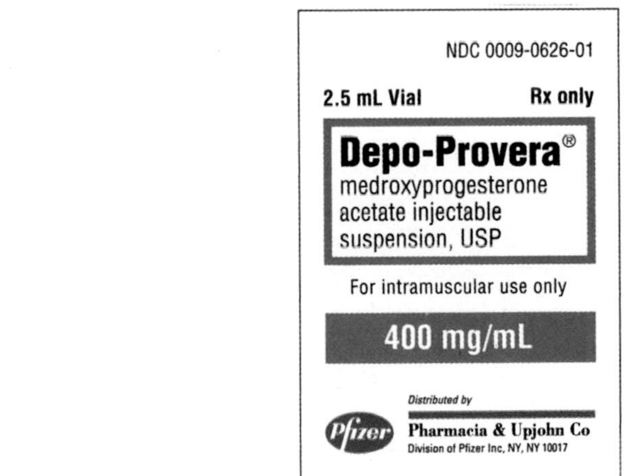

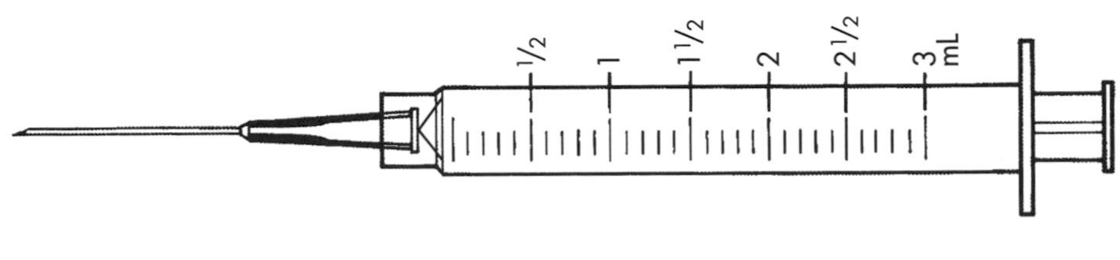

29. Order: Epogen 3,000 units subcut three times per week Monday, Wednesday, and Friday.

Available:

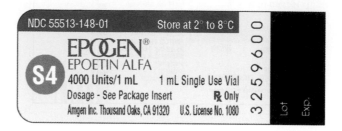

Express your answer in hundredths.

____

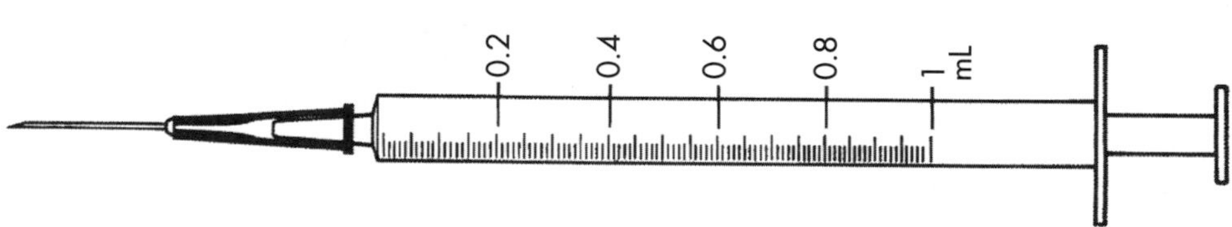

30. Order: Metoclopramide (Reglan) 15 mg IV stat.

Available:

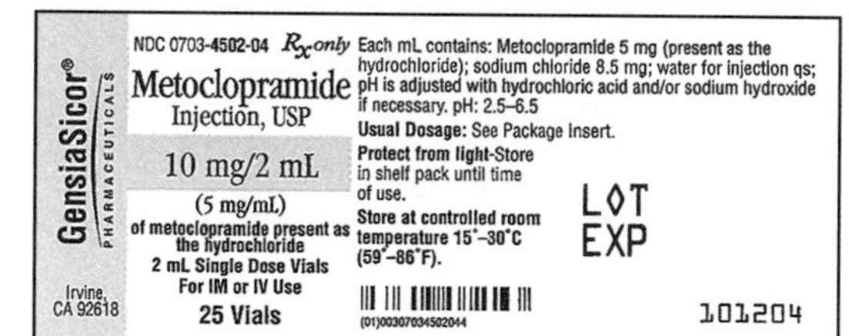

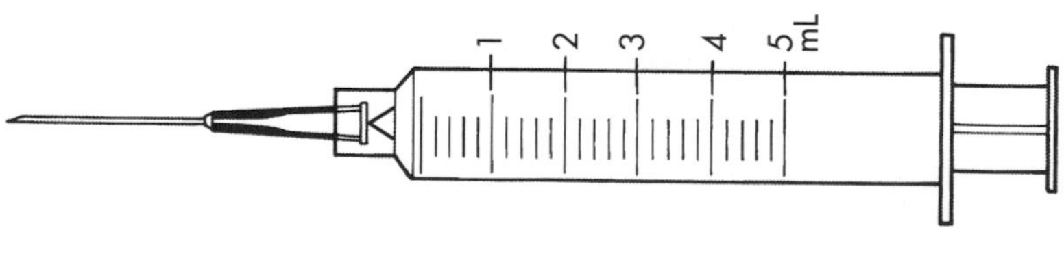

____

31. Order: Lovenox 30 mg subcut q12h.

Available:

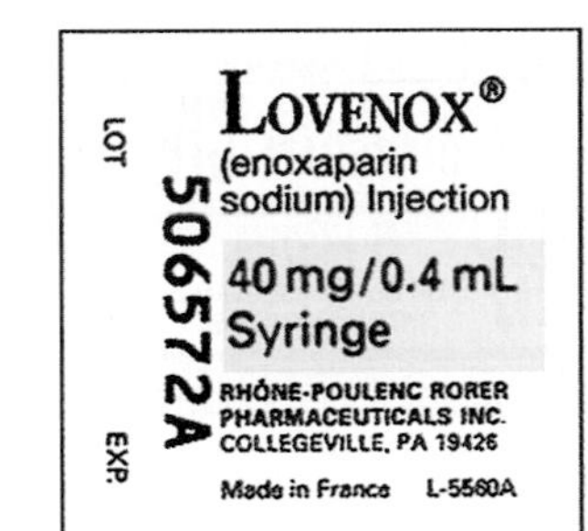

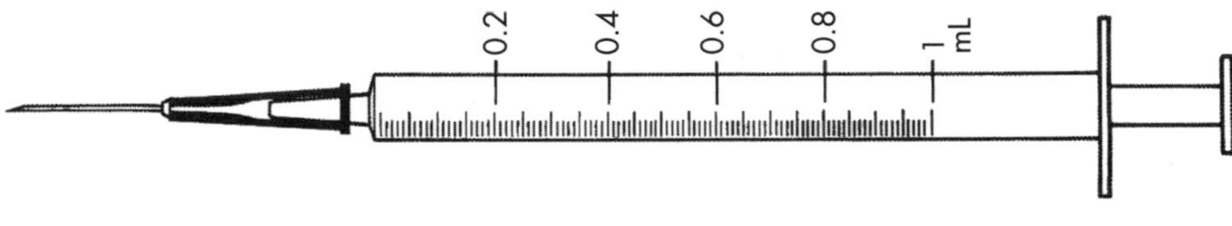

____

32. Order: Cimetidine 0.3 g IV t.i.d.

Available:

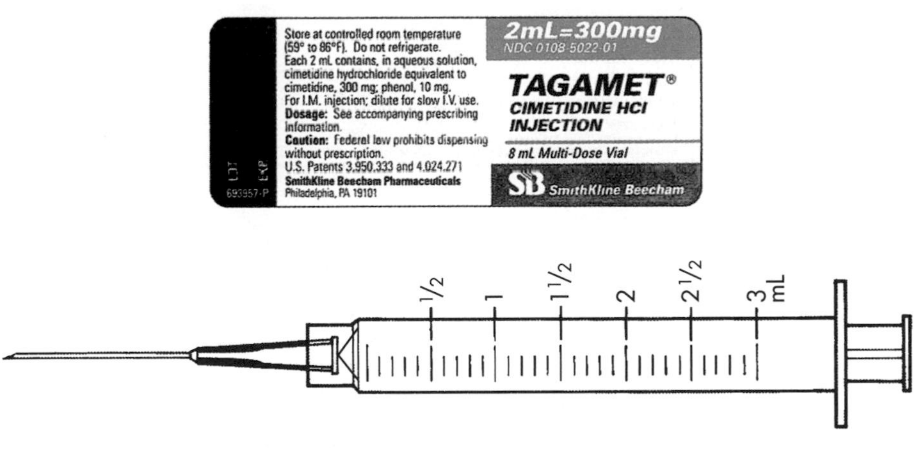

____

33. Order: Valium (diazepam) 7.5 mg IM stat.

Available:

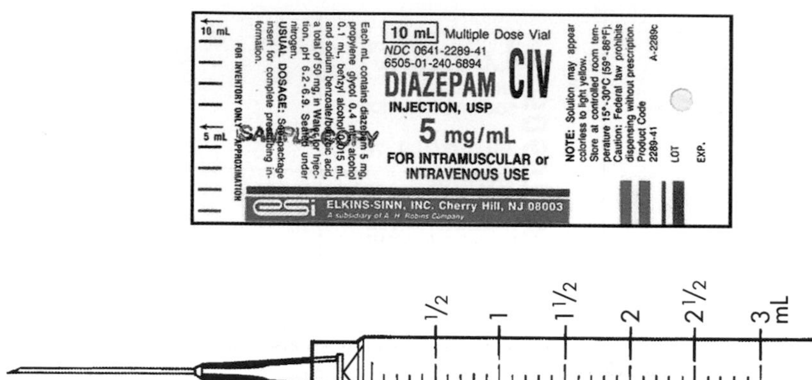

____

34. Order: Bumex (bumetanide) 1 mg IV daily.

Available:

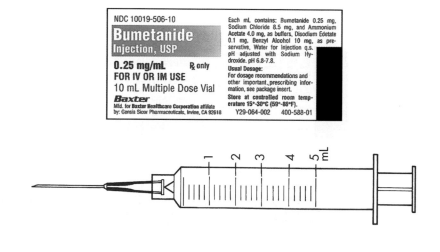

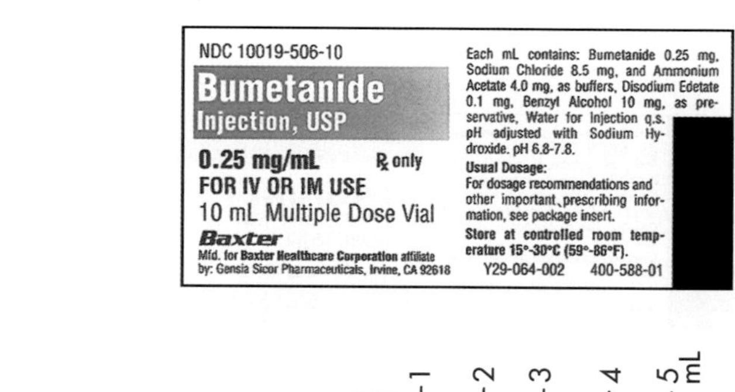

____

35. Order: gentamicin (Garamycin) 55 mg IV q8h.

Available:

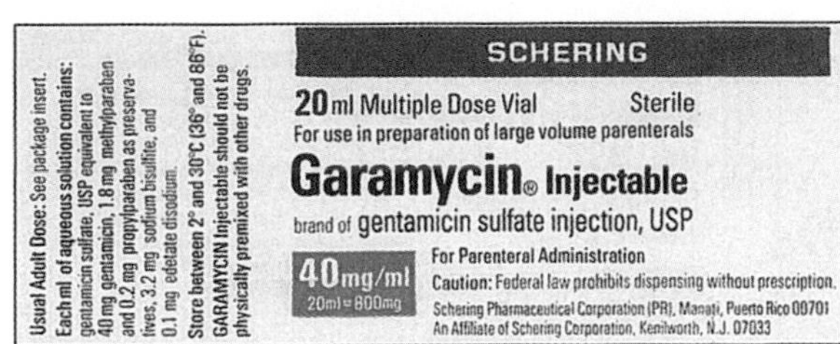

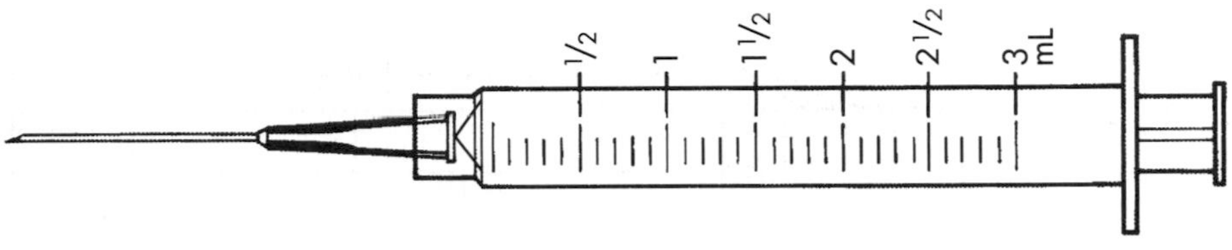

____

36. Order: Celestone, Soluspan (betamethasone) 12 mg IM q24h for 2 doses.

Available:

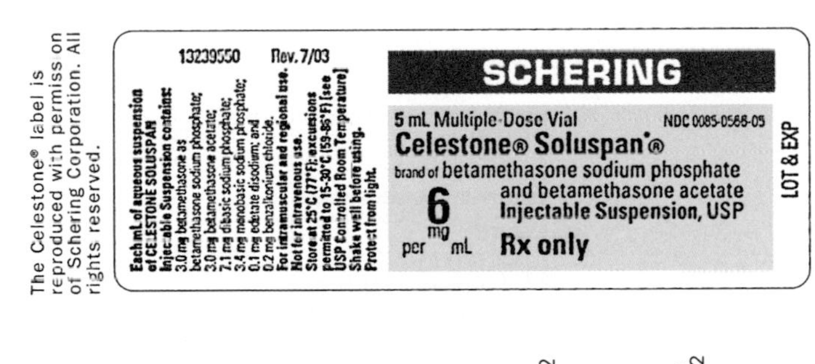

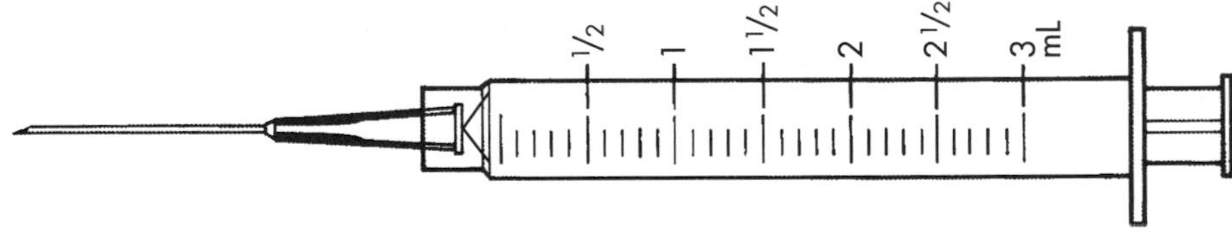

____

37. Order: Aminophylline 0.25 g IV q6h.

Available:

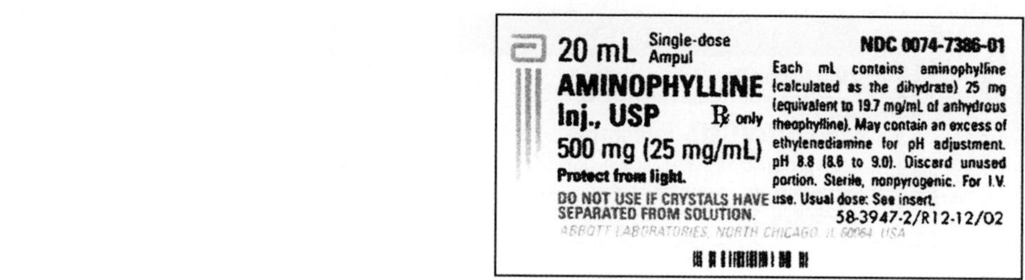

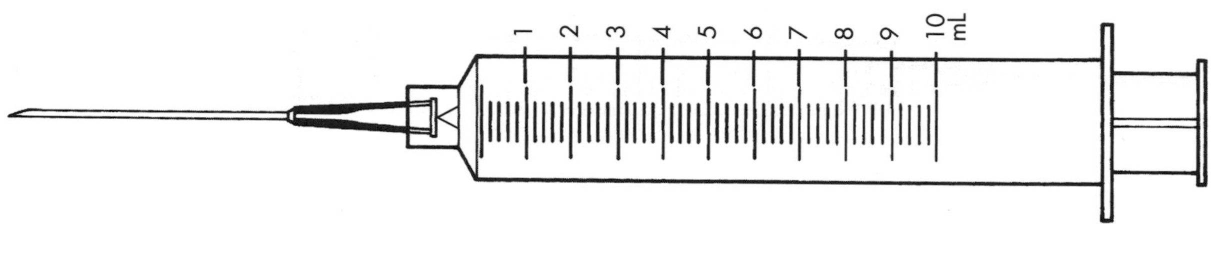

____

38. Order: Pronestyl 0.5 g IV stat.

Available:

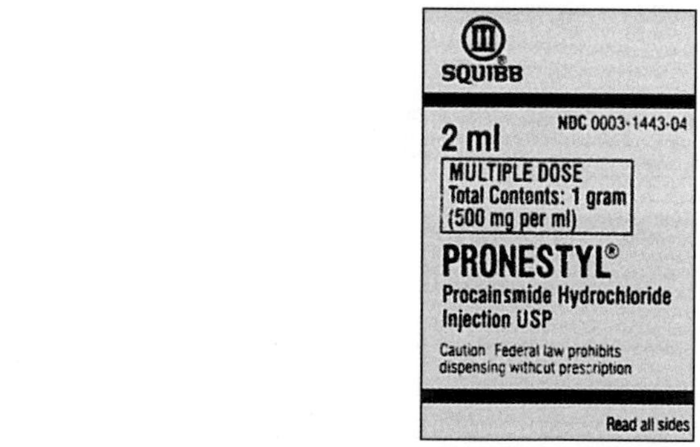

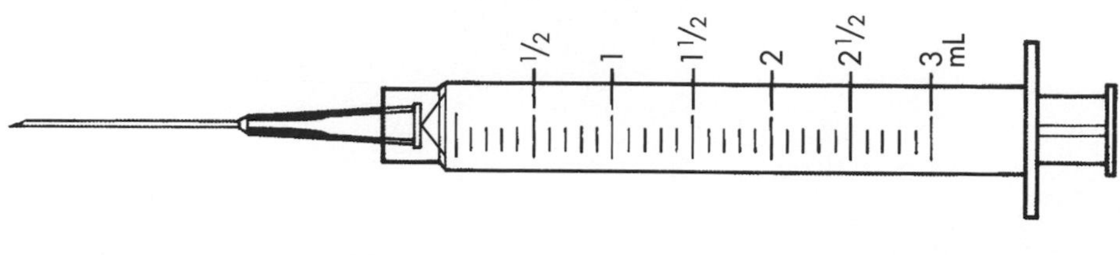

____

39. Order: Tigan 150 mg IM stat.

Available:

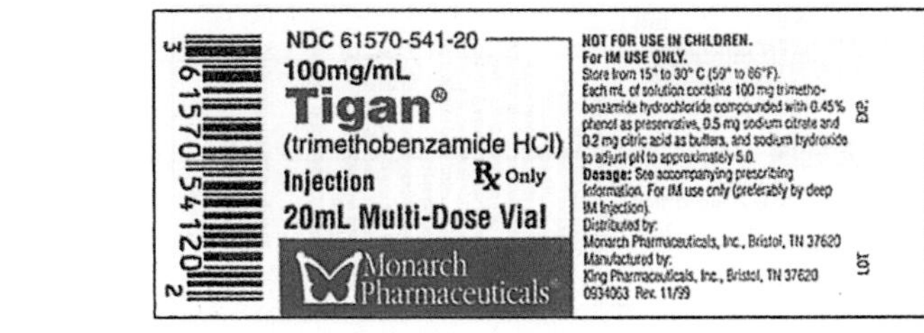

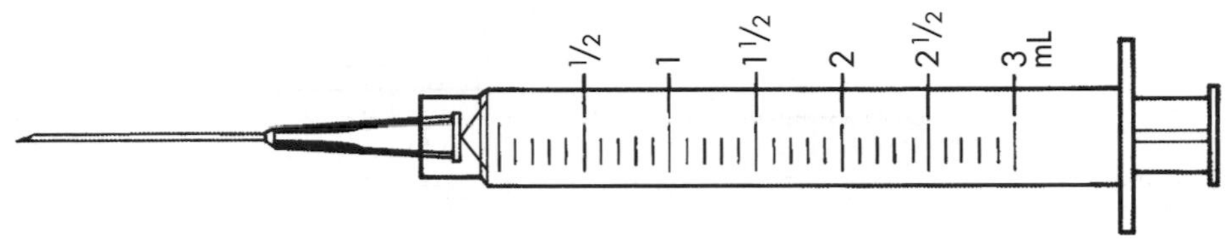

____

40. Order: Demerol (meperidine) 65 mg IM and Phenergan (promethazine) 25 mg IM q4h p.r.n. for pain.

Available:

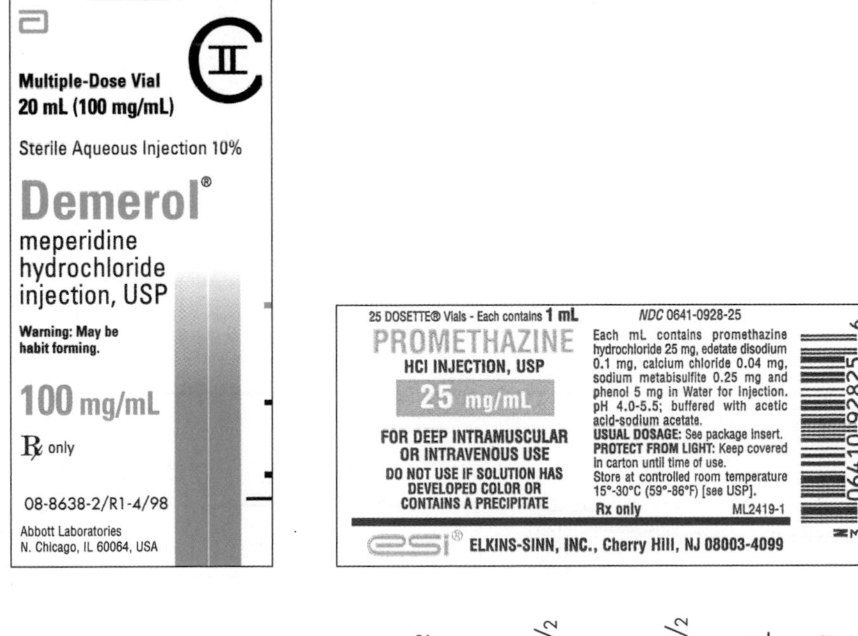

____

41. Order: Decadron (dexamethasone) 9 mg IV daily for 4 days.

Available:

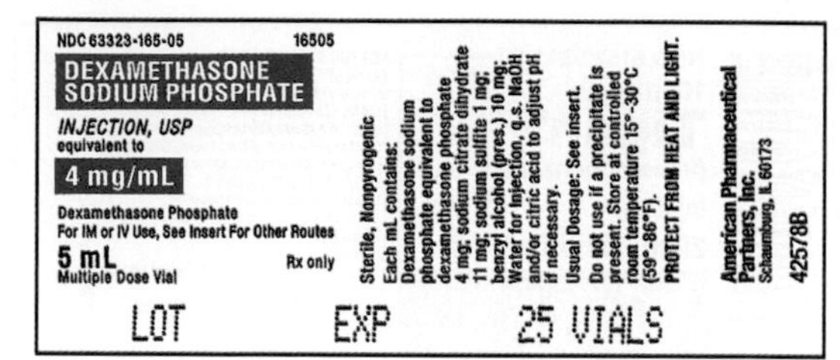

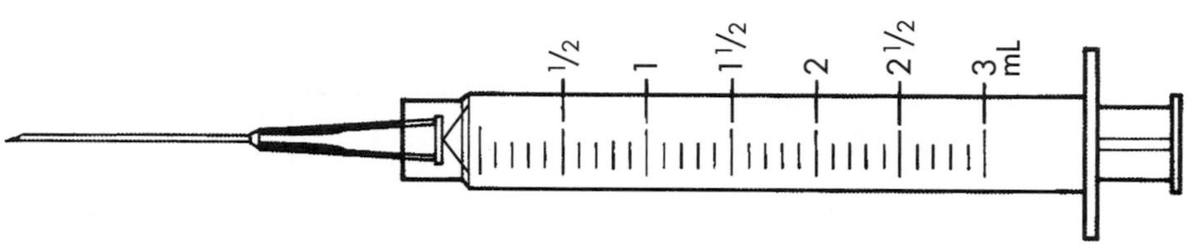

42. Order: Sublimaze (fentanyl) 60 mcg IM 30 minutes before surgery.

Available:

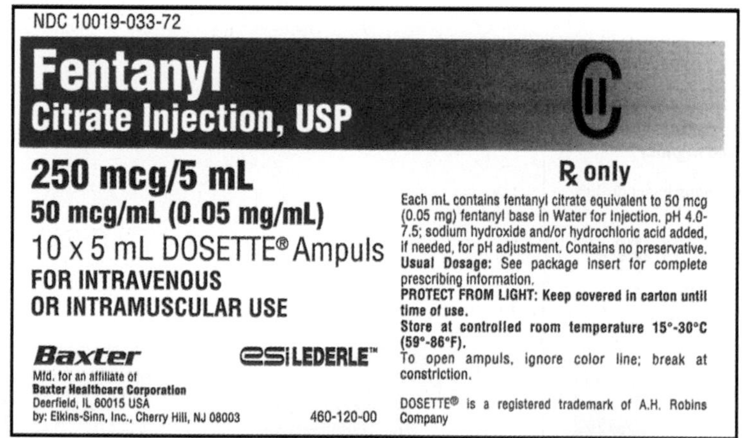

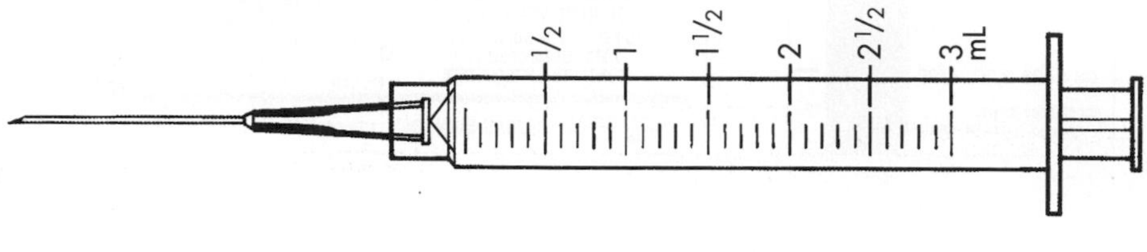

43. Order: Nubain 10 mg IV stat.

Available:

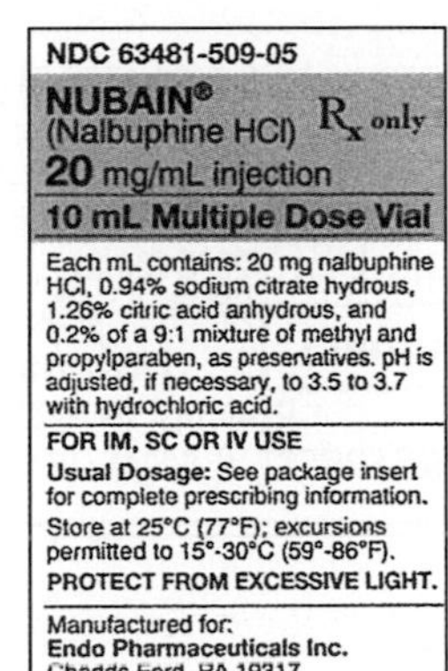

NDC 63481-509-05
NUBAIN®
(Nalbuphine HCl) Rx only
20 mg/mL injection
10 mL Multiple Dose Vial
Each mL contains: 20 mg nalbuphine HCl, 0.94% sodium citrate hydrous, 1.26% citric acid anhydrous, and 0.2% of a 9:1 mixture of methyl and propylparaben, as preservatives. pH is adjusted, if necessary, to 3.5 to 3.7 with hydrochloric acid.
FOR IM, SC OR IV USE
Usual Dosage: See package insert for complete prescribing information.
Store at 25°C (77°F); excursions permitted to 15°-30°C (59°-86°F).
PROTECT FROM EXCESSIVE LIGHT.
Manufactured for:
Endo Pharmaceuticals Inc.
Chadds Ford, PA 19317

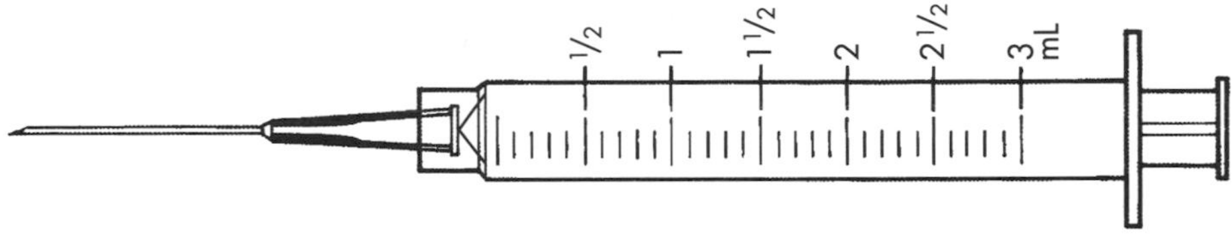

____

44. Order: Neupogen 175 mcg subcut every day for 2 weeks.

Available:

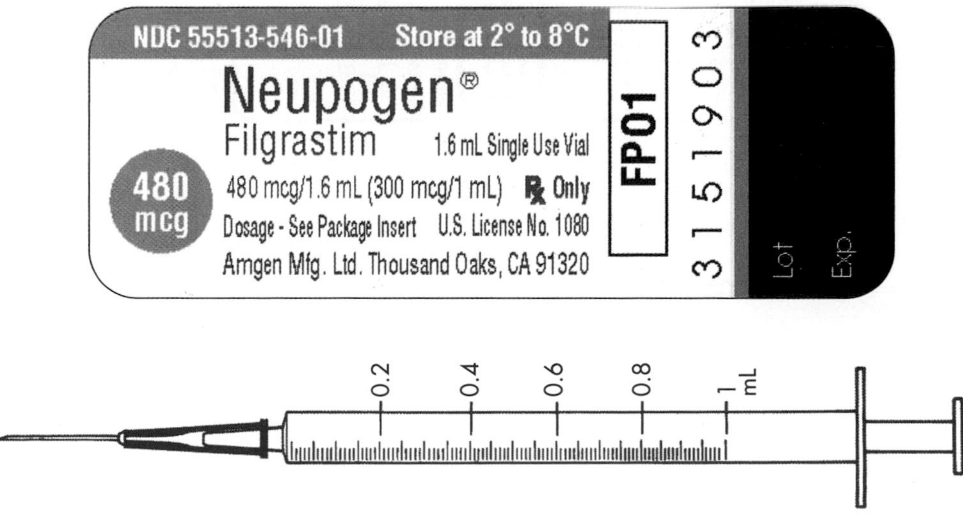

Express your answer to the hundredths.

____

45. Order: Butorphanol tartrate 1.5 mg IV q4h prn for pain.

Available:

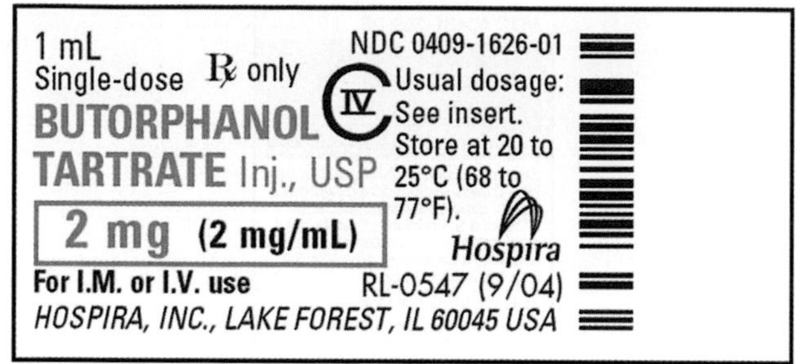

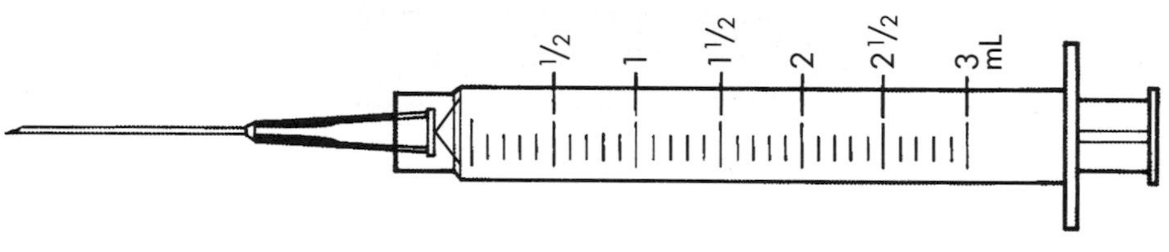

____

46. Order: Orphenadrine 60 mg IV q12h.

Available:

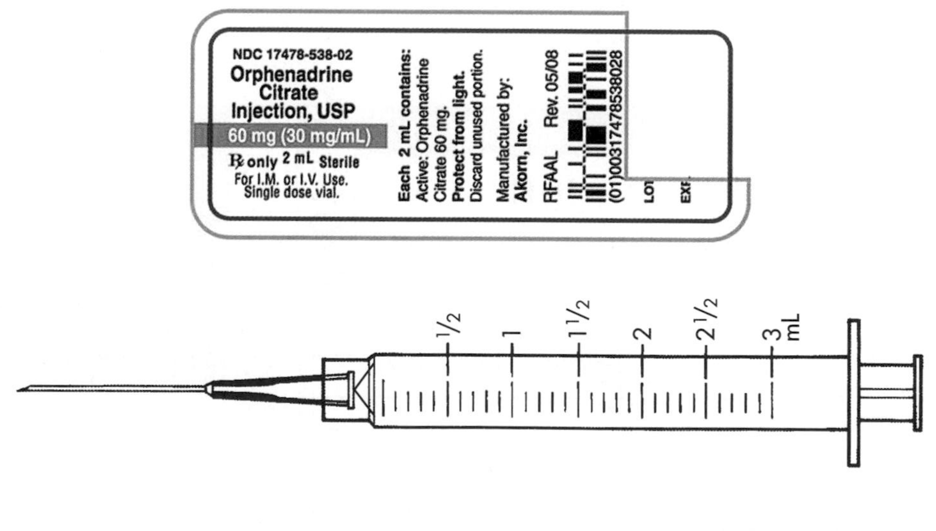

____

47. Order: Dexamethasone sodium phosphate 5 mg IV q12h.

Available:

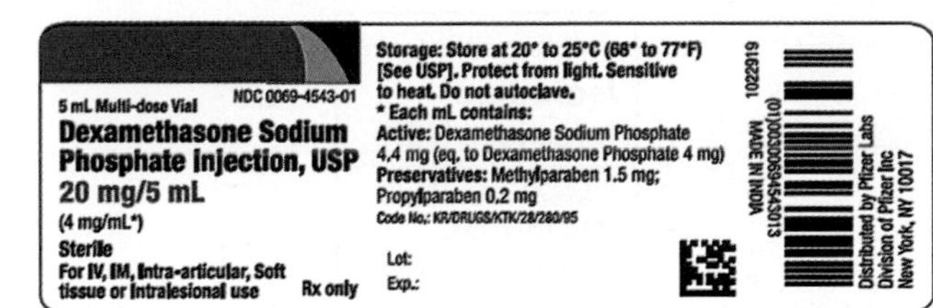

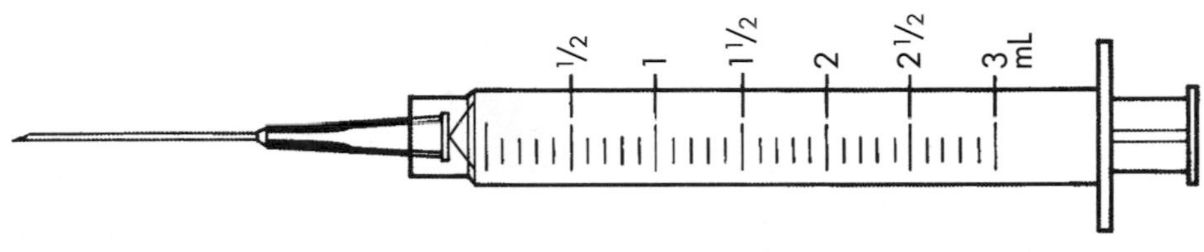

____

48. Order: Buprenorphine hydrochloride 0.6 mg IM as an initial dose, then 0.3 mg IM q6h prn.

Available:

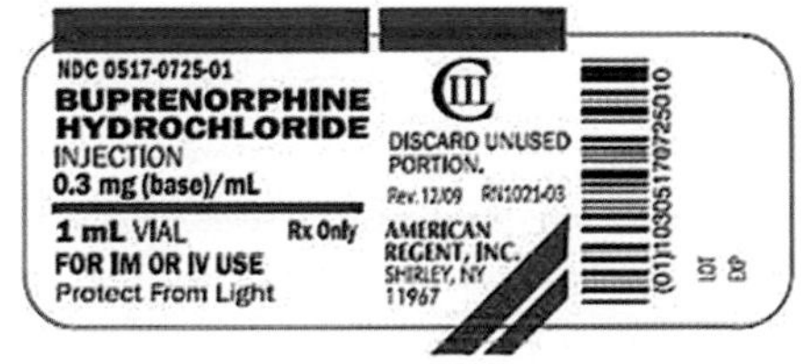

How many milliliters will you administer for the initial dose?

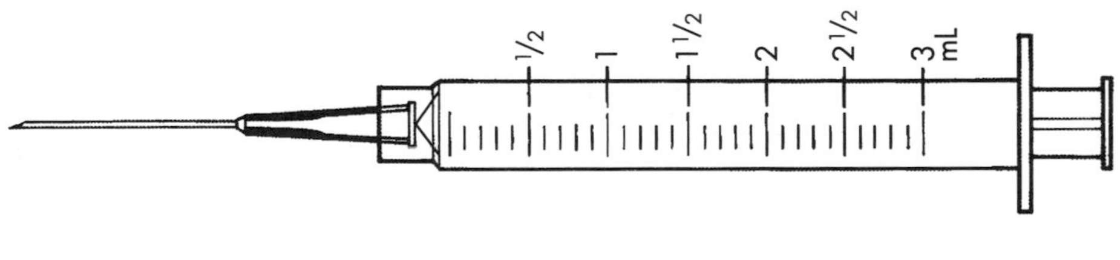

____

49. Order: Isoniazid 300 mg IM every third day.

Available:

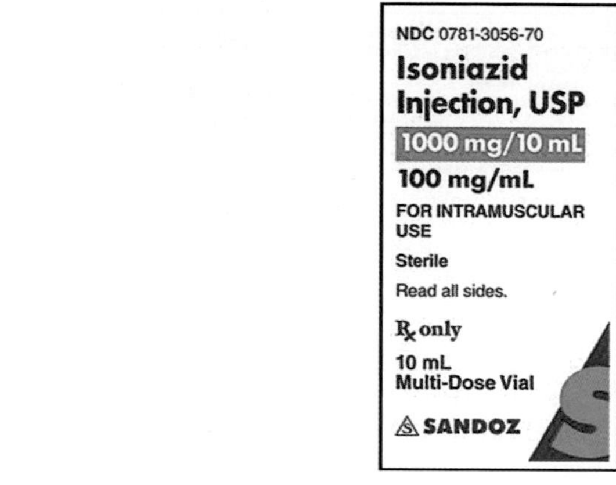

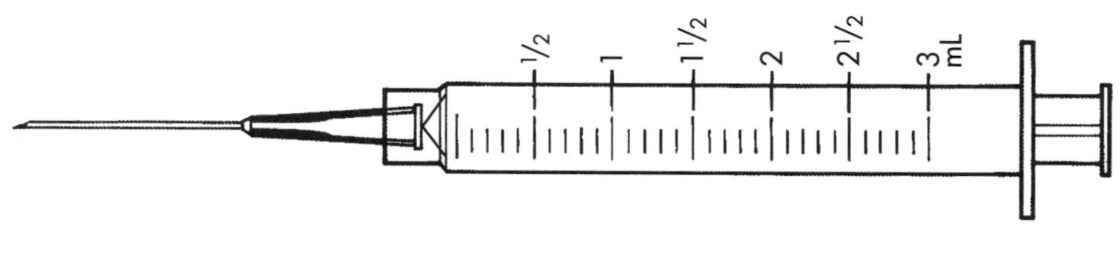

____

Answers on p. 419-426

ANSWERS

Chapter 18
Answers to Practice Problems

NOTE

Problems requiring conversion reflect conversion of what the prescriber ordered to what is available.

1. 3. 2. 4.

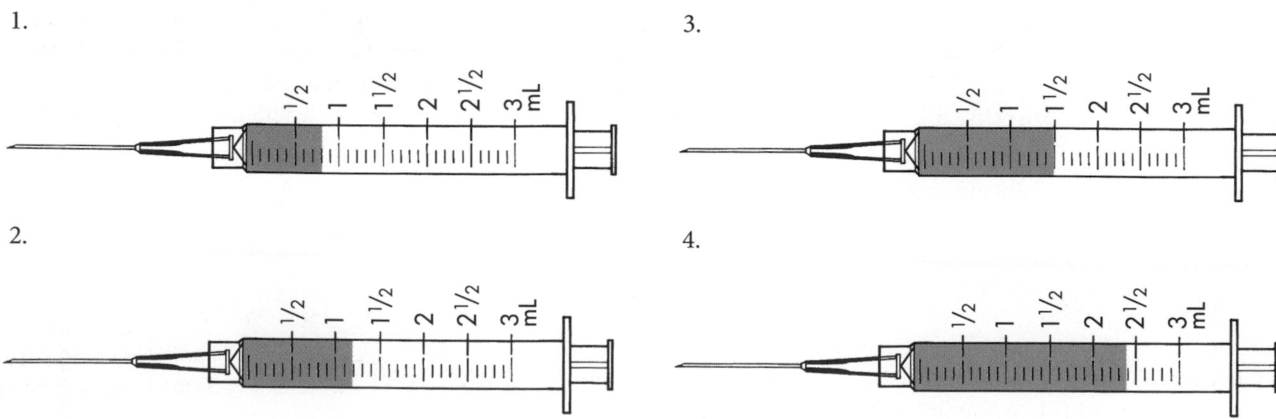

evolve

For additional practice problems, refer to the Parenteral Dosages section of the Elsevier's Interactive Drug Calculation Application, Version 1 on Evolve.

5. 1.4 mL
6. 1 mL
7. 0.9 mL
8. 0.4 mL
9. 4.4 mL
10. 7 mL
11. 3.2 mL
12. a. 10 mL
    b. 25 mg per mL
    c. 2 mL
13. a. 20 mL
    b. 100 mg per mL
    c. 0.5 mL
14. a. 2.8 mL
    b. 1 mg per 0.2 mL
    c. subcut
15. a. 20 mL
    b. 2 mg per mL
    c. 2
16. a. subcut
    b. 20 mg per 0.4 mL
17. a. 2 mL
    b. 20 mg per 2 mL, 10 mg per 1 mL
18. a. 200 mg per 100 mL, 2 mg per mL
    b. IV infusion only
19. a. 10 mL
    b. 10 mg per 10 mL, 1 mg per mL
20. a. 3 mL
    b. 150 mg per 3 mL, 50 mg per mL
    c. IV use only
21. a. 20 mL
    b. 2 mEq per mL
22. a. 1 mL
    b. 4,000 units per mL
23. a. 20 mL
    b. 500 units per mL
24. a. 10 mL
    b. 10 units per mL

25. $5\text{ mg}:1\text{ mL} = 10\text{ mg}:x\text{ mL}$

or

$$\frac{10\text{ mg}}{5\text{ mg}} \times 1\text{ mL} = x\text{ mL}$$

Answer: 2 mL. The dosage ordered is more than the available strength; therefore you will need more than 1 mL to administer the dosage.

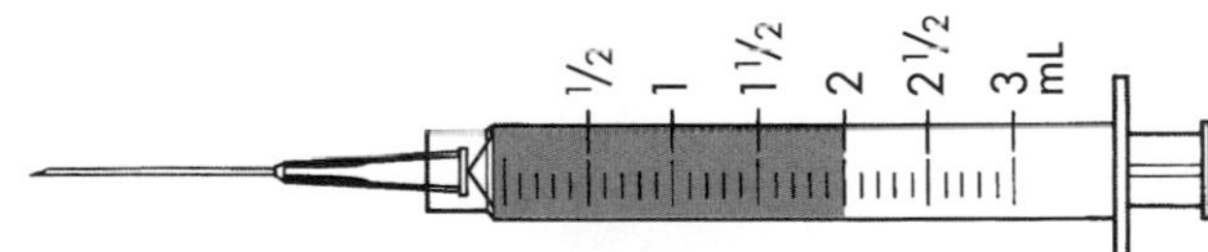

26. $100\text{ mg}:1\text{ mL} = 75\text{ mg}:x\text{ mL}$

or

$$\frac{75\text{ mg}}{100\text{ mg}} \times 1\text{ mL} = x\text{ mL}$$

Answer: 0.75 mL = 0.8 mL. The dosage ordered is less than the available strength; therefore you will need less than 1 mL to administer the dosage. Answer stated as decimal (0.8 mL); mL is a metric measure.

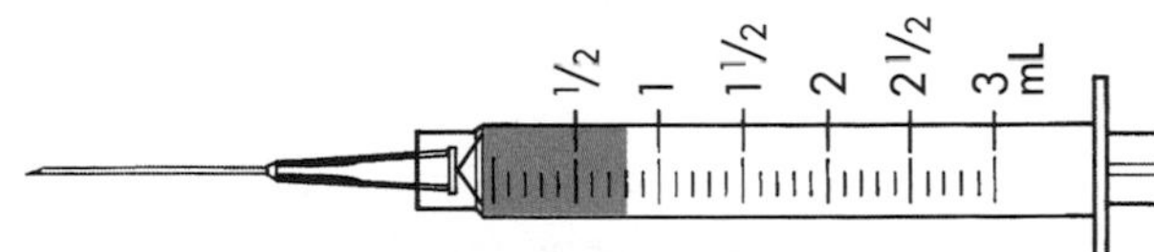

27. $130\text{ mg}:1\text{ mL} = 120\text{ mg}:x\text{ mL}$

or

$$\frac{120\text{ mg}}{130\text{ mg}} \times 1\text{ mL} = x\text{ mL}$$

Answer: 0.92 mL = 0.9 mL. The dosage ordered is less than the available strength; therefore you will need less than 1 mL to administer the dosage.

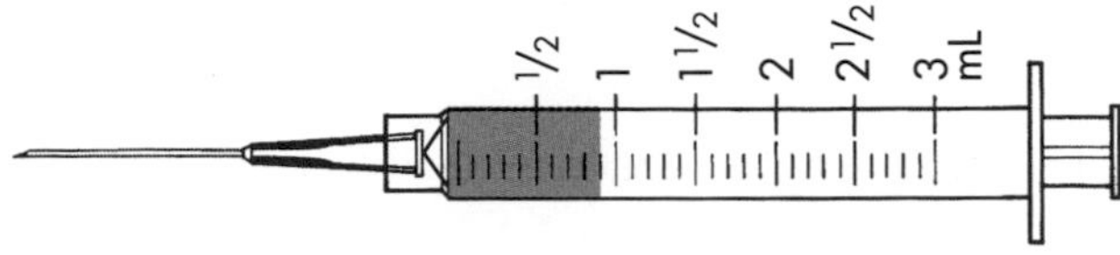

28. $5\text{ mg}:1\text{ mL} = 8\text{ mg}:x\text{ mL}$

or

$$\frac{8\text{ mg}}{5\text{ mg}} \times 1\text{ mL} = x\text{ mL}$$

Answer: 1.6 mL. The dosage ordered is more than the available strength; therefore you will need more than 1 mL to administer the dosage.

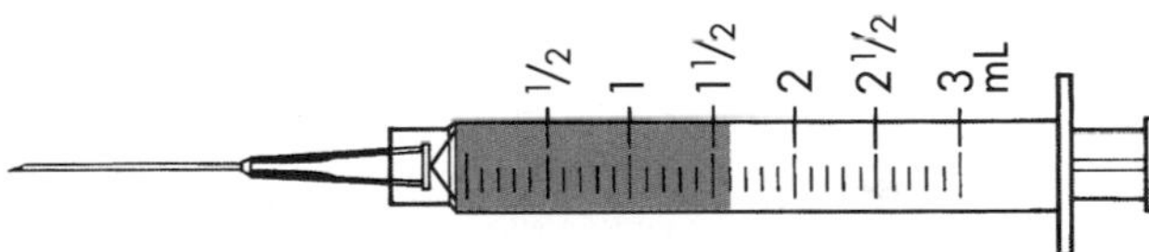

29. Conversion is required. Equivalent: 1,000 mcg = 1 mg. Therefore 0.05 mg = 50 mcg.

$100\text{ mcg}:1\text{ mL} - 50\text{ mcg}:x\text{ mL}$

or

$$\frac{50\text{ mcg}}{100\text{ mcg}} \times 1\text{ mL} = x\text{ mL}$$

Answer: 0.5 mL. The dosage ordered is less than what is available. Therefore you will need less than 1 mL to administer the dosage. Milliliter (mL) is metric, and answer is expressed as decimal. Problem could have also been done without a conversion by using the dosage indicated on the label in mg (0.1 mg per mL)

$0.1\text{ mg}:1\text{ mL} = 0.05\text{ mg}:x\text{ mL}$

or

$0.05\text{ mg} \times 1\text{ mL} = x\text{ mL}$

0.1 mg

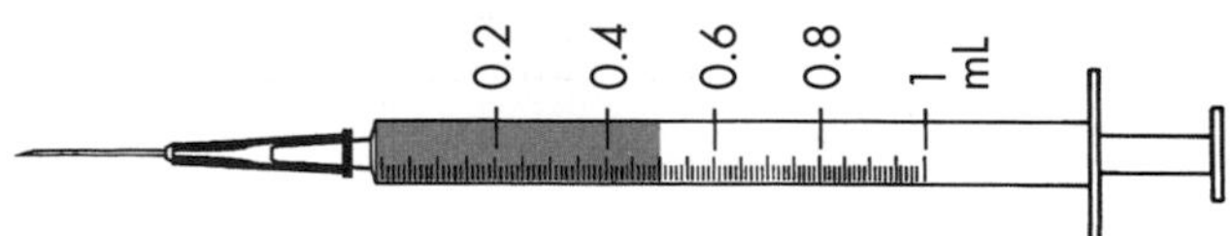

30. Demerol:

$$75 \text{ mg} : 1 \text{ mL} = 50 \text{ mg} : x \text{ mL}$$

or

$$\frac{50 \text{ mg}}{75 \text{ mg}} \times 1 \text{ mL} = x \text{ mL}$$

Answer: 0.66 mL = 0.7 mL. The dosage ordered is less than the available strength. Therefore less than 1 mL would be required to administer the dosage.

Vistaril:

$$50 \text{ mg} : 1 \text{ mL} = 25 \text{ mg} : x \text{ mL}$$

or

$$\frac{25 \text{ mg}}{50 \text{ mg}} \times 1 \text{ mL} = x \text{ mL}$$

Answer: 0.5 mL. The dosage ordered is less than the available strength. Therefore you will need less than 1 mL to administer the dosage. The total number of milliliters you will prepare to administer is 1.2 mL. This dosage is measurable on the small hypodermics. These two medications are often administered in the same syringe (0.7 mL Demerol + 0.5 mL Vistaril = 1.2 mL). Medications may be administered in the same syringe as long as they are compatible.

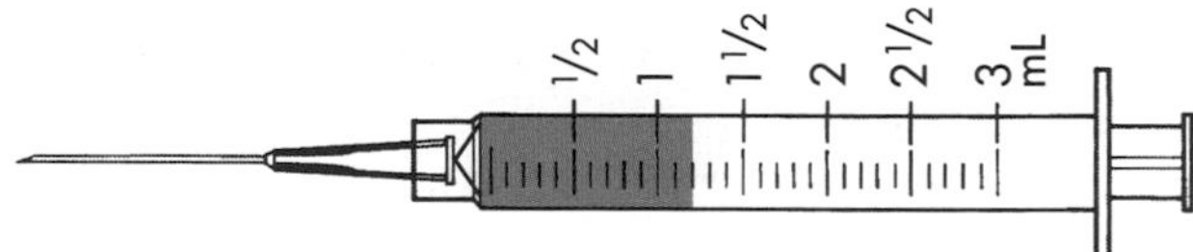

31. $$100 \text{ mg} : 1 \text{ mL} = 125 \text{ mg} : x \text{ mL}$$

or

$$\frac{125 \text{ mg}}{100 \text{ mg}} \times 1 \text{ mL} = x \text{ mL}$$

Answer: 1.25 mL = 1.3 mL. The dosage ordered is more than the available strength. Therefore you will need more than 1 mL to administer the dosage.

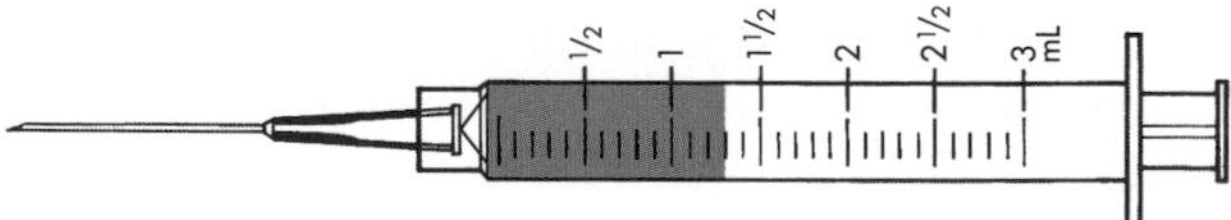

32. $$20{,}000 \text{ units} : 1 \text{ mL} = 5{,}000 \text{ units} : x \text{ mL}$$

or

$$\frac{5{,}000 \text{ units}}{20{,}000 \text{ units}} \times 1 \text{ mL} = x \text{ mL}$$

Answer: 0.25 mL. The dosage ordered is less than the available strength. Therefore you will need less than 1 mL to administer the dosage. This dosage can be measured accurately on the 1-mL (tuberculin) syringe, because it is measured in hundredths of a milliliter. The dosage you are administering is 0.25 mL, which is $\frac{25}{100}$.

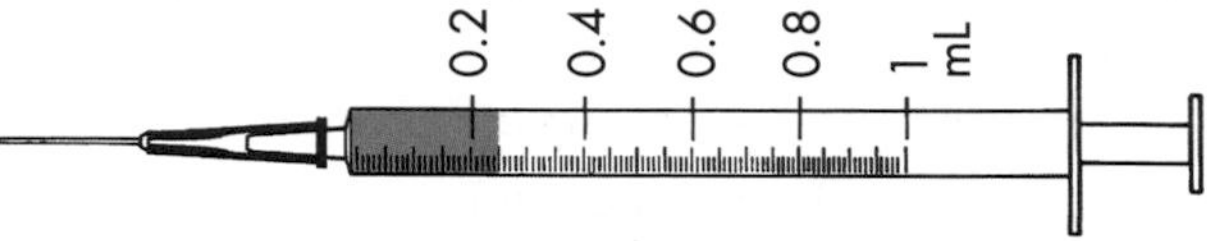

33. $$15 \text{ mg} : 1 \text{ mL} = 15 \text{ mg} : x \text{ mL}$$

or

$$\frac{15 \text{ mg}}{15 \text{ mg}} \times 1 \text{ mL} = x \text{ mL}$$

Answer: 1 mL. The label indicates that the dosage ordered is contained in 1 mL.

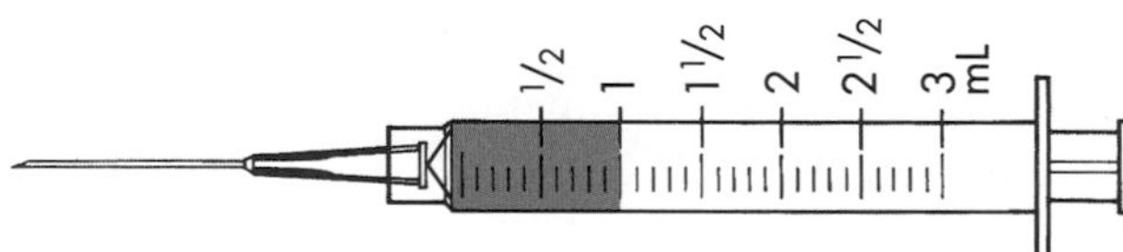

34. $$10 \text{ mg} : 1 \text{ mL} = 20 \text{ mg} : x \text{ mL}$$

or

$$\frac{20 \text{ mg}}{10 \text{ mg}} \times 1 \text{ mL} = x \text{ mL}$$

Answer: 2 mL. The dosage ordered is more than the available strength. Therefore you will need more than 1 mL to administer the required dosage (if dosage strength used is 10 mg per mL as indicated on the label).

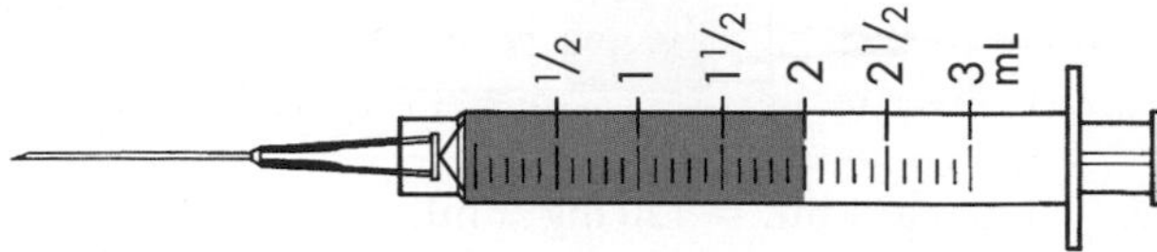

Alternate solution:

$$40 \text{ mg} : 4 \text{ mL} = 20 \text{ mg} : x \text{ mL}$$

or

$$\frac{20 \text{ mg}}{40 \text{ mg}} \times 4 \text{ mL} = x \text{ mL}$$

This setup still gives an answer of 2 mL.

Answers to Clinical Reasoning Questions

a. The right medication. Hydroxyzine and hydralazine have similar names but are two different medications.

b. Not reading the medication labels carefully and comparing them with the order, or medication administration record (MAR).

c. Hydralazine is an antihypertensive and could cause a fatal drop in the client's blood pressure.

d. Carefully comparing the medication label and dosage with the order or MAR three times while preparing the medication. Perhaps if the nurse had consulted a reliable drug reference, it may have alerted the nurse to the fact that hydralazine is used to treat hypertension and hydroxyzine is used for anxiety, which is what the medication was prescribed for.

Answers to Chapter Review

1. Conversion is required. Equivalent: 1,000 mg = 1 g. Therefore 0.3 g = 300 mg.

$$600 \text{ mg} : 4 \text{ mL} = 300 \text{ mg} : x \text{ mL}$$

or

$$\frac{300 \text{ mg}}{600 \text{ mg}} \times 4 \text{ mL} = x \text{ mL}$$

Answer: 2 mL. The dosage ordered is less than the available strength if you use the dosage strength 600 mg per 4 mL; therefore you will need less than 4 mL to administer the dosage.

Alternate solution:

$$150 \text{ mg} : 1 \text{ mL} = 300 \text{ mg} : x \text{ mL}$$

or

$$\frac{300 \text{ mg}}{150 \text{ mg}} \times 1 \text{ mL} = x \text{ mL}$$

This would net the same answer, 2 mL.

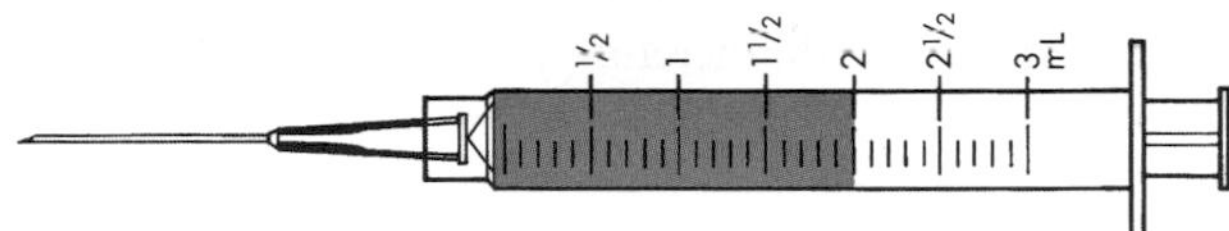

2.

$$500 \text{ mcg} : 1 \text{ mL} = 175 \text{ mcg} : x \text{ mL}$$

or

$$\frac{175 \text{ mcg}}{500 \text{ mcg}} \times 1 \text{ mL} = x \text{ mL}$$

Answer: 0.35 mL. The dosage ordered is less than the available strength. Therefore you will need less than 1 mL to administer the dosage.

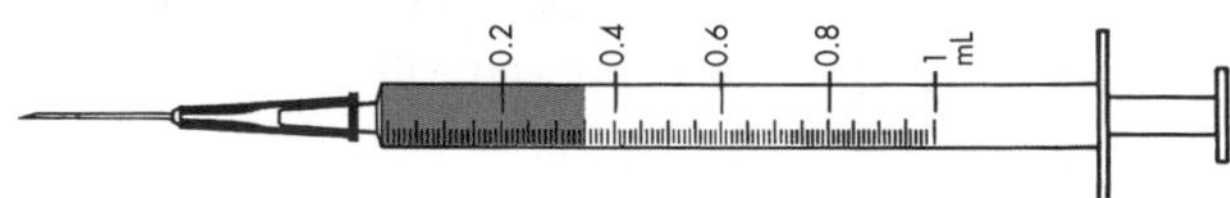

3.

$$30 \text{ mg} : 1 \text{ mL} = 25 \text{ mg} : x \text{ mL}$$

or

$$\frac{25 \text{ mg}}{30 \text{ mg}} \times 1 \text{ mL} = x \text{ mL}$$

Answer: 0.83 mL = 0.8 mL. The dosage ordered is less than what is available. Therefore you will need less than 1 mL to administer the dosage.

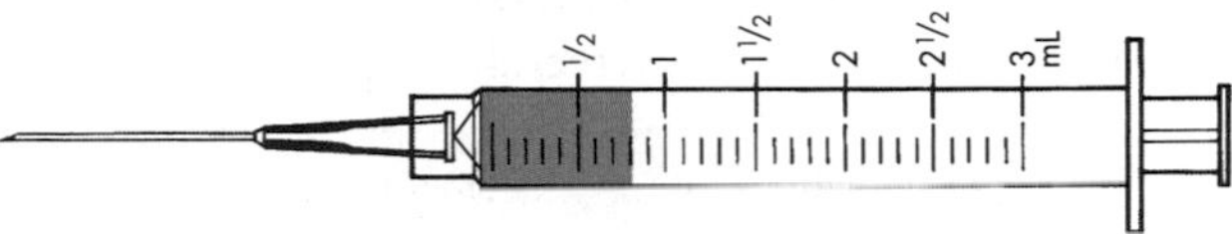

4. No conversion is required. Label indicates dosage in micrograms.

$$500 \text{ mcg} : 2 \text{ mL} = 100 \text{ mcg} : x \text{ mL}$$

or

$$\frac{100 \text{ mcg}}{500 \text{ mcg}} \times 2 \text{ mL} = x \text{ mL}$$

Answer: 0.4 mL. The dosage ordered is less than the available strength. The dosage required would be less than 2 mL.

Alternate solution:

$$250 \text{ mcg} : 1 \text{ mL} = 100 \text{ mcg} : x \text{ mL}$$

or

$$\frac{100 \text{ mcg}}{250 \text{ mcg}} \times 1 \text{ mL} = x \text{ mL}$$

This would net the same answer, 0.4 mL.

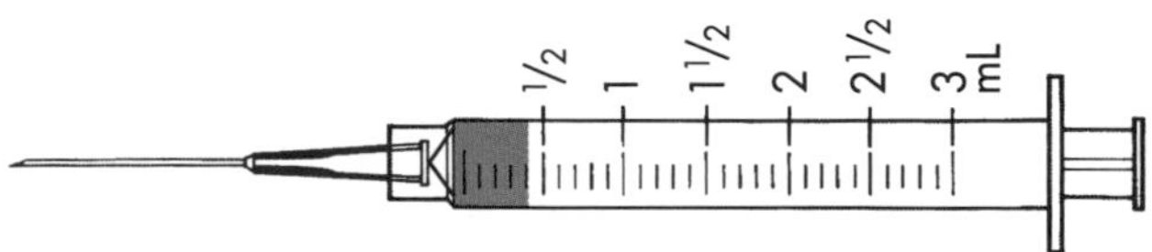

5. $10\text{ mg}:1\text{ mL} = 4\text{ mg}:x\text{ mL}$

or

$$\frac{4\text{ mg}}{10\text{ mg}} \times 1\text{ mL} = x\text{ mL}$$

Answer: 0.4 mL. The dosage ordered is less than the available strength; therefore less than 1 mL is required to administer the dosage.

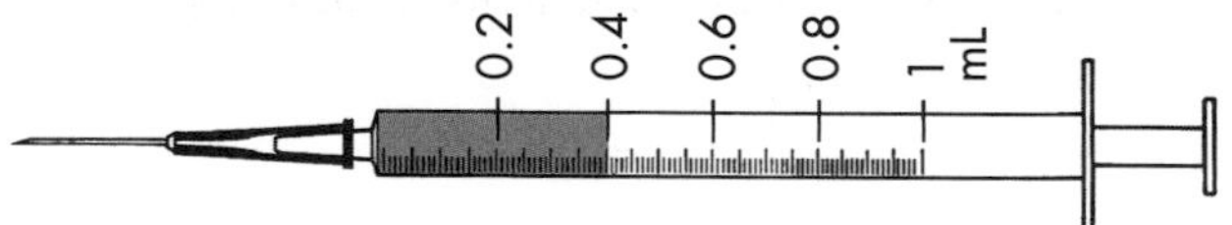

6. $1{,}200{,}000\text{ units}:2\text{ mL} = 1{,}200{,}000\text{ units}:x\text{ mL}$

or

$$\frac{1{,}200{,}000\text{ units}}{1{,}200{,}000\text{ units}} \times 2\text{ mL} = x\text{ mL}$$

Answer: 2 mL. The dosage ordered is contained in 2 mL; therefore you will need 2 mL to administer the dosage.

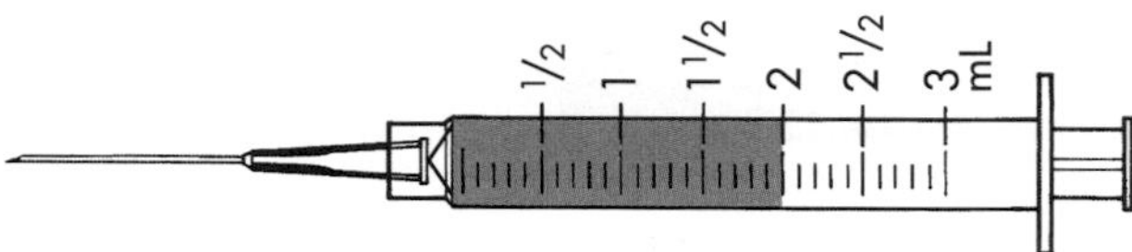

7. $40\text{ mg}:1\text{ mL} = 100\text{ mg}:x\text{ mL}$

or

$$\frac{100\text{ mg}}{40\text{ mg}} \times 1\text{ mL} = x\text{ mL}$$

Answer: 2.5 mL. The amount ordered is more than the available strength; therefore you will need more than 1 mL to administer the required dosage.

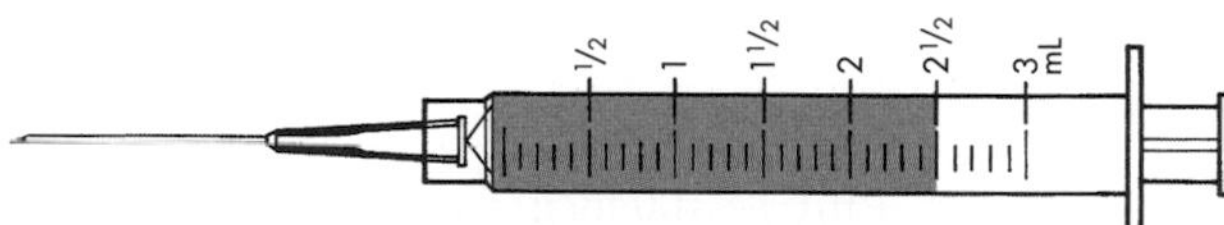

NOTE

You would need three (3) vials of the medication to obtain the indicated dose. The total volume available in the vial is 1.2 mL, which contains 40 mg.

8. $0.2\text{ mg}:1\text{ mL} = 0.4\text{ mg}:x\text{ mL}$

or

$$\frac{0.4\text{ mg}}{0.2\text{ mg}} \times 1\text{ mL} = 0.4\text{ mg}:x\text{ mL}$$

Answer: 2 mL. The dosage ordered is more than the available strength; therefore you will need more than 1 mL to administer the required dosage.

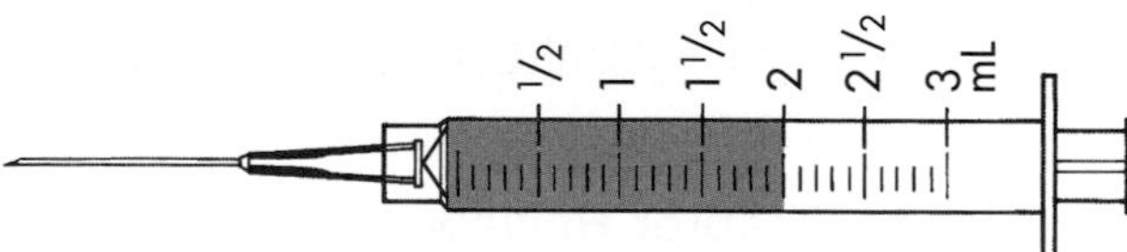

9. $10{,}000\text{ units}:1\text{ mL} = 8{,}000\text{ units}:x\text{ mL}$

or

$$\frac{8{,}000\text{ units}}{10{,}000\text{ units}} \times 1\text{ mL} = x\text{ mL}$$

Answer: 0.8 mL. The dosage ordered is less than the available strength. You will need less than 1 mL to administer the dosage.

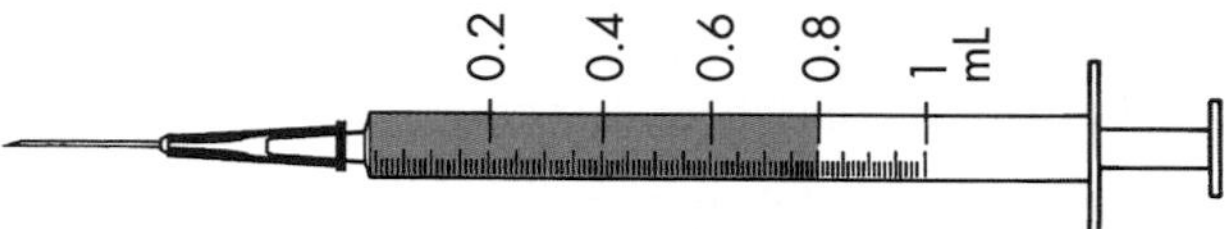

10. $250\text{ mg}:5\text{ mL} = 200\text{ mg}:x\text{ mL}$

or

$$\frac{200\text{ mg}}{250\text{ mg}} \times 5\text{ mL} = x\text{ mL}$$

Answer: 4 mL. The dosage ordered is less than the available strength; therefore you will need less than 5 mL to administer the dosage.

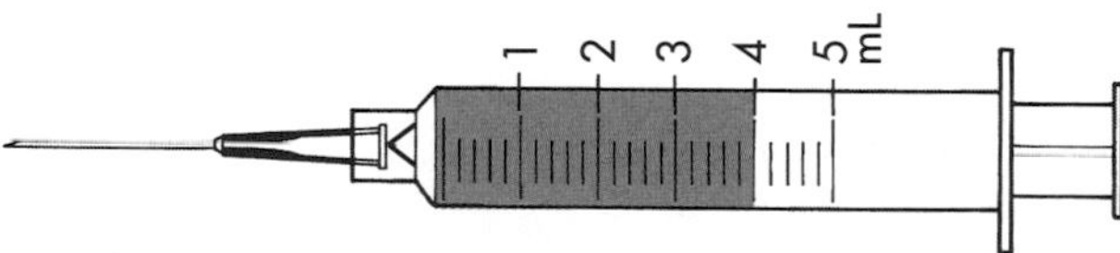

11. $10\text{ mg}:1\text{ mL} = 10\text{ mg}:x\text{ mL}$

or

$$\frac{10\text{ mg}}{10\text{ mg}} \times 1\text{ mL} = x\text{ mL}$$

Answer: 1 mL. The dosage ordered is the same as the available strength; therefore you will need 1 mL to administer the dosage.

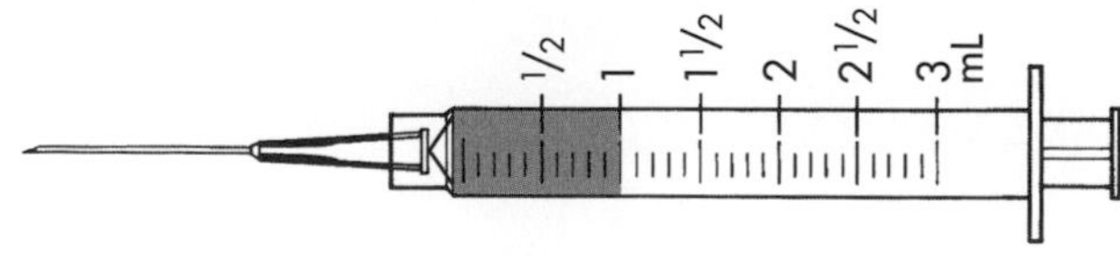

12. $20\text{ mg} : 2\text{ mL} = 40\text{ mg} : x\text{ mL}$

or

$$\frac{40\text{ mg}}{20\text{ mg}} \times 2\text{ mL} = x\text{ mL}$$

Answer: 4 mL. The dosage ordered is more than the available strength. Therefore you will need more than 2 mL to administer the dosage.

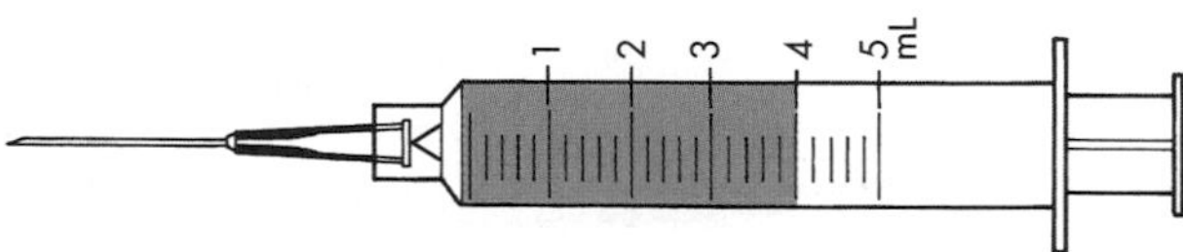

NOTE

You would need two (2) vials of the medication to administer the ordered dose. The total volume available in the vial is 2 mL, which is equal to 20 mg.

13. $50\text{ mg} : 1\text{ mL} = 25\text{ mg} : x\text{ mL}$

or

$$\frac{25\text{ mg}}{50\text{ mg}} \times 1\text{ mL} = x\text{ mL}$$

Answer: 0.5 mL. The dosage ordered is less than the available strength; therefore you will need less than 1 mL to administer the dosage. (The preferred answer is 0.5 mL. mL is a metric measure.)

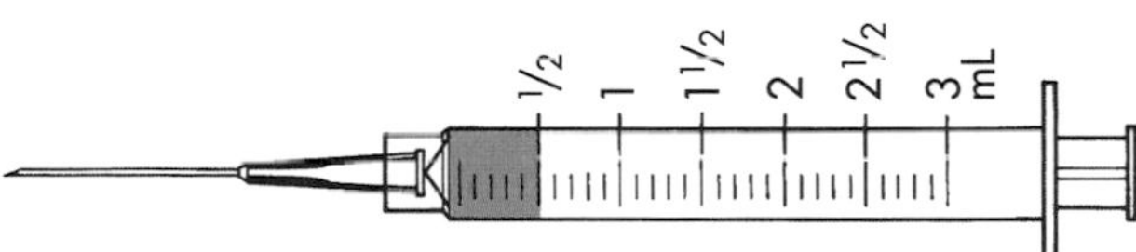

14. $2\text{ mg} : 1\text{ mL} = 1.5\text{ mg} : x\text{ mL}$

or

$$\frac{1.5\text{ mg}}{2\text{ mg}} \times 1\text{ mL} = x\text{ mL}$$

Answer: 0.8 mL. 0.75 mL is rounded to nearest tenth. The dosage ordered is less than the available strength. You will need less than 1 mL to administer the dosage.

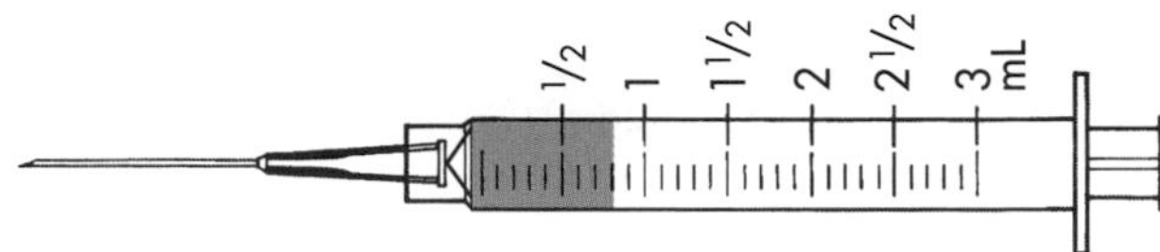

15. $40\text{ mg} : 1\text{ mL} = 50\text{ mg} : x\text{ mL}$

or

$$\frac{50\text{ mg}}{40\text{ mg}} \times 1\text{ mL} = x\text{ mL}$$

Answer: 1.3 mL. 1.25 mL is rounded to nearest tenth. The dosage ordered is more than the available strength per mL if you use 40 mg per mL. You will need more than 1 mL to administer the dosage.

Alternate solution:

$80\text{ mg} : 2\text{ mL} = 50\text{ mg} : x\text{ mL}$

or

$$\frac{50\text{ mg}}{80\text{ mg}} \times 2\text{ mL} = x\text{ mL}$$

This setup still gives an answer of 1.3 mL.

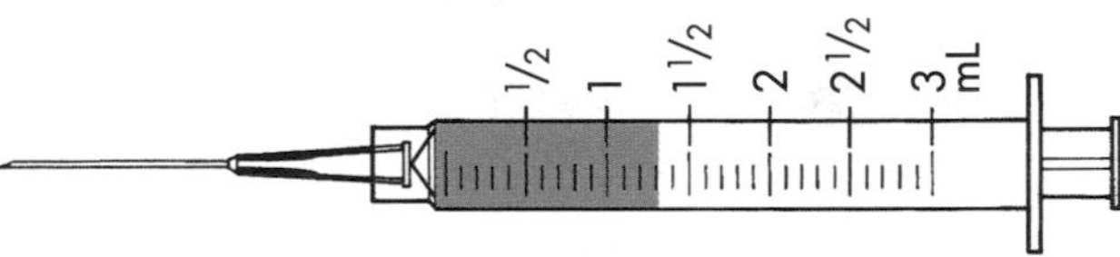

16. $50\text{ mg} : 1\text{ mL} = 25\text{ mg} : x\text{ mL}$

or

$$\frac{25\text{ mg}}{50\text{ mg}} \times 1\text{ mL} - x\text{ mL}$$

Answer: 0.5 mL. The dosage ordered is less than the available strength; therefore you will need less than 1 mL to administer the dosage. (Preferred answer: 0.5 mL because mL is a metric measure.)

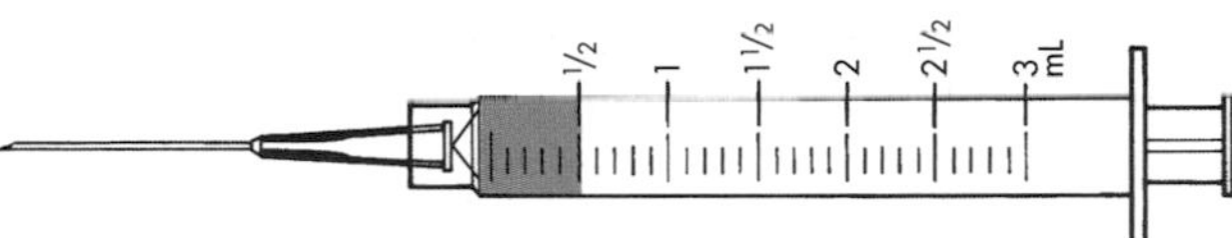

17. $4\text{ mg} : 2\text{ mL} = 3\text{ mg} : x\text{ mL}$

or

$$\frac{3\text{ mg}}{4\text{ mg}} \times 2\text{ mL} = x\text{ mL}$$

Answer: 1.5 mL. The dosage ordered is less than the available strength; therefore you will need less than 2 mL to administer the dosage.

Alternate solution:

$2\text{ mg} : 1\text{ mL} = 3\text{ mg} : x\text{ mL}$

or

$$\frac{3\text{ mg}}{2\text{ mg}} \times 1\text{ mL} = x\text{ mL}$$

This setup still gives an answer of 1.5 mL.

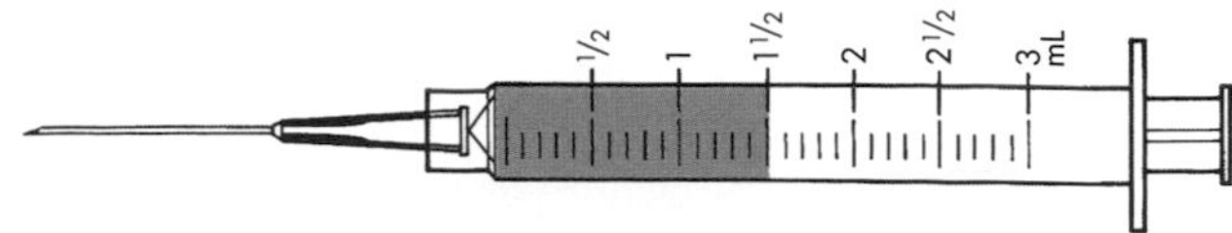

18. 250 mg : 2 mL = 400 mg : x mL

or

$$\frac{400 \text{ mg}}{250 \text{ mg}} \times 2 \text{ mL} = x \text{ mL}$$

Answer: 3.2 mL. The dosage ordered is more than the available strength. You will need more than 2 mL to administer the dosage.

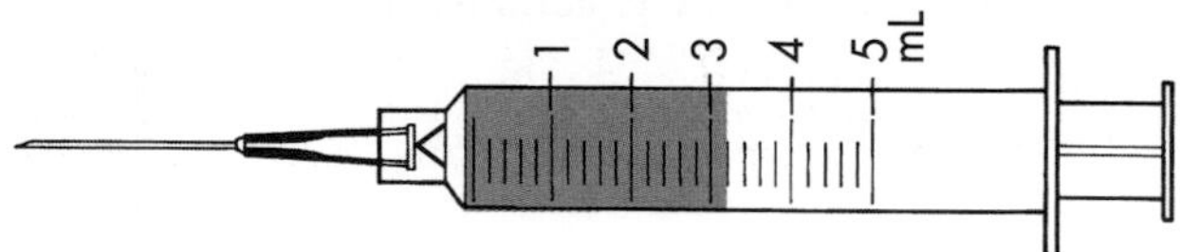

19. Use the dosage indicated on the label in mg; no conversion required.

0.4 mg : 1 mL = 0.2 mg : x mL

or

$$\frac{0.2 \text{ mg}}{0.4 \text{ mg}} \times 1 \text{ mL} = x \text{ mL}$$

Answer: 0.5 mL. The dosage ordered is less than the available strength. You will need less than 1 mL to administer the dosage.

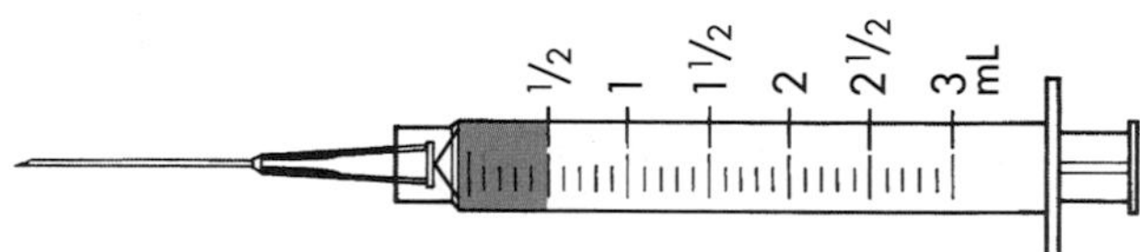

20. Conversion is required. Equivalent: 1,000 mcg = 1 mg. Therefore 200 mcg = 0.2 mg.

0.2 mg : 1 mL = 0.2 mg : x mL

or

$$\frac{0.2 \text{ mg}}{0.2 \text{ mg}} \times 1 \text{ mL} = x \text{ mL}$$

Answer: 1 mL. Because 200 mcg = 0.2 mg, you will need 1 mL to administer the required dosage.

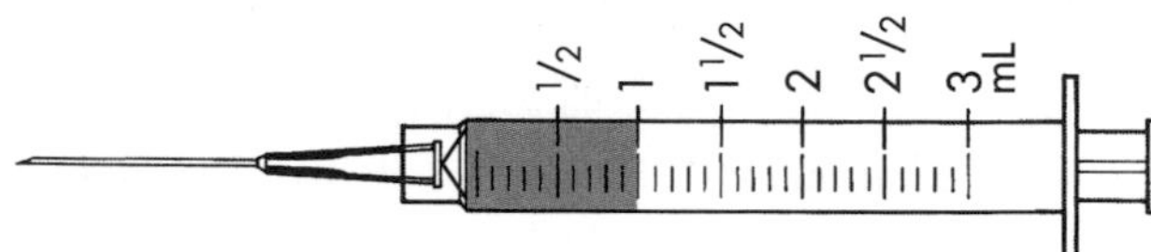

21. 40 mcg : 1 mL = 30 mcg : x mL

or

$$\frac{30 \text{ mcg}}{40 \text{ mcg}} \times 1 \text{ mL} = x \text{ mL}$$

Answer: 0.75 mL. The dosage ordered is less than the available strength. You will need less than 1 mL to administer the dosage.

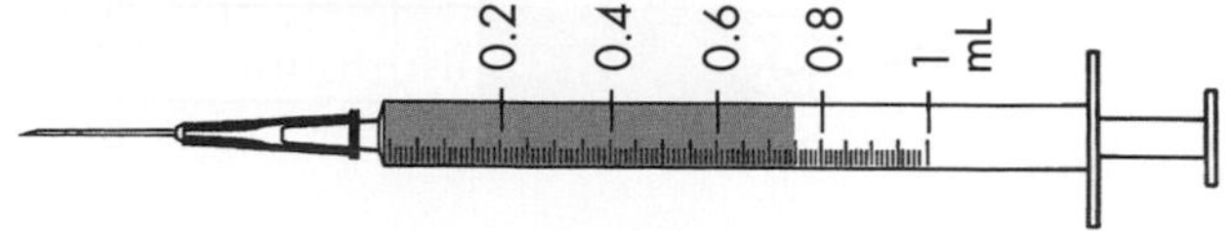

22. 50 mg : 1 mL = 35 mg : x mL

or

$$\frac{35 \text{ mg}}{50 \text{ mg}} \times 1 \text{ mL} = x \text{ mL}$$

Answer: 0.7 mL. The dosage ordered is less than the available strength. You will need less than 1 mL to administer the required dosage.

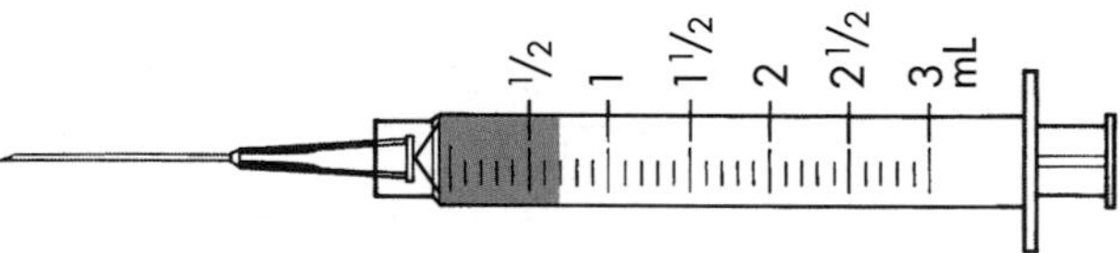

23. 100 mg : 1 mL = 60 mg : x mL

or

$$\frac{60 \text{ mg}}{100 \text{ mg}} \times 1 \text{ mL} = x \text{ mL}$$

Answer: 0.6 mL. The dosage ordered is less than the available strength. You will need less than 1 mL to administer the required dosage.

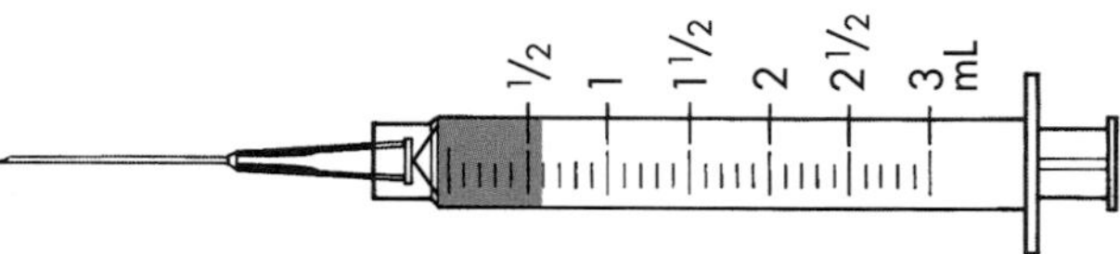

24. 50 mg : 2 mL = 50 mg : x mL

or

$$\frac{50 \text{ mg}}{50 \text{ mg}} \times 2 \text{ mL} = x \text{ mL}$$

Answer: 2 mL. The dosage ordered is contained in 2 mL; therefore you will need 2 mL to administer the dosage.

Alternate solution:

25 mg : 1 mL = 50 mg : x mL

or

$$\frac{50 \text{ mg}}{25 \text{ mg}} \times 1 \text{ mL} = x \text{ mL}$$

This setup will still give an answer of 2 mL.

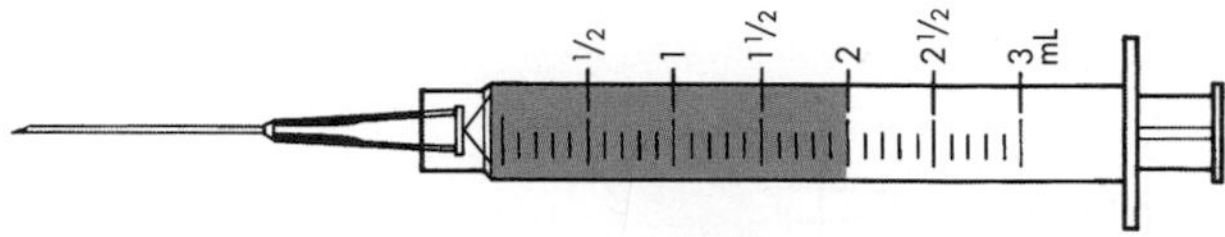

25. 0.5 mg : 2 mL = 0.4 mg : x mL

or

$$\frac{0.4 \text{ mg}}{0.5 \text{ mg}} \times 2 \text{ mL} = x \text{ mL}$$

Answer: 1.6 mL. The dosage ordered is less than the available strength. You will need less than 2 mL to administer the required dosage.

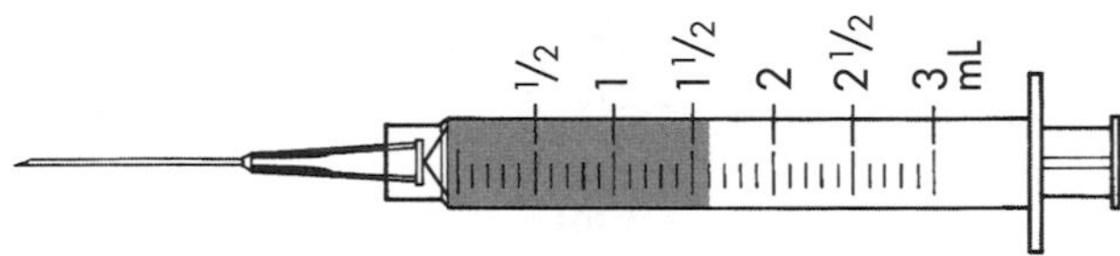

26. 300 mg : 1 mL = 500 mg : x mL

or

$$\frac{500 \text{ mg}}{300 \text{ mg}} \times 1 \text{ mL} = x \text{ mL}$$

Answer: 1.7 mL. 1.66 mL is rounded to the nearest tenth. The dosage ordered is more than the available strength. You will need more than 1 mL to administer the dosage.

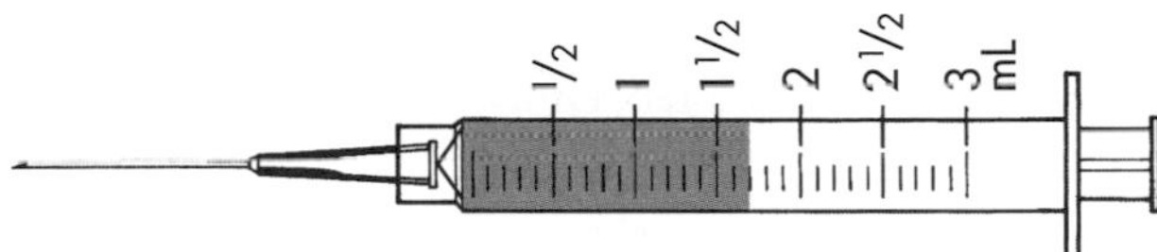

27. 2 mg : 1 mL = 1.5 mg : x mL

or

$$\frac{1.5 \text{ mg}}{2 \text{ mg}} \times 1 \text{ mL} = x \text{ mL}$$

Answer: 0.75 mL = 0.8 mL. The dosage ordered is less than the available strength; therefore you will need less than 1 mL to administer the dosage.

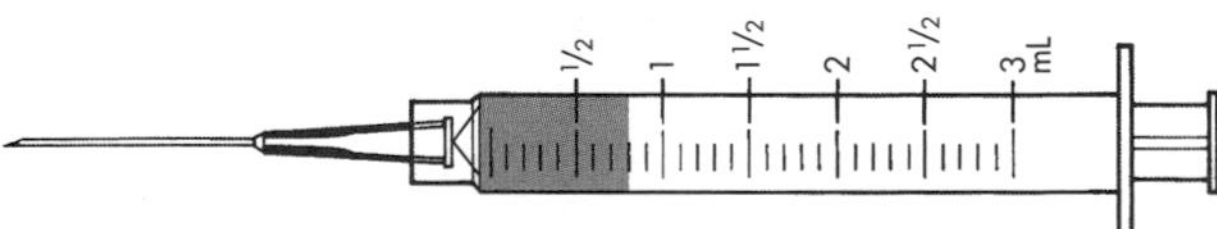

28. Conversion is required. Equivalent: 1,000 mg = 1 g Therefore 0.65 g = 650 mg

400 mg : 1 mL = 650 mg : x mL

or

$$\frac{650 \text{ mg}}{400 \text{ mg}} \times 1 \text{ mL} = x \text{ mL}$$

Answer: 1.6 mL; 1.62 rounded to the nearest tenth. The dosage ordered is greater than the available strength. You will need more than 1 mL to administer the dosage.

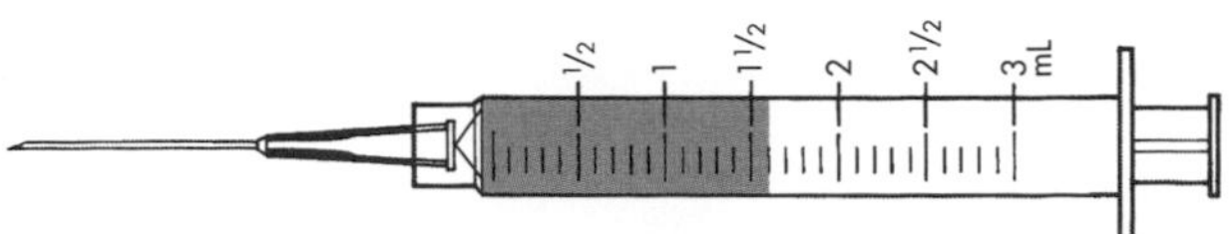

29. 4,000 units : 1 mL = 3,000 units : x mL

or

$$\frac{3{,}000 \text{ units}}{4{,}000 \text{ units}} \times 1 \text{ mL} = x \text{ mL}$$

Answer: 0.75 mL. The dosage ordered is less than the available strength. Therefore you will need less than 1 mL to administer the dosage.

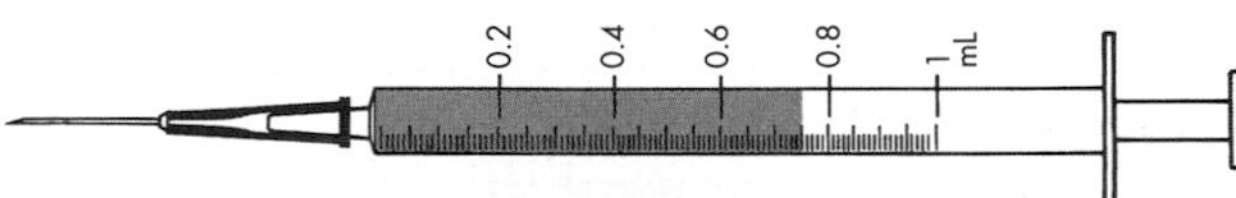

30. 10 mg : 2 mL = 15 mg : x mL

or

$$\frac{15 \text{ mg}}{10 \text{ mg}} \times 1 \text{ mL} = x \text{ mL}$$

Answer: 3 mL. The dosage ordered is greater than the available strength. Therefore you will need more than 2 mL to administer the dosage.

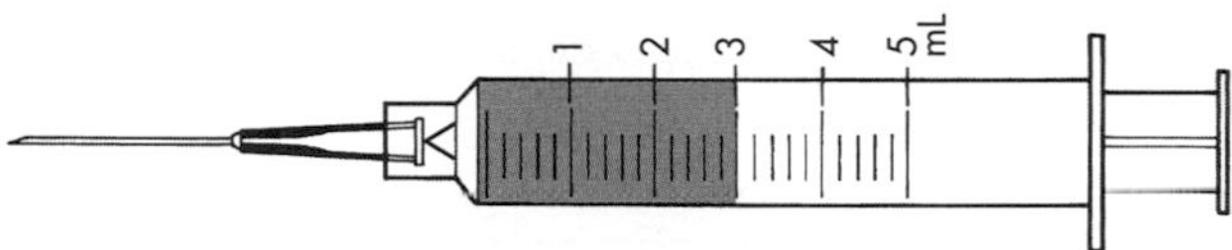

31. 40 mg : 0.4 mL = 30 mg : x mL

or

$$\frac{30 \text{ mg}}{40 \text{ mg}} \times 0.4 \text{ mL} = x \text{ mL}$$

Answer: 0.3 mL. The dosage ordered is less than the available strength. You will need less than 0.4 mL to administer the dosage.

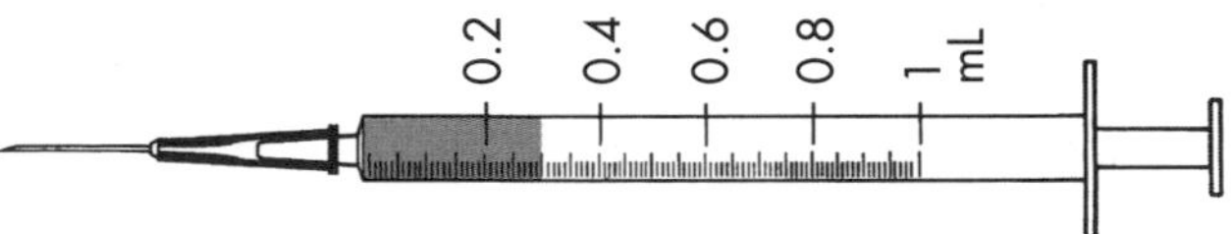

32. Conversion is required. Equivalent: 1,000 mg = 1 g. Therefore 0.3 g = 300 mg.

300 mg : 2 mL = 300 mg : x mL

or

$$\frac{300 \text{ mg}}{300 \text{ mg}} \times 2 \text{ mL} = x \text{ mL}$$

Answer: 2 mL. The label indicates that the dosage ordered, 300 mg, is contained in a volume of 2 mL.

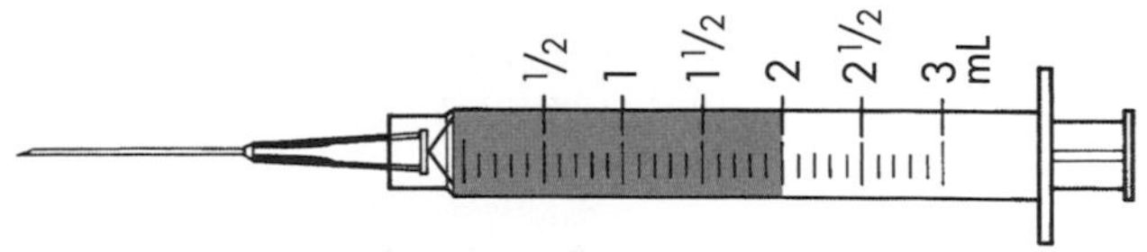

33. 5 mg : 1 mL = 7.5 mg : x mL

or

$$\frac{7.5 \text{ mg}}{5 \text{ mg}} \times 1 \text{ mL} = x \text{ mL}$$

Answer: 1.5 mL. (State the answer as a decimal; mL is a metric measure.) The dosage ordered is greater than the available strength. Therefore you will need more than 1 mL to administer the dosage.

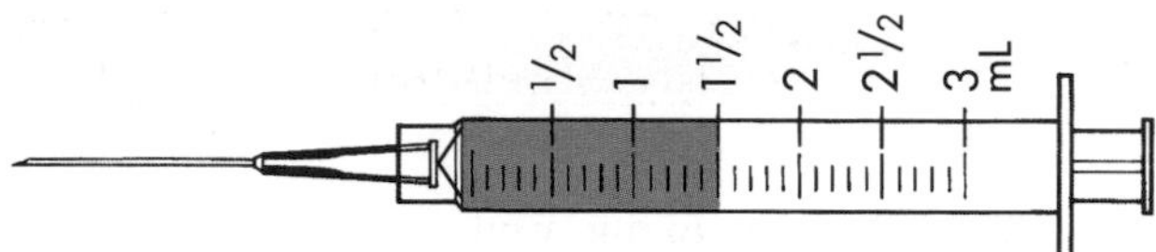

34. 0.25 mg : 1 mL = 1 mg : x mL

or

$$\frac{1 \text{ mg}}{0.25 \text{ mg}} \times 1 \text{ mL} = x \text{ mL}$$

Answer: 4 mL. The dosage ordered is more than the available strength. Therefore you will need more than 1 mL to administer the dosage.

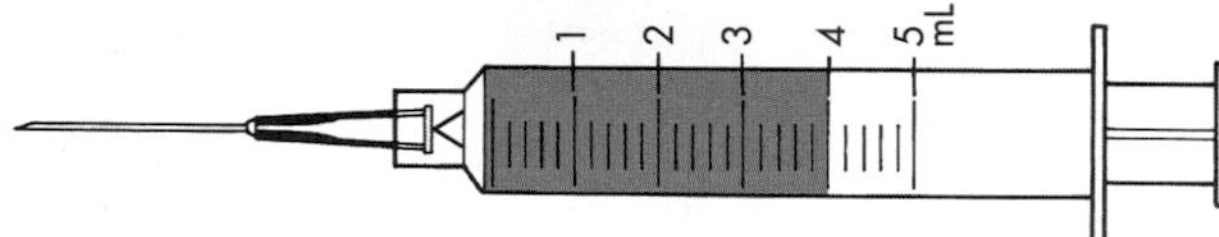

35. 40 mg : 1 mL = 55 mg : x mL

or

$$\frac{55 \text{ mg}}{40 \text{ mg}} \times 1 \text{ mL} = x \text{ mL}$$

Answer: 1.4 mL; 1.37 rounded to the nearest tenth. The dosage ordered is more than the available strength. Therefore you will need more than 1 mL to administer the dosage.

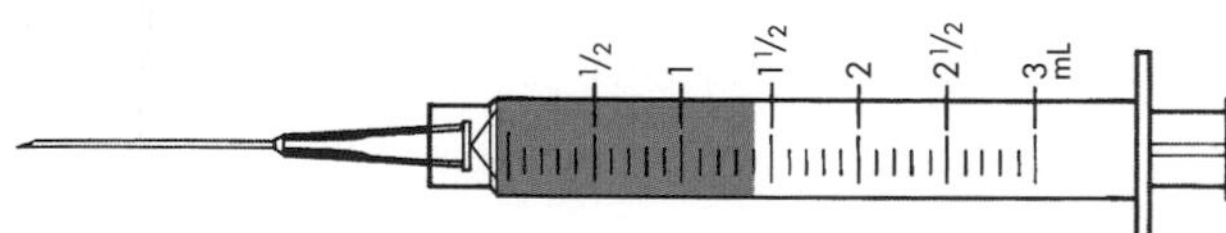

36. 6 mg : 1 mL = 12 mg : x mL

or

$$\frac{12 \text{ mg}}{6 \text{ mg}} \times 1 \text{ mL} = x \text{ mL}$$

Answer: 2 mL. The dosage ordered is greater than the available strength. Therefore you will need more than 1 mL to administer the dosage.

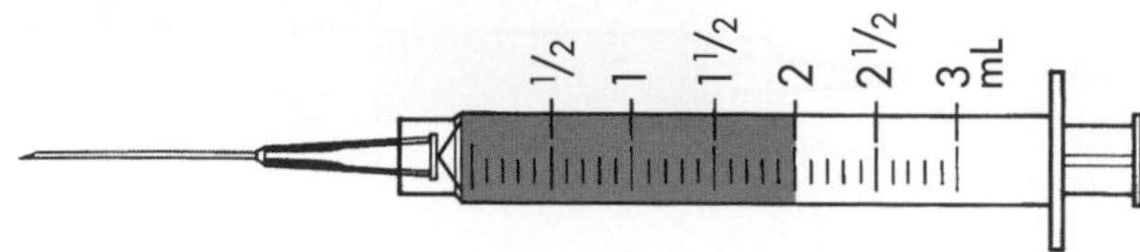

37. Conversion is required. Equivalent: 1,000 mg = 1 g. Therefore 0.25 g = 250 mg.

25 mg : 1 mL = 250 mg : x mL

or

$$\frac{250 \text{ mg}}{25 \text{ mg}} \times 1 \text{ mL} = x \text{ mL}$$

Alternate solution:

500 mg : 20 mL = 250 mg : x mL

or

$$\frac{250 \text{ mg}}{500 \text{ mg}} \times 20 \text{ mL} = x \text{ mL}$$

This setup will still give an answer of 10 mL.

Answer: 10 mL. The dosage ordered is greater than the available strength when using 25 mg per mL. Therefore you will need more than 1 mL to administer the dosage.

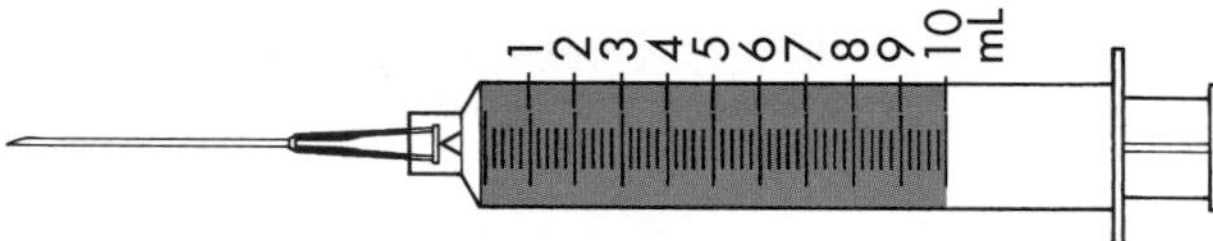

38. Conversion is required. Equivalent: 1,000 mg = 1 g. Therefore 0.5 g = 500 mg.

500 mg : 1 mL = 500 mg : x mL

or

$$\frac{500 \text{ mg}}{500 \text{ mg}} \times 1 \text{ mL} = x \text{ mL}$$

Answer: 1 mL. The dosage ordered, 500 mg, is contained in a volume of 1 mL.

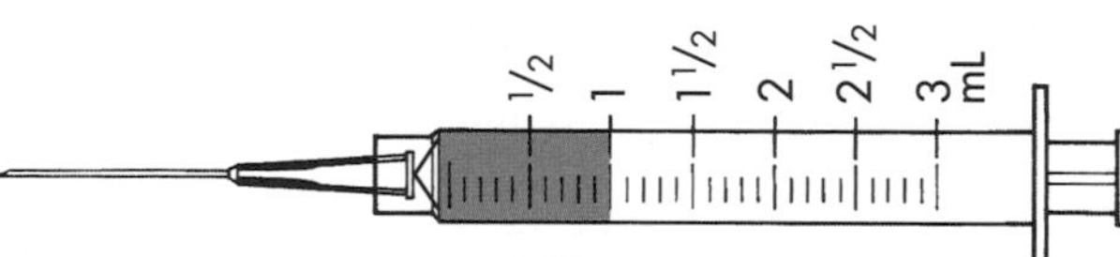

39. 100 mg : 1 mL = 150 mg : x mL

or

$$\frac{150 \text{ mg}}{100 \text{ mg}} \times 1 \text{ mL} = x \text{ mL}$$

Answer: 1.5 mL. (Answer stated as a decimal; mL is a metric measure.) The dosage ordered is greater than the available strength; therefore you will need more than 1 mL to administer the dosage.

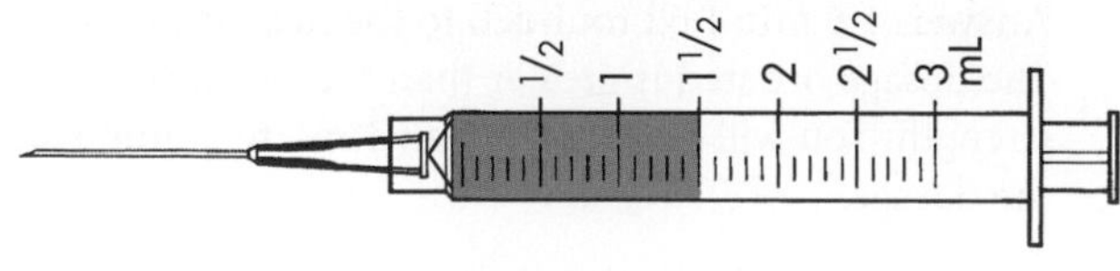

40. Demerol:

$$100 \text{ mg} : 1 \text{ mL} = 65 \text{ mg} : x \text{ mL}$$

or

$$\frac{65 \text{ mg}}{100 \text{ mg}} \times 1 \text{ mL} = x \text{ mL}$$

Answer: 0.7 mL; 0.65 mL rounded to the nearest tenth. The dosage ordered is less than the available strength. Therefore less than 1 mL would be required to administer the dosage.

Promethazine:

$$25 \text{ mg} : 1 \text{ mL} = 25 \text{ mg} : x \text{ mL}$$

or

$$\frac{25 \text{ mg}}{25 \text{ mg}} \times 1 \text{ mL} = x \text{ mL}$$

Answer: 1 mL. The label indicates that the dosage ordered, 25 mg, is contained in the volume of 1 mL. These two medications are often administered in the same syringe (0.7 mL of Demerol + 1 mL of promethazine = 1.7 mL).

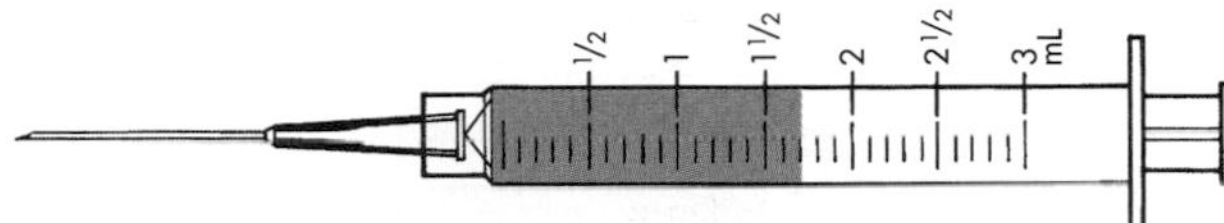

41. $4 \text{ mg} : 1 \text{ mL} = 9 \text{ mg} : x \text{ mL}$

or

$$\frac{9 \text{ mg}}{4 \text{ mg}} \times 1 \text{ mL} = x \text{ mL}$$

Answer: 2.3 mL; 2.25 mL rounded to the nearest tenth. The dosage ordered is greater than the available strength. You would need more than 1 mL to administer the dosage.

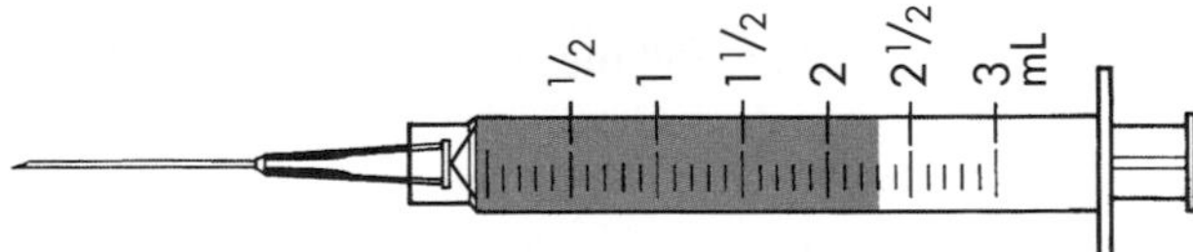

42. $50 \text{ mcg} : 1 \text{ mL} = 60 \text{ mcg} : x \text{ mL}$

or

$$\frac{60 \text{ mcg}}{50 \text{ mcg}} \times 1 \text{ mL} = x \text{ mL}$$

Answer: 1.2 mL. The dosage ordered is greater than the available strength when using 50 mcg per mL. You will need more than 1 mL to administer the dosage.

Alternate solution:

$$250 \text{ mcg} : 5 \text{ mL} = 60 \text{ mcg} : x \text{ mL}$$

or

$$\frac{60 \text{ mcg}}{250 \text{ mcg}} \times 5 \text{ mL} = x \text{ mL}$$

This setup will still give an answer of 1.2 mL.

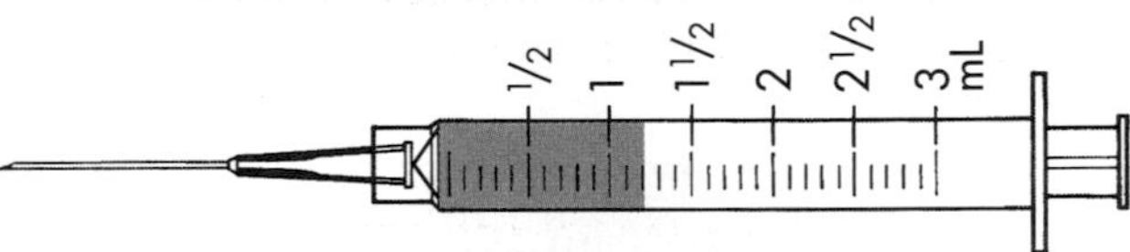

43. $20 \text{ mg} : 1 \text{ mL} = 10 \text{ mg} : x \text{ mL}$

or

$$\frac{10 \text{ mg}}{20 \text{ mg}} \times 1 \text{ mL} = x \text{ mL}$$

Answer: 0.5 mL. (Stated as 0.5 mL; mL is a metric measure.) The dosage ordered is less than the available strength. You will need less than 1 mL to administer the dosage.

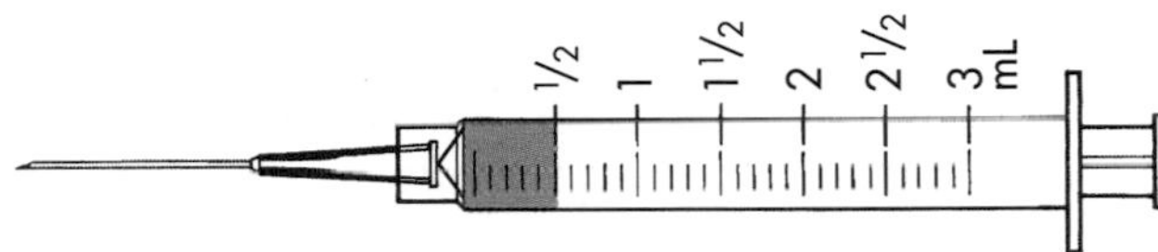

44. $300 \text{ mcg} : 1 \text{ mL} = 175 \text{ mcg} : x \text{ mL}$

or

$$\frac{175 \text{ mcg}}{300 \text{ mcg}} \times 1 \text{ mL} = x \text{ mL}$$

Answer: 0.58 mL. The dosage ordered is less than the available strength. You will need less than 1 mL to administer the dosage.

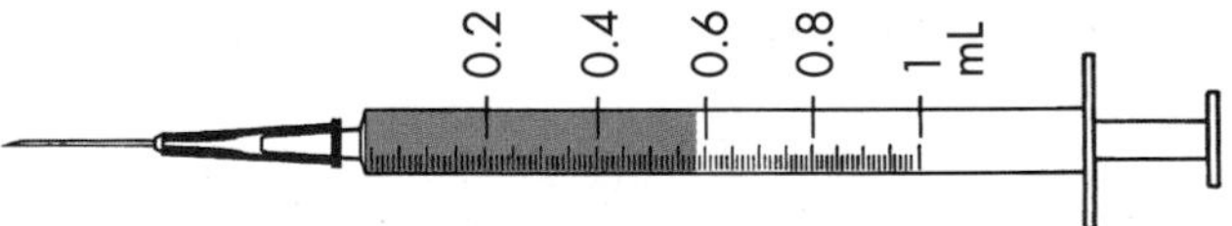

Alternate solution:

$$480 \text{ mcg} : 1.6 \text{ mL} = 175 \text{ mcg} : x \text{ mL}$$

or

$$\frac{175 \text{ mcg}}{480 \text{ mcg}} \times 1.6 \text{ mL} = x \text{ mL}$$

This setup would give the same answer of 0.58 mL.

45. 2 mg : 1 mL = 1.5 mg : x mL

or

$$\frac{1.5 \text{ mg}}{2 \text{ mg}} \times 1 \text{ mL} = x \text{ mL}$$

Answer: 0.8 mL; 0.75, rounded to the nearest tenth. The dosage ordered is less than the available strength. You will need less than 1 mL to administer the dosage.

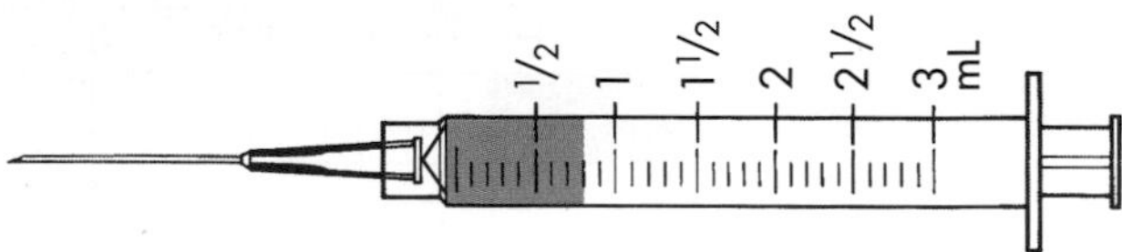

46. 60 mg : 2 mL = 60 mg : x mL

or

$$\frac{60 \text{ mg}}{60 \text{ mg}} \times 2 \text{ mL} = x \text{ mL}$$

Answer: 2 mL. The dosage ordered is contained in 2 mL; therefore, you will need 2 mL to administer the dosage.

Alternate solution:

30 mg : 1 mL = 60 mg : x mL

or

$$\frac{60 \text{ mg}}{30 \text{ mg}} \times 1 \text{ mL} = x \text{ mL}$$

This setup will still give an answer of 2 mL.

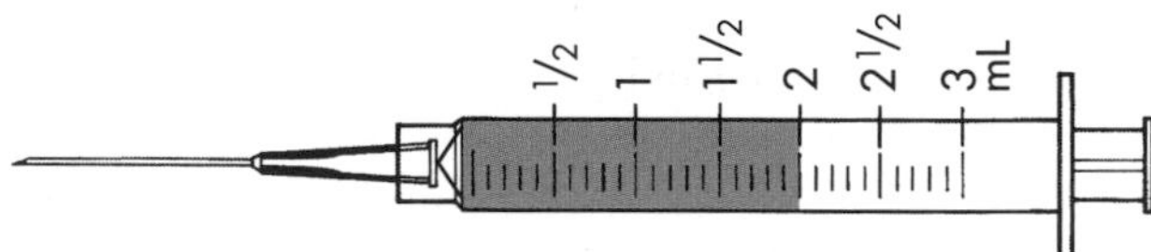

47. 20 mg : 5 mL = 5 mg : x mL

or

$$\frac{5 \text{ mg}}{20 \text{ mg}} \times 5 \text{ mL} = x \text{ mL}$$

Answer: 1.3 mL; 1.25, rounded to the nearest tenth. The dosage ordered is less than the available strength. You will need less than 5 mL to administer the dosage.

Alternate solution:

4 mg : 1 mL = 5 mL : x mL

or

$$\frac{5 \text{ mg}}{4 \text{ mg}} \times 1 \text{ mL} = x \text{ mL}$$

This setup will still give an answer of 1.3 mL; 1.25, rounded to the nearest tenth.

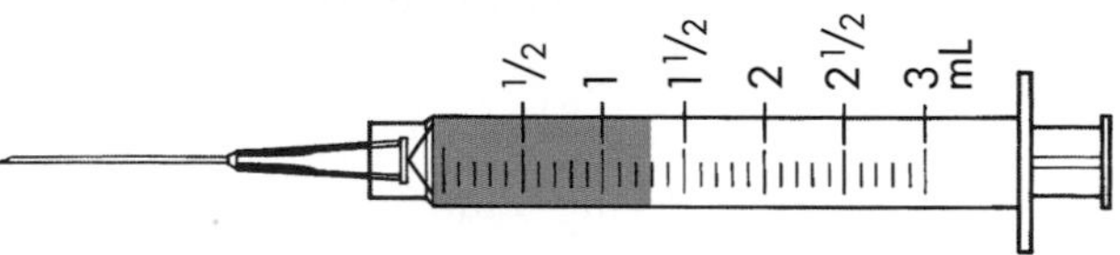

48. 0.3 mg : 1 mL = 0.6 mg : x mL

or

$$\frac{0.6 \text{ mg}}{0.3 \text{ mg}} \times 1 \text{ mL} = x \text{ mL}$$

Answer: 2 mL. The dosage ordered is more than the available strength. You will need more than 1 mL to administer the dosage.

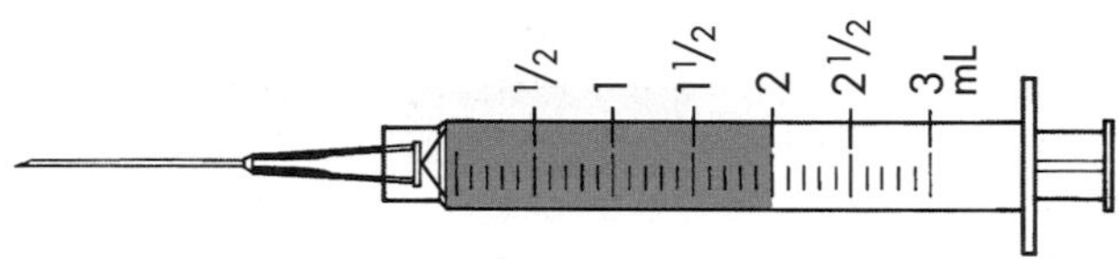

49. 1,000 mg : 10 mL = 300 mg : x mL

or

$$\frac{300 \text{ mg}}{1{,}000 \text{ mg}} \times 10 \text{ mL} = x \text{ mL}$$

Answer: 3 mL. The dosage ordered is less than the available strength. You will need less than 10 mL to administer the dosage.

Alternate solution:

100 mg : 1 mL = 300 mg : x mL

or

$$\frac{300 \text{ mg}}{100 \text{ mg}} \times 1 \text{ mL} = x \text{ mL}$$

This setup will still give an answer of 3 mL.

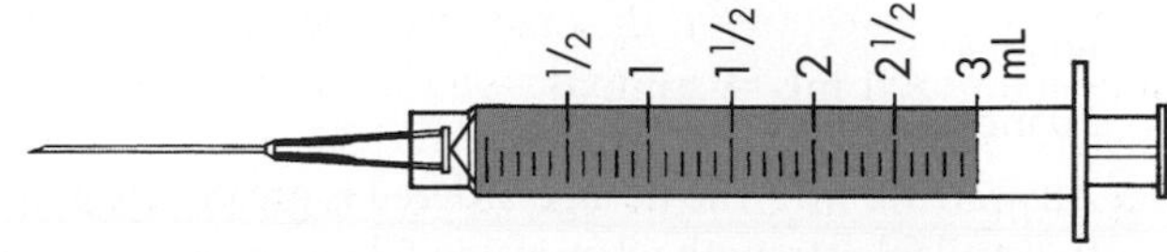

CHAPTER 19
Reconstitution of Solutions

Objectives

After reviewing this chapter, you should be able to:

1. Prepare a solution from a powdered medication according to directions on the vial or other resources
2. Identify essential information to be placed on the vial of a medication after it is reconstituted
3. Determine the best concentration strength for medications ordered when there are several directions for mixing
4. Identify the varying directions for reconstitution and select the correct directions to prepare the dosage ordered
5. Calculate dosages from reconstituted medications
6. Determine the rate in milliliters per hour for enteral feedings
7. Calculate the amount of solute and solvent needed to prepare a desired strength for enteral feedings, irrigations, and soaks

Some medications are unstable when stored in liquid form for long periods of time and therefore are packaged in powdered form. When medications come in powdered form, they must be diluted with a liquid referred to as a *diluent* or *solvent* before they can be administered to a client. Once a liquid is added to a powdered medication, some solutions may need to be used within an hour, 1 to 14 days, or longer, depending on the medication. For example, ampicillin must be used within an hour after reconstitution; EryPed, an oral suspension, is good for 35 days after reconstitution. The process of adding a solvent or diluent to a medication in powdered form to dissolve it and form a solution is referred to as *reconstitution.* Reconstitution is necessary for medications that come in powdered form before they can be measured and administered. If you think about it, this process is something you do in everyday situations. For example, when you make iced tea (powdered form), in essence you are reconstituting it. The iced tea, for example, is the powder, and the water you add to it is considered the diluent, or solvent.

As a safety precaution in some institutions, the pharmacy reconstitutes most medications. However, the nurse must understand the process of reconstitution because some medications may have to be reconstituted just before administration. Medications requiring reconstitution can be for oral or parenteral use; these are not always injectable medications. With emphasis being placed on home care, nurses and other health care providers may have to dilute things such as oral medications, irrigating solutions, and nutritional feedings. Sterile solutions are always used to reconstitute medications for injectable use. Special diluents, when required for reconstitution, are usually packaged with the powdered medication, but oral medications can often be, but are not always, reconstituted with tap water. Thus the nurse **must** know how the reconstitution process works. Understanding the terminology relating to reconstitution enables the nurse to understand the process:

- **Solute**—A powdered medication or liquid concentrate to be dissolved or diluted.
- **Solvent (diluent)**—A liquid that is added to the powder or liquid concentrate. The nurse must identify the solvent (diluent) to use. The type of solvent (diluent) varies according

to the medication. The package insert or the medication label will indicate the solvent (diluent) to be used and the amount. If the information is not indicated on the label, or the package insert is unavailable, consult the pharmacy or a medication reference such as the *Physician's Desk Reference (PDR),* a medication reference, or the hospital formulary.

- **Solution**—The liquid that results when the solvent (diluent) dissolves the solute (powdered medication or liquid concentrate).

Basic Principles for Reconstitution

The first step in reconstitution is to find the directions and carefully read the information on the vial or the package insert. Medications labeled and packaged with reconstitution directions may indicate "oral, IM, or IV use only." Always verify the route of administration ordered **before** reconstituting a medication. Different routes may require different directions for reconstitution. Follow the reconstitution directions specific to the route of administration and medication being administered.

Examples of the several directions for reconstitution are shown in this chapter.

> **SAFETY ALERT!**
>
> Before reconstituting a medication, read and follow the directions on the label or package insert. This includes checking the expiration date on the medication and diluent. Never assume the type or amount of diluent to be used. If the information is not available, consult appropriate resources, such as a reliable medication text, the *PDR,* a pharmacist, or the manufacturer's website, before reconstituting the medication.

1. The drug manufacturer provides directions for reconstitution, including information regarding the number of milliliters of diluent or solvent that should be added, as well as the type of solution that should be used to reconstitute the medication. The concentration (or strength) of the medication after it has been reconstituted according to the directions is also indicated on some medications. The directions for reconstitution must be read and followed carefully.
2. The diluent (solvent, liquid) commonly used for reconstitution is sterile water or sterile 0.9% sodium chloride (normal saline) solution, for injection. Sterile water and normal saline for injection is available in preservative-free diluent used for single-use reconstitution and in bacteriostatic form with preservatives that prevent the growth of microorganisms for multiple dose vials. Use only the diluent recommended. Using the wrong diluent can result in an incompatibility that can cause crystallization and/or clumping of the medication in solution. Some medications that require reconstitution may indicate they can be mixed with lidocaine, a local anesthetic, to reduce pain. Some medications may cause pain when injected (e.g., antibiotics). The label or package insert indicates when lidocaine can be used and the percentage. Always check with the prescriber before reconstituting a medication with lidocaine. Because lidocaine is a medication, it may necessitate an order from the prescriber. If lidocaine is used, make certain to use only lidocaine. Lidocaine can come combined with epinephrine. Epinephrine causes vasoconstriction (tightening of blood vessels), which delays the absorption of the medication. Some powdered medications for oral use may be reconstituted with tap water. The manufacturer's directions will tell you which solution to use. If the medication requires a special solution for reconstitution, it is usually supplied by the drug manufacturer and packaged with the medication (e.g., Librium).

> **SAFETY ALERT!**
>
> Always use a sterile solution for injection and for mixing to administer a medication by the parenteral route.

3. Once you have located the reconstitution directions on the label or package insert, you need to identify the following information:
   a. The type of diluent to use for reconstitution.
   b. The amount of diluent to add. This is essential because directions relating to the amount can vary according to the route of administration. There may be different dilution instructions for intravenous (IV) versus intramuscular (IM) administration.

c. The length of time the medication is good once it is reconstituted. The length of time a medication can be stored once reconstituted can vary depending on how it is stored. When medications are reconstituted, the solution must be used in a timely fashion. The potency (stability) of the medication may be several hours to several days or even a week or longer. Check the medication label, package insert, or appropriate resources for how long a medication may be used after reconstitution.

d. Directions for storing the medication after mixing. Medications must be stored appropriately once reconstituted per manufacturer's instructions to ensure optimal potency of the medication. Medications can become unstable when stored incorrectly and for long periods. Example: A label may state a medication maintains its potency 96 hours at room temperature or 7 days when refrigerated.

e. The strength or concentration of the medication after it has been reconstituted.

Refer to Figure 19-1 showing the Ceftriaxone reconstitution procedure for IM. Note that directions on the label say to add 2.1 mL 1% lidocaine hydrochloride injection or sterile water for injection and that each 1 mL contains 350 mg. The available dosage after reconstitution is 350 mg of Ceftriaxone per 1 mL of solution. **(Remember to check with the prescriber before reconstituting a medication with lidocaine.)**

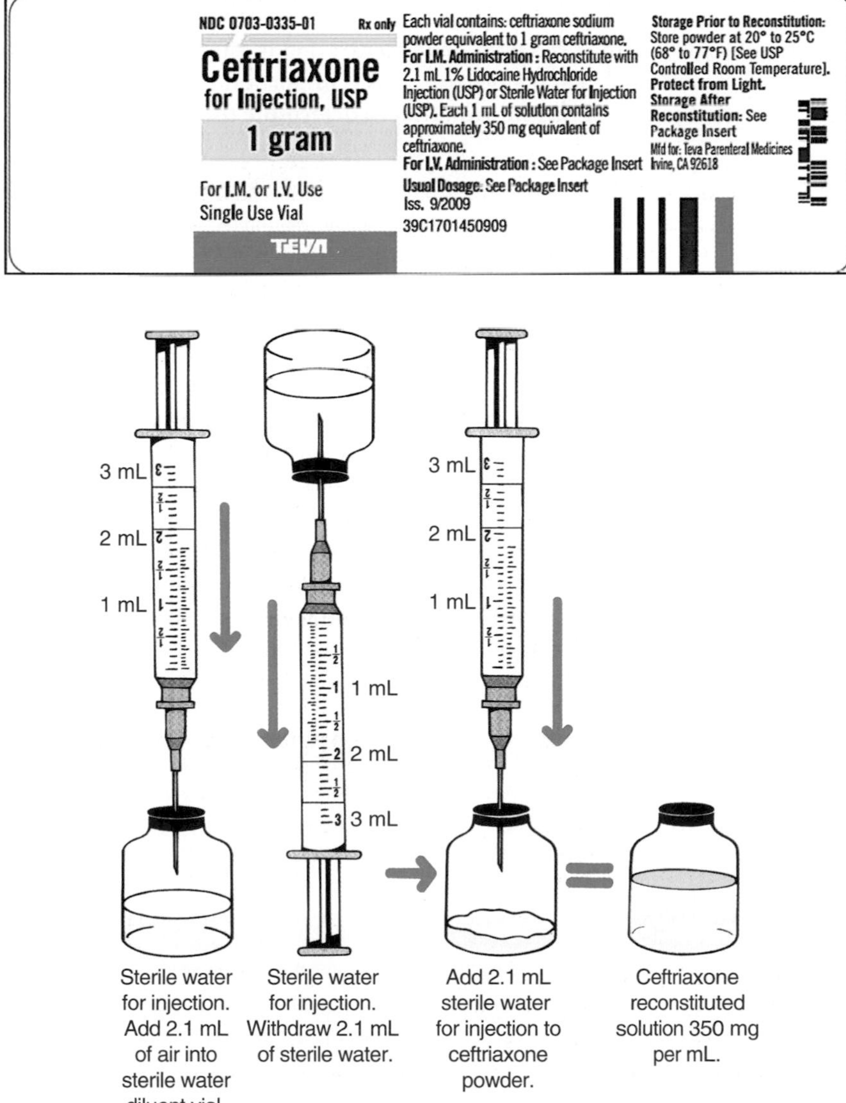

Figure 19-1 Ceftriaxone 1-g vial reconstitution.

4. If there are no directions for reconstitution on the label or on a package insert, or if any of the information (listed in number 3) is missing, consult appropriate resources such as the *Physician's Desk Reference (PDR)*, a pharmacology text, the hospital drug formulary, the pharmacy, or the manufacturer's website.
5. Injectable medications for reconstitution can come in a single-dose vial or a multiple-dose vial. When medications are in single-dose vials, there is only enough medication for **one** dose, and the contents are administered after reconstitution. In the case where the nurse reconstitutes a multiple-dose vial, there is enough medication for more than one dose. Therefore, when a multiple-dose vial is reconstituted, it is important to clearly label the vial after reconstitution with the following information:
   a. The date and time prepared, dosage strength prepared, the expiration date for the medication once reconstituted, and the time. *Note:* If all of the solution that is mixed is used, this information is not necessary. Information regarding the date and time of preparation and date and time of expiration is crucial when all of the medication is not used.
   b. Storage directions such as "Refrigerate."
   c. Your initials.

   If the medication label does not have room to clearly write the required information, add a label to the vial and indicate important information. Make certain the label is applied so that it does not obscure the medication name and dosage.
6. When reconstituting medications that are in multiple-dose vials or have several directions for preparation, **information regarding the dosage strength or final concentration (what the medication's strength or concentration is after you mixed it) must be on the label; for example, 500 mg per mL. This is important because others using the medication after you need this information to determine the dosage.**

TIPS FOR CLINICAL PRACTICE

When reconstituting a multiple-dose medication vial, label it with the required information and store it appropriately. If the vial is not labeled with a date and time the medication was reconstituted and the dosage strength after reconstitution and expiration date, the medication must be discarded. The nurse should never use an unlabeled reconstituted vial.

7. After the diluent is added to a powder, some medications completely dissolve and there is no additional volume added. Often, however, the powdered medication adds volume to the solution. The powdered medication takes up space as it dissolves and results in an increase in the amount of total (fluid) volume once it has dissolved. This is sometimes referred to as the *displacement factor,* or just *displacement.* The reconstituted material represents the diluent and powder. For example, directions for 1 g of powdered medication may state to add 2.5 mL sterile water for injection to provide an approximate volume of 3 mL (330 mg per mL). When the 2.5 mL of diluent is added, the 1 g of powdered medication displaces an additional 0.5 mL, for a total volume of 3 mL. The available dosage after reconstitution is 330 mg per milliliter of solution.

SAFETY ALERT!

Always determine both the type and amount of diluent to be used for reconstituting medications. Read and follow the label or package insert directions carefully to ensure that your client receives the intended dosage. Consult a pharmacist or other appropriate resources if there are any questions. Never assume!

TIPS FOR CLINICAL PRACTICE

If the powder displaces the liquid as it dissolves and increases the volume as illustrated in the example, the resulting volume and concentration must be considered when the correct dosage of medication is calculated. Whether a medication causes an increase in volume when it is reconstituted will be indicated on the medication label or the package insert.

The two types of reconstituted parenteral solutions are single strength and multiple strength. A single-strength solution has the directions for reconstitution printed on the label, as shown on the 1 g Ceftriaxone label in Figure 19-1. A multiple-strength solution usually has several directions for reconstitution and requires the nurse be even more attentive to the directions to select the best concentration to administer the required dosage. We will discuss reconstitution of multiple strength solutions.

Let's do some practice problems answering questions relating to single-strength solutions.

PRACTICE **PROBLEMS**

Using the label for Gemzar, answer the following questions.

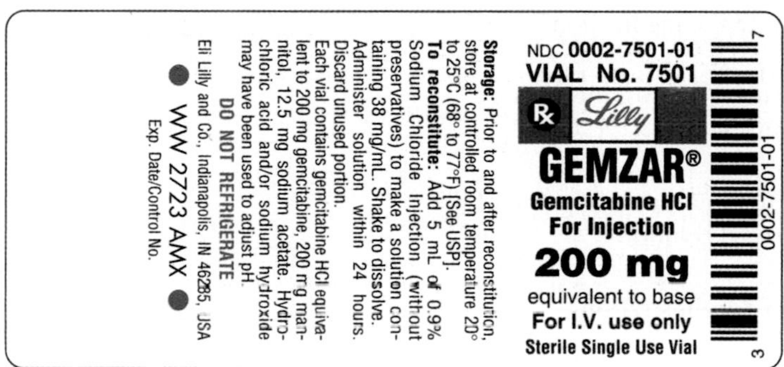
NDC 0002-7501-01
VIAL No. 7501
℞ Lilly
GEMZAR®
Gemcitabine HCl
For Injection
200 mg
equivalent to base
For I.V. use only
Sterile Single Use Vial
Storage: Prior to and after reconstitution, store at controlled room temperature 20° to 25°C (68° to 77°F) [See USP].
To reconstitute: Add 5 mL of 0.9% Sodium Chloride Injection (without preservatives) to make a solution containing 38 mg/mL. Shake to dissolve. Administer solution within 24 hours. Discard unused portion.
Each vial contains gemcitabine HCl equivalent to 200 mg gemcitabine, 200 mg mannitol, 12.5 mg sodium acetate. Hydrochloric acid and/or sodium hydroxide may have been used to adjust pH.
DO NOT REFRIGERATE
Eli Lilly and Co., Indianapolis, IN 46285, USA
WW 2723 AMX
Exp. Date/Control No.
0002-7501-01

1. What is the total dosage strength of Gemzar in this vial? ________________

2. How much diluent is added to the vial to prepare the medication for IV use? ________________

3. What diluent is recommended for reconstitution? ________________

4. What is the final concentration of the prepared solution for IV administration? ________________

5. How long will the reconstituted material retain its potency? ________________

6. 100 mg IV is ordered for day one of treatment. How many milliliters will you give? Shade the dosage in on the syringe provided. ________________

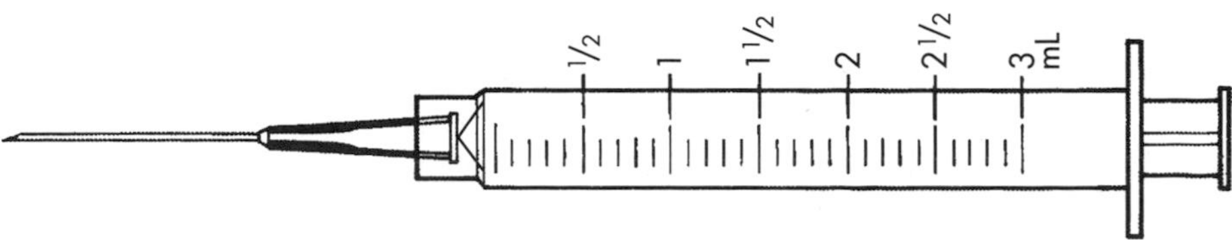

Using the label for Leucovorin calcium, answer the following questions.

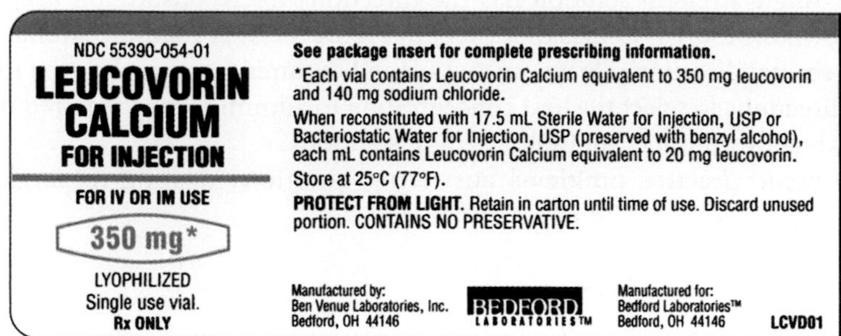

7. What is the total dosage strength of Leucovorin calcium in the vial? ________________

8. How much diluent is added to the vial to reconstitute the medication? ________________

9. What diluent is recommended for reconstitution? ________________

10. What is the final concentration of the reconstituted solution? ________________

11. Routes of administration ________________

12. Where can you find directions for complete prescribing information? ________________

13. 15 mg IM q6h is ordered. How many milliliters will you give? Shade the dosage on the syringe provided. ________________

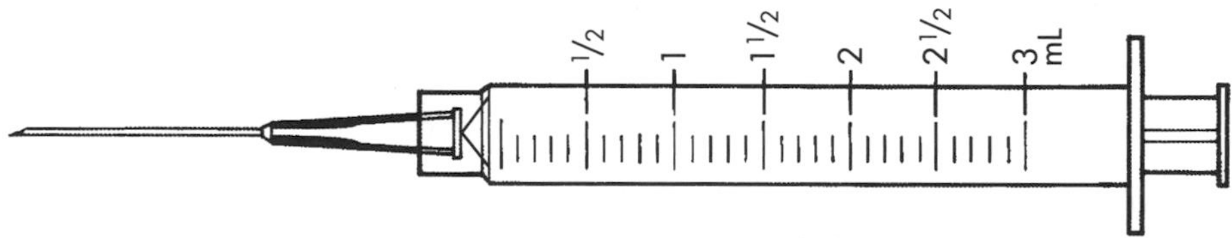

Using the label for Methylprednisolone sodium succinate, answer the following questions.

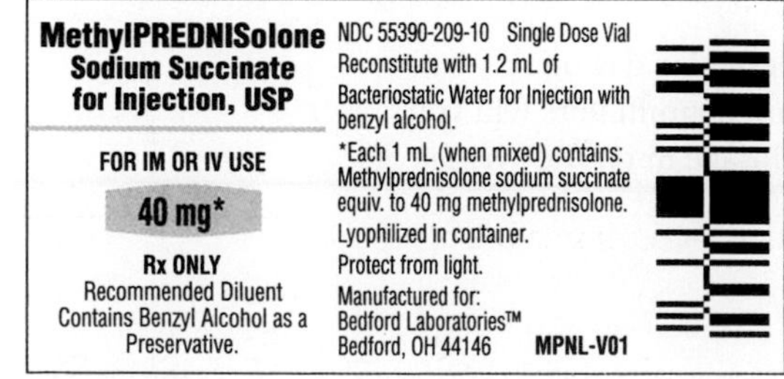

14. What is the total dosage strength of Methylprednisolone sodium succinate in the vial? ________________

15. What diluent is recommended to prepare an IV dosage? ______________________

16. How many milliliters of diluent are needed to prepare an IV dosage? ______________________

17. What is the final concentration of the solution prepared for IV administration? ______________________

18. Methylprednisolone sodium succinate 35 mg IV daily is ordered. How many milliliters will you give? Shade the dosage on the syringe provided. ______________________

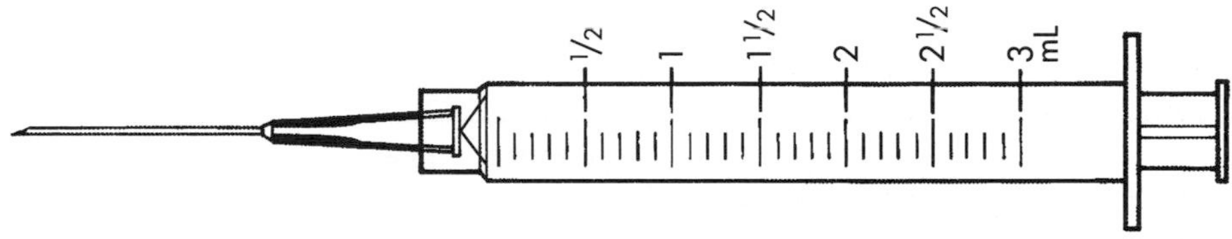
1/2
1
1 1/2
2
2 1/2
3
mL

Using the label for Rocephin, answer the following questions.

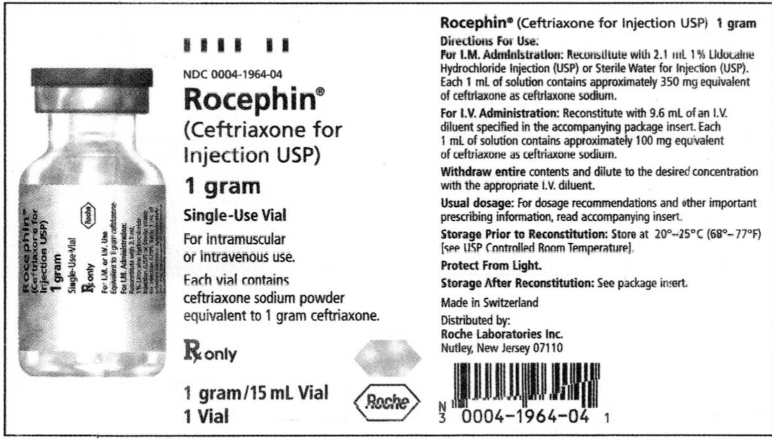
NDC 0004-1964-04
Rocephin®
(Ceftriaxone for Injection USP)
1 gram
Single-Use Vial
For intramuscular or intravenous use.
Each vial contains ceftriaxone sodium powder equivalent to 1 gram ceftriaxone.
℞ only
1 gram/15 mL Vial
1 Vial
Roche
Rocephin® (Ceftriaxone for Injection USP) 1 gram
Directions For Use:
For I.M. Administration: Reconstitute with 2.1 mL 1% Lidocaine Hydrochloride Injection (USP) or Sterile Water for Injection (USP). Each 1 mL of solution contains approximately 350 mg equivalent of ceftriaxone as ceftriaxone sodium.
For I.V. Administration: Reconstitute with 9.6 mL of an I.V. diluent specified in the accompanying package insert. Each 1 mL of solution contains approximately 100 mg equivalent of ceftriaxone as ceftriaxone sodium.
Withdraw entire contents and dilute to the desired concentration with the appropriate I.V. diluent.
Usual dosage: For dosage recommendations and other important prescribing information, read accompanying insert.
Storage Prior to Reconstitution: Store at 20°–25°C (68°–77°F) [see USP Controlled Room Temperature].
Protect From Light.
Storage After Reconstitution: See package insert.
Made in Switzerland
Distributed by:
Roche Laboratories Inc.
Nutley, New Jersey 07110
N 3 0004-1964-04 1

19. What is the total dosage strength of Rocephin in this vial? ______________________

20. For what routes of administration is the medication indicated? ______________________

21. How much diluent must be added to the vial to prepare the medication for IV use? ______________________

22. What kind of diluent is recommended for IV reconstitution? ______________________

23. What is the final concentration of the prepared solution for IV use? ______________________

24. How much diluent must be added to the vial to prepare the medication for IM use? ______________________

25. What kind of diluent is recommended for IM reconstitution? ________________

26. 1 g IV q12h is ordered. How many milliliters will you give? Shade the dosage on the syringe provided. ________________

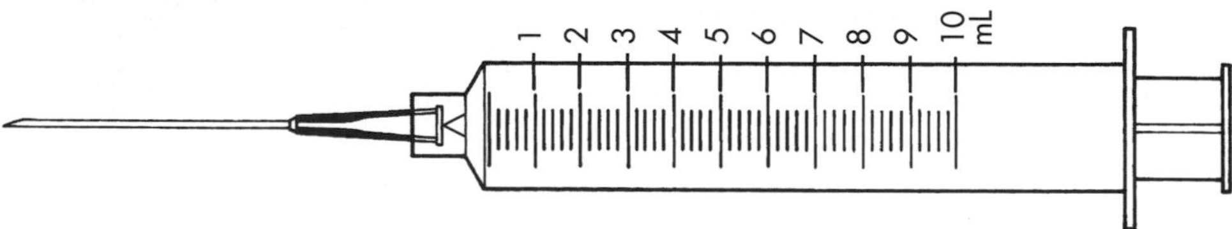

Using the label for Amoxicillin, answer the following questions.

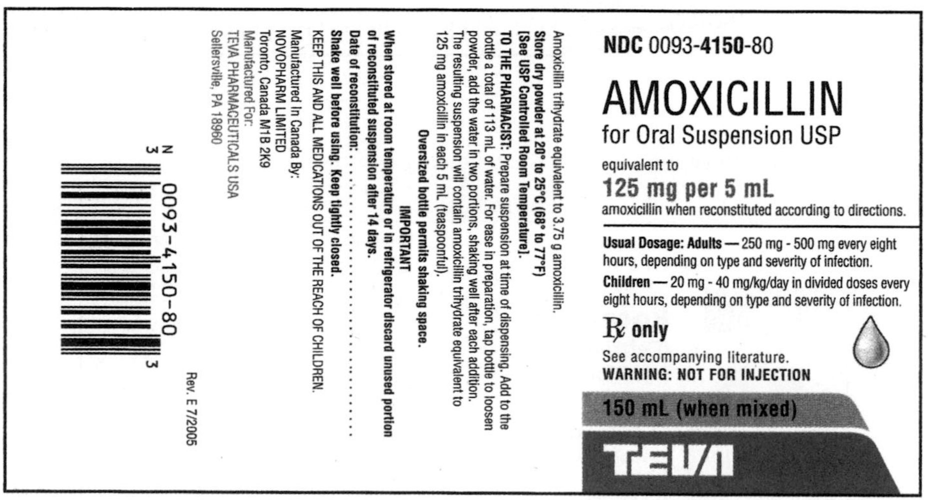

27. How much diluent must be added to prepare the solution? ________________

28. What type of solution is used for the diluent? ________________

29. What is the final concentration of the prepared solution? ________________

30. How should the medication be stored after it is reconstituted? ________________

Using the label for Acyclovir and a portion of the package insert, answer the following questions.

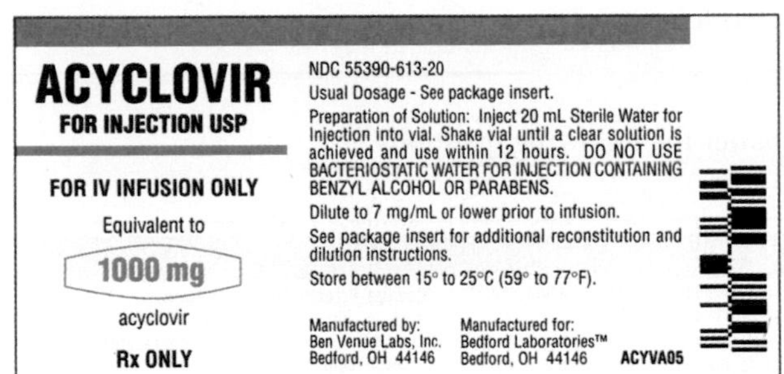

Method of Preparation: Each 10 mL vial contains acyclovir sodium equivalent to 500 mg of acyclovir. Each 20 mL vial contains acyclovir sodium equivalent to 1000 mg of acyclovir. The contents of the vial should be dissolved in Sterile Water for Injection as follows:

Contents of Vial	Amount of Diluent
500 mg	10 mL
1000 mg	20 mL

The resulting solution in each case contains 50 mg acyclovir per mL (pH approximately 11). Shake the vial well to assure complete dissolution before measuring and transferring each individual dose. DO NOT USE BACTERIOSTATIC WATER FOR INJECTION CONTAINING BENZYL ALCOHOL OR PARABENS.

31. What is the total dosage strength of Acyclovir in this vial? __________

32. How much diluent must be added to prepare the solution? __________

33. What diluent is recommended for reconstitution? __________

34. What is the final concentration of the prepared solution? __________

35. What is the route of administration? __________

Using the label for EES (Erythromycin Ethylsuccinate), answer the following questions.

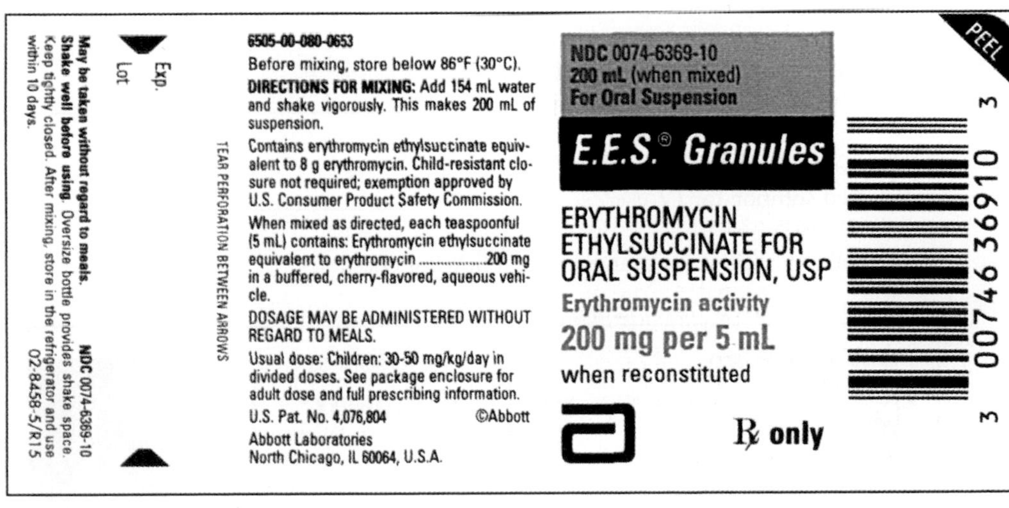

36. How much diluent must be added to prepare the solution? __________

37. What is the volume of the solution after it is mixed? __________

38. What is the final concentration of the prepared solution? ______________

39. For how long is the reconstituted solution good? ______________

Using the label for Ceftriaxone, answer the following questions.

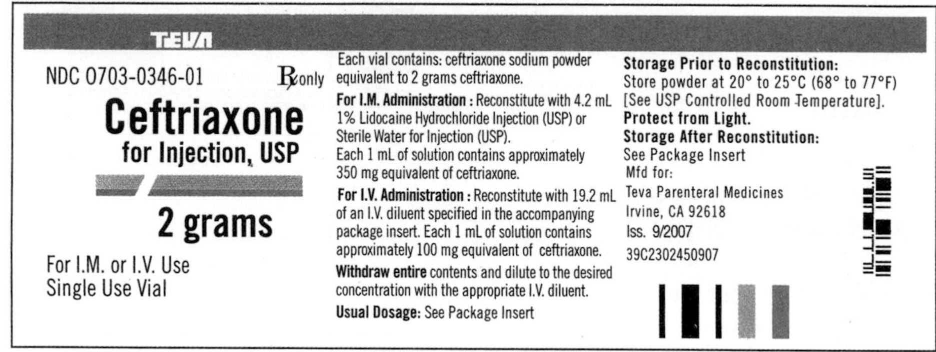

40. What is the total dosage strength of Ceftriaxone in this vial? ______________

41. How much diluent must be added to the vial to prepare the medication for IM use? ______________

42. How much diluent must be added to the vial to prepare the medication for IV use? ______________

43. What diluent is recommended for IV reconstitution? ______________

44. What is the final concentration of the prepared solution for IV use? ______________

Using the label for Zithromax, answer the following questions.

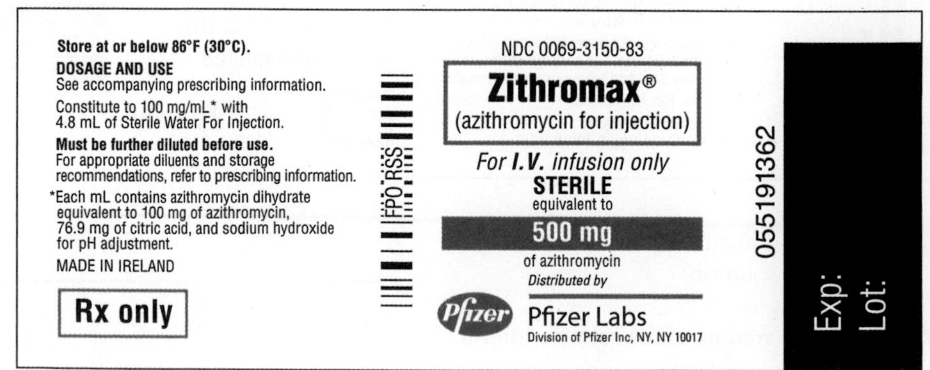

45. What is the total dosage strength of Zithromax in this vial? ______________

46. How many milliliters of diluent are needed to prepare an IV dosage? ____________________

47. What diluent is recommended for reconstitution? ____________________

48. What is the final concentration of the prepared solution? ____________________

49. Directions for use? ____________________

Using the label for Fluconazole, answer the following questions.

FOR ORAL USE ONLY

NDC 0049-3440-19

35 mL when reconstituted

STORAGE
Before Reconstitution: Store below 86°F (30°C).
After Reconstitution: Store suspension between 41°F (5°C) and 86°F (30°C). Protect from freezing.

DOSAGE AND USE
See accompanying prescribing information.

This package contains **350 mg** fluconazole in a natural orange-flavored mixture.*

*When reconstituted as directed, **each teaspoonful (5 mL) contains 50 mg of fluconazole.**

Rx only

DIFLUCAN®
(Fluconazole for Oral Suspension)

ORANGE FLAVORED

10 mg/mL
when reconstituted

Pfizer Roerig
Division of Pfizer Inc, NY, NY 10017

EXP

To the Pharmacist:

1. Mixing Directions:
   Tap bottle lightly to loosen powder. Add 24 mL of distilled water or Purified Water (USP) to the bottle. Shake well.
2. Store reconstituted suspension between 41°F (5°C) and 86°F (30°C). Protect from freezing.

Shake well before each use. Discard unused portion after 2 weeks.

50. How much diluent must be added to prepare the solution? ____________________

51. What diluent is recommended for reconstitution? ____________________

52. What is the final concentration of the prepared solution? ____________________

53. How should the medication be stored after it is reconstituted? ____________________

Answers on p. 473

Calculation of Medications When the Final Concentration (Dosage Strength) Is Not Stated

Sometimes a medication comes with directions for only one way to reconstitute it, and the label does not indicate the final dosage strength after it is mixed, such as "becomes 250 mg per mL." Example: A particular medication is available in 1 g in powder. Directions tell you that adding 2.5 mL of sterile water for injection yields 3 mL of solution. When you add 2.5 mL of sterile water to the powder, the volume expands to 3 mL. The concentration is not changing; you will get 3 mL of solution; however, it will be equal to 1 g.

Therefore, the problem is calculated by using 1 g = 3 mL.

Reconstituting Medications with More Than One Direction for Mixing (Multiple Strength)

Remember, the directions for reconstitution can be on the label or a package insert. At times, the vial will contain minimal information. It may only include the dosage strength and state, "see package insert for directions for reconstitution or storage."

Some medications, in addition to giving the route of administration, may come with several directions for preparing different solution strengths. In this case, the nurse must choose the concentration or dosage strength appropriate for the dosage ordered. A common medication that has a choice of dosage strengths is penicillin. When a medication comes with several directions for preparation or offers a choice of dosage strengths, you must choose the strength most appropriate for the dosage ordered. The following guidelines may be used.

Guidelines for Choosing Appropriate Concentrations

1. Route of administration. It is essential to verify the route of administration before reconstituting.
   a. IM—You are concerned that the amount does not exceed the maximum allowed for IM administration. However, you do not want to choose a concentration that will result in irritation when injected into a muscle. When a choice of strengths can be made, do not choose an amount that would exceed the amount allowed for IM administration or one that is very concentrated. Consider the muscle site being used and the age of the client.
   b. IV—Keep in mind that this medication is usually further diluted because, once reconstituted, the medication is then placed in additional fluid of 50 to 100 mL or more, depending on the medication being administered. Example: Erythromycin requires that the reconstituted solution be placed in 250 mL of fluid before administration to a client. In pediatrics, a medication may be given in a smaller volume of fluid, depending on the child's age, the child's size, and the medication.
2. Choose the concentration or dosage strength that comes closest to what the prescriber has ordered. The dosage strengths are given for the amount of diluent used. Example: If the prescriber orders 300,000 units of a particular medication IM, and the choices of strength are 200,000 units per mL, 250,000 units per mL, and 500,000 units per mL, the strength closest to 300,000 units per mL is 250,000 units per mL. It allows you to administer a dosage within the range allowed for IM administration, and it is not the most concentrated.

SAFETY ALERT!

When multiple directions are given for reconstituting medications, the smaller the amount of diluent used to reconstitute the medication, the more concentrated the resulting solution will be. Consider the route of administration when reconstituting medications. Always check the route and the directions related to reconstitution.

3. The word *respectively* may sometimes be used on a medication label for directions on reconstitution. For example, reconstitute with 23 mL, 18 mL, 8 mL of diluent to

provide concentrations of 200,000 units per mL, 250,000 units per mL, 500,000 units per mL, respectively. The word *respectively* means in the order given. In terms of the directions for reconstitution, this means that if you add 23 mL diluent, it will provide 200,000 units per mL, 18 mL diluent will provide 250,000 units per mL, etc. In other words, the amounts of diluent correspond to the order in which the concentrations are written. Remember: **When you are mixing a medication that is a multiple-strength solution, the dosage strength that you prepare must be written on the vial.**

Let's look at a sample label that shows a multiple-strength solution.

Some medications for parenteral use come with several directions for mixing to obtain several different solution strengths and require that you select a particular dosage strength. The dosage strength chosen should result in a reasonable amount of solution administered to the client. Remember that the route of administration is an essential consideration. Refer to the label for Pfizerpen (penicillin G potassium).

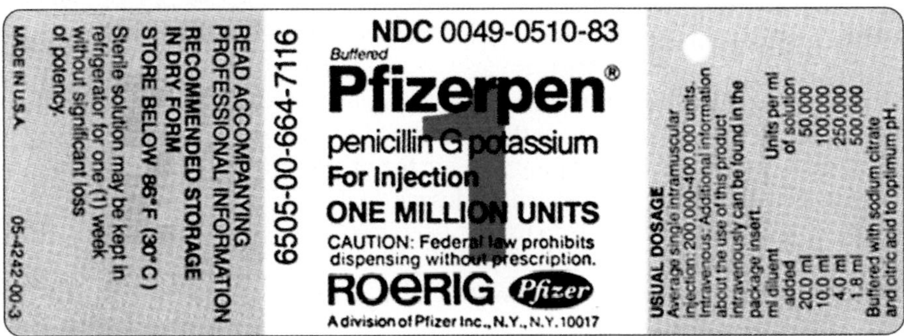

Notice that the label states one million units. This means a total of 1,000,000 units of penicillin is in the vial. The directions for reconstitution and the dosage strengths that can be obtained are listed on the label. The left column indicates the choices for diluent volume that can be used to reconstitute the medication. The right column indicates the final dosage strengths in units per mL that will be made based on the amount of diluent added. If the dosage ordered for the client was, for example, 250,000 units q6h, the most appropriate strength to mix would be 250,000 units per mL. If you look next to the dosage strength in the directions, you will notice that 4 mL of diluent must be added to obtain a concentration of 250,000 units per mL.

Let's assume the order is for 300,000 units IM for an adult. The best concentration in this case would be 250,000 units per mL. Refer to the label and notice that to make this concentration, you will need to add 4 mL of diluent. When calculated, the client would receive 1.2 mL (3 mL is the maximum for a large adult muscle). Remember that the condition of the intramuscular site and the client (age and muscle mass) must be considered. Depending on the status of the client, a different dosage strength may be a better choice. Notice also that when you reconstitute the medication using 4 mL, the total volume will be 4 mL, which means you have enough for approximately two additional doses. Because this is a multiple-strength solution, the dosage strength you choose must be indicated on the vial after you reconstitute it. Since the type of diluent is not indicated on the label, other resources, such as those recommended previously, must be consulted.

SAFETY ALERT!

If a multiple-strength solution is prepared and not used in its entirety, the dosage strength (final concentration) you mixed must be indicated on the label to verify the dosage strength of the reconstituted solution. Proper labeling is a crucial detail.

PRACTICE PROBLEMS

Using the label for penicillin G potassium, answer the following questions.

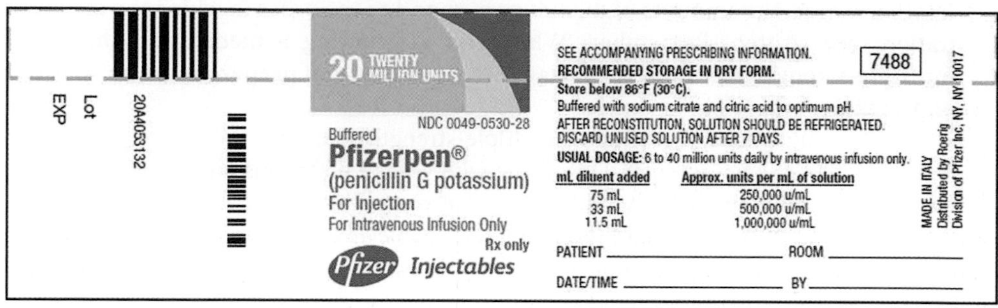

54. What is the total number of units of penicillin contained in the vial? (Write out in numbers.) ______________________

55. If you add 33 mL of diluent to the vial, what dosage strength will you print on the label? ______________________

56. If 2,000,000 units IV is ordered, which dosage strength would be appropriate to use? ______________________

57. How many milliliters will you administer if 2,000,000 units are ordered? ______________________

58. How long will the medication maintain its potency if refrigerated? ______________________

Using the label for penicillin G potassium, answer the following questions.

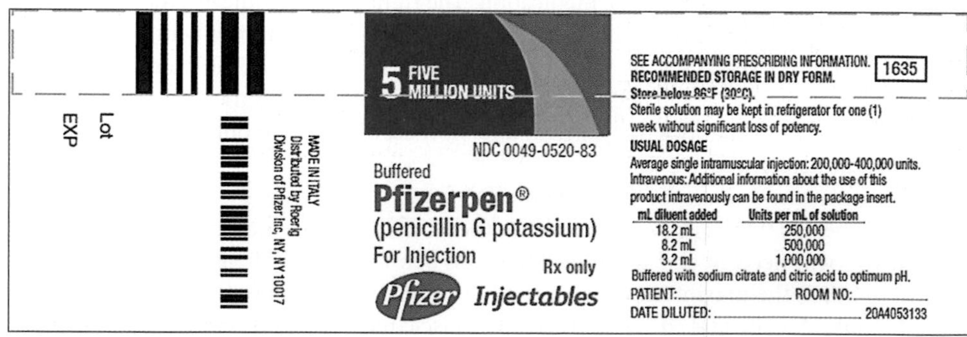

59. What is the total number of units of penicillin contained in the vial? (Write out in numbers.) ______________________

60. If 700,000 units IM is ordered, which dosage strength would be appropriate to use? ______________________

61. How many milliliters will you administer if 700,000 units are ordered? ______________________

62. Where will you store any unused medication? ______________________

63. How long will the medication maintain its potency? ______________________

64. What concentration strength would be obtained if you added 18.2 mL of diluent? (Write out in numbers.) ____________

65. Where would the usual dosage for IV administration be found? ____________

Answers on p. 473

Reconstitution from Package Insert Directions and Medications with Different Reconstitution Directions Depending on Route of Administration

If the label does not contain reconstitution directions, you must obtain directions from the information insert that accompanies the vial. Pay attention to the amount in the vial and the route; there may be different directions based on these factors. Refer to the Ceftazidime (Tazicef) label (Figure 19-2) and insert that follow. For example, note that the directions for Ceftazidime IV infusion are different for reconstitution for a 1 gram vial and a 2 gram vial. Also, note that the Ceftazidime label has different directions for IM injection and IV infusion. Always carefully check the route ordered, and follow the directions corresponding to the route.

SAFETY ALERT!

Carefully check the route ordered before reconstituting a medication and follow the directions corresponding to that route. Do not interchange the dilution instructions for IM or IV because you can harm a client.

Medications with Instructions to "See Accompanying Literature" (Package Insert) for Reconstitution and Administration

Some medications that require reconstitution may indicate the dosage strength contained in the vial and do not provide the information necessary to reconstitute the medication or information relating to administration. To prepare the powdered medication, you must see the package insert or accompanying literature. Refer to the Zyprexa label (Figure 19-3, *A*) and the accompanying package insert information (Figure 19-3, *B*). The label instructs you to "see accompanying literature for dosage, reconstitution instructions, and method of administration."

A

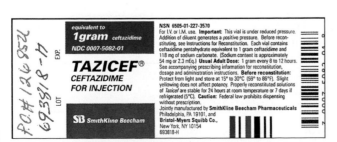

B

RECONSTITUTION

Single Dose Vials:
For I.M. injection, I.V. direct (bolus) injection, or I.V. infusion, reconstitute with Sterile Water for injection according to the following table. The vacuum may assist entry of the diluent. SHAKE WELL.

Table 5

Vial Size	Diluent to Be Added	Approx. Avail. Volume	Approx. Avg. Concentration
Intramuscular or Intravenous Direct (bolus) Injection			
1 gram	3.0 ml.	3.6 ml.	280 mg./ml.
Intravenous Infusion			
1 gram	10 ml.	10.6 ml.	95 mg./ml.
2 gram	10 ml.	11.2 ml.	180 mg./ml.

Withdraw the total volume of solution into the syringe (the pressure in the vial may aid withdrawal). The withdrawn solution may contain some bubbles of carbon dioxide.

NOTE: As with the administration of all parenteral products, accumulated gases should be expressed from the syringe immediately before injection of 'Tazicef'.

These solutions of 'Tazicef' are stable for 18 hours at room temperature or seven days if refrigerated (5°C.). Slight yellowing does not affect potency.

For I.V. infusion, dilute reconstituted solution in 50 to 100 ml. of one of the parenteral fluids listed under COMPATIBILITY AND STABILITY.

Figure 19-2 **A,** Tazicef 1 gram label. **B,** Tazicef package insert.

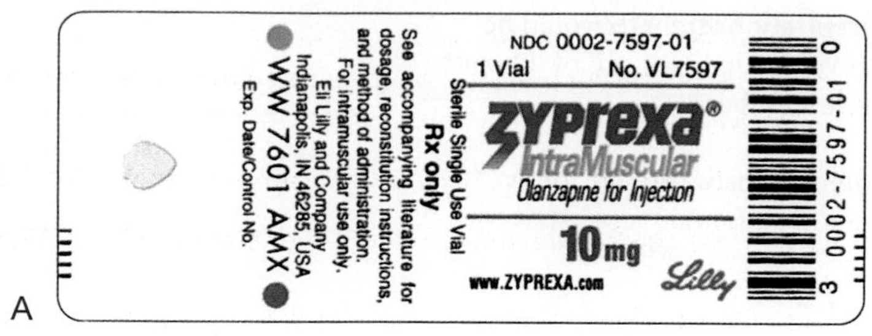

A

ZYPREXA® IntraMuscular (olanzapine for injection) Dosing

ZYPREXA IntraMuscular is approved for the treatment of agitation associated with schizophrenia and bipolar mania.

Dose (mg)	Injection volume (mL)
10.0 mg	Withdraw total contents of vial
7.5 mg	1.5 mL
5.0 mg	1.0 mL
2.5 mg	0.5 mL

10 mg is the recommended dose for agitation associated with bipolar mania and schizophrenia.

Follow the steps below to reconstitute and use ZYPREXA IntraMuscular:

1. Inject 2.1 mL of Sterile Water for Injection into single-packaged vial for up to 10-mg dose.
2. Dissolve contents of vial completely; resulting solution should be clear and yellow.
3. Use solution within 1 hour; discard any unused portion.
4. Refer to table for injection volumes and corresponding doses of ZYPREXA IntraMuscular.
5. Immediately after use, dispose of syringe in approved sharps box.

B

Figure 19-3 **A,** Zyprexa 10 mg label. **B,** Zyprexa package insert.

To reconstitute the medication and calculate a dosage you need to refer to the package insert. The directions instruct you to add 2.1 mL of sterile water for injection for dosages up to 10 mg, and indicate the number of mL to withdraw to administer specific dosages of the medication IM. Notice for example that if you had to administer 5 mg of Zyprexa IM, when the medication has been reconstituted, you would withdraw 1 mL of the medication to administer the ordered dosage of 5 mg. Use the Zyprexa label in Figure 19-3, *A* and *B*, to answer Practice Problems 66 through 71.

66. What is the dosage strength of the total vial? ______________

67. How much diluent must be added to this vial to prepare the medication for IM use? ______________

68. What diluent is recommended for reconstitution? ______________

69. How long will the reconstituted solution be good for? ______________

70. How much would you withdraw for a 7.5-mg dose? ______________

71. How much would you withdraw for a 2.5-mg dose? ______________

Answers on p. 473

Calculation of Dosages

If you are using ratio and proportion, the known ratio is also the dosage strength obtained after you mix the medication.

- In $\frac{D}{H} \times Q = x$, Q is the volume of solution that contains the dosage strength.
- In dimensional analysis, the first fraction written is the solution (volume) that contains the dosage strength.

Before we proceed to calculate dosages, let's review the steps to use with medications that have been reconstituted.

1. Ratio and proportion, the formula method, or dimensional analysis may be used to calculate the dosage. However, the H (have or what is available) is the dosage strength you obtain after you mix the medication according to directions.
2. Powdered medications may increase in volume after a liquid is added (diluent + powder). The volume to which the medication expands must be considered when calculations are made.
3. When the final concentration is not stated, the total weight of the medication in powdered form is used, and the number of milliliters produced after the solvent or liquid has been added.
4. As with all calculation problems, check to make sure that the ordered and the available medications are in the same system of measurement and the same units.
5. Do not forget to label your answer.

Example 1: To illustrate, let's calculate the dosage you would administer if you mixed penicillin and made a solution containing 1,000,000 units per mL. Order: 2,000,000 units IM q6h.

✓ Solution Using Ratio and Proportion

$$1{,}000{,}000 \text{ units} : 1 \text{ mL} = 2{,}000{,}000 \text{ units} : x \text{ mL}$$

(known) (unknown)

$$\frac{1{,}000{,}\cancel{000}\,x}{\cancel{1{,}000{,}000}} = \frac{2{,}\cancel{000{,}000}}{1{,}\cancel{000{,}000}}$$

Note cancellation of zeros to make numbers smaller.)

$$x = \frac{2}{1}$$

$$x = 2 \text{ mL}$$

Answer: 2 mL

✓ Solution Using the Formula Method

$$\frac{D}{H} \times Q = x$$

$$\frac{2{,}000{,}000 \text{ units}}{1{,}000{,}000 \text{ units}} \times 1 \text{ mL} = x \text{ mL}$$

$$x = \frac{2{,}\cancel{000{,}000}}{1{,}\cancel{000{,}000}}$$

$$x = 2 \text{ mL}$$

Answer: 2 mL

✓ Solution Using Dimensional Analysis

$$x \text{ mL} = \frac{1 \text{ mL}}{1{,}000{,}000 \cancel{\text{units}}} \times \frac{2{,}000{,}000 \cancel{\text{units}}}{1}$$

$$x = \frac{2{,}\cancel{000{,}000}}{1{,}\cancel{000{,}000}}$$

$$x = \frac{2}{1}$$

$$x = 2 \text{ mL}$$

Answer: 2 mL

Example 2: Order: 0.2 g of a medication IV q6h

Available: 500 mg of the medication in powdered form that states add 8 mL of diluent to yield a solution 500 mg per 8 mL.

✓ PROBLEM SETUP

1. A conversion is necessary. Equivalent: 1,000 mg = 1 g. Convert what is ordered into the available units. This will eliminate a decimal point. Therefore 0.2 g = 200 mg.
2. Think: What would a logical answer be?
   You will need more than 1 mL but less than 8 mL.

✓ Solution Using Ratio and Proportion

$$500 \text{ mg} : 8 \text{ mL} = 200 \text{ mg} : x \text{ mL}$$

(known) (unknown)

$$\frac{\cancel{500}x}{\cancel{500}} = \frac{200 \times 8}{500}$$

$$x = \frac{1{,}600}{500}$$

$$x = 3.2 \text{ mL}$$

Answer: 3.2 mL

✓ Solution Using the Formula Method

$$\frac{D}{H} \times Q = x$$

$$\frac{200 \text{ mg}}{500 \text{ mg}} \times 8 \text{ mL} = x \text{ mL}$$

$$x = \frac{200 \times 8}{500}$$

$$x = \frac{1{,}600}{500}$$

$$x = 3.2 \text{ mL}$$

Answer: 3.2 mL

✓ Solution Using Dimensional Analysis

$$x \text{ mL} = \frac{8 \text{ mL}}{500 \cancel{\text{mg}}} \times \frac{1{,}000 \cancel{\text{mg}}}{1 \cancel{\text{g}}} \times \frac{0.2 \cancel{\text{g}}}{1}$$

$$x = \frac{8{,}000 \times 0.2}{500}$$

$$x = \frac{1{,}600}{500}$$

$$x = 3.2 \text{ mL}$$

Answer: 3.2 mL

POINTS TO REMEMBER

- Directions for reconstituting medications are provided by the drug manufacturer.
- The directions for reconstituting medications can be found on the vial, the medication container, or a package insert. If there are no instructions on the vial, container, or the package insert is not available, consult other reliable resources (pharmacy, medication reference book, *PDR*).
- Read directions carefully for reconstitution, and reconstitute the medication specific to the route of administration ordered (e.g., IM or IV). Interchanging dilution instructions for routes can have serious outcomes for client.
- The type and amount of diluent to be used for reconstitution must be followed exactly.
- Lidocaine should not be used to reconstitute a medication without an order from the prescriber.
- Read directions relating to storage and the time period for maintaining potency of medication once it is reconstituted.
- If a medication is not used in its entirety after it is reconstituted and medication remains for future use, clearly label medication with the following:
  1. Date and time of preparation
  2. Date and time of expiration
  3. Initials of the preparer
  4. Dosage strength or concentration of reconstituted solution

Reconstitution of Noninjectable Solutions

The principles of reconstitution can be applied to nutritional liquids. Enteral feeding solutions are formulated to be administered in full strength; however, the nurse may, on occasion, need to dilute the enteral solution before administering it. Before beginning calculations, let's discuss enteral feedings.

Enteral Feeding

Enteral nutrition involves the provision of nutrients to the gastrointestinal tract. This nutrition is provided to clients who are unable to ingest food safely or have eating difficulties. Enteral nutrition may be provided with a nasogastric, jejunal, or gastric tube. It may consist of blended foods or tube feeding formulas. Tube feedings can be administered in several ways. Depending on the client's needs, they may be given as a bolus (administration of a single large dose) by means of gravity several times per day by using a large-volume syringe, as a continuous gravity drip over a period of $\frac{1}{2}$ to 1 hour several times per day by using a pouch to hang the feeding, or as a continuous drip by infusion pump. When clients are receiving a continuous feeding, the feeding is placed in a special pouch or container and attached to a feeding pump. A common feeding pump is the Kangaroo pump (Figure 19-4). When the feeding pump is used, the feeding is delivered at a rate expressed in milliliters per hour. For the purpose of this chapter, we will focus on administering a feeding by the continuous drip method with an enteral infusion pump.

When an order is written for feedings by continuous infusion, the nurse attaches the feeding to a special pump and administers it at the prescribed rate in milliliters per hour. A sample order is Jevity at 65 mL per hour by PEG (percutaneous endoscopic gastrostomy) or by NG (nasogastric) tube. The feeding order also includes a certain volume of water with feeding (100 to 250 mL). The amount of water given with a tube feeding and how it is administered vary from one institution to the next. Check the institution's policy relating to administering enteral feedings. Some orders may be written as follows: Pulmo Care 400 mL over 8 hours followed by 100 mL of water after each feed. When the prescriber does not indicate milliliters per hour, the nurse divides the number of milliliters ordered by the number of hours, and rounds answer to the nearest whole number, to determine the milliliters per hour to set the pump. In pediatrics, the order often specifies the formula and the rate. Example: Similac 24 at 20 mL per hr continuously by NG tube.

Example 1: Order: Pulmocare 400 mL over 8 hours followed by 100 mL of water after each feed. Determine the rate in milliliters per hour.

$$\frac{400 \text{ mL}}{8 \text{ hr}} = 50 \text{ mL/hr}$$

The pump would be set at 50 mL/hr.

Example 2: Order: Nepro 1,200 mL over 16 hours. Determine the rate in milliliters per hour.

$$\frac{1{,}200 \text{ mL}}{16 \text{ hr}} = 75 \text{ mL/hr}$$

The pump would be set to deliver 75 mL/hr.

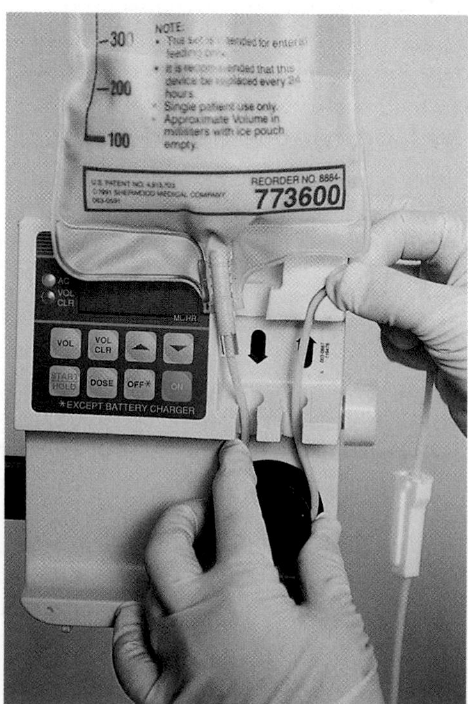

Figure 19-4 Kangaroo pump. (Potter PA, Perry AG, Stockert P, Hall A: *Fundamentals of nursing,* ed 9, St Louis, 2016, Mosby.)

In addition to nutrients, medications may be given through a tube. Liquid medications are preferred; however, some tablets may be crushed, dissolved in water, and administered.

Never assume. Not all medications are designed for administration through a tube, so check with the pharmacist or other appropriate resources. A medication's effectiveness could depend on the location of the tube (e.g., stomach, jejunum).

SAFETY ALERT!

Always verify that the medications to be administered are not sublingual, enteric-coated, or timed-release medications because such medications are absorbed differently and the effects of the medication may be altered. Consult the pharmacist or medication guide before tablets are crushed and before capsules are opened and dissolved for tube feeding administration.

PRACTICE **PROBLEMS**

Determine the rate in milliliters per hour for the following continuous feedings. Round answers to the nearest whole number.

72. Ensure 480 mL by NG tube over 8 hr. Follow with 100 mL of water after each feeding. ______________

73. Perative 1,600 mL over 24 hr by gastrostomy. Follow with 250 mL of water. ______________

Answers on p. 473

Determining the Strength of a Solution

Nurses or other health care professionals may be required to dilute a concentrated liquid or powder (solute) with a solution such as water or saline (solvent) so as to make a less concentrated solution. Water is a common solvent used to dilute solutions and has been referred to as the **universal solvent.** This may include preparation of irrigating solutions, soaks, and nutritional liquids. When reconstituting solutions that are noninjectable, it is essential to understand that the amount of liquid (solvent) that is used to make a substance less concentrated is determined by the desired strength of the solution.

Therefore, if you add more solvent, the final solution strength will be less concentrated; the less solvent that is added, the more concentrated the final solution strength will be. An example to illustrate this concept is the directions for making one quart of ice tea from a powder. Directions call for 4 cups of water to 1 packet of powdered ice tea. If you prefer a stronger tea taste, you might add 2 cups of water (solvent) to the powder (solute) making it more concentrated. However, if you add 4 cups of water (solvent) to the powder (solute), the final solution will be more diluted and less concentrated because you added more water (solvent).

The strength of a solution can be expressed using ratios, fractions, or percents. The fraction format is usually preferred to explain the ratio of solute to the total solution. For example, a $\frac{1}{3}$ strength solution indicates 1 part solute for 3 parts of the total solution. This could be expressed as 1 : 3 solution or $33\frac{1}{3}\%$ solution.

Calculation of Solutions

Because of special circumstances in both adults and children, nutritional liquids may require dilution before they are used. These nutritional liquids may be administered orally or through feeding tubes. Nutritional solutions can be supplied in ready-to-use form, powder for reconstitution, or liquid concentrate. Nutritional formulas may be diluted with sterile or tap water. **Always consult a reference or institutional policy regarding what should be used to reconstitute a nutritional formula.**

To prepare a prescribed solution of a certain strength from a solute, first let's review some basic terms.

Solute—A concentrated liquid or solid substance to be dissolved or diluted
Solvent—A liquid substance that dissolves another substance. Commonly used solvents are sterile water and normal saline.
Solution—A solute plus a solvent
To prepare a solution of a specific strength, use the following steps:

1. $\text{Desired solution strength} \times \frac{\text{Amount of}}{\text{desired solution}} = \text{Solute (substance/concentrated liquid to be dissolved)}$

Note: The strength of the desired solution is written as a fraction; the amount of desired solution is expressed in milliliters or ounces, depending on the problem. This will give you the amount of solute you will need to add to the solvent to prepare the desired solution.

2. $\text{Amount of desired solution} - \text{Solute} = \frac{\text{Amount of liquid needed to}}{\text{dissolve substance (solvent)}}$

Example 1: Order: ⅓-strength Ensure 900 mL by NG tube over 8 hr

Solution:

$$\underset{\text{(desired strength)}}{\tfrac{1}{3}} \times \underset{\text{(amount of solution)}}{900 \text{ mL}} = \underset{\text{(solute)}}{x}$$

Step 1:

$$x = \frac{900}{3}$$

$$x = 300 \text{ mL}$$

You need 300 mL of the formula (solute).

Step 2:

$$\underset{\text{(amount of solution)}}{900 \text{ mL}} - \underset{\text{(solute)}}{300 \text{ mL}} = \underset{\text{(amount needed to dissolve) (solvent)}}{600 \text{ mL}}$$

Therefore, you would add 600 mL water to 300 mL of Ensure to make 900 mL of ⅓-strength Ensure.

Example 2: ¾-strength Isomil 4 oz p.o. q4h for 24 hr

Note: 4 oz q4h = 6 feedings; 4 oz × 6 = 24 oz

1 oz = 30 mL; therefore 24 oz = 720 mL

$$\frac{3}{4} \times 720 \text{ mL} = x \text{ mL}$$

$$x = \frac{2{,}160}{4}$$

$x = 540$ mL of the formula (solute)

$$\underset{\text{(amount of solution)}}{720 \text{ mL}} - \underset{\text{(solute)}}{540 \text{ mL}} = \underset{\text{(amount needed to dissolve solvent)}}{180 \text{ mL}}$$

Therefore, you would add 180 mL water to 540 mL of Isomil to make 720 mL of ¾-strength Isomil for a 24-hour period.

Irrigating Solutions and Soaks

Nurses or other health care professionals may need to dilute solutions for use as a topical solution, or for irrigating body cavities or wounds. Normal saline is the preferred solution for cleaning wounds, for the application of moist dressings and packing of wounds. The use of cytotoxic solutions is discouraged. Current practice for wound irrigation recommends the use of non-cytotoxic wound cleaners such as normal saline, potable (tap) water, and sterile water. Normal saline solution is the preferred and frequently used solution for wound irrigation. Normal saline is the common term for 0.9% NaCl (full-strength) and is an isotonic solution (the same tonicity or osmolarity as blood and other body serums) and does not harm tissues. According to *Fundamentals of Nursing, 9th edition* (Potter, Perry, Stockert, Hall, 2017), agents such as Dakin's Solution (sodium hypochlorite solution), acetic acid, povidone-iodine, and hydrogen peroxide are cytotoxic solutions. Cytotoxic solutions are toxic to cells and may interfere with healing. However, the healthcare provider providing wound care must always take into account the solution ordered and the nature of the wound.

Example 1: Using full-strength normal saline (0.9%), prepare 180 mL of $\frac{1}{4}$ strength normal saline solution diluted with sterile water for wound care.

Solution: The fraction represents the desired solution strength: $\frac{1}{4}$ strength means 1-part solute (normal saline) to 4 total parts solution.

1. No conversion required.
2. $\frac{1}{4}$ (desired strength) $\times$ 180 mL (amount of solution) $=$ x mL (solute)

$$x = \frac{180}{4}$$

$$x = 45 \text{ mL}$$

You need 45 mL of solute (normal saline) to prepare the desired solution (180 mL of ¼ strength). The total you want to make is 180 mL. The amount of solvent you need is therefore:

180 mL − 45 mL = 135 mL (solvent/sterile water)

To make 180 mL of $\frac{1}{4}$ strength normal saline, mix 45 mL of full-strength normal saline and 135 mL of sterile water.

Think: 45 mL is $\frac{1}{4}$ of the total volume (180 mL) and 135 mL + 45 mL = 180 mL.

Example 2: The prescriber orders a sacral wound irrigated with $\frac{1}{3}$ strength normal saline and sterile water tid. 75 mL is needed for each irrigation (tid means three times a day). You will need to prepare 75 mL $\times$ 3 irrigations = 225 mL total solution.

How much normal saline (full-strength) and sterile water will you need?

Solution: The fraction represents the desired solution strength: $\frac{1}{3}$ means 1-part solute (normal saline) to 3 total parts solutions.

1. No conversion required.
2. $\frac{1}{3}$ (desired strength) $\times$ 225 mL (amount of solution) $=$ x mL (solute)

$$x = \frac{225}{3}$$

$$x = 75 \text{ mL}$$

You need 75 mL of solute (normal saline) to prepare the desired solution (225 mL of $\frac{1}{3}$ strength). The total you want to make is 225 mL. The amount of solvent you need is therefore:

225 mL − 75 mL = 150 mL (solvent/sterile water)

To make 225 mL of $\frac{1}{3}$ strength normal saline, mix 75 mL of full-strength normal saline and 150 mL of sterile water.

Think: 75 mL is $\frac{1}{3}$ of the total volume (225 mL) and 150 mL + 75 mL = 225 mL.

SAFETY ALERT!

Think and calculate with accuracy. Errors can be made in determining the dilution for a solution if you incorrectly calculate the amount of solute and solvent for a required solution strength.

PRACTICE **PROBLEMS**

Prepare the following strength solutions. (Express answers in mL.)

74. $\frac{2}{3}$-strength Sustacal 300 mL p.o. q.i.d. ________________

75. $\frac{3}{4}$-strength Ensure 16 oz by nasogastric (NG) tube over 8 hr ________________

76. $\frac{1}{2}$-strength Ensure 20 oz by gastrostomy tube (GT) over 5 hr ________________

For each of the following, indicate how you would prepare the following solutions using full-strength normal saline as the solute and sterile water as the solvent.

77. 8 oz of $\frac{1}{4}$ strength for wound cleansing ________________

78. 480 mL of $\frac{1}{3}$ strength for wound irrigation ________________

79. 120 mL of $\frac{3}{4}$ strength for skeletal pain care ________________

80. 160 mL of $\frac{5}{8}$ strength solution ________________

Answers on p. 474

POINTS TO REMEMBER

- Enteral feedings (continuous) are placed on an infusion pump and administered at a rate expressed in milliliters per hour. The prescriber usually orders the feeding rate in milliliters per hour. If not, the nurse must calculate the rate at which to deliver the feeding.
- To prepare a solution of a specific strength, write the desired solution strength as a fraction and multiply it by the amount of desired solution. This will give you the amount of solute needed.
- The amount of desired solution − solute = amount of liquid needed to dissolve the substance (solvent).
- Think and calculate with accuracy to avoid making errors in determining the dilution for a required solution strength.

CLINICAL REASONING

1. **Scenario:** Order: Ceftazidime 250 mg IM q8h.

   The nurse had the package insert below and a 1-g vial.

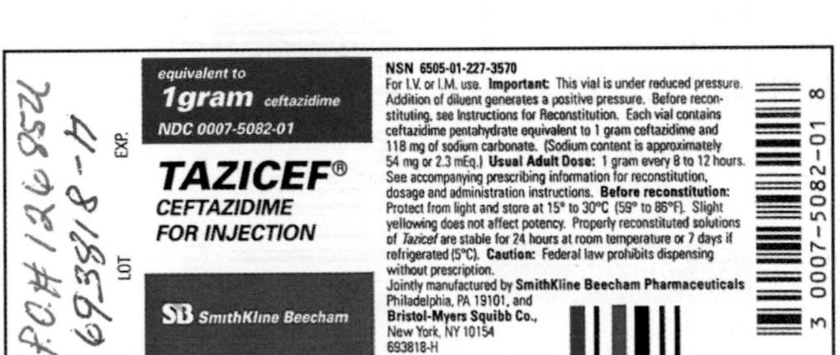
equivalent to
1gram ceftazidime
NDC 0007-5082-01
TAZICEF®
CEFTAZIDIME
FOR INJECTION
SB SmithKline Beecham
EXP.
LOT
NSN 6505-01-227-3570
For I.V. or I.M. use. Important: This vial is under reduced pressure. Addition of diluent generates a positive pressure. Before reconstituting, see Instructions for Reconstitution. Each vial contains ceftazidime pentahydrate equivalent to 1 gram ceftazidime and 118 mg of sodium carbonate. (Sodium content is approximately 54 mg or 2.3 mEq.) Usual Adult Dose: 1 gram every 8 to 12 hours. See accompanying prescribing information for reconstitution, dosage and administration instructions. Before reconstitution: Protect from light and store at 15° to 30°C (59° to 86°F). Slight yellowing does not affect potency. Properly reconstituted solutions of Tazicef are stable for 24 hours at room temperature or 7 days if refrigerated (5°C). Caution: Federal law prohibits dispensing without prescription.
Jointly manufactured by SmithKline Beecham Pharmaceuticals Philadelphia, PA 19101, and Bristol-Myers Squibb Co., New York, NY 10154
693818-H
3 0007-5082-01 8

RECONSTITUTION

Single Dose Vials:
For I.M. injection, I.V. direct (bolus) injection, or I.V. infusion, reconstitute with Sterile Water for injection according to the following table. The vacuum may assist entry of the diluent. SHAKE WELL.

Table 5

Vial Size	Diluent to Be Added	Approx. Avail. Volume	Approx. Avg. Concentration
Intramuscular or Intravenous Direct (bolus) Injection			
1 gram	3.0 ml.	3.6 ml.	280 mg./ml.
Intravenous Infusion			
1 gram	10 ml.	10.6 ml.	95 mg./ml.
2 gram	10 ml.	11.2 ml.	180 mg./ml.

Withdraw the total volume of solution into the syringe (the pressure in the vial may aid withdrawal). The withdrawn solution may contain some bubbles of carbon dioxide.

NOTE: **As with the administration of all parenteral products, accumulated gases should be expressed from the syringe immediately before injection of 'Tazicef'.**

These solutions of 'Tazicef' are stable for 18 hours at room temperature or seven days if refrigerated (5°C.). Slight yellowing does not affect potency.

For I.V. infusion, dilute reconstituted solution in 50 to 100 ml. of one of the parenteral fluids listed under COMPATIBILITY AND STABILITY.

The nurse reconstituted the medication (Ceftazidime) with 10.6 mL of diluent and administered 2.6 mL to the client.

a. What error occurred here? ______________________

b. What concentration should have been made? ______________________

c. What concentration did the nurse make and for which route? ______________________

d. What is the potential outcome of the error? ______________________

e. What measures could have been taken to prevent the error? ______________________

Answers on p. 474

CHAPTER REVIEW

Use the labels where provided to obtain the necessary information; shade the dosage on syringes where provided. Round the answers to the nearest tenth where indicated.

1. Order: methylprednisolone sodium succinate 165 mg IV daily.

   Available:

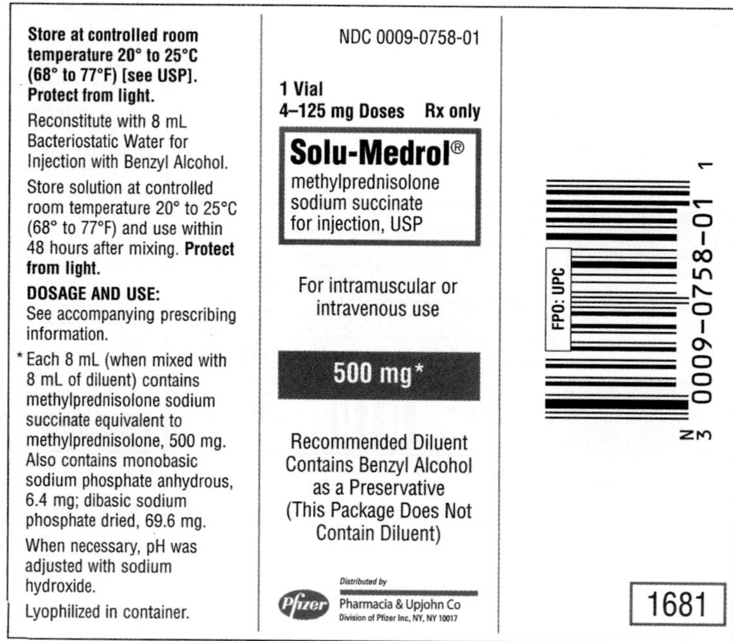

   a. How many milliliters will you administer? ______________

   b. Shade the dosage calculated on the syringe provided.

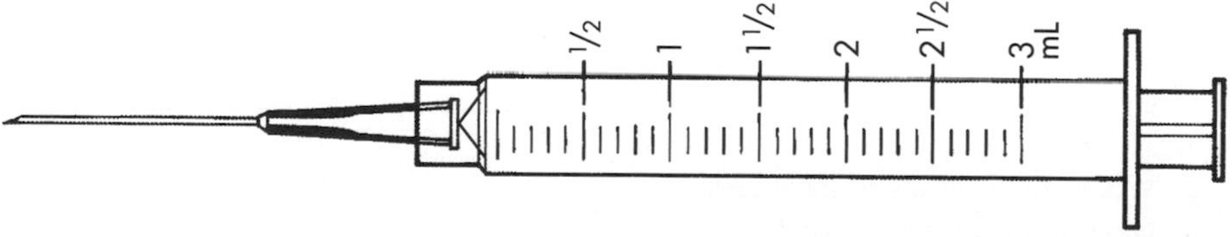

2. Order: Ampicillin 375 mg IM q6h

Available:

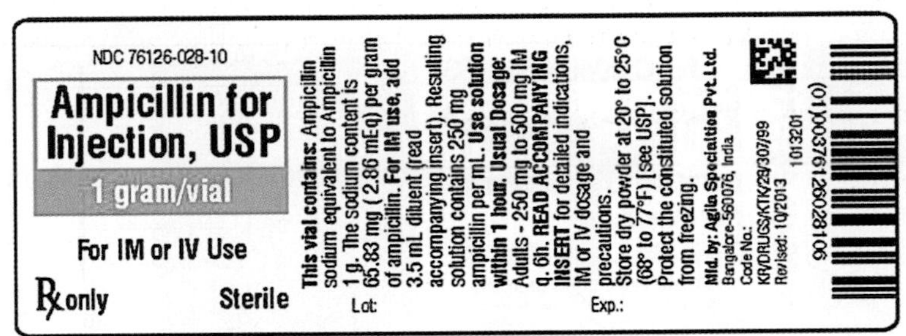

a. How much diluent must be added to the vial for IM administration? ____________________

b. What is the final concentration of the solution prepared for IM administration? ____________________

c. How many milliliters will you administer? ____________________

d. Shade the dosage calculated on the syringe provided.

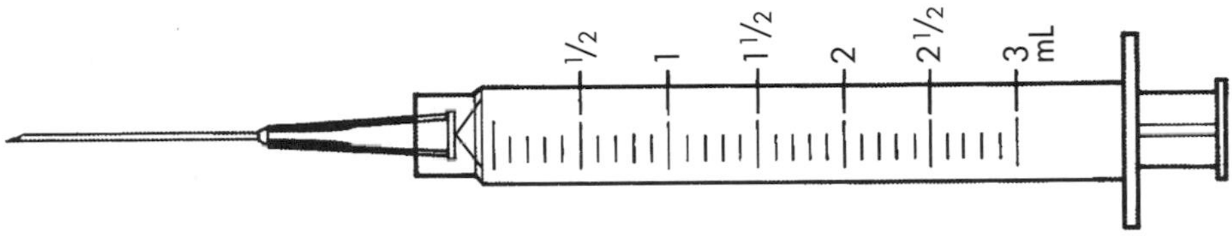

3. Order: Amoxicillin 0.4 g p.o. q8h.

Available:

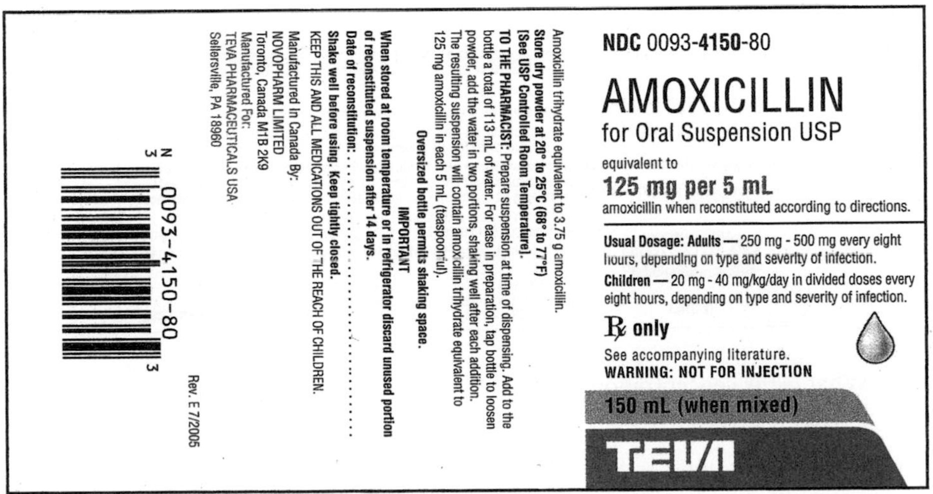

a. How much diluent must be added to prepare the solution? ____________________

b. What diluent is recommended for reconstitution? ____________________

c. What is the dosage strength of the reconstituted solution? ____________________

d. How many milliliters will you administer? ____________________

e. How long will the medication maintain its potency? ____________________

4. Order: penicillin G potassium 275,000 units IM q6h.

   Available:

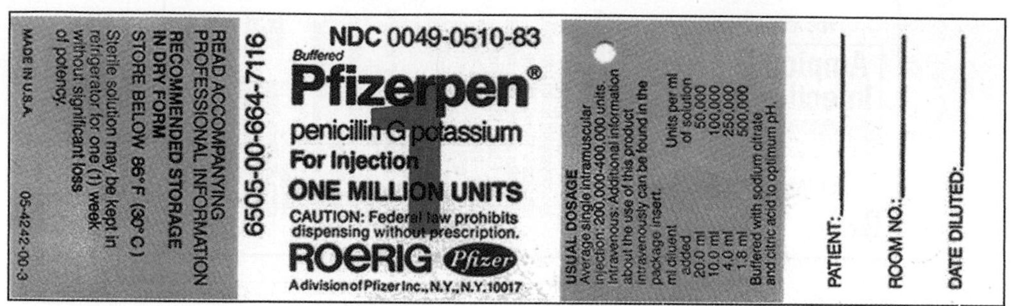

   a. Which dosage strength would be best to choose? ____________

   b. How many milliliters of diluent would be needed to make the dosage strength? ____________

   c. How many milliliters will you administer? ____________

   d. Shade the dosage calculated on the syringe provided.

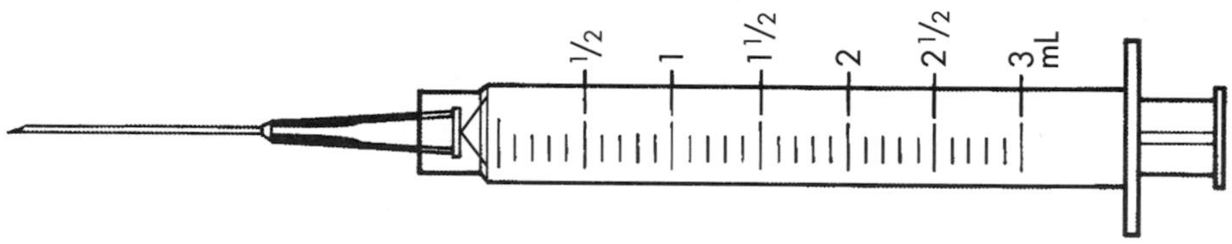

5. Order: Cytarabine 200 mg IV daily for 1 week.

   Available:

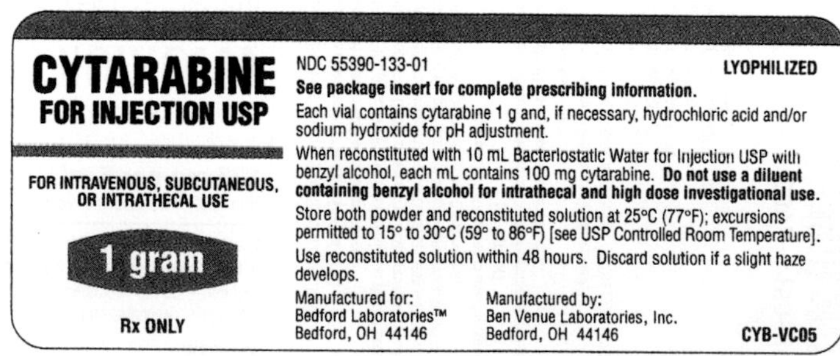

   a. What is the concentration of the reconstituted material? ____________

   b. How many milliliters will you add to the IV? ____________

   c. Shade the dosage calculated on the syringe provided.

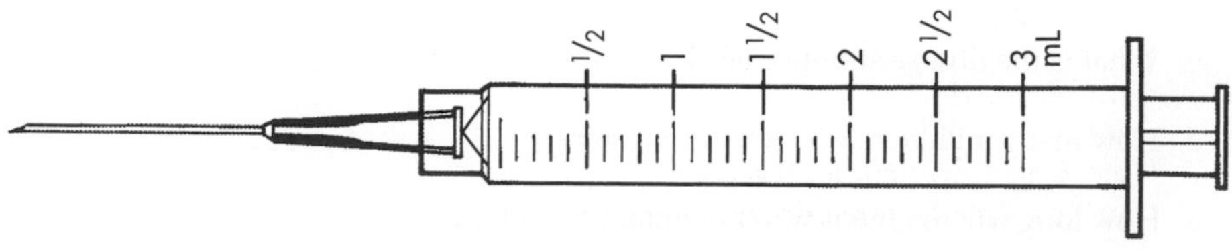

6. Order: Methylprednisolone Sodium Succinate 175 mg IV q6h.

   Available:

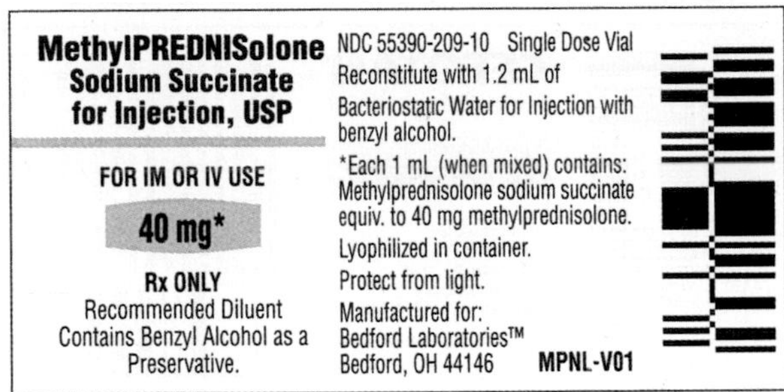

   a. What is the total dosage strength of Methylprednisolone Sodium Succinate in this vial? ____________________

   b. What diluent is recommended for reconstitution? ____________________

   c. How many milliliters will you add to the IV? ____________________

   d. Shade the dosage calculated on the syringe provided.

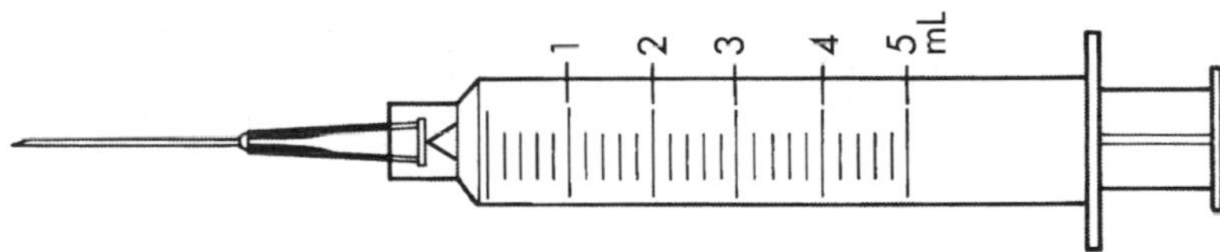

7. Order: Amoxicillin/clavulanate 0.5 g p.o. q12h (calculation based on Amoxicillin).

   Available:

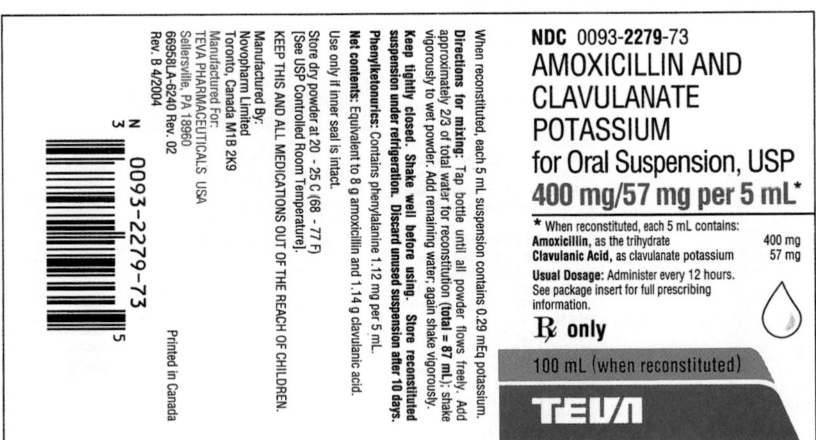

   a. How many milliliters of diluent must be added? ____________________

   b. What is the dosage strength after reconstitution? ____________________

   c. How many milliliters are needed to administer the required dosage? ____________________

8. Order: Cefotan 1.2 g IM q12h.

   Available: Read the medication label and portion of the package insert.

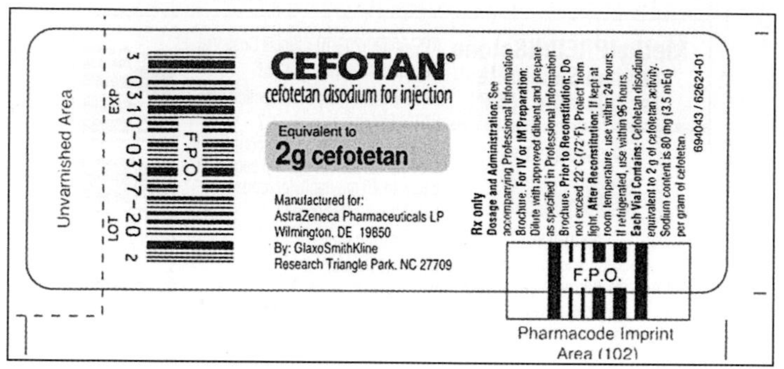

Vial Size	Amount of Diluent Added (mL)	Approximate Withdrawable Vol (mL)	Approximate Average Concentration (mg/mL)
1 gram	2	2.5	400
2 gram	3	4	500

   a. How many milliliters will you administer? ____________

   b. Shade the dosage calculated on the syringe provided.

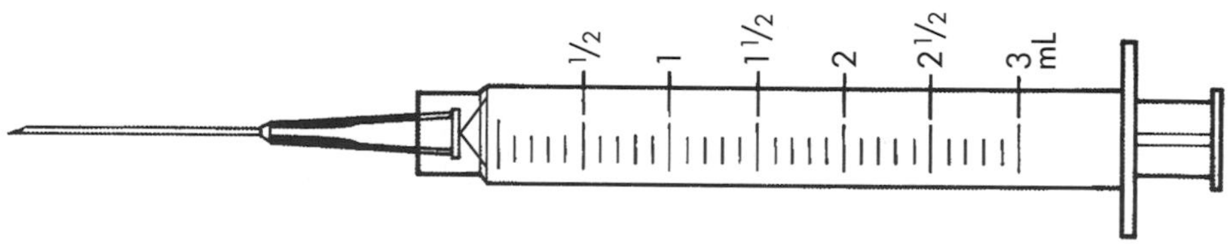

9. Order: Biaxin 350 mg p.o. q12h for 10 days.

   Available:

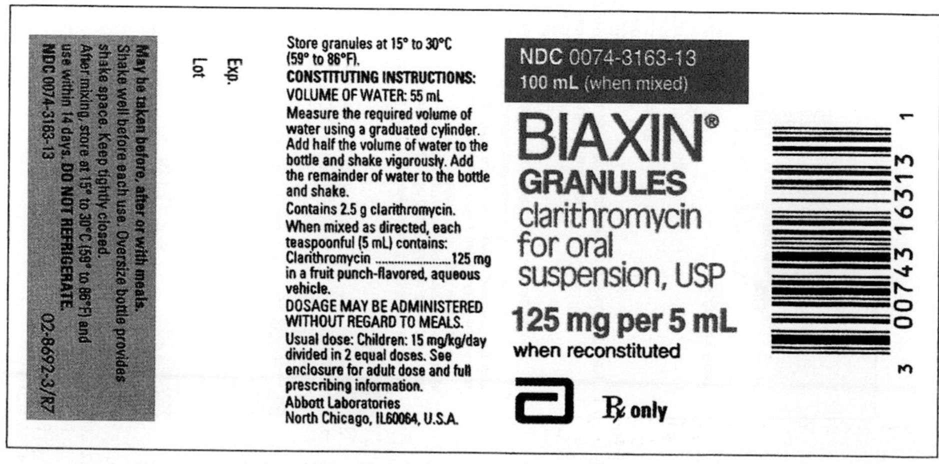

   a. How many milliliters of diluent must be added? ____________

   b. What is the dosage strength after reconstitution? ____________

   c. How many milliliters will you administer? ____________

10. Order: Penicillin G potassium 400,000 units IM q4h.

    Available:

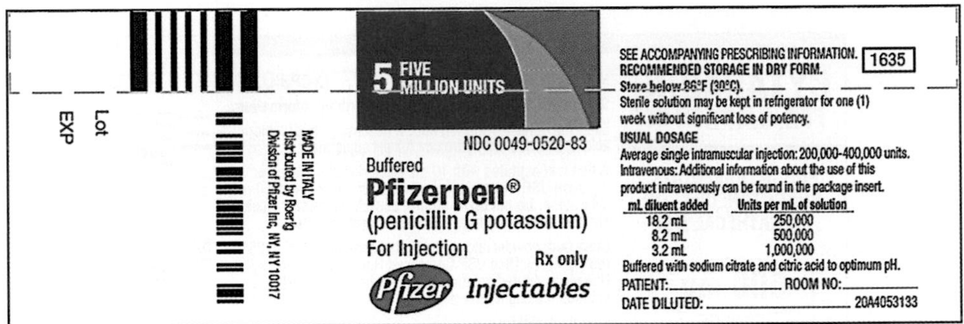

a. How many milliliters will you administer? ______________________

b. Shade the dosage calculated on the syringe provided.

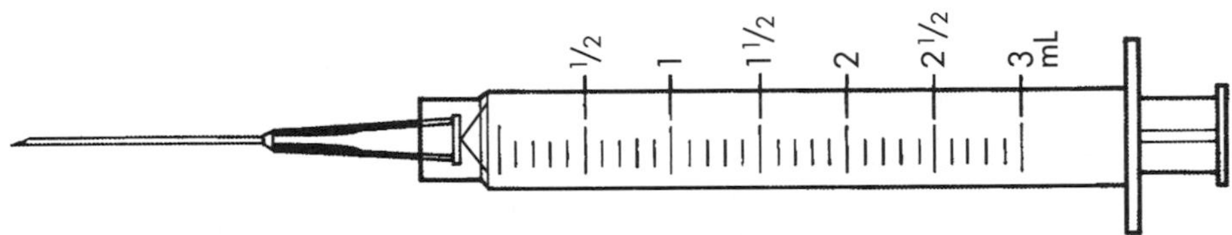

11. Order: Ceftazidime 250 mg IM q12h.

    Available:

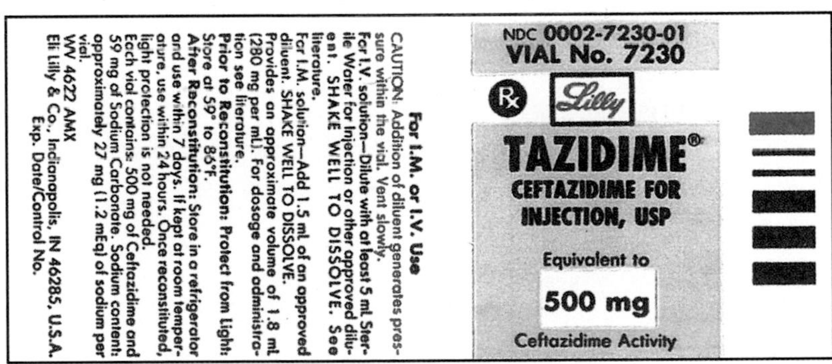

a. How many milliliters will you administer? ______________________

b. Shade the dosage calculated on the syringe provided.

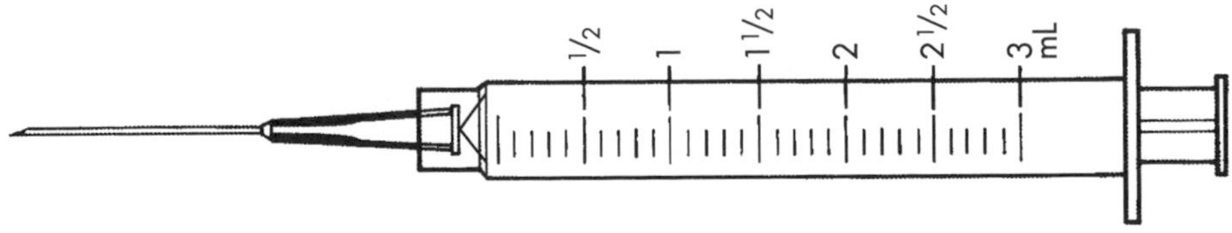

12. Order: Cytarabine 150 mg IV daily for 7 days.

Available:

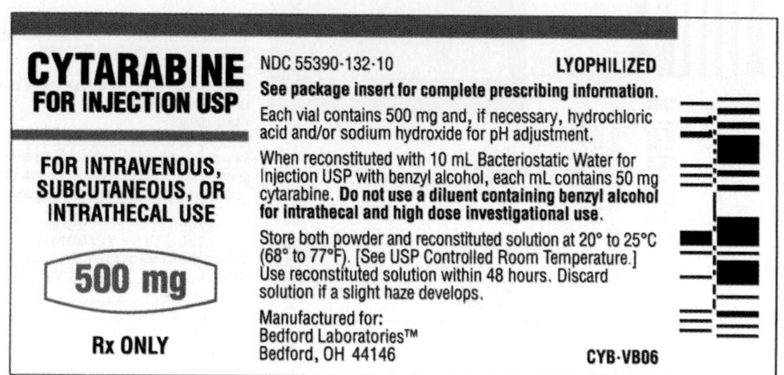
CYTARABINE FOR INJECTION USP

NDC 55390-132-10 LYOPHILIZED

See package insert for complete prescribing information.

Each vial contains 500 mg and, if necessary, hydrochloric acid and/or sodium hydroxide for pH adjustment.

FOR INTRAVENOUS, SUBCUTANEOUS, OR INTRATHECAL USE

When reconstituted with 10 mL Bacteriostatic Water for Injection USP with benzyl alcohol, each mL contains 50 mg cytarabine. **Do not use a diluent containing benzyl alcohol for intrathecal and high dose investigational use.**

Store both powder and reconstituted solution at 20° to 25°C (68° to 77°F). [See USP Controlled Room Temperature.] Use reconstituted solution within 48 hours. Discard solution if a slight haze develops.

500 mg

Manufactured for:
Bedford Laboratories™
Bedford, OH 44146

Rx ONLY

CYB-VB06

a. How many milliliters will you administer? ____________

b. Shade the dosage calculated on the syringe provided.

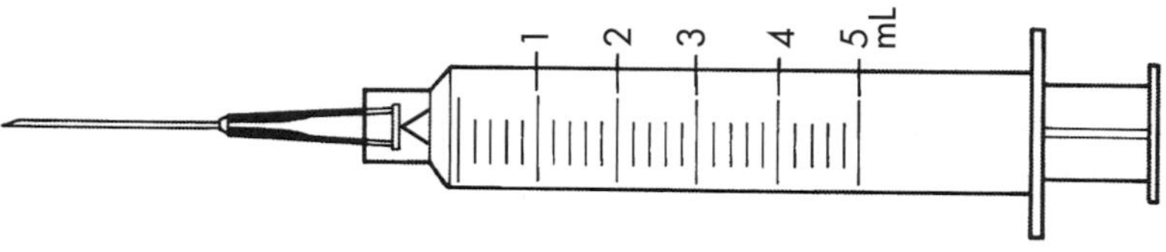

13. Order: Vancomycin 0.45 g IV q8h.

Use the directions from the insert below.

Available:

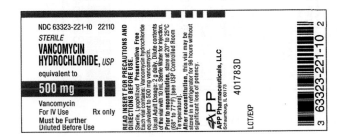

PREPARATION AND STABILITY

At the time of use, reconstitute by adding either 10 mL of Sterile Water for Injection to the 500-mg vial or 20 mL of Sterile Water for Injection to the 1-g vial of dry, sterile vancomycin powder. Vials reconstituted in this manner will give a solution of 50 mg/mL. FURTHER DILUTION IS REQUIRED.

After reconstitution, the vials may be stored in a refrigerator for 14 days without significant loss of potency. Reconstituted solutions containing 500 mg of vancomycin must be diluted with at least 100 mL of diluent. Reconstituted solutions containing 1 g of vancomycin must be diluted with at least 200 mL of diluent. The desired dose, diluted in this manner, should be administered by intermittent intravenous infusion over a period of at least 60 minutes.

a. How many milliliters of diluent must be added to the vial? ________________

b. What is the final concentration of the prepared solution? ________________

c. How many milliliters will you add to the IV? ________________

d. Shade the dosage calculated on the syringe provided.

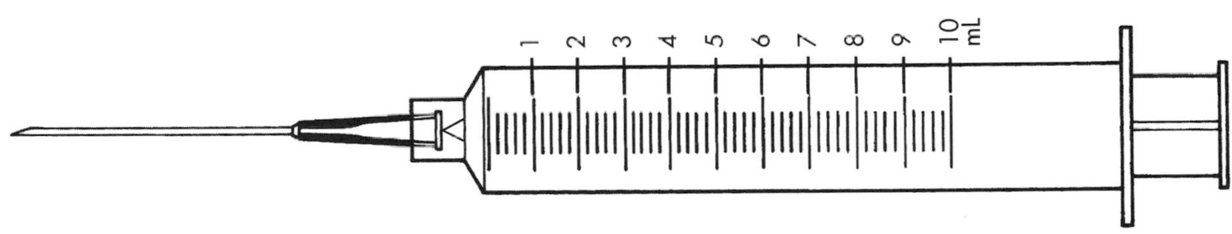

14. Order: Levothyroxine sodium 0.05 mg IV daily.

    Available:

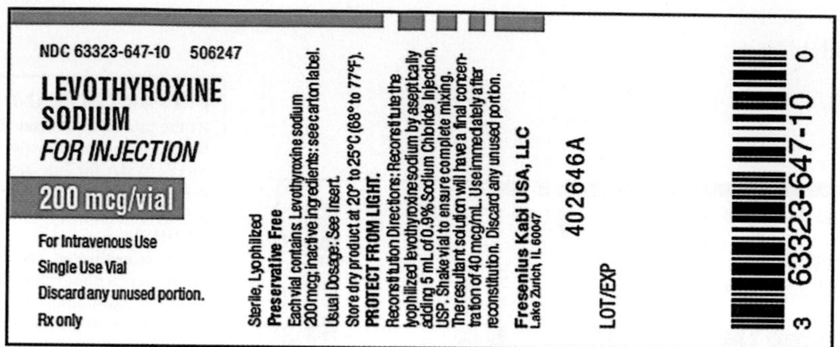

    a. How many milliliters will you add to the IV? ____________________

    b. Shade the dosage calculated on the syringe provided.

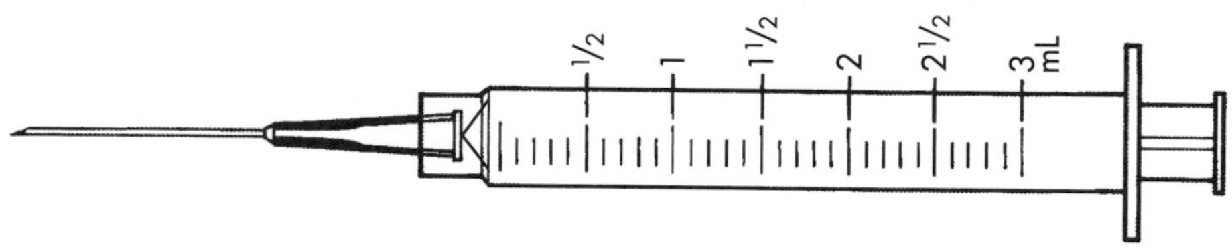

15. Order: Acyclovir 0.25 g IV q8h for 5 days.

    Use the directions from the insert below.

    Available:

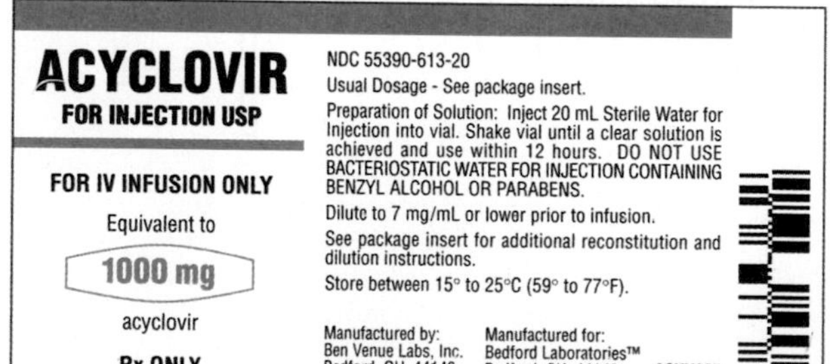

Method of Preparation: Each 10 mL vial contains acyclovir sodium equivalent to 500 mg of acyclovir. Each 20 mL vial contains acyclovir sodium equivalent to 1000 mg of acyclovir. The contents of the vial should be dissolved in Sterile Water for Injection as follows:

Contents of Vial	Amount of Diluent
500 mg	10 mL
1000 mg	20 mL

The resulting solution in each case contains 50 mg acyclovir per mL (pH approximately 11). Shake the vial well to assure complete dissolution before measuring and transferring each individual dose. DO NOT USE BACTERIOSTATIC WATER FOR INJECTION CONTAINING BENZYL ALCOHOL OR PARABENS.

    a. How many milliliters will you add to the IV? ____________________

    b. Shade the dosage calculated on the syringe provided.

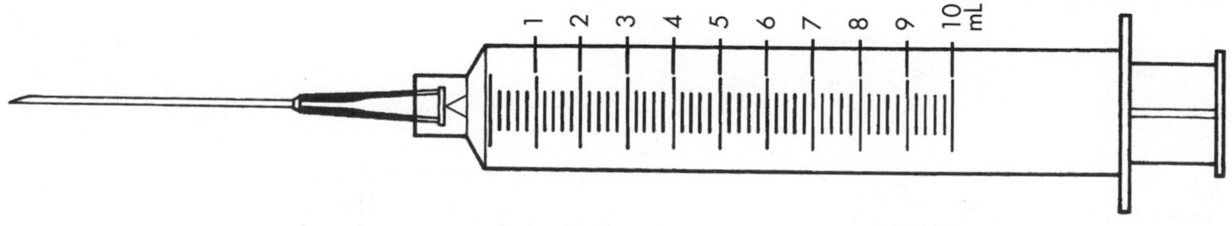

16. Order: Vantin 200 mg p.o. q12h.

Available:

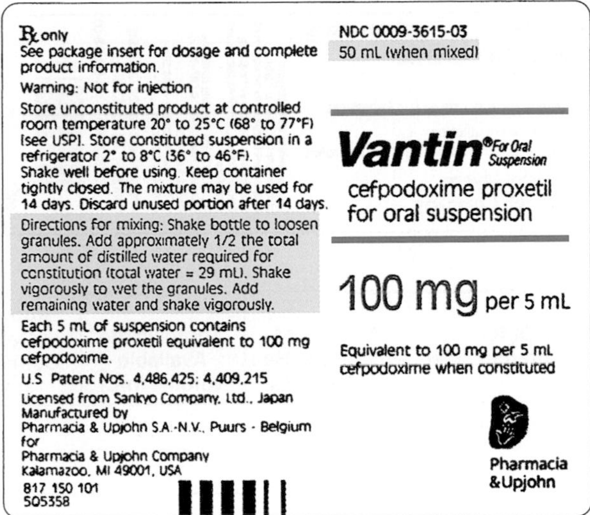
℞ only
See package insert for dosage and complete product information.
Warning: Not for injection
Store unconstituted product at controlled room temperature 20° to 25°C (68° to 77°F) [see USP]. Store constituted suspension in a refrigerator 2° to 8°C (36° to 46°F). Shake well before using. Keep container tightly closed. The mixture may be used for 14 days. Discard unused portion after 14 days.
Directions for mixing: Shake bottle to loosen granules. Add approximately 1/2 the total amount of distilled water required for constitution (total water = 29 mL). Shake vigorously to wet the granules. Add remaining water and shake vigorously.
Each 5 mL of suspension contains cefpodoxime proxetil equivalent to 100 mg cefpodoxime.
U.S. Patent Nos. 4,486,425; 4,409,215
Licensed from Sankyo Company, Ltd., Japan
Manufactured by
Pharmacia & Upjohn S.A.-N.V., Puurs - Belgium
for
Pharmacia & Upjohn Company
Kalamazoo, MI 49001, USA
817 150 101
505358

NDC 0009-3615-03
50 mL (when mixed)
Vantin® For Oral Suspension
cefpodoxime proxetil for oral suspension
100 mg per 5 mL
Equivalent to 100 mg per 5 mL cefpodoxime when constituted
Pharmacia & Upjohn

How many milliliters will you administer using an oral syringe? ______________

17. Order: Cefazolin 0.5 g IM q8h.

Available:

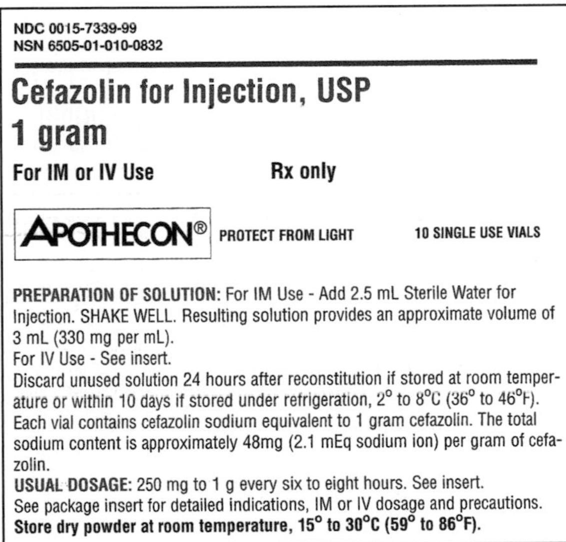
NDC 0015-7339-99
NSN 6505-01-010-0832
Cefazolin for Injection, USP
1 gram
For IM or IV Use **Rx only**
APOTHECON® PROTECT FROM LIGHT 10 SINGLE USE VIALS
PREPARATION OF SOLUTION: For IM Use - Add 2.5 mL Sterile Water for Injection. SHAKE WELL. Resulting solution provides an approximate volume of 3 mL (330 mg per mL).
For IV Use - See insert.
Discard unused solution 24 hours after reconstitution if stored at room temperature or within 10 days if stored under refrigeration, 2° to 8°C (36° to 46°F).
Each vial contains cefazolin sodium equivalent to 1 gram cefazolin. The total sodium content is approximately 48mg (2.1 mEq sodium ion) per gram of cefazolin.
USUAL DOSAGE: 250 mg to 1 g every six to eight hours. See insert.
See package insert for detailed indications, IM or IV dosage and precautions.
Store dry powder at room temperature, 15° to 30°C (59° to 86°F).

a. How many milliliters will you administer? ______________

b. Shade the dosage on the syringe provided.

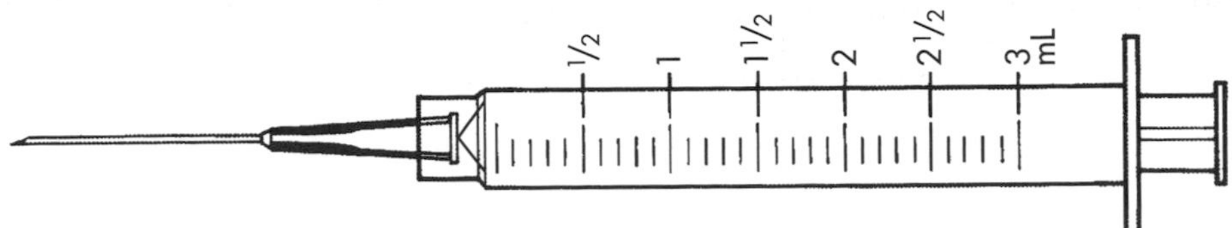

18. Order: Maxipime (Cefepime Hydrochloride) 1.5 g IV q12h.

Available:

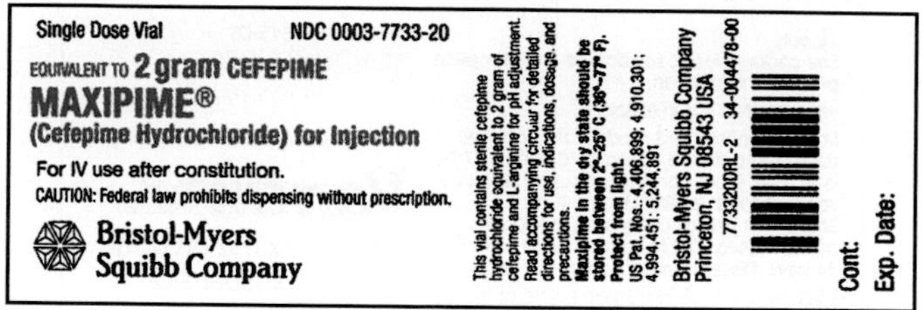

Single-Dose Vials for Intravenous/Intramuscular Administration	Amount of Diluent to Be Added (mL)	Approximate Available Volume (mL)	Approximate Cefepime Concentration (mg/mL)
cefepime vial content			
1 g (IV)	10	11.3	100
1 g (IM)	2.4	3.6	280
2 g (IV)	10	12.5	160

a. How many milliliters will you add to the IV? ______________

b. Shade the dosage on the syringe provided.

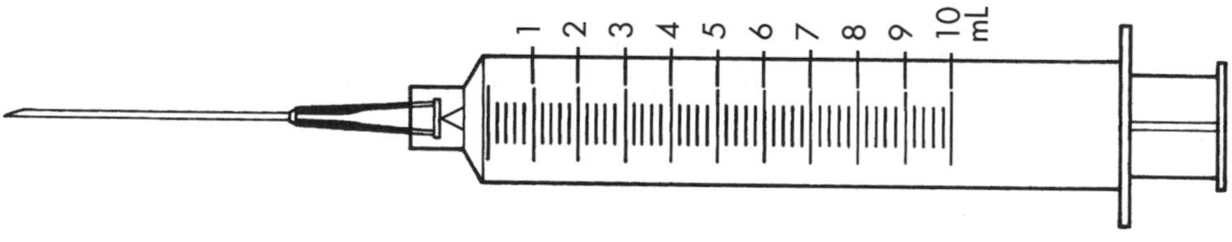

19. Order: Penicillin G Sodium 425,000 units IV daily.

Available:

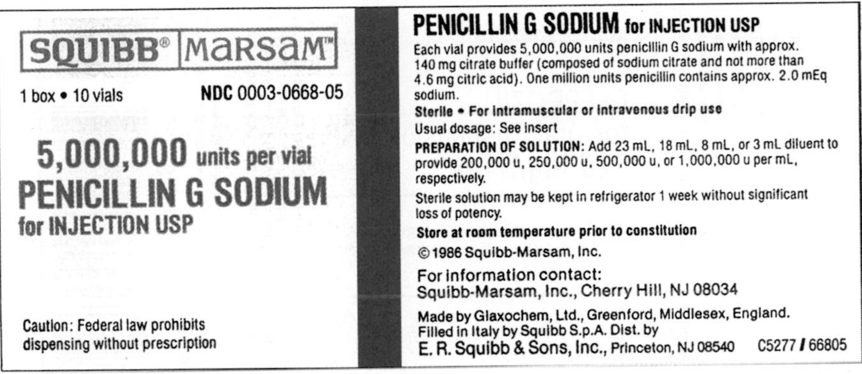

a. Which dosage strength would be best to choose? ______________

b. How many mL of diluent would be needed to make the dosage strength? ______________

c. How many milliters will you add to the IV? ______________

d. Shade the dosage calculated on the syringe provided.

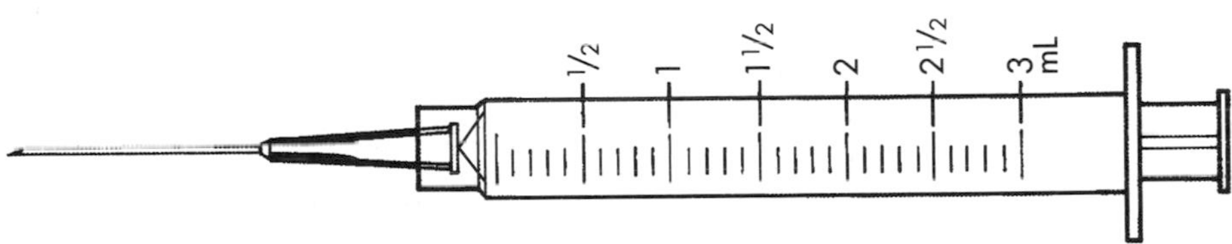

20. Order: Vfend 200 mg IV q12h.

Available:

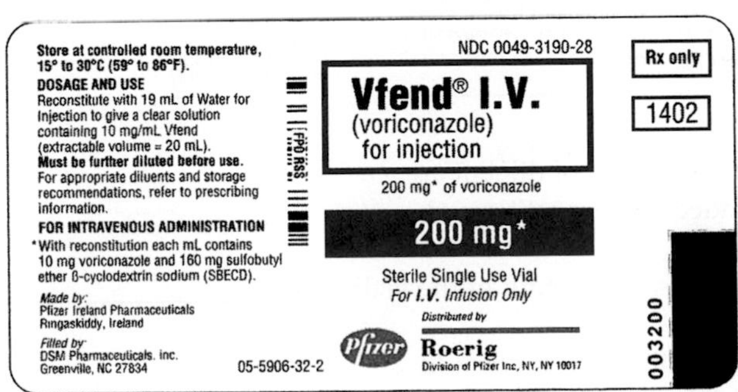

a. How many milliliters of diluent must be added to the vial? ______________

b. How many milliliters will you add to the IV? ______________

21. Order: Cefprozil 500 mg p.o. q12h for 10 days.

    Available:

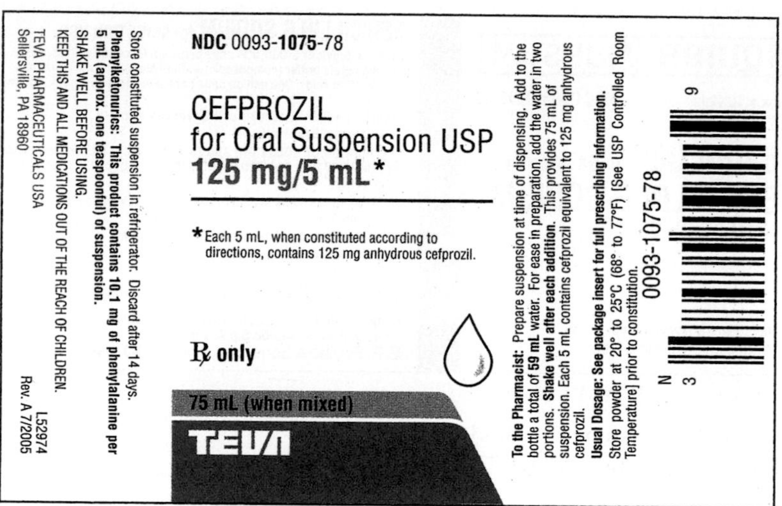

   a. How many milliliters of diluent are recommended for reconstitution? __________

   b. How many milliliters will the bottle contain after reconstitution? __________

   c. How many milliliters will you administer? __________

22. Order: Zosyn 2.25 g q8h IV.

    Available:

NDC 0206-8620-11

40.5 GRAM

ZOSYN™ Sterile Piperacillin Sodium and Tazobactam Sodium

PHARMACY BULK VIAL

Contains no preservative. Reconstitute with exactly 152 mL of a suitable diluent to achieve a concentration of 200 mg/mL of piperacillin and 25 mg/mL of tazobactam. Discard any unused portion after 24 hours if stored at room temperature or after 48 hours if refrigerated. See package circular for complete directions for use.

Control No. Exp. Date

Date Prepared _____
Diluent Used _____
Prepared by _____

Prior to Reconstitution: Store at Controlled Room Temperature 15-30°C (59-86°F). After Reconstitution: DO NOT FREEZE RECONSTITUTED SOLUTION. See package circular for stability of reconstituted solution.

Lederle

Each vial provides sterile piperacillin sodium and tazobactam sodium cryodesiccated powders equivalent to 36 grams of piperacillin, 4.5 grams of tazobactam and 84.54 mEq (1,944 mg) of sodium.
CAUTION: Federal law prohibits dispensing without prescription.

For IV Use

32324-93 D1
LEDERLE PIPERACILLIN, INC.
Carolina, Puerto Rico 00987

   a. How many milliliters of diluent are recommended for reconstitution? __________

   b. What is the dosage strength of the vial? __________

   c. How many milliliters will you add to the IV? (The dosage is based on the two medications together.) __________

23. Order: Zithromax 500 mg p.o. stat for 1 dose.

Available:

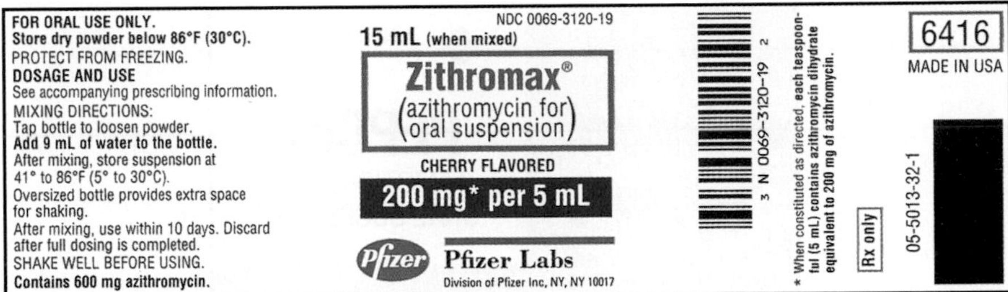

How many milliliters will you administer? ______________

24. Order: Cefobid 1 g IM q12h for 5 days.

Available: Cefobid 1 g with directions to add 1.4 mL of sterile water for injection. Each 2 mL yields 1 g.

a. How many milliliters will you administer? ______________

b. Shade the dosage on the syringe provided.

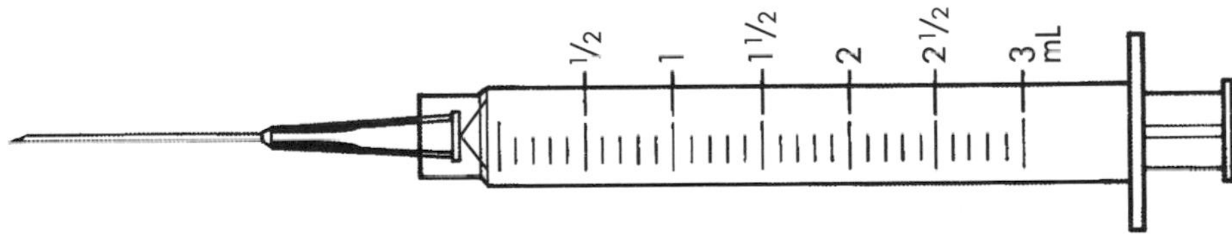

25. Order: Unasyn 1.5 g IV q6h.

Available:

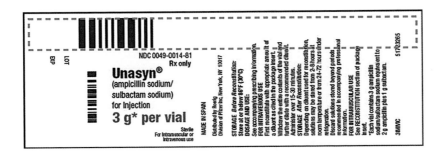

Refer to portion of package insert.

Unasyn Vial Size	Volume of Diluent to Be Added	Withdrawal Volume
1.5 g	3.2 mL	4 mL
3 g	6.4 mL	8 mL

How many milliliters will you add to the IV? ______________

26. Order: Pepcid 20 mg p.o. b.i.d.

    Available:

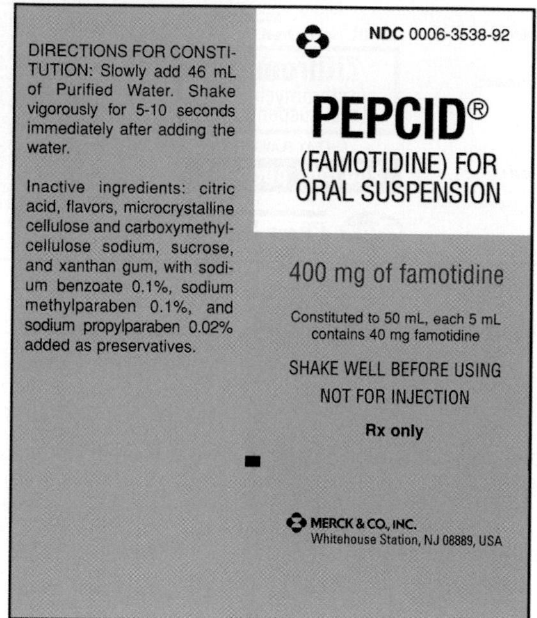

How many milliliters will you administer using an oral syringe? ____________________

27. Order: Rocephin 125 mg IM stat.

Available:

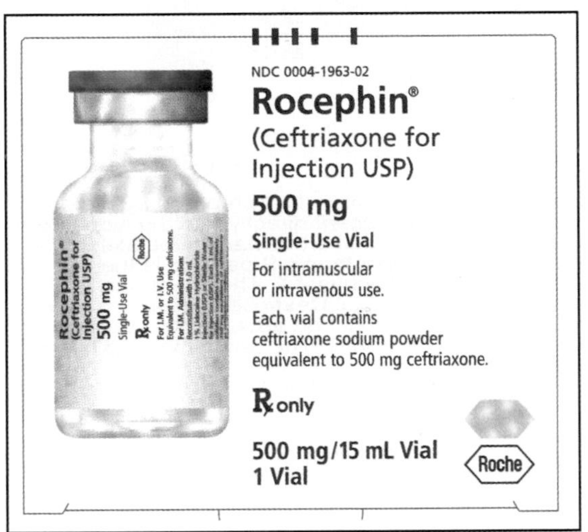

NDC 0004-1963-02
Rocephin®
(Ceftriaxone for Injection USP)
500 mg
Single-Use Vial
For intramuscular or intravenous use.
Each vial contains ceftriaxone sodium powder equivalent to 500 mg ceftriaxone.
℞ only
500 mg/15 mL Vial
1 Vial
Roche

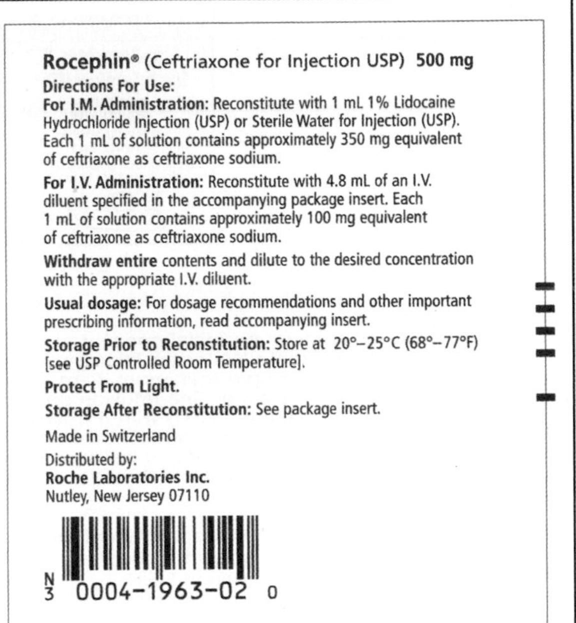

Rocephin® (Ceftriaxone for Injection USP) 500 mg
Directions For Use:
For I.M. Administration: Reconstitute with 1 mL 1% Lidocaine Hydrochloride Injection (USP) or Sterile Water for Injection (USP). Each 1 mL of solution contains approximately 350 mg equivalent of ceftriaxone as ceftriaxone sodium.
For I.V. Administration: Reconstitute with 4.8 mL of an I.V. diluent specified in the accompanying package insert. Each 1 mL of solution contains approximately 100 mg equivalent of ceftriaxone as ceftriaxone sodium.
Withdraw entire contents and dilute to the desired concentration with the appropriate I.V. diluent.
Usual dosage: For dosage recommendations and other important prescribing information, read accompanying insert.
Storage Prior to Reconstitution: Store at 20°–25°C (68°–77°F) [see USP Controlled Room Temperature].
Protect From Light.
Storage After Reconstitution: See package insert.
Made in Switzerland
Distributed by:
Roche Laboratories Inc.
Nutley, New Jersey 07110
N 3 0004-1963-02 0

a. How many milliliters will you administer? ________________

b. Shade the dosage on the syringe provided.

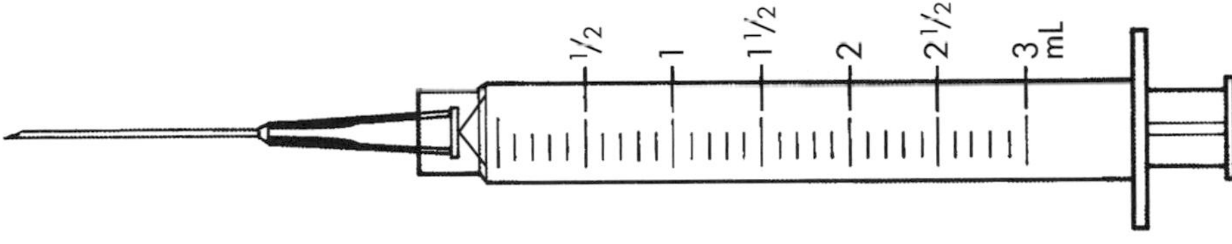

28. Order: Amphotericin B 45.5 mg IV every day.

Available:

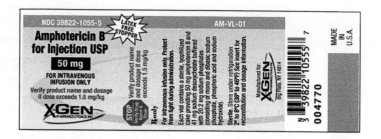

Preparation of Solutions
Reconstitute as follows: An initial concentrate of 5 mg amphotericin B per mL is first prepared by rapidly expressing 10 mL Sterile Water for Injection USP *without a bacteriostatic agent* directly into the lyophilized cake, using a sterile needle (minimum diameter: 20 gauge) and syringe. Shake the vial immediately until the colloidal solution is clear. The infusion solution, providing 0.1 mg amphotericin B per mL, is then obtained by further dilution (1:50) with 5% Dextrose Injection USP *of pH above 4.2*. The pH of each container of Dextrose Injection should be ascertained before use. Commercial Dextrose Injection usually has a pH above 4.2; however, if it is below 4.2, then 1 or 2 mL of buffer should be added to the Dextrose Injection before it is used to dilute the concentrated solution of amphotericin B. The recommended buffer has the following composition:

Dibasic sodium phosphate (anhydrous)	1.59 g
Monobasic sodium phosphate (anhydrous)	0.96 g
Water for Injection USP	qs 100.0 mL

Use the information from the partial package insert to answer the questions and calculate the number of milliliters you will administer.

a. How many milliliters of diluent must be added for the initial concentration? ______________

b. What is the recommended diluent? ______________

c. What is the final concentration of the prepared solution per milliliter? ______________

d. How many milliliters will you administer (initial dose)? ______________

29. Order: Omnicef 300 mg p.o. q12h for 5 days.

Available:

Usual Dosage: Children-14 mg/kg/day in a single dose or in two divided doses, depending on age, weight, and type of infection. See package enclosure for full prescribing information.

This bottle contains 2.5 g cefdinir.

Keep this and all drugs out of the reach of children.

Store dry powder and reconstituted suspension at 25°C (77°F); excursions permitted to 15°-30°C (59°-86°F) [see USP Controlled Room Temperature].

DIRECTIONS FOR RECONSTITUTION
Prepare suspension at time of dispensing by adding a total of **63 mL** water to the bottle. Tap bottle to loosen the powder, then add about half the water, and shake. Add the remaining water and shake to complete suspension. This provides 100 mL of suspension. Each 5 mL contains 125 mg cefdinir after reconstitution.

See bottom of carton for expiration date and lot number.

NDC 0074-3771-13

Omnicef®

(Cefdinir) for Oral Suspension

125 mg/5 mL

℞ only

SHAKE WELL BEFORE USING.

Keep bottle tightly closed.
Any unused portion must be discarded 10 days after mixing.

RECONSTITUTE WITH 63 mL WATER

100 mL (when reconstituted)

a. How many milliliters of diluent must be added to the bottle for reconstitution? ________________

b. What is the final concentration of the prepared solution? ________________

c. How many milliliters will you administer? ________________

30. Order: Ceftriaxone 0.5 g IV q12 h

Available:

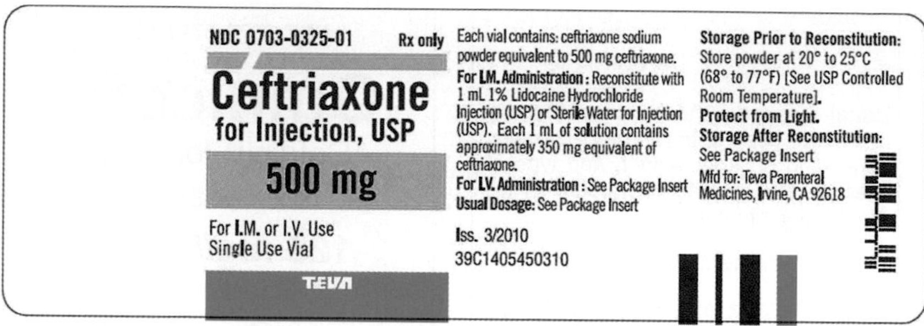

Intravenous Administration

Ceftriaxone for injection, USP should be administered intravenously by infusion over a period of 30 minutes. Concentrations between 10 mg/mL and 40 mg/mL are recommended; however, lower concentrations may be used if desired. Reconstitute vials with an appropriate IV diluent. After reconstitution, each 1 mL of solution contains approximately 100 mg equivalent of ceftriaxone. Withdraw entrire contents and dilute to the desired concentration with the appropriate IV diluent.

Vial Dosage Size	Amount of Diluent to Be Added
250 mg	2.4 mL
500 mg	4.8 mL
1 g	9.6 mL
2 g	19.2 mL

a. How many milliliters will you add to the IV? ______________________

b. Shade the dosage calculated on the syringe provided.

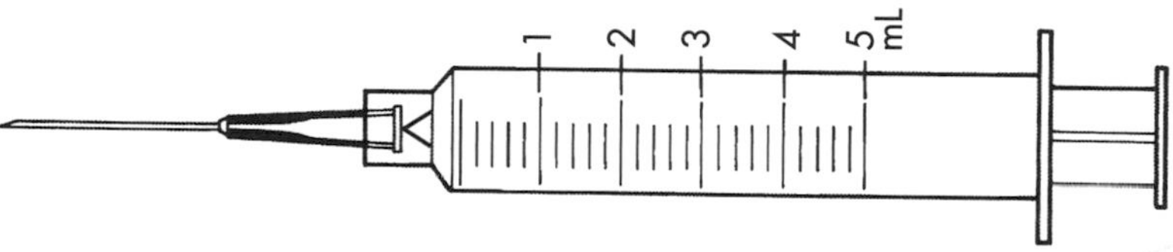

31. Order: Oxacillin 0.35 g IM q6h.

Available:

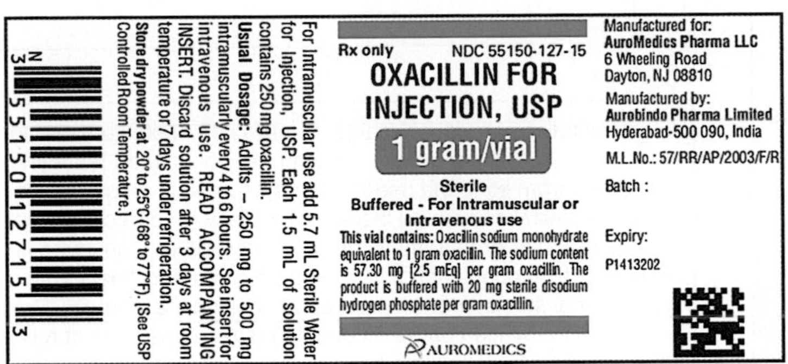

a. How many milliliters will you administer IM? ______________________

b. Shade the dosage calculated on the syringe provided.

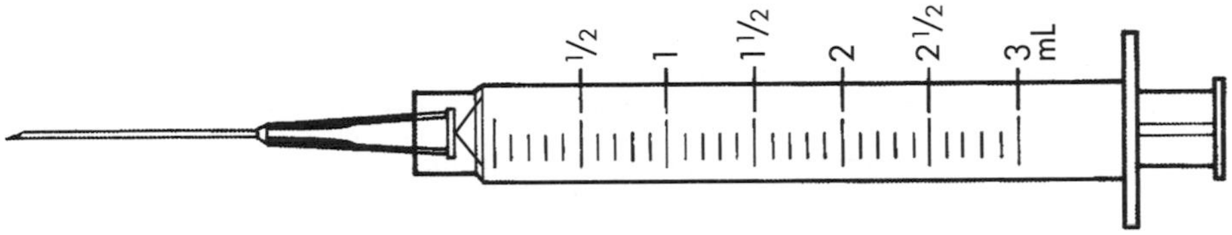

32. Order: Streptomycin 0.75 g IM daily for 1 week.

Available:

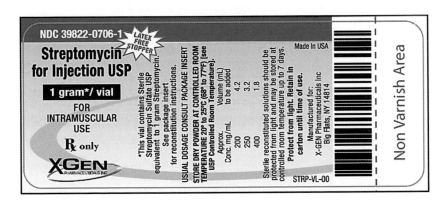

Directions: dilute with 1.8 mL of sterile water for injection.

a. How many milliliters will you administer IM? ______________________

b. Shade the dosage calculated on the syringe provided.

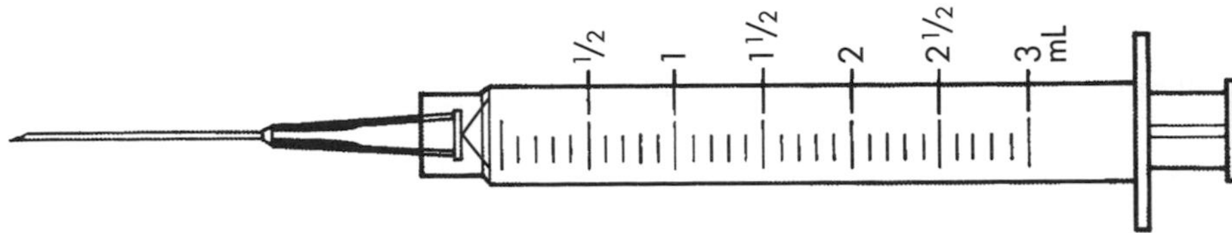

33. Order: Visudyne 10 mg IV × 1 dose.

Available:

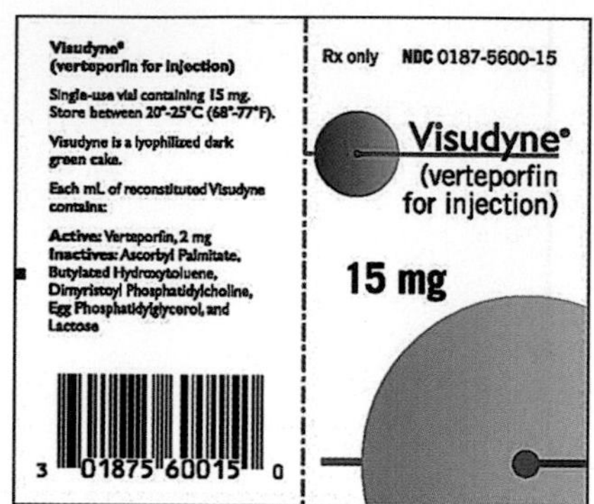

Reconstitute each vial of Visudyne with 7 mL of sterile water for Injection to provide 7.5 mL containing 2 mg/mL. Reconstituted Visudyne must be protected from light and used within 4 hours. It is recommended that reconstituted Visudyne be inspected visually for particulate matter and discoloration prior to administration. Reconstituted Visudyne is an opaque dark green solution. Visudyne may precipitate in saline solutions. Do not use normal saline or other parenteral solutions, except 5% Dextrose for Injection, for dilution of the reconstituted Visudyne. Do not mix Visudyne in the same solution with other drugs.

a. How many milliliters will you administer IV? ______________________

b. Shade the dosage calculated on the syringe provided.

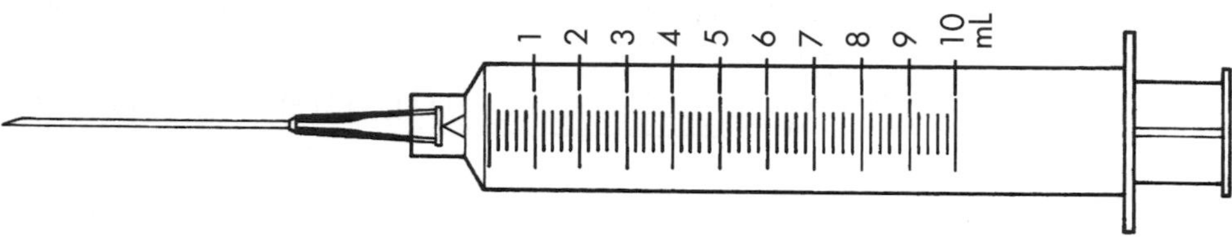

Prepare the following solutions from the nutritional formulas. (Express answers in mL.)

34. Order: ¼-strength Ensure 12 oz by nasogastric tube over 6 hr. ______________

35. Order: ⅔-strength Isomil 6 oz p.o. q4h for 24 hr.
(State answer for single feeding.) ______________________

36. A client has an order for Jevity 1,000 mL by continuous feeding through a gastrostomy tube over 16 hours, followed by 250 mL of free water. The feeding is placed on an infusion pump. Calculate the mL per hr to set the pump at. (Round answer to nearest whole number.) ______________________

37. Order: ⅛-strength Ensure 4 oz by nasogastric tube q4h for 24h. (State answer for single feeding.) ______________________

Indicate how you would prepare each of the following using full-strength normal saline (solute) and sterile water (solvent).

38. Clean sacral wound with 4 oz of ½ strength normal saline q6h. You make enough solution for 24 hours. ______________________

39. Irrigate foot wound with 0.24 L of ¼ strength daily. ______________

40. 18 oz of ⅔ strength solution for wound irrigation ______________

41. 0.5 L of ¼ strength solution for wound irrigation ______________

Answers on pp. 475-481

ANSWERS

Chapter 19

Answers to Practice Problems

1. 200 mg per vial
2. 5 mL
3. 0.9% sodium chloride injection without preservatives
4. 38 mg per mL
5. 24 hours
6. 2.6 mL

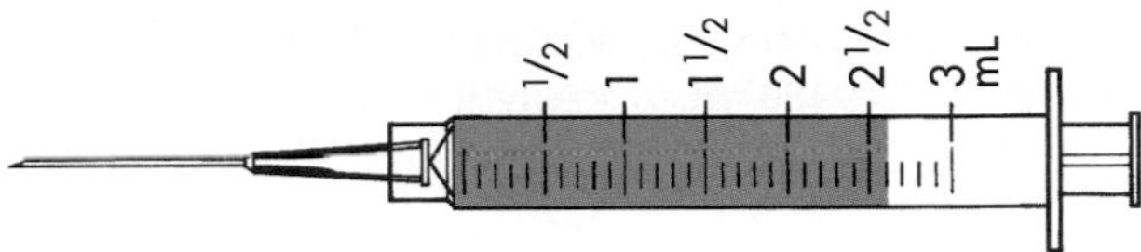

7. 350 mg per vial
8. 17.5 mL
9. Sterile water for injection or Bacteriostatic water for injection preserved with benzyl alcohol
10. 20 mg per mL
11. IV or IM use
12. see package insert
13. 0.8 mL

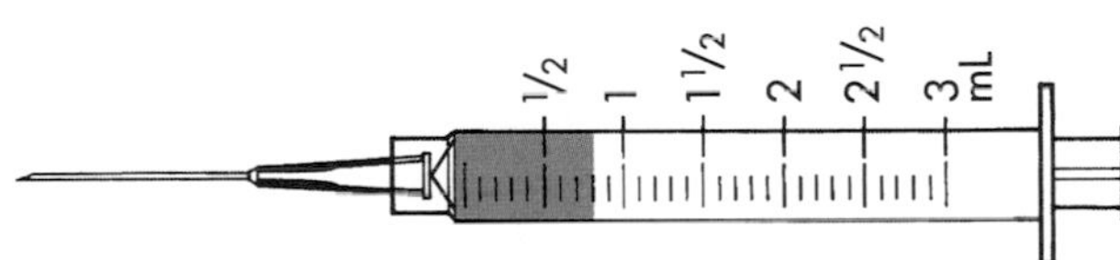

14. 40 mg per vial
15. Bacteriostatic water for injection with benzyl alcohol
16. 1.2 mL
17. 40 mg per mL
18. 0.9 mL

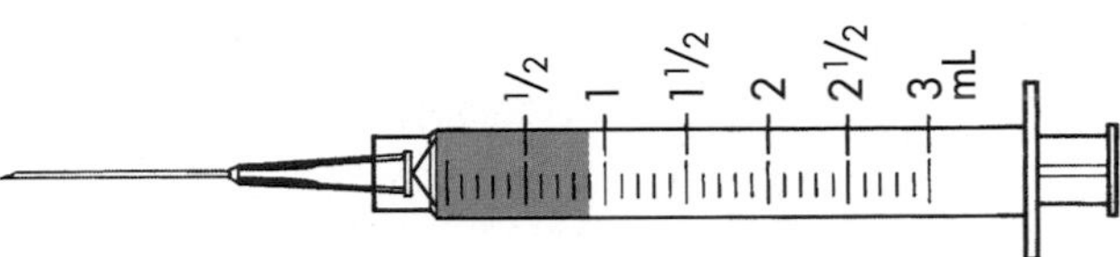

19. 1 g per vial (1 gram per vial)
20. IM or IV use
21. 9.6 mL
22. IV diluent specified in the accompanying package insert
23. 100 mg per mL
24. 2.1 mL
25. 1% Lidocaine hydrochloride injection or sterile water for injection
26. 10 mL

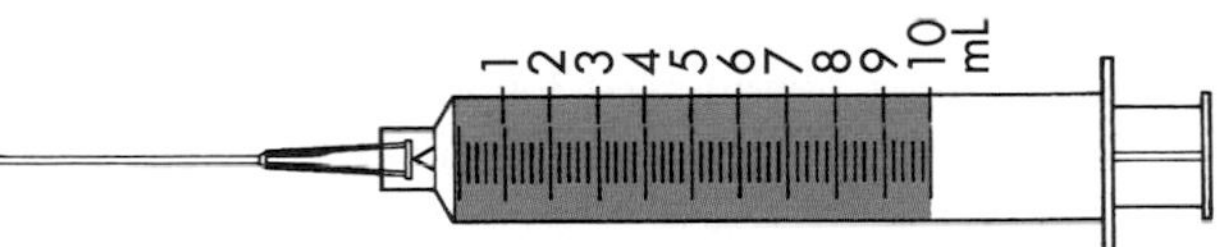

27. 113 mL
28. water
29. 125 mg per 5 mL
30. Store at room temperature or refrigerate and keep tightly closed.
31. 1,000 mg (1 g) per vial
32. 20 mL
33. sterile water for injection
34. 50 mg per mL
35. IV infusion only
36. 154 mL
37. 200 mL
38. 200 mg per 5 mL (1 tsp)
39. 10 days (refrigerated)
40. 2 g per vial
41. 4.2 mL
42. 19.2 mL
43. IV diluents specified in the accompanying package insert
44. 100 mg per mL
45. 500 mg per vial
46. 4.8 mL
47. sterile water for injection
48. 100 mg per mL
49. IV infusion only
50. 24 mL
51. distilled water *or* purified water
52. 50 mg per 5 mL (1 tsp); 10 mg per mL
53. Store reconstituted suspension between 41° F (5° C) and 86° F (30° C). Protect from freezing.
54. 20,000,000 units
55. 500,000 units per mL
56. 1,000,000 units per mL; this strength is closest to what is ordered.
57. 2 mL
58. 7 days (1 week)
59. 5,000,000 units
60. 500,000 units per mL
61. 1.4 mL
62. refrigerator
63. 7 days (1 week)
64. 250,000 units per mL
65. package insert
66. 10 mg per vial
67. 2.1 mL
68. sterile water for injection
69. 1 hour
70. 1.5 mL
71. 0.5 mL
72. $\frac{480 \text{ mL}}{8 \text{ hr}} = 60 \text{ mL/hr}$
73. $\frac{1{,}600 \text{ mL}}{24 \text{ hr}} = 66.6 = 67 \text{ mL/hr}$

74. 300 mL qid $= 300 \text{ mL} \times 4 = 1{,}200 \text{ mL}$

$\frac{2}{3} \times 1{,}200 \text{ mL} = x \text{ mL}$

$$x = \frac{2{,}400}{3}$$

$x = 800$ mL of formula needed

$1{,}200 \text{ mL} - 800 \text{ mL} = 400$ mL (water)

Therefore, you will add 400 mL of water to 800 mL of Sustacal to make 1,200 mL of $\frac{2}{3}$-strength Sustacal.

75. 1 oz = 30 mL; therefore 16 oz = 480 mL

$\frac{3}{4} \times 480 \text{ mL} = x \text{ mL}$

$$x = \frac{1{,}440}{4}$$

$$x = 360 \text{ mL}$$

$x = 360$ mL of formula needed.

$480 \text{ mL} - 360 \text{ mL} = 120$ mL. You would need 360 mL of formula and 120 mL of water to make 480 mL of $\frac{3}{4}$ strength Ensure.

76. 1 oz = 30 mL; therefore 20 oz = 600 mL

$\frac{1}{2} \times 600 \text{ mL} = x \text{ mL}$

$$x = \frac{600}{2}$$

$$x = 300 \text{ mL}$$

$x = 300$ mL

$600 \text{ mL} - 300 \text{ mL} = 300$ mL (10 oz of water)

Answer: You would need 300 mL of Ensure and 300 mL of water to make 600 mL of 1/2 strength Ensure.

77. 1 oz = 30 mL; therefore 8 oz = 240 mL

$\frac{1}{4} \times 240 \text{ mL} = x \text{ mL}$

$$x = \frac{240}{4}$$

$x = 60$ mL

60 mL normal saline (solute) + 180 mL sterile water (solvent) = 240 mL $\frac{1}{4}$ strength solution.

78. $\frac{1}{3} \times 480 \text{ mL} = x \text{ mL}$

$$x = \frac{480}{3}$$

$x = 160$ mL

160 mL normal saline (solute) + 320 mL sterile water (solvent) = 480 mL $\frac{1}{3}$ strength solution.

79. $\frac{3}{4} \times 120 \text{ mL} = x \text{ mL}$

$$x = \frac{360}{4}$$

$x = 90$ mL

90 mL normal saline (solute) + 30 mL sterile water (solvent) = 120 mL $\frac{3}{4}$ strength solution.

80. $\frac{5}{8} \times 160 \text{ mL} = x \text{ mL}$

$$x = \frac{800}{8}$$

$x = 100$ mL

100 mL normal saline (solute) + 60 mL sterile water (solvent) = 160 mL $\frac{5}{8}$ strength solution.

Answers to Clinical Reasoning Questions

1. a. The wrong dosage was administered because the nurse chose the incorrect dilution instructions. The dilution instructions used were for IV instead of IM.

   b. The concentration for IM should have been made (add 3 mL of diluents to give a concentration of 280 mg per mL).

   c. The nurse added 10.6 mL of a diluent and made the concentration for IV administration 95 mg per mL.

   d. The client received three times the mL of medication IM (2.6 mL instead of 0.9 mL). Interchanging dilution instructions for IV and IM administration can have serious outcomes ranging from irritation of muscles to formation of a sterile abscess.

   e. This type of error could have been prevented by the nurse by reading the label carefully for the correct amount of diluents for the route ordered. Nurses must always check the route ordered and follow the directions that correspond to that route. The dilution instructions for IV and IM should never be interchanged.

NOTE

For problems in which conversion is indicated, answers are shown with order converted to what is available. Calculations could also be performed using dimensional analysis.

Answers to Chapter Review

1. $500 \text{ mg} : 8 \text{ mL} = 165 \text{ mg} : x \text{ mL}$

$$\frac{500x}{500} = \frac{1{,}320}{500}$$

$$x = 2.64 = 2.6 \text{ mL}$$

or

$$\frac{165 \text{ mg}}{500 \text{ mg}} \times 8 \text{ mL} = x \text{ mL}$$

a. Answer: 2.6 mL. The dosage ordered is less than the available strength. You will need less than 8 mL to administer the dosage.

b.

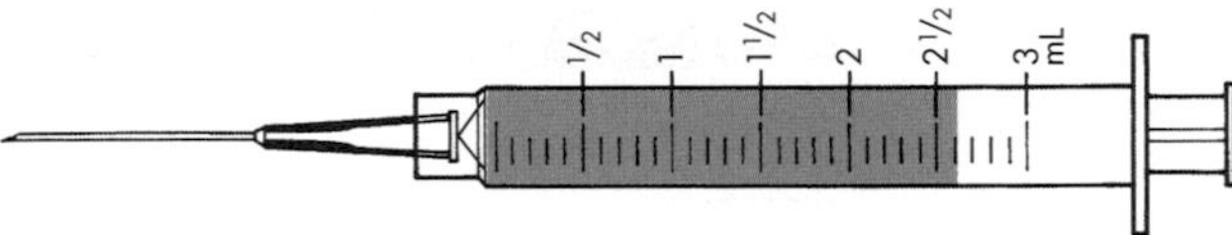

2. a. 3.5 mL

b. 250 mg per 1 mL

c. $250 \text{ mg} : 1 \text{ mL} = 375 \text{ mg} : x \text{ mL}$

$$\frac{250x}{250} = \frac{375}{250}$$

$$x = 1.5 \text{ mL}$$

or

$$\frac{375 \text{ mg}}{250 \text{ mg}} \times 1 \text{ mL} = x \text{ mL}$$

d. Answer: 1.5 mL. The dosage ordered is greater than the available strength; you will need more than 1 mL to administer the dosage.

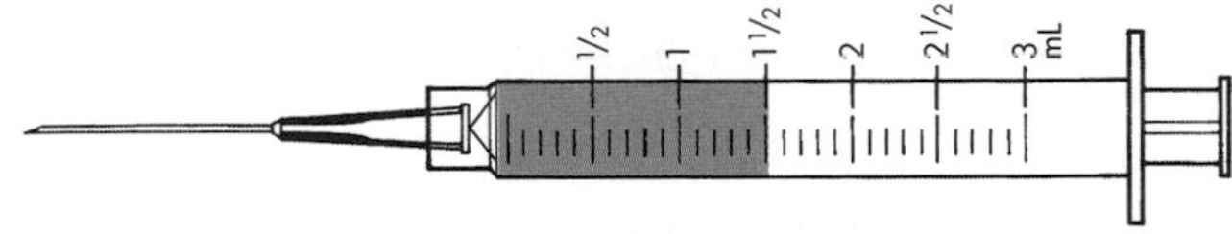

3. Conversion required 1 g = 1,000 mg; therefore 0.4 g = 400 mg

a. 113 mL

b. water

c. 125 mg per 5 mL

$125 \text{ mg} : 5 \text{ mL} = 400 \text{ mg} : x \text{ mL}$

$$\frac{125x}{125} = \frac{2{,}000}{125}$$

$$x = 16 \text{ mL}$$

or

$$\frac{400 \text{ mg}}{125 \text{ mg}} \times 5 \text{ mL} = x \text{ mL}$$

d. Answer: 16 mL. The dosage ordered is more than the available strength. You will need more than 5 mL to give the dosage. 16 mL p.o. can be administered; sometimes large volumes are administered p.o.

e. 14 days

4. a. 250,000 units per mL

b. 4 mL

c. $250{,}000 \text{ units} : 1 \text{ mL} = 275{,}000 \text{ units} : x \text{ mL}$

$$\frac{250{,}000x}{250{,}000} = \frac{275{,}\cancel{000}}{250{,}\cancel{000}}$$

$$x = \frac{275}{250}$$

$$x = 1.1 \text{ mL}$$

or

$$\frac{275{,}000 \text{ units}}{250{,}000 \text{ units}} \times 1 \text{ mL} = x \text{ mL}$$

d. Answer: 1.1 mL. The dosage ordered is more than what is available; therefore you will need more than 1 mL to administer the dosage.

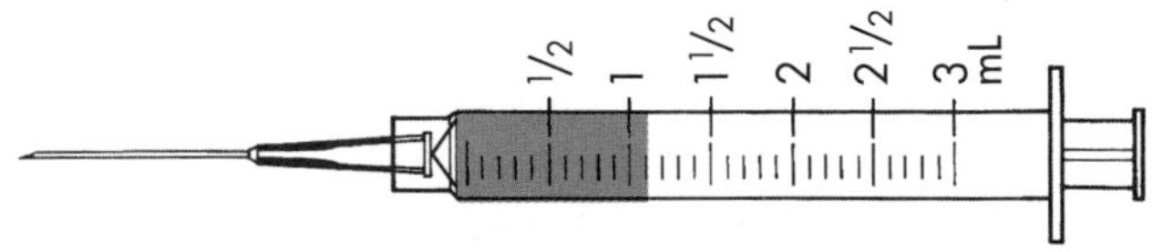

5. a. 100 mg per mL
   b. $100 \text{ mg} : 1 \text{ mL} = 200 \text{ mg} : x \text{ mL}$

$$\frac{100x}{100} = \frac{200}{100}$$

$$x = 2 \text{ mL}$$

or

$$\frac{200 \text{ units}}{100 \text{ units}} \times 1 \text{ mL} = x \text{ mL}$$

   Answer: 2 mL. The dosage ordered is more than what is available; therefore you will need more than 1 mL to administer the dosage.

   c.

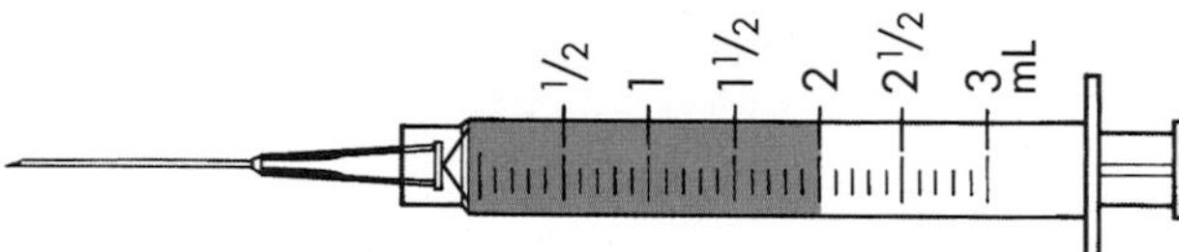

6. a. 40 mg per vial
   b. bacteriostatic water for injection with benzyl alcohol
   c. $40 \text{ mg} : 1 \text{ mL} = 175 \text{ mg} : x \text{ mL}$

$$\frac{40x}{40} = \frac{175}{40}$$

$$x = 4.37 = 4.4 \text{ mL}$$

or

$$\frac{175 \text{ mg}}{40 \text{ mg}} \times 1 \text{ mL} = x \text{ mL}$$

   Answer: 4.4 mL. When mixed according to directions the dosage is 40 mg per mL. You will need more than 1 mL to administer the dosage ordered.

   d.

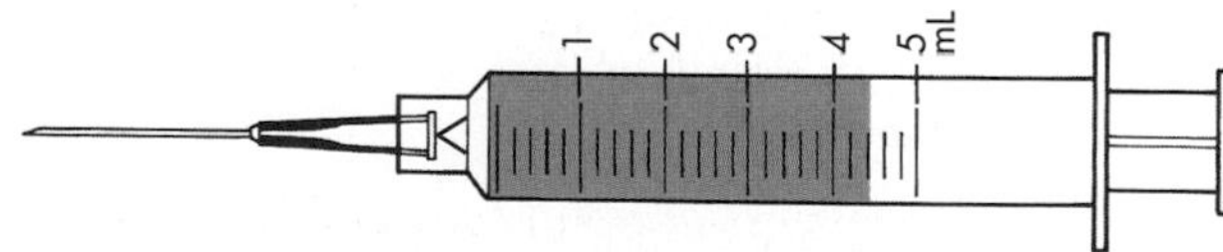

7. Conversion required. Equivalent: 1,000 mg = 1 g; therefore 0.5 g = 500 mg
   a. 87 mL
   b. 400 mg per 5 mL
   c. 6.3 mL

$$400 \text{ mg} : 5 \text{ mL} = 500 \text{ mg} : x \text{ mL}$$

$$\frac{400x}{400} = \frac{2{,}500}{400}$$

$$x = 6.25 = 6.3 \text{ mL}$$

or

$$\frac{500 \text{ mg}}{400 \text{ mg}} \times 5 \text{ mL} = x \text{ mL}$$

   Answer: 6.3 mL. The dosage ordered is more than the available strength. You will need more than 5 mL to give the dosage.

8. Conversion is required. Equivalent: 1,000 mg = 1 g; therefore 1.2 g = 1,200 mg.
   a. $500 \text{ mg} : 1 \text{ mL} = 1{,}200 \text{ mg} : x \text{ mL}$

$$\frac{500x}{500} = \frac{1{,}200}{500}$$

$$x = 2.4 \text{ mL}$$

or

$$\frac{1{,}200 \text{ mg}}{500 \text{ mg}} \times 1 \text{ mL} = x \text{ mL}$$

   b. Answer: 2.4 mL. The dosage ordered is greater than the available strength; therefore you will need more than 1 mL to administer the dosage.

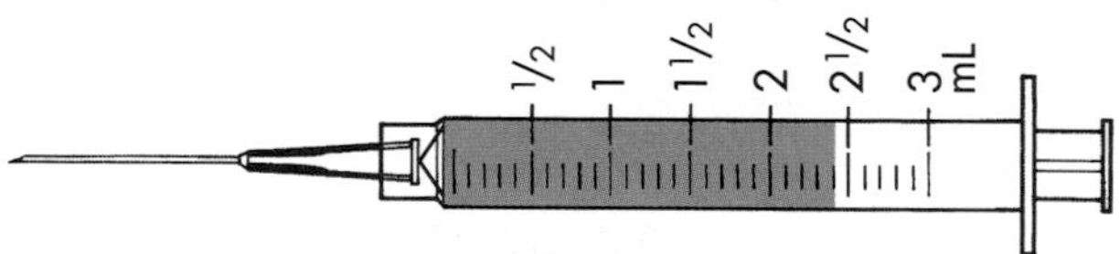

9. a. 55 mL
   b. 125 mg per 5 mL
   c. $125 \text{ mg} : 5 \text{ mL} = 350 \text{ mg} : x \text{ mL}$

$$\frac{125x}{125} = \frac{1{,}750}{125}$$

$$x = 14 \text{ mL}$$

or

$$\frac{350 \text{ mg}}{125 \text{ mg}} \times 5 \text{ mL} = x \text{ mL}$$

   Answer: 14 mL. The dosage ordered is more than the available strength. Therefore you will need more than 5 mL to administer the dosage.

10. a. $500{,}000 \text{ units} : 1 \text{ mL} = 400{,}000 \text{ units} : x \text{ mL}$

or

$$\frac{400{,}000 \text{ units}}{500{,}000 \text{ units}} \times 1 \text{ mL} = x \text{ mL}$$

   Answer: 0.8 mL. The dosage ordered is less than the available strength; therefore you will need less than 1 mL to administer the dosage. *Note:* 500,000 units per mL was used because it is closest to the ordered dose.

   b.

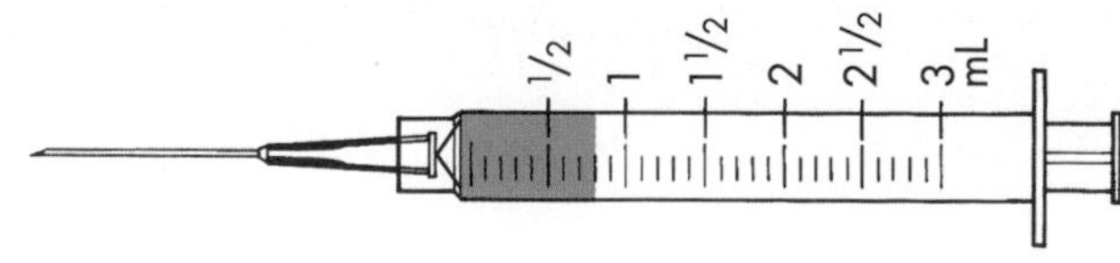

11. a. $280\text{ mg} : 1\text{ mL} = 250\text{ mg} : x\text{ mL}$

or

$$\frac{2500\text{ mg}}{280\text{ mg}} \times 1\text{ mL} = x\text{ mL}$$

Answer: 0.9 mL; 0.89 mL rounded to the nearest tenth. The dosage ordered is less than the available strength; therefore you will need less than 1 mL to administer the dosage.

b.

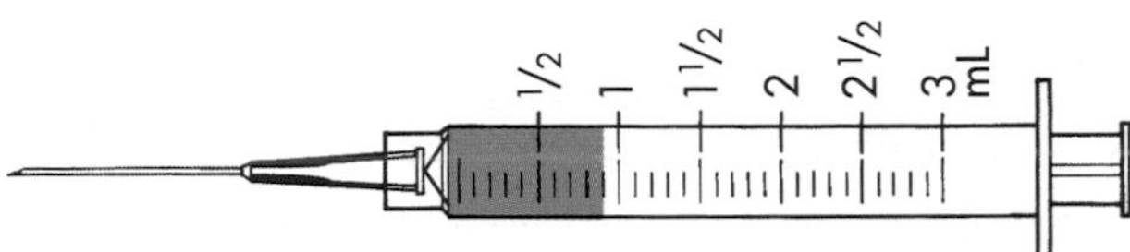

12. a. $50\text{ mg} : 1\text{ mL} = 150\text{ mg} : x\text{ mL}$

or

$$\frac{150\text{ mg}}{50\text{ mg}} \times 1\text{ mL} = x\text{ mL}$$

Answer: 3 mL. The dosage ordered is greater than the available strength; you will need more than 1 mL to administer the dosage.

b.

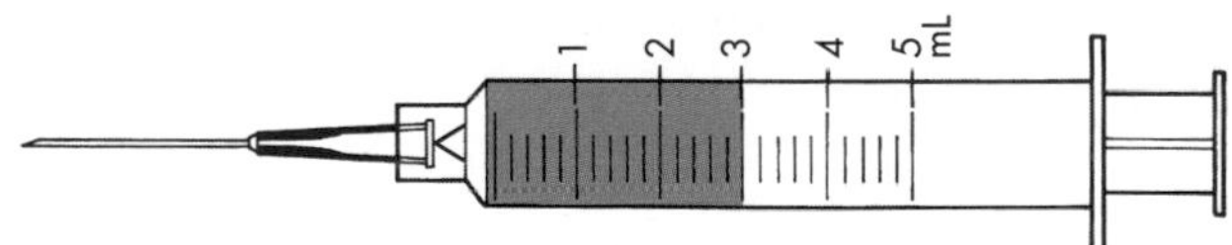

13. Conversion is required. Equivalent: 1,000 mg = 1 g; therefore 0.45 g = 450 mg.

a. 10 mL

b. 50 mg per mL

c. $50\text{ mg} : 1\text{ mL} = 450\text{ mg} : x\text{ mL}$

$x = 9\text{ mL}$

or

$$\frac{450\text{ mg}}{50\text{ mg}} \times 1\text{ mL} = x\text{ mL}$$

Answer: 9 mL. The dosage ordered is greater than the available strength; therefore you will need more than 1 mL to administer the dosage.

d.

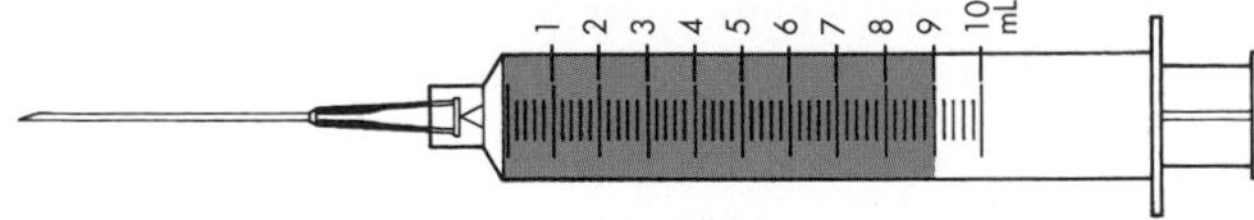

14. Conversion is required. Equivalent: 1,000 mcg = 1 mg; therefore 0.05 mg = 50 mcg.

a. $40\text{ mcg} : 1\text{ mL} = 50\text{ mcg} : x\text{ mL}$

$$\frac{40x}{40} = \frac{50}{40}$$

$$x = 1.3\text{ mL}$$

or

$$\frac{50\text{ mcg}}{40\text{ mcg}} \times 5\text{ mL} = x\text{ mL}$$

Answer: 1.3 mL; 1.25 mL rounded to the nearest tenth. The dosage ordered is less than the available strength; therefore you will need less than 5 mL to administer the dosage.

b.

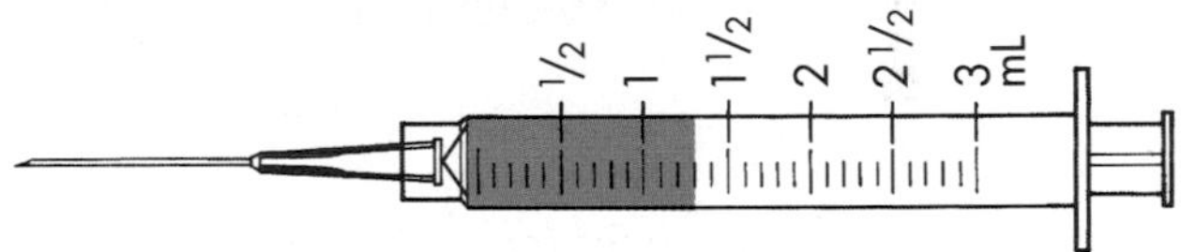

15. Conversion is required. Equivalent: 1,000 mg = 1 g; therefore 0.25 g = 250 mg.

a. $50\text{ mg} : 1\text{ mL} = 250\text{ mg} : x\text{ mL}$

$$\frac{50x}{50} = \frac{250}{50}$$

$$x = 5\text{ mL}$$

or

$$\frac{250\text{ mg}}{50\text{ mg}} \times 1\text{ mL} = x\text{ mL}$$

Answer: 5 mL. The dosage ordered is more than the available strength; therefore you will need more than 1 mL to administer the dosage.

b.

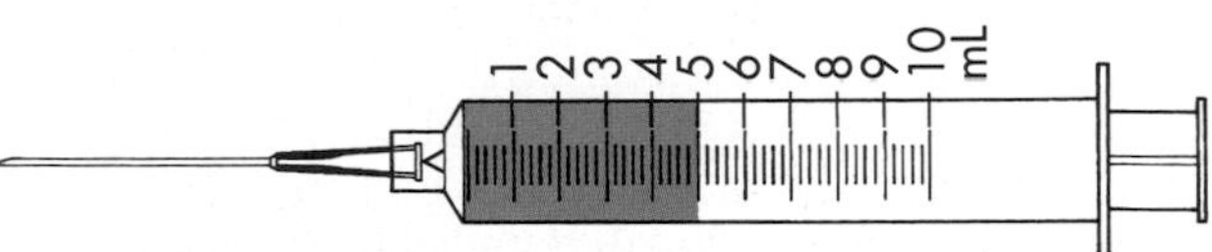

16. $100\text{ mg} : 5\text{ mL} = 200\text{ mg} : x\text{ mL}$

or

$$\frac{200\text{ mg}}{100\text{ mg}} \times 5\text{ mL} = x\text{ mL}$$

Answer: 10 mL. The dosage ordered is greater than the available strength; therefore you will need more than 5 mL to administer the dosage.

17. Conversion is required. Equivalent: 1,000 mg = 1 g; therefore 0.5 g = 500 mg.

$$330 \text{ mg} : 1 \text{ mL} = 500 \text{ mg} : x \text{ mL}$$

or

$$\frac{500 \text{ mg}}{330 \text{ mg}} \times 1 \text{ mL} = x \text{ mL}$$

a. Answer: 1.5 mL. The dosage ordered is more than what is available; therefore you will need more than 1 mL to administer the dosage.

b.

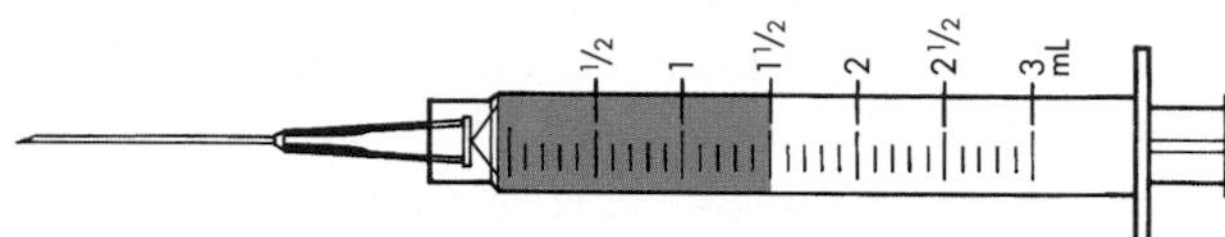

18. Conversion is required. Equivalent: 1,000 mg = 1 g; therefore 1.5 g = 1,500 mg.

$$160 \text{ mg} : 1 \text{ mL} = 1{,}500 \text{ mg} : x \text{ mL}$$

or

$$\frac{1{,}500 \text{ mg}}{160 \text{ mg}} \times 1 \text{ mL} = x \text{ mL}$$

a. Answer: 9.4 mL; 9.37 mL rounded to the nearest tenth. The dosage ordered is more than the available strength; therefore you will need more than 1 mL to administer the dosage.

b.

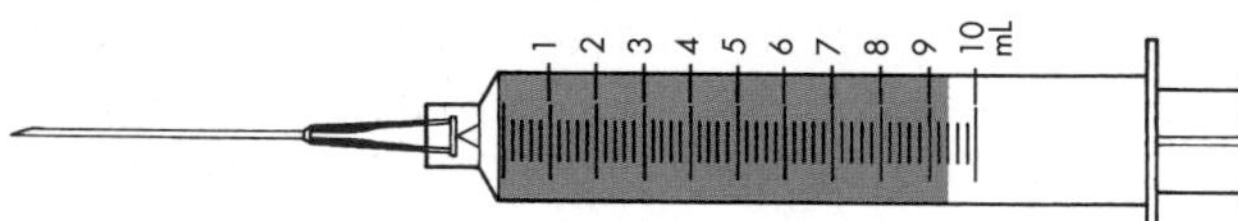

19. a. 500,000 units per mL

b. 8 mL

c. $500{,}000 \text{ units} : 1 \text{ mL} = 425{,}000 \text{ units} : x \text{ mL}$

or

$$\frac{425{,}000 \text{ units}}{500{,}000 \text{ units}} \times 1 \text{ mL} = x \text{ mL}$$

Answer: 0.9 mL; 0.85 mL rounded to the nearest tenth. The dosage ordered is less than the available dosage strength. Therefore you will need less than 1 mL to administer the dosage. 500,000 units per mL is closer to what prescriber ordered.

d.

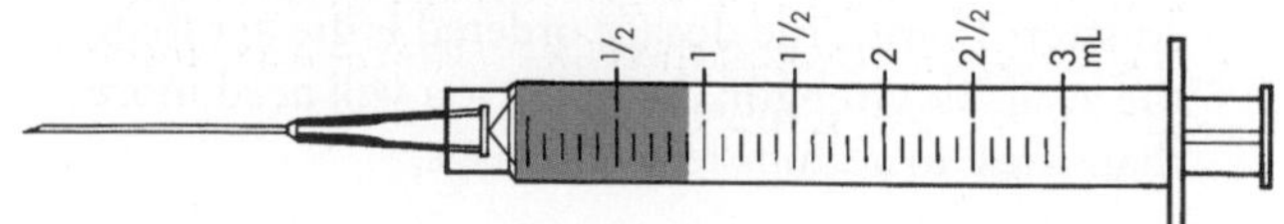

20. a. 19 mL

b. $10 \text{ mg} : 1 \text{ mL} = 200 \text{ mg} : x \text{ mL}$

$$\frac{10x}{10} = \frac{200}{10}$$

$$x = 20 \text{ mL}$$

or

$$\frac{200 \text{ units}}{10 \text{ units}} \times 1 \text{ mL} = x \text{ mL}$$

Answer: 20 mL. The dosage ordered is more than the available strength; therefore you will need more than 1 mL to administer the dosage.

21. a. 59 mL

b. 75 mL

c. $125 \text{ mg} : 5 \text{ mL} = 500 \text{ mg} : x \text{ mL}$

$$\frac{125x}{125} = \frac{2{,}500}{125}$$

$$x = 20 \text{ mL}$$

or

$$\frac{500 \text{ mg}}{125 \text{ mg}} \times 5 \text{ mL} = x \text{ mL}$$

Answer: 20 mL. The dosage ordered is greater than the available strength; therefore you will need more than 5 mL to administer the dosage.

22. a. 152 mL

b. 40.5 g per vial

c. Conversion is required. 1,000 mg = 1 g; 2.25 g = 2,250 mg

The piperacillin and tazobactam are added together for calculation. When reconstituted, the result is 200 mg per mL of piperacillin and 25 mg per mL of tazobactam.

200 mg per mL + 25 mg per mL = 225 mg per mL.

$$225 \text{ mg} : 1 \text{ mL} = 2{,}250 \text{ mg} : x \text{ mL}$$

$$\frac{225x}{225} = \frac{2{,}250}{225}$$

$$x = 10 \text{ mL}$$

or

$$\frac{2{,}250 \text{ mg}}{225 \text{ mg}} \times 1 \text{ mL} = x \text{ mL}$$

Answer: 10 mL. The dosage ordered is greater than the available strength; therefore more than 1 mL is needed to administer the dosage.

23. $200\text{ mg}:5\text{ mL} = 500\text{ mg}:x\text{ mL}$

$$\frac{200x}{200} = \frac{2{,}500}{200}$$

$$x = 12.5\text{ mL}$$

or

$$\frac{500\text{ mg}}{200\text{ mg}} \times 5\text{ mL} = x\text{ mL}$$

Answer: 12.5 mL. The dosage ordered is more than what is available; therefore you will need more than 5 mL to administer the dosage.

24. a. $1\text{ g}:2\text{ mL} = 1\text{ g}:x\text{ mL}$

$$x = 2\text{ mL}$$

or

$$\frac{1\text{ g}}{1\text{ g}} \times 2\text{ mL} = x\text{ mL}$$

b. Answer: 2 mL. When mixed according to directions, the solution gives 1 g in 2 mL; therefore you will need to give 2 mL to administer the ordered dosage.

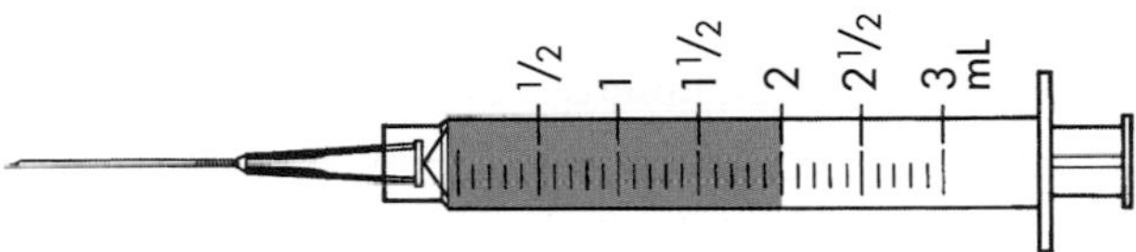

25. $3\text{ g}:8\text{ mL} = 1.5\text{ g}:x\text{ mL}$

or

$$\frac{1.5\text{ g}}{3\text{ g}} \times 8\text{ mL} = x\text{ mL}$$

Answer: 4 mL. The dosage ordered is less than the available strength; therefore you will need less than 8 mL to administer the dosage. (Ordered dosage is half of the available strength.)

26. $40\text{ mg}:5\text{ mL} = 20\text{ mg}:x\text{ mL}$

$$\frac{40x}{40} = \frac{100}{40}$$

$$x = 2.5\text{ mL}$$

or

$$\frac{20\text{ mg}}{40\text{ mg}} \times 5\text{ mL} = x\text{ mL}$$

Answer: 2.5 mL. The dosage ordered is less than the available strength; you will need less than 5 mL to administer the dosage.

27. $350\text{ mg}:1\text{ mL} = 125\text{ mg}:x\text{ mL}$

$$\frac{350x}{350} = \frac{125}{350}$$

$$x = 0.4\text{ mL}$$

$$\frac{125\text{ mg}}{350\text{ mg}} \times 1\text{ mL} = x\text{ mL}$$

Answer: 0.4 mL; 0.35 mL rounded to the nearest tenth. The dosage ordered is less than what is available; therefore you need less than 1 mL to administer the dosage.

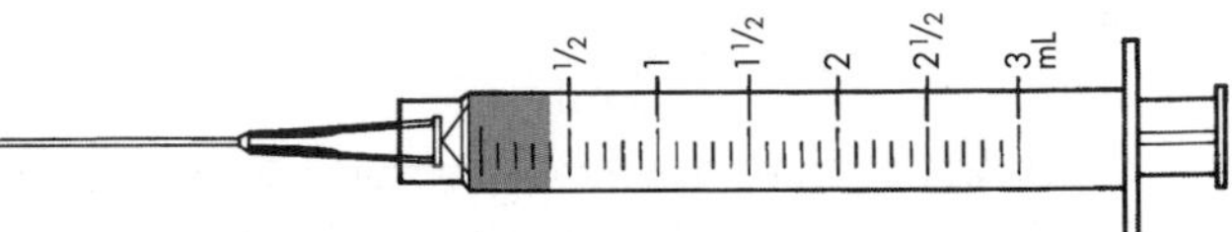

28. a. 10 mL

b. sterile water for injection without a bacteriostatic agent

c. 5 mg per mL

d. $5\text{ mg}:1\text{ mL} = 45.5\text{ mg}:x\text{ mL}$

or

$$\frac{45.5\text{ mg}}{5\text{ mg}} \times 1\text{ mL} = x\text{ mL}$$

Alternate solution

$$0\text{ mg}:10\text{ mL} = 45.5\text{ mg}:x\text{ mL}$$

or

$$\frac{45.5\text{ mg}}{50\text{ mg}} \times 10\text{ mL} = x\text{ mL}$$

This set-up would net the same answer of 9.1 mL

Answer: 9.1 mL is the dose for the initial concentration (before further dilution). The dosage ordered is more than the available strength; therefore you need more than 1 mL to administer the dosage. This medication would have to be further diluted according to the instructions as follows: The infusion solution, providing 0.1 mg amphotericin B per mL, is then obtained by further dilution (1:50) with 5% dextrose injection. This may be accomplished by adding 49 mL dextrose and water injection to each 1 mL (5 mg) of amphotericin B solution. The concentrated amphotericin solution to dilute is the 9.1 mL. Therefore we need to add it. 9.1 × 49 mL = 445.9 = 446 mL of IV solution before administering the medication IV.

29. a. 63 mL

b. 125 mg per 5 mL

c. $125\text{ mg}:1\text{ mL} = 300\text{ mg}:x\text{ mL}$

or

$$\frac{300\text{ mg}}{125\text{ mg}} \times 5\text{ mL} = x\text{ mL}$$

Answer: 12 mL. The dosage ordered is greater than the available strength; therefore you will need more than 5 mL to administer the dosage.

30. Conversion is required. Equivalent: 1,000 mg = 1 g; therefore 0.5 g = 500 mg

a. 100 mg : 1 mL = 500 mg : x mL

or

$$\frac{500 \text{ mg}}{100 \text{ mg}} \times 1 \text{ mL} = x \text{ mL}$$

Answer: 5 mL. The dosage ordered is more than the available strength; therefore you will need more than 1 mL to administer the dosage.

b.

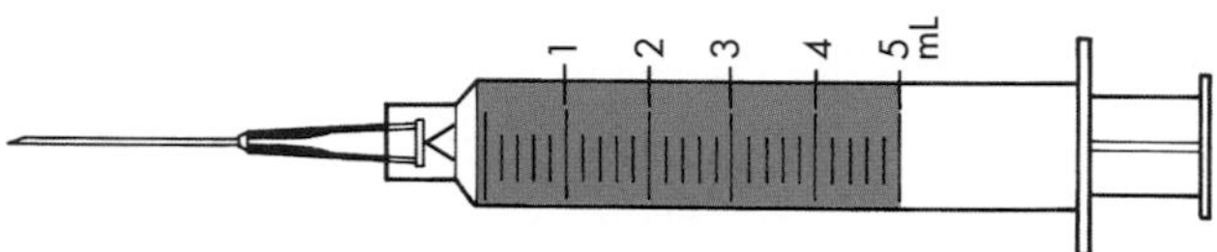

31. Conversion is required. Equivalent: 1,000 mg = 1 g; therefore 0.35 g = 350 mg

a. 250 mg : 1.5 mL = 350 mg : x mL

or

$$\frac{350 \text{ mg}}{250 \text{ mg}} \times 1.5 \text{ mL} = x \text{ mL}$$

Answer: 2.1 mL. The dosage ordered is more than the available strength; therefore you will need more than 1.5 mL to administer the dosage.

b.

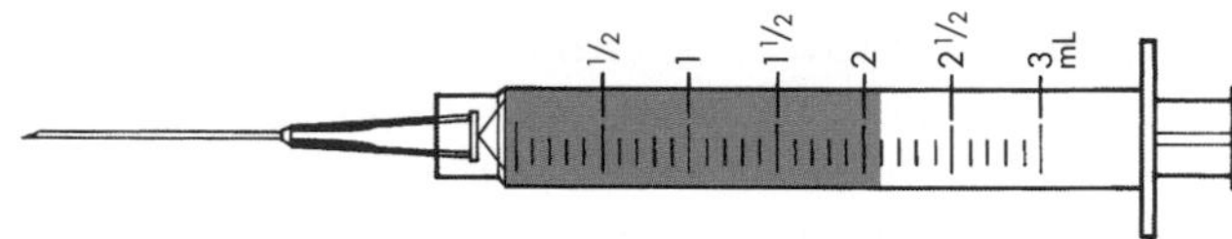

32. Conversion is required. Equivalent: 1 g = 1,000 mg; therefore 0.75 g = 750 mg

a. 400 mg : 1 mL = 750 mg : x mL

or

$$\frac{750 \text{ mg}}{400 \text{ mg}} \times 1 \text{ mL} = x \text{ mL}$$

Answer: 1.9 mL; 1.87 rounded to the nearest tenth. The dosage ordered is more than the available strength. Therefore you will need more than 1 mL to administer the dosage.

b.

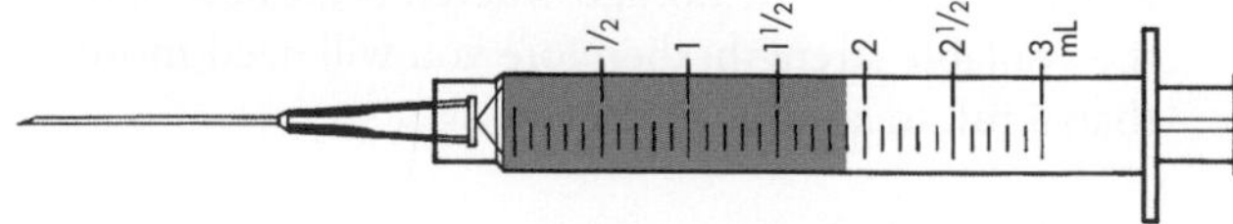

33. a. 2 mg : 1 mL = 10 mg : x mL

or

$$\frac{10 \text{ mg}}{2 \text{ mg}} \times 1 \text{ mL} = x \text{ mL}$$

Answer: 5 mL. The dosage ordered is more than the available strength. Therefore you will need more than 1 mL to administer the dosage.

b.

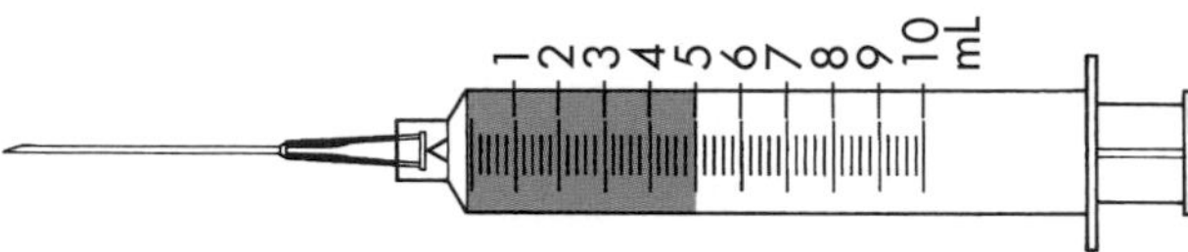

34. 1 oz = 30 mL; therefore 12 oz = 360 mL

$$\frac{1}{4} \times 360 \text{ mL} = x \text{ mL}$$

$$\frac{360}{4} = x$$

$$x = 90 \text{ mL}$$

x = 90 mL; you need 90 mL of Ensure.

360 mL − 90 mL Ensure = 270 mL of water.

Answer: 90 mL Ensure + 270 mL water = 360 mL ¼ strength Ensure.

35. 1 oz = 30 mL; therefore 6 oz = 180 mL

$$\frac{2}{3} \times \frac{180}{1} = \frac{360}{3} = 120 \text{ mL Isomil}$$

180 mL − 120 mL = 60 mL water

You would add 60 mL of water to 120 mL Isomil to make 180 mL of ⅔ strength Isomil for each feeding po q4h.

36. $$\frac{1{,}000 \text{ mL}}{16 \text{ hr}} = 62.5 \text{ mL/hr}$$

Answer: 63 mL/hr (62.5 rounded to nearest whole number)

37. 1 oz = 30 mL; therefore 4oz = 120 mL

$$\frac{1}{8} \times \frac{120}{1} = \frac{120}{8} = 15 \text{ mL Ensure}$$

120 mL − 15 mL = 105 mL water

You would add 105 mL of water to 15 mL Ensure to make 120 mL of ⅛ strength Ensure for each feeding by nasogastric tube q4h.

38. q6h = 4 times in 24 hours; therefore 4 oz × 4 = 16 oz.

1 oz = 30 mL; therefore 16 oz = 480 mL

480 mL × ½ = x mL

$$x = \frac{480}{2}$$

x = 240 mL

240 mL normal saline (solute) + 240 mL sterile water (solvent) = 480 mL ½ strength solution.

39. Conversion required. Equivalent: 1 L = 1,000 mL.

    therefore; 0.24 L = 240 mL

    240 mL × $\frac{1}{4}$ = x mL

    $x = \frac{240}{4}$

    $x = 60$ mL

    60 mL normal saline (solute) + 180 mL sterile water (solvent) = 240 mL $\frac{1}{4}$ strength solution.

40. 1 oz = 30 mL; therefore 18 oz = 540 mL

    540 mL × $\frac{2}{3}$ = x mL

    $x = 540 \times \frac{2}{3}$

    $x = \frac{1{,}080}{3}$

    $x = 360$ mL

    360 mL normal saline (solute) + 180 mL sterile water (solvent) = 540 mL 2 strength solution.

41. Conversion required. Equivalent: 1 L = 1,000 mL.

    Therefore; 0.5 L = 500 mL

    500 mL × $\frac{1}{4}$ = x mL

    $x = \frac{500}{4}$

    $x = 125$ mL

    125 mL normal saline (solute) + 375 mL sterile water (solvent) = 500 mL $\frac{1}{4}$ strength solution.

CHAPTER 20
Insulin

Objectives

After reviewing this chapter, you should be able to:

1. Identify important information on insulin labels
2. Identify various methods for insulin administration
3. Read calibrations on 30-, 50-, and 100-unit syringes
4. Measure insulin in single dosages
5. Measure combined insulin dosages
6. Calculate doses for U-500 insulin using a 1 mL syringe
7. Calculate doses for U-500 insulin to measure using U-100 insulin syringe

Insulin, which is used in the treatment of diabetes mellitus (DM), is a hormone secreted by the islets of Langerhans in the pancreas. It is a necessary hormone for glucose use by the body. Individuals who do not produce adequate insulin experience an increase in their blood sugar (glucose) level. These individuals may require the administration of insulin. Accuracy in insulin administration is extremely important because inaccurate dosages can lead to serious or life-threatening effects. Any error that occurs in medication administration, regardless of the reason for it, may result in harm to a client; however, there are some medications that have been designated *high-alert medications.* Medications that are considered high-alert medications have a high risk of causing injury or death to a client and are also identified as those with which health care providers often make errors. The Institute for Safe Medication Practices (ISMP) defines high-alert medications as "drugs that bear a heightened risk of causing significant patient harm when they are used in error" (ISMP, 2014). The consequences associated with errors with these medications are usually more devastating than those that occur with other medications. High-alert medications require that safeguards be in place to ensure that when they are used, there is a focus on safely using them and preventing harm to those who receive them.

The ISMP has published a list of high-alert medications that require safeguards to decrease the risk of errors and fatal outcomes. This list includes high-alert medications administered in the acute care setting as well as medications administered in the community and ambulatory settings. Nurses as well as other health care providers need to be highly attentive when calculating dosages and administering high-alert medications. Insulin (anti-diabetic agent) and heparin (anti-thrombotic agent), along with other medications, have been identified as high-alert medications by the Institute for Safe Medication Practices (ISMP). See Appendix E, "High-Alert Medications." Heparin will be discussed in Chapter 23. This chapter will focus on basic concepts related to the safe administration of insulin. Always follow the policy of the institution for administering high-alert medications to decrease the chance of error and harm to the client.

In addition to dosage calculation errors, ISMP has identified other causes of errors that have occurred with insulin, including the following:

- Knowledge deficits regarding insulin concentrations (specifically that "U-100" means the concentration is 100 units per mL) and the differences between insulin syringes and other parenteral syringes

- Reading medication labels incorrectly
- Incorrect preparation of insulin for IV infusion
- Mental slips leading to confusion between heparin and insulin, because both are measured in units, administered subcutaneously or intravenously, and are supplied in multidose vials that may look similar

This is just a sample of the causes of errors with insulin. There have been numerous reports to ISMP of misadministration of insulin. This has serious implications for nurses as well as other health care providers.

SAFETY ALERT!

Nurses **must** correctly interpret insulin orders and use the correct syringe to measure insulin for administration. Accuracy in insulin preparation and administration is crucial to prevent administration of inaccurate dosages, which can result in serious or life-threatening effects.

Insulin dosages are measured in units and administered with syringes that correspond to insulin U-100; U-100 insulin means 100 units per milliliter. The most common types of insulin are supplied in 10-mL vials and labeled U-100. Insulin is also available as U-500 (500 units per mL). U-500 is a more concentrated strength and is used for diabetic clients who have blood sugars that fluctuate to extremely high levels.

SAFETY ALERT!

It is crucial that the nurse use **extreme caution** when administering U-500 insulin to prevent unintentional overdose, which can result in irreversible insulin shock and death for a client.

U-500 insulin, 500 units per mL, is five (5) times as concentrated as U-100, which is 100 units per mL.

Types of Insulin

Insulins distributed in the United States are synthetic "human insulins" or their analogs, which are chemically altered DNA. Insulin from a human source is designated on the label as recombinant DNA (rDNA origin). Recombinant DNA insulin causes fewer reactions.

Humalog insulin (lispro), also known as recombinant DNA, is a fast-acting insulin analog. Lispro acts within 5 to 15 minutes. Lispro can be administered 5 minutes before meals, whereas regular insulin can be administered 30 to 60 minutes before meals. Like regular human insulin, Lispro is clear and can be administered intravenously as well as subcutaneously. Errors have occurred from the timing of lispro as well as its similarity to regular insulin; both are clear. Other rapid-acting insulin analogs include aspart (NovoLog) and glulisine (Apidra). Like lispro and regular insulin, these analogs are clear and can also be administered intravenously as well as subcutaneously.

Lantus (insulin glargine) is an analog of human insulin, classified as long-acting, and permits once-daily dosing. It can be administered at any time during the day for 24-hour coverage without a peak; however, it must be administered at the same time every day. In addition, it is clear in appearance, intended for subcutaneous use only, and cannot be mixed with other insulins. The packaging is distinct; the vial is tall, narrow, and the name Lantus is printed in purple letters. Levemir (detemir), which is also long acting, is also generally given once daily. However, it does not last as long as Lantus, so clients may require a nighttime dose. Like Lantus, Levemir cannot be mixed with other insulins. According to the American Diabetes Association, most people with type I diabetes should use insulin analogs to reduce hypoglycemic risk (American Diabetes Association, 2013).

Tresiba (insulin degludec injection), a long-acting insulin analog, was approved in 2015 by the U.S. Food and Drug Administration (FDA). Tresiba is administered subcutaneously once daily at any time of day. It should not be diluted or mixed with other insulins and is available in the FlexTouch pen in two concentrations: 100 units per mL and 200 units per mL.

Labels

It is essential that the nurse know the essential information on an insulin label and where to locate it. Information such as the origin of insulin, type, brand and generic names, the dosage strength or concentration, and storage information is indicated on the label.

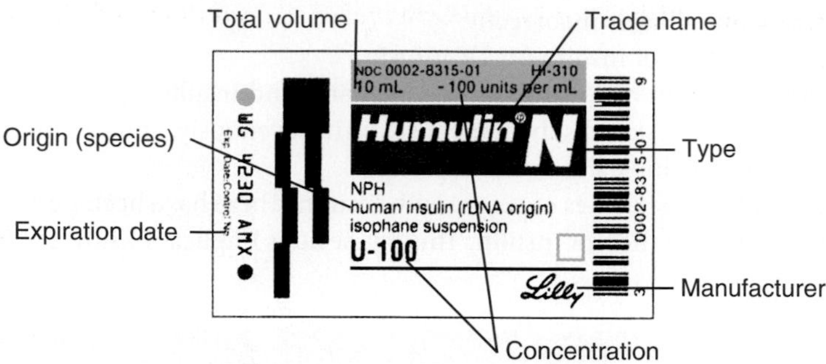

Figure 20-1 Label for U-100 insulin.

Figure 20-1 shows information that can be found on an insulin label. Notice the following:

- The letter that follows the trade name Humulin, N identifies the type of insulin by action and time. Notice the label shows Humulin (trade name), followed by the letter N. N = NPH (intermediate-acting). These letters are important identifiers for insulin.
- Notice the use of uppercase letters for the letter N for NPH. You will see R for regular insulin.
- Concentration (dosage strength) of the insulin is also indicated; notice U-100 (100 units per mL)

The expiration date is also indicated on insulin labels and is important to check.

Review the important information identified on the label in Figure 20-1.

Refer to the label in Figure 20-2 for U-500 insulin.

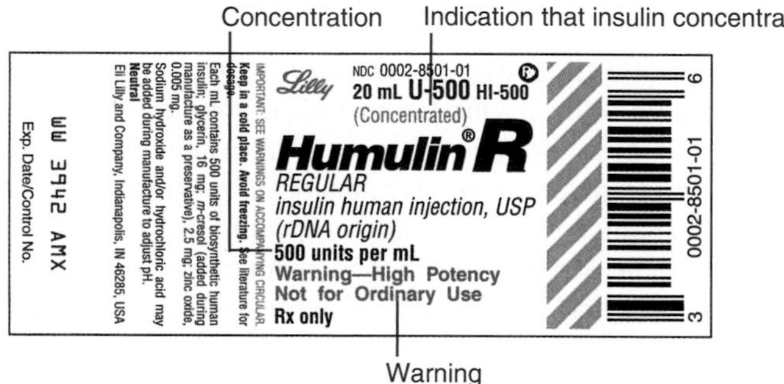

Figure 20-2 Label for U-500 insulin.

Notice the following on the U-500 insulin label:

- Indication that U-500 is concentrated in red.
- Concentration (dosage strength) U-500 (500 units per mL).
- Warning in red: "High potency, not for ordinary use."

SAFETY ALERT!

Careful reading of insulin labels is essential to avoid a medication error that could be life-threatening. Always read the label carefully and compare it with the medication order to ensure selection of the right type of insulin, correct action time, and concentration (strength).

Insulin Action Times

Insulins are classified by their actions as rapid-acting, short-acting, intermediate-acting, or long-acting. Intermediate- and long-acting insulins can only be administered subcutaneously. Nurses must be familiar with the action times of insulins. Figure 20-3 shows samples of labels grouped by action times. As stated, note the use of N for NPH Insulin and R for Regular, indicated in bold uppercase letters. Regular and NPH insulin are the two types that have traditionally been used most frequently, and they are often mixed.

Below are samples of labels for insulin types grouped according to their action times.

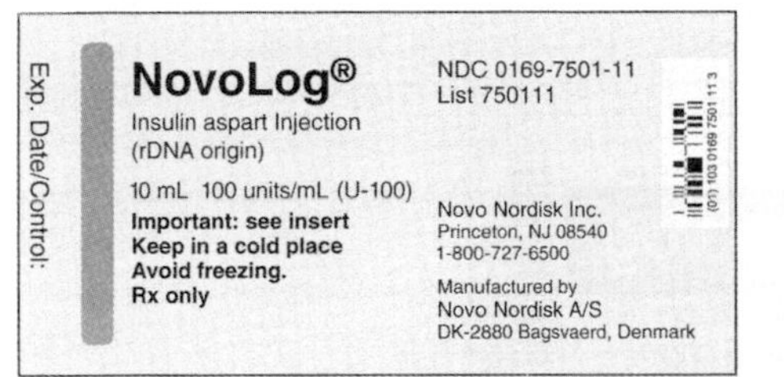

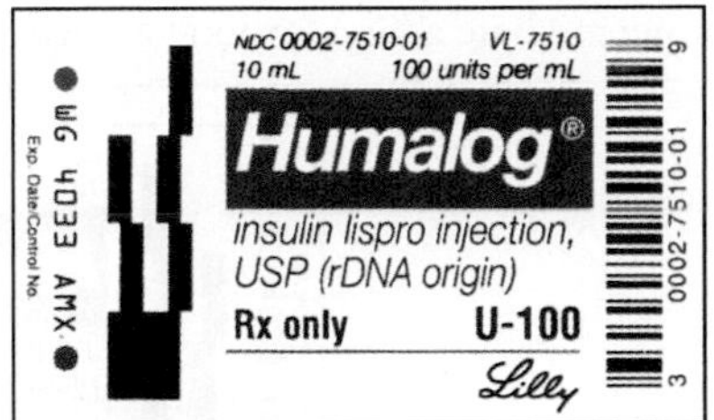

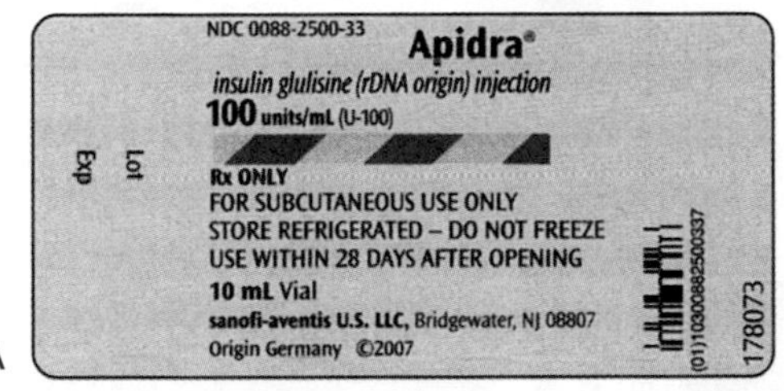

A

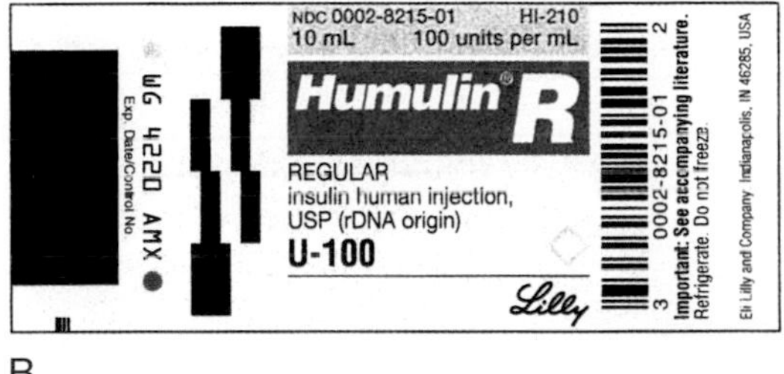

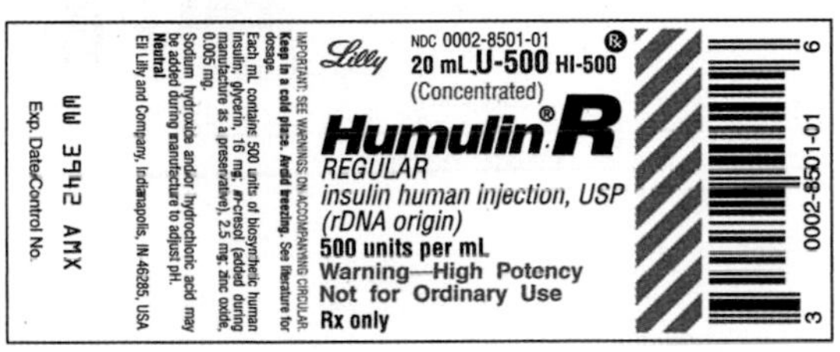

B

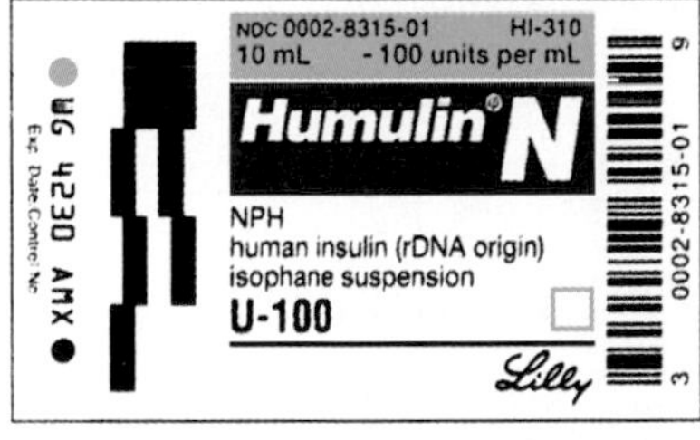

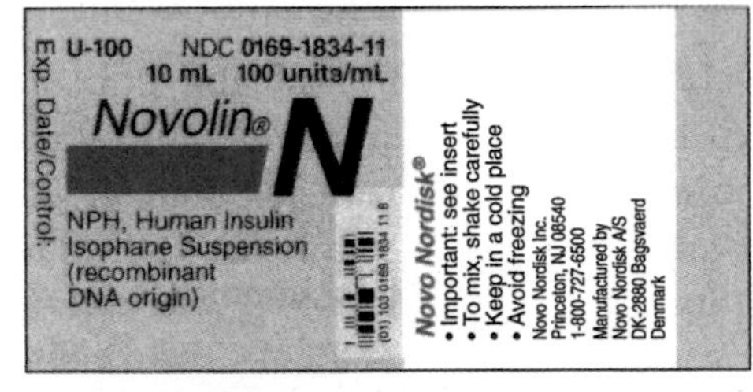

C

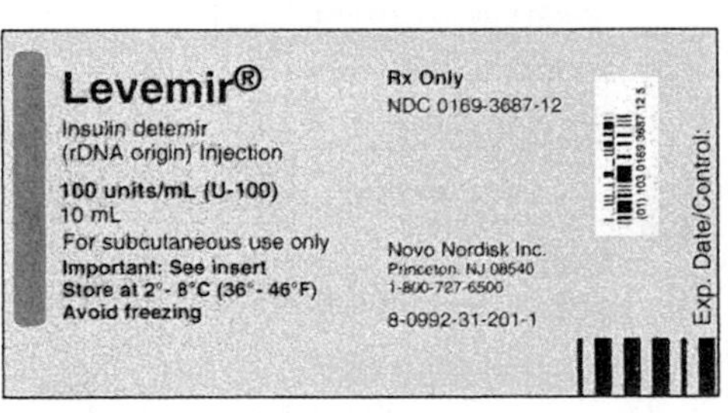

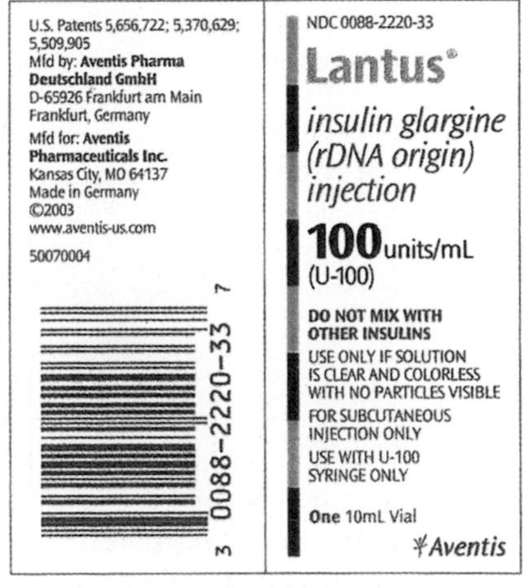

D

Figure 20-3 **A,** Rapid acting (fast acting). **B,** Short acting. **C,** Intermediate acting. **D,** Long acting.

PRACTICE PROBLEMS

Using the labels below, identify the insulin trade name and action time (short acting, rapid acting, intermediate acting, or long acting).

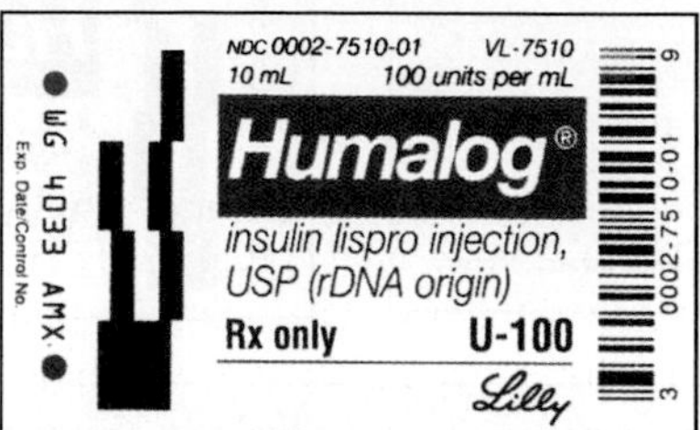

1. Trade name ____________ Action time ____________

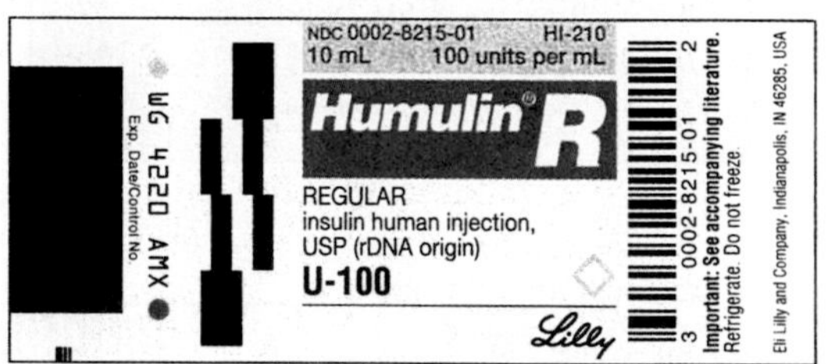

2. Trade name ____________ Action time ____________

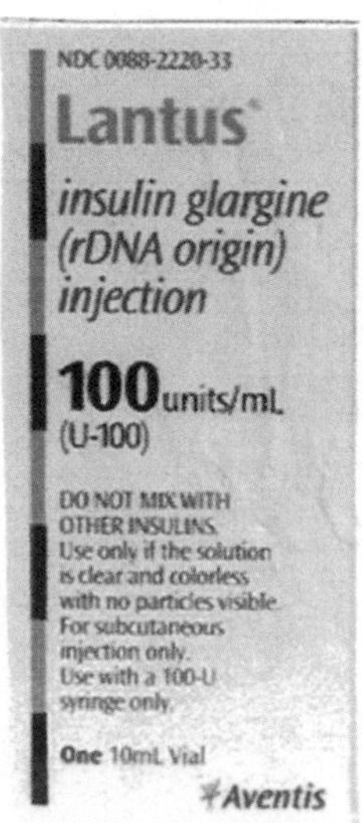

3. Trade name ____________ Action time ____________

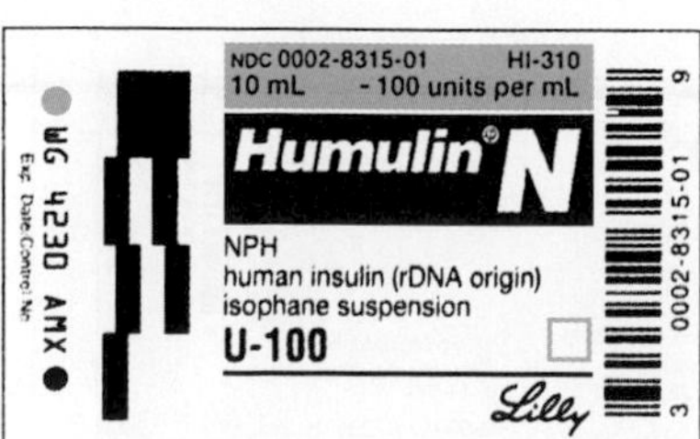

4. Trade name ____________ Action time ____________

Answers on p. 509-510

Appearance of Insulin

Regular insulin, Humalog (lispro), Lantus (insulin glargine), Apidra (insulin glulisine), aspart (Novolog), and Levemir (insulin detemir) insulin are clear. All other insulin is cloudy. They include NPH and fixed-combination insulins such as Humulin 70/30, 50/50, and Humalog 75/25.

Premixed, Fixed, and Combination Insulins

Fixed-combination insulins are shown in Figure 20-4. These insulins have become popular for clients who must mix fast-acting and intermediate-acting insulins. The purpose of the fixed-combination insulins is to simulate the varying levels of insulin within the bodies of diabetic persons. The availability of the premixed-combination insulins has also decreased the need for clients to mix insulins, as well as decreased the number of required injections. Premixed combination insulins are available in vials and pens for administration and contain both mealtime and basal insulin. This combination can only be administered subcutaneously or by insulin pen. Read labels carefully on combination insulins to identify differences. Selecting the incorrect combination could result in a serious or life-threatening error. Always read an insulin label carefully and compare it to the medication order to avoid errors in administration.

> **SAFETY ALERT!**
>
> Carefully read all insulin labels to ensure selection of the correct type of insulin. The action of insulin varies according to the type of insulin and combination.

To understand fixed-combination insulin orders, it is important for the nurse to read the labels to understand what types of insulin are included in the combination and that they have different action times. For example, Humulin 50/50 concentration in (Figure 20-4, *A*) means there is 50% NPH insulin and 50% regular insulin in each unit. Therefore, if the order was 20 units of Humulin 50/50, the client would receive 10 units of NPH (50%, or 0.5 × 20 units = 10 units) and 10 units of regular. Humalog Mix 75/25 (Figure 20-4, *B*) contains 75% lispro protamine insulin (intermediate-acting) and 25% lispro, or "rapid insulin."

Note that Novolin 70/30 (Figure 20-4, *D*) concentration means there is 70% NPH insulin (isophane) and 30% regular insulin in each unit. Therefore, if the order was 30 units of Novolin U-100 70/30 insulin, the client would receive 21 units of NPH (70%, or 0.7 × 30 units = 21 units) and 9 units of regular insulin (30%, or 0.3 × 30 units = 9 units).

Note the label for NovoLog Mix 70/30 (Figure 20-4, *C*) and the difference in combination from Novolin 70/30 (Figure 20-4, *D*). NovoLog Mix 70/30 is a combination of aspart protamine (70%) and aspart (30%). Novolin is a combination of 70% NPH and 30% regular.

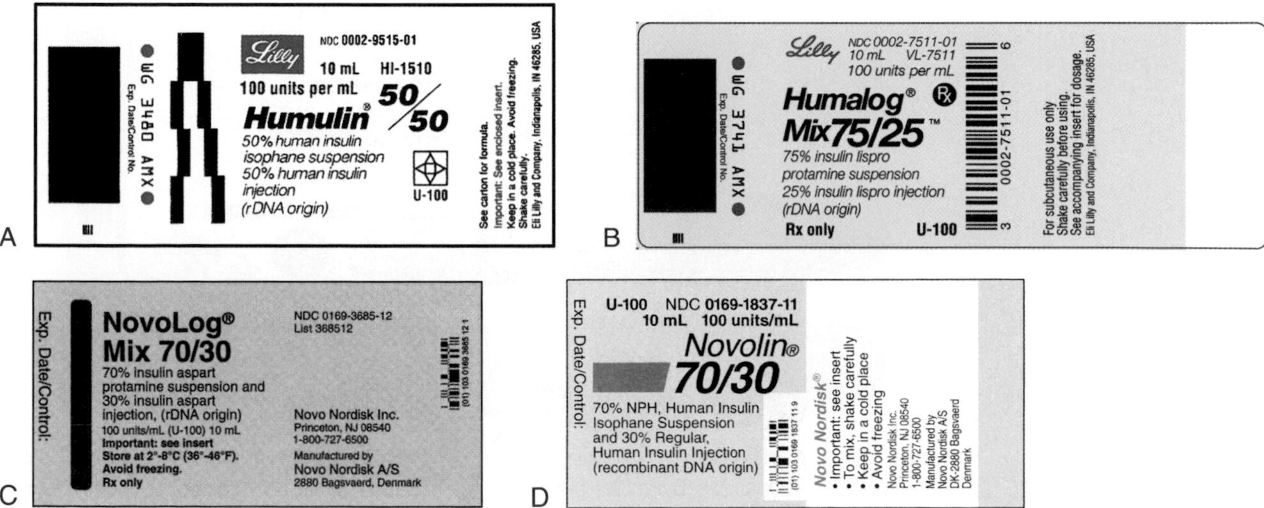

Figure 20-4 Fixed-combination insulins.

In 2015 the FDA approved Ryzodeg 70/30 (insulin degludec and insulin aspart). Ryzodeg is available in a flex pen in a concentration of 100 units per mL and has a unique blend of 70% insulin degludec (long-acting insulin), and 30% insulin aspart (rapid-acting insulin). It can be administered once or twice daily with any main meal.

Insulin Administration

The major route of administration of insulin is by subcutaneous injection; it is never administered intramuscularly. Regular U-100 insulin, aspart, and glulisine can be administered intravenously.

Insulin Pumps

Insulin can also be administered by a pump. A CSII pump (continuous subcutaneous insulin infusion) is an insulin pump. An insulin pump is not an IV pump. Figure 20-5, *A*, shows an insulin pump and a blood glucose monitor. Insulin pumps deliver rapid- or short-acting insulin continuously for 24 hours a day through a catheter placed under the skin. This eliminates the need for multiple daily injections of insulin. Pumps can be programmed to deliver a basal rate and/or a bolus dose. Basal insulin is delivered continuously over 24 hours to keep blood glucose levels in range between meals and overnight. The basal rate can be programmed to deliver different rates at different times. Bolus doses can be delivered at meal time to provide control for additional food intake. The two types of pumps are implantable and external (portable).

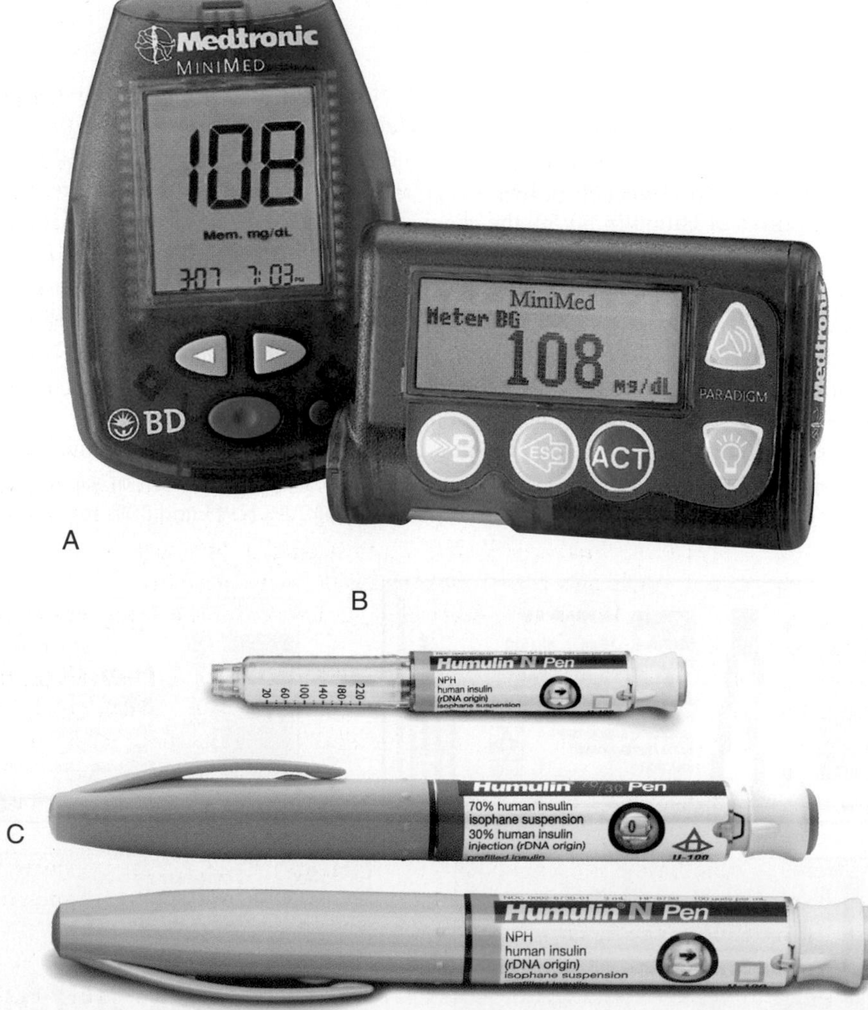

Figure 20-5 A, Paradigm® 515 insulin pump and Paradigm Link™ blood glucose monitor. **B,** Humulin N pen with no cap. **C,** Prefilled pens, Humulin 70/30 and Humulin N. (**A** and **C,** Copyright © Eli Lilly and Company. All rights reserved. Used with permission. ® Humalog and Humulin are registered trademarks of Eli Lilly and Company. **B,** From Medtronic, Minneapolis, MN.)

Insulin Pen

Insulin can also be delivered by an insulin pen. When capped, the insulin pen looks very much like an ink pen. Use of the insulin pens affords clients an easy and accurate method for self-administration of insulin. Insulin pens come in two forms, disposable and reusable. Disposable pens contain a prefilled cartridge and are thrown out after they are emptied. Reusable pens require replacement of the insulin cartridge each time it is emptied. The needles in insulin pens are extremely short and thin. Figure 20-5, *B*, shows the parts of an insulin pen. Figure 20-5, *C*, shows examples of prefilled insulin pens. The insulin pen has a dose selector knob that is used to "dial" the desired dose of units. The dose dial is turned until the correct number of units is displayed in the dose window. Some of the newer pens have a digital dose display that can be easily misinterpreted if the pen is held upside down. For example, a dose of 27 units looks like 72 units on the digital display if the pen is held incorrectly and read upside down. Client education on the use of the insulin pen (correct way to hold the pen and read the display) is a **must.** This will help in the prevention of dosing errors. Once the pen has been cleared of any air in the cartridge (primed) and the dose set, the insulin is injected by pressing on the injection button. When the injection is completed, the needle is removed and cap replaced. Insulin pens are available in many styles and colors. All insulin pens are designed for single client use and cannot be shared with other clients, even if a new needle is attached.

Although insulin pens were designed for client self-administration of insulin, in an effort to decrease errors with insulin and improve medication safety, many hospitals are also switching from the administration of insulin from vials to pens. Many hospital pharmacies are also supplying insulin pens for nurses to administer insulin (ISMP, 2015).

Measuring Insulin in a U-100 Syringe

The insulin syringes and their calibration was introduced in Chapter 18. Recall from Chapter 18 that insulin syringes are available in three sizes (100 unit, 1 mL; 50 unit, 0.5 mL; and 30 unit, 0.3 mL). These syringes are calibrated exclusively for U-100 insulin (100 units per mL) and marked U-100. U-100 insulin should be measured in U-100 insulin syringes and **not** in syringes calibrated in milliliters, such as a 1-mL or 3-mL syringe. U-500 insulin is measured in a 1-mL syringe. Correct dosage requires a calculation, which will be discussed later in this chapter.

Measuring U-100 insulin with the insulin syringe makes it easy to obtain a correct dosage without mathematical calculation. To prepare the U-100 insulin when only one dosage is required, the U-100 insulin syringe is used to draw up the ordered U-100 insulin to the unit calibration that corresponds to the ordered dose. The nurse **must** carefully select the correct insulin and withdraw the correct amount. It is not necessary to use dosage calculation formulas or ratio and proportion to calculate the volume for administering U-100 insulin. The insulin syringe is designed to measure insulin in units, and insulin is ordered in units. After drawing up insulin, the nurse should provide the order, vial, and syringe to another nurse to verify the insulin dosage before administering to client to avoid errors. In other words, the dosage should always be double-checked by another nurse.

Let's look at the U-100 insulin syringes. An essential skill is correctly reading the syringe calibrations on U-100 syringes.

1. **Lo-Dose syringe**—It has a capacity of 50 units (0.5 mL). Each calibration on the syringe measures 1 unit. There is also a 30-unit (0.3 mL) syringe, which is used to accurately measure very small amounts of insulin. It is marked in units up to 30 units. Each calibration is 1 unit.
2. **1-mL (100-unit) capacity syringe**—The 100-unit syringe comes with even and odd numbers on it. There are two types of 1-mL syringes in current use.
   a. The single-scale syringe is calibrated in 2-unit increments. Any dosage measured in an odd number of units is measured between the even calibrations. This would not be the desired syringe for clients with vision problems.
   b. The double-scale syringe (dual syringe) has odd-numbered units on the left in 2-unit increments (1, 3 etc.) and even-numbered units on the right in 2-unit increments (2, 4 etc.). To avoid confusion, the scale on the left should be used for odd numbers of units (e.g., 13 units) and the scale on the right for even numbers of units (e.g., 26 units). When even numbers of units are measured, each calibration is then measured as 2 units.

> **SAFETY ALERT!**
>
> Administer insulin in an insulin syringe used only for the administration of U-100 insulin. Do not use an insulin syringe to measure other medications that are measured in units. Syringes of 30 and 50 units measure a smaller volume of insulin but are intended for the measurement of U-100 insulin only. Use the smallest capacity insulin syringe available to ensure the accuracy of dosage preparation.

To review what the four types of insulin syringes look like, see Figure 20-6.

Lo-Dose Syringe

Let's look at some insulin dosages measured in the syringes to help you visualize the amounts in a syringe. Syringe *A* shows 30 units and syringe *B* shows 37 units in a Lo-Dose syringe.

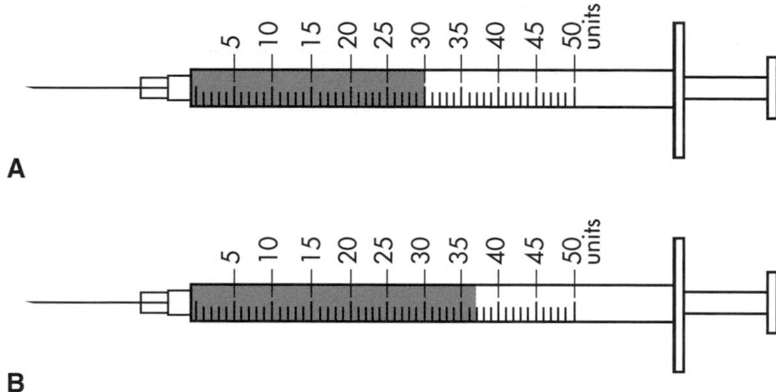

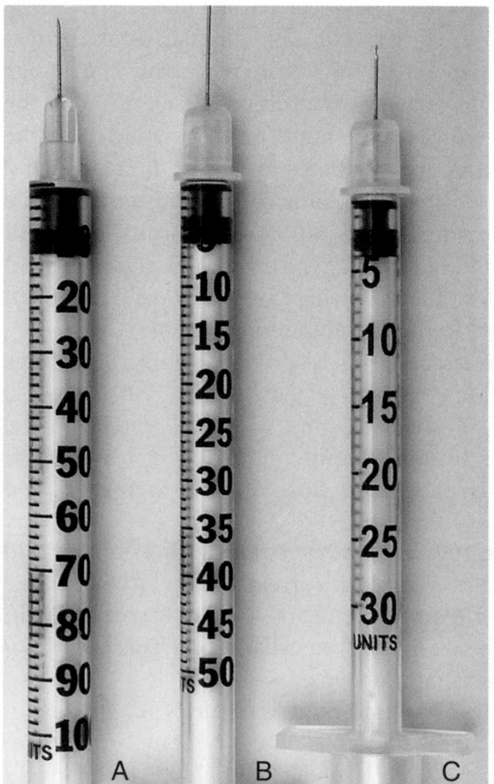

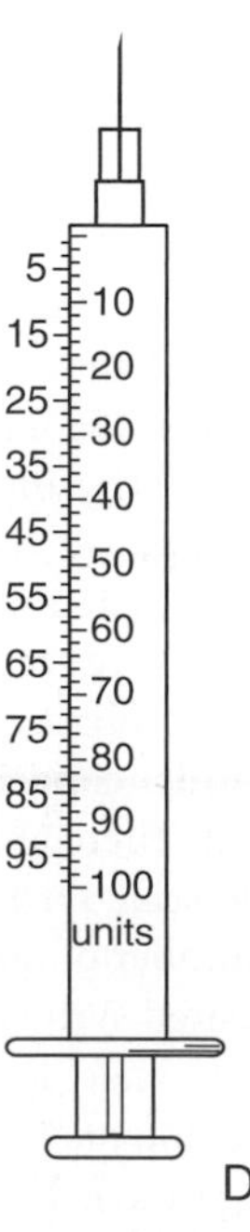

Figure 20-6 Types of insulin syringes. **A,** Single-scale (100 units). **B,** Lo-Dose insulin syringe (50 units). **C,** Lo-Dose insulin syringe (30 units). **D,** Double-scale syringe (100 units).

PRACTICE PROBLEMS

Using the syringes below, indicate the dosages shown by the arrows.

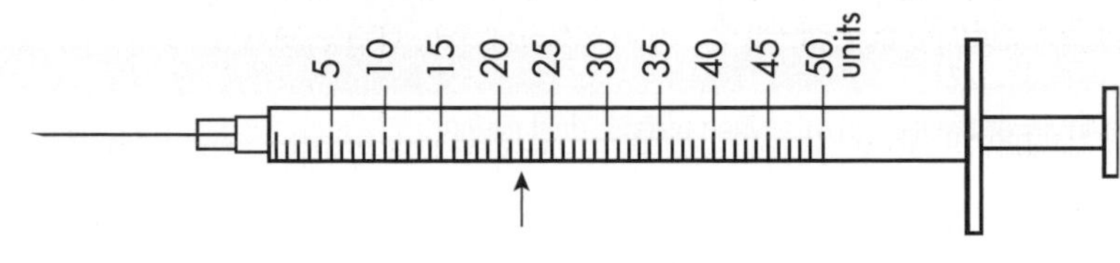

5. ______________________________

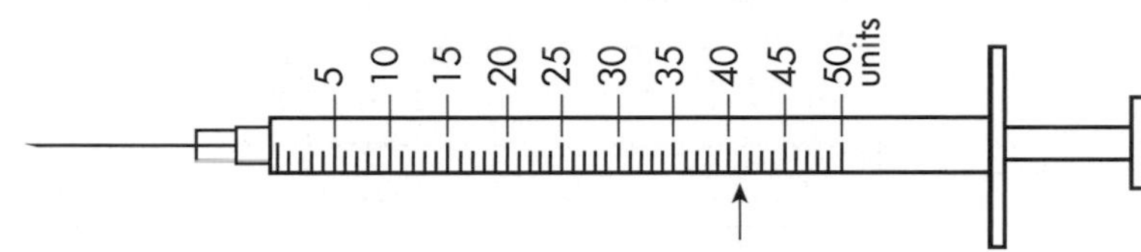

6. ______________________________

Using the syringes below, shade in the dosages indicated.

7. 17 units

8. 47 units

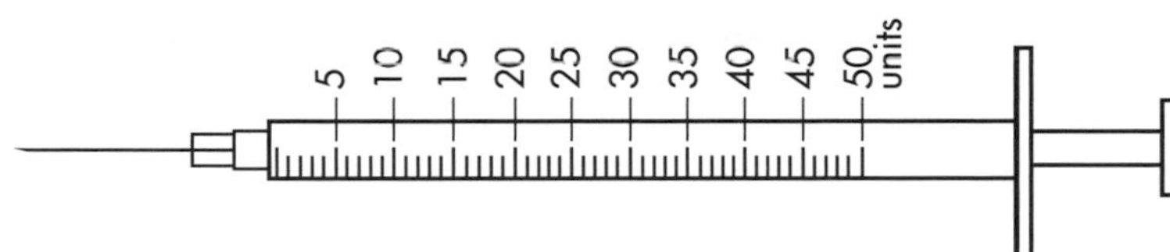

Answers on p. 509-510

Single-Scale 1-mL Syringe

Now let's look at what dosages would look like on a single-scale 1-mL syringe. The syringes below show 25 units in syringe *A* and 55 units in syringe *B*. Notice that the dosages are drawn up between the even calibrations.

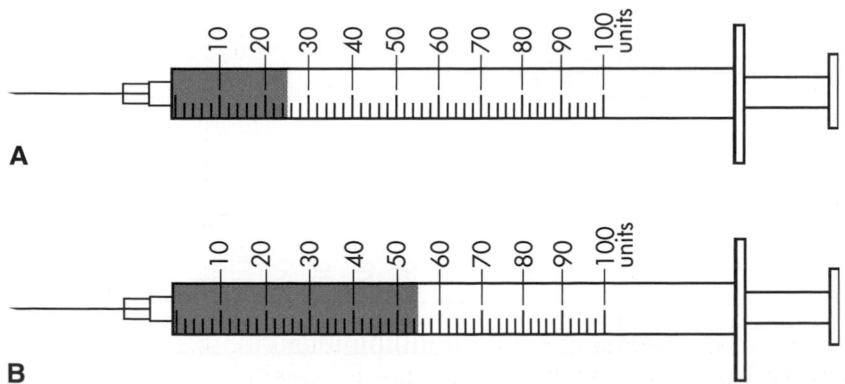

Double-Scale 1-mL Syringe

Now let's look at the dosage indicated on a double-scale (100-unit) 1-mL syringe. Syringe *C* shows 37 units; notice that the scale on the left is used. Syringe *D* shows 54 units; notice that the scale on the right is used.

SAFETY ALERT!

Look carefully at the increments when using a dual syringe.

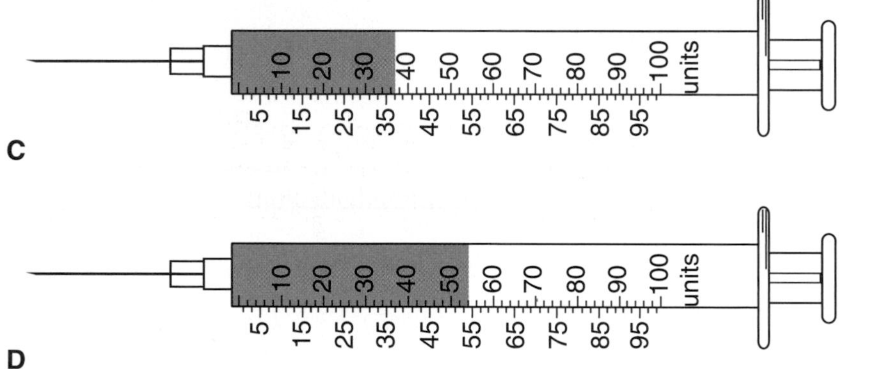

PRACTICE PROBLEMS

Indicate the following dosages shaded on the 100-unit (1-mL) syringes.

9. ______________________

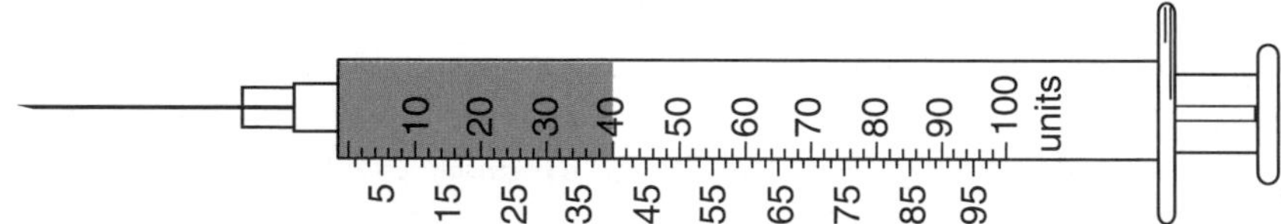

10. ______________________

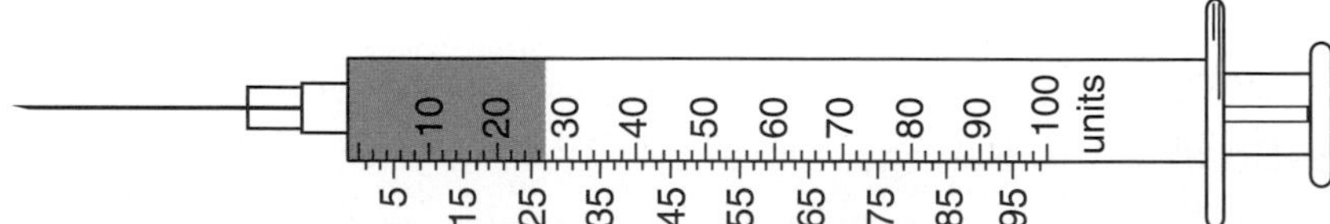

11. ______________________

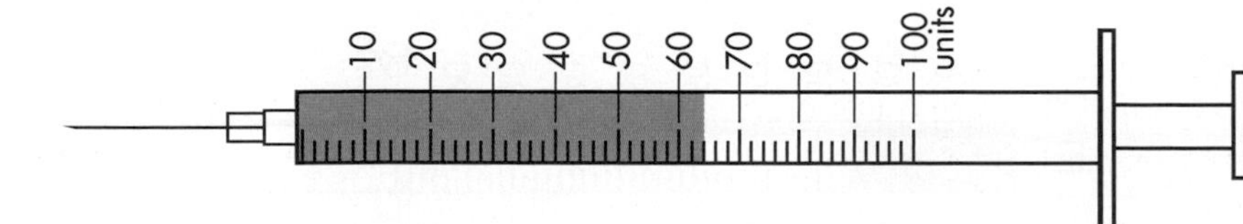

12. ______________________

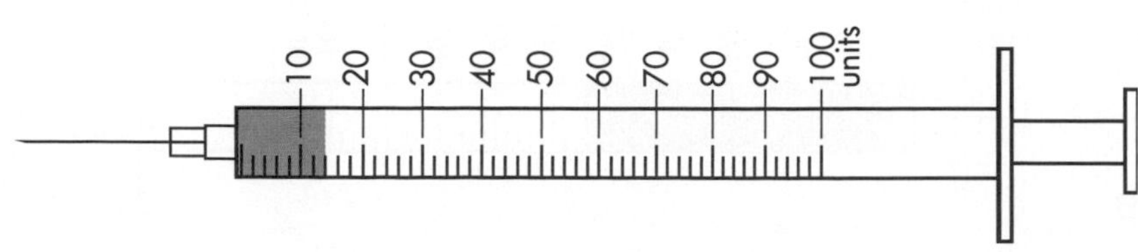

Shade the specified dosages on each of the U-100 syringes below.

13. 88 units

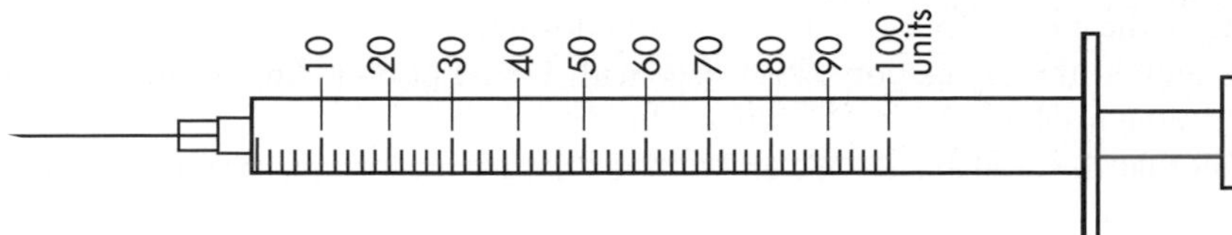

14. 44 units

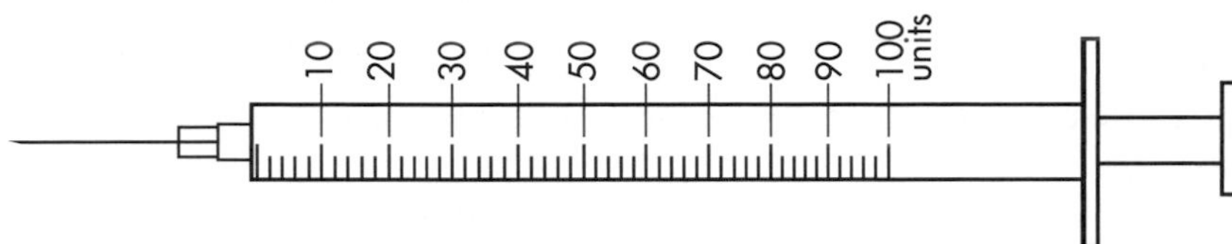

15. 30 units

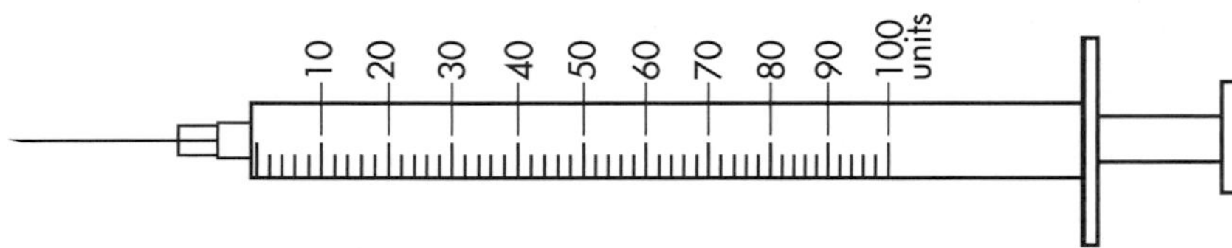

Answers on p. 509-510

U-500 Insulin

As previously discussed, U-500 insulin means 500 units per mL, which means it is five (5) times more potent than U-100 (100 units per mL). Always check how many units are in 1 mL, because **accidental substitution of U-500 for U-100 insulin could result in a fatal overdose.** The label on U-500, as discussed, also has a warning in red. A syringe to measure U-500 insulin has not been developed, despite recommendations by safety experts. Therefore the standard 1-mL syringe is used in the hospital to measure U-500 insulin doses.

According to ISMP, as the obesity epidemic continues and insulin resistance problems worsen, larger doses of insulin are more frequently required to meet glycemic needs and have led to an increased use of U-500 insulin. To prevent dosage errors with U-500 insulin, The Joint Commission (TJC) and the Institute for Safe Medication Practices (ISMP) recommend that a 1-mL syringe be used to administer U-500 insulin. They also recommend that the prescriber write both the number of units and the volume in milliliters of insulin required to administer the dose (ISMP, 2011).

Example: Humulin® R U-500 regular insulin 175 units (0.35 mL) subcut daily before breakfast.

Although the prescriber specifies the volume to be administered in the order, the nurse **must** always calculate and double-check the volume ordered before administering to a client. Because of the consequences that can occur with dosing errors with U-500 insulin, the following should be done:

- Read the label carefully—note the concentration is 500 units per mL.
- If there is uncertainty regarding the order, clarify it. **Do not assume!**
- Perform the required calculation.
- Measure U-500 insulin in a 1-mL syringe.

- Two nurses must check calculations and preparations before administration to the client. This should be done using independent verification. The check by the second nurse must occur away from the first nurse, with no knowledge of the first nurse's calculations. The calculation of the dosage is done independently.
- Educate the client about U-500 insulin and dosing.

Let's look at the calculation of a dosage with U-500 insulin. Any of the methods presented can be used to calculate U-500 insulin dosages.

- Recall that the available dosage and ordered dosage are in units, and the volume is ordered in milliliters (mL).
- It is essential to check that the ordered volume is correct before administering.

Example: Humulin Regular U-500 insulin 155 units (0.31 mL) subcut stat.

Solution:

1. Convert: No conversion needed. The dosage ordered is the same as the dosage available (units).
2. Think: 155 units of U-500 insulin (500 units per mL) is less than ½ of 1 mL of U-500 insulin.
3. Calculate to determine the amount.

✓ Formula Method

$$\frac{155 \text{ units}}{500 \text{ units}} \times 1 \text{ mL} = x \text{ mL}$$

$$x = \frac{155}{500}$$

$$x = 0.31 \text{ mL}$$

(verifies the amount in order of the number of mL required)

✓ Solution Using Ratio and Proportion

$$500 \text{ units} : 1 \text{ mL} = 155 \text{ units} : x \text{ mL}$$

$$\frac{500x}{500} = \frac{155}{500}$$

$$x = \frac{155}{500}$$

$$x = 0.31 \text{ mL}$$

✓ Solution Using Dimensional Analysis

$$x \text{ mL} = \frac{1 \text{ mL}}{500 \cancel{\text{units}}} \times 155 \cancel{\text{units}}$$

$$x = \frac{155}{500}$$

$$x = 0.31 \text{ mL}$$

Remember that before administering, have another nurse perform an independent verification. Remember that an error could be fatal.

See the amount measured in a 1-mL syringe:

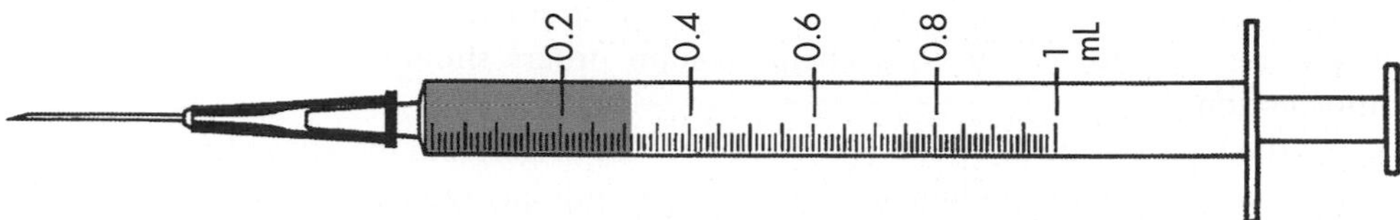

0.31 mL of U-500 insulin measured in a 1-mL syringe.

Note: For clients taking U-500 insulin at home you may need to provide teaching related to measuring U-500 insulin at home. The following rule can be used:

- To measure U-500 insulin doses at home, divide the prescribed U-500 insulin dose by 5. This will give the volume (unit markings on a U-100 insulin syringe).

Let's look at the example problem to illustrate this rule:

Order: 155 units of U-500 insulin. (The client needs to draw up the insulin using a U-100 syringe.) U-500 insulin is 5× more concentrated than U-100 insulin; therefore, the equivalent amount in a U-100 syringe will be $\frac{1}{5}$ the amount (volume) that the U-100 would measure.

$$155 \text{ units} \times \frac{1}{5} = \frac{155}{5} = 31 \text{ units}$$

or

$$\frac{155 \text{ units}}{500 \text{ units}} = \frac{x \text{ units}}{100 \text{ units}}$$

$$500x = 15{,}500$$

$$\frac{500x}{500} = \frac{15{,}500}{500}$$

$x = 31$ units (of U-500 insulin in a U-100 insulin syringe)

or

155 units: 500 units = x units: 100 units

Remember: A ratio format can be written in different formats.

See amount drawn up in a Lo-Dose 50 unit syringe and U-100 dual syringe.

31 units (U-100) = 155 units (U-500)

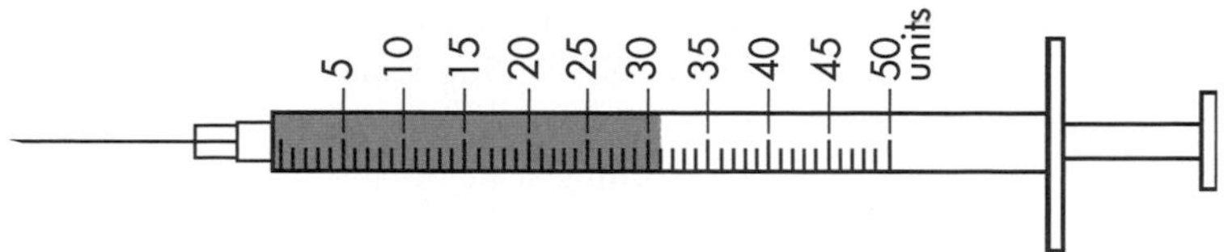

31 units (U-100) = 155 units (U-500)

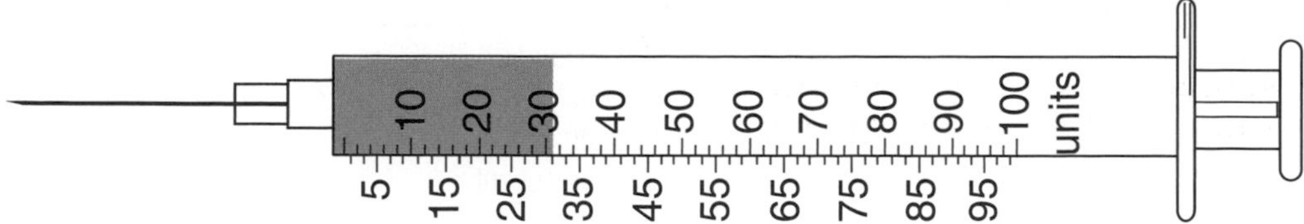

Insulin Orders

Like any written medication order, an insulin order must be written clearly and contain certain information to prevent errors in administration. An error in administration can cause harmful effects to a client. Insulin orders should contain the following information:

a. The brand name of insulin (which implies the origin) and the action time. Example: Humulin R indicates human origin. Regular indicates rapid action. Some orders may be written simply as Humulin Regular.
b. The number of units to be administered. Example: 20 units, Humulin Regular.
c. The route (subcut). Insulin is usually administered subcutaneously; however, regular insulin, aspart, and glulisine can be administered intravenously, as well.
d. The time it should be given. Example: ½ hour before meals.
e. The strength of the insulin to be administered. Example: U-100.

Example of Insulin Order: Regular Humulin insulin U-100 20 units subcut ½ hr ā breakfast.

SAFETY ALERT!

To avoid misinterpretation, the abbreviation "U," which stands for units, should not be used when insulin orders are written. The word *units* should be written out. Errors have occurred as a result of the "U" being mistaken for a "0" in a handwritten order. Example: 6U subcut stat of Humulin Regular. The U is almost completely closed and could be misread as 60 units. The recommendation to write out the word *units* has also been issued by the Institute for Safe Medication Practices (ISMP) and should be included on each accredited organization's "do not use" list approved by The Joint Commission (TJC).

Insulin Coverage

Sometimes, in addition to standing insulin orders, clients may require additional insulin "to cover" their increased blood glucose (sugar) level. Traditionally, the use of the sliding scale has been used for glycemic control. The sliding scale is a set of orders that indicate a certain dosage of insulin based on the client's blood glucose (BG) level (the amount of glucose in a given amount of blood recorded in mg in a deciliter, or mg/dL). Orders for the sliding scale may also indicate capillary blood glucose (CBG) to indicate the checking of blood glucose for the sliding scale. Most sliding scale orders use regular (short-acting) or lispro (rapid-acting) insulin. The prescriber specifies the dosage of insulin based on a specific blood glucose level range. Sliding scales are individualized to the client.

When orders for a sliding scale are written, the amount of insulin to be administered and the blood glucose range should be specific. A sample coverage order (sliding scale) is shown on the next page. Using the sliding scale, if the blood glucose level for the client is 135 mg/dL, you would not administer any insulin because 135 mg/dL is less than 180 mg/dL. However, if the client's blood glucose level is 200 mg/dL, you would administer 2 units of regular insulin immediately because 200 mg/dL is between 181 and 240 mg/dL. Abbreviations that denote sliding scale include SSI (sliding scale insulin), SSRI (sliding scale regular insulin), and SS (sliding scale). According to Cohen (2010), the abbreviation SSRI should not be used as an abbreviation for sliding scale because it can also be interpreted as selective serotonin reuptake inhibitor.

Sample Insulin Sliding Scale

Humulin Regular U-100 according to finger stick q8h	
0-180 mg/dL	No coverage
181-240 mg/dL	2 units subcut
241-300 mg/dL	4 units subcut
301-400 mg/dL	6 units subcut
Greater than 400 mg/dL	8 units subcut stat and notify doctor Repeat finger stick in 2 hr

TIPS FOR CLINICAL PRACTICE

When orders are written for sliding scale, the abbreviation "SS" should not be used to mean sliding scale. In the apothecary system, ss means 1/2, and ss could also be mistaken for the number 55. Write out sliding scale.

Note that the process for documenting the insulin administered varies among institutions. Know the institution's policies and protocols regarding the use of the sliding scale.

Despite current evidence cited in the literature indicating the sliding scale as not being effective in achieving glycemic control, and discouragement regarding its use by the American Diabetes Association (ADA), the sliding scale is still in use in some health care institutions.

According to an article by DeYoung and colleagues (2011) entitled "Controlling blood glucose levels in hospital patients: current recommendations," the sliding scale insulin regimen is largely ineffective because it treats hyperglycemia after it occurs; it does not prevent elevated blood glucose (BG) or its recurrence. The article also indicates the following in regard to use of the sliding scale insulin regimen:

- It can be dangerous.
- The sliding scale regimen prescribed on admission is likely to remain unmodified throughout the patient's hospital stay.
- The exacerbation of hyperglycemia and hypoglycemia caused by rapid BG alterations has increased the risk of poor clinical outcomes and even death.

Current Recommendations for Use of the Sliding Scale Protocol

"Controlling blood glucose levels in hospital patients: current recommendations," (DeYoung et al, 2011) a consensus statement on inpatient glycemic control management from the American Association of Clinical Endocrinologists and the American Diabetes Association, calls for scheduled subcutaneous insulin administration with basal insulin, nutritional (meal), and correctional components—an approach that promotes the best outcomes in noncritically ill clients. In addition to improved client outcomes, the management program has proved to be safe and effective in managing hyperglycemia in noncritical hospital patients. Prolonged use of the sliding insulin scale as the sole regimen is discouraged.

The basal insulin component uses a long-acting insulin analogue to control the fasting plasma glucose level, and the nutritional component uses rapid-acting insulin to cover nutritional intake and correct hyperglycemia. The basal plus rapid-acting insulin is referred to as *basal/bolus insulin therapy,* which closely approximates normal physiological insulin production and controls hyperglycemia. The correction dose is determined by the patient's insulin sensitivity and current blood glucose level. Insulin sensitivity is calculated by adding up the patient's total daily insulin requirement and dividing that amount into 1,500 (for type 2 DM) or 1,700 (for type 1 DM). The use of this management combines the basal insulin with mealtime (prandial insulin).

In summary, the basal-prandial insulin therapy is a physiological approach to insulin therapy that uses multiple daily injections to cover both basal and prandial therapy. The basal prandial insulin therapy is a regimen that has evidence to support it as being optimal to achieving glycemic control in clients with diabetes.

Preparing a Single Dosage of Insulin in an Insulin Syringe

Measuring insulin in an insulin syringe is different from the administration of most other injectable medications. There is no calculation or conversion required because the syringe measures units of insulin, rather than volume of solution. An order must be written following the previously stated guidelines. Frequent errors have occurred with insulin dosages, and insulin is considered a high-alert medication. Because of this, special attention should be used when preparing dosages of insulin. Insulin dosage errors can be avoided by following two important rules to ensure safe administration of insulin.

RULE

Avoiding Insulin Dosage Errors

- Insulin dosages **MUST** be checked by two nurses. To be considered an independent verification, the check by the second nurse must occur independently, away from the first nurse, with no prior knowledge of calculations to verify the dosage.
- In the preparation of combination dosages (two insulins), two nurses must verify each step of the process.

Example 1: Order: Humulin R U-100 40 units subcut in AM ½ hr before breakfast

Available: Humulin R labeled U-100

To measure 40 units, withdraw U-100 insulin to the 40-unit mark on the U-100 syringe. A Lo-Dose syringe can also be used to draw up this dose, as shown below.

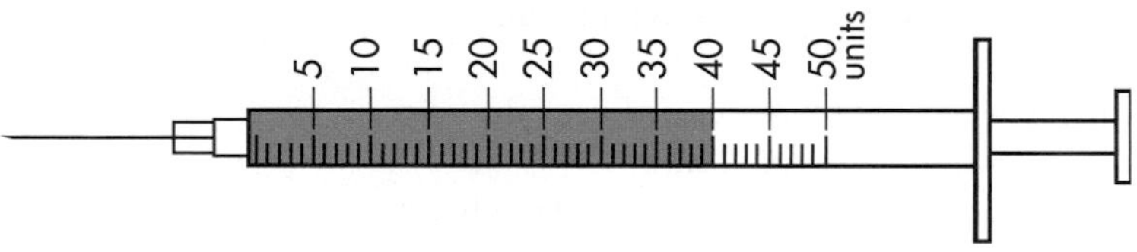

Example 2: Order: Humulin N U-100 70 units subcut daily at 7:30 AM

Available: Humulin N labeled U-100

There is no calculation or conversion required here. Draw up the required amount using a U-100 (1-mL) syringe.

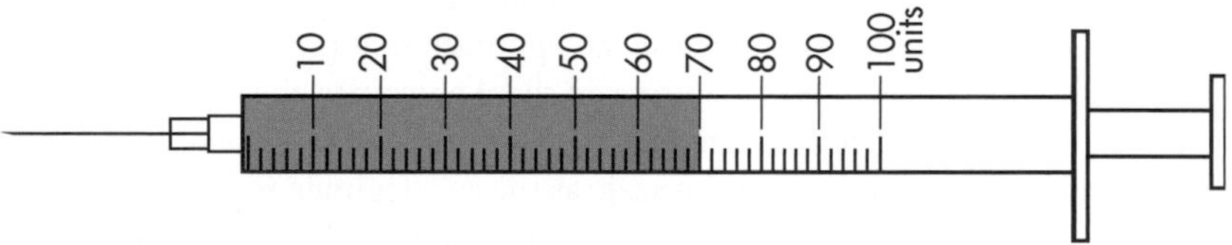

Example 3: Order: Humulin R U-100 5 units subcut stat

Available: Humulin R labeled U-100

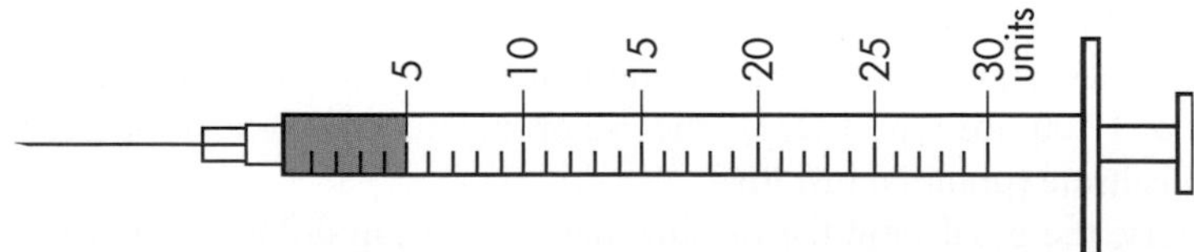

Measuring Two Types of Insulin in the Same Syringe

Sometimes individuals may require two different types of insulin for control of their blood sugar levels: for example, NPH and regular. To decrease the number of injections, it is common to mix two insulins in a single syringe. To mix insulin in one syringe, remember:

RULE

Safety When Combining Two Insulins in Same Syringe

Draw up clear insulin first, and then draw up cloudy insulin. Rapid- and short-acting insulins are clear (regular, aspart, lispro). Intermediate-acting (NPH) insulin is cloudy.
THINK: First rapid-acting or short-acting insulin, then intermediate-acting insulin.
THINK: The insulin that acts **first** is drawn up **first.**

Drawing regular insulin up first prevents contamination of the regular insulin with other insulin. This sequence is extremely important.

To prepare insulin in one syringe (mixing insulin), complete the following steps (Figures 20-7 and 20-8):

1. Cleanse tops of both vials with an alcohol wipe.
2. Inject air equal to the amount being withdrawn into the vial of cloudy insulin first. When the air is injected, the tip of the needle should not touch the solution.
3. Remove the needle from the vial of cloudy insulin.
4. Using the same syringe, inject an amount of air into the regular insulin (clear) equal to the amount to be withdrawn, invert or turn the bottle up in the air, and draw up the desired amount.
5. Remove the syringe from the regular insulin, and check for air bubbles. If air bubbles are present, gently tap the syringe to remove them.
6. Next, withdraw the desired dosage from the vial of cloudy insulin.
7. The total number of units in the syringe will be the sum of the two insulin orders.

Note: Provide the order, vial of insulin, and syringe to another nurse for independent verification each time you draw up an insulin dose.

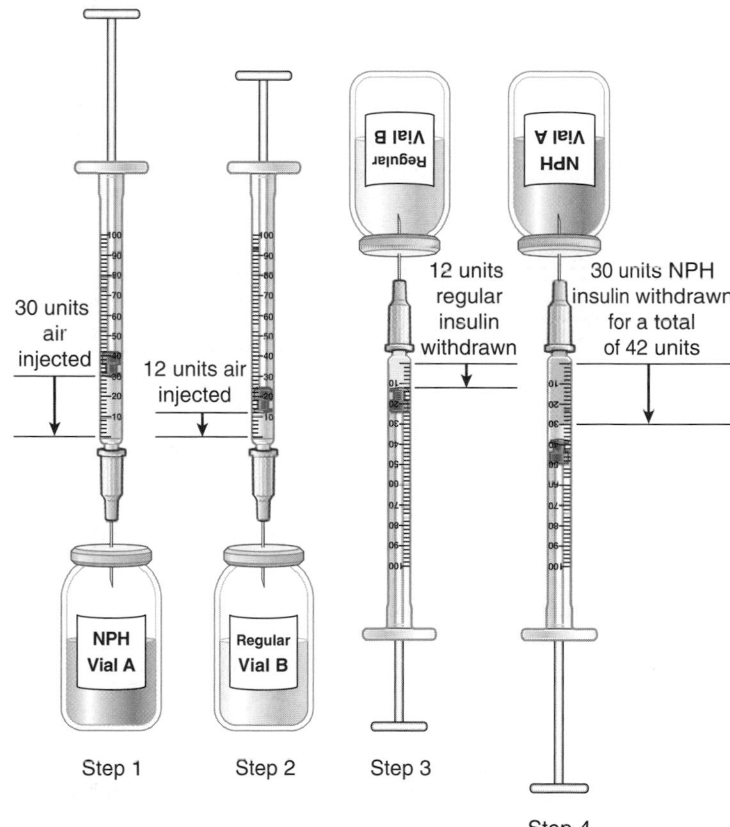

Figure 20-7 Mixing insulins. Order: Humulin N (NPH) U-100 30 units subcut, Humulin R (Regular) U-100, 12 units subcut. **Step 1,** Inject 30 units of air into Humulin N first; do not allow needle to touch insulin. **Step 2,** Inject 12 units of air into Humulin R. **Step 3,** Withdraw 12 units; withdraw needle. **Step 4,** Insert needle into vial of Humulin N and withdraw 30 units. Total 30 units Humulin N (NPH) + 12 units Humulin R (Regular) = 42 units. (Modified from Harkreader H, Hogan MA: *Fundamentals of nursing: caring and clinical judgment,* ed 3, St. Louis, 2007, Saunders.)

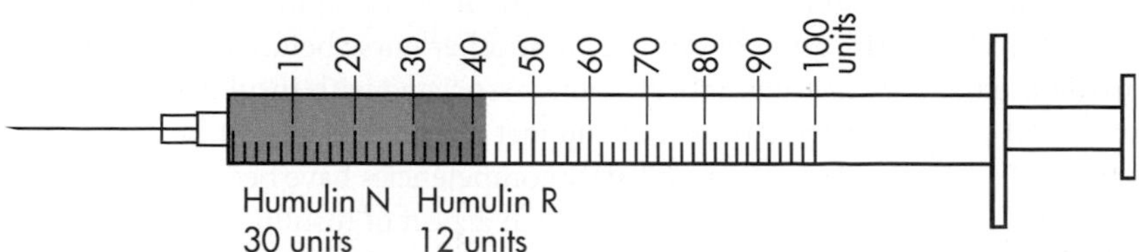

Figure 20-8 Total of two insulins combined. Total = 42 units (30 units Humulin NPH + 12 units Humulin R).

SAFETY ALERT!

DO NOT combine long-acting insulin types or dilute them with any other insulin preparation. The effects can be life threatening.

TIPS FOR CLINICAL PRACTICE

- Cloudy insulin should be rolled gently between the palms of the hands to mix it before it is drawn up. *Do not* shake insulin. Shaking creates bubbles in addition to breaking down the particles and causing clumping.
- Insulins mix instantly; they do not remain separated. Therefore, insulin that has been overdrawn cannot be returned to the vial. You must discard the entire medication and start over.

Example 1: The order is to administer 18 units of regular U-100 subcut and 22 units subcut of NPH U-100.

The total amount of insulin is 40 units (18 units [regular] + 22 units [NPH] = 40 units).

To administer this dosage, a Lo-Dose syringe or a U-100 (1-mL) syringe can be used. However, because the dosage is 40 units, the Lo-Dose would be more desirable. (See the syringes that follow, illustrating this dosage.)

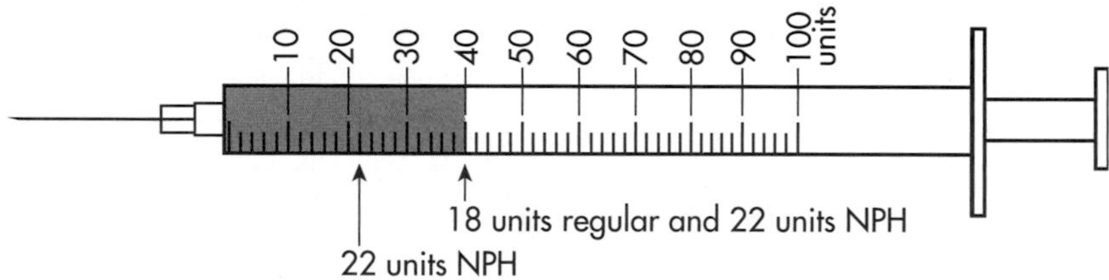

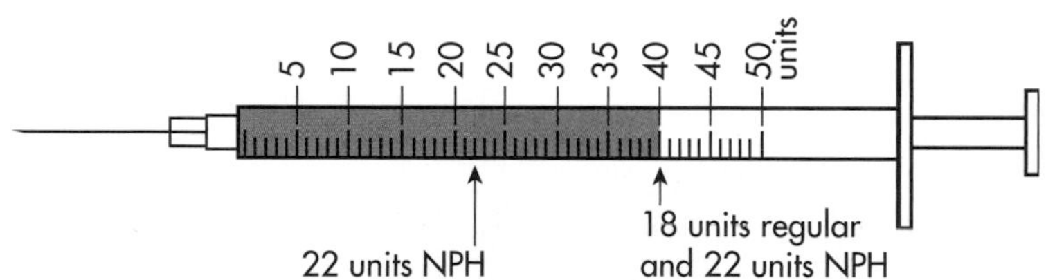

TIPS FOR CLINICAL PRACTICE

When mixing insulins, it is important to follow the steps outlined. Committing one of the following phrases to memory may help you remember the steps: (1) last injected is **first** drawn up; (2) run fast first (regular), then slow down (NPH); (3) clear to cloudy; or (4) it is alphabetical: clear, cloudy. Also remember, when mixing insulins, only the same type should be mixed together – for example, Humulin and Humulin.

As nurses, we need to remember the importance of taking steps to prevent errors that can occur in dosage administration. Extra care must be taken to prevent errors with high-alert medications. The results can be fatal to a client. Reading insulin labels carefully, obtaining independent verification of dosages by another nurse before administering insulin, recognizing the use of dangerous abbreviations associated with insulin and the errors they can cause, and performing practices that support safety and prevent harm to a client are part of the QSEN competency of safety. Safety competencies have been incorporated in this chapter to ensure that you consider safety in each aspect of insulin administration.

POINTS TO REMEMBER

- U-100 means 100 units per mL.
- Carefully read the prescriber's orders.
- To ensure accuracy, U-100 insulin should be given only with an insulin syringe. Insulin syringes should not be used to measure other medications measured in units.
- U-100 insulin is designed to be given with syringes marked U-100.
- Insulin dosages must be exact. Read the calibration on the insulin syringes carefully.
- Lo-Dose syringes are desirable for small dosages up to 50 units. The Lo-Dose 30-unit syringe may be used for dosages up to 30 units. Although Lo-Dose insulin syringes (30 units and 50 units) can hold a smaller volume, they are intended for U-100 insulin only.
- A U-100 (1-mL capacity) syringe is desirable when the dosage exceeds 50 units.
- Drawing up insulin correctly is critical to safe administration of insulin to clients.
- When insulins are mixed, regular insulin (clear) is always drawn up first, then cloudy.
- Do not shake insulin. Roll the insulin gently between the palms of the hands to mix.
- When insulins are mixed, the total volume is the sum of the two insulin amounts.
- Regular insulin, aspart, and glulisine are approved for IV administration.
- Read insulin labels to ensure that you have the correct type of insulin, to avoid medication errors. Only mix the same types of insulin (e.g., Humulin R and Humulin N).
- Use the smallest-capacity syringe possible to ensure accuracy.
- Insulin orders should be written with units spelled out, not abbreviated U.
- Do not mix long-acting insulin with any other insulin or dilute with any other insulin preparation.
- Avoid insulin dosage errors; always obtain an independent verification by a second nurse.
- U-500 insulin means 500 units per mL.
- In the hospital, measure U-500 insulin in a 1-mL syringe.
- Be prepared to teach a client how to measure U-500 insulin with a U-100 insulin syringe upon discharge.
- Errors with U-500 insulin can be fatal. Make careful calculations.
- Current evidence supports basal-prandial insulin therapy, which improves client outcomes and is an optimal strategy for achieving glycemic control in diabetic clients.

CLINICAL **REASONING**

1. **Scenario:** The prescriber wrote the following insulin order:
   Humulin U-100 10 U subcut ā breakfast.
   The nurse assumed the order was for regular insulin 100 units and administered the insulin to the client.
   Later, it was discovered the insulin dose desired was NPH 10 units.
   a. What error occurred here? __________
   b. What client medication rights were violated? __________
   c. What is the potential outcome of the error? __________
   d. What measures could have been taken to prevent the error that occurred? ________

2. **Scenario:** A client is to receive Humulin R U-100 10 units subcut and Humulin N U-100 14 units subcut before breakfast. In drawing up the insulins in the same syringe, the nurse used the following technique:
   a. Injected 10 units of air into the regular vial.
   b. Injected 14 units of air into the NPH vial.
   c. Withdrew 14 units of NPH insulin, then the 10 units of regular insulin.
      (a) What is the error in the technique of drawing up the two insulins? __________
      (b) What is the potential outcome from the technique used? __________

Answers on p. 510

CHAPTER REVIEW

Using the syringes below and the labels where provided, indicate the dosage you would prepare and shade the dosage on the syringe provided.

1. Order: Humulin N U-100 56 units subcut daily every AM ½ hour before breakfast.

   Available:

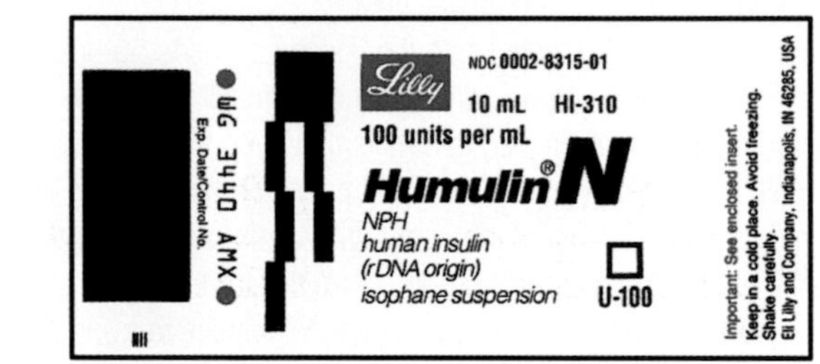

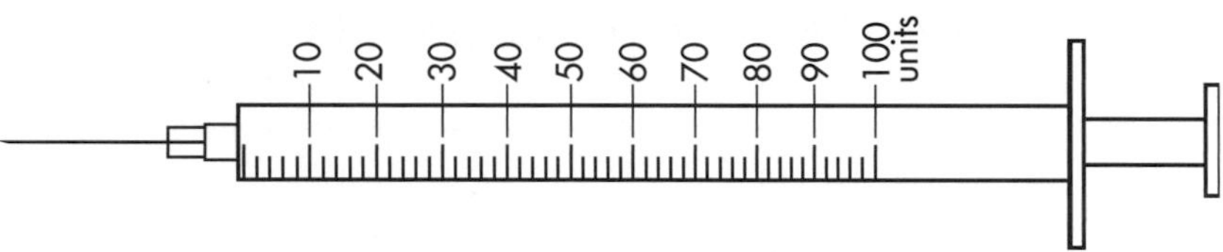

2. Order: Humulin R U-100 18 units subcut and Humulin N U-100 40 units subcut daily at 7:30 AM. (Indicate the total insulin dosage.)

   Available:

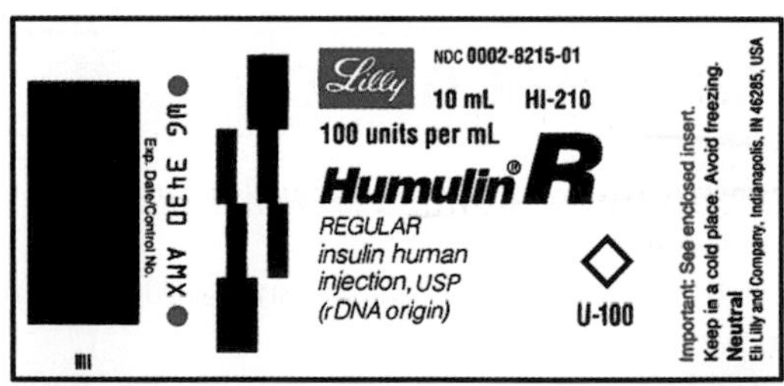

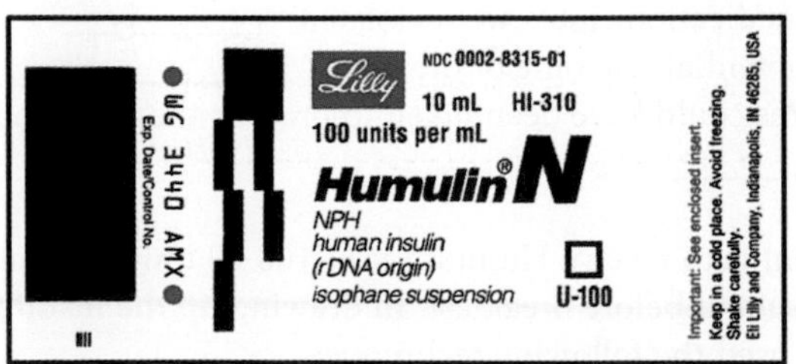

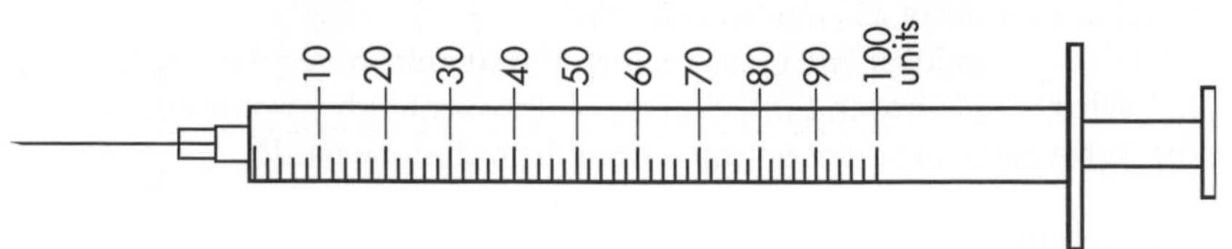

3. Order: Novolin R U-100 9 units subcut daily.

Available:

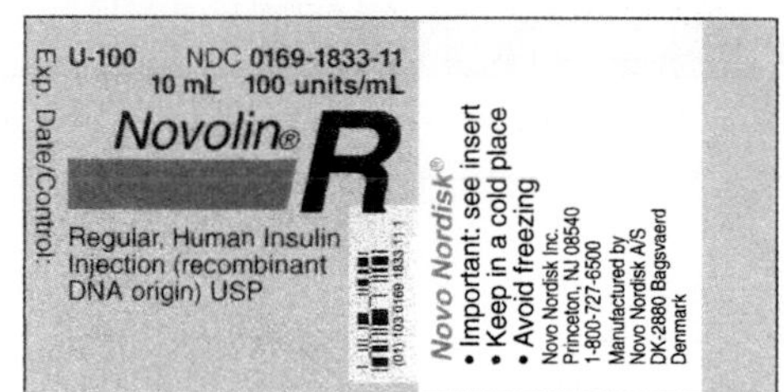

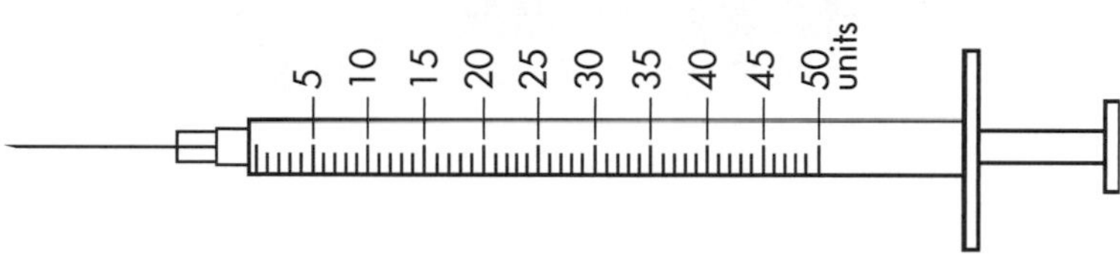

Indicate the number of units measured in the following syringes.

4. Units measured ______________________

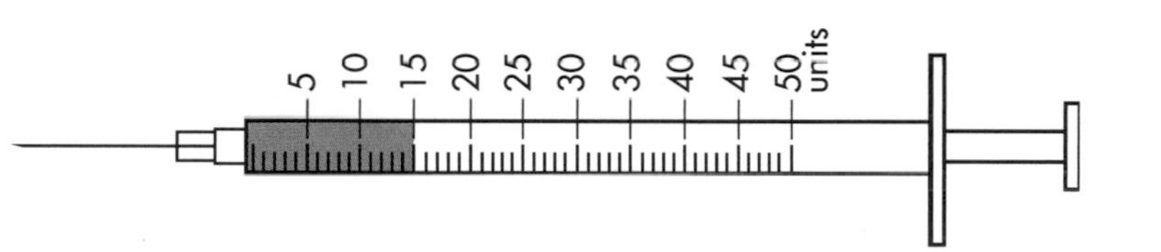

5. Units measured ______________________

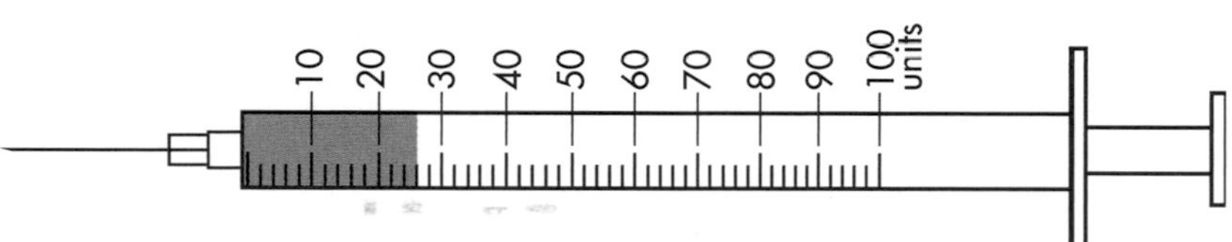

6. Units measured ______________________

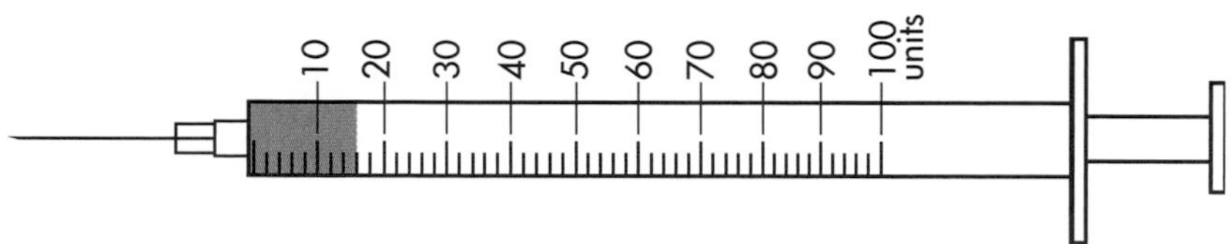

7. Units measured ______________________

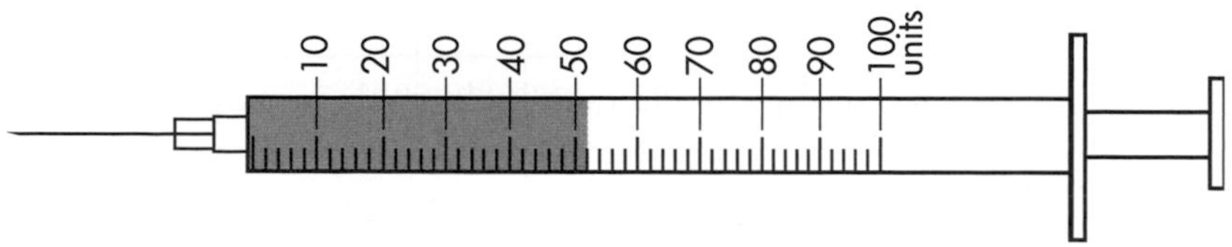

8. Units measured ____________

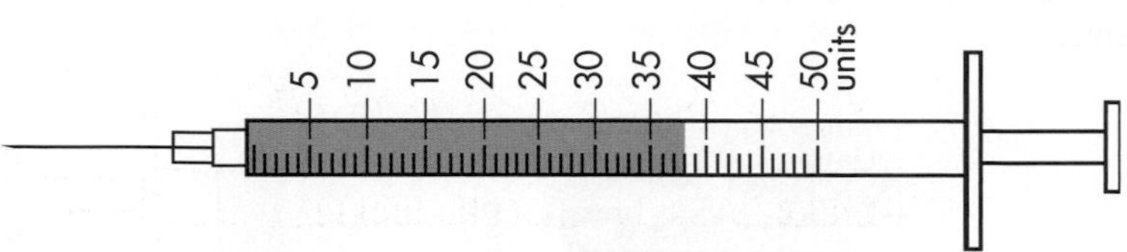

9. Units measured ____________

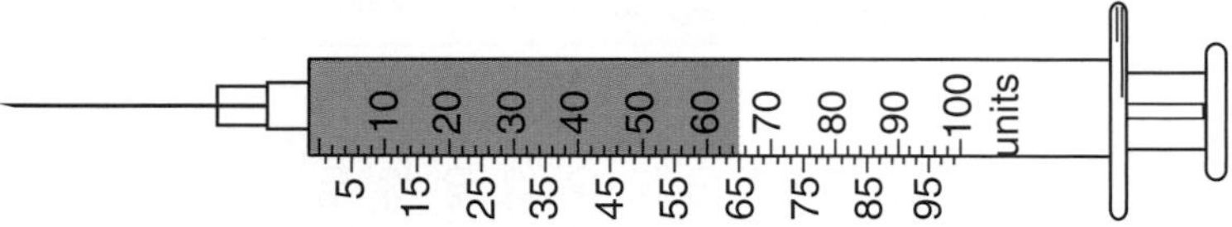

10. Units measured ____________

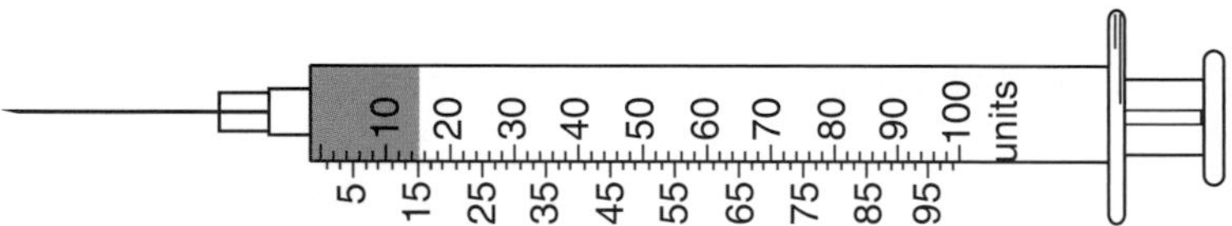

Calculate the dosage of insulin where necessary, and shade the dosage on the syringe provided. Labels have been provided for some problems.

11. Order: Humulin R U-100 10 units subcut at 7:30 AM.

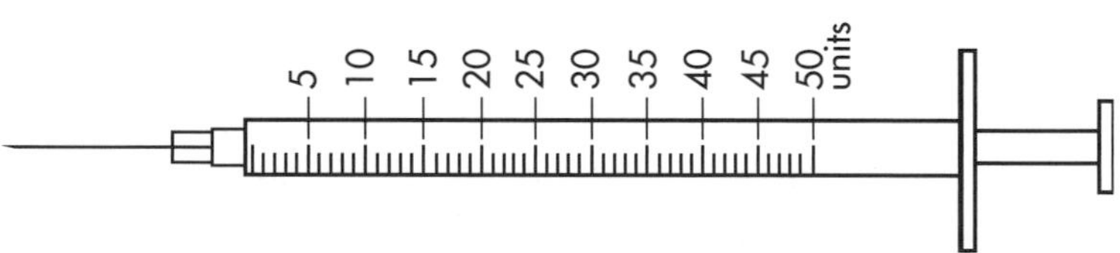

12. Order: Humulin R U-100 16 units subcut and Humulin N U-100 24 units subcut a.c. 7:30 AM. (Indicate the total insulin dosage.)

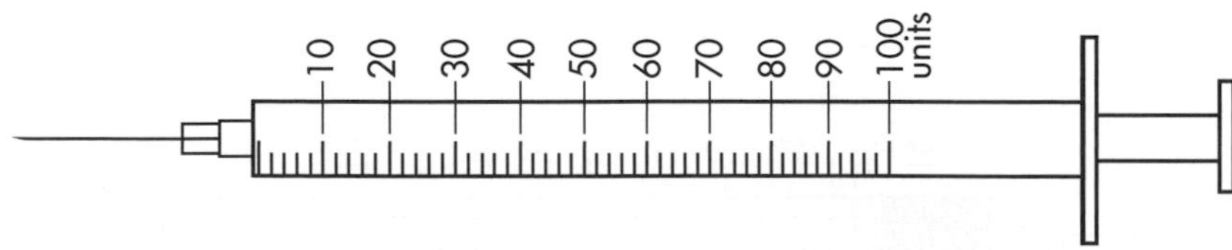

13. Order: Humulin R U-100 10 units subcut and Humulin N U-100 15 units subcut a.c. 7:30 AM. (Indicate the total insulin dosage.)

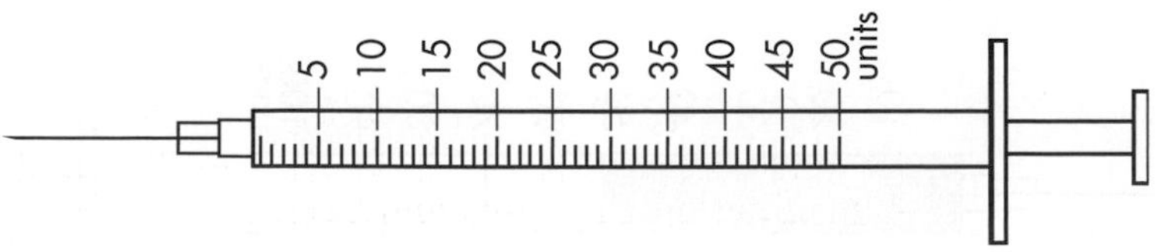

14. Order: Humulin R U-100 5 units subcut and Humulin N U-100 25 units subcut a.c. 7:30 AM. (Indicate the total insulin dosage.)

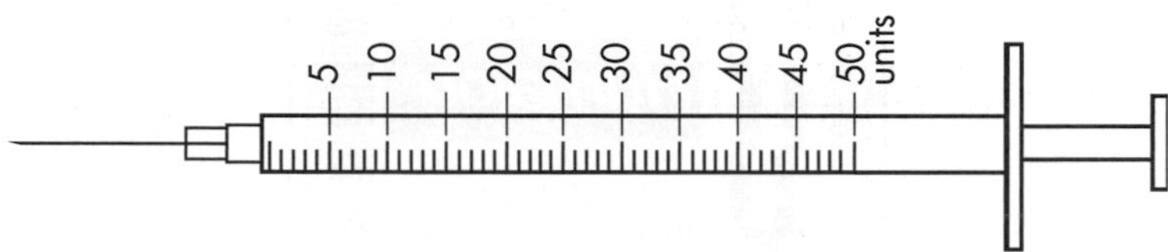

15. Order: Novolin R U-100 40 units subcut and Novolin N U-100 10 units subcut at 7:30 AM. (Indicate the total insulin dosage.)

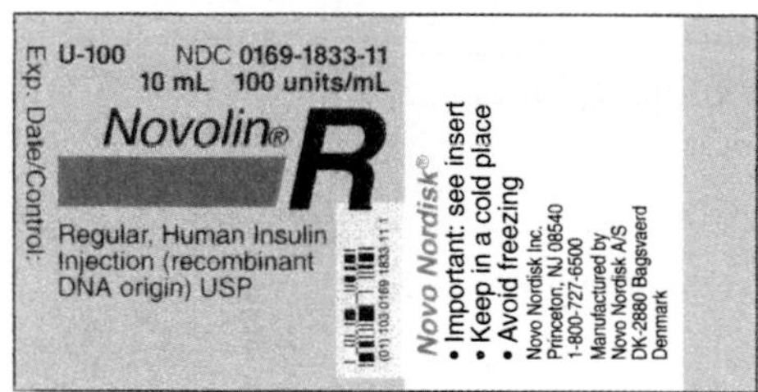

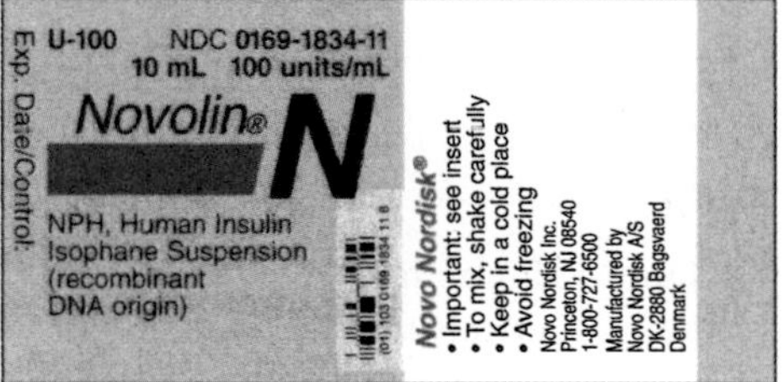

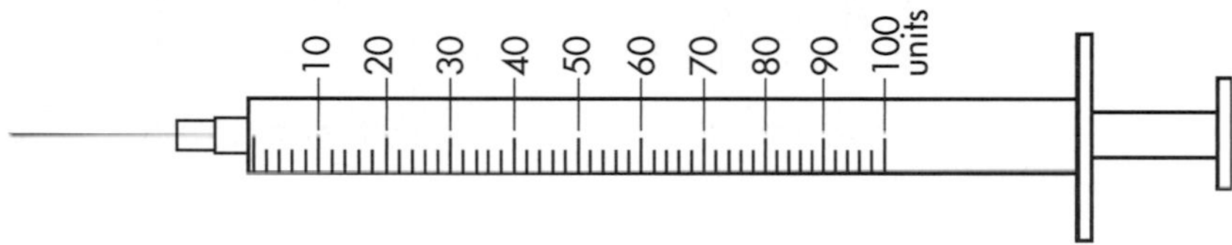

16. Order: Humulin N U-100 48 units subcut and Humulin R U-100 30 units subcut a.c. 7:30 AM. (Indicate the total insulin dosage.)

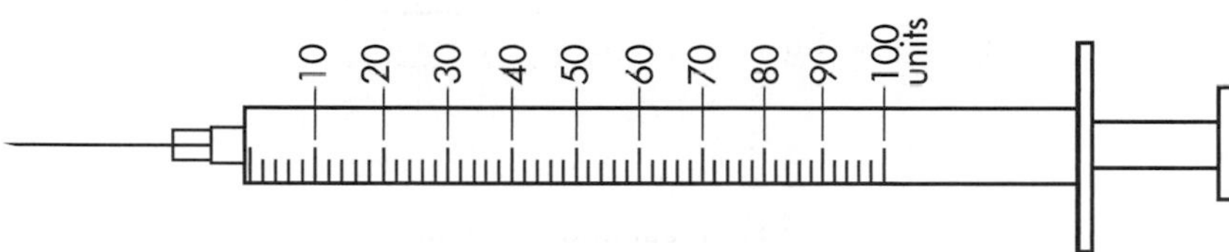

17. Order: Novolin R U-100 16 units subcut and Novolin N U-100 12 units subcut 7:30 AM. (Indicate the total insulin dosage.)

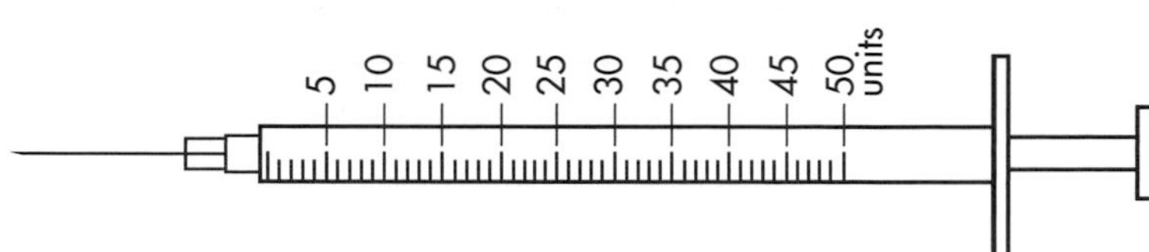

18. Order: Novolin R U-100 17 units subcut 5 PM.

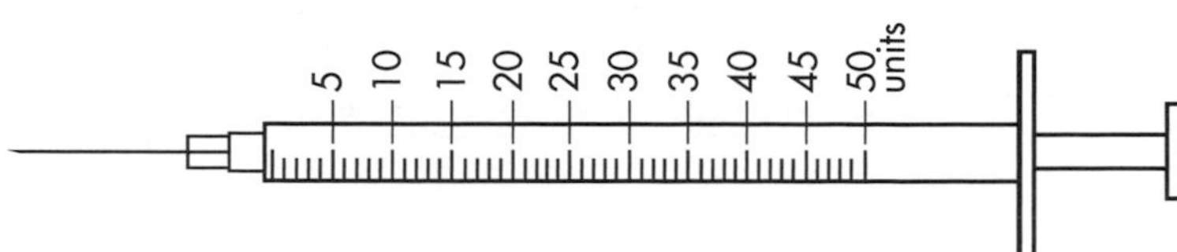

19. Order: Humalog U-100 15 units subcut daily at 7:30 AM.

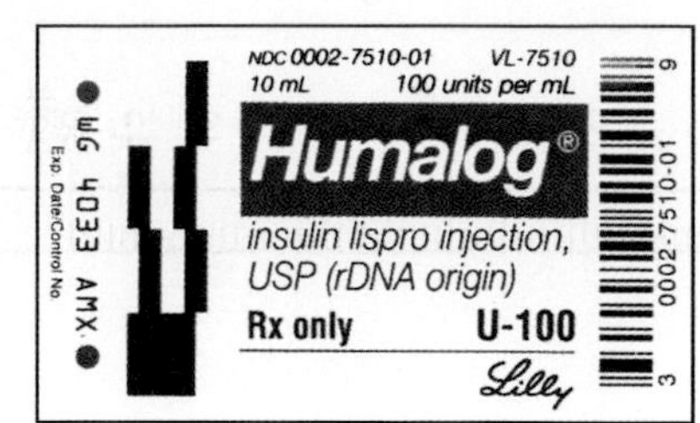

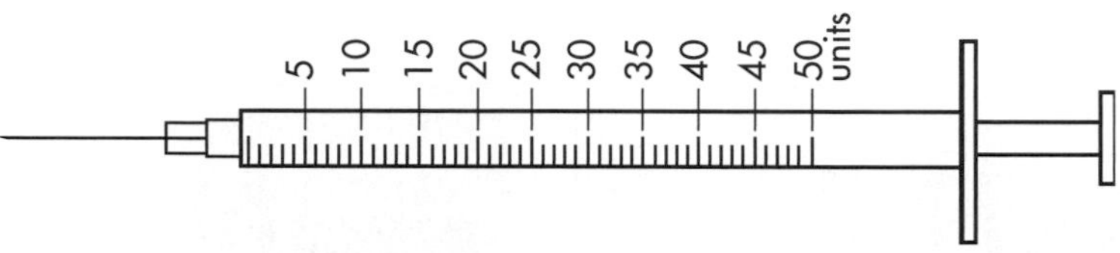

20. Order: Humulin R U-100 26 units subcut and Humulin N U-100 48 units subcut daily. (Indicate the total insulin dosage.)

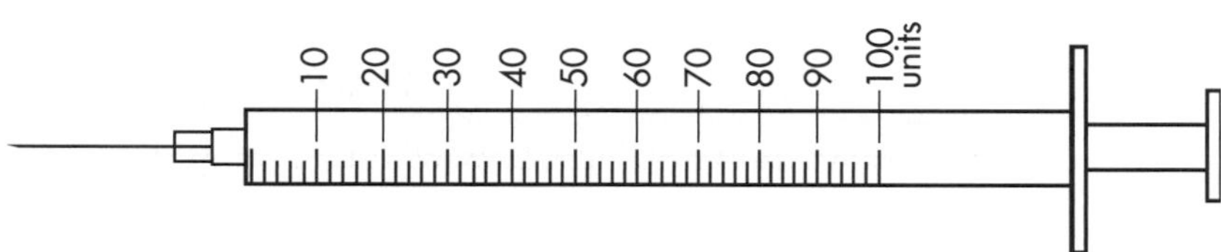

21. Order: Humulin 70/30 U-100 27 units subcut at 5 PM.

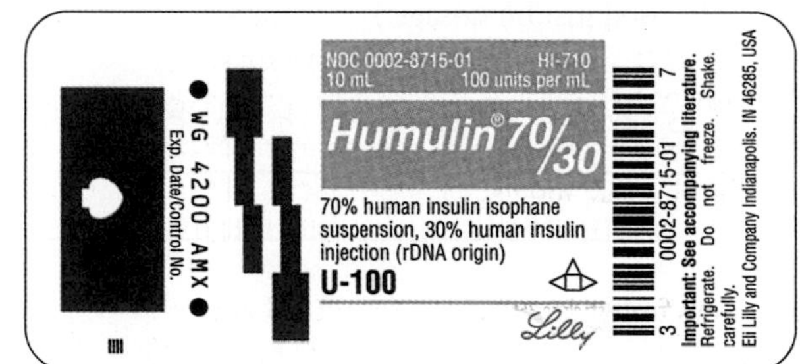

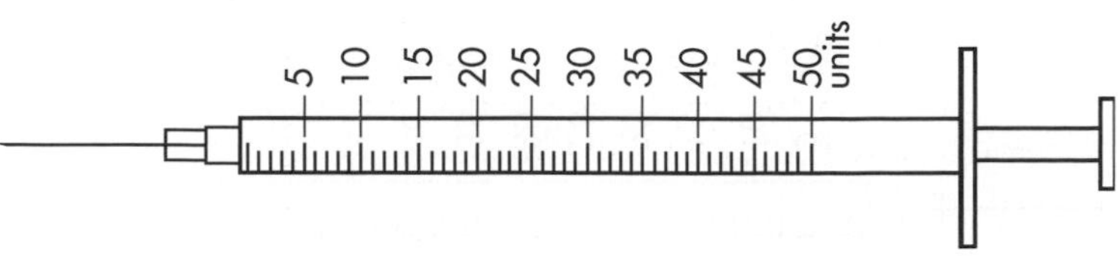

22. Order: Novolin R U-100 21 units subcut and Novolin N U-100 35 units subcut daily at 7:30 AM. (Indicate the total insulin dosage.)

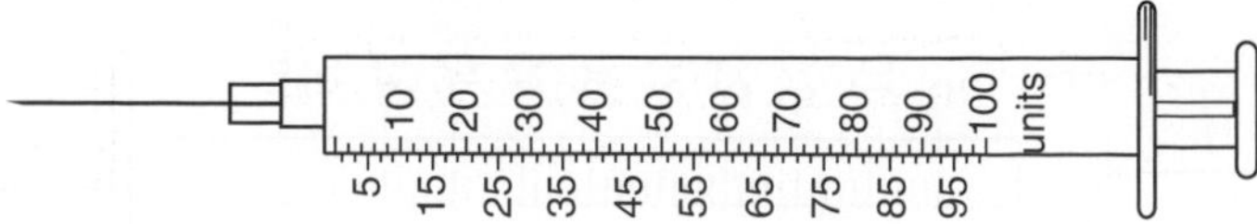

23. Order: Novolin Regular U-100 5 units subcut and Novolin N U-100 35 units subcut 7:30 AM. (Indicate the total insulin dosage.)

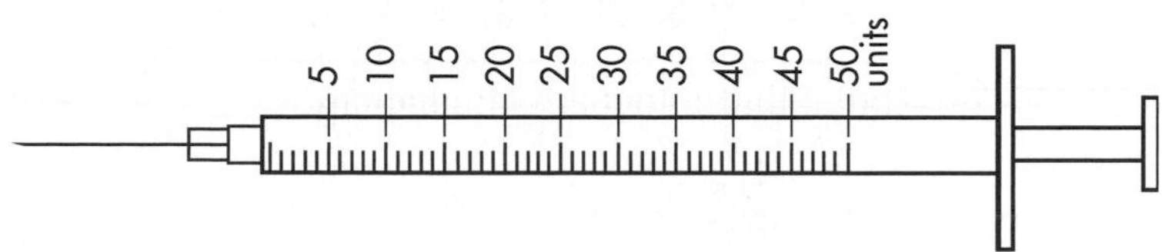

24. Order: NovoLog U-100 36 units subcut 7:30 AM before breakfast.

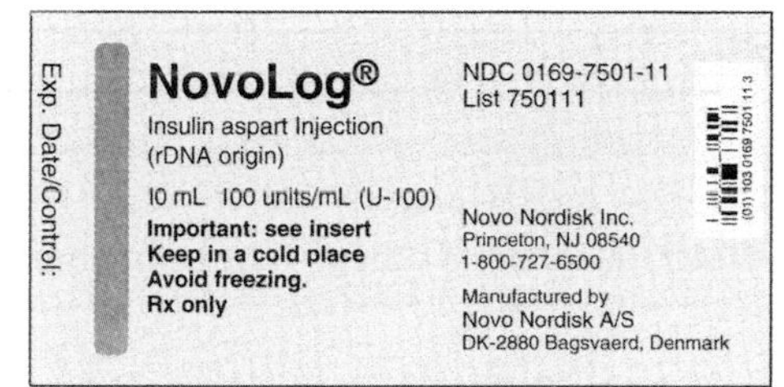

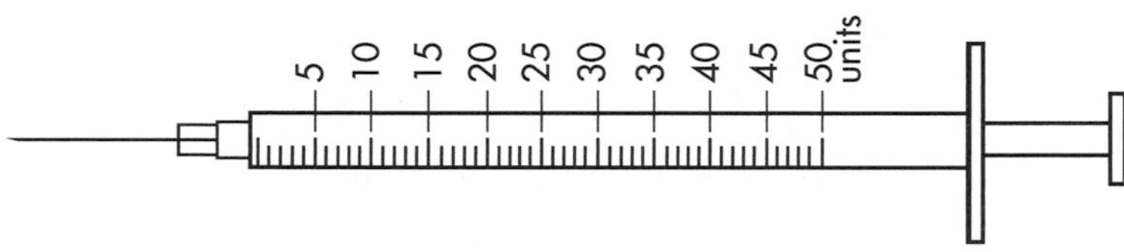

25. A client has a sliding scale for insulin dosages. The order is for Humulin Regular insulin U-100 q6h as follows:

Finger stick	0-180 mg/dL	no coverage
Blood sugar	181-240 mg/dL	2 units subcut
	241-300 mg/dL	4 units subcut
	301-400 mg/dL	6 units subcut
	Greater than 400 mg/dL	8 units subcut and repeat finger stick in 2 hr

At 11:30 AM, the client's finger stick is 364 mg/dL. Shade the syringe to indicate the dosage that should be given.

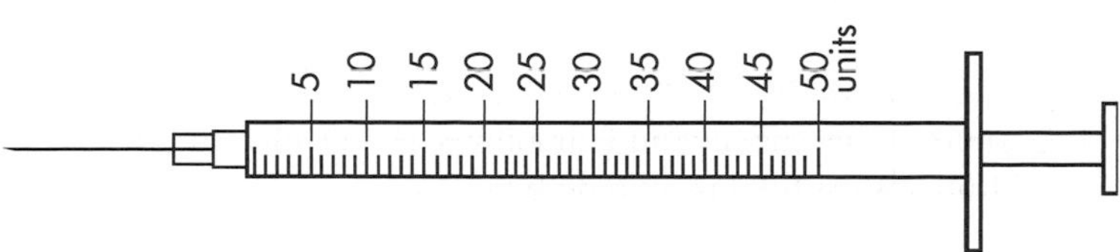

26. Order: Humulin R U-100 32 units subcut every morning at 7:30 AM.

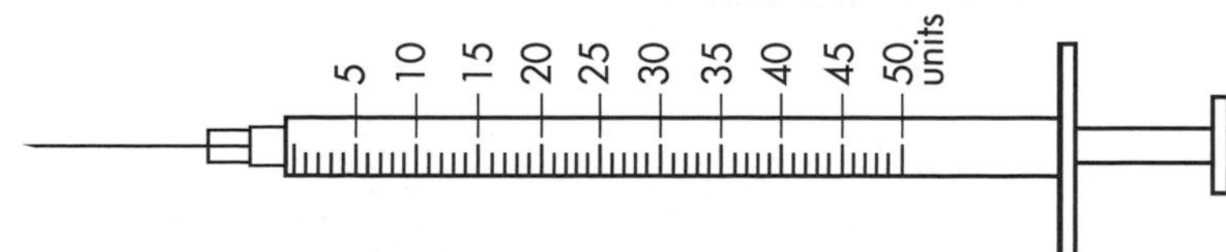

27. Order: Humulin R U-100 9 units subcut 5 PM.

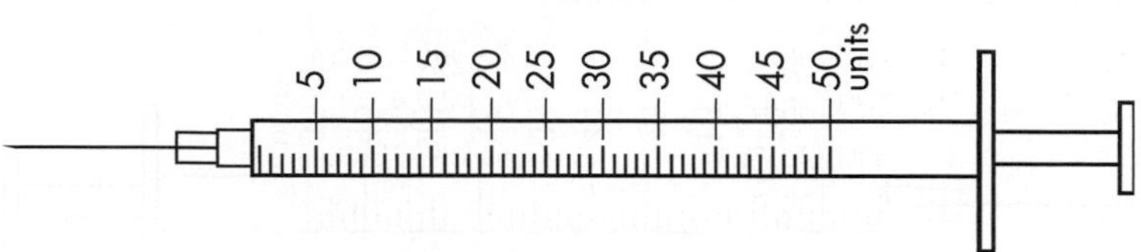

28. Order: Humulin N U-100 11 units subcut at bedtime.

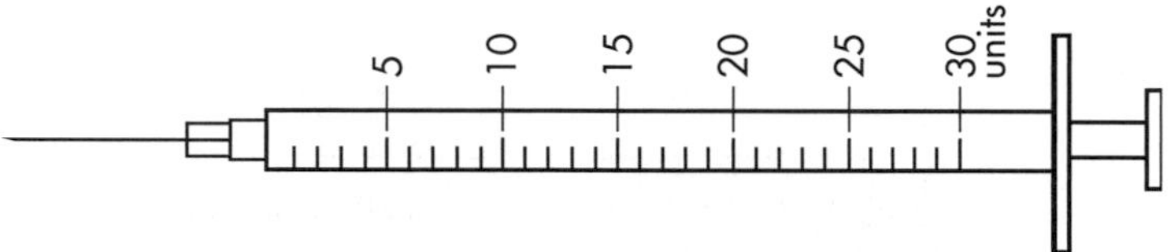

29. Order: Humulin 70/30 U-100 20 units subcut ½ hr before breakfast.

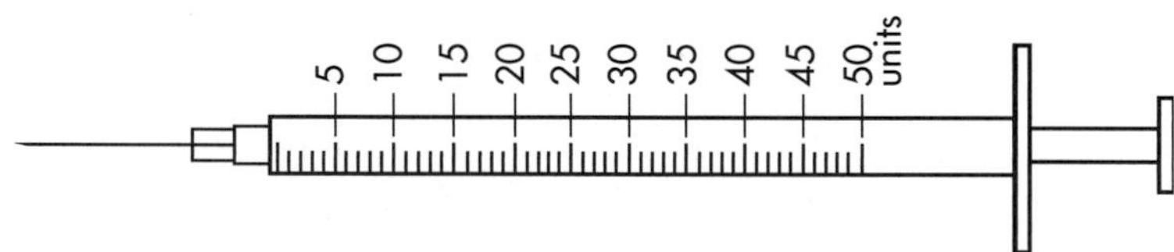

30. Order: Humulin R U-100 10 units subcut and Humulin N U-100 42 units subcut at 4:30 PM. (Indicate the total insulin dosage.)

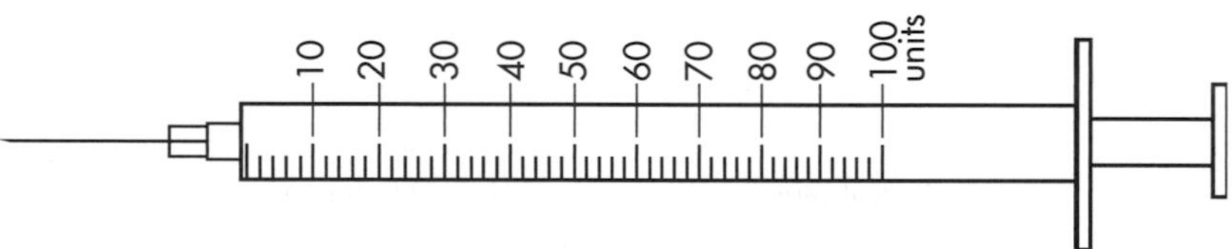

31. Order: Novolin R U-100 8 units subcut and Novolin N U-100 15 units subcut at 7:30 AM. (Indicate the total insulin dosage.)

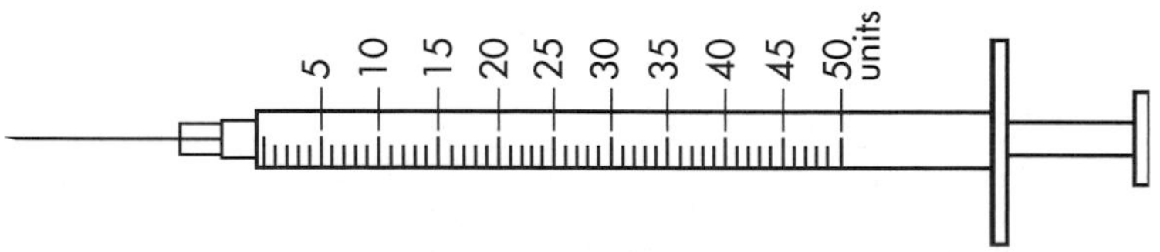

32. Order: Humulin R U-100 30 units subcut and Humulin N U-100 40 units subcut every day at 8:00 AM. (Indicate the total insulin dosage.)

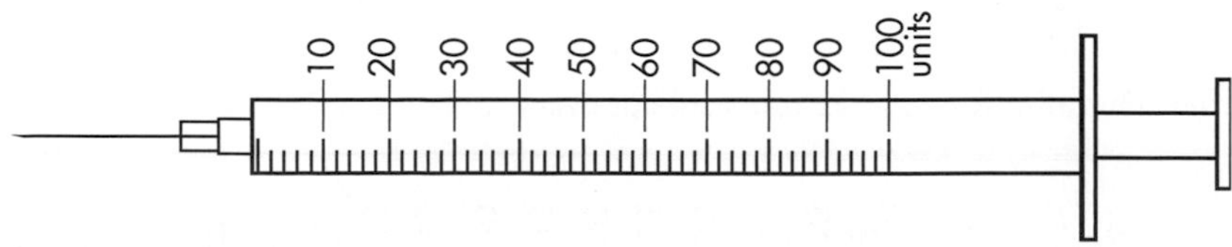

33. A client has a sliding scale for insulin dosages. The order is for Humulin R U-100 q6h as follows:

Finger stick	201-250 mg/dL	4 units subcut
Blood sugar	251-300 mg/dL	6 units subcut
(mg/dL)	301-350 mg/dL	8 units subcut
	351-400 mg/dL	10 units subcut
	Greater than 400 mg/dL	call MD

At 6:00 PM, the client's blood sugar is 354 mg/dL. Shade the syringe to indicate the dosage that should be administered.

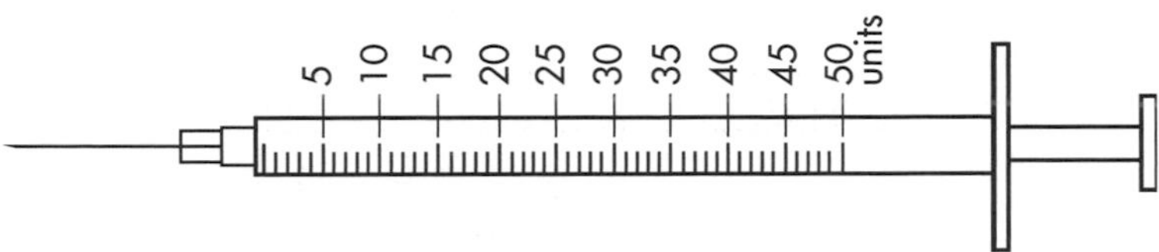

34. Order: Humulin R regular U-500 insulin 200 units subcut stat.

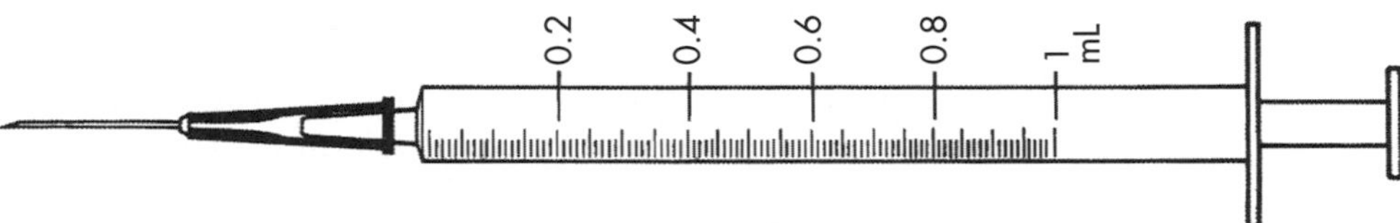

35. Order: Humulin R regular U-500 insulin 250 units subcut stat.

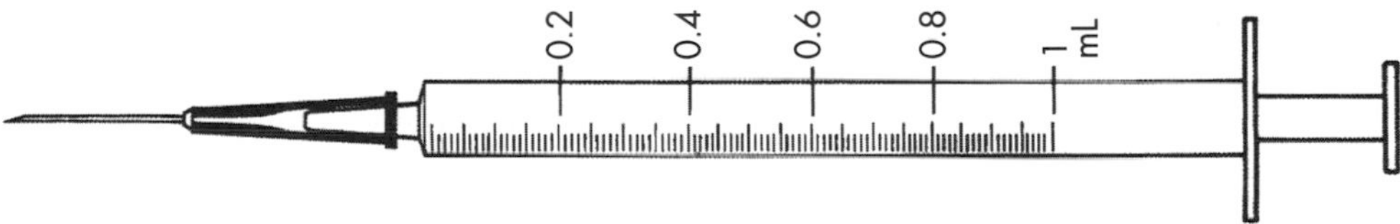

36. Order: Humulin R regular U-500 insulin 225 units subcut stat. (Show calculation that would be done for client teaching to administer medication at home.)

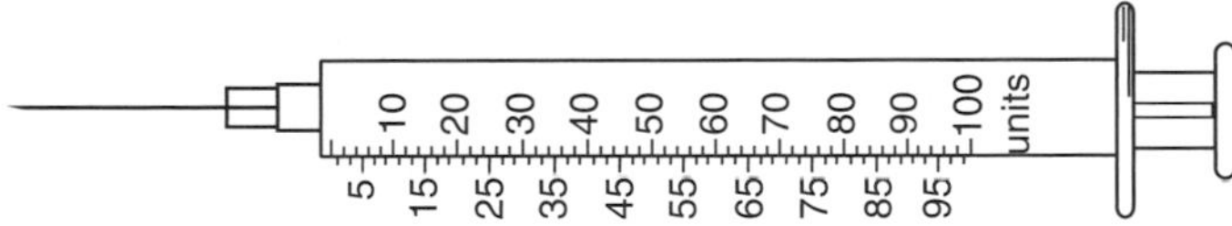

Answers on pp. 511-512

ANSWERS

Chapter 20

Answers to Practice Problems

1. Humalog, rapid acting (fast acting)
2. Humulin R Regular, short acting
3. Lantus, long acting
4. Humulin N, NPH, intermediate acting
5. 22 units

evolve

For additional practice problems, refer to the the Dosages Measured in Units section of the Elsevier's Interactive Drug Calculation Application, Version 1 on Evolve.

6. 41 units

7.

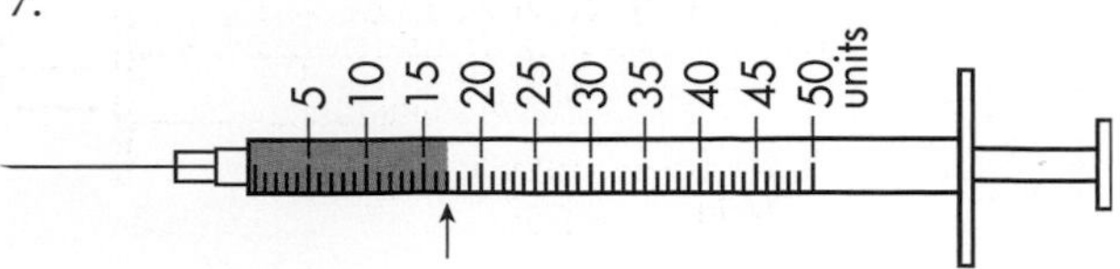

8.

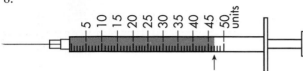

9. 40 units

10. 27 units

11. 64 units

12. 14 units

13.

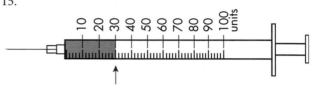

14.

15.

Answers to Clinical Reasoning Questions

1. a. The wrong insulin was administered. Failure to clarify an insulin order when the type of insulin was not specified, and the dosage was not clear because the U for units was used. U almost closed caused the "U" to be mistaken for "0."

   b. The right medication, the right dosage.

   c. The client received 10 times the dose of an insulin (regular) that was not ordered. Regular insulin is short acting, and NPH is intermediate acting and was desired. Administering the insulin would likely cause a dangerously low glucose level (hypoglycemia). Results could be tremors, confusion, sweating, and death. This incident constitutes malpractice.

   d. The error could have been prevented by remembering that all the essential components of an insulin order should have been in the order (name of insulin, number of units to be administered, route, frequency, and strength). When one element is missing, never assume. The order should have been clarified with the prescriber. Further, the dosage should have been double-checked with another nurse. In addition, units should have been written out in the order to avoid misinterpretation of "U" as a zero (0). Many insulin errors occur when the nurse fails to clarify an incomplete order or misinterprets the dosage when units is abbreviated.

2. a. The nurse should have injected the 14 units of air into the NPH vial and then injected 10 units of air into the regular vial and drawn up the 10 units of regular insulin first. First regular, then NPH. Another nurse should have been present during the mixing and to verify the dosage drawn.

   b. Contamination of insulins. Regular (rapid acting) is drawn up first to prevent it from becoming contaminated with the intermediate-acting insulin. This can also result in reversing the doses of the two insulins being drawn up and result in incorrect insulin dosages.

Answers to Chapter Review

1.

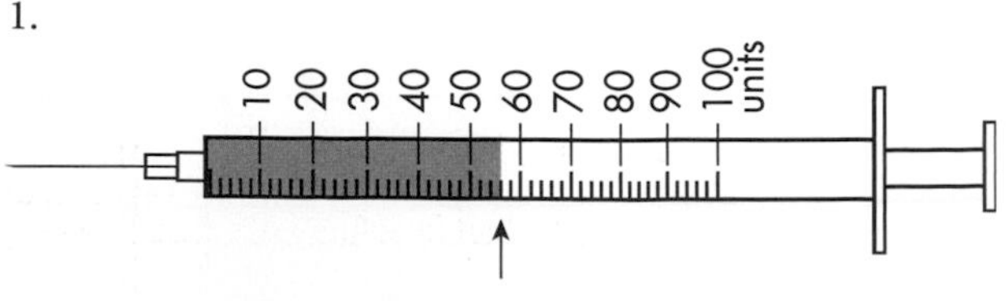

2.

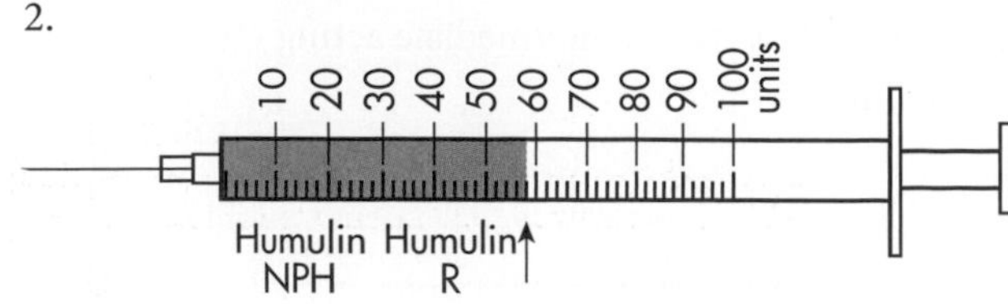

3.

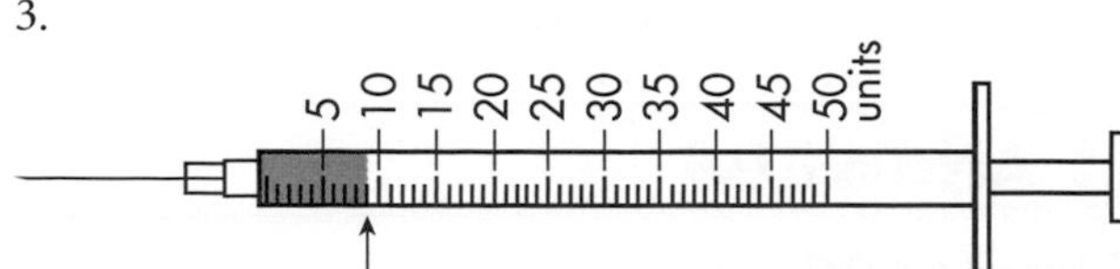

4. 15 units

5. 26 units

6. 16 units

7. 52 units

8. 38 units

9. 65 units

10. 15 units

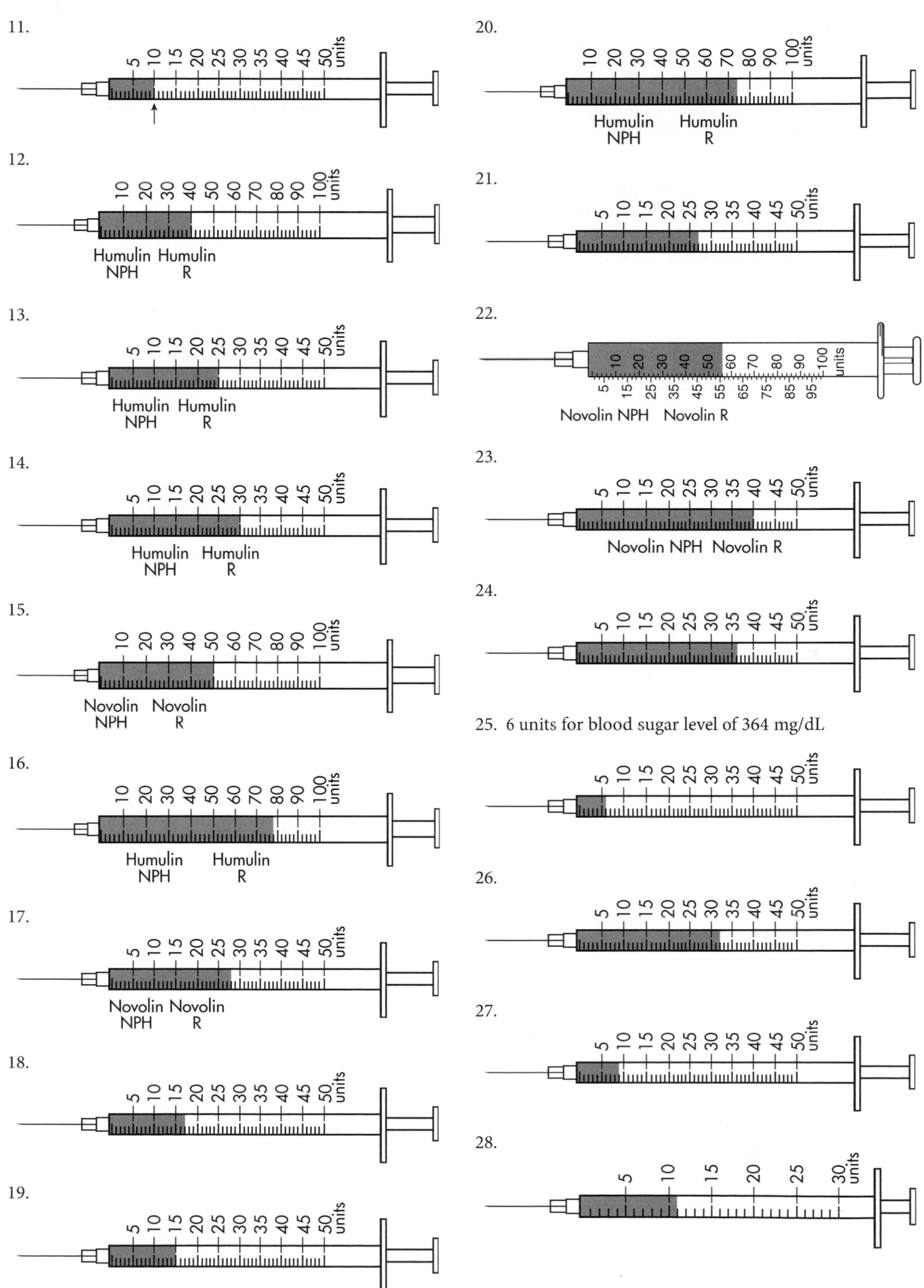
11.
12.
Humulin NPH Humulin R
13.
Humulin NPH Humulin R
14.
Humulin NPH Humulin R
15.
Novolin NPH Novolin R
16.
Humulin NPH Humulin R
17.
Novolin NPH Novolin R
18.
19.
20.
Humulin NPH Humulin R
21.
22.
Novolin NPH Novolin R
23.
Novolin NPH Novolin R
24.
25. 6 units for blood sugar level of 364 mg/dL
26.
27.
28.

29.

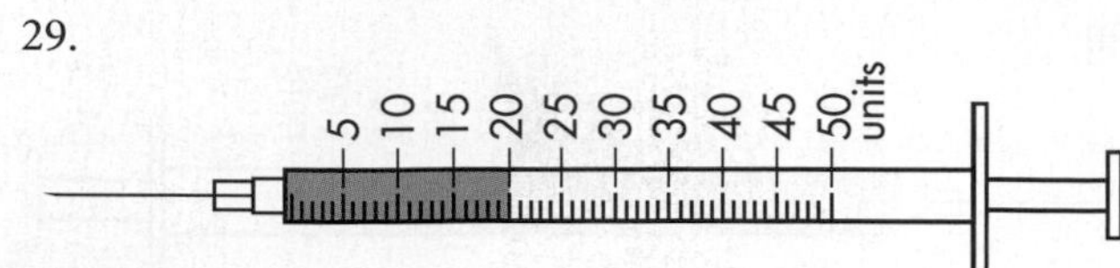

30.

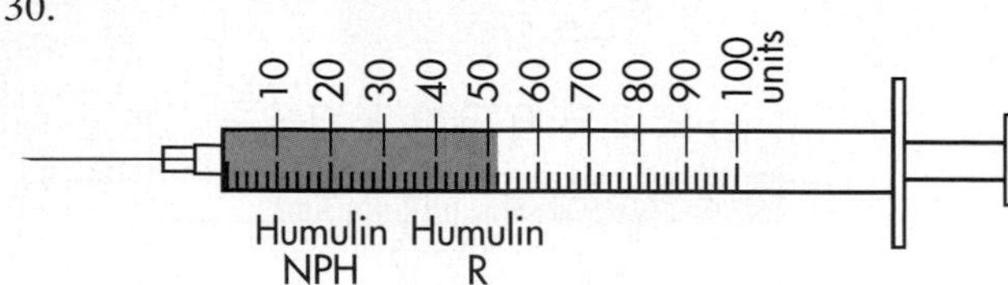

31.

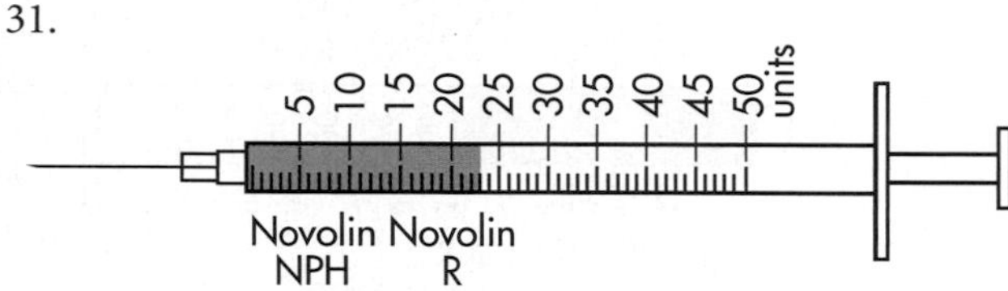

32.

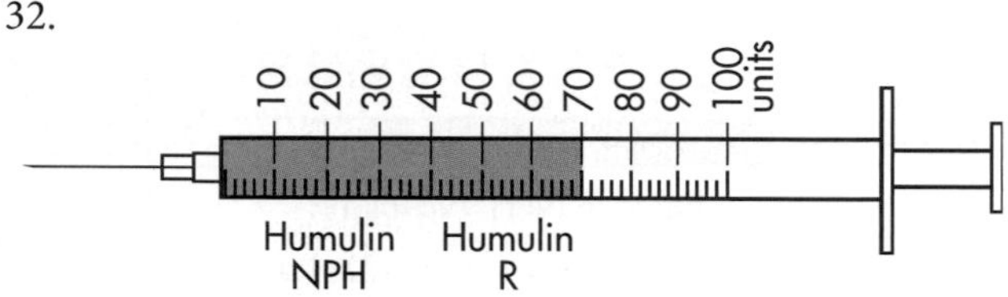

33. 10 unit blood sugar 354 mg/dL

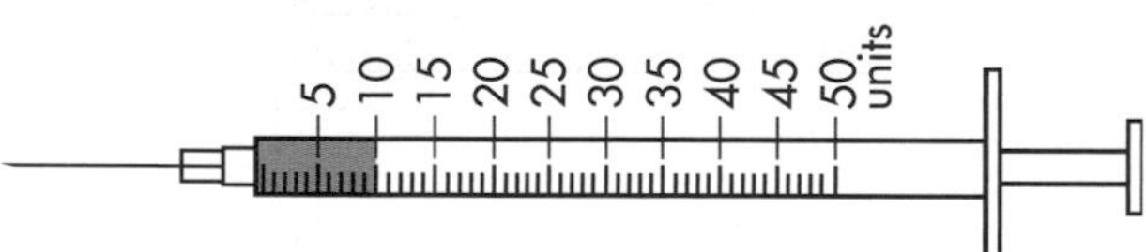

34. $\dfrac{200 \text{ units}}{500 \text{ units}} \times 1 \text{ mL} = x \text{ mL}$

$x = \dfrac{200}{500}$

$$x = \begin{array}{r}0.4\\5\overline{)200.0}\end{array}$$

$x = 0.4 \text{ mL}$

$500 \text{ units} : 1 \text{ mL} = 200 \text{ units} : x \text{ mL}$

or

$\dfrac{500 \text{ units}}{1 \text{ mL}} = \dfrac{200 \text{ units}}{x \text{ mL}}$

Answer: 0.4 mL of U-500 insulin measured in a 1-mL syringe.

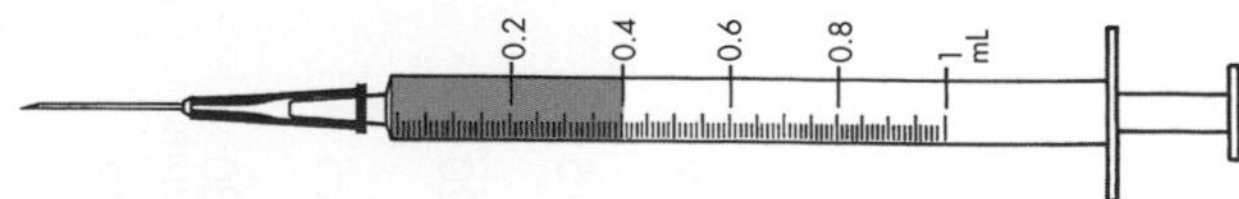

35. $\dfrac{250 \text{ units}}{500 \text{ units}} \times 1 \text{ mL} = x \text{ mL}$

$x = \dfrac{250}{500}$

$$x = \begin{array}{r}0.5\\500\overline{)250.0}\end{array}$$

$x = 0.5 \text{ mL}$

or

$500 \text{ units} : 1 \text{ mL} = 250 \text{ units} : x \text{ mL}$

or

$\dfrac{500 \text{ units}}{1 \text{ mL}} = \dfrac{250 \text{ units}}{x \text{ mL}}$

Answer: 0.5 mL of U-500 insulin measured in a 1-mL syringe.

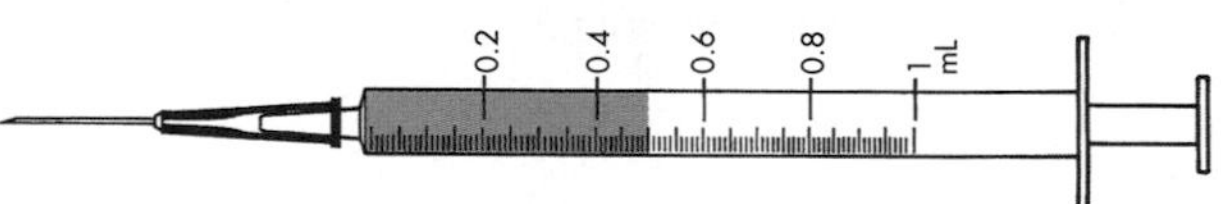

36. U-500 insulin is five times more concentrated than U-100 insulin; therefore, the amount in a U-100 syringe would be $\frac{1}{5}$ the amount U-100 insulin would measure.

$225 \text{ units} \times \dfrac{1}{5} = \dfrac{225}{5} = 45 \text{ units}$

or

$\dfrac{225 \text{ units}}{500 \text{ units}} = \dfrac{x \text{ units}}{100 \text{ units}}$

$\dfrac{500x}{500} = \dfrac{22{,}500}{500}$

$x = 45 \text{ units}$

or

$225 \text{ units} : 500 \text{ units} = x \text{ units} : 100 \text{ units}$

Answer: 45 units (of U-500 insulin measured in a U-100 insulin syringe). The calculation verifies the estimate. Instruct the client to draw up 45 units in the U-100 syringe, which is equivalent to 225 units of U-500 insulin.

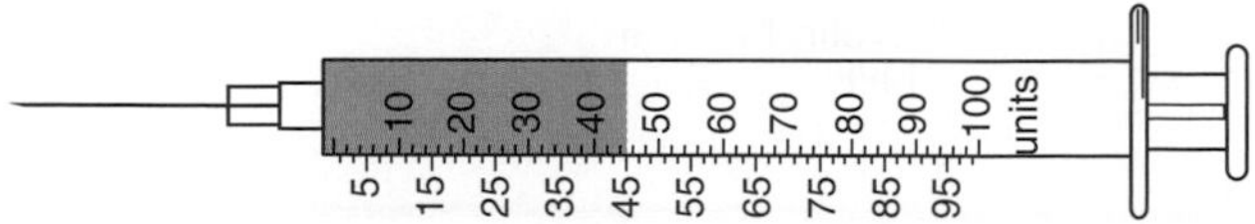

UNIT FIVE

Intravenous, Heparin, and Critical Care Calculations and Pediatric and Adult Calculations Based on Weight

The ability to accurately calculate flow rates for intravenous medications is essential to both heparin administration and critical care calculations.

Chapter 21 Intravenous Solutions and Equipment

Chapter 22 Intravenous Calculations

Chapter 23 Heparin Calculations

Chapter 24 Critical Care Calculations

Chapter 25 Pediatric and Adult Dosage Calculations Based on Weight

CHAPTER 21 Intravenous Solutions and Equipment

Objectives

After reviewing this chapter, you should be able to:

1. Identify common intravenous (IV) solutions and abbreviations
2. Calculate the amount of specific components in IV solutions
3. Define the following terms associated with IV therapy: peripheral line, central line, primary line, secondary line, saline/heparin locks, IV piggyback (IVPB), and IV push
4. Differentiate among various devices used to administer IV solutions (e.g., patient-controlled analgesia [PCA] pumps, syringe pumps, volumetric pumps)
5. Identify best practices that prevent IV administration errors and ensure client safety
6. Identify how technology related to IV therapy can enhance client safety

A general discussion of intravenous therapy will make it easier to understand the calculations associated with IV therapy, which will be discussed in Chapter 22. Intravenous (IV) therapy is the infusion of fluids, nutrients (i.e., vitamins, electrolytes, carbohydrates, fatty acids), blood or blood products, or medications through a vein. The reasons for the ordering and administration of IV fluids are varied and include:

- To maintain fluid and electrolyte balance. Fluids that are given to help sustain normal levels of fluids and electrolytes are called *maintenance fluids.*
- To replace lost fluids—when a client has lost fluids as a result of vomiting, diarrhea, or hemorrhage, IV fluids are administered to replenish fluid volume, and referred to as *replacement fluids.*
- To prevent depletion in clients who has the potential to become depleted, such as a client who is allowed nothing by mouth (NPO) for surgery or prior to the administration of chemotherapy.
- Act as a medium for administering medications directly into the bloodstream.

Fluids administered directly into the bloodstream have a rapid effect that is necessary during emergencies or other critical care situations when medications are needed. The advantage of administering medications by this route is the immediate availability of the medication to the body and the rapidity of action. However, IV administration of medications can be rapidly fatal to the client if the incorrect medication or dosage is administered. There are numerous medications available for IV use. Each medication has guidelines relating to its use. Health care providers are responsible to know about the medications they administer and the protocol relating to IV administration of medications.

IV medication protocols are valuable references, often posted in the medication room of an institution. They provide nurses with specifics about usual medication dosage, dilution for IV administration, compatibility, and specific observations of a client that need to be made during medication administration. **Always adhere to the protocol for administering IV medications.**

IV Delivery Methods

IV fluids and medications can be administered by continuous and intermittent infusion.

- *Continuous IV infusions* replace or maintain fluids and electrolytes. As the name implies, a continuous infusion is an IV solution that flows continuously until it is changed.
- *Intermittent IV infusions* (e.g., IV piggyback [IVPB], IV push) are used to administer medications and supplemental fluids. Intermittent peripheral infusion devices, known as saline or heparin locks, are used to maintain venous access without the need for continuous infusion.
- Hypodermoclysis (HDC), or clysis, is the subcutaneous infusion of fluids. It is considered to be an easy hydration technique suitable for mildly to moderately dehydrated adult clients, especially the elderly; for clients who are unable to take adequate fluids orally; and for clients for whom it is difficult or impractical to insert an intravenous line. The advantages of hypodermocylsis include: it can be administered at home by family members or a nurse; it is simple to insert; and it lessens the need for hospitalization of a client for hydration.

SAFETY ALERT!

Administration of IV fluids to the **correct client at the right rate** and **monitoring** the client during the therapy is a safety priority and are essential nursing responsibilities. If a client receives an IV infusion too rapidly and is not monitored closely, reactions can vary from mild to severe (death). Follow the same six rights of medication administration when administering IV therapy to clients. IV fluids are considered to be medications.

IV Solutions

There are several types of IV fluids. The type of fluid used is individualized according to the client and the reason for its use. IV solutions come prepared in plastic bags or glass bottles ranging from 50 mL (bags only) to 1,000 mL. IV plastic bags are more commonly used. IV solutions are clearly labeled with the exact components and amount of solution. When IV solutions are written in orders and charts, abbreviations are used. You may encounter various abbreviations; however, the percentage and initials, regardless of how they are written, have the same meaning: "D" is for dextrose, "W" is for water, "S" is for saline, and "NS" is for normal saline. Ringer's lactate (lactated Ringer's), a commonly used electrolyte solution, is abbreviated "RL" or "LR" and occasionally "RLS." Refer to Box 21-1, and learn the common abbreviations for IV solutions. Figures 21-1 to 21-6 show various IV solutions. Abbreviations are often used when health care providers discuss IV solutions. It is important for nurses to know the common IV solution components and the solution concentration strengths represented by such abbreviations. Refer to Box 21-1 and learn the common abbreviations for IV solutions.

BOX 21-1 Abbreviations for Common IV Solutions

NaCl	Sodium chloride
NS	Normal saline (0.9% NaCl)
$\frac{1}{2}$ NS	$\frac{1}{2}$ Normal saline (0.45% NaCl)
D5W or 5% D/W	Dextrose 5% in water
D5RL	Dextrose 5% and lactated Ringer's (Ringer's lactate)
RL or RLS	Lactated Ringer's solution (electrolytes)
D5NS	Dextrose 5% in Normal saline (0.9% NaCl)
D5 and $\frac{1}{2}$ NS (0.45%)	Dextrose 5% in $\frac{1}{2}$ Normal saline (0.45% NaCl)

Note: IV bags are labeled as sodium chloride (NaCl) but frequently referred to as normal saline (NS).

IV Solution Components

Intravenous fluids generally contain glucose (dextrose), sodium chloride (NaCl), water, and/or electrolytes. The components of IV fluids are indicated on the label of the IV fluid.

Solution Strength

The abbreviation letters indicate the components in the IV solution, and the numbers indicate the solution strength or concentration of the components in the IV fluid. The numbers may be written as subscripts; for example, D_5W (dextrose 5% in water).

Normal saline solutions are written with 0.9 and the percent sign included (e.g., D_5 0.9% NS). NS is the abbreviation used for normal saline. Normal saline is also referred to as sodium chloride (NaCl). Saline is available in different percentages. Normal saline is the common term used for 0.9% sodium chloride.

Another common saline IV concentration is 0.45% NaCl, often written as 1/2 NS (0.45% is half of 0.9%). Other saline solution strengths include 0.33% NaCl, also abbreviated as 1/3 NS, and 0.225% NaCl, also abbreviated as 1/4 NS. Some IV orders, therefore, may be written as 1/2 NS, 1/4 NS, 1/3 NS. IV solutions can contain saline only (see Figure 21-6) or saline mixed with dextrose, which would be indicated with percentage of dextrose (e.g., D_5 0.9% sodium chloride) (see Figures 21-3 and 21-4).

> **SAFETY ALERT!**
>
> Pay close attention to IV abbreviations. The letters indicate the solution components, whereas the numbers indicate the solution strength.

Let's examine some IV labels (see Figures 21-1 to 21-6). Recall from Chapter 5 that solution strength expressed as percent (%) indicates the number of grams (g) per 100 milliliters (mL).

- D_5W. This abbreviation means dextrose 5% in water, which means each 100 mL of solution contains 5 g dextrose (Figure 21-1).
- D_5 RL. This abbreviation means 5% dextrose in lactated Ringer's. Lactated Ringer's is a solution containing electrolytes, including potassium chloride and calcium chloride (Figure 21-2).
- 5% Dextrose and 0.9% sodium chloride. This solution contains 5 g of dextrose and 0.9 g (or 900 mg) of sodium chloride per 100 mL solution (Figure 21-3).
- 5% Dextrose and 0.45% sodium chloride. This solution contains 5 g of dextrose and 0.45 g (or 450 mg) of sodium chloride per 100 mL solution (Figure 21-4).

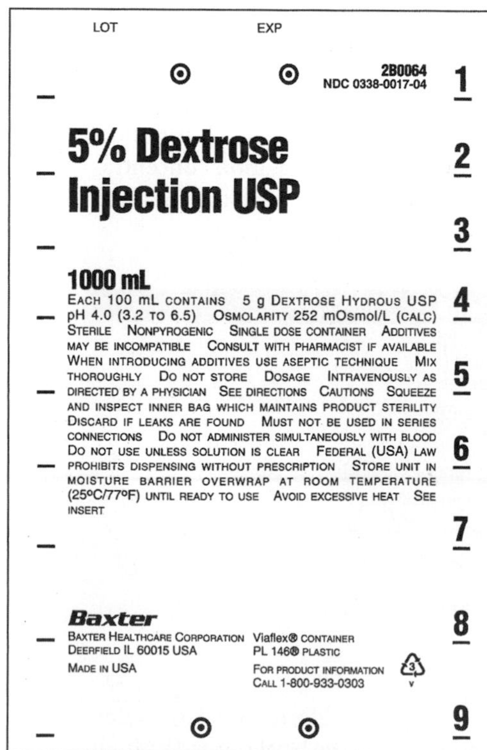

Figure 21-1 5% Dextrose (D5W).

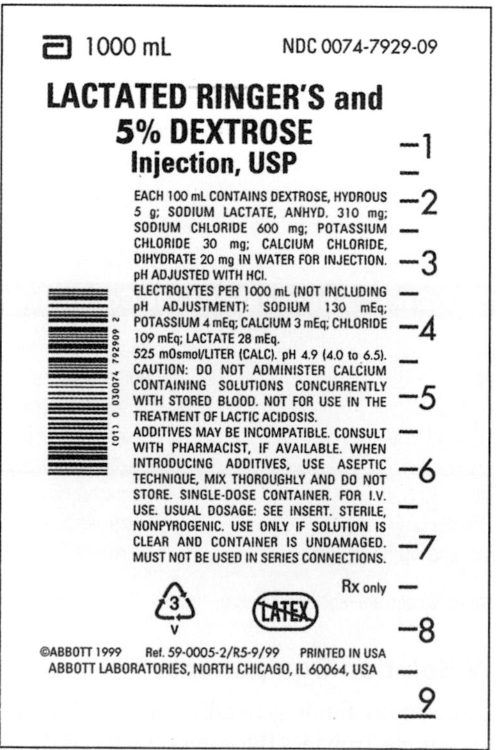

Figure 21-2 Lactated Ringer's and 5% dextrose (D5LR).

Notice Figure 21-5 also contains 5% dextrose and 0.45% sodium chloride like the IV label shown in Figure 21-4, but it also contains 20 mEq of potassium chloride. Potassium chloride is a high-alert medication. Notice the label on the IV has the "20 mEq potassium" indicated in red. **Do not confuse these two solutions. Always read labels carefully.**

- NS or 0.9% NaCl. This solution contains 0.9 g (or 900 mg) of sodium chloride per 100 mL (Figure 21-6).

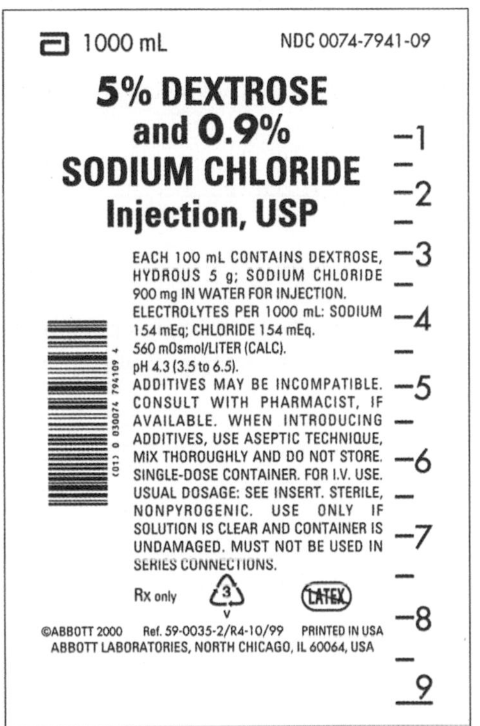

Figure 21-3 5% Dextrose in 0.9% sodium chloride.

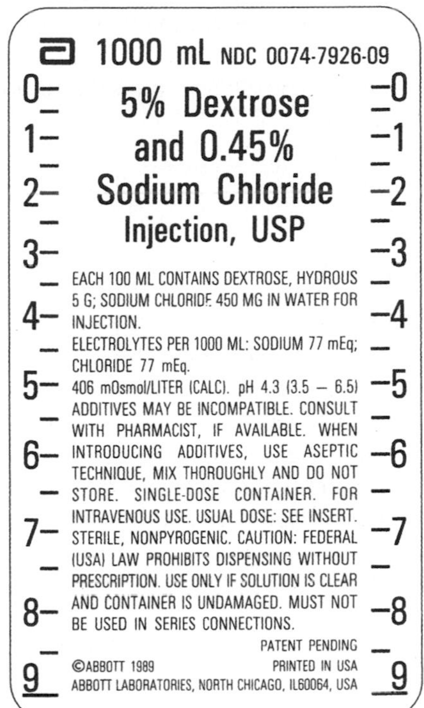

Figure 21-4 5% Dextrose in 0.45% sodium chloride.

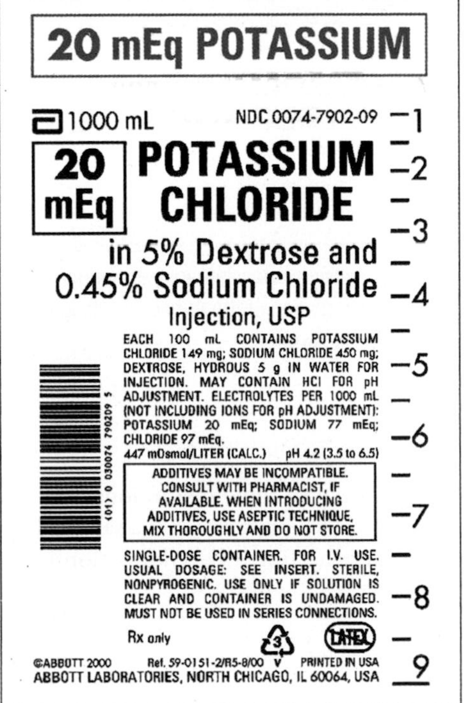

Figure 21-5 20 mEq Potassium chloride in 5% dextrose in 0.45% sodium chloride.

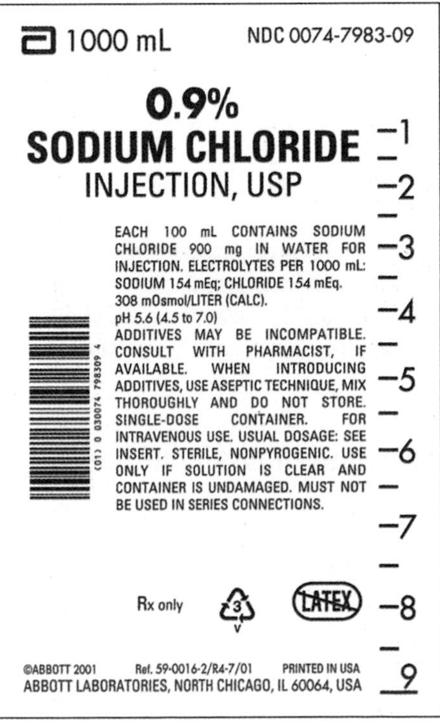

Figure 21-6 0.9% Sodium chloride.

IV Solution Additives

Some IV solutions are available, premixed by the manufacturer, with additives such as medications or electrolytes. Figure 21-5 shows an IV solution premixed with potassium chloride (KCl), a commonly prescribed additive to IV fluids. In many institutions, IV solutions are available premixed with potassium. Premixed additives are clearly marked on IV solution as shown in Figure 21-5. Additives can also be inserted into IV solution by the nurse or pharmacist. If this is done, a label indicating the name and amount of additive must be applied to the solution container.

SAFETY ALERT!

Before placing any additives in an IV solution (vitamins, medications, electrolytes), be sure the additives are compatible with the solution. Some incompatible additives may cause the solution to become cloudy or crystallize. Always verify the compatibility of the additive and solution.

IV Orders

The prescriber is responsible for writing the order. However, administering and monitoring an IV is a nursing responsibility. An IV order (Figure 21-7, shows sample IV orders) **must** specify the following:

- Name of the IV solution
- Name of medication to be added, if any
- Amount (volume) to be administered
- Time period during which the IV is to infuse

Order	Interpretation
D_5W 1,000 mL IV q8h	Infuse 1,000 mL 5% dextrose in water intravenously every 8 hours.
0.9% NS 1,000 mL IV with 20 mEq KCl per L q8h.	Infuse 1,000 mL 0.9% normal saline IV solution with 20 milliequivalents of potassium chloride added per liter every 8 hours.

Figure 21-7 Sample IV orders.

SAFETY ALERT!

Remember the following when adding potassium to an IV:

- It should be compatible with the solution and well diluted.
- Monitor client during infusion; rapid infusion of potassium can cause death due to cardiac depression, arrhythmias, and arrest.
- Check IV site frequently; medication is extremely irritating.
- Administer IV using an infusion control device.
- Never administer potassium concentrate IV push.
- **DO NOT** add potassium to an IV bag that is already infusing. Injecting potassium into an upright infusing IV solution causes the medication to concentrate in the lower portion of the IV bag, resulting in the client receiving a concentrated medication solution, which can be harmful.

Charting of IV Solution

IV fluids are charted on the intake and output (I&O) sheet; in some institutions, they are also charted on the medication administration record (MAR). Figure 21-8 is a sample I&O charting record. In institutions where there is computer charting, this information is entered into the electronic record.

Juice glass – 180 mL	Small water cup – 120 mL
Water glass – 210 mL	Jello cup – 150 mL
Coffee cup – 240 mL	Ice cream – 120 mL
Soup bowl – 180 mL	Creamer – 30 mL

Client information

Date: 8/17/17

INTAKE						OUTPUT			
Time	Type	Amt	Time	IV/ Blood type	Amount absorbed	Time	Urine	Stool	Other
			7A	1,000 mL D5W	800 mL	9A	400 mL		
			12P	IVPB	100 mL	1P	500 mL		
8 hr total					900 mL		900 mL		

Figure 21-8 Sample of charting IV fluids on I&O record.

Calculating Percentage of Solute in IV Fluids

The amount of each ingredient in an IV fluid can be calculated; however, it is not necessary because the label on the IV solution indicates the amount of each ingredient. Calculation of the percentage of solutions was presented in Chapter 5, which deals with percentages.

As you may recall, it is possible to determine the percentage of substances such as dextrose in IV solutions. It is important to remember that **solution strength expressed as a percentage means grams of solute per 100 mL of fluid.** Therefore, 5% dextrose solution will have 5 g of dextrose in each 100 mL. In addition to the amount of dextrose in the solution, amounts of other components, such as sodium chloride, can be determined. To calculate the amount of a specific component in an IV solution, a ratio and proportion or dimensional analysis can be used.

Example 1: Calculate the amount of dextrose in 500 mL D5W. Remember % = g per 100 mL; therefore, 5% dextrose = 5 g dextrose per 100 mL.

✓ Solution Using Ratio and Proportion

$$5 \text{ g}:100 \text{ mL} = x \text{ g}:500 \text{ mL} \quad or \quad \frac{5 \text{ g}}{100 \text{ mL}} = \frac{x \text{ g}}{500 \text{ mL}}$$

$$\frac{100x}{100} = \frac{2{,}500}{100}$$

$$x = 25 \text{ g}$$

500 mL D5W contains 25 g of dextrose

Remember that ratios and proportions can be stated in various formats.

✔ Solution Using Dimensional Analysis

5% dextrose = 5 g dextrose per 100 mL. Enter it as the starting fraction, and determine the number of grams in the solution.

$$x\text{ g} = \frac{5\text{ g}}{\underset{1}{\cancel{100\text{ mL}}}} \times \frac{\overset{5}{\cancel{500\text{ mL}}}}{1}$$

$$x = 25\text{ g dextrose}$$

500 mL D5W contains 25 g dextrose

Example 2: Calculate the amount of sodium chloride (NaCl) in 1,000 mL NS.

0.9% = 0.9 g NaCl per 100 mL

✔ Solution Using Ratio and Proportion

$$0.9\text{ g}:100\text{ mL} = x\text{ g}:1{,}000\text{ mL} \quad or \quad \frac{0.9\text{ g}}{100\text{ mL}} = \frac{x\text{ g}}{1{,}000\text{ mL}}$$

$$\frac{100x}{100} = \frac{900}{100}$$

$$x = 9\text{ g NaCl}$$

1,000 mL of NS contains 9 g of sodium chloride

✔ Solution Using Dimensional Analysis

0.9% = 0.9 g NaCl per 100 mL. Use the grams of solute per 100 mL of fluid as the starting fraction.

$$x\text{ g} = \frac{0.9\text{ g}}{\underset{1}{\cancel{100\text{ mL}}}} \times \frac{\overset{10}{\cancel{1{,}000\text{ mL}}}}{1}$$

$$x = 9\text{ g NaCl}$$

1,000 mL of NS contains 9 g of NaCl

Example 3: Calculate the amount of dextrose and sodium chloride in 1,000 mL of 5% dextrose and 0.45% normal saline (D5 and ½ NS).

✔ Solution Using Ratio and Proportion

D5 = dextrose 5% = 5 g dextrose per 100 mL

0.45% NS = 0.45 g NaCl per 100 mL

$$\text{Dextrose: } 5\text{ g}:100\text{ mL} = x\text{ g}:1{,}000\text{ mL} \quad or \quad \frac{5\text{ g}}{100\text{ mL}} = \frac{x\text{ g}}{1{,}000\text{ mL}}$$

$$\frac{100x}{100} = \frac{5{,}000}{100}$$

$$x = 50\text{ g dextrose}$$

$$\text{NaCl: } 0.45\text{ g}:100\text{ mL} = x\text{ g}:1{,}000\text{ mL} \quad or \quad \frac{0.45\text{ g}}{100\text{ mL}} = \frac{x\text{ g}}{1{,}000\text{ mL}}$$

$$\frac{100x}{100} = \frac{450}{100}$$

$$x = 4.5\text{ g NaCl}$$

1,000 mL D5 0.45% NS contains 50 g of dextrose and 4.5 g of NaCl

✓ Solution Using Dimensional Analysis

5% dextrose = 5 g dextrose per 100 mL

0.45% NS = 0.45 g NaCl per 100 mL

$$\text{Dextrose: } x\text{ g} = \frac{5\text{ g}}{\cancel{100\text{ mL}}_{1}} \times \frac{\cancel{1{,}000\text{ mL}}^{10}}{1}$$

$$x = 50\text{ g dextrose}$$

$$\text{NaCl: } x\text{ g} = \frac{0.45\text{ g}}{\cancel{100\text{ mL}}_{1}} \times \frac{\cancel{1{,}000\text{ mL}}^{10}}{1}$$

$$x = 4.5\text{ g NaCl}$$

1,000 mL D5 0.45% NS contains 50 g of dextrose and 4.5 g of NaCl

IV Sites

IV fluids may be administered through a peripheral line or central line.

- **Peripheral line**—is generally used for short-term therapy. The infusion site of a peripheral line is a vein in the arm, hand, or scalp in an infant; or if other sites are not accessible, and on rare occasions, a vein in the leg.
- **Central line**—provides direct access to large major veins. Used for long-term therapy. For a central line, a special catheter is used to access a large vein such as the subclavian or jugular vein. A central line is used for infusion of large amounts of fluids and for infusion of highly concentrated electrolyte replacements, chemotherapy (infusion of medications for cancer), and total parenteral nutrition (TPN). TPN is an IV solution that provides nutrients. Parenteral nutrition solutions consist of glucose, amino acids, minerals, vitamins, and/or fat emulsions. Examples of central catheters include triple lumen, Hickman, Broviac, and Groshong catheters. When a peripheral vein is used to access a central vein, you may see the term *peripherally inserted central catheter* or **PICC line.** A PICC line is inserted into the antecubital vein in the arm and is advanced into the superior vena cava. A **Port-A-Cath** is used to deliver medication to a central vein. It is surgically placed under the skin and accessed through the skin to intermittently administer IV medications.

Monitoring IVs

The nurse is responsible for monitoring the client during an IV infusion. IV site and the infusion should be checked according to hospital policy for the volume of remaining fluid, the correct infusion rate, and for signs of complications. It is the nurse's responsibility to maintain and regulate IV infusions.

Administration of IV Fluids

IV fluids are administered by an IV infusion set, which includes a sealed bag containing the fluids. A drip chamber is connected to the IV bottle or bag. The flow rate is adjusted to drops per minute (gtt/min) by use of a roller clamp. Some IV tubings have a sliding clamp attached, which can be used to temporarily stop the IV infusion. Injection ports are located on the IV tubing and on most IV solution bags. Injection ports allow for injection of medications directly into the bag of solution or line. The injection ports also allow for attachment of secondary IV lines that contain fluids or medications to the primary line. Figure 21-9 shows a primary line infusion set. IV fluids infuse by gravity flow. This means that for the IV solution to infuse, it must be hung above the level of the client's heart, which will allow for adequate pressure to be exerted for the IV to infuse. The height of the IV bag, therefore, has a relationship to the rate of flow. The higher the IV bag is hung, the greater the pressure; therefore, the IV will infuse at a more rapid rate.

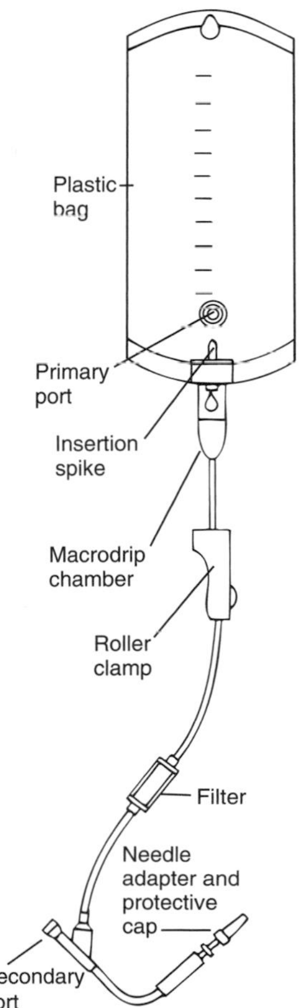

Figure 21-9 Intravenous infusion set. (From Clayton BD, Willihnganz M: *Basic pharmacology for nurse,* ed 17, St Louis, 2017, Mosby.)

Primary and Secondary Lines

Medications may be added to a primary line either before the IV is started or after it has been infusing. Examples of medications added include electrolytes, such as potassium chloride, and vitamins, such as multivitamins (MVI). These medications are usually diluted in a large volume of fluid (1,000 mL), particularly potassium chloride, because of the side effects and untoward reactions that can occur. In some institutions IV solutions containing potassium chloride are stocked by the pharmacy and obtained on request by the unit, eliminating the need to add it to an IV bag. **Secondary lines** attach to the primary line at an injection port. The main purpose of secondary lines is to infuse medications on an intermittent basis (e.g., antibiotics every 6 hr). They can also be used to infuse other IV fluids, as long as they are compatible with the fluid on the primary line. A secondary line is referred to as an IV piggyback (IVPB). Notice that the IVPB is hanging higher than the primary line (Figure 21-10, *A*).

The IVPB is hanging higher than the primary line so that it gives it greater pressure than the primary, thereby allowing it to infuse first. Most secondary administration sets come with an extender that allows the nurse to lower the primary bag. Notice that the secondary bags are smaller than the primary. Amounts of 50 to 100 mL are seen most often. The amount of solution used for the IVPB is determined by the medication being added. Some medications may have to be mixed in 250 mL of fluid for administration. IVPB medications can come premixed by the manufacturer or pharmacist, depending on the institution, or the nurse may have to prepare them. The rate for an IVPB to infuse should be checked. The manufacturer's insert provides recommended times for infusion if not stated in the prescriber's order.

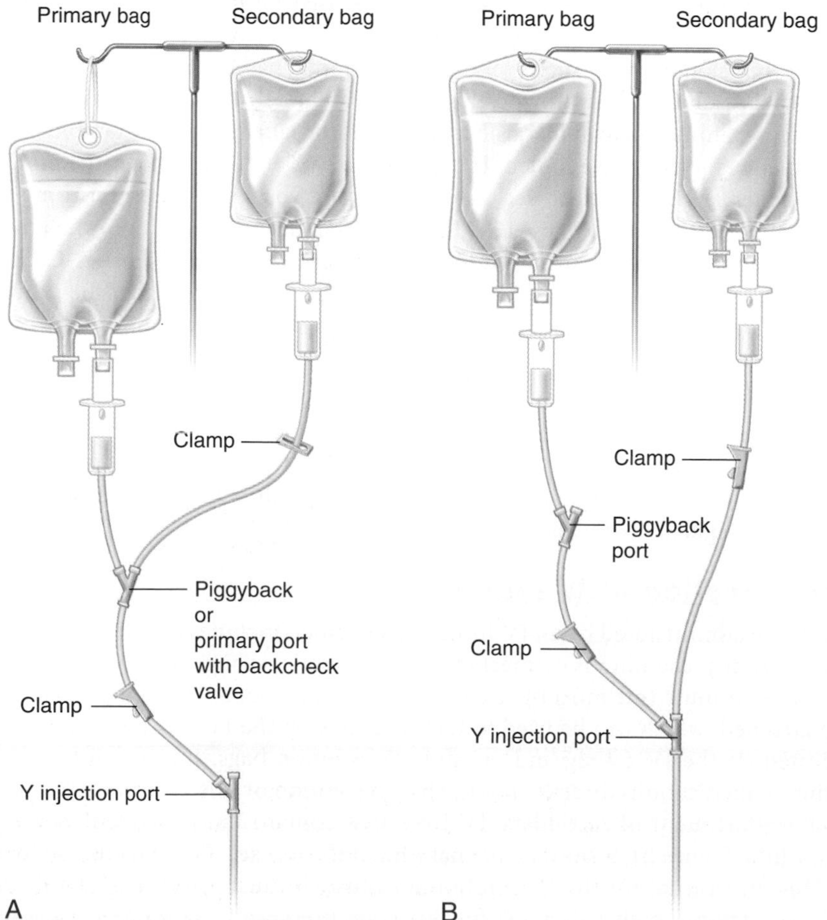

Figure 21-10 **A,** Piggyback. **B,** Tandem. (From Harkreader H, Hogan MA: *Fundamentals of nursing: caring and clinical judgment,* ed 3, St. Louis, 2007, Saunders.)

Blood Administration Tubing

The administration of blood and blood products is commonly done with a special tubing called Y-tubing. The "Y" refers to two spikes above the drip chamber of the IV tubing. One spike is attached to the blood container, and the other is attached to a container of normal saline (NaCl) solution. Normal saline is used to flush the IV tubing before and after the transfusion. Tubing for blood administration has an in-line filter (to remove small clots (micro emboli) and particles from the blood before it's infused into the client). Blood may be administered by gravity or electronic pump (Figure 21-11). Blood transfusions and blood products are regulated in the same manner as any other intravenous infusion and also involve calculation of flow rates and infusion times.

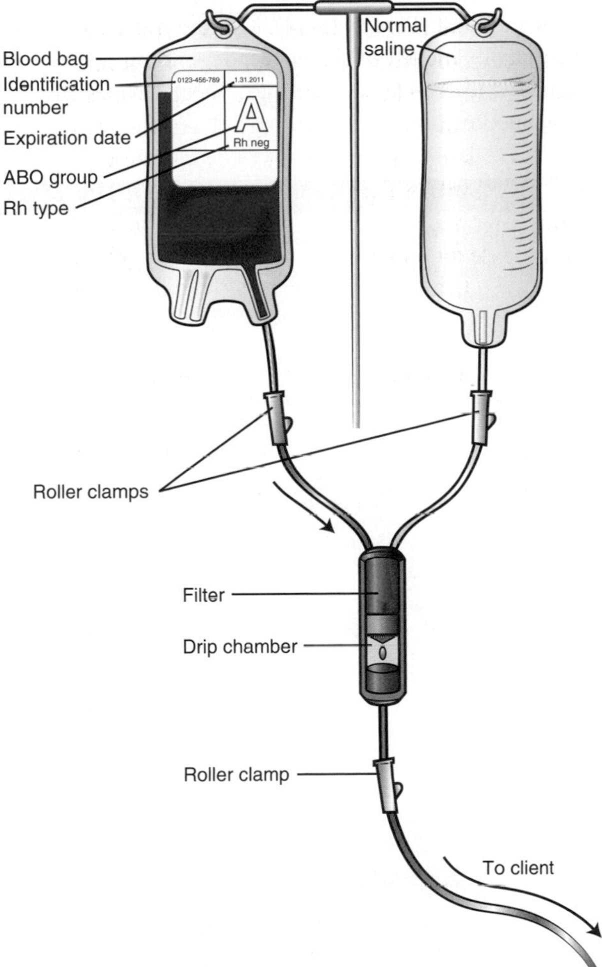

Figure 21-11 Setup for blood administration.

Systems for Administering Medications by Intravenous Piggyback

Tandem Piggyback Setup. The tandem piggyback setup is a small IV bag connected to the port of a primary infusion line or to an intermittent venous access. Unlike the piggyback setup, however, the small IV bag that is to infuse is placed at the same height as the primary infusion bag or bottle. In this setup the tandem and primary IV solution infuse simultaneously (see Figure 21-10, *B*). The nurse must monitor the tandem system closely and clamp the tandem setup immediately once the medication has infused to prevent the IV solution from the primary line from backing up into the tandem line.

Another type of secondary medication setup used in some institutions is called the **ADD-Vantage system.** This system requires a special type of IV bag that has a port for inserting the medication (usually in powder form and mixed with the IV solution as a diluent). The contents of the vial are therefore mixed into the total solution and then infused (Figure 21-12).

The Baxter Mini-Bag Plus is also used to administer piggyback medication. The mini-bag, which is dispensed by the pharmacy, has a vial of unreconstituted medication attached to a special port. You break an internal seal and mix the medication and diluent just before administration. The medication vial remains attached to the mini-bag (Figure 21-13).

Volume control devices are used for accurate measurement of small-volume medications and fluids. Most volume control devices have a capacity of 100 to 150 mL and can be used with secondary or primary lines. They are also used intermittently for medication purposes. They have a port that allows medication to be injected and a certain amount of IV fluid to be added as a diluent (Figure 21-14). Volume control devices are referred to by their trade names (Volutrol, Soluset, or Buretrol), depending on the institution. They are used mostly in pediatrics and critical care settings. These devices allow for precise control of the infusion and the medication.

SAFETY ALERT!

When an infusion time is not stated for IVPB, check appropriate resources, such as a medication book or the hospital pharmacy. The nurse is responsible for any error that occurs in reference to IV administration, including incorrect rate of administration.

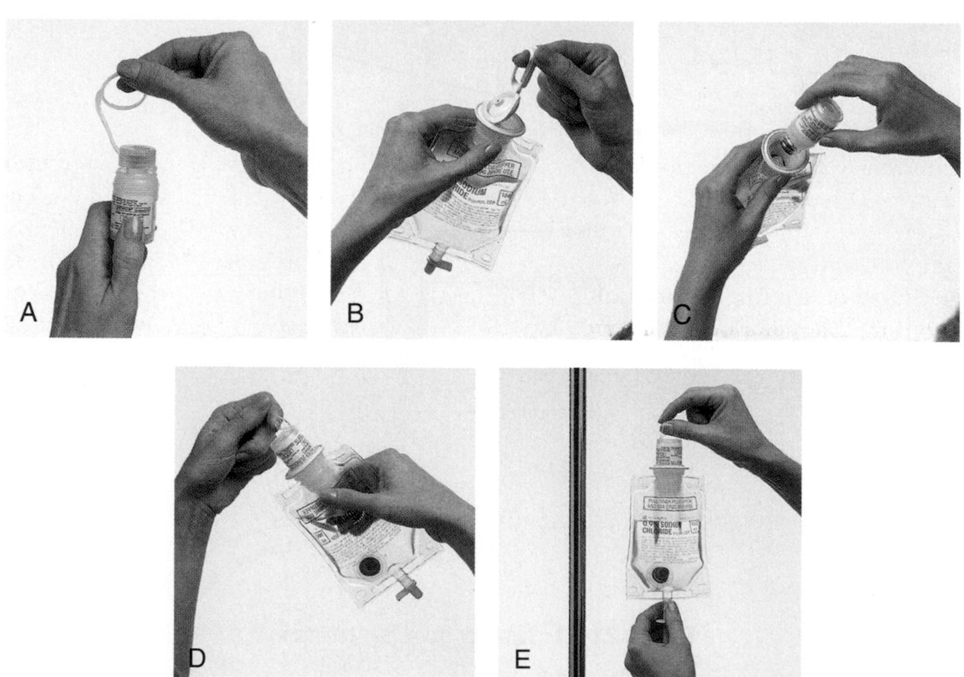

Figure 21-12 Assembling and administering medication with the ADD-VANTAGE® system. **A,** Swing the pull ring over the top of the vial, and pull down far enough to start the opening. Then pull straight up to remove the cap. Avoid touching the rubber stopper and vial threads. **B,** Hold diluent container and gently grasp the tab on the pull ring. Pull up to break the tie membrane. Pull back to remove the cover. Avoid touching the inside of the vial port. **C,** Screw the vial into the vial port until it will go no further. Recheck the vial to ensure that it is tight. Label appropriately. **D,** Mix container contents thoroughly to ensure complete dissolution. Look through bottom of vial to verify complete mixing. Check for leaks by squeezing container firmly. If leaks are found, discard unit. **E,** When ready to administer, remove the white administration port cover and pierce the container with the piercing pin. (From Hospira, Inc., Lake Forest, IL.)

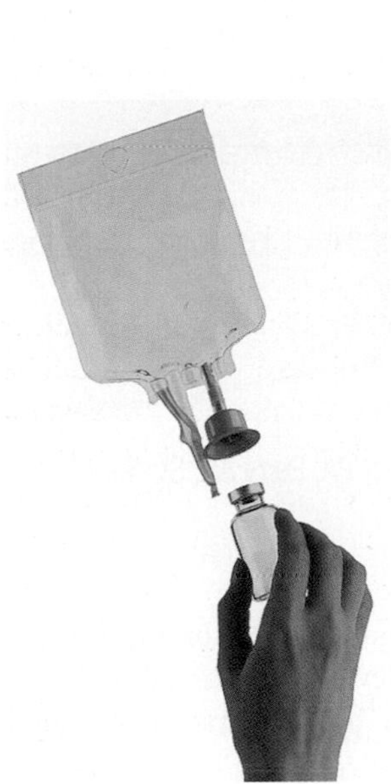

Figure 21-13 Mini-Bag Plus. (From Baxter Healthcare Corporation, Deerfield, IL.)

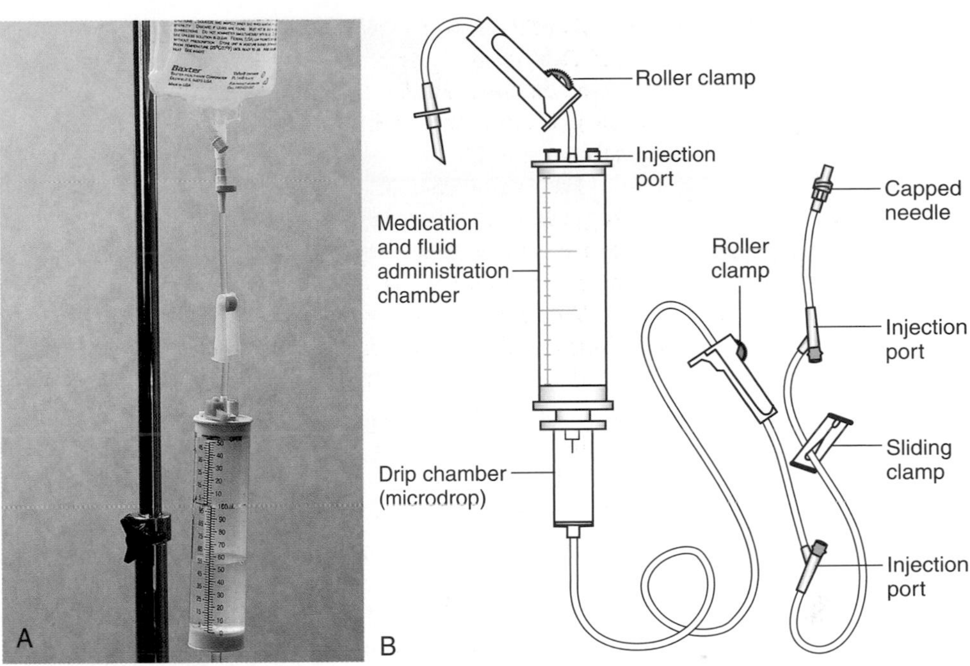

Figure 21-14 **A,** Volume-controlled device. **B,** Parts of a volume control set. (**A,** From Potter PA, Perry AG, Stockert P, Hall A: *Essentials for Nursing Practice,* ed 8, St Louis, 2015, Mosby.)

Saline and Heparin IV Locks

Intermittent venous access devices (Figure 21-15) are used for the purpose of administering IV medication intermittently or for access to a vein in an emergency situation. Intermittent venous access devices are referred to as *medlocks, saline locks, heplocks,* and *intermittent peripheral infusion devices* (IPIDs). The line is usually kept free from blockage or clotting by irrigating it with heparin (anticoagulant) or sterile saline solution. The solution used and the amount of solution vary from institution to institution.

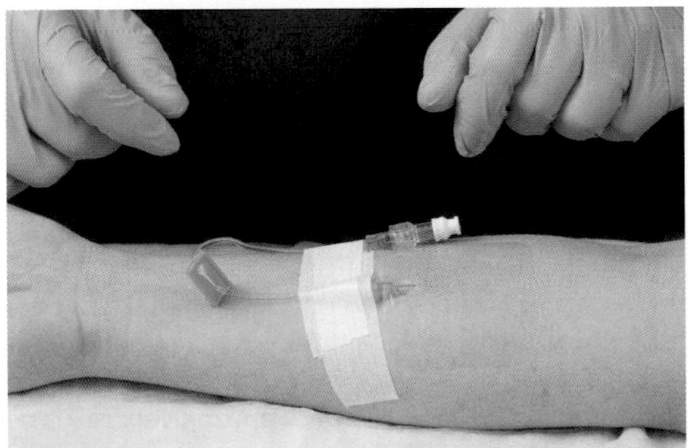

Figure 21-15 Intermittent lock covered with a rubber diaphragm. (From Potter PA, Perry AG, Stockert P, Hall A: *Fundamentals of nursing,* ed 9, St Louis, 2016, Mosby.)

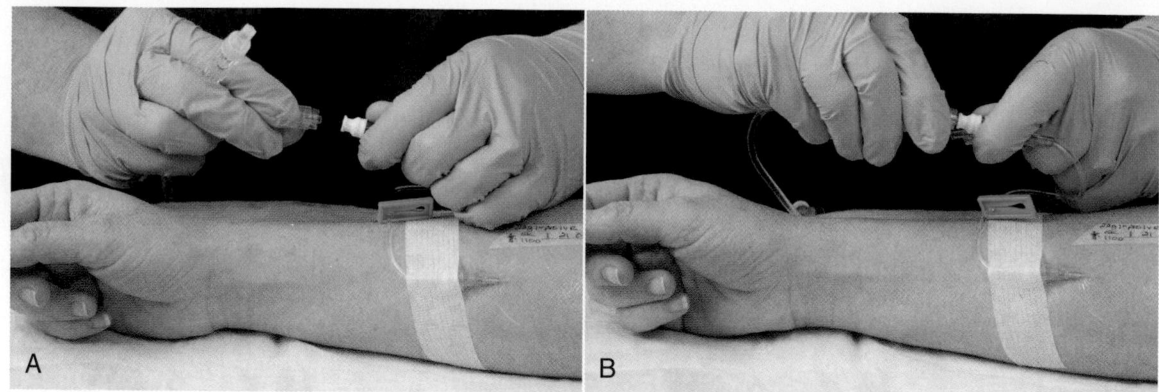

Figure 21-16 **A,** Needleless infusion system. **B,** Connection into an injection port. (From Potter PA, Perry AG, Stockert P, Hall A: *Fundamentals of nursing,* ed 9, St Louis, 2016, Mosby.)

Various institutions have purchased a needleless system (Figure 21-16) for administration of medications through the primary line and for access devices such as saline locks. The needleless system does not require attachment of a needle by the nurse. The system allows for administration by IV push, bolus, or piggyback.

When medications are administered through intermittent venous access devices (also called *access devices*), they must be periodically flushed to maintain patency. Due to bolusing of clients when heparin is used, heparin (a potent anticoagulant despite its use in dilute forms) is now used only on the initial insertion of the catheter. For subsequent flushings of the port, normal saline solution is used (1 to 3 mL, depending on institution policy).

SAFETY ALERT!

Remember that heparin is a high-alert medication that comes in many dosage strengths (concentrations). The concentration for a heparin lock flush is 10 units per mL or 100 units per mL. The average heparin flush dosage is 10 units and **never** exceeds 100 units. Always check the concentration of heparin carefully.

When medications are administered through an intermittent access device, the device must be flushed before and after medication is given. The letters used in most institutions to remember the technique for medication administration are S, I, S (saline, IV medications, saline). Some institutions use the acronym SAS (saline, administer medication, saline). With early discharge and an increased number of home care clients discharged with access devices in place, it is imperative that clients be taught about the care of the intermittent access device.

SAFETY ALERT!

Always refer to the policy at your institution or health care agency regarding the frequency, volume, and concentration of saline or heparin to be used to maintain the IV lock.

Medications can be administered through a port used for direct injection of medication by syringe or directly into the vein by venipuncture. This is referred to as IV **push** or **bolus.** IV *push* indicates that a syringe is attached to the lock and the medication is pushed in. IV *bolus* indicates that a volume of IV fluid is infused over a specific period of time through an IV administration set attached to the lock. There are guidelines, however, relating to the acceptable rate for IV push administration. **Check appropriate references for the rate for IV push medication administration.** Also check the institution's policy and a pharmacology reference regarding administration by IV push or bolus.

Electronic Infusion Devices

There are several electronic infusion devices on the market to regulate intravenous fluid and/or medication infusions (e.g., an IV Pump). See Figure 21-17. Each device can be set

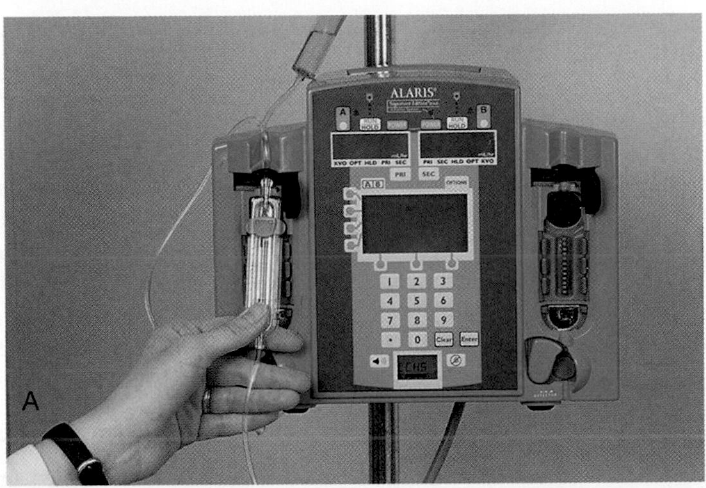

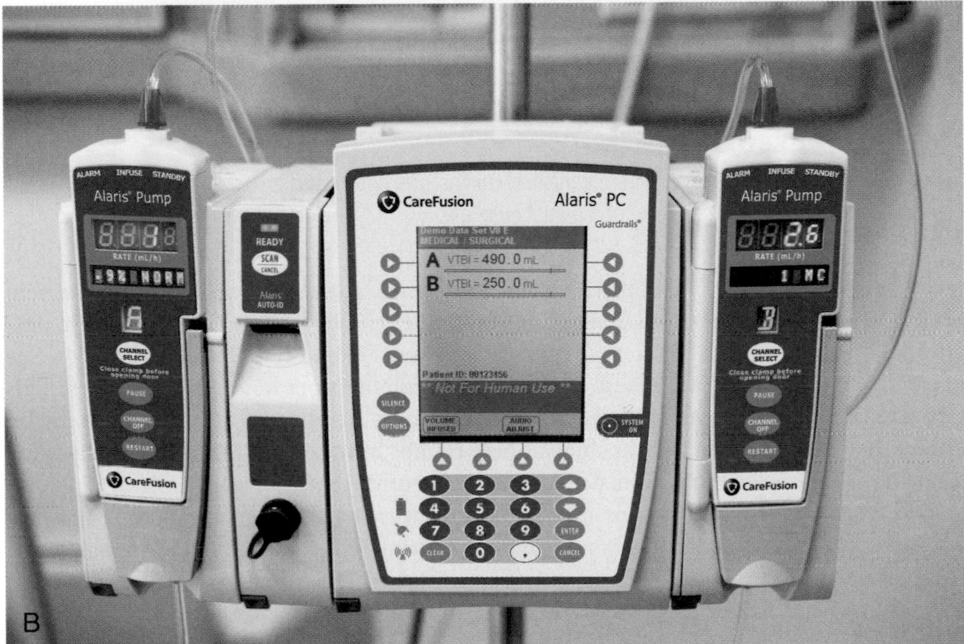

Figure 21-17 **A,** Dual-channel infusion pump. **B,** Alaris® System. (**A,** From Potter PA, Perry AG, Stockert P, Hall A: *Fundamentals of nursing,* ed 9, St Louis, 2016, Mosby. **B,** From CareFusion.)

for a specific flow rate and generally emits an alarm if the rate is interrupted. The use of electronic infusion devices is based on the need to strictly regulate the IV. Electronic infusion devices are essential in pediatrics and the critical care setting, where they provide for infusion of small amounts of fluid or medications with precision. Manufacturers supply special tubing that must be used with their infusion devices. Most of the electronic infusion devices in current use are powered by direct current (from a wall unit) as well as having an internal rechargeable battery. When unplugged (e.g., to allow client ambulation), the battery becomes the power source.

While infusion pumps were designed to improve client safety and provide more precise and accurate delivery of IV therapy, infusion pumps are not without dangers and present significant threats to client safety, with various performance problems that have resulted in both over- and underinfusion. Pump efficacy is a primary and continual concern of the U.S. Food and Drug Administration (FDA). Problems with infusion pumps that have been cited by the FDA include alarm errors, battery failures, and inadequate interface design (FDA 2014). There are several strategies recommended by the FDA (2010b) to reduce client risk when using infusion pumps, which include planning ahead, labeling, and frequent checking. Planning ahead includes having a backup plan for the replacement of IV pumps with electrical or mechanical failure.

Other strategies that have been documented to increase safety during the use of infusion pumps include, when using multiple-channel pumps, labeling each infusion line and conducting frequent rounds to double-check IV solutions and detect device programming errors. Infusions of high-alert medications should undergo independent double-checking before administration. It is also recommended that IV fluid and medication labels be prominently displayed on the infusion pump and the tubing at the port of entry. Because of the errors that have occurred with infusion devices because of incorrect programming, it is mandatory that all programming of infusion devices be double-checked. Hospital or clinical in-service education is required for the use of all infusion devices. Nurses need to apply the six "rights" of safe medication administration to IV pumps. The right client should always receive the right fluid and/or medication by the appropriate IV pump programmed to deliver the right dosage and volume with the right documentation and continual monitoring. Do not rely solely on the pump. The nurse is still responsible for ensuring client safety.

Available on the market today are programmable infusion pumps, called smart pumps, that have safety features designed to help in the prevention of medication errors. Smart pumps have customized software that has a reference library of medications indicating the minimum and maximum rates at which medications should safely infuse.

SAFETY ALERT!

An institution may use many different infusion pumps. The health care provider must know how to use them correctly to prevent client harm and a fatal outcome.

Electronic Volumetric Pumps. Electronic volumetric pumps infuse fluids into the vein under pressure and against resistance and do not depend on gravity. The pumps are programmed to deliver a set amount of fluid per hour (see Figure 21-17). There is a wide range of electronic pumps. Because these pumps deliver milliliters per hour (mL/hr), any milliliter calculation that results in a decimal fraction must be rounded to a whole milliliter, unless the pump has decimal capability. These pumps may be seen in some intensive care units and are also used to administer chemotherapeutic agents.

Syringe Pumps. Syringe pumps are electronic devices that deliver medications or fluids by use of a syringe. The medication is measured in a syringe and attached to the special pump, and the medication is infused at a set rate (Figure 21-18). These pumps are useful in pediatrics and intensive care units, as well as in labor and delivery areas, hospice, and critical care.

Patient-Controlled Analgesia Devices. Patient-controlled analgesia is a form of pain management that allows the client to self-administer IV analgesics. This is accomplished by using a computerized infuser pump attached to the IV line (Figure 21-19, *B*). The patient-controlled analgesia (PCA) pump is programmed to allow dosages of narcotics only within specific limits to be delivered to prevent overdosage. The dosage and frequency of administration are ordered by the prescriber and set on the pump. The client self-medicates by use of a control button. The pump also keeps a record of the number of times the client uses it. The display on the pump lets clients know when they are able to medicate themselves and when it is impossible to give themselves another dosage. The pump therefore has what is called a lockout interval. This is an interval during which no medications are delivered. A medication commonly administered by PCA is morphine (30 mg morphine per 30 mL). Portable PCA pumps are also available and are battery operated (see Figure 21-19, *A*).

Nurses must be familiar with the infusion devices used at their institution; in-service education is essential in the use of all infusion devices.

The Joint Commission's (TJC) 2005 National Patient Safety Goals established a goal designed to improve client safety when using infusion pumps. Health care organizations are required to ensure free-flow protection on all infusion devices and PCA pumps. Free-flow protection means that the tubing has a built-in mechanism similar to a clamp that is mobilized when the tubing is removed from the pump, therefore preventing flow of fluid into the client when the pump is stopped or the tubing is taken out of the infusion pump.

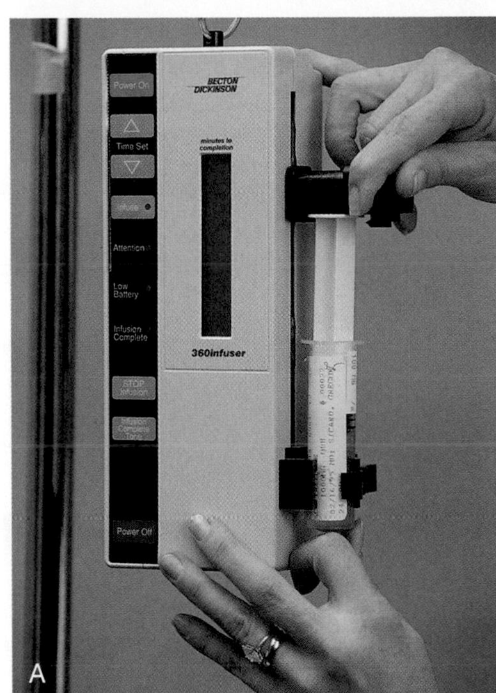

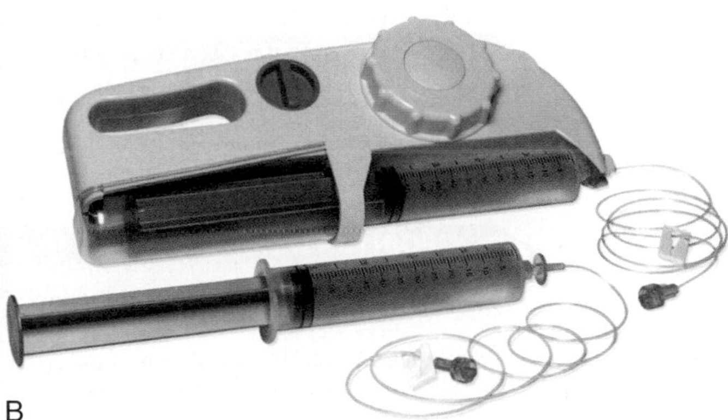

Figure 21-18 **A,** Syringe inserted into syringe pump. **B,** Freedom 60 syringe infusion pump system. (**A,** From Perry AG, Potter PA, Elkin MK, Ostendorf WR: *Nursing interventions and clinical skills,* ed 6, St Louis, 2016, Mosby. **B,** From Repro-Med Systems, Inc., Chester, NY.)

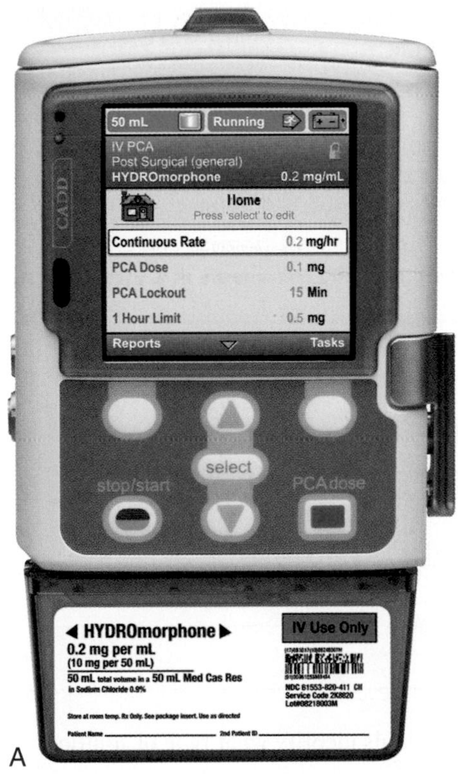

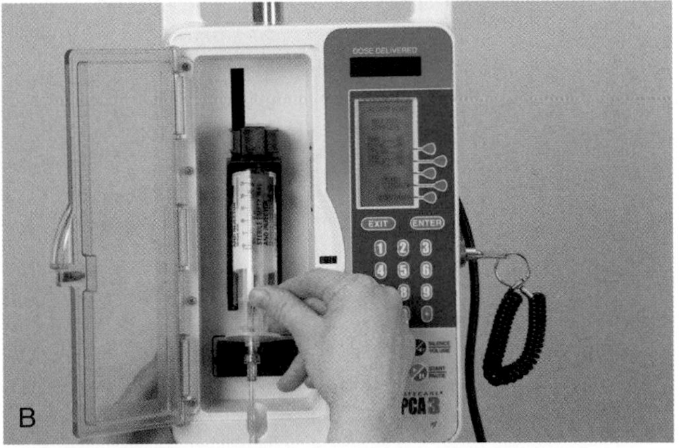

Figure 21-19 **A,** CADD®-Solis pain management pump. **B,** Patient-controlled analgesia (PCA) ambulatory infusion pump. (**A,** From Smiths Medical ASD, Inc., St. Paul, MN. **B,** From Perry AG, Potter PA, Elkin MK, Ostendorf WR: *Nursing interventions and clinical skills,* ed 6, St Louis, 2016, Mosby.)

Infusion Devices for the Home Care Setting

Another type of infusion device is the balloon device, which is used mainly in outpatient and home care settings to administer single-dose infusion therapies. One such device is the elastometric balloon device, which is made of soft, rubberized, disposable material that inflates to a predetermined volume to hold and dispense a single dose of IV medication. Baxter manufactures this type of IV system. Med Flo, an ambulatory infusion device, is another system developed for ambulatory use. This device can be placed in a pocket to conceal it. Other infusion sets available include battery-operated pumps.

SAFETY ALERT!

Clients must be educated about any electronic device they will use. Both devices and clients must be monitored to ascertain proper functioning.

POINTS TO REMEMBER

- IV orders are written by the doctor or other prescriber certified to do so (e.g., nurse practitioner, physician's assistant).
- IV orders must specify the name of the solution, medications (if any are to be added), the amount to be administered, and the infusion time.
- Several electronic devices are on the market for infusing IV solutions. Always familiarize yourself with the equipment before use.
- Follow the institution's protocol for IV administration.
- Nurses have the primary responsibility for monitoring the client during IV therapy.
- Nurses are responsible for any errors that occur in administration of IV fluids (e.g., inadequate dilution, too rapid infusion).
- Pay close attention to IV abbreviations. The letters indicate the solution components, and the numbers indicate the solution strength.
- Solution strength expressed as a percentage (%) indicates grams of solute per 100 mL of fluid.
- Principles relating to flow rate and infusion times are also applicable to parenteral nutrition solutions and blood and blood products.
- Apply the six rights of medication administration to IV infusion pumps. The nurse is responsible to ensure client safety when a client is receiving fluids and/or medications by an infusion pump.

PRACTICE **PROBLEMS**

Answer the following questions as briefly as possible.

1. What does PCA stand for? ____________________

2. An IV initiated in a client's lower arm is called what type of line?

   ____

3. IVPB is an abbreviation for ____________________.

4. A client has an IV of 1,000 mL 0.9% NS. The initials identify what type of solution?

   ____

5. A secondary line is hung ____________________ than the primary line.

6. Volumetric pumps infuse fluids into the vein by ____________________.

Identify the components and percentage strength of the following IV solutions:

7. D20W ______________________________

8. D5W 10 mEq KCl ______________________________

9. How many grams of dextrose does 500 mL D10W contain? ______________

Calculate the amount of dextrose and/or sodium chloride in the following IV solutions:

10. 750 mL D5 NS

dextrose ______________________________

NaCl ______________________________

11. 250 mL D10W

dextrose ______________________________

12. 1,000 mL D5 0.33% NS

dextrose ______________________________

NaCl ______________________________

13. 500 mL D5 ½ NS

dextrose ______________________________

NaCl ______________________________

Answers on p. 534

CLINICAL **REASONING**

Scenario: A client returned to the unit after surgery connected to a patient-controlled analgesia (PCA) pump. An order was written to attach a solution of 100 mL 0.9% normal saline (NS) with morphine 100 mg to the pump and infuse at a rate of 1 mg per 6 min. The ordered solution was inserted into the device and the rate set. The client had been instructed on the use of the PCA pump. The client continued to complain of severe pain on each shift despite the pump indicating that medication was being received at the set rate. The client received intermittent boluses of morphine to relieve pain.

Twenty-four hours later a nurse opened the PCA pump, found the full bag of IV solution in place, and noticed that the tubing had not been primed.

What should have been done in this situation?

____

____

____

Answer on p. 534

CHAPTER REVIEW

For each of the following IV solutions labeled *A* to *D* specify the letter of the illustration corresponding to the fluid abbreviation.

1. D5 ½ NS ______________________

2. D5W ______________________

3. RL ______________________

4. D5NS ______________________

5. A client has a PCA in use following surgery. What is this device used to control?
____

6. When an IV medication is injected directly into the vein through a port, it is called an IV ______________ or ______________.

LOT EXP

2B2324
NDC 0338-0117-04
DIN 00061085

Lactated Ringer's Injection USP

1000 mL

Each 100 mL contains 600 mg Sodium Chloride USP 310 mg Sodium Lactate 30 mg Potassium Chloride USP 20 mg Calcium Chloride USP pH 6.5 (6.0 to 7.5) mEq/L Sodium 130 Potassium 4 Calcium 2.7 Chloride 109 Lactate 28 Osmolarity 273 mOsmol/L (calc) Sterile Nonpyrogenic Single dose container **Not for use in the treatment of lactic acidosis** Additives may be incompatible Consult with pharmacist if available When introducing additives use aseptic technique Mix thoroughly Do not store Dosage intravenously as directed by a physician See directions Cautions Squeeze and inspect inner bag which maintains product sterility Discard if leaks are found Must not be used in series connections Do not administer simultaneously with blood Do not use unless solution is clear Federal (USA) law prohibits dispensing without prescription Store unit in moisture barrier overwrap at room temperature (25°C/77°F) until ready to use Avoid excessive heat See insert

Baxter
Baxter Healthcare Corporation
Deerfield IL 60015 USA
Made in USA
Distributed in Canada by
Baxter Corporation
Toronto Ontario Canada
Viaflex® container
PL 146® plastic
For product information
Call 1-800-933-0303

A

LOT EXP

2B1073
NDC 0338-0085-03

5% Dextrose and 0.45% Sodium Chloride Injection USP

500 mL

Each 100 mL contains 5 g Dextrose Hydrous USP 450 mg Sodium Chloride USP pH 4.0 (3.2 to 6.5) mEq/L Sodium 77 Chloride 77 Hypertonic Osmolarity 406 mOsmol/L (calc) Sterile Nonpyrogenic Single dose container Additives may be incompatible Consult with pharmacist if available When introducing additives use aseptic technique Mix thoroughly Do not store Dosage intravenously as directed by a physician See directions Cautions Squeeze and inspect inner bag which maintains product sterility Discard if leaks are found Must not be used in series connections Do not use unless solution is clear Federal (USA) law prohibits dispensing without prescription Store unit in moisture barrier overwrap at room temperature (25°C/77°F) until ready to use Avoid excessive heat See insert

Baxter
Baxter Healthcare Corporation
Deerfield IL 60015 USA
Made in USA
Viaflex® container
PL 146® plastic
For product information
Call 1-800-933-0303

B

LOT EXP
2B0064
NDC 0338-0017-04
5% Dextrose Injection USP
1000 mL
EACH 100 mL CONTAINS 5 g DEXTROSE HYDROUS USP pH 4.0 (3.2 TO 6.5) OSMOLARITY 252 mOsmol/L (CALC) STERILE NONPYROGENIC SINGLE DOSE CONTAINER ADDITIVES MAY BE INCOMPATIBLE CONSULT WITH PHARMACIST IF AVAILABLE WHEN INTRODUCING ADDITIVES USE ASEPTIC TECHNIQUE MIX THOROUGHLY DO NOT STORE DOSAGE INTRAVENOUSLY AS DIRECTED BY A PHYSICIAN SEE DIRECTIONS CAUTIONS SQUEEZE AND INSPECT INNER BAG WHICH MAINTAINS PRODUCT STERILITY DISCARD IF LEAKS ARE FOUND MUST NOT BE USED IN SERIES CONNECTIONS DO NOT ADMINISTER SIMULTANEOUSLY WITH BLOOD DO NOT USE UNLESS SOLUTION IS CLEAR FEDERAL (USA) LAW PROHIBITS DISPENSING WITHOUT PRESCRIPTION STORE UNIT IN MOISTURE BARRIER OVERWRAP AT ROOM TEMPERATURE (25ºC/77ºF) UNTIL READY TO USE AVOID EXCESSIVE HEAT SEE INSERT
Baxter
BAXTER HEALTHCARE CORPORATION
DEERFIELD IL 60015 USA
MADE IN USA
Viaflex® CONTAINER
PL 146® PLASTIC
FOR PRODUCT INFORMATION
CALL 1-800-933-0303
1 2 3 4 5 6 7 8 9

C

LOT EXP
2B1064
NDC 0338-0089-04
5% Dextrose and 0.9% Sodium Chloride Injection USP
1000 mL
EACH 100 mL CONTAINS 5 g DEXTROSE HYDROUS USP 900 mg SODIUM CHLORIDE USP pH 4.0 (3.2 TO 6.5) mEq/L SODIUM 154 CHLORIDE 154 HYPERTONIC OSMOLARITY 560 mOsmol/L (CALC) STERILE NONPYROGENIC SINGLE DOSE CONTAINER ADDITIVES MAY BE INCOMPATIBLE CONSULT WITH PHARMACIST IF AVAILABLE WHEN INTRODUCING ADDITIVES USE ASEPTIC TECHNIQUE MIX THOROUGHLY DO NOT STORE DOSAGE INTRAVENOUSLY AS DIRECTED BY A PHYSICIAN SEE DIRECTIONS CAUTIONS SQUEEZE AND INSPECT INNER BAG WHICH MAINTAINS PRODUCT STERILITY DISCARD IF LEAKS ARE FOUND MUST NOT BE USED IN SERIES CONNECTIONS DO NOT USE UNLESS SOLUTION IS CLEAR FEDERAL (USA) LAW PROHIBITS DISPENSING WITHOUT PRESCRIPTION STORE UNIT IN MOISTURE BARRIER OVERWRAP AT ROOM TEMPERATURE (25ºC/77ºF) UNTIL READY TO USE AVOID EXCESSIVE HEAT SEE INSERT
Baxter
BAXTER HEALTHCARE CORPORATION
DEERFIELD IL 60015 USA
MADE IN USA
Viaflex® CONTAINER
PL 146® PLASTIC
FOR PRODUCT INFORMATION
CALL 1-800-933-0303
1 2 3 4 5 6 7 8 9

D

7. The two major intravenous access sites are ______________ and ______________.

8. A client is to receive an antibiotic IVPB. In order for the antibiotic to infuse first, how must it be hung in relation to the existing IV solution bag? ______________

Calculate the amount of dextrose and/or sodium chloride in each of the following IV solutions:

9. 0.5 L D5 1/4 NS

dextrose ______________ g

NaCl ______________ g

10. 750 mL D5 1/2 NS

dextrose ______________ g

NaCl ______________ g

Answers on p. 535

evolve

For additional practice problems, refer to the Intravenous Flow Rates section of the Elsevier's Interactive Drug Calculation Application, Version 1 on Evolve.

ANSWERS

Chapter 21

Answers to Practice Problems

1. patient-controlled analgesia
2. peripheral
3. intravenous piggyback
4. 0.9% normal saline, 0.9% sodium chloride (NaCl)
5. higher
6. pressure
7. 20% dextrose in water
8. 5% dextrose in water with 10 mEq potassium chloride (KCl)
9. 50 g
10. Dextrose: $5\text{ g} : 100\text{ mL} = x\text{ g} : 750\text{ mL}$

$$\frac{100x}{100} = \frac{3{,}750}{100}$$

$$x = 37.5\text{ g dextrose}$$

or

$$\frac{5\text{ g}}{100\text{ mL}} = \frac{x\text{ g}}{750\text{ mL}}$$

NaCl: $0.9\text{ g} : 100\text{ mL} = x\text{ g} : 750\text{ mL}$

$$\frac{100x}{100} = \frac{675}{100}$$

$$x = 6.75\text{ g NaCl}$$

or

$$\frac{0.9\text{ g}}{100\text{ mL}} = \frac{x\text{ g}}{750\text{ mL}}$$

750 mL D5NS contains 37.5 g of dextrose and 6.75 g NaCl (saline).

11. $10\text{ g} : 100\text{ mL} = x\text{ g} : 250\text{ mL}$

$$\frac{100x}{100} = \frac{2{,}500}{100}$$

$$x = 25\text{ g dextrose}$$

or

$$\frac{10\text{ g}}{100\text{ mL}} = \frac{x\text{ g}}{250\text{ mL}}$$

250 mL D10W contains 25 g dextrose.

12. Dextrose: $5\text{ g} : 100\text{ mL} = x\text{ g} : 1{,}000\text{ mL}$

$$\frac{100x}{100} = \frac{5{,}000}{100}$$

$$x = 50\text{ g dextrose}$$

or

$$\frac{5\text{ g}}{100\text{ mL}} = \frac{x\text{ g}}{1{,}000\text{ mL}}$$

NaCl: $0.33\text{ g} : 100\text{ mL} = x\text{ g} : 1{,}000\text{ mL}$

$$\frac{100x}{100} = \frac{330}{100}$$

$$x = 3.3\text{ g NaCl}$$

or

$$\frac{0.33\text{ g}}{100\text{ mL}} = \frac{x\text{ g}}{1{,}000\text{ mL}}$$

1,000 mL D5 0.33% NS contains 50 g dextrose and 3.3 g NaCl (saline).

13. Dextrose: $5\text{ g} : 100\text{ mL} = x\text{ g} : 500\text{ mL}$

$$\frac{100x}{100} = \frac{2{,}500}{100}$$

$$x = 25\text{ g dextrose}$$

or

$$\frac{5\text{ g}}{100\text{ mL}} = \frac{x\text{ g}}{500\text{ mL}}$$

NaCl: $0.45\text{ g} : 100\text{ mL} = x\text{ g} : 500\text{ mL}$

$$\frac{100x}{100} = \frac{225}{100}$$

$$x = 2.25\text{ g NaCl}$$

or

$$\frac{0.45\text{ g}}{100\text{ mL}} = \frac{x\text{ g}}{500\text{ mL}}$$

500 mL D5 1/2 NS contains 25 g dextrose and 2.25 g of NaCl (saline).

Answer to Clinical Reasoning Question

Troubleshooting should have been done by the nurses caring for the client. If the client's pain was not being relieved, the device should have been checked for possible malfunctioning and to determine whether the machine had been set up properly. It is mandatory that all programming be double-checked by nurses and the pump be monitored frequently to ensure that it is functioning. The client's continual complaint of severe pain with no relief should have been a key to the nurses caring for the client.

Answers to Chapter Review

1. B
2. C
3. A
4. D
5. pain
6. push *or* bolus
7. peripheral and central
8. higher
9. 25 g dextrose; 1.125 g NaCl

   Equivalent: 1 L = 1,000 mL

   Therefore 0.5 L = 500 mL

   Dextrose:

   $$5\text{ g}:100\text{ mL} = x\text{ g}:500\text{ mL}$$
   $$\frac{100x}{100} = \frac{2{,}500}{100}$$
   $$x = 25\text{ g dextrose}$$

   or

   $$\frac{5\text{ g}}{100\text{ mL}} = \frac{x\text{ g}}{500\text{ mL}}$$

   NaCl:

   $$0.225\text{ g}:100\text{ mL} = x\text{ g}:500\text{ mL}$$
   $$\frac{100x}{100} = \frac{112.5}{100}$$
   $$x = 1.125\text{ g NaCl}$$

   or

   $$\frac{0.225\text{ g}}{100\text{ mL}} = \frac{x\text{ g}}{500\text{ mL}}$$

   500 mL D5 1/4 NS contains 25 g dextrose and 1.125 g NaCl (saline).

10. 37.5 g dextrose; 3.375 g NaCl

    Dextrose:

    $$5\text{ g}:100\text{ mL} = x\text{ g}:750\text{ mL}$$
    $$\frac{100x}{100} = \frac{3{,}750}{100}$$
    $$x = 37.5\text{ g of dextrose}$$

    or

    $$\frac{5\text{ g}}{100\text{ mL}} = \frac{x\text{ g}}{750\text{ mL}}$$

    NaCl:

    $$0.45\text{ g}:100\text{ mL} = x\text{ g}:750\text{ mL}$$
    $$\frac{100x}{100} = \frac{337.5}{100}$$
    $$x = 3.375\text{ g NaCl}$$

    or

    $$\frac{0.45\text{ g}}{100\text{ mL}} = \frac{x\text{ g}}{750\text{ mL}}$$

    750 mL D5 1/2 NS contains 37.5 g dextrose and 3.375 g NaCl (saline).

CHAPTER 22
Intravenous Calculations

Objectives

After reviewing this chapter, you should be able to:

1. Calculate milliliters per hour (mL/hr)
2. Identify the two types of administration tubing
3. Identify from intravenous (IV) tubing packages the drop factor in drops per milliliter (gtt/mL)
4. Calculate IV flow rate in drops per minute (gtt/min) using a formula method and dimensional analysis
5. Calculate IV flow rate in gtt/min using a shortcut method (mL/hr and constant drop factor)
6. Calculate the flow rate for medications ordered IV over a specified time period
7. Calculate infusion times and completion times
8. Recalculate IV flow rates and determine the percentage (%) of increase or decrease
9. Calculate the rate for medications administered IV push

This chapter will present the calculations performed with intravenous therapy. As stated previously, nurses have the responsibility to make sure that clients are receiving the correct rate. Several methods to calculate IV rates are presented in the chapter: ratio and proportion, dimensional analysis, the formula, and division factor method. Let's now begin our calculations with determining IV rates in milliliters per hour (mL/hr).

IV Flow Rate Calculation

IV fluids are usually ordered to be administered at rates expressed in mL/hr. Examples: 3,000 mL in 24 hr, 1,000 mL in 8 hr. Small volumes of fluid are often used when the IV fluid contains medications such as antibiotics. Rates for IV fluids are usually expressed in drops per minute (gtt/min) when an infusion device is not used. When an infusion device is used, the rate must be expressed in mL/hr.

Calculating Flow Rates for Infusion Pumps in mL/hr

When a client is using an electronic infuser such as a volumetric pump, the prescriber orders the volume, and the nurse is responsible for programming the pump to deliver the ordered volume. The prescriber may order the IV volume in mL/hr; however, if not, the nurse must calculate it and program the pump.

SAFETY ALERT!

With technological advances, there are some IV pumps that are capable of delivering IV fluids in tenths of a milliliter. Always be familiar with the IV equipment being used at the institution before rounding milliliters per hour (mL/hr) to the nearest whole mL/hr.

For most electronic devices that regulate the flow of IV solutions, the rate is expressed in milliliters per hour (mL/hr). For the purpose of this text, the equipment being used is programmable in whole mL/hr; therefore, mL/hr should be rounded to a whole number unless indicated that the infusion pump has decimal capability. Let's begin with the calculation of IV flow rates in mL/hr. Identify the following:

- Volume (amount) of solution in milliliters
- Time expressed in hours
- Round flow rate to nearest whole number or tenths, depending on the equipment

$$x \text{ mL/hr} = \frac{\text{Amount of solution (mL)}}{\text{Time in hours}}$$ (rounded to whole number or tenths, depending on the equipment)

✓ Solution Using Formula Method

Example 1: Client with an infusion pump has an order for 3,000 mL D5W over 24 hours.

1. Think: pump is regulated in mL/hr.
2. Set up in formula:

$$x \text{ mL/hr} = \frac{3{,}000 \text{ mL}}{24 \text{ hr}}$$

$$x = 125 \text{ mL/hr}$$

The pump would be set to deliver 125 mL/hr.

✓ Solution Using Ratio and Proportion

An alternative to the above formula would be to set up a ratio and proportion as follows:

$$3{,}000 \text{ mL} : 24 \text{ hr} = x \text{ mL} : 1 \text{ hr}$$

$$\frac{24x}{24} = \frac{3{,}000}{24}$$

$$x = 125 \text{ mL/hr}$$

Remember, as stated in the chapter on ratio and proportion, that a ratio and proportion can be set up in several formats. This could have been set up with the desired time for the infusion (usually 1 hr) over the total time ordered in hours, and the other side would be the hourly amount in milliliters labeled "x" over the total volume to be infused in milliliters:

$$\frac{1 \text{ hr}}{24 \text{ hr}} = \frac{x \text{ mL}}{3{,}000 \text{ mL}} \quad or \quad 1 \text{ hr} : 24 \text{ hr} = x \text{ mL} : 3{,}000 \text{ mL}$$

When medications are added to an IV, such as IVPB, it may be ordered to infuse in less than an hour, which often occurs when antibiotics are administered. When the time period is less than an hour by an electronic infusion device, the time must still be determined in mL/hr. Use a ratio proportion to determine mL/hr or use the formula:

$$x \text{ mL/hr} = \frac{\text{Total mL to infuse}}{\text{Number of min to infuse}} \times 60 \text{ min/hr}$$

Let's look at an example illustrating this.

Example 2: A client on an infusion pump is to receive an antibiotic in 50 mL of 0.9% NS over 30 minutes.

1. Think: The pump infuses in mL/hr. Use a ratio and proportion to determine mL/hr. Remember: 1 hr = 60 min.
2. Set up proportion:

✓ Solution Using Ratio and Proportion

$$50 \text{ mL} : 30 \text{ min} = x \text{ mL} : 60 \text{ min} \quad or \quad \frac{50 \text{ mL}}{30 \text{ min}} = \frac{x \text{ mL}}{60 \text{ min}}$$

$$30x = 50 \times 60$$

$$\frac{30x}{30} = \frac{3{,}000}{30}$$

$$x = 100 \text{ mL/hr}$$

The pump must be set to deliver 100 mL/hr for 50 mL to infuse within 30 minutes.

An alternate to using the ratio proportion to determine mL/hr for a time period less than an hour by infusion pump is to use the following formula:

$$x \text{ mL/hr} = \frac{\text{Total mL to infuse}}{\text{Number of min to infuse}} \times 60 \text{ min/hr}$$

Let's look at example #2 using this formula

$$x \text{ mL/hr} = \frac{50 \text{ mL}}{\overset{}{\cancel{30}}\ \cancel{\text{min}}_{1}} \times \frac{\overset{2}{\cancel{60}}\ \cancel{\text{min}}/\text{hr}}{1}$$

Notice minutes can be cancelled here:

$$x = \frac{100}{1}$$

$$x = 100 \text{ mL/hr}$$

Calculating mL/hr Using Dimensional Analysis

Calculation of mL/hr using dimensional analysis is similar to the formula method.

Steps:

- Identify what you are looking for, and write it to the left of the equation in a fraction format.
- Write the starting fraction using the information from the problem.

Example 1: Client with an infusion pump has an order for 3,000 mL of D5W over 24 hr.

Label factor: $\frac{x \text{ mL}}{\text{hr}} =$

Starting fraction: $\frac{3{,}000 \text{ mL}}{24 \text{ hr}}$

$$\frac{x \text{ mL}}{\text{hr}} = \frac{3{,}000 \text{ mL}}{24 \text{ hr}}$$

Note: No cancellation of units is required here.

$$x = 125 \text{ mL/hr}$$

Example 2: A client with an infusion pump is to receive an antibiotic in 50 mL of 0.9% NS over 30 minutes.

Notice here that the time is less than an hour. The pump delivers mL/hr. Therefore, the fraction 1 hr = 60 min is added to the equation.

$$\frac{x \text{ mL}}{\text{hr}} = \frac{50 \text{ mL}}{\cancel{30}\ \cancel{\text{min}}_{1}} \times \frac{\overset{2}{\cancel{60}}\ \cancel{\text{min}}}{1 \text{ hr}}$$

Note: Minutes are cancelled here so that you are left with mL/hr.

$$x = 100 \text{ mL/hr}$$

SAFETY ALERT!

The usual rate in mL/hr ranges from 50 to 200 mL/hr. If the rate exceeds this amount, double check the order and your calculation before programming the rate into an infusion pump.

POINTS TO REMEMBER

- Electronic infusion device = mL/hr.
- To determine flow rates for an electronic infusion device, pump or controller, determine mL/hr using the following formula:

$$x \text{ mL/hr} = \frac{\text{Total mL ordered}}{\text{Total hours ordered}}$$ (rounded to whole number or tenths, depending on the equipment)

- If the infusion time is less than 1 hr, use a ratio and proportion or dimensional analysis to determine mL/hr.
- Remember 60 min = 1 hr.
- An alternate method to determine the rate for infusion time expressed in a time period less than an hour is as follows:

$$x \text{ mL/hr} = \frac{\text{Total mL to infuse}}{\text{Number of minutes to infuse}} \times 60 \text{ min/hr}$$

- Round mL/hr to a whole number or the nearest tenth, depending on equipment used.
- Always be familiar with the equipment being used by the institution before rounding to a whole number.

PRACTICE **PROBLEMS**

Calculate the flow rate in mL/hr. (Equipment used is programmable in whole mL/hr)

1. 1,800 mL of D5W in 24 hr by infusion pump ______________
2. 2,000 mL D5W in 24 hr by infusion pump ______________
3. 500 mL RL in 12 hr by infusion pump ______________
4. 100 mL 0.45% NS in 45 min by infusion pump ______________
5. 1,500 mL D5RL in 24 hr by infusion pump ______________
6. 750 mL D5W in 16 hr by infusion pump ______________
7. 30 mL of antibiotic in 0.9% NS in 20 min by infusion pump ______________

Answers on p. 587

Manually Regulated IVs

When an electronic infusion device is not used, the nurse uses a gravity-flow system and must manually regulate the IV flow rate. To do this the nurse must calculate the ordered IV flow rate as the number of drops per minute (gtt/min).

IV flow rates in gtt/min are based on the IV tubing calibration, referred to as the *drop factor.* The drop factor is the number of drops per milliliter (gtt/mL) that a particular IV tubing delivers. The drop size is determined by the size of the tubing or the small needle inside the drop chamber releasing the drops into the drip chamber. (The larger the tubing, the larger the drops.) See Figure 22-1. Note that in the larger tubing in Figure 22-1, *A*, the drops are large (macrodrops). The drops delivered by the small needle in Figure 22-1, *B*, are very small drops (microdrops). The *drop factor* of the IV tubing is stated on the IV

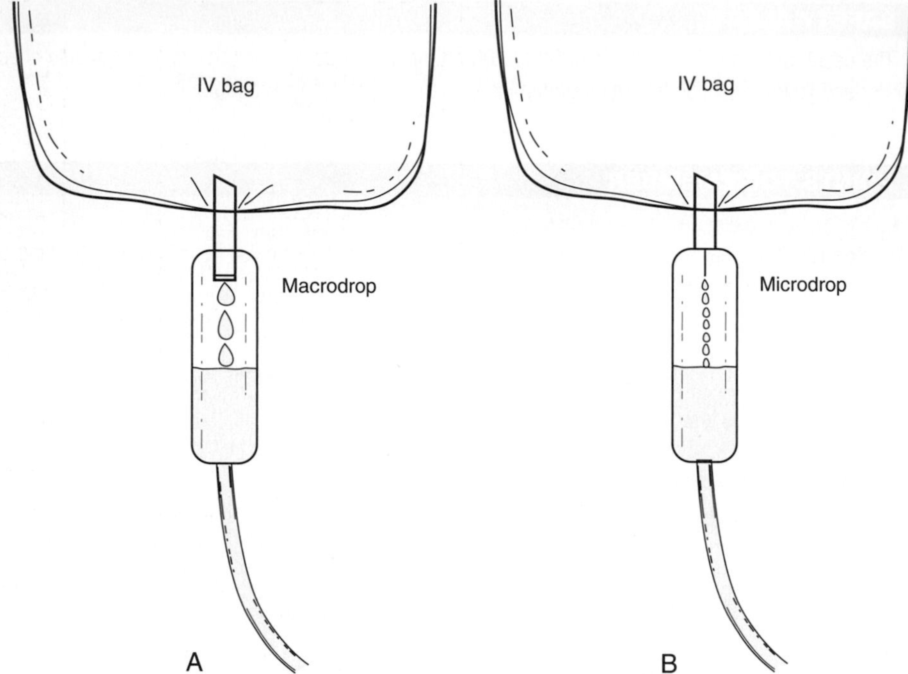

Figure 22-1 Comparison of **(A)** macrodrops and **(B)** microdrops.

tubing package (Figure 22-2). The first step in calculating gtt/min is to identify the *drop factor* of the tubing.

IV tubing has a drip chamber (sometimes referred to as a drop chamber). The drip chamber is located at the site of the entrance of the tubing into the container of intravenous solution. The nurse determines the IV flow rate in gtt/min and counts the drops of IV fluid falling into the drip chamber per minute or fraction of a minute. This is accomplished by placing a watch that has a second hand close to the drip chamber and counting the drops. The flow rate is regulated by a hand-operated slide clamp or a roller clamp that is opened or closed so the drops fall at the desired rate (Figure 22-3).

SAFETY ALERT!

IV infusions under manual control need to be monitored regularly. The flow rate of a manually regulated IV can be affected by the height of the IV infusion, the location of the infusion site, and changes in the client position, which can result in impediment of the IV flow rate or excessive amounts of fluid being delivered to the client.

IV Tubing

The two common types of tubing used to administer IV fluids are *macrodrop tubing* and *microdrop tubing.*

Macrodrop Tubing

Macrodrop is the standard type of tubing used for general IV administration. This type of tubing delivers a certain number of gtt/mL, as specified by the manufacturer. Macrodrop tubing delivers 10, 15, or 20 drops per mL (gtt/mL). Macrodrops are large drops; therefore, large amounts of fluid are administered in macrodrops and there are fewer drops in 1 mL (see Figure 22-1, *A*). Most institutions stock one macrodrop tubing for routine IV adult administration. Always read the IV tubing package and identify the drop factor of the tubing.

SAFETY ALERT!

The nurse must be aware of the drop factor to accurately administer IV fluids at the correct rate to a client. Never assume the drop factor for macrodrop tubing; it can be 10, 15, or 20 gtt/mL. Knowing the drop factor of the IV tubing used can prevent an error in IV rate determination and the client receiving IV fluid at the incorrect rate.

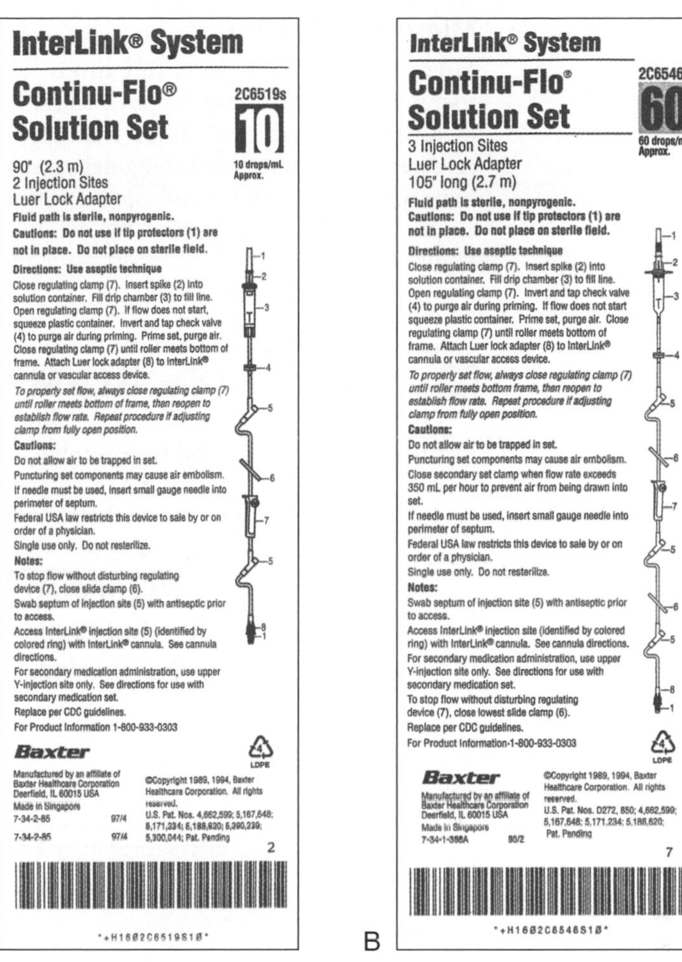

Figure 22-2 Administration sets (package). **A,** Set with drop factor of 10 (10 gtt = 1 mL). **B,** Set with drop factor of 60 (60 gtt = 1 mL).

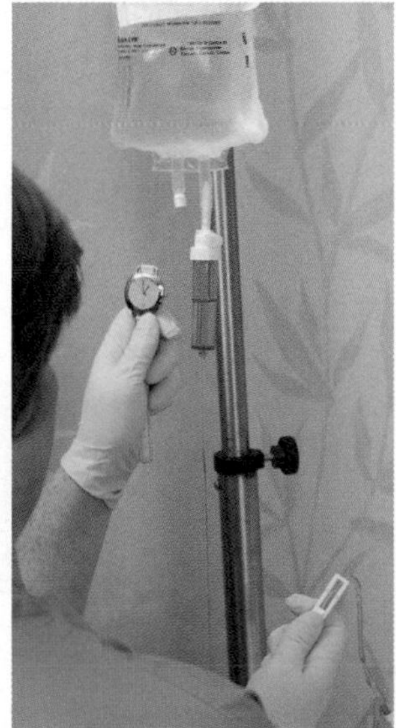

Figure 22-3 Observing the drip chamber to count drops per minute. (From Potter PA, Perry AG, Stockert P, Hall A: *Fundamentals of nursing,* ed 9, St Louis, 2016, Mosby.)

Microdrop Tubing

Microdrop tubing delivers tiny drops, which can be inferred from the prefix *micro;* therefore there are many drops in 1 mL. It is used when small amounts and more exact measurements are needed, for example, in pediatrics, for the elderly, and in critical care settings. Microdrop tubing delivers 60 gtt/mL. Because there are 60 minutes in an hour, the number of microdrops per minute is equal to the number of mL/hr. For example, if clients are receiving 100 mL/hr, they are receiving 100 microdrops/min (see Figure 22-1, *B*).

PRACTICE PROBLEMS

Identify the drop factor and type of tubing for the IV tubing pictured below.

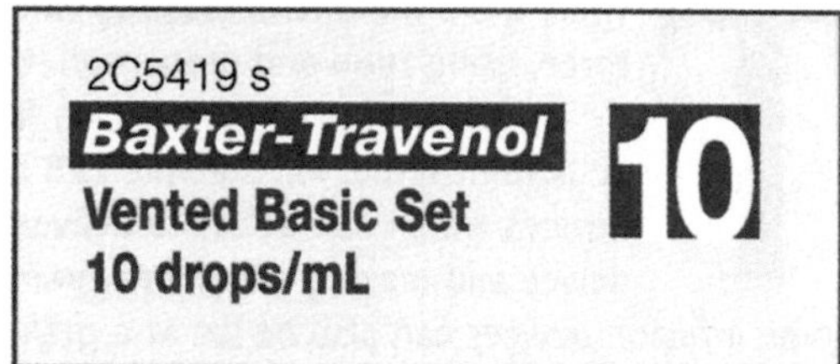

8. ______________________

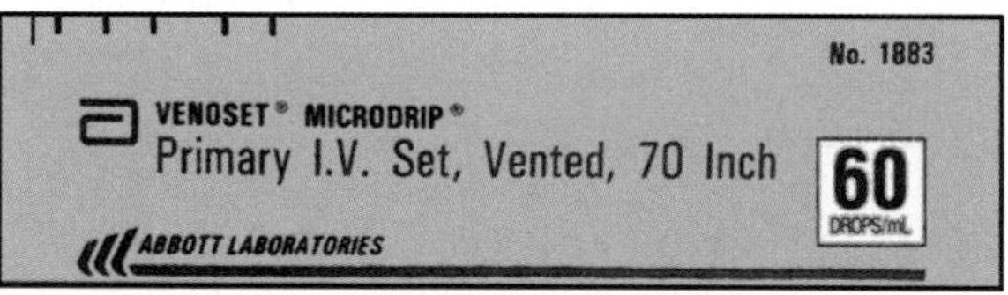

9. ______________________

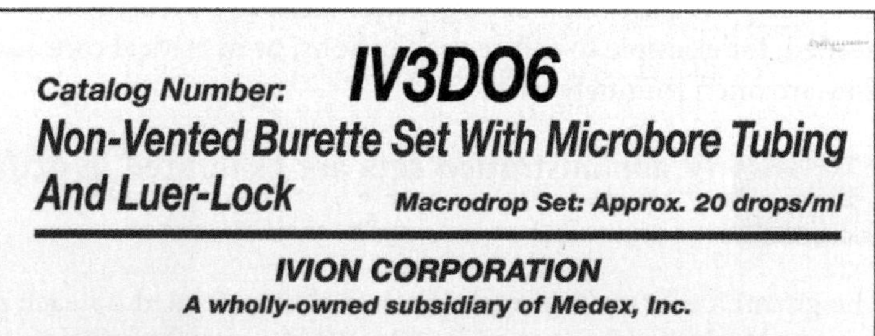

10. ______________________

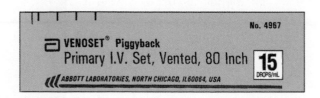

11. ______________________

Answers on p. 587

POINTS TO REMEMBER

- Knowing the drop factor is the ***FIRST*** step in accurate administration of IV fluids, in gtt/min.
- The drop factor always appears on the package of the IV tubing.
- Macrodrops are large and deliver 10, 15, or 20 gtt/mL.
- Microdrops are small and deliver 60 gtt/mL.
- Drop factor = gtt/mL.

Calculating Flow Rates in Drops Per Minute Using a Formula

The calculation of IV flow rate in gtt/min can be done by using a formula method or dimensional analysis. Several formulas can be used; this text will focus on the most popular formula used. Calculation of the rate in gtt/min by using dimensional analysis will also be demonstrated in this chapter.

To calculate the flow rate at which an IV is to infuse, regardless of the method used (formula or dimensional analysis), the nurse needs to know the following:

1. The volume or number of milliliters to infuse
2. The drop factor (gtt/mL) of the IV tubing
3. The time element (minutes or hours)

Formula Method

The information is placed into a formula. Let's examine a formula that might be used. This formula is the most popular when calculating flow rate, and the rate can be expressed as 60 minutes or less.

$$x \text{ gtt/min} = \frac{\text{Amount of solution (mL)} \times \text{Drop factor}}{\text{Time (min)}}$$

Before calculating, let's review some basic principles:

1. Drops per minute are always expressed in whole numbers. Think: You cannot regulate an IV to half a drop, **you can only count whole drops;** therefore, drops are expressed in whole numbers.
2. Principles of rounding are applied if calculation for gtt/min does not result in a whole number. Carry calculation one decimal place and round gtt/min to the nearest whole number. For example, 19.5 is rounded to 20 gtt/min.
3. Answers must be labeled. The label is usually drops per minute unless otherwise specified. Examples: 100 gtt/min or 17 gtt/min. To reinforce the differences in drop factor, the type of tubing is sometimes included as part of the label. Examples: 100 microgtt/min or 17 macrogtt/min.

Let's look at some sample problems and a step-by-step method of using the formula to obtain answers.

Example 1: Order: D5W to infuse at 100 mL/hr. Drop factor: 10 gtt/mL. At what rate in gtt/min should the IV be regulated?

1. Set up the problem, placing the information given in the correct position in the formula.

$$x \text{ gtt/min} = \frac{100 \text{ mL} \times 10 \text{ gtt/mL}}{60 \text{ min}}$$

2. Reduce where possible to make numbers smaller and easier to manage. Note that the labels are dropped when starting to perform mathematical steps.

$$x = \frac{100 \times \overset{1}{\cancel{10}}}{\underset{6}{\cancel{60}}} = \frac{100 \times 1}{6} = \frac{100}{6}$$

3. Divide $\frac{100}{6}$ to obtain rate in gtt/min. Carry division one decimal place and round off to the nearest whole number.

$$x = \frac{100}{6} = 16.6 = 17$$

$$x = 17 \text{ gtt/min; } 17 \text{ macrogtt/min}$$

To deliver 100 mL/hr with a drop factor of 10 gtt/mL, the IV rate should be adjusted to 17 gtt/min. This answer can also be expressed with the type of tubing as part of the label, for example, 17 macrogtt/min.

Example 2: Order: IV medication in 50 mL NS in 20 minutes. Drop factor: microdrop (60 gtt/mL). At what rate in gtt/min should the IV be regulated?

$$x \text{ gtt/min} = \frac{50 \text{ mL} \times \overset{3}{\cancel{60}} \text{ gtt/mL}}{\underset{1}{\cancel{20}} \text{ min}}$$

$$x = \frac{50 \times 3}{1} = \frac{150}{1} = 150$$

$$x = 150 \text{ gtt/min; } 150 \text{ microgtt/min}$$

To deliver 50 mL in 20 minutes with a drop factor of 60 gtt/mL, the IV should be adjusted to 150 gtt/min. This may sound like a lot; however, remember the type of tubing used is a microdrop.

Dimensional Analysis Method

Let's look at calculating rate in gtt/min using the process of dimensional analysis. Remember that IV fluids are ordered in small volumes of fluid that usually contain medication or in large volumes to infuse over several hours. Let's look at the previous examples by using dimensional analysis.

Example 1: Order: D5W to infuse at 100 mL/hr. Drop factor: 10 gtt/mL. At what rate in gtt/min should the IV be regulated?

1. You are calculating gtt/min, so write gtt/min to the left of the equation, followed by the equals sign (=), and label gtt/min x since that is what you're looking for:

$$\frac{x \text{ gtt}}{\text{min}} =$$

2. Extract the information that contains gtt from the problem; the drop factor is 10 gtt/1 mL. Write this factor into the equation, placing gtt in the numerator.

$$\frac{x \text{ gtt}}{\text{min}} = \frac{10 \text{ gtt}}{1 \text{ mL}}$$

3. The next fraction is written so that the denominator matches the previous fraction (what you are looking for). Go back to the problem, and you will see that the order is to infuse 100 mL in 1 hr. Enter the 1 hr as 60 min in the denominator because you are calculating gtt/min (100 mL/60 min).

$$\frac{x \text{ gtt}}{\text{min}} = \frac{10 \text{ gtt}}{1 \text{ mL}} \times \frac{100 \text{ mL}}{60 \text{ min}}$$

4. Now that you have the completed equation, cancel the units and notice that you are left with the desired gtt/min.

$$\frac{x\text{ gtt}}{\text{min}} = \frac{10\text{ gtt}}{1\text{ }\cancel{\text{mL}}} \times \frac{100\text{ }\cancel{\text{mL}}}{60\text{ min}}$$

$$x = \frac{100 \times \overset{1}{\cancel{10}}}{\underset{6}{\cancel{60}}} = \frac{100}{6} = 16.6 = 17$$

$$x = 17\text{ gtt/min; 17 macrogtt/min}$$

Note: Example 1 could have been done without changing the hourly rate to 60 min, but it would have required the addition of a 1 hr = 60 min conversion factor to the equation.

$$\frac{x\text{ gtt}}{\text{min}} = \frac{10\text{ gtt}}{1\text{ mL}} \times \frac{100\text{ mL}}{1\text{ hr}} \times \frac{1\text{ hr}}{60\text{ min}}$$

The next step would be to cancel the denominator/numerator mL and hr, leaving the desired gtt and min.

$$\frac{x\text{ gtt}}{\text{min}} = \frac{10\text{ gtt}}{1\text{ }\cancel{\text{mL}}} \times \frac{100\text{ }\cancel{\text{mL}}}{1\text{ }\cancel{\text{hr}}} \times \frac{1\text{ }\cancel{\text{hr}}}{60\text{ min}}$$

$$x = \frac{100 \times \overset{1}{\cancel{10}}}{\underset{6}{\cancel{60}}} = \frac{100}{6} = 16.6 = 17$$

$$x = 17\text{ gtt/min; 17 macrogtt/min}$$

Example 2: Order: An IV medication of 50 mL NS in 20 min. Drop factor: microdrop (60 gtt/mL). At what rate in gtt/min should the IV be regulated?

1. You are calculating gtt/min, so write gtt/min to the left of the equation, followed by the equals sign (=), and label gtt/min *x*, since that is what you're looking for,

$$\frac{x\text{ gtt}}{\text{min}} =$$

2. Extract the information that contains gtt from the problem; the drop factor is 60 gtt/1 mL. Write this factor in the equation, placing gtt in the numerator.

$$\frac{x\text{ gtt}}{\text{min}} = \frac{60\text{ gtt}}{1\text{ mL}}$$

3. The next fraction is written so that the denominator matches the previous fraction (what you are looking for). Go back to the problem, and you will see that the order is to infuse 50 mL in 20 minutes. Enter the third fraction so that 50 mL is in the numerator and 20 minutes is in the denominator.

$$\frac{x\text{ gtt}}{\text{min}} = \frac{60\text{ gtt}}{1\text{ mL}} \times \frac{50\text{ mL}}{20\text{ min}}$$

4. Now that you have the completed equation, cancel the units and notice that you are left with the desired gtt/min.

$$\frac{x \text{ gtt}}{\text{min}} = \frac{60 \text{ gtt}}{1 \cancel{\text{mL}}} \times \frac{50 \cancel{\text{mL}}}{20 \text{ min}}$$

$$x = \frac{60 \times \overset{5}{\cancel{50}}}{\underset{2}{\cancel{20}}} = \frac{300}{2} = 150$$

$$x = 150 \text{ gtt/min; } 150 \text{ microgtt/min}$$

Answer: $x = 150$ gtt/min; 150 microdrops/min

Calculating Drops per Minute with Large Volumes of Fluid

Remember that IV fluids can be ordered in large volumes to infuse over several hours, for example, 1,000 mL over 8 hr; or the large volume can be ordered by total volume to infuse and the mL/hr rate of infusion (125 mL/hr). Example: 1,000 mL D5W at a rate of 125 mL/hr. Remember that when a large volume to infuse over several hours is ordered, a preliminary step can be done to change it to mL/hr. Example: 1,000 mL D5W to infuse in 8 hr. Divide the total volume by the number of hours to get mL/hr. In this case, 1,000 mL ÷ 8 hr = 125 mL/hr. Then proceed to calculate gtt/min.

$$x \text{ mL/hr} = \frac{\text{Amount of solution (mL)}}{\text{Time (hr)}}$$

The formula method or dimensional analysis may be used to calculate gtt/min for a volume of fluid to be administered in more than 1 hour. Now let's look at some examples where a large volume of fluid will infuse over more than 1 hour.

Example 1: Order: 1,000 mL D5W to infuse in 8 hr. Drop factor: 20 gtt/mL. At what rate in gtt/min should the IV be regulated?

✔ Solution Using the Formula Method

1. Calculate the mL/hr.

$$x \text{ mL/hr} = \frac{1{,}000 \text{ mL}}{8 \text{ hr}}$$

$$x = 125 \text{ mL/hr}$$

2. Calculate the gtt/min.

$$x \text{ gtt/min} = \frac{125 \text{ mL} \times 20 \text{ gtt/mL}}{60 \text{ min}}$$

3. Reduce.

$$x = \frac{125 \times \overset{1}{\cancel{20}}}{\underset{3}{\cancel{60}}} = \frac{125 \times 1}{3} = \frac{125}{3}$$

$$x = \frac{125}{3} = 41.6 = 42$$

$$x = 42 \text{ gtt/min; } 42 \text{ macrogtt/min}$$

✓ Solution Using Dimensional Analysis

1. Begin by determining mL/hr, converting the time in hours to minutes. 1 hr = 60 min. Now proceed to set up the problem in the dimensional analysis equation.
2. Enter the gtt/min being calculated first, followed by the equals sign (=).

$$\frac{x \text{ gtt}}{\text{min}} =$$

3. Enter the drop factor (20 gtt/mL) with gtt in the numerator.

$$\frac{x \text{ gtt}}{\text{min}} = \frac{20 \text{ gtt}}{1 \text{ mL}}$$

4. Take from the problem the amount to be administered over 1 hr (60 min), and write the fraction so that it matches the denominator of the fraction immediately before it.

$$\frac{x \text{ gtt}}{\text{min}} = \frac{20 \text{ gtt}}{1 \text{ mL}} \times \frac{125 \text{ mL}}{60 \text{ min}}$$

5. Now that you have completed the equation, cancel the units, and proceed with the mathematical process to obtain the answer.

$$\frac{x \text{ gtt}}{\text{min}} = \frac{\overset{1}{\cancel{20}} \text{ gtt}}{1 \cancel{\text{mL}}} \times \frac{125 \cancel{\text{mL}}}{\underset{3}{\cancel{60}} \text{ min}}$$

$$x = \frac{125}{3} = 41.6 = 42$$

$$x = 42 \text{ gtt/min; } 42 \text{ macrogtt/min}$$

Note: The above example could have been done without changing 1 hr to 60 min; however, if it is left as 1 hr, you will need to add the additional fraction (1 hr = 60 min). With the same example, the equation would be stated as follows:

$$\frac{x \text{ gtt}}{\text{min}} = \frac{20 \text{ gtt}}{1 \text{ mL}} \times \frac{125 \text{ mL}}{1 \text{ hr}} \times \frac{1 \text{ hr}}{60 \text{ min}}$$

Notice that the conversion factor 1 hr = 60 min is written so the numerator matches the denominator of the fraction immediately before it. To solve the equation, cancel units and proceed as follows:

$$\frac{x \text{ gtt}}{\text{min}} = \frac{20 \text{ gtt}}{1 \cancel{\text{mL}}} \times \frac{125 \cancel{\text{mL}}}{1 \cancel{\text{hr}}} \times \frac{1 \cancel{\text{hr}}}{60 \text{ min}}$$

$$x = \frac{\overset{1}{\cancel{20}} \times 125 \times 1}{\underset{3}{\cancel{60}}} = \frac{125}{3} = 41.6 = 42$$

$$x = 42 \text{ gtt/min; } 42 \text{ macrogtt/min}$$

Remember that determining mL/hr before calculating gtt/min helps keep the numbers smaller. However, using dimensional analysis also allows you to determine gtt/min without this step by writing one equation; but you would need the conversion factor 1 hr = 60 min. The equation would be stated as follows:

$$\frac{x \text{ gtt}}{\text{min}} = \frac{20 \text{ gtt}}{1 \text{ mL}} \times \frac{1{,}000 \text{ mL}}{8 \text{ hr}} \times \frac{1 \text{ hr}}{60 \text{ min}}$$

Notice that the volume ordered is written to match the denominator of the fraction immediately before it and that the conversion factor 1 hr = 60 min is written, so the numerator matches the denominator before it.

$$\frac{x \text{ gtt}}{\text{min}} = \frac{20 \text{ gtt}}{1 \cancel{\text{mL}}} \times \frac{1{,}000 \cancel{\text{mL}}}{8 \cancel{\text{hr}}} \times \frac{1 \cancel{\text{hr}}}{60 \text{ min}}$$

$$x = \frac{20 \times 1{,}000 \times 1}{480} = \frac{\overset{1{,}000}{\cancel{20{,}000}}}{\underset{24}{\cancel{480}}}$$

$$x = \frac{1{,}000}{24} = 41.6 = 42$$

$$x = 42 \text{ gtt/min; } 42 \text{ macrogtt/min}$$

Example 2: Order: 1,500 mL 0.9% NS in 10 hr. Drop factor: 15 gtt/mL. At what rate in gtt/min should the IV infuse?

✔ Solution Using the Formula Method

1. Calculate mL/hr.

$$x \text{ mL/hr} = \frac{1{,}500 \text{ mL}}{10 \text{ hr}}$$

$$x = 150 \text{ mL/hr}$$

2. Calculate gtt/min.

$$x \text{ gtt/min} = \frac{150 \text{ mL} \times 15 \text{ gtt/mL}}{60 \text{ min}}$$

3. $$x = \frac{150 \times \overset{1}{\cancel{15}}}{\underset{4}{\cancel{60}}} = \frac{150}{4}$$

4. $$x = \frac{150}{4} = 37.5 = 38$$

$$x = 38 \text{ gtt/min; } 38 \text{ macrogtt/min}$$

✔ Solution Using Dimensional Analysis

1. Calculate mL/hr (1,500 mL ÷ 10 hr = 150 mL/hr); convert the time in hours to minutes. Proceed using the steps outlined in Example 1.

$$\frac{x \text{ gtt}}{\text{min}} = \frac{15 \text{ gtt}}{1 \text{ mL}} \times \frac{150 \text{ mL}}{60 \text{ min}}$$

$$\frac{x \text{ gtt}}{\text{min}} = \frac{\overset{1}{\cancel{15}} \text{ gtt}}{1 \cancel{\text{mL}}} \times \frac{150 \cancel{\text{mL}}}{\underset{4}{\cancel{60}} \text{ min}}$$

$$x = \frac{150}{4} = 37.5 = 38$$

$$x = 38 \text{ gtt/min; } 38 \text{ macrogtt/min}$$

or

Set up the equation without changing 1 hr to 60 min.

$$\frac{x\text{ gtt}}{\text{min}} = \frac{15\text{ gtt}}{1\text{ mL}} \times \frac{150\text{ mL}}{1\text{ hr}} \times \frac{1\text{ hr}}{60\text{ min}}$$

$$\frac{x\text{ gtt}}{\text{min}} = \frac{15\text{ gtt}}{1\text{ }\cancel{\text{mL}}} \times \frac{150\text{ }\cancel{\text{mL}}}{1\text{ }\cancel{\text{hr}}} \times \frac{1\text{ }\cancel{\text{hr}}}{60\text{ min}}$$

$$x = \frac{\overset{1}{\cancel{15}} \times 150 \times 1}{\underset{4}{\cancel{60}}} = \frac{150}{4} = 37.5 = 38$$

$x = 38$ gtt/min; 38 macrogtt/min

or

Set up the equation without finding mL/hr first.

$$\frac{x\text{ gtt}}{\text{min}} = \frac{15\text{ gtt}}{1\text{ mL}} \times \frac{1{,}500\text{ mL}}{10\text{ hr}} \times \frac{1\text{ hr}}{60\text{ min}}$$

$$\frac{x\text{ gtt}}{\text{min}} = \frac{15\text{ gtt}}{1\text{ }\cancel{\text{mL}}} \times \frac{1{,}500\text{ }\cancel{\text{mL}}}{10\text{ }\cancel{\text{hr}}} \times \frac{1\text{ }\cancel{\text{hr}}}{60\text{ min}}$$

$$x = \frac{\overset{1}{\cancel{15}} \times 1{,}500 \times 1}{\underset{40}{\cancel{600}}} = \frac{1{,}500}{40} = 37.5 = 38$$

$x = 38$ gtt/min; 38 macrogtt/min

PRACTICE PROBLEMS

Calculate the flow rate in gtt/min using the formula method or dimensional analysis.

12. Administer D5RL at 75 mL/hr. The drop factor is 10 gtt/mL. ____________

13. Administer D5 $\frac{1}{2}$ NS at 30 mL/hr. The drop factor is a microdrop. ____________

14. Administer RL at 125 mL/hr. The drop factor is 15 gtt/mL. ____________

15. Administer 1,000 mL D5 0.33% NS in 6 hr. The drop factor is 15 gtt/mL. ____________

16. An IV medication in 60 mL of 0.9% NS is to be administered in 45 min. The drop factor is a microdrop. ____________

17. 1,000 mL of Ringer's lactate solution (RL) is to infuse in 16 hr. The drop factor is 15 gtt/mL. ____________

18. Infuse 150 mL of D5W in 2 hr. The drop factor is 20 gtt/mL. ____________

19. Administer 3,000 mL D5 and ½ NS in 24 hr. The drop factor is 10 gtt/mL. ______

20. Infuse 2,000 mL D5W in 12 hr. The drop factor is 15 gtt/mL. ______

21. An IV medication in 60 mL D5W is to be administered in 30 minutes. The drop factor is a microdrop. ______

Answers on pp. 587-588

Calculation of IV Flow Rates Using a Shortcut Method

This shortcut method can be used where the IV sets all have the same drop factor. Example: an institution where all the macrodrop sets deliver 10 gtt/mL. This method can also be used with microdrop sets (60 gtt/mL). It is important to note that this method can be used only if the rate of the IV infusion is expressed in mL/hr (mL/60 min). It is imperative that nurses become very familiar with the administration equipment at the institution where they work.

To use this method, you must know the drop factor constant for the administration set you are using. The drop factor constant is sometimes referred to as the *division factor*. To obtain the drop factor constant (division factor) for the IV administration set being used, divide 60 by the drop factor calibration. Box 22-1 shows the constant calculated based on the drop factor for the tubing.

BOX 22-1 Drop Factor Constants

Drop Factor of Tubing	Drop Factor Constant
10 gtt/mL	$\frac{60}{10} = 6$
15 gtt/mL	$\frac{60}{15} = 4$
20 gtt/mL	$\frac{60}{20} = 3$
60 gtt/mL	$\frac{60}{60} = 1$

Example: The drop factor for an IV administration set is 15 gtt/mL. To obtain the drop factor constant:

$$\frac{60}{15} = 4 \text{ (drop factor constant } = 4)$$

RULE

After the drop factor constant is determined, the gtt/min can be calculated in one step:

$$x \text{ gtt/min} = \frac{\text{mL/hr}}{\text{gtt factor constant}}$$

PRACTICE PROBLEMS

Calculate the drop factor constant for the following IV sets.

22. 20 gtt/mL ______________________

23. 10 gtt/mL ______________________

24. 60 gtt/mL ______________________

Answers on pp. 588-589

Now that you know how to determine the drop factor constant, let's look at examples of using a shortcut method to calculate gtt/min.

Example 1: Administer 0.9% NS at 100 mL/hr. The drop factor is 20 gtt/mL. The drop factor constant is 3.

✓ Solution Using the Shortcut Method

Therefore, this problem could be done by using the shortcut method once you know the drop factor constant (division factor).

$$x \text{ gtt/min} = \frac{100 \text{ mL/hr}}{3} = 33.3 = 33$$

$$x = 33 \text{ gtt/min; } 33 \text{ macrogtt/min}$$

Notice that the 100 mL/hr rate divided by the drop factor constant gives the same answer.

✓ Solution Using Dimensional Analysis

Step 1: State mL/hr as mL/60 min.

$$\frac{x \text{ gtt}}{\text{min}} = \frac{\overset{1}{\cancel{20}} \text{ gtt}}{1 \cancel{\text{mL}}} \times \frac{100 \cancel{\text{mL}}}{\underset{3}{\cancel{60}} \text{ min}}$$

Note: In the equation, because time is stated as 60 min, the administration set calibration (20) will be divided into 60 (min) to obtain a constant number (3). 3 is the drop factor constant for 20 gtt/mL administration set. Using the drop factor constant, you can calculate gtt/min in one step (divide mL/hr by the drop factor constant).

$$\frac{x \text{ gtt}}{\text{min}} = \frac{\overset{1}{\cancel{20}} \text{ gtt}}{1 \cancel{\text{mL}}} \times \frac{100 \cancel{\text{mL}}}{\underset{3}{\cancel{60}} \text{ min}} = 33.3 = 33$$

$$\text{or } 100 \text{ mL/hr} \div 3 = 33.3 = 33$$

$$x = 33 \text{ gtt/min; } 33 \text{ macrogtt/min}$$

Example 2: Administer D5W at 125 mL/hr. The drop factor is 15 gtt/mL. The drop factor constant is 4.

✓ Solution Using the Shortcut Method

Calculate the gtt/min.

$$x \text{ gtt/min} = \frac{125 \text{ mL/hr}}{4} = 31.2 = 31$$

$$x = 31 \text{ gtt/min; } 31 \text{ macrogtt/min}$$

✓ Solution Using Dimensional Analysis

Administer D5W at 125 mL/hr. The drop factor is 15 gtt/mL. The drop factor constant is 4.

$$\frac{x \text{ gtt}}{\text{min}} = \frac{\overset{1}{\cancel{15}} \text{ gtt}}{1 \cancel{\text{mL}}} \times \frac{125 \cancel{\text{mL}}}{\underset{4}{\cancel{60}} \text{ min}} = 31.2 = 31$$

$$or \ 125 \text{ mL} \div 4 = 31.2 = 31$$

$$x = 31 \text{ gtt/min; } 31 \text{ macrogtt/min}$$

Example 3: Administer 0.9% NS at 75 mL/hr. The drop factor is 60 gtt/mL. The drop factor constant is 1.

✓ Solution Using the Shortcut Method

Calculate the gtt/min.

$$x \text{ gtt/min} = \frac{75 \text{ mL/hr}}{1} = 75$$

$$x = 75 \text{ gtt/min; } 75 \text{ microgtt/min}$$

✓ Solution Using Dimensional Analysis

$$\frac{x \text{ gtt}}{\text{min}} = \frac{\overset{1}{\cancel{60}} \text{ gtt}}{1 \cancel{\text{mL}}} \times \frac{75 \cancel{\text{mL}}}{\underset{1}{\cancel{60}} \text{ min}} = 75$$

$$x = 75 \text{ gtt/min; } 75 \text{ microgtt/min}$$

Answer: $x = 75$ gtt/min; 75 microgtt/min

PRACTICE **PROBLEMS**

Calculate the rate in gtt/min using the shortcut method.

25. Order: D5W 200 mL/hr.
    Drop factor: 10 gtt/mL ______________

26. Order: RL 50 mL/hr.
    Drop factor: 15 gtt/mL ______________

27. Order: 0.45% NS 80 mL/hr.
    Drop factor: 60 gtt/mL ______________

28. Order: 0.9% NS 140 mL/hr.
    Drop factor: 20 gtt/mL ______________

Answers on p. 589

Remember that the shortcut method discussed (using the drop factor constant) can be used to calculate the gtt/min for any volume of fluid that can be stated in mL/hr or mL/60 min.

RULE

The shortcut method can be used if the volume is large; however, an additional step of changing mL/hr first must be done. You can then proceed to calculate the gtt/min using the shortcut method.

Example 1: Order: RL 1,500 mL in 12 hr. Drop factor: 15 gtt/mL. Drop factor constant: 4.

$$1{,}500 \text{ mL} \div 12 = 125 \text{ mL/hr}$$

✓ Solution Using the Shortcut Method

Now that you have mL/hr, you can proceed with the shortcut method, using the drop factor constant.

$$x \text{ gtt/min} = \frac{125 \text{ mL}}{4} = 31.2 = 31 \text{ gtt/min}$$

Answer: $x = 31$ gtt/min; 31 macrogtt/min

✓ Solution Using Dimensional Analysis

Step 1: Determine mL/hr expressed as mL/60 min.

$$\frac{x \text{ gtt}}{\text{min}} = \frac{\overset{1}{\cancel{15}} \text{ gtt}}{1 \cancel{\text{mL}}} \times \frac{125 \cancel{\text{mL}}}{\underset{4}{\cancel{60}} \text{ min}} = \frac{125}{4} = 31.2 = 31 \text{ gtt/min}$$

Answer: $x = 31$ gtt/min; 31 macrogtt/min

Example 2: Order: 20 mL D5W in 30 min. Drop factor: 15 gtt/mL. Drop factor constant: 4.

✓ Solution Using the Shortcut Method

If the volume of fluid to be infused is small, the volume and the time must each be multiplied to get mL/hr. To express this in mL/hr, you multiply by 2.

$$20 \text{ mL/30 min} = (20 \times 2)/(2 \times 30 \text{ min}) = 40 \text{ mL/hr}$$

$$x \text{ gtt/min} = \frac{40 \text{ mL}}{4} = 10$$

$$x = 10 \text{ gtt/min; 10 macrogtt/min}$$

✓ Solution Using Dimensional Analysis

Step 1: Change 20 mL/30 min to 40 mL/hr as shown above.

Step 2: Express 40 mL/hr as 40 mL/60 min.

$$\frac{x \text{ gtt}}{\text{min}} = \frac{\overset{1}{\cancel{15}} \text{ gtt}}{1 \cancel{\text{mL}}} \times \frac{40 \cancel{\text{mL}}}{\underset{4}{\cancel{60}} \text{ min}} = \frac{40}{4} = 10$$

$$x = 10 \text{ gtt/min; 10 macrogtt/min}$$

PRACTICE PROBLEMS

Calculate the gtt/min using the shortcut method.

29. Order: 1,000 mL D5W in 10 hr.
    Drop factor: 10 gtt/mL __________

30. Order: 1,500 mL RL in 12 hr.
    Drop factor: 15 gtt/mL __________

31. Order: 40 mL D5W in 20 min.
    Drop factor: 10 gtt/mL __________

Answers on p. 589

Calculating IV Flow Rates When Several Solutions Are Ordered

IV orders are often written for different amounts or types of fluid to be given in a certain time period. These orders are frequently written for a 24-hour interval and are usually split over three shifts. IV solutions may have medications added, such as potassium chloride or multivitamins.

Steps to calculating:

1. Add up the total amount of fluid.
2. Proceed as with other IV problem calculations.

Note: When medications such as potassium chloride and vitamins are added to IV solutions, they are generally not considered in the total volume. (At some institutions, to consider the medication in the volume, it must be 10 mL or more. Always check the policy of the institution.)

Example 1: Order: The following IVs for 24 hours. Drop factor: 15 gtt/mL.

a. 1,000 mL D5W with 10 mEq potassium chloride (KCl)

b. 500 mL D5NS c̄ 1 ampule multivitamin (MVI)

c. 500 mL D5W

1. Calculate mL/hr.

$$x \text{ mL/hr} = \frac{2{,}000 \text{ mL}}{24 \text{ hr}} = 83.3 = 83$$

$$x = 83 \text{ mL/hr}$$

2. Calculate gtt/min.

$$x \text{ gtt/min} = \frac{83 \text{ mL} \times 15 \text{ gtt/mL}}{60 \text{ min}}$$

3. Reduce.

$$x = \frac{83 \times \overset{1}{\cancel{15}}}{\underset{4}{\cancel{60}}} = \frac{83 \times 1}{4} = 20.7 = 21$$

$$x = 21 \text{ gtt/min; 21 macrogtt/min}$$

Answer: $x = 21$ gtt/min; 21 macrogtt/min

Example 2: IV orders are as follows:

a. 1,000 mL D5W

b. 1,000 mL D5 0.9%

c. 500 mL D5 and $\frac{1}{2}$ NS

Drop factor: 10 gtt/mL to infuse at 150 mL/hr.

The hourly rate is 150 mL/hr. Calculation is done based on this:

$$x \text{ gtt/min} = \frac{150 \text{ mL} \times 10 \text{ gtt/mL}}{60 \text{ min}}$$

$$x = \frac{150 \times \overset{1}{\cancel{10}}}{\underset{6}{\cancel{60}}} = \frac{150 \times 1}{6} = 25$$

$x = 25$ gtt/min; 25 macrogtt/min

Note: Use the previous examples to set up using dimensional analysis.

PRACTICE **PROBLEMS**

Calculate the flow rate in gtt/min.

32. Order: Dextrose 5% with Ringer lactate solution (D5RL) c̄ 20 units Pitocin for 2 L at 125 mL/hr. Drop factor: 15 gtt/mL ________________

33. Order: To infuse in 16 hr. Drop factor: 10 gtt/mL

    a. D5W 500 mL c̄ 10 mEq KCl

    b. D5W 1,000 mL

    c. D5W 1,000 mL c̄ 1 ampule MVI ________________

34. Order: 1,000 mL D5 0.9% NS for 3 L at 100 mL/hr. Drop factor: microdrop. ________________

35. Order: D5W 1,000 mL + 20 mEq KCl for 2 L to infuse in 10 hr. Drop factor: 15 gtt/mL ________________

Answers on pp. 589-590

POINTS TO REMEMBER

- To calculate the IV flow rate in gtt/min, the nurse must have the volume of solution, the time factor for the IV to infuse, and the drop factor of the tubing.
- Drop factor is expressed as gtt/mL and indicated on the package of the IV tubing.
- Calculation of gtt/min can be done by using the formula method or dimensional analysis.
  Formula:

$$x \text{ gtt/min} = \frac{\text{Amount of solution (mL)} \times \text{gtt factor (gtt/mL)}}{\text{Time (min)}}$$

- Formula is used for any time period that can be expressed as 60 min or less.
- For time periods greater than 60 min, find mL/hr first, and then use the formula to determine gtt/min.

continued

- Round gtt/min to the nearest whole number (division carried one decimal place).
- A shortcut method can be used to calculate flow rates infusing mL/hr. It cannot be used if time period is less than 1 hr and calculated in minutes.
- To determine the drop constant factor for an IV set, divide 60 by the calibration of the set.

Calculating IV Flow Rates Using a Dial-Flow Controller

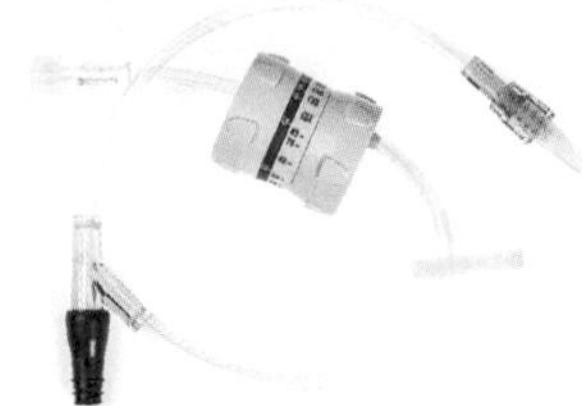

Figure 22-4 Dial-a-Flow™. (Photo courtesy of ICU Medical Inc.)

Dial-flow controllers are also known as IV manual regulators. There are a wide variety of dial-flow controllers available for use and are either part of IV tubing or added on. (Figure 22-4). These devices are regulated manually, and it is important to know that they are not infusion pumps. Use of the device is based on several factors, including severity of illness, type of therapy, and the setting. Dial-flow devices are designed to regulate the flow of IV fluid instead of using the roller clamp on the IV tubing. The flow rate can be adjusted from 5 to 250 mL/hr. To operate the device, you set or dial the desired flow rate in mL/hr, which is an estimate, and then the rate must be verified by counting drops per minute. Drops per minute would be calculated using one of the methods presented in the chapter. Although use of the dial-flow controller may allow for more consistent flow than a roller clamp, its accuracy is about the same as a roller clamp.

If used, it is important to understand that it does not relinquish the nurse from his or her responsibility to monitor the IV to ensure that there is accurate delivery of the ordered infusion rate. Let's look at examples using this device.

Example: Order: D_5W 1,000 mL at 100 mL/hr. Drop factor of IV tubing: 10 gtt/mL

1. Turn the dial of the controller to 100 mL/hr
2. Use the formula to determine gtt/min

$$x \text{ gtt/min} = \frac{100 \text{ mL} \times \cancel{10} \text{ gtt/mL}}{\cancel{60} \text{ min}} = \frac{100}{6}$$

$$x = \frac{100}{6} = 16.6$$

$$x = 17 \text{ gtt/min; } 17 \text{ macrogtt/min}$$

3. Verify accuracy of controller by counting the drops either for a minute or a fraction, such as 20 seconds (17 gtt ÷ 3 = 5.6 = 6 gtt). You find the number of drops is 6; the controller is delivering the correct rate. If the rate is not correct for 20 seconds, the controller dial can be adjusted. The rate will need to be monitored periodically during the infusion.

SAFETY ALERT!

The flow rate on the controller is in **mL/hr, not gtt/min.** Failure to verify the drop rate can result in client not receiving the correct rate and receiving insufficient or excessive IV fluid. To ensure client safety, the controller as well as the client **must** be monitored during administration of IV therapy.

Calculating Intermittent IV Infusions Piggyback

Medications such as antibiotics can also be given by adding a secondary container of solution that contains the medication. The administration of medication by attaching it to a port on the primary line is referred to as *piggyback.* The volume of the piggyback container is usually 50 to 100 mL and should infuse over 20, 30, or 60 minutes, depending on the type and amount of medication added. If the volume of fluid in which the antibiotic is to be infused is not stated in the order, check a medication reference guide. The formula method or dimensional analysis is used to determine the rate in gtt/min at which the medication should be infused. Note: At some institutions the medication being added has to be 10 mL or more to be considered in the volume of IV fluid; check policy of the institution.

Example: Order: Keflin 2 g IVPB (piggyback) over 30 min. The Keflin is placed in 100 mL of fluid after it is dissolved. The drop factor is 15 gtt/mL. At what rate in gtt/min should the IV be regulated?

To calculate this, the 100 mL of fluid in which the medication is dissolved is used as the volume.

✓ Solution Using the Formula Method

$$x \text{ gtt/min} = \frac{100 \text{ mL} \times 15 \text{ gtt/mL}}{30 \text{ min}}$$

$$x = \frac{100 \times \overset{1}{\cancel{15}}}{\underset{2}{\cancel{30}}} = \frac{100 \times 1}{2} = \frac{100}{2}$$

$$x = \frac{100}{2} = 50$$

$$x = 50 \text{ gtt/min; } 50 \text{ macrogtt/min}$$

The IV would be regulated at 50 gtt/min; 50 macrogtt/min.

✓ Solution Using Dimensional Analysis

$$\frac{x \text{ gtt}}{\text{min}} = \frac{\overset{1}{\cancel{15}} \text{ gtt}}{1 \cancel{\text{mL}}} \times \frac{100 \cancel{\text{mL}}}{\underset{2}{\cancel{30}} \text{ min}}$$

$$x = \frac{100}{2} = 50$$

$$x = 50 \text{ gtt/min; } 50 \text{ macrogtt/min}$$

PRACTICE **PROBLEMS**

Calculate the rate in gtt/min for the following medications being administered IVPB. Use the labels where provided. (Add volume of medication being added to IV solutions, where indicated.)

36. Order: Doxycycline 50 mg IVPB in D_5W 100 mL over 1 hr. Drop factor: 15 gtt/mL ________________

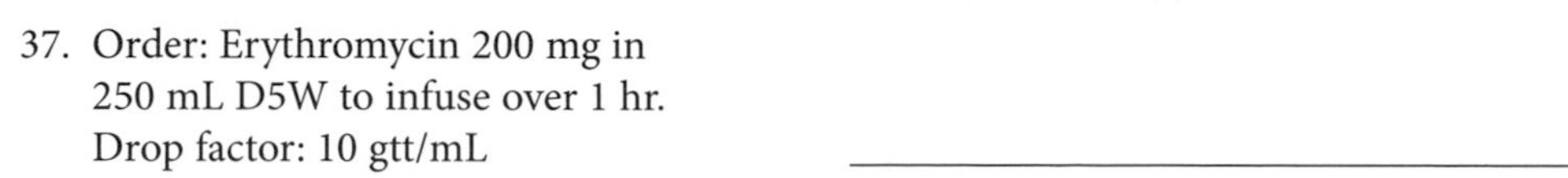

37. Order: Erythromycin 200 mg in 250 mL D5W to infuse over 1 hr. Drop factor: 10 gtt/mL ________________

38. Order: Ampicillin 1 g is added to 50 mL D5W to infuse over 45 minutes. Drop factor: 10 gtt/mL. For IV reconstitute with 10 mL of diluent to get 1 g per 10 mL. (Consider the medication added in the volume of fluid.)

    a. How many milliliters of medication must be added to the solution? ________________

    b. Calculate the rate in gtt/min at which the IV should infuse. ________________

39. Order: Clindamycin 900 mg in 75 mL D5W over 30 minutes. Drop factor: 10 gtt/mL

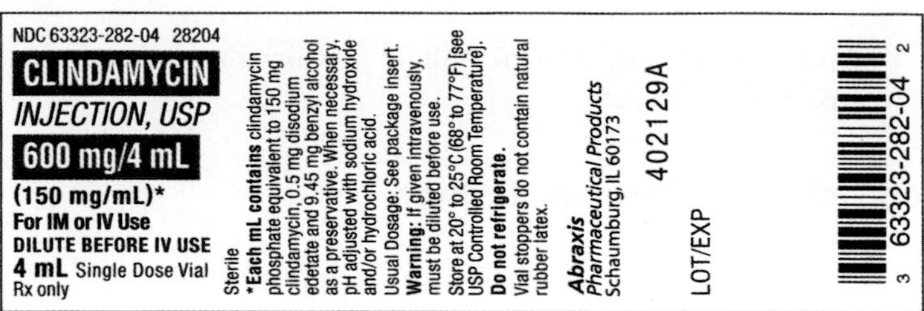

a. How many milliliters of medication must be added to the solution? __________

b. Calculate the rate in gtt/min at which the IV should infuse. __________

40. Order: Tagamet 300 mg IVPB q8hr. The medication has been added to 50 mL D5W to infuse over 30 minutes. Drop factor: 10 gtt/mL

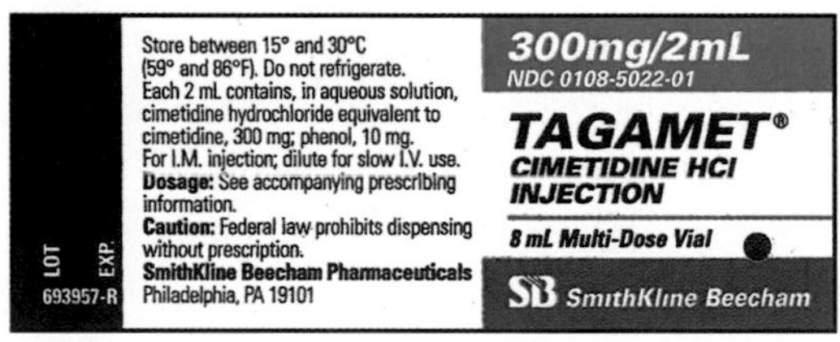

a. How many milliliters of medication must be added to the solution? __________

b. Calculate the rate in gtt/min at which the IV should infuse. __________

41. Order: Vancomycin 500 mg IVPB q24hr. The reconstituted vancomycin provides 50 mg per mL. The medication is placed in 100 mL of D5W to infuse over 60 minutes. Drop factor: 15 gtt/mL. (Consider the medication added in the volume of fluid.)

a. How many milliliters of medication must be added to the solution? __________

b. Calculate the rate in gtt/min at which the IV should infuse. __________

42. Order: Fungizone (amphotericin B) 20 mg IV Soluset (IVSS) in 300 mL D5W over 6 hr. The reconstituted material contains 50 mg per 10 mL. Drop factor: 60 gtt/per mL

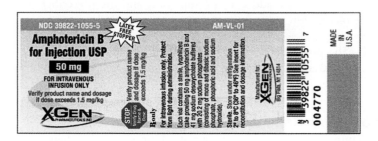

a. How many milliliters will you add to the IV solution? __________

b. At what rate in gtt/min should the IV infuse? __________

43. Order: Septra (sulfamethoxazole and trimethoprim) 300 mg in 300 mL D5W over 1 hr q6h. Drop factor: 10 gtt/mL. Calculate the dose using trimethoprim.

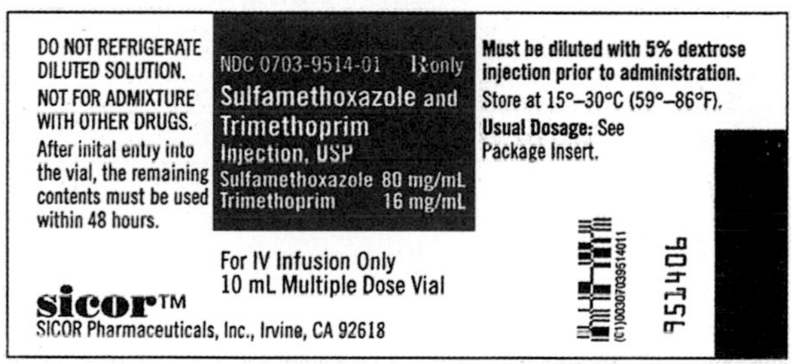

a. How many milliliters of medication will be added to the IV? (Round the answer to the nearest tenth.) __________

b. Consider the medication added to the volume of IV fluid. Calculate the rate in gtt/min at which the IV should infuse. __________

44. Order: Retrovir (zidovudine) 100 mg IV q4h over 1 hr. Available medication states each mL contains 10 mg of zidovudine.

The medication is placed in 100 mL of D5W. Drop factor: 10 gtt/mL (Consider the medication added to the volume of IV fluid.) __________

Answers on pp. 590-591

Determining the Amount of Medication in a Specific Amount of Solution

Sometimes medications are added to IV solutions, and the prescriber orders a certain amount of the medication to be given in a certain time period.

Example 1: The prescriber may order 20 mEq of potassium chloride to be placed in 1,000 mL of fluid to be administered at a rate of 2 mEq of potassium per hour.

✔ Solution Using Ratio and Proportion

Calculate the number of milliliters per hour of solution needed to deliver 2 mEq of potassium chloride per hour.

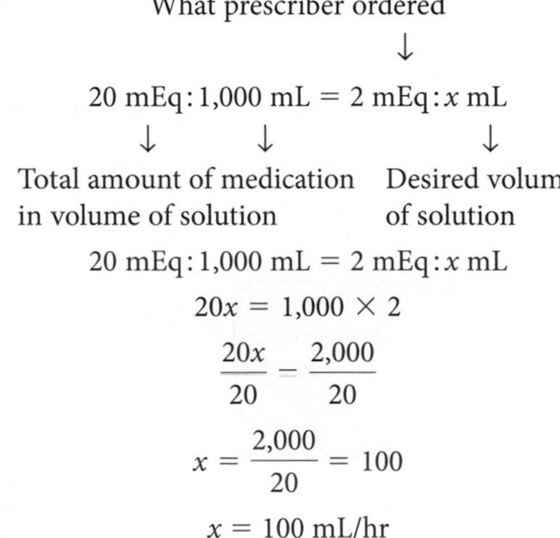

What prescriber ordered
20 mEq : 1,000 mL = 2 mEq : x mL
Total amount of medication in volume of solution
Desired volume of solution
20 mEq : 1,000 mL = 2 mEq : x mL
20x = 1,000 × 2
20x/20 = 2,000/20
x = 2,000/20 = 100
x = 100 mL/hr

Thus 100 mL per hour of fluid would be needed to administer 2 mEq of potassium chloride per hour.

✔ Solution Using Dimensional Analysis

Step 1: Determine the amount of solution in milliliters per hour needed to administer 2 mEq of potassium chloride per hour. Enter mL/hr being calculated first.

$$\frac{x\text{ mL}}{\text{hr}} =$$

Step 2: Enter the 1,000 mL per 20 mEq as the starting fraction.

$$\frac{x\text{ mL}}{\text{hr}} = \frac{1{,}000\text{ mL}}{20\text{ mEq}}$$

Step 3: Enter the 2 mEq/1 hr rate ordered with mEq as the numerator.

$$\frac{x\text{ mL}}{\text{hr}} = \frac{1{,}000\text{ mL}}{20\text{ mEq}} \times \frac{2\text{ mEq}}{1\text{ hr}}$$

Step 4: Cancel the units so you are left with mL/hr.

$$\frac{x \text{ mL}}{\text{hr}} = \frac{1{,}000 \text{ mL}}{\underset{10}{\cancel{20}} \cancel{\text{mEq}}} \times \frac{\overset{1}{\cancel{2}} \cancel{\text{mEq}}}{1 \text{ hr}}$$

$$x = \frac{1{,}000}{10} = 100$$

$$x = 100 \text{ mL/hr}$$

100 mL/hr would deliver 2 mEq of potassium chloride per hour.

Example 2: The prescriber orders 100 units of Humulin regular insulin to be added to 500 mL of 0.45% saline ($\frac{1}{2}$ NS) to infuse at 10 units per hour. The IV flow rate should be how many milliliters per hour?

✔ Using Ratio and Proportion

Set up a proportion with the known on one side and the unknown on the other.

$$100 \text{ units} : 500 \text{ mL} = 10 \text{ units} : x \text{ mL}$$

$$100x = 500 \times 10$$

$$\frac{100x}{100} = \frac{5{,}000}{100}$$

$$x = \frac{5{,}000}{100} = 50$$

$$x = 50 \text{ mL/hr}$$

For the client to receive 10 units of insulin per hour, 50 mL/hr must be administered.

✔ Solution Using Dimensional Analysis

Follow the steps outlined in Example 1.

$$\frac{x \text{ mL}}{\text{hr}} = \frac{\overset{5}{\cancel{500}} \text{ mL}}{\underset{1}{\cancel{100}} \cancel{\text{units}}} \times \frac{10 \cancel{\text{units}}}{1 \text{ hr}}$$

$$x = \frac{50}{1} = 50$$

$$x = 50 \text{ mL/hr}$$

POINTS TO REMEMBER

- To determine the amount of medication in a specific amount of solution, use ratio proportion or dimensional analysis.
- Determine the amount (volume) of IV fluid to administer the prescribed medication in mL/hr.
- When preparing medications for intermittent infusion:
  - Reconstitute the medication using the label or package insert if needed.
  - Calculate the amount to administer.
  - Determine the IV flow rate using the IV formula.

PRACTICE PROBLEMS

Solve the following problems using the steps indicated.

45. Order: 15 mEq of potassium chloride in 1,000 mL of D5 ½ NS to be administered at a rate of 2 mEq/hr.

    How many mL/hr should the IV infuse at? ________________

46. Order: 10 units of Humulin regular insulin per hour. 50 units of insulin is placed in 250 mL NS.

    How many mL/hr should the IV infuse at? ________________

47. Order: 15 units of Humulin regular insulin per hour. 40 units of insulin is placed in 250 mL of NS.

    How many mL/hr should the IV infuse at? ________________

Answers on p. 591

Determining Infusion Times and Volumes

You may need to calculate the following:

a. **Time in hours**—How long it will take a certain amount of fluid to infuse or how long it may last.

b. **Volume**—The total number of milliliters a client will receive in a certain time period

These unknown elements can be determined by the use of the formula method or dimensional analysis.

Formula

$$x \text{ gtt/min} = \frac{\text{Amount of solution (mL)} \times \text{Drop Factor}}{\text{Time (min)}}$$

Steps to Calculating a Problem with an Unknown with the Formula Method

1. Take the information given in the problem and place it in the formula.
2. Place an x in the formula in the position of the unknown. If you are trying to determine time in hours, place x in the position for minutes; once you find the minutes, divide the number of minutes by 60 (60 minutes = 1 hr) to get the number of hours. If you are trying to determine the volume the client would receive, place an x in the position for amount of solution, and label x mL.
3. Set up an algebraic equation so that you can solve for x.
4. Solve the equation.
5. Label the answer in hours or milliliters for volume.

Sample Problem 1: Determining hours:

An IV is regulated at 20 microgtt/min. How many hours will it take for 100 mL to infuse?

✓ Problem Setup in Formula Method

1. $20 \text{ microgtt/min} = \dfrac{100 \text{ mL} \times 60 \text{ gtt/mL}}{x \text{ min}}$

2. Reduce:

$$\frac{20x}{20} = \frac{100 \times \overset{3}{\cancel{60}}}{\underset{1}{\cancel{20}}} = \frac{100 \times 3}{1}$$

$$x = 300 \text{ min}$$

3. Change minutes to hours:

$$60 \text{ minutes} = 1 \text{ hr}$$

$$\text{Therefore } \frac{300 \text{ min}}{60} = 5 \text{ hr}$$

$$x = 5 \text{ hr}$$

Note: Placing 20 gtt/min over 1 does not alter the value.

$$\frac{20 \text{ microgtt/min}}{1} = \frac{100 \text{ mL} \times 60 \text{ gtt/mL}}{x \text{ min}}$$

✔ Problem Setup in Dimensional Analysis

1. Write x hr being calculated first. Now enter 1 hr = 60 min as the starting fraction, placing 1 hr as the numerator to match the hr being calculated.

$$x \text{ hr} = \frac{1 \text{ hr}}{60 \text{ min}}$$

2. Refer to the problem; the numerator min must match the denominator in the starting fraction. This is provided by the 20 microgtt/min. Place the rate as a fraction with 1 min as the numerator and 20 gtt as the denominator.

$$x \text{ hr} = \frac{1 \text{ hr}}{60 \text{ min}} \times \frac{1 \text{ min}}{20 \text{ gtt}}$$

3. Check the problem; the third fraction is entered, so the numerator matches the denominator in the fraction before it. This is provided by the drop factor 60 gtt/mL. Place 60 in the numerator; and use 1 mL as the denominator.

$$x \text{ hr} = \frac{1 \text{ hr}}{60 \text{ min}} \times \frac{1 \text{ min}}{20 \text{ gtt}} \times \frac{60 \text{ gtt}}{1 \text{ mL}}$$

4. The last fraction written has to match mL in the fraction before it. The mL entry is provided by the 100 mL of fluid.

$$x \text{ hr} = \frac{1 \text{ hr}}{60 \text{ min}} \times \frac{1 \text{ min}}{20 \text{ gtt}} \times \frac{60 \text{ gtt}}{1 \text{ mL}} \times \frac{100 \text{ mL}}{1}$$

5. Cancel the units; notice that you are left with hours. Reduce if possible, and perform mathematical process.

$$x \text{ hr} = \frac{1 \text{ hr}}{\underset{1}{\cancel{60} \cancel{\text{min}}}} \times \frac{1 \cancel{\text{min}}}{\underset{1}{\cancel{20} \cancel{\text{gtt}}}} \times \frac{\overset{1}{\cancel{60}} \cancel{\text{gtt}}}{1 \cancel{\text{mL}}} \times \frac{\overset{5}{\cancel{100}} \cancel{\text{mL}}}{1}$$

$$x = 5 \text{ hr}$$

When you are calculating time intervals, and the time or the answer comes out in hours and minutes, express the entire time in hours. For example, 1 hour and 30 minutes = 1.5 hr or $1\frac{1}{2}$ hr; $1\frac{1}{2}$ hr is the preferred term.

When calculating volume, proceed with the problem in the same way as calculating time interval except x is placed in a different position and labeled mL.

Sample Problem 2: Determining volume:
An IV is regulated at 17 macrogtt/min. The drop factor is 15 gtt/mL. How much fluid volume in milliliters will the client receive in 8 hr?

✔ Problem Setup in Formula Method

1. $$17 \text{ macrogtt/min} = \frac{x \text{ mL} \times 15 \text{ gtt/mL}}{480 \text{ min}}$$

2. Reduce:

$$17 = \frac{x \times \overset{1}{\cancel{15}}}{\underset{32}{\cancel{480}}}$$

$$\frac{17}{1} = \frac{x}{32}$$

3. $x = 17 \times 32 = 544$ mL
   $x = 544$ mL

Note: Formula uses minutes. In problem, 8 hours was changed to 480 minutes.

✔ Problem Setup in Dimensional Analysis

1. Write x mL being calculated first. Now enter the drop factor as the starting fraction, placing 1 mL as the numerator to match the mL being calculated.

$$x \text{ mL} = \frac{1 \text{ mL}}{15 \text{ gtt}}$$

2. Refer to the problem; the numerator gtt must match the denominator in the starting fraction. This is provided by the IV rate; 17 macrogtt/min. Place the rate as a fraction with 17 gtt as the numerator and 1 min as the denominator.

$$x \text{ mL} = \frac{1 \text{ mL}}{15 \text{ gtt}} \times \frac{17 \text{ gtt}}{1 \text{ min}}$$

3. Refer to the problem; this fraction is entered so that it matches the denominator in the fraction before it. You could change 8 hr to minutes by using 60 min = 1 hr (8 hr = 480 min), or enter the conversion 60 min = 1 hr since the time here is in hours. Entering 60 min = 1 hr eliminates a pre-step of converting 8 hr to minutes. Enter 60 min = 1 hr; 60 min in the numerator and 1 hr in the denominator.

If the time in the problem is converted to minutes, this eliminates the need for 60 min = 1 hr and shortens the equation by one fraction.

$$x \text{ mL} = \frac{1 \text{ mL}}{15 \text{ gtt}} \times \frac{17 \text{ gtt}}{1 \text{ min}} \times \frac{480 \text{ min}}{1}$$

$$x \text{ mL} = \frac{1 \text{ mL}}{\underset{1}{\cancel{15}} \cancel{\text{gtt}}} \times \frac{17 \cancel{\text{gtt}}}{1 \cancel{\text{min}}} \times \frac{\overset{32}{\cancel{480}} \cancel{\text{min}}}{1}$$

$$x = \frac{17 \times 32}{1}$$

$$x = 544 \text{ mL}$$

Some of the problems illustrated in calculating an unknown may be solved without using the formula method or dimensional analysis; however, the use of one or the other is recommended.

POINTS TO REMEMBER

Determining the Unknown

- Use the IV formula and place the information given into the position of the formula.

$$x \text{ gtt/min} = \frac{\text{Amount of solution (mL)} \times \text{drop factor}}{\text{Time (min)}}$$

Use x for unknown values.

1. For determining time—place an x in the minutes position, and then divide the minutes by 60 to determine the time in hours.
2. For volume—place an x in the position for amount of solution and label x mL. Convert the hours to minutes.

- Set up an algebraic equation and solve for x.
- Answers for time are labeled in hours, with mL for volume, unless instructed otherwise.

PRACTICE **PROBLEMS**

Solve for the unknown in the following problems as indicated.

48. You find that there is 150 mL of D5W left in an IV. The IV is infusing at 60 microgtt/min. How many hours will the fluid last? ____________

49. 0.9% NS is infusing at 35 macrogtt/min. The drop factor is 15 gtt/mL. How many milliliters of fluid will the client receive in 5 hours? ____________

50. 180 mL of D5 RL is left in an IV that is infusing at 45 macrogtt/min. The drop factor is 15 gtt/mL. How many hours will the fluid last? ____________

51. D5 $\frac{1}{2}$ NS is infusing at 45 macrogtt/min. The drop factor is 15 gtt/mL. How many milliliters will the client receive in 8 hr? ____________

52. There is 90 mL of D5 0.33% NS left in an IV that is infusing at 60 microgtt/min. The drop factor is 60 gtt/mL. How many hours will the fluid last? ____________

Answers on p. 592

Recalculating an IV Flow Rate

Flow rates on IVs change when a client stands, sits, or is repositioned in bed if IVs are infusing by gravity. Therefore, nurses must frequently check the flow rates. IVs are generally labeled with a start and finish time as well as markings with specific time periods. Sometimes IVs infuse ahead of schedule, or they may be behind schedule if they are not monitored closely. When this happens, the IV flow rate must be recalculated. To recalculate the flow rate, the nurse uses the volume remaining and the time remaining. Recalculation may be done with uncomplicated infusions. IVs that require exact infusion rates should be monitored by an electronic infusion device.

SAFETY ALERT!

Never arbitrarily increase or decrease an IV to get it back on schedule without assessing a client and checking with the prescriber. Increasing or decreasing the rate without thought can result in serious harm to a client, including overhydration or underhydration. Check the policy of the institution. Avoid off-schedule IV rates by regularly monitoring the IV at least every 30 to 60 minutes.

When an IV is significantly ahead of or behind schedule, you may need to notify the prescriber, depending on the client's condition and the use of appropriate nursing judgment. **Always assess the client** before making any change in an IV rate. Changes depend on the client's condition. Check the institution's policy regarding the percentage of adjustment that can be made. Each situation must be individually evaluated, and appropriate action must be taken.

A safe rule is that the recalculated flow rate should not vary from the original rate by more than 25%. If the recalculated rate varies by more than 25% from the original rate, the prescriber should be notified. The order may require revision. If a client is stable, recalculate the IV rate, using the remaining volume and time, and then proceed to calculate gtt/min using the formula method or dimensional analysis. Refer to content in the chapter (calculating gtt/min) if necessary. Let's go over the steps to recalculate an IV rate if allowed by your institution policy, and the client is stable.

To recalculate an IV flow rate:

- Use the remaining volume and remaining hours, and calculate the rate in mL/hr.

$$x \text{ mL/hr} = \frac{\text{Remaining volume}}{\text{Remaining time (hr)}}$$

- Use the mL/hr to calculate gtt/min, using the formula:

$$x \text{ gtt/min} = \frac{\text{Number of mL} \times \text{drop factor}}{\text{Time in minutes}}$$

- Determine whether the new rate calculation is greater or lesser than 25%. Use the amount of increase or decrease divided by the original rate.

$$\frac{\text{Amount of} \uparrow \text{or} \downarrow}{\text{Original rate}} = \text{\% of variation of original rate (round to nearest whole percent)}$$

Let's look at some examples. Note: All examples assume the institution allows a 25% IV flow variation, and the clients are stable.

Example 1: 1,000 mL of D5 RL was to infuse in 8 hr at 31 gtt/min (31 macrogtt/min). The drop factor is 15 gtt/mL. After 4 hr, you notice 700 mL of fluid left in the IV. Recalculate the flow rate for the remaining solution. *Note:* The infusion is behind schedule. After 4 hr, half of the volume (or 500 mL) should have infused.

✔ Solution Using the Shortcut Method

Time remaining: 8 hr − 4 hr = 4 hr

Volume remaining: 1,000 mL − 300 mL = 700 mL

700 mL ÷ 4 = 175 mL/hr

Drop factor is 15 gtt/mL.

Drop factor constant therefore is 4.

$$x \text{ gtt/min} = \frac{175 \text{ mL/hr}}{4} = 43.7 = 44 \text{ gtt/min}$$

x = 44 gtt/min; 44 macrogtt/min (recalculated rate)

To determine the percentage of the change:

$$\frac{44 - 31}{31} = \frac{13}{31} = 0.419 = 42\%$$

✓ Solution Using Dimensional Analysis

$$\text{Time remaining: } 8 \text{ hr} - 4 \text{ hr} = 4 \text{ hr}$$

$$\text{Volume remaining: } 700 \text{ mL}$$

$$\frac{x \text{ gtt}}{\text{min}} = \frac{\overset{1}{\cancel{15}} \text{ gtt}}{1 \cancel{\text{mL}}} \times \frac{700 \cancel{\text{mL}}}{4 \cancel{\text{hr}}} \times \frac{1 \cancel{\text{hr}}}{\underset{4}{\cancel{60}} \text{ min}} = 43.7 = 44$$

$$x = 44 \text{ gtt/min; } 44 \text{ macrogtt/min}$$

Note: As shown in the earlier discussion relating to gtt/min, shortcut methods could be used in a dimensional analysis setup as well.

Course of Action: Assess the client; notify the prescriber. This increase could result in serious consequences for the client. Do not increase the rate. The increase is greater than 25%.

In this situation, the flow rate must be increased from 31 gtt/min (31 macrogtt/min) to 44 gtt/min (44 macrogtt/min), which is more than 25% of the original. Always assess the client first to determine the client's ability to tolerate an increase in fluid. In addition to assessing the client's status, you should notify the prescriber. A new order is needed since the recalculated rate is greater than 25%.

Example 2: IV Ahead of Schedule. An IV of 1,000 mL D5W is to infuse from 8 AM to 4 PM (8 hr). The drop factor is 10 gtt/mL. The rate is set at 20 gtt/min (20 macrogtt/min). In 5 hr, you notice that 700 mL has infused. Recalculate the flow rate for the remaining solution.

✓ Solution Using the Shortcut Method

$$\text{Time remaining: } 8 \text{ hr} - 5 \text{ hr} = 3 \text{ hr}$$

$$\text{Volume remaining: } 1{,}000 \text{ mL} - 700 \text{ mL} = 300 \text{ mL}$$

$$300 \text{ mL} \div 3 = 100 \text{ mL/hr}$$

Drop factor is 10 gtt/mL; therefore the drop factor constant is 6.

$$x \text{ gtt/min} = \frac{100 \text{ mL/hr}}{6} = 16.6 = 17$$

$$x = 17 \text{ gtt/min; } 17 \text{ macrogtt/min}$$

Determine the percentage of change:

$$\frac{17 - 20}{20} = \frac{-3}{20} = -0.15 = -15\%$$

✓ Solution Using Dimensional Analysis

$$\text{Time remaining: } 8 \text{ hr} - 5 \text{ hr} = 3 \text{ hr}$$

$$\text{Volume remaining: } 1{,}000 \text{ mL} - 700 \text{ mL} = 300 \text{ mL}$$

$$\frac{x \text{ gtt}}{\text{min}} = \frac{\overset{1}{\cancel{10}} \text{ gtt}}{1 \cancel{\text{mL}}} \times \frac{\overset{100}{\cancel{300}} \cancel{\text{mL}}}{\underset{1}{\cancel{3}} \cancel{\text{hr}}} \times \frac{1 \cancel{\text{hr}}}{\underset{6}{\cancel{60}} \text{ min}} = 16.6 = 17$$

$$x = 17 \text{ gtt/min; } 17 \text{ macrogtt/min}$$

In this situation, the flow rate must be decreased from 20 gtt/min (20 macrogtt/min) to 17 gtt/min (17 macrogtt/min), but this is not a change greater than 25% of the original; −15% is within the acceptable 25% of change. However, the client's condition must still be assessed to determine the ability to tolerate the change, and the prescriber may still require notification.

Course of Action: This is an acceptable decrease; it is less than 25%. Assess the client, adjust the rate, if allowed by institutional policy, and assess during the remainder of the infusion.

✓ Alternate to Determining the Percentage of Variation

As already stated, you can adjust the flow rate as much as (+) or (−) 25%. Think: 25% = $\frac{1}{4}$. Therefore, you can verify the safety of the recalculated rate you obtained by using a method that eliminates the need to use percents. To do this, do the following:

- Divide the original rate by 4, then add, and subtract the result from the original rate. This will provide a range for the acceptable rate adjustment. Let's use the two examples we just did.
- **In example 1,** the original rate is 31 gtt/min (macrogtt/min), and the recalculated rate is 44 gtt/min.

Original rate ± (original rate ÷ 4) = Acceptable IV rate adjustment

$$31 + (31 \div 4) = 31 + 7.75 = 38.75 = 39 \text{ gtt/min (macrogtt/min).}$$
$$31 - (31 \div 4) = 31 - 7.75 = 23.25 = 23 \text{ gtt/min (macrogtt/min).}$$

The safe acceptable IV rate adjustment is 23 to 39 gtt/min (macrogtt/min).

NO, 44 gtt/min is above 25%, so the prescriber needs to provide a new IV order. Increase in the rate above 25% could cause harm to the client.

- **In example 2,** the original rate is 20 gtt/min, and the recalculated rate is 17 gtt/min.
  Original rate ± (original rate ÷ 4) = Acceptable IV rate adjustment

$$20 + (20 \div 4) = 20 + 5 = 25 \text{ gtt/min (macrogtt/min).}$$
$$20 - (20 \div 4) = 20 - 5 = 15 \text{ gtt/min (macrogtt/min).}$$

The safe acceptable IV rate adjustment is 15 to 25 gtt/min (macrogtt/min). It is safe to slow the rate to 17 gtt/min (macrogtt/min), which is less than 25%.

POINTS TO REMEMBER

- Monitor IV therapy every 30 to 60 min to maintain the ordered IV rate.
- Do not arbitrarily speed up or slow down an IV that is behind or ahead of schedule.
- Know the hospital policy regarding recalculation of IV flow rate. An IV should not vary more than 25% from its original rate.
- To recalculate an IV rate:
- Determine mL/hr:

$$x \text{ mL/hr} = \frac{\text{Remaining volume}}{\text{Remaining time (hrs)}}$$

- Use mL/hr and recalculate the rate in gtt/min.

$$x \text{ gtt/min} = \frac{\text{Number of mL} \times \text{drop factor}}{\text{Time in minutes}}$$

- Determine the % of variation

$$\frac{\text{Amount of} \uparrow \text{or} \downarrow}{\text{Original rate}} = \text{\% of variation}$$

- Alternate to use of percent: Divide the original rate by 4, then add and subtract the result from the original rate to get the acceptable IV rate adjustment.
- Contact the prescriber for a new IV order, if the recalculated rate exceeds 25%.

PRACTICE PROBLEMS

For each of the problems, recalculate the IV flow rates in gtt/min rates using either method presented, determine the percentage of change, and state your course of action. *Note:* The institution allows 25% variation and clients are stable.

53. 500 mL of 0.9% NS was ordered to infuse in 8 hr at the rate of 16 gtt/min (16 macrogtt/min). The drop factor is 15 gtt/mL. After 5 hr, you find 250 mL of fluid left.

a. ______________ gtt/min

b. ______________ % variation

c. ______________ Course of action

54. 250 mL of D5W was to infuse in 3 hr at the rate of 21 gtt/min (21 macrogtt/min). Drop factor: 15 gtt/mL. With $1\frac{1}{2}$ hr remaining, you find 200 mL left.

a. ______________ gtt/min

b. ______________ % variation

c. ______________ Course of action

55. 1,500 mL D5 RL to infuse in 12 hr at 42 gtt/min (42 macrogtt/min). After 6 hr, 650 mL has infused. Drop factor: 20 gtt/mL.

a. ______________ gtt/min

b. ______________ % variation

c. ______________ Course of action

56. 1,000 mL D5 0.33% NS was to infuse in 12 hr at 28 gtt/min (28 macrogtt/min). After 4 hr, 250 mL has infused. Drop factor: 20 gtt/mL.

a. ______________ gtt/min

b. ______________ % variation

c. ______________ Course of action

57. 500 mL D5 0.9% NS to infuse in 5 hr at 100 gtt/min (100 microgtt/min). After 2 hr, 250 mL has infused. Drop factor: 60 gtt/mL.

a. ______________ gtt/min

b. ______________ % variation

c. ______________ Course of action

Answers on pp. 592-593

Calculating Total Infusion Times

IV fluids are ordered by the prescriber for administration at a certain rate in mL/hr, such as 1,000 mL D5W to infuse at 100 mL/hr. **The nurse needs to be able to determine the number of hours that an IV solution takes to infuse.** When the nurse calculates the total time for a certain volume of solution to infuse intravenously, this is referred to as **determining total infusion time.** To calculate infusion time, it is necessary for the nurse to have knowledge of the amount (volume) to infuse and the set calibration (drop factor) in gtt/mL.

Knowing the length of time for an infusion helps the nurse monitor IV therapy and prepare for the hanging of a new solution as the one infusing is being completed. Determining infusion times helps avoid things such as a line clotting off as a result of not knowing when an IV was to be completed. A nurse who knows the infusion time can anticipate when to start a new IV infusion and when to determine lab values that may have to be obtained after a certain amount of fluid has infused.

Calculating Infusion Time From Volume and Hourly Rate Ordered

Infusion time is determined by taking the total number of milliliters to infuse and dividing it by the rate in mL/hr at which the solution is infusing. This can also be done by using a ratio and proportion, in which the known ratio is the ordered rate in mL/hr and would be the first ratio (on one side) and the unknown ratio for total milliliters to infuse in *x* hours would be the second ratio. In addition, this can be done by using dimensional analysis.

Formula

$$\frac{\text{Total number of mL to infuse}}{\text{mL/hr infusion rate}} = \text{Total infusion time}$$

Example 1: Calculate the infusion time for an IV of 1,000 mL D5W infusing at a rate of 125 mL/hr.

✔ Solution Using the Formula Method

1,000 mL (total number of mL to infuse)

125 mL/hr (mL/hr to infuse)

$$\frac{1{,}000 \cancel{\text{mL}}}{125 \cancel{\text{mL}}/\text{hr}} = 1000 \div 125 = 8 \text{ hr}$$

Infusion time = 8 hr

✔ Solution Using Dimensional Analysis

1. Write the hr being calculated to the left of the equals sign.

$$x \text{ hr} =$$

2. Use the problem information that contains hr, and enter it as the starting fraction (125 mL/hr). Place 1 hr in the numerator and 125 mL in the denominator.

$$x \text{ hr} = \frac{1 \text{ hr}}{125 \text{ mL}}$$

3. Refer to the problem for mL (1,000 mL to be infused). Place 1,000 mL as the next numerator to match mL in the first denominator.

$$x \text{ hr} = \frac{1 \text{ hr}}{125 \text{ mL}} \times \frac{1{,}000 \text{ mL}}{1}$$

4. Cancel the units, reducing if possible; the unit hr remains and is calculated.

$$x \text{ hr} = \frac{1 \text{ hr}}{\overset{}{\cancel{125}}_{1} \cancel{\text{mL}}} \times \frac{\overset{8}{\cancel{1000}} \cancel{\text{mL}}}{1}$$

$$x = 8 \text{ hr}$$

Example 2: 1,000 mL of D5 ½ NS is ordered to infuse at 150 mL/hr. Calculate the infusion time to the nearest hundredth.

✔ Solution Using the Formula Method

$$\frac{1{,}000 \cancel{\text{mL}}}{150 \cancel{\text{mL}}/\text{hr}} = 6.66 \text{ hr}$$

Fractions of hours can be changed to minutes: 6 represents the total number of hours; 0.66 represents a fraction of an hour and can be converted to minutes. This is done by multiplying 0.66 by 60 min (60 min = 1 hr) and then rounding off to the nearest whole number.

$$0.66 \cancel{\text{hr}} \times 60 \text{ min}/\cancel{\text{hr}} = 39.6 = 40 \text{ min}$$

Infusion time = 6 hr and 40 minutes

✔ Solution Using Dimensional Analysis

Use the same steps as outlined in Example 1.

$$x \text{ hr} = \frac{1 \text{ hr}}{150 \cancel{\text{mL}}} \times \frac{1{,}000 \cancel{\text{mL}}}{1}$$

$$x = 6.66 \text{ hr}$$

Convert 0.66 hr to minutes by multiplying by 60 min (1 hr); then round off to the nearest whole number.

$$0.66 \cancel{\text{hr}} \times 60 \text{ min}/\cancel{\text{hr}} = 39.6 = 40 \text{ min}$$

or

$$x \text{ min} = \frac{60 \text{ min}}{1 \cancel{\text{hr}}} \times \frac{0.66 \cancel{\text{hr}}}{1}$$

Once infusion time has been calculated, the nurse can use this information to determine the time an IV would be completed. For Example 2 this would be determined as follows: add the calculated infusion time to the time the infusion was started. If the IV in Example 2 was hung at 7:00 AM, add the 6 hours and 40 minutes to that time. The IV would be completed at 1:40 PM.

An easy way to do this is by using military time to determine the time it would be completed.

Example: 7:00 AM = 0700

After converting 7:00 AM to military time, add 6 hours and 40 minutes to arrive at your answer of 1340.

0700 + 640 = 1340 = 1:40 PM

Note: Converting traditional time to military time is covered in Chapter 9. Refer to that chapter to refresh your memory on how to do this.

PRACTICE PROBLEMS

Determine infusion time for the following IVs. State time in traditional and military time.

58. An IV of 500 mL NS is to infuse at 60 mL/hr.

    a. Determine the infusion time. __________

    b. The IV was started at 10:00 PM. When would the IV infusion be completed? __________

59. An IV of 250 mL D5W is to infuse at 80 mL/hr.

    a. Determine the infusion time. __________

    b. The IV was started at 2:00 AM. When would the IV infusion be completed? __________

60. 1,000 mL of D5W is to infuse at 40 mL/hr.

    a. Determine the infusion time. __________

    b. The IV was started at 2:10 PM on August 26. When would the IV infusion be completed? __________

61. An IV of 1,000 mL D5 RL is to infuse at 60 mL/hr.

    a. Determine the infusion time. __________

    b. The IV was started at 6:00 AM. At what time would this IV infusion be completed? __________

62. An IV of 500 mL D5W is to infuse at 75 mL/hr.

    a. Determine the infusion time. __________

    b. The IV was started at 2:00 PM. At what time would the IV infusion be completed? __________

Answers on p. 594

Calculating Infusion Time When Rate in mL/hr Is Not Indicated for Large Volumes of Fluid

There are situations in which the prescriber may order the IV solution and not indicate the rate in mL/hr. The only information may be the total number of milliliters to infuse, the flow rate (gtt/min) of the IV, and the number of gtt/mL that the tubing delivers. In this situation, before the infusion time is calculated, the following must be done:

1. Convert gtt/min to mL/min.
2. Convert mL/min to mL/hr.

After completing these steps, you are ready to calculate the infusion time for the IV using the same formula:

$$\frac{\text{Total number of mL to infuse}}{\text{mL/hr infusion rate}}$$

Example: A client is receiving 1,000 mL of RL. The IV is infusing at 21 macrogtt/min (21 gtt/min). The administration set delivers 10 gtt/mL. Calculate the infusion time.

Step 1: Use a ratio and proportion to change gtt/min to mL/min.

$$10 \text{ gtt} : 1 \text{ mL} = 21 \text{ gtt} : x \text{ mL}$$

$$\frac{10x}{10} = \frac{21}{10}$$

$$x = 2.1 \text{ mL/min}$$

Step 2: Convert mL/min to mL/hr.

$$2.1 \text{ mL}/\cancel{\text{min}} \times 60\ \cancel{\text{min}}/\text{hr} = 126 \text{ mL/hr}$$

Step 3: Determine infusion time as already shown.

a. $\dfrac{1{,}000\ \cancel{\text{mL}}}{126\ \cancel{\text{mL}}/\text{hr}} = 7.93 \text{ hr}$

b. $0.93\ \cancel{\text{hr}} \times 60 \text{ min}/\cancel{\text{hr}} = 55.8 = 56 \text{ minutes}$

Infusion time = 7 hr and 56 minutes

Note: To determine the time the infusion would be completed, you would add the infusion time to the time the IV was started.

✓ Solution Using Dimensional Analysis

1. Write the hr being calculated first to the left of the equals sign, then write 1 hr = 60 min as the first fraction. Place 1 hr in the numerator and 60 min in the denominator.

$$x \text{ hr} = \frac{1 \text{ hr}}{60 \text{ min}}$$

2. Refer to the problem for information that contains min, and place it as the second fraction, placing min in the numerator (21 gtt/min).

$$x \text{ hr} = \frac{1 \text{ hr}}{60 \text{ min}} \times \frac{1 \text{ min}}{21 \text{ gtt}}$$

3. Refer to the problem again; you need gtt to match the denominator of the second fraction. This is indicated in the drop factor (10 gtt/mL). Write the fraction with 10 gtt in the numerator and mL in the denominator.

$$x \text{ hr} = \frac{1 \text{ hr}}{60 \text{ min}} \times \frac{1 \text{ min}}{21 \text{ gtt}} \times \frac{10 \text{ gtt}}{1 \text{ mL}}$$

4. The final fraction must match the denominator of the preceeding fraction. The mL is provided by the volume of fluid to infuse (1,000 mL).

$$x \text{ hr} = \frac{1 \text{ hr}}{\underset{6}{\cancel{60}}\ \cancel{\text{min}}} \times \frac{1\ \cancel{\text{min}}}{21\ \cancel{\text{gtt}}} \times \frac{\overset{1}{\cancel{10}}\ \cancel{\text{gtt}}}{1\ \cancel{\text{mL}}} \times \frac{1{,}000\ \cancel{\text{mL}}}{1} = 7.93 \text{ hr}$$

$$0.93\ \cancel{\text{hr}} \times 60 \text{ min}/\cancel{\text{hr}} = 55.8 = 56 \text{ min}$$

or

$$x \text{ min} = \frac{60 \text{ min}}{1\ \cancel{\text{hr}}} \times \frac{0.93\ \cancel{\text{hr}}}{1} = 55.8 = 56 \text{ min}$$

$$x = 56 \text{ min}$$

Infusion time = 7 hr and 56 min

PRACTICE PROBLEMS

Determine the infusion time for the following IVs.

63. A client is receiving 1,000 mL D5W at 25 microgtt/min. Drop factor is microdrop. ______________

64. A client is receiving 250 mL of NS at 17 macrogtt/min. Drop factor: 15 gtt/mL. ______________

65. A client is receiving 1,000 mL D5W. The IV is infusing at 30 macrogtt/min. Drop factor: 20 gtt/mL. ______________

66. A client is receiving 1,000 mL D5W at 20 macrogtt/min. Drop factor: 10 gtt/mL. ______________

67. A client is receiving 100 mL D5W at 10 macrogtt/min. Drop factor: 15 gtt/mL. ______________

Answers on p. 594

Calculating Infusion Time for Small Volumes of Fluid

There may be times when it is necessary for the nurse to determine the infusion time for small volumes of fluid that will infuse in less than an hour. To do this the nurse must first do the following:

1. Calculate the mL/min.
2. Divide the total volume by the mL/min to obtain the infusion time. The infusion time will be in minutes.

Example: An IV antibiotic of 30 mL is infusing at 20 macrogtt/min. Drop factor is 10 gtt/mL. Determine the infusion time.

Step 1: Calculate the mL/min.

$$10 \text{ gtt} : 1 \text{ mL} = 20 \text{ gtt} : x \text{ mL}$$

$$\frac{10x}{10} = \frac{20}{10}$$

$$x = 2 \text{ mL/min}$$

Step 2: Divide the total volume by mL/min.

$$30 \cancel{\text{mL}} \div 2 \cancel{\text{mL}}/\text{min} = 15 \text{ minutes}$$

The infusion time is 15 minutes.

✔ Solution Using Dimensional Analysis

Place min to the left of the equals sign. (Since a small volume is being infused in less than 1 hr, the time will be in minutes.) Therefore, the conversion factor 60 min = 1 hr is not necessary.

$$x \text{ min} =$$

The remaining steps are the same as for calculating infusion time for large volumes.

$$x \text{ min} = \frac{1 \text{ min}}{\overset{}{\cancel{20}} \cancel{\text{gtt}}_{2}} \times \frac{\overset{1}{\cancel{10}} \cancel{\text{gtt}}}{1 \cancel{\text{mL}}} \times \frac{30 \cancel{\text{mL}}}{1}$$

$$x = \frac{30}{2} = 15 \text{ min}$$

$$x = 15 \text{ min}$$

The infusion time is 15 minutes.

PRACTICE PROBLEMS

Determine the infusion times for the following:

68. An IV medication of 35 mL is infusing at 30 macrogtt/min. Drop factor: 15 gtt/mL. ____________

69. An IV medication of 20 mL is infusing at 35 microgtt/min. Drop factor: 60 gtt/mL. ____________

Answers on p. 594

Charting IV Therapy

At some institutions, continuous IV therapy may be charted on a special IV record or IV flow sheet. Medications that are administered intermittently by piggyback are charted on other medication sheets according to the order (e.g., standing medication sheet, p.r.n., or single, stat medication record). Forms used to chart IV therapy (whether a client is receiving IV solution that contains medications or solution without medications) vary from institution to institution. At institutions where a computerized system is used, IVs are charted directly into the computer. Appropriate assessments relating to IV sites are also charted on either a form for IV therapy or in the computer.

Labeling Solution Bags

The markings on IV solution bags are not as precise as, for example, those on a syringe. Most IV bags are marked in increments of 50 to 100 mL. After calculating the amount of solution to infuse in 1 hour, the nurse may mark the bag to indicate where the level of fluid should be at each hour. Marking the IV bag allows the nurse to check that the fluid is infusing on time. Many institutions have commercially prepared labels for this purpose.

POINTS TO REMEMBER

- To calculate infusion time, use dimensional analysis or divide the total volume to infuse expressed in mL/hr.

$$\frac{\text{Total number of mL to infuse}}{\text{mL/hr infusion rate}}$$

- Express fractional hours in minutes by multiplying by 60; round to nearest whole number.
- To obtain the completion time for an IV, add the infusion time calculated to the time IV was started. (Time can be stated in traditional or military time.)
- Calculation of completion times provides the nurse with the opportunity to plan ahead. (Have the next IV bag ready to hang once solution is completed, to prevent the line from clotting off.)
- Labeling IV solution bags provides a visual record of the infusion status.

Administration of Medications by IV Push

Injection ports on IV tubing can be used for direct injection of medication with a syringe, which is called an IV push. When using the primary line, the medication should be administered through the port closest to the client. An IV push medication can also be administered using a saline or heparin lock, which can be attached to the IV catheter. A saline lock indicates that saline is used to flush or maintain IV catheter patency whereas a heparin lock indicates that heparin is used to maintain the IV catheter patency. Medications can be administered with an IV push by attaching the syringe to the lock and pushing in the medication. The lock is usually flushed after administration of the medication.

> **SAFETY ALERT!**
>
> Remember that heparin is a **high-alert medication.** Heparin lock flush is usually in dosage strengths of 10 or 100 units per mL. Always read the label carefully. Know the agency policy for the use of heparin to maintain an IV lock.

When medication is administered by IV push, the client experiences rapid results from the medication. Direct IV administration is used to deliver diluted or undiluted medication over a brief period (seconds or minutes). Medication literature and institutional guidelines provide the acceptable rate for IV push medication administration. Because of the rapidity of action, an error in calculation can result in a serious outcome. Medications can be administered by IV push by registered nurses who have been specially trained in this practice at some institutions. An IV bolus usually indicates a quantity of fluid can be infused over a specified period of time through an IV set-up attached to the lock.

Most IV push medications should be administered over a period of 1 to 5 minutes (or longer). The volume of the prescribed medication should be calculated in increments of 15 to 30 seconds. This allows the use of a watch to provide accurate administration. The actual administration of IV push medications is beyond the scope of this text. For a detailed description of the technique, consult a clinical skills textbook.

> **SAFETY ALERT!**
>
> Never infuse IV medications more rapidly than recommended. Carefully read literature for dilution and time for administration. IV medications are potent and rapid acting.

When administering medications by direct IV infusion, it is necessary to remember the following:

- **The compatibility of the IV solution and the medication must be verified.**
- The tubing will require a flush after direct administration to ensure that all the medication has been given and none remains in the tubing.
- The amount of time needed to administer a medication by direct IV infusion can be determined by using ratio and proportion or dimensional analysis. Let's look at some examples.

Example 1: Order: Tagamet 200 mg IV push now

Available: Tagamet 300 mg per 2 mL

The literature recommends diluting the Tagamet to a total of 20 mL. Compatible solution recommended is sodium chloride injection (0.9%). Inject over a period of not less than 2 minutes. An injection time of 5 minutes is ordered.

a. How many mL of Tagamet will you administer?
b. How many mL of sodium chloride must you add to obtain the desired volume?
c. To administer the infusion in 5 minutes, how many mL should you infuse every minute?
d. How much should you infuse every 15 seconds?

a. **Ratio and Proportion:**

$$300\text{ mg} : 2\text{ mL} = 200\text{ mg} : x\text{ mL} \quad \textit{or} \quad \frac{300\text{ mg}}{2\text{ mL}} = \frac{200\text{ mg}}{x\text{ mL}}$$

$$\frac{300x}{300} = \frac{400}{300} = 1.33$$

$$x = 1.3\text{ mL}$$

Formula Method: $$\frac{200\text{ mg}}{300\text{ mg}} \times 2\text{ mL} = x\text{ mL}$$

Dimensional Analysis: $$x\text{ mL} = \frac{2\text{ mL}}{300\text{ }\cancel{\text{mg}}} \times \frac{200\text{ }\cancel{\text{mg}}}{1}$$

1.3 mL Tagamet would equal 200 mg.

b. According to the literature, the total volume of the diluent and medication is 20 mL. If the literature stated to dilute in 20 mL, then the total volume would be the medication and diluent

$$\begin{array}{l} 20\text{ mL desired} \\ \underline{-1.3\text{ mL dosage}} \\ 18.7\text{ mL amount to add} \end{array}$$

c. **Ratio and Proportion:** (1 minute)

$$20\text{ mL} : 5\text{ minutes} = x\text{ mL} : 1\text{ minute}$$

$$\frac{5x}{5} = \frac{20}{5}$$

$$x = 4\text{ mL per minute}$$

d. **Ratio and Proportion:** (15 sec)

$$4\text{ mL} : 60\text{ seconds} = x\text{ mL} : 15\text{ sec}$$

$$\frac{60x}{60} = \frac{60}{60}$$

$$x = 1\text{ mL every 15 seconds}$$

Dimensional Analysis:

Steps:

1. The desired unit is mL; place it to the left of the equals sign.

$$x\text{ mL} =$$

2. Refer to the problem, and place the mL ordered as the first fraction (20 mL in 5 min); place mL in the numerator to match the mL desired.

$$x\text{ mL} = \frac{20\text{ mL}}{5\text{ min}}$$

3. Place 1 min in the numerator of the next fraction.

$$x \text{ mL} = \frac{\overset{4}{\cancel{20}} \text{ mL}}{\underset{1}{\cancel{5}} \cancel{\text{min}}} \times \frac{1 \cancel{\text{min}}}{1} = 4$$

$$x = 4 \text{ mL per minute}$$

4 mL per minute

Notice that in this question you are asked to determine seconds. (Express 4 mL per minute as 4 mL per 60 seconds.) 60 seconds = 1 minute. The starting fraction would be 4 mL/60 sec:

$$x \text{ mL} = \frac{4 \text{ mL}}{60 \cancel{\text{sec}}} \times \frac{15 \cancel{\text{sec}}}{1}$$

$$x = \frac{60}{60} = 1$$

This could also be done using the 4 mL/min; however, you would need an additional fraction to be added to the equation. The equation would be as follows:

$$x \text{ mL} = \frac{4 \text{ mL}}{1 \cancel{\text{min}}} \times \frac{1 \cancel{\text{min}}}{60 \cancel{\text{sec}}} \times \frac{15 \cancel{\text{sec}}}{1}$$

$$x = 1 \text{ mL every 15 seconds}$$

Example 2: Order: Ativan 3 mg IV push stat

Available: Ativan 4 mg per mL

The literature states not to exceed 2 mg/min. Determine the time to administer the medication as ordered.

a. How many mL of Ativan will you prepare? (Express in hundredths.)
b. How many min would administer the medication as ordered?

a. **Ratio and Proportion:** $4 \text{ mg} : 1 \text{ mL} = 3 \text{ mg} : x \text{ mL}$ *or* $\frac{4 \text{ mg}}{1 \text{ mL}} = \frac{3 \text{ mg}}{x \text{ mL}}$

$$\frac{4x}{4} = \frac{3}{4}$$

$$x = 0.75 \text{ mL}$$

Formula Method: $\frac{3 \text{ mg}}{4 \text{ mg}} \times 1 \text{ mL} = x \text{ mL}$

Dimensional Analysis: $x \text{ mL} = \frac{1 \text{ mL}}{4 \cancel{\text{mg}}} \times \frac{3 \cancel{\text{mg}}}{1}$

b. **Ratio and Proportion:** $2 \text{ mg} : 1 \text{ min} = 3 \text{ mg} : x \text{ min}$ *or* $\frac{2 \text{ mg}}{1 \text{ min}} = \frac{3 \text{ mg}}{x \text{ min}}$

$$\frac{2x}{2} = \frac{3}{2}$$

$$x = 1\frac{1}{2} \text{ min}$$

$1\frac{1}{2}$ min to administer the medication as ordered

Dimensional Analysis: Use the steps outlined in Example 1 to determine the time.

$$x \text{ min} = \frac{1 \text{ min}}{2 \cancel{\text{mg}}} \times \frac{3 \cancel{\text{mg}}}{1}$$

POINTS TO REMEMBER

IV Push Medications

- Always verify the compatibility of the medication and the IV solution when administering medications by IV push.
- Never administer a medication by IV push at a rate faster than recommended. Always read package inserts and reputable medication resources for minimum time for IV administration and dilution.
- Use ratio and proportion or dimensional analysis to determine the IV push time as recommended by a reputable reference.

PRACTICE **PROBLEMS**

Calculate the IV push rate as indicated for Problems 70 to 72.

70. Order: Valium 20 mg IV push stat at 5 mg/min for a client with seizures.

    Available: Valium 5 mg per mL

    a. How many milliliters will be needed to administer the dosage? __________

    b. Determine the time it would take to infuse the dosage. __________

    c. How many milligrams would you administer every 15 seconds? __________

71. Order: Dilantin 150 mg IV push stat.

    Available: Dilantin 250 mg per 5 mL. Literature states IV infusion not to exceed 50 mg/min.

    a. How much should you prepare to administer? __________

    b. How much time is needed to administer the required dosage? __________

72. Order: AquaMEPHYTON 5 mg IV push stat.

    Available: AquaMEPHYTON 10 mg per mL. The literature states that the medication should be diluted in at least 10 mL of NS and administered at a rate of 1 mg or fraction thereof per minute.

    a. How much diluent should you add to the medication? __________

    b. How much medication should you inject every 30 seconds to infuse the medication at a rate of 1 mg/min? __________

Answers on p. 595

CLINICAL REASONING

Scenario: An elderly client has an order for 1,000 mL D5W at 100 mL/hr. The nurse assigned to the client attached IV tubing to the IV with a drop factor of 10 gtt/mL without checking the package of IV tubing. As a habit from a previous institution where she worked, the IV flow rate was calculated based on the drop factor of 20 gtt/mL. At the beginning of the next shift, the nurse making rounds noticed that the client was having difficulty breathing and seemed restless. When the nurse checked the IV rate, she discovered the rate was 33 macrogtt/min instead of 17 macrogtt/min.

a. What factors contributed to the error? ______________________________

b. How did the IV rate contribute to the problem and why? ______________________________

c. What should have been the action of the nurse who attached the IV tubing in relation to IV administration? ______________________________

Answers on p. 595

CHAPTER REVIEW

Calculate the IV flow rate in gtt/min for the following IV administrations, unless another unit of measure is stated.

1. 1,000 mL D5RL to infuse in 8 hr.
   Drop factor: 20 gtt/mL ______________________________

2. 2,500 mL D5NS to infuse in 24 hr.
   Drop factor: 10 gtt/mL ______________________________

3. 500 mL D5W to infuse in 4 hr.
   Drop factor: 15 gtt/mL ______________________________

4. 300 mL NS to infuse in 6 hr.
   Drop factor: 60 gtt/mL ______________________________

5. 1,000 mL D5W for 24 hr KVO (keep vein open). Drop factor: 60 gtt/mL ______________________________

6. 500 mL D5 $\frac{1}{2}$ NS over 12 hr.
   Drop factor: 20 gtt/mL ______________________________

7. 1,000 mL RL to infuse in 10 hr.
   Drop factor: 20 gtt/mL ______________________________

8. 1,500 mL NS to infuse in 12 hr.
   Drop factor: 10 gtt/mL ______________________________

9. A unit of whole blood (500 mL) to infuse in 4 hr. Drop factor: 10 gtt/mL ______________________________

10. A unit of packed cells (250 mL) to infuse in 4 hr. Drop factor: 10 gtt/mL ______________________________

11. 1,500 mL D5W in 8 hr.
    Drop factor: 20 gtt/mL ______________________________

12. 3,000 mL RL in 24 hr.
    Drop factor: 15 gtt/mL ______________________________

13. Infuse 2 L RL in 24 hr.
Drop factor: 15 gtt/mL ______

14. 500 mL D5W in 4 hr.
Drop factor: 60 gtt/mL ______

15. 1,000 mL D5 0.45% NS in 6 hr.
Drop factor: 20 gtt/mL ______

16. 250 mL D5W in 8 hr.
Drop factor: 60 gtt/mL ______

17. 1 L of D5W to infuse at 50 mL/hr.
Drop factor: 60 gtt/mL ______

18. 2 L D5RL at 150 mL/hr.
Drop factor: 15 gtt/mL ______

19. 500 mL D5W in 6 hr.
Drop factor: 15 gtt/mL ______

20. 1,500 mL NS in 12 hr.
Drop factor: 10 gtt/mL ______

21. 1,500 mL D5W in 24 hr.
Drop factor: 15 gtt/mL ______

22. 2,000 mL D5W in 16 hr.
Drop factor: 20 gtt/mL ______

23. 500 mL D5W in 8 hr.
Drop factor: 15 gtt/mL ______

24. 250 mL D5W in 10 hr.
Drop factor: 60 gtt/mL ______

25. Infuse 300 mL of D5W at 75 mL/hr.
Drop factor: 60 gtt/mL ______

26. Infuse 125 mL/hr of D5RL.
Drop factor: 20 gtt/mL ______

27. Infuse 40 mL/hr of D5W.
Drop factor: 60 gtt/mL ______

28. Infuse an IV medication with a volume of 50 mL in 45 minutes.
Drop factor: 60 gtt/mL ______

29. Infuse 90 mL/hr of NS.
Drop factor: 15 gtt/mL ______

30. Infuse 150 mL/hr of D5RL.
Drop factor: 10 gtt/mL ______

31. Infuse 2,500 mL of D5W in 24 hr.
Drop factor: 15 gtt/mL ______

32. Infuse an IV medication in 50 mL of 0.9% NS in 40 minutes. Drop factor: 10 gtt/mL __________

33. Infuse an IV medication in 100 mL D5W in 30 minutes. Drop factor: 20 gtt/mL __________

34. Infuse 250 mL 0.45% NS in 5 hr. Drop factor: 20 gtt/mL __________

35. Infuse 1,000 mL of D5W at 80 mL/hr. Drop factor: 20 gtt/mL __________

36. Infuse 150 mL of D5RL in 30 minutes. Drop factor: 10 gtt/mL __________

37. Infuse Kefzol 0.5 g in 50 mL D5W in 30 minutes. Drop factor: 60 gtt/mL __________

38. Infuse Plasmanate 500 mL over 3 hr. Drop factor: 10 gtt/mL __________

39. Infuse albumin 250 mL over 2 hr. Drop factor: 15 gtt/mL __________

40. The prescriber orders the following IVs for 24 hr. Drop factor: 10 gtt/mL
    a. 1,000 mL D5W with 1 ampule MVI (multivitamin)
    b. 500 mL D5W
    c. 250 mL D5W __________

41. Infuse vancomycin 1 g IVPB in 150 mL D5W in 1.5 hr. Drop factor: 60 gtt/mL __________

42. If 2 L D5W is to infuse in 16 hr, how many milliliters are to be administered per hour? __________

43. If 500 mL of RL is to infuse in 4 hr, how many milliliters are to be administered per hour? __________

44. If 200 mL of NS is to infuse in 2 hr, how many milliliters are to be administered per hour? __________

45. If 500 mL of D5W is to infuse in 8 hr, how many milliliters are to be administered per hour? __________

46. Infuse a TPN solution of 1,100 mL in 12 hr. How many milliliters are to be administered per hour? __________

47. Infuse 500 mL Intralipids IV in 6 hr.
Drop factor: 10 gtt/mL ______________________

48. Infuse 3,000 mL D5W in 20 hr.
Drop factor: 20 gtt/mL ______________________

49. An IV of 500 mL D5W with 200 mg of minocycline is to infuse in 6 hr.
Drop factor: 15 gtt/mL ______________________

50. An IV of D5W 500 mL was ordered to infuse over 10 hr at a rate of 13 gtt/min (13 macrogtt/min).
Drop factor: 15 gtt/mL
After 3 hr, you notice that 300 mL of IV solution is left. Recalculate the rate in gtt/min for the remaining solution ______________________ gtt/min
Determine the percentage of change in IV rate, and state your course of action. ______________________ %

51. An IV of D5W 1,000 mL was ordered to infuse over 8 hr at a rate of 42 gtt/min (42 macrogtt/min).
Drop factor: 20 gtt/mL
After 4 hr, you notice that only 400 mL has infused. Recalculate the rate in gtt/min for the remaining solution. ______________________ gtt/min
Determine the percentage of change, and state your course of action. ______________________ %

52. An IV of 1,000 mL D5 1/2 NS has been ordered to infuse at 125 mL/hr.
Drop factor: 15 gtt/mL
The IV was hung at 7 AM. At 11 AM, you check the IV, and there is 400 mL left. Recalculate the rate in gtt/min for the remaining solution. ______________________ gtt/min
Determine the percentage of change, and state your course of action. ______________________ %

53. An IV of 500 mL of 0.9% NS is to infuse in 12 hr at a rate of 42 gtt/min (42 microgtt/min).
Drop factor: 60 gtt/mL
The IV was hung at 7 AM. You check the IV in $2\frac{1}{2}$ hours and find 300 mL remaining. Recalculate the rate in gtt/min for the remaining solution. ______________________ gtt/min
Determine the percentage of change, and state your course of action. ______________________ %

54. An IV of 1,000 mL D5W is to infuse in 10 hr. Drop factor: 15 gtt/mL
The IV was started at 4 AM. At 10 AM, 600 mL remains in the bag.
Is the IV on schedule? __________
If not, recalculate the rate in gtt/min for the remaining solution. __________ gtt/min
Determine the percentage of change and state your course of action. __________ %

55. 900 mL of RL is infusing at a rate of 80 gtt/min (80 macrodrops/min).
Drop factor: 15 gtt/mL
How long will it take for the IV to infuse? (Express time in hours and minutes.) __________

56. A client is receiving 1,000 mL of D5W at 100 mL/hr. How many hours will it take for the IV to infuse? __________

57. 1,000 mL of D5W is infusing at 20 gtt/min (20 macrogtt/min).
Drop factor: 10 gtt/mL
How long will it take for the IV to infuse? (Express time in hours and minutes.) __________

58. 450 mL of NS is infusing at 25 gtt/min (25 macrogtt/min).
Drop factor: 20 gtt/mL
How many hours will it take for the IV to infuse? __________

59. 100 mL of D5W is infusing at 10 gtt/min (10 macrogtt/min).
The administration set delivers 15 gtt/mL. How many hours will it take for the IV to infuse? __________

60. An IV is regulated at 25 gtt/min (25 macrogtt/min).
Drop factor: 15 gtt/mL
How many milliliters of fluid will the client receive in 8 hr? __________

61. An IV is regulated at 40 gtt/min (40 microdrop/min).
Drop factor: 60 gtt/mL
How many milliliters of fluid will the client receive in 10 hr? __________

62. An IV is regulated at 30 gtt/min (30 macrogtt/min).
Drop factor: 15 gtt/mL
How many milliliters of fluid will the client receive in 5 hr? __________

63. 10 mEq of potassium chloride is placed in 500 mL of D5W to be administered at the rate of 2 mEq/hr. At what rate in mL/hr should the IV infuse? ____________________

64. 25 mEq of potassium chloride is added to 1,000 mL of D5W to be administered at the rate of 4 mEq/hr. At what rate in mL/hr should the IV infuse? ____________________

65. Order: Humulin regular U-100 7 units/hr. The IV solution contains 50 units of Humulin regular insulin in 250 mL of 0.9% NS. At what rate in mL/hr should the IV infuse? ____________________

66. Order: Humulin regular U-100 18 units/hr. The IV solution contains 100 units of Humulin regular insulin in 250 mL of 0.9% NS. At what rate in mL/hr should the IV infuse? ____________________

67. Order: Humulin regular U-100 11 units/hr. The IV solution contains 100 units of Humulin regular insulin in 100 mL of 0.9% NS. At what rate in mL/hr should the IV infuse? ____________________

68. Infuse gentamicin 65 mg in 150 mL 0.9% NS IVPB over 1 hr.
Drop factor: 10 gtt/mL
At what rate in gtt/min should the IV infuse? ____________________

69. Infuse ampicillin 1 g that has been diluted in 40 mL 0.9% NS to infuse in 40 minutes.
Drop factor: 60 gtt/mL
At what rate in gtt/min should the IV infuse? ____________________

70. Administer IV medication with a volume of 35 mL in 30 minutes.
Drop factor: 60 gtt/mL
At what rate in gtt/min should the IV infuse? ____________________

71. Administer IV medication with a volume of 80 mL in 40 minutes.
Drop factor: 15 gtt/mL
At what rate in gtt/min should the IV infuse? ____________________

72. Administer 50 mL of an antibiotic in 25 minutes.
Drop factor: 10 gtt/mL
At what rate in gtt/min would you regulate the IV? ____________________

73. An IV is to infuse at 65 mL/hr.
Drop factor: 15 gtt/mL
At what rate in gtt/min should the IV infuse? ______________

74. 50 mL of 0.9% NS with 1 g ampicillin is infusing at 50 microgtt/min (50 gtt/min).
Drop factor: 60 gtt/mL
Determine the infusion time. ______________

75. 500 mL RL is to infuse at a rate of 80 mL/hr. If the IV was started at 7 PM, what time will the IV be completed? ______________
State time in military and traditional time. ______________

76. A volume of 150 mL of NS is to infuse at 25 mL/hr.
   a. Calculate the infusion time. ______________
   b. The IV was started at 3:10 AM. What time will the IV be completed? State time in traditional and military time. ______________

77. The doctor orders 2.5 L of D5W to infuse at 150 mL/hr. Determine the infusion time. ______________

78. Order: Lasix 120 mg IV stat.
Available: 10 mg per mL. The literature states IV not to exceed 40 mg/min.
   a. How many milliliters will you prepare? ______________
   b. Calculate the time required to administer the medication as ordered. ______________

79. Order: Inocor 60 mg IV push over 2 min.
Available: Inocor 100 mg per 20 mL
   a. How many milliliters will you prepare? ______________
   b. Determine the amount that should be infused per minute. ______________

80. Order: Levaquin 500 mg IVPB in 100 mL 0.9% NS q12h over 1 hr.
Drop factor: 10 gtt/mL
Determine rate in gtt/min. ______________

81. Order: Zosyn 1.3 g in 100 mL D5W IVPB q8h to infuse over 30 min.
Drop factor: 60 gtt/mL
Determine rate in gtt/min. ______________

82. 500 mL D5W with 30,000 units of heparin to infuse at 1,500 units per hour.
Determine rate in mL/hr. ______________

83. Order: Humulin regular U-100 20 units per hr. The IV solution contains 100 units of Humulin Regular in 500 mL of 0.9% NS.
At what rate in mL/hr should the IV infuse? ______________

84. Order: Humulin regular U-100 15 units per hr. The IV solution contains 100 units of Humulin Regular in 250 mL of 0.9% NS.
At what rate in mL/hr should the IV infuse? ______________

Answers on pp. 595-602

ANSWERS

Chapter 22

Answers to Practice Problems

1. $x \text{ mL/hr} = \dfrac{1{,}800 \text{ mL}}{24 \text{ hr}}; x = 75 \text{ mL/hr}$

2. $x \text{ mL/hr} = \dfrac{2{,}000 \text{ mL}}{24 \text{ hr}} = 83.3; x = 83 \text{ mL/hr}$

3. $x \text{ mL/hr} = \dfrac{500 \text{ mL}}{12 \text{ hr}} = 41.6; x - 42 \text{ mL/hr}$

4. *Remember:* When infusion time is less than an hour, use a ratio and proportion to determine the rate in mL/hr or the formula.

   $100 \text{ mL} : 45 \text{ min} = x \text{ mL} : 60 \text{ min}$

   $\dfrac{45x}{45} = \dfrac{6{,}000}{45} = 133.3; x = 133 \text{ mL/hr}$

   or

   $x \text{ mL/hr} = \dfrac{100 \text{ mL}}{\underset{3}{\cancel{45}} \cancel{\text{min}}} \times \dfrac{\overset{4}{\cancel{60}} \cancel{\text{min}}/\text{hr}}{1}$

   $x = \dfrac{400}{3} = 133.3; x = 133 \text{ mL/hr}$

5. $x \text{ mL/hr} = \dfrac{1{,}500 \text{ mL}}{24 \text{ hr}} = 62.5; x = 63 \text{ mL/hr}$

6. $x \text{ mL/hr} = \dfrac{750 \text{ mL}}{16 \text{ hr}} = 46.8; x = 47 \text{ mL/hr}$

7. *Remember:* When infusion time is less than an hour, use a ratio and proportion to determine the rate in mL/hr or the formula.

   $30 \text{ mL} : 20 \text{ min} - x \text{ mL} : 60 \text{ min}$

   $\dfrac{20x}{20} = \dfrac{1{,}800}{20} = 90; x = 90 \text{ mL/hr}$

   or

   $x \text{ mL/hr} = \dfrac{30 \text{ mL}}{\underset{1}{\cancel{20}} \cancel{\text{min}}} \times \dfrac{\overset{3}{\cancel{60}} \cancel{\text{min}}/\text{hr}}{1}$

   $x = \dfrac{90}{1} = x = 90 \text{ mL/hr}$

8. 10 gtt/mL, macrodrop
9. 60 gtt/mL, microdrop
10. 20 gtt/mL, macrodrop
11. 15 gtt/mL, macrodrop
12. $x \text{ gtt/min} = \dfrac{75 \text{ mL} \times 10 \text{ gtt/mL}}{60 \text{ min}} =$

    $\dfrac{75 \times 10}{60} = \dfrac{75 \times 1}{6} = \dfrac{75}{6}$

    $x = \dfrac{75}{6} = 12.5$

    $x = 13$ gtt/min; 13 macrogtt/min

Evolve

For additional practice problems, refer to the Intravenous Flow Rates section of the Elsevier's Interactive Drug Calculation Application, Version 1 on Evolve.

13. $x \text{ gtt/min} = \dfrac{30 \text{ mL} \times 60 \text{ gtt/mL}}{60 \text{ min}} =$

$$\frac{30 \times 60}{60} = \frac{30 \times 1}{1} = \frac{30}{1}$$

$x = \dfrac{30}{1}; x = 30$

$x = 30$ gtt/min; 30 microgtt/min

14. $x \text{ gtt/min} = \dfrac{125 \text{ mL} \times 15 \text{ gtt/mL}}{60 \text{ min}} =$

$$\frac{125 \times 15}{60} = \frac{125 \times 1}{4} = \frac{125}{4}$$

$x = \dfrac{125}{4} = 31.2$

$x = 31$ gtt/min; 31 macrogtt/min

15. Step 1: Calculate mL/hr.

$x \text{ mL/hr} = \dfrac{1{,}000 \text{ mL}}{6 \text{ hr}} = 166.6$

$x = 167$ mL/hr

Step 2: Calculate gtt/min

$x \text{ gtt/min} = \dfrac{167 \text{ mL} \times 15 \text{ gtt/mL}}{60 \text{ min}} =$

$$\frac{167 \times 15}{60} = \frac{167 \times 1}{4} = \frac{167}{4}$$

$x = \dfrac{167}{4} = 41.7$

$x = 42$ gtt/min; 42 macrogtt/min

16. $x \text{ gtt/min} = \dfrac{60 \text{ mL} \times 60 \text{ gtt/mL}}{45 \text{ min}} =$

$$\frac{60 \times 60}{45} = \frac{60 \times 4}{3} = \frac{240}{3}$$

$x = \dfrac{240}{3}; x = 80$

$x = 80$ gtt/min; 80 microgtt/min

NOTE

These problems could also be done by first determining rate in mL/min to be administered and then calculating rate in gtt/min or by using dimensional analysis.

17. Step 1: Calculate mL/hr.

$x \text{ mL/hr} = \dfrac{1{,}000 \text{ mL}}{16 \text{ hr}} = 62.5; x = 63 \text{ mL/hr}$

Step 2: Calculate gtt/min.

$x \text{ gtt/min} = \dfrac{63 \text{ mL} \times 15 \text{ gtt/mL}}{60 \text{ min}} =$

$$\frac{63 \times 15}{60} = \frac{63 \times 1}{4} = \frac{63}{4}$$

$x = \dfrac{63}{4} = 15.7 = 16$

$x = 16$ gtt/min; 16 macrogtt/min

18. Step 1: Calculate mL/hr.

$x \text{ mL/hr} = \dfrac{150 \text{ mL}}{2 \text{ hr}}; x = 75 \text{ mL/hr}$

Step 2: Calculate gtt/min.

$x \text{ gtt/min} = \dfrac{75 \text{ mL} \times 20 \text{ gtt/mL}}{60 \text{ min}} =$

$$\frac{75 \times 20}{60} = \frac{75 \times 1}{3} = \frac{75}{3}$$

$x = \dfrac{75}{3}$

$x = 25$ gtt/min; 25 macrogtt/min

19. Step 1: Calculate mL/hr.

$x \text{ mL/hr} = \dfrac{3{,}000 \text{ mL}}{24 \text{ hr}}; x = 125 \text{ mL/hr}$

Step 2: Calculate gtt/min.

$x \text{ gtt/min} = \dfrac{125 \text{ mL} \times 10 \text{ gtt/mL}}{60 \text{ min}} =$

$$\frac{125 \times 10}{60} = \frac{125 \times 1}{6} = \frac{125}{6}$$

$x = \dfrac{125}{6} = 20.8 = 21$

$x = 21$ gtt/min; 21 macrogtt/min

20. Step 1: Calculate mL/hr.

$x \text{ mL/hr} = \dfrac{2{,}000 \text{ mL}}{12 \text{ hr}} = 166.6 = 167$

$x = 167$ mL/hr

Step 2: Calculate gtt/min.

$x \text{ gtt/min} = \dfrac{167 \text{ mL} \times 15 \text{ gtt/mL}}{60 \text{ min}} =$

$$\frac{167 \times 15}{60} = \frac{167 \times 1}{4} = \frac{167}{4}$$

$x = \dfrac{167}{4} = 41.7 = 42$

$x = 42$ gtt/min; 42 macrogtt/min

21. $x \text{ gtt/min} = \dfrac{60 \text{ mL} \times 60 \text{ gtt/mL}}{30 \text{ min}} =$

$$\frac{60 \times 60}{30} = \frac{60 \times 2}{1} = \frac{120}{1}$$

$x = \dfrac{120}{1} = 120$

$x = 120$ gtt/min; 120 microgtt/min

22. 20 gtt/mL

$\dfrac{60}{20}$

Answer: 3

23. 10 gtt/mL

$$\frac{60}{10}$$

Answer: 6

24. 60 gtt/mL

$$\frac{60}{60}$$

Answer: 1

25. Step 1: Determine the drop factor constant.

$$60 \div 10 = 6$$

Step 2: Calculate gtt/min.

$$x \text{ gtt/min} = \frac{200 \text{ mL/hr}}{6} = 33.3 = 33$$

$x = 33$ gtt/min; 33 macrogtt/min

26. Step 1: Determine the drop factor constant.

$$60 \div 15 = 4$$

Step 2: Calculate gtt/min.

$$x \text{ gtt/min} = \frac{50 \text{ mL/hr}}{4} = 12.5 = 13$$

$x = 13$ gtt/min; 13 macrogtt/min

27. Step 1: Determine the drop factor constant.

$$60 \div 60 = 1$$

Step 2: Calculate gtt/min.

$$x \text{ gtt/min} = \frac{80 \text{ mL/hr}}{1} = 80$$

$x = 80$ gtt/min; 80 microgtt/min

28. Step 1: Determine the drop factor constant.

$$60 \div 20 = 3$$

Step 2: Calculate gtt/min.

$$x \text{ gtt/min} = \frac{140 \text{ mL/hr}}{3} = 46.6 = 47$$

$x = 47$ gtt/min; 47 macrogtt/min

29. Step 1: Determine mL/hr.

$$x \text{ mL/hr} = \frac{1{,}000 \text{ mL}}{10 \text{ hr}}; x = 100 \text{ mL/hr}$$

Step 2: Determine the drop factor constant.

$$60 \div 10 = 6$$

Step 3: Calculate gtt/min.

$$x \text{ gtt/min} = \frac{100 \text{ mL/hr}}{6} = 16.6 = 17$$

$x = 17$ gtt/min; 17 macrogtt/min

30. Step 1: Determine mL/hr.

$$x \text{ mL/hr} = \frac{1{,}500 \text{ mL}}{12 \text{ hr}}; x = 125 \text{ mL/hr}$$

Step 2: Determine the drop factor constant.

$$60 \div 15 = 4$$

Step 3: Calculate gtt/min.

$$x \text{ gtt/min} = \frac{125 \text{ mL/hr}}{4} = 31.2 = 31$$

$x = 31$ gtt/min; 31 macrogtt/min

31. Remember that small volumes are multiplied and expressed in mL/hr.

Step 1: Determine mL/hr.

$$40 \text{ mL/20 min} = 40 \times 3 \ (3 \times 20 \text{ min}) = 120 \text{ mL/hr}$$

Step 2: Determine the drop factor constant.

$$60 \div 10 = 6$$

Step 3: Calculate gtt/min.

$$x \text{ gtt/min} = \frac{120 \text{ mL/hr}}{6} = 20$$

$x = 20$ gtt/min; 20 macrogtt/min

32. $$x \text{ gtt/min} = \frac{125 \text{ mL} \times 15 \text{ gtt/mL}}{60 \text{ min}} = \frac{125 \times 15}{60} = \frac{125 \times 1}{4} = \frac{125}{4}$$

$$x = \frac{125}{4} = 31.2 = 31$$

$x = 31$ gtt/min; 31 macrogtt/min

33. Step 1: Determine mL/hr.

$$x \text{ mL/hr} = \frac{2{,}500 \text{ mL}}{16 \text{ hr}} = 156.2 = 156$$

Step 2: Calculate gtt/min.

$$x \text{ gtt/min} = \frac{156 \text{ mL} \times 10 \text{ gtt/mL}}{60 \text{ min}} = \frac{156 \times 10}{60} = \frac{156 \times 1}{6} = \frac{156}{6}$$

$$x = \frac{156}{6} = 26$$

$x = 26$ gtt/min; 26 macrogtt/min

34. $$x \text{ gtt/min} = \frac{100 \text{ mL} \times 60 \text{ gtt/mL}}{60 \text{ min}} = \frac{100 \times 60}{60} = \frac{100 \times 1}{1} = \frac{100}{1}$$

$$x = \frac{100}{1} = 100$$

$x = 100$ gtt/min; 100 microgtt/min

35. 1 L = 1,000 mL

2 L = 2,000 mL

Step 1: Determine mL/hr.

$$x \text{ mL/hr} = \frac{2{,}000 \text{ mL}}{10 \text{ hr}}; x = 200 \text{ mL/hr}$$

Step 2: Calculate gtt/min.

$$x \text{ gtt/min} = \frac{200 \text{ mL} \times 15 \text{ gtt/mL}}{60 \text{ min}} =$$

$$\frac{200 \times 15}{60} = \frac{200 \times 1}{4} = \frac{200}{4}$$

$$x = \frac{200}{4} = 50$$

$x = 50$ gtt/min; 50 macrogtt/min

NOTE

Practice Problems 32-35 could also have been done by using the shortcut method (determining drop factor constant and then calculating gtt/min). This method would give the same answers.

36. $$x \text{ gtt/min} = \frac{100 \text{ mL} \times 15 \text{ gtt/mL}}{60 \text{ min}} =$$

$$\frac{100 \times 15}{60} = \frac{100 \times 1}{4} = \frac{100}{4}$$

$$x = \frac{100}{4} = 25$$

$x = 25$ gtt/min; 25 macrogtt/min

37. $$x \text{ gtt/min} = \frac{250 \text{ mL} \times 10 \text{ gtt/mL}}{60 \text{ min}} =$$

$$\frac{250 \times 10}{60} = \frac{250 \times 1}{6} = \frac{250}{6}$$

$$x = \frac{250}{6} = 41.6 = 42$$

$x = 42$ gtt/min; 42 macrogtt/min

38. a. 1 g : 10 mL = 1 g : x mL

or

$$\frac{1 \text{ g}}{1 \text{ g}} \times 10 \text{ mL} = x \text{ mL}$$

$x = 10$ mL

Answer: 10 mL. The dosage ordered is contained in a volume of 10 mL. 10 mL of medication is added to the 50 mL of IV solution to give a total of 60 mL.

b. $$x \text{ gtt/min} = \frac{60 \text{ mL} \times 10 \text{ gtt/mL}}{45 \text{ min}} =$$

$$\frac{60 \times 10}{45} = \frac{60 \times 2}{9} = \frac{120}{9}$$

$$x = \frac{120}{9} = 13.3 = 13$$

$x = 13$ gtt/min; 13 macrogtt/min

39. a. 150 mg : 1 mL = 900 mg : x mL

or

$$x = \frac{900 \text{ mg}}{150 \text{ mg}} \times 1 \text{ mL} = x \text{ mL}$$

$x = 6$ mL

Answer: 6 mL. The dosage ordered is more than the available strength; therefore more than 1 mL is needed to administer the dosage ordered.

Alternate solution:

600 mg : 4 mL = 900 mg : x mL

or

$$\frac{900 \text{ mg}}{600 \text{ mg}} \times 4 \text{ mL} = x \text{ mL}$$

This set-up would net the same answer.

b. $$x \text{ gtt/min} = \frac{75 \text{ mL} \times 10 \text{ gtt/mL}}{30 \text{ min}} =$$

$$\frac{75 \times 10}{30} = \frac{75 \times 1}{3} = \frac{75}{3}$$

$$x = \frac{75}{3} = 25$$

$x = 25$ gtt/min; 25 macrogtt/min

40. a. 300 mg : 2 mL = 300 mg : x mL

or

$$x = \frac{300 \text{ mg}}{300 \text{ mg}} \times 2 \text{ mL} = x \text{ mL}$$

$x = 2$ mL

Answer: 2 mL. The dosage ordered is contained in a volume of 2 mL. Label indicates 300 mg per 2 mL.

b. $$x \text{ gtt/min} = \frac{50 \text{ mL} \times 10 \text{ gtt/mL}}{30 \text{ min}} =$$

$$\frac{50 \times 10}{30} = \frac{50 \times 1}{3} = \frac{50}{3}$$

$$x = \frac{50}{3} = 16.6 = 17$$

$x = 17$ gtt/min; 17 macrogtt/min

41. a. 50 mg : 1 mL = 500 mg : x mL

or

$$\frac{500 \text{ mg}}{50 \text{ mg}} \times 1 \text{ mL} = x \text{ mL}$$

$x = 10$ mL

Answer: 10 mL. The dosage ordered is greater than the available strength; therefore you will need more than 1 mL to administer the ordered dosage. The volume of medication is added to the 100 mL of IV solution to get a total of 110 mL.

b. $x \text{ gtt/min} = \dfrac{110 \text{ mL} \times 15 \text{ gtt/mL}}{60 \text{ min}} =$

$$\frac{110 \times 15}{60} = \frac{110 \times 1}{4} = \frac{110}{4}$$

$$x = \frac{110}{4} = 27.5 = 28$$

$x = 28$ gtt/min; 28 macrogtt/min

42. a. 50 mg : 10 mL = 20 mg : x mL

or

$$\frac{20 \text{ mg}}{50 \text{ mg}} \times 10 \text{ mL} = x \text{ mL}$$

Answer: 4 mL. The dosage ordered is less than the available strength; therefore you will need less than 10 mL to administer the ordered dosage.

Step 1: Calculate mL/hr.

$$x \text{ mL/hr} = \frac{300 \text{ mL}}{6 \text{ hr}}; x = 50 \text{ mL/hr}$$

Step 2: Calculate gtt/min.

b. $x \text{ gtt/min} = \dfrac{50 \text{ mL} \times 60 \text{ gtt/mL}}{60 \text{ min}} =$

$$\frac{50 \times 60}{60} = \frac{50 \times 1}{1} = \frac{50}{1}$$

$$x = \frac{50}{1} = 50$$

$x = 50$ gtt/min; 50 microgtt/min

43. a. 16 mg : 1 mL = 300 mg : x mL

or

$$\frac{300 \text{ mg}}{16 \text{ mg}} \times 1 \text{ mL} = x \text{ mL}$$

Answer: 18.8 mL (18.75 mL rounded to the nearest tenth). The dosage ordered is more than the available strength; therefore you will need more than 1 mL to administer the ordered dosage.

b. $x \text{ gtt/min} = \dfrac{318.8 \text{ mL} \times 10 \text{ gtt/mL}}{60 \text{ min}} =$

$$\frac{318.8 \times 10}{60} = \frac{318.8 \times 1}{6} = \frac{318.8}{6}$$

$$x = \frac{318.8}{6} = 53.1 = 53$$

$x = 53$ gtt/min; 53 macrogtt/min

44. The available solution indicates each milliliter contains 10 mg of the medication. To administer the ordered dose, you will need to add 10 mL of medication to the IV volume. 100 mL of IV fluid and medication volume gives a total of 110 mL.

$$x \text{ gtt/min} = \frac{110 \text{ mL} \times 10 \text{ gtt/mL}}{60 \text{ min}} =$$

$$\frac{110 \times 10}{60} = \frac{110 \times 1}{6} = \frac{110}{6}$$

$$x = \frac{110}{6} = 18.3 = 18$$

$x = 18$ gtt/min; 18 macrogtt/min

45. 15 mEq : 1,000 mL = 2 mEq : x mL

$$\frac{15x}{15} = \frac{2{,}000}{15} = 133.3$$

$$x = 133 \text{ mL/hr}$$

or

$$\frac{15 \text{ mEq}}{1{,}000 \text{ mL}} = \frac{2 \text{ mEq}}{x \text{ mL}}$$

Answer: 133 mL/hr to deliver 2 mEq of potassium chloride per hour.

46. 50 units : 250 mL = 10 units : x mL

$$\frac{50x}{50} = \frac{2{,}500}{50}$$

$$x = 50 \text{ mL/hr}$$

or

$$\frac{50 \text{ units}}{250 \text{ mL}} = \frac{10 \text{ units}}{x \text{ mL}}$$

Answer: 50 mL/hr must be administered for the client to receive 10 units/hr.

47. 40 units : 250 mL = 15 units : x mL

$$\frac{40x}{40} = \frac{3{,}750}{40} = 93.7$$

$$x = 94 \text{ mL/hr}$$

or

$$\frac{40 \text{ units}}{250 \text{ mL}} = \frac{15 \text{ units}}{x \text{ mL}}$$

Answer: 94 mL/hr must be administered for the client to receive 15 units/hr.

NOTE

Problem 48 asks for time in hours, so minutes are changed to parts of hours.

48. $60 \text{ microgtt/min} = \dfrac{150 \text{ mL} \times 60 \text{ gtt/mL}}{x \text{ min}}$

$$60 = \frac{150 \times 60}{x}$$

$$60 = \frac{9{,}000}{x}$$

$$\frac{60x}{60} = \frac{9{,}000}{60}$$

$$x = 150 \text{ minutes}$$

60 min = 1 hr; 150 min ÷ 60 = 2.5 hr

Answer: $2\frac{1}{2}$ hr

NOTE

Because the formula is time in minutes, 5 hours was changed to minutes by multiplying 5 × 60 (60 min = 1 hr).

49. $35 \text{ macrogtt/min} = \dfrac{x \text{ mL} \times 15 \text{ gtt/mL}}{300 \text{ min}}$

$$35 = x\,(\times)\,\frac{\cancel{15}\;1}{\cancel{300}\;20}$$

$$35 = \frac{x}{20}$$

$$x = 35 \times 20 = 700$$

$$x = 700 \text{ mL}$$

NOTE

Problem 50 asks for time in hours, so minutes are changed to parts of hours.

50. $45 \text{ macrogtt/min} = \dfrac{180 \text{ mL} \times 15 \text{ gtt/mL}}{x \text{ min}}$

$$45 = \frac{180 \times 15}{x}$$

$$45 = \frac{2{,}700}{x}$$

$$\frac{45x}{45} = \frac{2{,}700}{45}$$

$$x = 60 \text{ min}$$

60 min = 1 hr; 60 min ÷ 60 = 1 hr

Answer: 1 hr

NOTE

Formula is in minutes; therefore, 8 hr × 60 = 480 min.

51. $45 \text{ macrogtt/min} = \dfrac{x \text{ mL} \times 15 \text{ gtt/mL}}{480 \text{ min}}$

$$45 = x\,(\times)\,\frac{\cancel{15}\;1}{\cancel{480}\;32}$$

$$45 = \frac{x}{32}$$

$$x = 45 \times 32 = 1{,}440$$

$$x = 1{,}440 \text{ mL}$$

NOTE

Problem 52 asks for time in hours, so minutes are changed to parts of hours.

52. $60 \text{ microgtt/min} = \dfrac{90 \text{ mL} \times 60 \text{ gtt/mL}}{x \text{ min}}$

$$60 = \frac{90 \times 60}{x}$$

$$60 = \frac{5{,}400}{x}$$

$$\frac{60x}{60} = \frac{5{,}400}{60}$$

$$x = 90 \text{ minutes}$$

60 min = 1 hr; 90 min ÷ 60 = 1.5 hr = $1\frac{1}{2}$ hr

53. Step 1: Determine mL/hr for the remaining solution.

$x \text{ mL/hr} = \dfrac{250 \text{ mL}}{3 \text{ hr}}$; $x = 83.3 = 83$ mL/hr

Step 2: Calculate gtt/min.

$$x \text{ gtt/min} = \frac{83 \text{ mL} \times 15 \text{ gtt/mL}}{60 \text{ min}} =$$

$$\frac{83 \times 15}{60} = \frac{83 \times 1}{4} = \frac{83}{4} = 20.7 = 21$$

$x = 21$ gtt/min; 21 macrogtt/min

a. $x = 21$ gtt/min; 21 macrogtt/min

b. Determine the percentage of change.

$$\frac{21 - 16}{16} = \frac{5}{16} = 0.312 = 31\%$$

c. Percentage of change is greater than 25%. Assess client. Consult prescriber; order may need to be revised.

Determine the acceptable range for variation.

16 + (16 ÷ 4) = 16 + 4 = 20 gtt/min (macrogtt/min)

16 − (16 ÷ 4) = 16 − 4 = 12 gtt/min (macrogtt/min)

The safe range is 12–20 gtt/min (macrodrop/min). The recalculated rate is 21, although only out of range by 1 gtt. It is greater than 25%.

54. Step 1: Determine mL/hr for the remaining solution.

$$x \text{ mL/hr} = \frac{200 \text{ mL}}{1.5 \text{ hr}} = 133.3 = 133 \text{ mL/hr}$$

Step 2: Calculate gtt/min.

$$x \text{ gtt/min} = \frac{133 \text{ mL} \times 15 \text{ gtt/mL}}{60 \text{ min}} = \frac{133 \times 15}{60} = \frac{133 \times 1}{4} = \frac{133}{4}$$

$$x = \frac{133}{4} = 33.2 = 33$$

a. $x = 33$ gtt/min; 33 macrogtt/min

b. Determine the percentage of change.

$$\frac{33 - 21}{21} = \frac{12}{21} = 0.571 = 57\%$$

c. Percentage of change is greater than 25%. Assess client. Consult prescriber; order may need to be revised.

Determine the acceptable range for variation.

$21 + (21 \div 4) = 21 + 5.25 = 26.25 = 26$ gtt/min (macrogtt/min)

$21 - (21 \div 4) = 21 - 5.25 = 15.75 = 16$ gtt/min (macrogtt/min)

The safe range is 16–20 gtt/min (macrogtt/min). The recalculated rate is 33 gtt/min (macrogtt). No, increasing the IV rate is greater than 25%.

55. Step 1: Determine mL/hr for the remaining solution.

$$x \text{ mL/hr} = \frac{850 \text{ mL}}{6 \text{ hr}} = 141.6 = 142$$

$x = 142$ mL/hr

Step 2: Calculate gtt/min.

$$x \text{ gtt/min} = \frac{142 \text{ mL} \times 20 \text{ gtt/mL}}{60 \text{ min}} = \frac{142 \times 20}{60} = \frac{142 \times 1}{3} = \frac{142}{3}$$

$$x = \frac{142}{3} = 47.3 = 47$$

a. $x = 47$ gtt/min; 47 macrogtt/min

b. Determine the percentage of change.

$$\frac{47 - 42}{42} = \frac{5}{42} = 0.119 = 12\%$$

c. This is an acceptable increase. Assess if client can tolerate adjustment in rate. Check hospital policy.

Determine the acceptable range of variation.

$42 + (42 \div 4) = 42 + 10.5 = 52.5 = 53$ gtt/min (macrogtt/min)

$42 - (42 \div 4) = 42 - 10.5 = 31.5 = 32$ gtt/min (macrogtt/min)

The safe range is 32–53 gtt/min (macrogtt/min). The recalculated rate is 47 gtt/min (macrogtt/min). It is safe to increase the rate to 47 gtt/min (macrogtt/min) which is within the safe ±25% range.

56. Step 1: Determine mL/hr for the remaining solution.

$$x \text{ mL/hr} = \frac{750 \text{ mL}}{8 \text{ hr}} = 93.7 = 94$$

$x = 94$ mL/hr

Step 2: Calculate gtt/min.

$$x \text{ gtt/min} = \frac{94 \text{ mL} \times 20 \text{ gtt/mL}}{60 \text{ min}} = \frac{94 \times 20}{60} = \frac{94 \times 1}{3} = \frac{94}{3}$$

$$x = \frac{94}{3} = 31.3 = 31$$

a. $x = 31$ gtt/min; 31 macrogtt/min

b. Determine the percentage of change.

$$\frac{31 - 28}{28} = \frac{3}{28} = 0.107 = 11\%$$

c. The percentage of change is 11%. This is an acceptable increase. Assess if client can tolerate adjustment in rate. Check if allowed by institution policy.

Determine the acceptable range of variation.

$28 + (28 \div 4) = 28 + 7 = 35$ gtt/min (macrogtt/min)

$28 - (28 \div 4) = 28 - 7 = 21$ gtt/min (macrogtt/min)

The safe range is 21–35 gtt/min (macrogtt/min). The recalculated rate is 31. It is safe to increase the IV rate, which falls within the safe ±25% range.

57. Step 1: Determine mL/hr for remaining solution.

$$x \text{ mL/hr} = \frac{250 \text{ mL}}{3 \text{ hr}} = 83.3 = 83$$

$$x = 83 \text{ mL/hr}$$

Step 2: Calculate gtt/min.

$$x \text{ gtt/min} = \frac{83 \text{ mL} \times 60 \text{ gtt/mL}}{60 \text{ min}} = \frac{83 \times 60}{60} = \frac{83 \times 1}{1} = \frac{83}{1}$$

a. $x = 83$ gtt/min; 83 microgtt/min

b. Determine the percentage of change.

$$\frac{83 - 100}{100} = \frac{-17}{100} = -0.17 = -17\%$$

c. The percentage of change is −17%. This is an acceptable decrease. Assess client to see if able to tolerate adjustment in rate. Check if allowed by institution policy.

$100 + (100 \div 4) = 100 + 25 = 125$ gtt/min (microdrop)

$100 - (100 \div 4) = 100 - 25 = 75$ gtt/min (microdrop)

The safe range is 75–125 gtt/min (microdrop). The recalculated rate is 83 gtt/min (microdrop). It is safe to decrease the rate to slow the rate to 83 gtt/min (microgtt), which is within the safe ±25% range.

58. $\frac{500 \text{ mL}}{60 \text{ mL/hr}} = 8.33 \text{ hr}$

$0.33 \text{ hr} \times 60 \text{ min/hr} = 19.8 = 20 \text{ min}$

a. Answer: 8 hr + 20 min = infusion time

b. Answer: 6:20 AM (10:00 PM + 8 hr + 20 min); military time: 0620

59. $\frac{250 \text{ mL}}{80 \text{ mL/hr}} = 3.12 \text{ hr}$

$0.12 \text{ hr} \times 60 \text{ min/hr} = 7.2 = 7 \text{ min}$

a. Answer: 3 hr + 7 min = infusion time

b. Answer: 5:07 AM (2:00 AM + 3 hr + 7 min); military time: 0507

60. $\frac{1{,}000 \text{ mL}}{40 \text{ mL/hr}} = 25 \text{ hr}$

a. Answer: 25 hr = infusion time

b. Answer: 3:10 PM August 27 (2:10 PM on August 26 + 25 hr); military time: 1510

(Most IV solutions are not considered sterile after 24 hr; therefore it should be changed after 24 hr.)

61. $\frac{1{,}000 \text{ mL}}{60 \text{ mL/hr}} = 16.66 \text{ hr}$

$0.66 \text{ hr} \times 60 \text{ min/hr} = 39.6 = 40 \text{ min}$

a. Answer: 16 hr + 40 min = infusion time

b. Answer: 10:40 PM (6:00 AM + 16 hr + 40 min); military time: 2240

62. $\frac{500 \text{ mL}}{75 \text{ mL/hr}} = 6.66 \text{ hr}$

$0.66 \text{ hr} \times 60 \text{ min/hr} = 39.6 = 40 \text{ min}$

a. Answer: 6 hr + 40 minutes = infusion time

b. Answer: 8:40 PM (2:00 PM + 6 hr + 40 min); military time: 2040

63. Step 1: 60 gtt : 1 mL = 25 gtt : x mL

$$\frac{60x}{60} = \frac{25}{60}$$

$x = 25 \div 60 = 0.41$ mL/min

Step 2: $0.41 \text{ mL/min} \times 60 \text{ min/hr} = 24.6 = 25 \text{ mL/hr}$

Step 3: $\frac{1{,}000 \text{ mL}}{25 \text{ mL/hr}} = 40 \text{ hr}$

Answer: 40 hr = infusion time (IV would be changed after 24 hrs)

64. Step 1: 15 gtt : 1 mL = 17 gtt : x mL

$$\frac{15x}{15} = \frac{17}{15}$$

$x = 17 \div 15 = 1.13 = 1.1$ mL/min

Step 2: $1.1 \text{ mL/min} \times 60 \text{ min/hr} = 66 \text{ mL/hr}$

Step 3: $\frac{250 \text{ mL}}{66 \text{ mL/hr}} = 3.78 \text{ hr}$

$60 \text{ min/hr} \times 0.78 \text{ hr} = 46.8 = 47 \text{ min}$

Answer: 3 hr + 47 min = infusion time

65. Step 1: 20 gtt : 1 mL = 30 gtt : x mL

$$\frac{20x}{20} = \frac{30}{20}$$

$x = 30 \div 20 = 1.5$ mL/min

Step 2: $1.5 \text{ mL/min} \times 60 \text{ min/hr} = 90 \text{ mL/hr}$

Step 3: $\frac{1{,}000 \text{ mL}}{90 \text{ mL/hr}} = 11.11 \text{ hr}$

$60 \text{ min/hr} \times 0.11 \text{ hr} = 6.6 = 7 \text{ min}$

Answer: 11 hr + 7 min = infusion time

66. Step 1: 10 gtt : 1 mL = 20 gtt : x mL

$$\frac{10x}{10} = \frac{20}{10}$$

$x = 2$ mL/min

Step 2: $2 \text{ mL/min} \times 60 \text{ min/hr} = 120 \text{ mL/hr}$

Step 3: $\frac{1{,}000 \text{ mL}}{120 \text{ mL/hr}} = 8.33 \text{ hr}$

$60 \text{ min/hr} \times 0.33 \text{ hr} = 19.8 = 20 \text{ min}$

Answer: 8 hr + 20 min = infusion time

67. Step 1: 15 gtt : 1 mL = 10 gtt : x mL

$$\frac{15x}{15} = \frac{10}{15} = 0.666 = 0.67$$

$x = 0.67$ mL/min

Step 2: $0.67 \text{ mL/min} \times 60 \text{ min/hr} = 40.2 \text{ mL/hr} = 40 \text{ mL/hr}$

Step 3: $\frac{100 \text{ mL}}{40 \text{ mL/hr}} = 2.5 \text{ hr}$

Answer: 2 hr + 30 min = infusion time

68. Step 1: 15 gtt : 1 mL = 30 gtt : x mL

$$\frac{15x}{15} = \frac{30}{15}$$

$x = 2$ mL/min

Step 2: $35 \text{ mL} \div 2 \text{ mL/min} = 17.5 = 18 \text{ min}$

Answer: 18 min = infusion time

69. Step 1: 60 gtt : 1 mL = 35 gtt : x mL

$$\frac{60x}{60} = \frac{35}{60}$$

$x = 0.58$ mL/min

Step 2: $20 \text{ mL} \div 0.58 \text{ mL/min} = 34.4 = 34 \text{ min}$

Answer: 34 min = infusion time

70. a. 5 mg : 1 mL = 20 mg : x mL

$$\frac{5x}{5} = \frac{20}{5}$$

$$x = 4 \text{ mL}$$

Answer: 4 mL. The dosage ordered is greater than the available strength; therefore more than 1 mL is needed to administer the dosage ordered.

or

$$\frac{20 \text{ mg}}{5 \text{ mg}} \times 1 \text{ mL} = x \text{ mL}$$

$$x \text{ mL} = \frac{1 \text{ mL}}{5 \cancel{\text{mg}}} \times \frac{20 \cancel{\text{mg}}}{1}$$

b. 5 mg : 1 min = 20 mg : x min

$$\frac{5x}{5} = \frac{20}{5}$$

$$x = 4 \text{ min}$$

c. 5 mg : 60 sec = x mg : 15 sec

$$\frac{60x}{60} = \frac{15}{60}$$

$$x = 1.25 \text{ mg per 15 sec}$$

71. a. 250 mg : 5 mL = 150 mg : x mL

$$\frac{250x}{250} = \frac{750}{250}$$

$$x = 3 \text{ mL}$$

or

$$\frac{150 \text{ mg}}{250 \text{ mg}} \times 5 \text{ mL} = x \text{ mL}$$

Answer: 3 mL. The dosage ordered is less than the available strength; therefore you would need less than 5 mL to administer the dosage ordered.

b. 50 mg : 1 min = 150 mg : x min

$$\frac{50x}{50} = \frac{150}{50}$$

$$x = 3 \text{ min}$$

72. a. 10 mL diluent

b. 1 mg : 60 sec = x mg : 30 sec

$$\frac{60x}{60} = \frac{30}{60}$$

$$x = 0.5 \text{ mg/30 sec}$$

Answers to Clinical Reasoning Questions

a. The nurse was accustomed to using 20 gtt/mL and calculated the IV rate using 20 gtt/mL. The tubing used at the institution delivered 10 gtt/mL, and the nurse did not check the drop factor on the IV set package. Failure to check the drop factor of the IV tubing resulted in an incorrect IV rate.

b. Because of the excessive IV rate, the client developed signs of fluid overload and could have developed congestive heart failure.

c. The nurse should never assume what the drop factor for IV tubing is for macrodrop administration sets because they can vary. The nurse should have checked the IV tubing package for the drop factor, which is printed on the package.

Answers to Chapter Review

NOTE

Many of the IV problems involving gtt/min could also be done by using the shortcut method or dimensional analysis.

NOTE

Some answers in the Chapter Review reflect the number of drops rounded to the nearest whole number and the rate in mL/hr.

1. a. Determine mL/hr

$$x \text{ mL/hr} = \frac{1{,}000 \text{ mL}}{8 \text{ hr}}; x = 125 \text{ mL/hr}$$

b. Calculate gtt/min.

$$x \text{ gtt/min} = \frac{125 \text{ mL} \times 20 \text{ gtt/mL}}{60 \text{ min}}$$

x = 42 gtt/min; 42 macrogtt/min

2. a. Determine mL/hr.

$$x \text{ mL/hr} = \frac{2{,}500 \text{ mL}}{24 \text{ hr}}; x = 104 \text{ mL/hr}$$

b. Calculate gtt/min.

$$x \text{ gtt/min} = \frac{104 \text{ mL} \times 10 \text{ gtt/mL}}{60 \text{ min}}$$

x = 17 gtt/min; 17 macrogtt/min

3. a. Determine mL/hr.

$$x \text{ mL/hr} = \frac{500 \text{ mL}}{4 \text{ hr}}; x = 125 \text{ mL/hr}$$

b. Calculate gtt/min.

$$x \text{ gtt/min} = \frac{125 \text{ mL} \times 15 \text{ gtt/mL}}{60 \text{ min}}$$

x = 31 gtt/min; 31 macrogtt/min

4. a. Determine mL/hr.

$x \text{ mL/hr} = \dfrac{300 \text{ mL}}{6 \text{ hr}}; x = 50 \text{ mL/hr}$

b. Calculate gtt/min.

$x \text{ gtt/min} = \dfrac{50 \text{ mL} \times 60 \text{ gtt/mL}}{60 \text{ min}}$

$x = 50$ gtt/min; 50 microgtt/min

5. a. Determine mL/hr.

$x \text{ mL/hr} = \dfrac{1{,}000 \text{ mL}}{24 \text{ hr}} = 41.6 = 42; x = 42 \text{ mL/hr}$

b. Calculate gtt/min.

$x \text{ gtt/min} = \dfrac{42 \text{ mL} \times 60 \text{ gtt/mL}}{60 \text{ min}}$

$x = 42$ gtt/min; 42 microgtt/min

6. a. Determine mL/hr.

$x \text{ mL/hr} = \dfrac{500 \text{ mL}}{12 \text{ hr}} = 41.6 = 42; x = 42 \text{ mL/hr}$

b. Calculate gtt/min.

$x \text{ gtt/min} = \dfrac{42 \text{ mL} \times 20 \text{ gtt/mL}}{60 \text{ min}}$

$x = 14$ gtt/min; 14 macrogtt/min

7. a. Determine mL/hr.

$x \text{ mL/hr} = \dfrac{1{,}000 \text{ mL}}{10 \text{ hr}}; x = 100 \text{ mL/hr}$

b. Calculate gtt/min.

$x \text{ gtt/min} = \dfrac{100 \text{ mL} \times 20 \text{ gtt/mL}}{60 \text{ min}}$

$x = 33$ gtt/min; 33 macrogtt/min

8. a. Determine mL/hr.

$x \text{ mL/hr} = \dfrac{1{,}500 \text{ mL}}{12 \text{ hr}}; x = 125 \text{ mL/hr}$

b. Calculate gtt/min.

$x \text{ gtt/min} = \dfrac{125 \text{ mL} \times 10 \text{ gtt/mL}}{60 \text{ min}}$

$x = 21$ gtt/min; 21 macrogtt/min

9. a. Determine mL/hr.

$x \text{ mL/hr} = \dfrac{500 \text{ mL}}{4 \text{ hr}}; x = 125 \text{ mL/hr}$

b. Calculate gtt/min.

$x \text{ gtt/min} = \dfrac{125 \text{ mL} \times 10 \text{ gtt/mL}}{60 \text{ min}}$

$x = 21$ gtt/min; 21 macrogtt/min

10. a. Determine mL/hr.

$x \text{ mL/hr} = \dfrac{250 \text{ mL}}{4 \text{ hr}}; x = 63 \text{ mL/hr}$

b. Calculate gtt/min.

$x \text{ gtt/min} = \dfrac{63 \text{ mL} \times 10 \text{ gtt/mL}}{60 \text{ min}}$

$x = 11$ gtt/min; 11 macrogtt/min

11. a. Determine mL/hr.

$x \text{ mL/hr} = \dfrac{1{,}500 \text{ mL}}{8 \text{ hr}}; x = 188 \text{ mL/hr}$

b. Calculate gtt/min.

$x \text{ gtt/min} = \dfrac{188 \text{ mL} \times 20 \text{ gtt/mL}}{60 \text{ min}}$

$x = 63$ gtt/min; 63 macrogtt/min

12. a. Determine mL/hr.

$x \text{ mL/hr} = \dfrac{3{,}000 \text{ mL}}{24 \text{ hr}}; x = 125 \text{ mL/hr}$

b. Calculate gtt/min.

$x \text{ gtt/min} = \dfrac{125 \text{ mL} \times 15 \text{ gtt/mL}}{60 \text{ min}}$

$x = 31$ gtt/min; 31 macrogtt/min

13. 1 L = 1,000 mL

2 L = 2,000 mL

a. Determine mL/hr.

$x \text{ mL/hr} = \dfrac{2{,}000 \text{ mL}}{24 \text{ hr}}; x = 83 \text{ mL/hr}$

b. Calculate gtt/min.

$x \text{ gtt/min} = \dfrac{83 \text{ mL} \times 15 \text{ gtt/mL}}{60 \text{ min}}$

$x = 21$ gtt/min; 21 macrogtt/min

14. a. Determine mL/hr.

$x \text{ mL/hr} = \dfrac{500 \text{ mL}}{4 \text{ hr}}; x = 125 \text{ mL/hr}$

b. Calculate gtt/min.

$x \text{ gtt/min} = \dfrac{125 \text{ mL} \times 60 \text{ gtt/mL}}{60 \text{ min}}$

$x = 125$ gtt/min; 125 microgtt/min

15. a. Determine mL/hr.

$x \text{ mL/hr} = \dfrac{1{,}000 \text{ mL}}{6 \text{ hr}}; x = 167 \text{ mL/hr}$

b. Calculate gtt/min.

$x \text{ gtt/min} = \dfrac{167 \text{ mL} \times 20 \text{ gtt/mL}}{60 \text{ min}}$

$x = 56$ gtt/min; 56 macrogtt/min

16. a. Determine mL/hr.

$x \text{ mL/hr} = \dfrac{250 \text{ mL}}{8 \text{ hr}}; x = 31 \text{ mL/hr}$

b. Calculate gtt/min.

$x \text{ gtt/min} = \dfrac{31 \text{ mL} \times 60 \text{ gtt/mL}}{60 \text{ min}}$

$x = 31$ gtt/min; 31 microgtt/min

17. $x \text{ gtt/min} = \dfrac{50 \text{ mL} \times 60 \text{ gtt/mL}}{60 \text{ min}}$

$x = 50$ gtt/min; 50 microgtt/min

18. $x \text{ gtt/min} = \dfrac{150 \text{ mL} \times 15 \text{ gtt/mL}}{60 \text{ min}}$

$x = 38$ gtt/min; 38 macrogtt/min

19. a. Determine mL/hr.

$x \text{ mL/hr} = \dfrac{500 \text{ mL}}{6 \text{ hr}}; x = 83 \text{ mL/hr}$

b. Calculate gtt/min.

$x \text{ gtt/min} = \dfrac{83 \text{ mL} \times 15 \text{ gtt/mL}}{60 \text{ min}}$

$x = 21$ gtt/min; 21 macrogtt/min

20. a. Determine mL/hr.

$x \text{ mL/hr} = \dfrac{1{,}500 \text{ mL}}{12 \text{ hr}}; x = 125 \text{ mL/hr}$

b. Calculate gtt/min.

$x \text{ gtt/min} = \dfrac{125 \text{ mL} \times 10 \text{ gtt/mL}}{60 \text{ min}}$

$x = 21$ gtt/min; 21 macrogtt/min

21. a. Determine mL/hr.

$x \text{ mL/hr} = \dfrac{1{,}500 \text{ mL}}{24 \text{ hr}}; x = 63 \text{ mL/hr}$

b. Calculate gtt/min.

$x \text{ gtt/min} = \dfrac{63 \text{ mL} \times 15 \text{ gtt/mL}}{60 \text{ min}}$

$x = 16$ gtt/min; 16 macrogtt/min

22. a. Determine mL/hr.

$x \text{ mL/hr} = \dfrac{2{,}000 \text{ mL}}{16 \text{ hr}}; x = 125 \text{ mL/hr}$

b. Calculate gtt/min.

$x \text{ gtt/min} = \dfrac{125 \text{ mL} \times 20 \text{ gtt/mL}}{60 \text{ min}}$

$x = 42$ gtt/min; 42 macrogtt/min

23. a. Determine mL/hr.

$x \text{ mL/hr} = \dfrac{500 \text{ mL}}{8 \text{ hr}}; x = 63 \text{ mL/hr}$

b. Calculate gtt/min.

$x \text{ gtt/min} = \dfrac{63 \text{ mL} \times 15 \text{ gtt/mL}}{60 \text{ min}}$

$x = 16$ gtt/min; 16 macrogtt/min

24. a. Determine mL/hr.

$x \text{ mL/hr} = \dfrac{250 \text{ mL}}{10 \text{ hr}}; x = 25 \text{ mL/hr}$

b. Calculate gtt/min.

$x \text{ gtt/min} = \dfrac{25 \text{ mL} \times 60 \text{ gtt/mL}}{60 \text{ min}}$

$x = 25$ gtt/min; 25 microgtt/min

25. $x \text{ gtt/min} = \dfrac{75 \text{ mL} \times 60 \text{ gtt/mL}}{60 \text{ min}}$

$x = 75$ gtt/min; 75 microgtt/min

26. $x \text{ gtt/min} = \dfrac{125 \text{ mL} \times 20 \text{ gtt/mL}}{60 \text{ min}}$

$x = 42$ gtt/min; 42 macrogtt/min

27. $x \text{ gtt/min} = \dfrac{40 \text{ mL} \times 60 \text{ gtt/mL}}{60 \text{ min}}$

$x = 40$ gtt/min; 40 microgtt/min

28. $x \text{ gtt/min} = \dfrac{50 \text{ mL} \times 60 \text{ gtt/mL}}{45 \text{ min}}$

$x = 67$ gtt/min; 67 microgtt/min

29. $x \text{ gtt/min} = \dfrac{90 \text{ mL} \times 15 \text{ gtt/mL}}{60 \text{ min}}$

$x = 23$ gtt/min; 23 macrogtt/min

30. $x \text{ gtt/min} = \dfrac{150 \text{ mL} \times 10 \text{ gtt/mL}}{60 \text{ min}}$

$x = 25$ gtt/min; 25 macrogtt/min

31. a. Determine mL/hr.

$x \text{ mL/hr} = \dfrac{2{,}500 \text{ mL}}{24 \text{ hr}}; x = 104 \text{ mL/hr}$

b. Calculate gtt/min.

$x \text{ gtt/min} = \dfrac{104 \text{ mL} \times 15 \text{ gtt/mL}}{60 \text{ min}}$

$x = 26$ gtt/min; 26 macrogtt/min

32. $x \text{ gtt/min} = \dfrac{50 \text{ mL} \times 10 \text{ gtt/mL}}{40 \text{ min}}$

$x = 13$ gtt/min; 13 macrogtt/min

33. $x \text{ gtt/min} = \dfrac{100 \text{ mL} \times 20 \text{ gtt/mL}}{30 \text{ min}}$

$x = 67$ gtt/min; 67 macrogtt/min

34. a. Determine mL/hr.

$x \text{ mL/hr} = \dfrac{250 \text{ mL}}{5 \text{ hr}}; x = 50 \text{ mL/hr}$

b. Calculate gtt/min.

$x \text{ gtt/min} = \dfrac{50 \text{ mL} \times 20 \text{ gtt/mL}}{60 \text{ min}}$

$x = 17$ gtt/min; 17 macrogtt/min

35. $x \text{ gtt/min} = \dfrac{80 \text{ mL} \times 20 \text{ gtt/mL}}{60 \text{ min}}$

$x = 27$ gtt/min; 27 macrogtt/min

36. $x \text{ gtt/min} = \dfrac{150 \text{ mL} \times 10 \text{ gtt/mL}}{30 \text{ min}}$

$x = 50$ gtt/min; 50 macrogtt/min

37. $x \text{ gtt/min} = \dfrac{50 \text{ mL} \times 60 \text{ gtt/mL}}{30 \text{ min}}$

$x = 100$ gtt/min; 100 microgtt/min

38. a. Determine mL/hr.

$x \text{ mL/hr} = \dfrac{500 \text{ mL}}{3 \text{ hr}}; x = 167 \text{ mL/hr}$

b. Calculate gtt/min.

$x \text{ gtt/min} = \dfrac{167 \text{ mL} \times 10 \text{ gtt/mL}}{60 \text{ min}}$

$x = 28$ gtt/min; 28 macrogtt/min

39. a. Determine mL/hr.

$x \text{ mL/hr} = \dfrac{250 \text{ mL}}{2 \text{ hr}}; x = 125 \text{ mL/hr}$

b. Calculate gtt/min.

$x \text{ gtt/min} = \dfrac{125 \text{ mL} \times 15 \text{ gtt/mL}}{60 \text{ min}}$

$x = 31$ gtt/min; 31 macrogtt/min

40. a. Determine mL/hr.

$x \text{ mL/hr} = \dfrac{1{,}750 \text{ mL}}{24 \text{ hr}}; x = 73 \text{ mL/hr}$

b. Calculate gtt/min.

$x \text{ gtt/min} = \dfrac{73 \text{ mL} \times 10 \text{ gtt/mL}}{60 \text{ min}}$

$x = 12$ gtt/min; 12 macrogtt/min

41. a. Determine mL/hr.

$x \text{ mL/hr} = \dfrac{150 \text{ mL}}{1.5 \text{ hr}}; x = 100 \text{ mL/hr}$

b. Calculate gtt/min.

$x \text{ gtt/min} = \dfrac{100 \text{ mL} \times 60 \text{ gtt/mL}}{60 \text{ min}}$

$x = 100$ gtt/min; 100 microgtt/min

42. 1 L = 1,000 mL

2 L = 2,000 mL

$x \text{ mL/hr} = \dfrac{2{,}000 \text{ mL}}{16 \text{ hr}}; x = 125 \text{ mL/hr}$

43. $x \text{ mL/hr} = \dfrac{500 \text{ mL}}{4 \text{ hr}}; x = 125 \text{ mL/hr}$

44. $x \text{ mL/hr} = \dfrac{200 \text{ mL}}{2 \text{ hr}}; x = 100 \text{ mL/hr}$

45. $x \text{ mL/hr} = \dfrac{500 \text{ mL}}{8 \text{ hr}}; x = 63 \text{ mL/hr}$

46. Determine mL/hr.

$x \text{ mL/hr} = \dfrac{1{,}100 \text{ mL}}{12 \text{ hr}}; x = 92 \text{ mL/hr}$

47. a. Determine mL/hr.

$x \text{ mL/hr} = \dfrac{500 \text{ mL}}{6 \text{ hr}}; x = 83 \text{ mL/hr}$

b. Calculate gtt/min.

$x \text{ gtt/min} = \dfrac{83 \text{ mL} \times 10 \text{ gtt/mL}}{60 \text{ min}}$

$x = 14$ gtt/min; 14 macrogtt/min

48. a. Determine mL/hr.

$x \text{ mL/hr} = \dfrac{3{,}000 \text{ mL}}{20 \text{ hr}}; x = 150 \text{ mL/hr}$

b. Calculate gtt/min.

$x \text{ gtt/min} = \dfrac{150 \text{ mL} \times 20 \text{ gtt/mL}}{60 \text{ min}}$

$x = 50$ gtt/min; 50 macrogtt/min

49. a. Determine mL/hr.

$x \text{ mL/hr} = \dfrac{500 \text{ mL}}{6 \text{ hr}}; x = 83 \text{ mL/hr}$

b. Calculate gtt/min.

$x \text{ gtt/min} = \dfrac{83 \text{ mL} \times 15 \text{ gtt/mL}}{60 \text{ min}}$

$x = 21$ gtt/min; 21 macrogtt/min

50. Time remaining = 7 hr

Volume remaining = 300 mL

a. Determine mL/hr for remaining solution.

$x \text{ mL/hr} = \dfrac{300 \text{ mL}}{7 \text{ hr}}; x = 43 \text{ mL/hr}$

b. Determine gtt/min (recalculated rate).

$x \text{ gtt/min} = \dfrac{43 \text{ mL} \times 15 \text{ gtt/mL}}{60 \text{ min}}$

$x = 11$ gtt/min

Answer: 11 macrogtt/min; 11 gtt/min

c. Determine the percentage change.

$\dfrac{11 - 13}{13} = \dfrac{-2}{13} = -0.153 = -15\%$

The −15% is within the acceptable 25% variation. Assess if client can tolerate adjustment in rate.

Negative percentage of variation (−15%) indicates the adjusted rate will be decreased. Assess client, check institution policy, and continue to assess client during rate change.

Determine accepted range of variation.

$13 + (13 \div 4) = 13 + 3.25 = 16.25 = 16$ gtt/min (macrogtt/min)

$13 - (13 \div 4) = 13 - 3.25 = 9.75 = 10$ gtt/min (macrogtt/min)

The acceptable range is 10–16 gtt/min (macrogtt/min). The recalculated rate is 11 gtt/min (macrogtt/min). It is safe to slow the IV rate to 11 gtt/min (macrogtt/min), which is in the safe range. It is below 25%.

51. Time remaining = 4 hr

Volume remaining = 600 mL

a. Determine mL/hr for remaining solution.

$$x \text{ mL/hr} = \frac{600 \text{ mL}}{4 \text{ hr}}; x = 150 \text{ mL/hr}$$

b. Determine gtt/min (recalculated rate).

$$x \text{ gtt/min} = \frac{150 \text{ mL} \times 20 \text{ gtt/mL}}{60 \text{ min}}$$

$x = 50$ gtt/min

Answer: 50 gtt/min; 50 macrogtt/min

c. Determine the percentage change.

$$\frac{50 - 42}{42} = \frac{8}{42} = 0.190 = 19\%$$

The percentage of change is 19%. This is an acceptable increase. Assess if client can tolerate the adjustment in rate (42 gtt/min to 50 gtt/min). Check if allowed by institution policy. Assess client during rate change.

Determine accepted range of variation.

$42 + (42 \div 4) = 42 + 10.5 = 52.5 = 53$ gtt/min (macrodrop)

$42 - (42 \div 4) = 42 - 10.5 = 31.5 = 32$ gtt/min (macrodrop)

The acceptable range is 32–53 gtt/min (macrodrop). The recalculated rate is 50 gtt/min (macrodrop). The IV increase to 50 gtt/min (macrogtt) is within the safe range of 25%.

52. Time remaining = 4 hr

Volume remaining = 400 mL

a. Determine mL/hr for remaining solution.

$$x \text{ mL/hr} = \frac{400 \text{ mL}}{4 \text{ hr}}; x = 100 \text{ mL/hr}$$

After determining mL/hr, gtt/min is recalculated.

b. Determine gtt/min (recalculated rate).

$$x \text{ gtt/min} = \frac{100 \text{ mL} \times 15 \text{ gtt/mL}}{60 \text{ min}}$$

$x = 25$ gtt/min

Answer: 25 gtt/min; 25 macrogtt/min

c. The IV was ahead. The original IV order was 125 mL/hr = 31 gtt/min (31 macrogtt/min). The IV would have to be decreased from 31 gtt/min (31 macrogtt/min) to 25 gtt/min (25 macrogtt/min). Determine the percentage change.

$$\frac{25 - 31}{31} = \frac{-6}{31} = -0.193 = -19\%$$

The −19% is within acceptable 25% variation. Assess if client can tolerate the adjustment in rate. Negative percentage of variation (−19%) indicates the adjusted rate will be decreased. Check institution policy. Assess client during rate change.

Determine accepted range of variation.

$31 + (31 \div 4) = 31 + 7.75 = 38.75 = 39$ gtt/min (macrogtt/min)

$31 - (31 \div 4) = 31 - 7.75 = 23.25 = 23$ gtt/min (macrogtt/min)

The accepted range is 23–39 gtt/min (macrogtt). The recalculated rate is 25 gtt/min (macrogtt/min). It is safe to slow the rate to 25 gtt/min (macrogtt/min) which is within the safe range of 25%.

53. Time remaining = $9\frac{1}{2}$ hr

Volume remaining = 300 mL

a. Determine mL/hr for remaining solution.

$$x \text{ mL/hr} = \frac{300 \text{ mL}}{9.5 \text{ hr}}; x = 31.5 = 32$$

$x = 32$ mL/hr

b. Determine gtt/min (recalculated rate).

$$x \text{ gtt/min} = \frac{32 \text{ mL} \times 60 \text{ gtt/mL}}{60 \text{ min}}$$

$x = 32$ gtt/min; 32 microgtt/min

c. The IV is ahead. The IV rate would need to be decreased from 42 gtt/min (42 microgtt/min) to 32 gtt/min (32 microgtt/min). Determine the percentage change.

$$\frac{32 - 42}{42} = \frac{-10}{42} = -0.238 = -24\%$$

The −24% is within the acceptable 25% variation. Assess whether the client can tolerate the adjustment in rate. The negative percentage of variation (−24%) indicates that the adjusted rate will be decreased. Check institution policy. Assess client during rate change. Determine accepted range of variation.

Determine accepted range of variation.

$42 + (42 \div 4) = 42 + 10.5 = 52.5 = 53$ gtt/min (microgtt/min)

$42 - (42 \div 4) = 42 - 10.5 = 31.5 = 32$ gtt/min (microgtt/min)

The accepted range is 32 to 53 gtt/min (microgtt/min). The recalculated rate is 32 gtt/min (microgtt/min). It is safe to slow the rate to 32 gtt/min (microgtt/min), which is within the safe range of 25%.

54. Time remaining = 4 hr

Volume remaining = 600 mL

a. Determine mL/hr for remaining solution.

$x \text{ mL/hr} = \frac{600 \text{ mL}}{4 \text{ hr}}; x = 150 \text{ mL/hr}$

b. Determine gtt/min (recalculated rate).

$x \text{ gtt/min} = \frac{150 \text{ mL} \times 15 \text{ gtt/mL}}{60 \text{ min}} = 38 \text{ gtt/min}$

$x = 38$ gtt/min; 38 macrogtt/min

c. IV is not on schedule. The original IV order was 100 mL/hr = 25 gtt/min (25 macrogtt/min). The IV would have to be increased from 25 gtt/min (25 macrogtt/min) to 38 gtt/min (38 macrogtt/min). Determine the percentage of increase.

$$\frac{38 - 25}{25} = \frac{13}{25} = 52\%$$

The percentage of change is greater than 25%. Assess client. Check with prescriber; order may need to be revised. (Do not increase.)

Determine accepted range of variation.

25 + (25 ÷ 4) = 25 + 6.25 = 31.25 = 31 gtt/min (macrogtt/min)

25 − (25 ÷ 4) = 25 − 6.25 = 18.75 = 19 gtt/min (macrogtt/min)

The accepted range is 19–31 gtt/min (macrogtt/min). The recalculated rate is 38 gtt/min (macrogtt/min). The IV is more than 25% which is not in the safe range.

55. 80 macrogtt/min (80 gtt/min) = $\frac{900 \text{ mL} \times 15 \text{ gtt/mL}}{x \text{ min}}$

$$80 = \frac{900 \times 15}{x}$$

$$\frac{80x}{80} = \frac{13{,}500}{80}$$

$$x = 168.75 \text{ minutes}$$

60 min = 1 hr; 168.75 ÷ 60 = 2.81 hr

Time: 2.81 hr. Since 0.81 represents a fraction of an additional hour, 0.81 ~~hr~~ × 60 min/~~hr~~ = 48.6 = 49 min.

Answer: 2 hr and 49 min

56. $\frac{1{,}000 \cancel{\text{mL}}}{100 \cancel{\text{mL}}/\text{hr}} = 10 \text{ hr}$

57. 20 macrogtt/min (20 gtt/min) = $\frac{1{,}000 \text{ mL} \times 10 \text{ gtt/mL}}{x \text{ min}}$

$$20 = \frac{1{,}000 \times 10}{x}$$

$$\frac{20x}{20} = \frac{10{,}000}{20}$$

$$x = 500 \text{ min}$$

60 min = 1 hr; 500 ÷ 60 = 8.33 hr

Time: 8.33 hr

0.33 ~~hr~~ × 60 min/~~hr~~ = 19.8 = 20 min

Answer: 8 hr and 20 min

58. 25 macrogtt/min (25 gtt/min) = $\frac{450 \text{ mL} \times 20 \text{ gtt/mL}}{x \text{ min}}$

$$25 = \frac{450 \times 20}{x}$$

$$\frac{25x}{25} = \frac{9{,}000}{25}$$

$$x = 360 \text{ min}$$

60 min = 1 hr; 360 ÷ 60 = 6 hr

Answer: 6 hr

59. 10 macrogtt/min (10 gtt/min) = $\frac{100 \text{ mL} \times 15 \text{ gtt/mL}}{x \text{ min}}$

$$10 = \frac{100 \times 15}{x}$$

$$\frac{10x}{10} = \frac{1{,}500}{10}$$

$$x = 150 \text{ min}$$

60 min = 1 hr; 150 ÷ 60 = 2.5 = 2 1/2 hr

Answer: 2 1/2 hr

60. 25 macrogtt/min (25 gtt/min) = $\frac{x \text{ mL} \times 15 \text{ gtt/mL}}{480 \text{ min}}$

$$25 = \frac{x \times 15}{480}$$

$$25 = \frac{15x}{480}$$

$$\frac{15x}{15} = \frac{25 \times 480}{15}$$

$$\frac{15x}{15} = \frac{12{,}000}{15}$$

$$x = 800 \text{ mL}$$

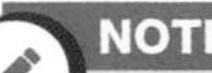

NOTE

For problems 60-62: Formula, time expressed in minutes (60 min = 1 hr).

61. $40 \text{ microgtt/min } (40 \text{ gtt/min}) = \dfrac{x \text{ mL} \times 60 \text{ gtt/mL}}{600 \text{ min}}$

$$40 = \frac{x \times 60}{600}$$
$$40 = \frac{60x}{600}$$
$$\frac{60x}{60} = \frac{40 \times 600}{60}$$
$$\frac{60x}{60} = \frac{24{,}000}{60}$$
$$x = 400 \text{ mL}$$

62. $30 \text{ macrogtt/min } (30 \text{ gtt/min}) = \dfrac{x \text{ mL} \times 15 \text{ gtt/mL}}{300 \text{ min}}$

$$30 = \frac{x \times 15}{300}$$
$$30 = \frac{15x}{300}$$
$$\frac{15x}{15} = \frac{30 \times 300}{15}$$
$$\frac{15x}{15} = \frac{9{,}000}{5}$$
$$x = 600 \text{ mL}$$

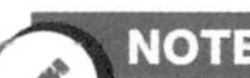

NOTE

For problems 63-67 a ratio and proportion could be set up in a format other than the one shown in the problems.

63. $10 \text{ mEq} : 500 \text{ mL} = 2 \text{ mEq} : x \text{ mL}$

$$10x = 500 \times 2$$
$$\frac{10x}{10} = \frac{1{,}000}{10}$$
$$x = 100 \text{ mL/hr}$$

Answer: 100 mL/hr of fluid would be needed to administer 2 mEq of potassium chloride.

64. $25 \text{ mEq} : 1{,}000 \text{ mL} = 4 \text{ mEq} : x \text{ mL}$

$$\frac{25x}{25} = \frac{4{,}000}{25} = 160$$
$$x = 160 \text{ mL/hr}$$

160 mL/hr would deliver 4 mEq of potassium chloride.

65. $50 \text{ units} : 250 \text{ mL} = 7 \text{ units} : x \text{ mL}$

$$\frac{50x}{50} = \frac{1{,}750}{50}; x = 35 \text{ mL/hr}$$

66. $100 \text{ units} : 250 \text{ mL} = 18 \text{ units} : x \text{ mL}$

$$\frac{100x}{100} = \frac{4{,}500}{100}; x = 45 \text{ mL/hr}$$

67. $100 \text{ units} : 100 \text{ mL} = 11 \text{ units} : x \text{ mL}$

$$\frac{100x}{100} = \frac{1{,}100}{100}; x = 11 \text{ mL/hr}$$

68. $x \text{ gtt/min} = \dfrac{150 \text{ mL} \times 10 \text{ gtt/mL}}{60 \text{ min}}$

$x = 25$ gtt/min; 25 macrogtt/min

69. $x \text{ gtt/min} = \dfrac{40 \text{ mL} \times 60 \text{ gtt/mL}}{40 \text{ min}}$

$x = 60$ gtt/min; 60 microgtt/min

70. $x \text{ gtt/min} = \dfrac{35 \text{ mL} \times 60 \text{ gtt/mL}}{30 \text{ min}}$

$x = 70$ gtt/min; 70 microgtt/min

71. $x \text{ gtt/min} = \dfrac{80 \text{ mL} \times 15 \text{ gtt/mL}}{40 \text{ min}}$

$x = 30$ gtt/min; 30 macrogtt/min

72. $x \text{ gtt/min} = \dfrac{50 \text{ mL} \times 10 \text{ gtt/mL}}{25 \text{ min}}$

$x = 20$ gtt/min; 20 macrogtt/min

73. $x \text{ gtt/min} = \dfrac{65 \text{ mL} \times 15 \text{ gtt/mL}}{60 \text{ min}}$

$x = 16$ gtt/min; 16 macrogtt/min

74. Step 1: $60 \text{ gtt} : 1 \text{ mL} = 50 \text{ gtt} : x \text{ mL}$

$$\frac{60x}{60} = \frac{50}{60}$$

$x = 50 \div 60$; $x = 0.83$ mL/min

Step 2: $0.83 \text{ mL}/\cancel{\text{min}} \times 60 \text{ } \cancel{\text{min}}/\text{hr} = 49.8 = 50 \text{ mL/hr}$

Step 3: $\dfrac{50 \text{ } \cancel{\text{mL}}}{50 \text{ } \cancel{\text{mL}}/\text{hr}} = 1 \text{ hr}$

Answer: 1 hr = infusion time

75. Step 1: $\dfrac{500 \text{ } \cancel{\text{mL}}}{80 \text{ } \cancel{\text{mL}}/\text{hr}} = 6.25 \text{ hr}$

Step 2: $60 \text{ min}/\cancel{\text{hr}} \times 0.25 \text{ } \cancel{\text{hr}} = 15 \text{ min}$

6 hr and 15 min = infusion time

Step 3: (7:00 PM + 6 hr + 15 min)

Answer: 1:15 AM; military time: 0115

76. $\dfrac{150 \text{ } \cancel{\text{mL}}}{25 \text{ } \cancel{\text{mL}}/\text{hr}} = 6 \text{ hr}$

a. 6 hr = infusion time

b. (3:10 AM + 6 hr = 9:10 AM). IV will be completed at 9:10 AM; military time: 0910.

77. Conversion is required. Equivalent:

1 L = 1,000 mL

Therefore 2.5 L = 2,500 mL

Step 1: $\dfrac{2{,}500 \text{ } \cancel{\text{mL}}}{150 \text{ } \cancel{\text{mL}}/\text{hr}} = 16.66 \text{ hr}$

Step 2: $60 \text{ min}/\cancel{\text{hr}} \times 0.66 \text{ } \cancel{\text{hr}} = 39.6 = 40 \text{ min}$

16 hr and 40 min = infusion time

78. a. 10 mg : 1 mL = 120 mg : x mL

$\frac{10x}{10} = \frac{120}{10}$; $x = 12$ mL

or

$\frac{120\text{ mg}}{10\text{ mg}} \times 1\text{ mL} = x\text{ mL}$

Answer: 12 mL. The dosage ordered is more than the available strength; therefore more than 1 mL would be required to administer the dosage ordered.

b. 40 mg : 1 min = 120 mg : x min

$\frac{40x}{40} = \frac{120}{40}$; $x = 3$ min

Answer: 3 min

79. a. 100 mg : 20 mL = 60 mg : x mL

$\frac{100x}{100} = \frac{1,200}{100}$; $x = 12$ mL

or

$\frac{60\text{ mg}}{100\text{ mg}} \times 20\text{ mL} = x\text{ mL}$

Answer: 12 mL. The dosage ordered is less than the available strength; therefore you will need less than 20 mL to administer the dosage ordered.

b. $\frac{12\text{ mL}}{2\text{ min}} = 6$ mL/min

80. $x\text{ gtt/min} = \frac{100\text{ mL} \times 10\text{ gtt/mL}}{60\text{ min}}$;

$x = 16.6 = 17$

$x = 17$ gtt/min; 17 macrogtt/min

81. $x\text{ gtt/min} = \frac{100\text{ mL} \times 60\text{ gtt/mL}}{30\text{ min}}$

$x = 200$ gtt/min; 200 microdrop/min

82. 30,000 units : 500 mL = 1,500 units : x mL

$\frac{30,000x}{30,000} = \frac{750,000}{30,000}$

$x = \frac{750,000}{30,000} = 25$

$x = 25$ mL/hr

83. 100 units : 500 mL = 20 units : x mL

$\frac{100x}{100} = \frac{10,000}{100} = 100$

$x = 100$ mL/hr

84. 100 units : 250 mL = 15 units : x mL

$\frac{100x}{100} = \frac{3,750}{100} = 37.5 = 38$

$x = 38$ mL/hr

CHAPTER 23
Heparin Calculations

Objectives

After reviewing this chapter, you should be able to:

1. State the importance of calculating heparin dosages accurately
2. Identify errors that have occurred with heparin administration
3. Calculate subcutaneous dosages of heparin
4. Calculate heparin dosages being administered intravenously (mL per hr, units per hr)
5. Calculate safe heparin dosages based on weight

Heparin Errors

Heparin, like insulin, is classified as a **high-alert** medication because it carries a significant risk of causing serious injuries or death to a client if misused. Heparin is one of the most commonly reported medications involved in errors that have caused harm to clients. The United States Pharmacopeial (USP) listed heparin as being in the top 10 medications most frequently involved in medication errors. Many errors associated with heparin occurred during the medication administration phase. The majority of heparin errors have occurred with preparation, dispensing, and dosing. Despite the identification of heparin as being a high-alert medication, publicizing of high-profile and fatal events that have occurred, heparin dosage errors continued to occur. The causes of errors that have been cited with heparin include:

- Calculation errors
- Mix-ups with concentrations of heparin
- Confusion with the total amount in a vial of heparin and the amount per mL (i.e., a 10 mL vial of heparin held a total of 1,000 units when the vial contained a total of 10,000 units, 1,000 units per mL) which have led to fatal heparin overdoses
- Insufficient monitoring of the client

The increase in the frequency of errors that have occurred with anticoagulants prompted focus of attention from the Institute for Safe Medication Practices (ISMP), The Joint Commission (TJC), and the Federal Drug Administration (FDA). According to ISMP, anticoagulant medications are more likely to cause harm resulting from complex dosing, insufficient monitoring, and inconsistent patient compliance. As a result of the adverse drug events associated with heparin, TJC's National Patient Safety goal (NPSG) 03.05.01 was developed to reduce the likelihood of client harm associated with the use of anticoagulant therapy. The NPSG delineates a hospital's responsibilities for the administration of anticoagulation therapy. These requirements can be viewed on TJC's website at www.jointcommission.org.

To reduce medication errors with heparin, new labeling requirements for heparin sodium injection was announced at the US Pharmacopeial Convention (USP) in 2013. The labeling standards for Heparin Sodium Injection, USP, and Heparin Lock Flush Solution, USP (including prefilled heparin flush syringes) were updated, requiring new heparin labels to clearly express the heparin amount per entire container followed by the amount per mL in parentheses. Other changes that have occurred (2009) include additional label enhancements to differentiate heparin sodium injection USP from other products, including heparin lock flush solution USP by indicating "Not for lock flush" on the vials of heparin sodium injection, and bolder and larger typeface. Labels on heparin solutions will be discussed further in this chapter with the discussion of sample heparin labels. **Despite the changes in labels, it is important for the nurse to correctly identify label dosage strengths and to understand that failure to do this will result in continual errors.**

Other recommendations to decrease heparin errors also include the use of weight-based protocol that uses the client's weight in kilograms (kg) as the basis for determining heparin bolus doses and infusion rates, which will be discussed in this chapter. Strategies to reduce errors and therefore reduce the risk of harm to clients incorporates the QSEN competency of safety.

Some heparin protocols also use the activated partial thromboplastin time (aPTT or APTT) to monitor the client's clotting values while receiving heparin. Another lab test being used is the measurement of anti-factor Xa levels. Heparin requires close monitoring of the client's blood work because of the bleeding potential associated with anticoagulant drugs.

Heparin can be administered subcutaneously or intravenously; it is never administered intramuscularly because of the danger of hematomas (collection of extravasated blood trapped in tissues of skin or in an organ). Heparin therapy frequently consists of a combination of prescribed intermittent IV boluses (large doses to achieve a rapid, therapeutic effect) followed by continuous IV infusion. When administered as a continuous IV infusion, the heparin dosage rate may be ordered in units/hr, mL/hr, or individualized by weight as units per kilogram per hour (units/kg/hr). To maintain a constant rate, accurate dosing, and safe administration, heparin is always administered by an electronic infusion device.

Heparin Dosage Strengths

Heparin is available in a variety of strengths. Heparin is available in single-dose and multidose vials as well as commercially prepared IV solutions and prepackaged syringes. Lovenox (enoxaparin) and Fragmin (dalteparin sodium) are examples of low molecular weight heparin prescribed for prevention and treatment of deep-vein thrombosis (DVT) following abdominal surgery, hip or knee replacement, unstable angina, and acute coronary syndromes. (See labels in Figure 23-1.)

Heparin sodium for injection is available in several dosage strengths (e.g., 1,000 units per mL; 5,000 units per mL; 10,000 units per mL). Heparin Lock Flush Solution, which is used for flushing (e.g., med-locks, specialized IV lines), is available in 10 and 100 units per mL. Heparin flush solution 10 units per mL and 100 units per mL is a different concentration of heparin than what is administered subcutaneously or intravenously.

SAFETY ALERT!

The average heparin flush dosage strength is 10 units per mL and never exceeds 100 units per mL. Heparin sodium for injection and heparin lock flush solution can never be used interchangeably.

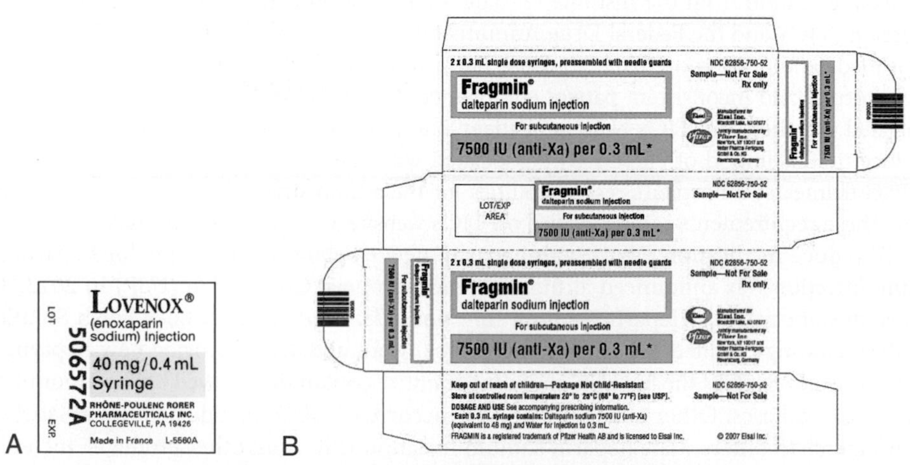

Figure 23-1 **A,** Lovenox label. **B,** Fragmin label.

Reading Heparin Labels

Heparin labels must always be read carefully to ensure that you have the correct concentrations.

> **SAFETY ALERT!**
>
> Careful reading of **heparin** labels is critical to the prevention of lethal dosage errors with heparin. Health care agencies may still be transforming from the old to new label regulations.
>
> Heparin labels must now express the strength (amount) per total volume as the primary and prominent expression on the label, followed in close proximity by the strength per milliliter (ISMP, 2013a).

Refer to the labels shown in Figure 23-2, A and B, for Heparin Sodium Injection, USP notice the following:

- Bolder and larger typeface
- The strength per total volume is expressed (e.g., Label A, 10,000 units per 10 mL, Label B, 50,000 units per 5 mL), followed by the dosage strength per mL in parenthesis for both (Label A, 1,000 units per mL, Label B, 10,000 units per mL)
- The statement "Not for lock flush"

Figure 23-3 shows a label for Heparin Lock Flush Solution USP, notice the strength per total volume (100 units per 10 mL) and the dosage strength per mL (10 units per mL).

> **SAFETY ALERT!**
>
> The nurse's primary responsibility is to administer the correct dosage and ensure that the dosage being administered is safe. When in doubt regarding a dosage a client is receiving, check with the prescriber before administering it. To avoid misinterpretation when orders are written or done by computer entry, the word *units* should not be abbreviated.

Remember that there are a number of available vial dosage strengths. Figure 23-2 shows sample labels of the various dosage strengths.

> **SAFETY ALERT!**
>
> Heparin is available in different strengths; read labels carefully before administering to ensure the client's safety. Verify the dosage, vial, and amount to be given. Obtain **independent verification** of the dosage to ensure accuracy. Heparin is a high alert medication and must be **double-checked** by another nurse. Continuous monitoring while the client is receiving heparin is essential because of the risk of hemorrhage or clots with an incorrect dose.

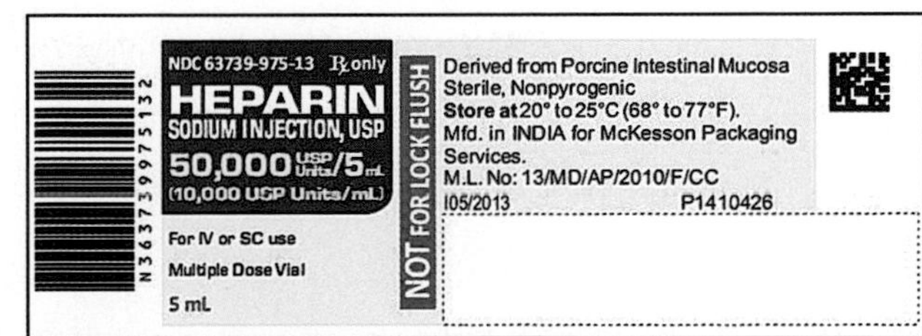

Figure 23-2 **A,** 10,000 units per 10 mL (1,000 units per mL). **B,** 50,000 units per 5 mL (10,000 units per mL).

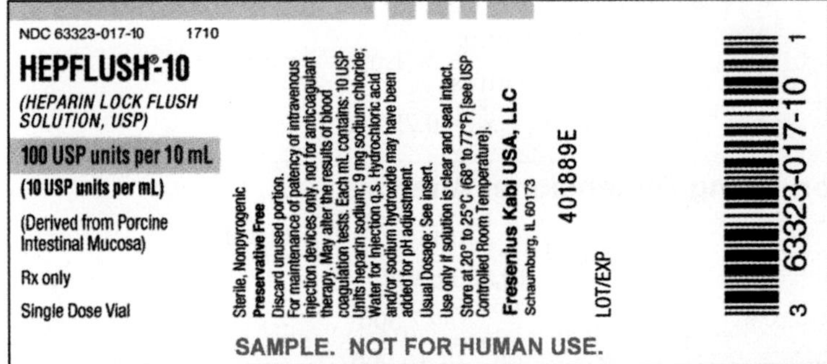

Figure 23-3 Heparin lock solution, 100 units per 10 mL (10 units per mL).

Commercially prepared IV solutions are also available from pharmaceutical companies in several strengths. The dosage written in red is for the purpose of attracting attention to the fact that the bag contains heparin. The use of premixed standardized bags of intravenous fluid with heparin assists in the prevention of some dosage errors with heparin. In some institutions, heparin for IV use is prepared in the pharmacy in various dosage strengths. If the dosage desired is not available in a commercially prepared solution or from the pharmacy, the nurse will be responsible for preparing the solution.

SAFETY ALERT!

Always carefully read heparin labels (three times) and the prescribed dose. Adherence to the "six rights" of medication administration is critical in preventing dosing errors with heparin. Careful reading of heparin labels is critical to prevent lethal dosage errors.

Now let's proceed with the calculation of heparin dosages.

Calculation of Subcutaneous Dosages

Because of its inherent dangers and the need to ensure an accurate and exact dosage, when heparin is administered subcutaneously, a tuberculin syringe (1 mL) is used. Heparin is also available for use in prepackaged syringes. Institutional policies differ regarding the administration of heparin, and the nurse is responsible for knowing and following the policies. The methods of calculating presented in previous chapters are used to calculate subcutaneous (subcut) heparin, except the dosage is never rounded and is administered with a tuberculin syringe. The prescriber will order heparin in units, and an order written in any other unit of measure should be questioned before administration.

Example: **Order:** Heparin 7,500 units subcut daily

Available: Heparin labeled 10,000 units per mL

What will you administer to the client?

Setup:

1. No conversion is necessary. There is no conversion for units.
2. Think—What would be a logical dosage?
3. Set up in ratio and proportion, the formula method, or dimensional analysis and solve.

✓ Solution Using Ratio and Proportion

$$10{,}000 \text{ units} : 1 \text{ mL} = 7{,}500 \text{ units} : x \text{ mL}$$

or

$$\frac{10{,}000 \text{ units}}{1 \text{ mL}} = \frac{7{,}500 \text{ units}}{x \text{ mL}}$$

$$\frac{10{,}000x}{10{,}000} = \frac{7{,}500}{10{,}000}$$

$$x = \frac{7{,}5\cancel{00}}{10{,}0\cancel{00}}$$

$$x = 0.75 \text{ mL}$$

✓ Solution Using the Formula Method

$$\frac{7{,}500 \text{ units}}{10{,}000 \text{ units}} \times 1 \text{ mL} = x \text{ mL}$$

$$x = 0.75 \text{ mL}$$

✓ Solution Using Dimensional Analysis

$$x \text{ mL} = \frac{1 \text{ mL}}{10{,}000 \cancel{\text{units}}} \times \frac{7{,}500 \cancel{\text{units}}}{1}$$

$$x = \frac{7{,}5\cancel{00}}{10{,}0\cancel{00}}$$

$$x = 0.75 \text{ mL}$$

The dosage of 0.75 mL is reasonable because the ordered dose is less than what is available. Therefore, less than 1 mL will be needed to administer the dosage. This dosage can be measured accurately only with a tuberculin syringe (calibrated in tenths and hundredths of a milliliter). This dosage would not be rounded to the nearest tenth of a milliliter. A tuberculin syringe illustrating the dosage to be administered is shown in Figure 23-4.

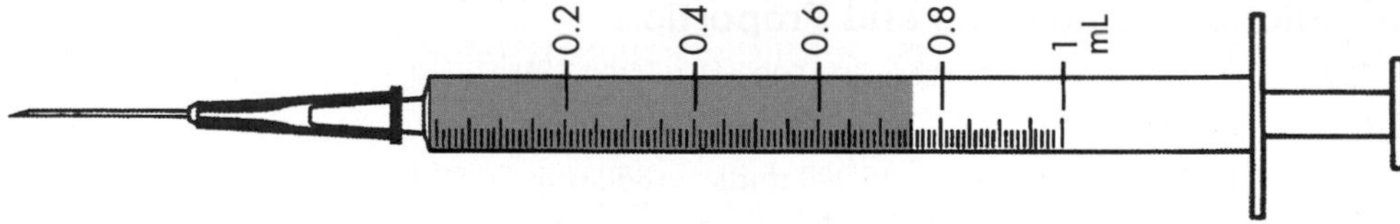

Figure 23-4 Tuberculin syringe illustrating 0.75 mL drawn up.

Calculation of IV Heparin Solutions

Using Ratio and Proportion to Calculate Units per Hour

Calculating the rate in units/hr can be done by using ratio and proportion or dimensional analysis.

Example: An IV solution of heparin is ordered for a client. D5W 1,000 mL containing 20,000 units of heparin is to infuse at 30 mL/hr. Calculate the dosage of heparin the client is to receive per hour.

Set up proportion:

$$20{,}000 \text{ units} : 1{,}000 \text{ mL} = x \text{ units} : 30 \text{ mL}$$

or

$$\frac{20{,}000 \text{ units}}{1{,}000 \text{ mL}} = \frac{x \text{ units}}{30 \text{ mL}}$$

$$1{,}000x = 20{,}000 \times 30$$

$$\frac{1{,}000x}{1{,}000} = \frac{600{,}\cancel{000}}{1{,}\cancel{000}}$$

$$x = 600 \text{ units/hr}$$

Using Dimensional Analysis to Calculate Units per Hour

Steps:

- Isolate units/hr being calculated first.
- Place the 20,000 units per 1,000 mL as the starting fraction with units in the numerator, to match the units in the numerator being calculated.
- Enter the 30 mL/hr rate with 30 mL as the numerator; notice that this matches the starting fraction mL denominator.
- Cancel the mL to obtain the desired unit (units/hr).
- Reduce if possible, and perform the necessary math operations.

$$\frac{x \text{ units}}{\text{hr}} = \frac{20{,}\cancel{000} \text{ units}}{1{,}\cancel{000} \cancel{\text{mL}}} \times \frac{30 \cancel{\text{mL}}}{1 \text{ hr}}$$

$$x = \frac{20 \times 30}{1}$$

$$x = \frac{600}{1}$$

$$x = 600 \text{ units/hr}$$

Calculating mL/hr from Units/hr

Because heparin is ordered in units/hr and infused with an electronic infusion device, it is necessary to do calculations in mL/hr.

SAFETY ALERT!

An infusion pump is required for the safe administration of all intravenous heparin infusions.

Example 1: **Order:** Infuse heparin 850 units/hr from a solution containing D5W 500 mL with heparin 25,000 units IV.

✓ Solution Using Ratio and Proportion

$$25{,}000 \text{ units} : 500 \text{ mL} = 850 \text{ units} : x \text{ mL}$$

or

$$\frac{25{,}000 \text{ units}}{500 \text{ mL}} = \frac{850 \text{ units}}{x \text{ mL}}$$

Solve:

$$25{,}000\,x = 500 \times 850$$

$$\frac{25{,}000x}{25{,}000} = \frac{425{,}\cancel{000}}{25{,}\cancel{000}}$$

$$x = \frac{425}{25}$$

$$x = 17 \text{ mL/hr}$$

✓ Solution Using Dimensional Analysis

Steps:

- Isolate mL/hr being calculated first.
- Enter the starting fraction 25,000 units per 500 mL, placing mL as the numerator. Notice that this will match the mL numerator of the units being calculated.
- Enter the 850 units/hr rate ordered with units in the numerator.
- Cancel units; the desired unit mL/hr is left.
- Reduce if possible, and perform the math operations.

$$\frac{x \text{ mL}}{\text{hr}} = \frac{\overset{1}{\cancel{500}} \text{ mL}}{\underset{50}{\cancel{25{,}000}} \cancel{\text{units}}} \times \frac{850 \cancel{\text{units}}}{1 \text{ hr}}$$

$$x = \frac{85\cancel{0}}{5\cancel{0}}$$

$$x = \frac{85}{5}$$

$$x = 17 \text{ mL/hr}$$

To infuse 850 units/hr from a solution of 25,000 units in D5W 500 mL, the flow rate would be 17 mL/hr.

Example 2: Infuse 1,200 units of heparin per hour from a solution containing 20,000 units in 250 mL D5W.

✓ Solution Using Ratio and Proportion

$$20{,}000 \text{ units} : 250 \text{ mL} = 1{,}200 \text{ units} : x \text{ mL}$$

or

$$\frac{20{,}000 \text{ units}}{250 \text{ mL}} = \frac{1{,}200 \text{ units}}{x \text{ mL}}$$

Solve:

$$20{,}000x = 1{,}200 \times 250$$

$$\frac{20{,}000x}{20{,}000} = \frac{30\cancel{0{,}000}}{2\cancel{0{,}000}}$$

$$x = \frac{30}{2}$$

$$x = 15 \text{ mL/hr}$$

✓ Solution Using Dimensional Analysis

Follow the same steps outlined in Example 1.

$$\frac{x \text{ mL}}{\text{hr}} = \frac{\overset{1}{\cancel{250}} \text{ mL}}{\underset{80}{\cancel{20{,}000}} \cancel{\text{units}}} \times \frac{1{,}200 \cancel{\text{units}}}{1 \text{ hr}}$$

$$x = \frac{1{,}20\cancel{0}}{8\cancel{0}}$$

$$x = 15 \text{ mL/hr}$$

Calculating Heparin Dosages Based on Weight

To prevent dosage and administration errors with heparin, many hospitals have established **heparin protocols** to guide the administration of IV heparin dosages. The dosages of heparin are individualized based on the client's weight. The protocols are based on the client's weight in kilograms and the client's activated partial thromboplastin time (APTT), a blood clotting value measured in seconds. APTT is used as the criterion to titrate the dosage, and adjustments are made accordingly (see sample protocol in Figure 23-5). Heparin protocols consist of:

- The bolus or loading dose, which is the initial bolus based on the client's weight in kilograms
- The initial infusion rate based on the client's weight in kilograms
- Directions on what additional bolus and rate alterations must be made based on APTT results

Heparin protocols consist of **three** steps in the administration process in the following sequence: (1) **bolus,** (2) **continuous infusion,** and (3) **rebolus** and /or adjust infusion rate (increase, decrease, or discontinue).

It is imperative that nurses be familiar with the protocol at their individual institutions. The bolus and infusion rate can vary among institutions. According to Clayton and Willihnganz's *Basic Pharmacology for Nurses* (2017), the bolus dosage is 70 to 100 units/kg, and the infusion rate is 15 to 25 units/kg/hr. These values can be different depending on the institution. At some institutions, the weight of the client is to the nearest tenth of a kilogram, or the exact number of kilograms. **Always be familiar with the values and protocol used for heparin administration at the institution to prevent errors and to ensure the safe administration of heparin.**

SAFETY ALERT!

In order for heparin to be therapeutically effective, the dosage **must** be accurate. A larger dosage than required can cause a client to hemorrhage, and an underdosage may not have the desired effect. Any questionable dosages should be verified with the prescriber.

Weight-Based Heparin Protocol

1. Bolus with heparin at 80 units/kg
2. Begin intravenous infusion of heparin at 18 units/kg/hr using 25,000 units heparin in 250 mL D_5W or a concentration of 100 units per mL.
3. APTT 6 hours after rate change and then daily at 7am
4. Adjust intravenous heparin daily based on APTT results
   - APTT less than 35 sec, Bolus with 80 units/kg and increase rate by 4 units/kg/hr.
   - APTT 35-45 sec, Bolus with 40 units/kg and increase rate by 2 units/kg/hr.
   - APTT 46-70 sec, **No Change.**
   - APTT 71-90 sec, Decrease rate by 2 units/kg/hr
   - APTT greater than 90 sec, **Stop** heparin infusion for 1 hour, and decrease rate by 3 units/kg/hr

Figure 23-5 Sample Heparin weight-based protocol. *Note:* This protocol is for calculation purposes only.

Remember, IV heparin is administered by infusion pump. There are some pumps as discussed in the IV Chapter (Chapter 22) that are capable of delivering IV fluids in tenths of a milliliter. Always check the equipment available at the institution before rounding IV flow rates to whole milliliters per hour (mL/hr). In this text, for the purpose of calculating, round mL/hr to a whole number unless provided information to do otherwise.

Let's work through some examples of calculation of heparin dosages based on weight. For the purpose of practice problems, the client's weight will be rounded to the nearest tenth of a kilogram.

Example 1: A client weighs 160 lb. Order: Administer a bolus of heparin sodium IV.

The hospital protocol is 80 units/kg. How many units will you give?

Step 1: Calculate the client's weight in kilograms.

Conversion factor: 1 kg = 2.2 lb

$$160 \text{ lb} \div 2.2 = 72.72 = 72.7 \text{ kg}$$

Step 2: Calculate the heparin bolus dosage.

$$80 \text{ units}/\cancel{\text{kg}} \times 72.7\ \cancel{\text{kg}} = 5{,}816 \text{ units}$$

The client should receive 5,816 units IV heparin as a bolus.

Example 2: A client weighs 165 lb.

Heparin infusion: Heparin 25,000 units in 1,000 mL 0.9% sodium chloride.

Bolus with heparin sodium at 80 units/kg, then initiate drip at 18 units/kg/hr.

Calculate the initial heparin bolus dosage.

Calculate the infusion rate, and determine the rate in mL/hr at which you will set the infusion device.

Step 1: Calculate the client's weight in kilograms.

Conversion factor: 1 kg = 2.2 lb

$$165 \text{ lb} \div 2.2 = 75 \text{ kg}$$

Step 2: Calculate the heparin bolus dosage.

$$80 \text{ units}/\cancel{\text{kg}} \times 75\ \cancel{\text{kg}} = 6{,}000 \text{ units}$$

The client should receive 6,000 units IV heparin as a bolus.

Step 3: Calculate the infusion rate for the IV dosage.

$$18 \text{ units}/\cancel{\text{kg}}/\text{hr} \times 75\ \cancel{\text{kg}} = 1{,}350 \text{ units/hr}$$

Step 4: Determine the rate in mL/hr at which to set the infusion device.

$$1{,}000 \text{ mL} : 25{,}000 \text{ units} = x \text{ mL} : 1{,}350 \text{ units}$$
$$25{,}000x = 1{,}350 \times 1{,}000$$

$$\frac{25{,}000x}{25{,}000} = \frac{1{,}350{,}\cancel{000}}{25{,}\cancel{000}}$$

$$x = 54 \text{ mL/hr}$$

or

Formula could be used:

$$\frac{D}{H} \times Q = x$$

$$\frac{1{,}350 \text{ units per hr}}{25{,}000 \text{ units}} \times 1{,}000 \text{ mL} = x \text{ mL per hr}$$

$$x = 54 \text{ mL/hr}$$

The pump would be set at 54 mL/hr to deliver 1,350 units/hr.

Now let's do a practice problem going through the steps of calculating the bolus, continuous infusion, rebolus, and/or adjust infusion rate using the protocol in Figure 25-3 for a client weighing 198 lb. Round weight to the nearest tenth as indicated.

Step 1: Convert the client's weight to kilograms.

Conversion factor: 1 kg = 2.2 lb

198 lb ÷ 2.2 = 90 kg

Step 2: Calculate the heparin bolus dosage.

80 units/$\cancel{\text{kg}}$ × 90 $\cancel{\text{kg}}$ = 7,200 units. The client should receive 7,200 units IV heparin as a bolus.

To determine the volume (mL) the client would receive, remember that the concentration of heparin was indicated as 100 units per mL. This can be done using ratio and proportion or dimensional analysis.

100 units : 1 mL= 7,200 units : x mL

$$\frac{100x}{100} = \frac{7{,}200}{100}$$

x = 72 mL (bolus is 72 mL)

Step 3: Calculate the infusion rate (18 units/kg/hr)

18 units/$\cancel{\text{kg}}$/hr × 90 $\cancel{\text{kg}}$ = 1,620 units/hr

Determine the rate in mL/hr at which to set the infusion device (using the concentration of 100 units per mL)

100 units : 1 mL = 1,620 units : x mL

$$\frac{100x}{100} = \frac{1{,}620}{100} = 16.2$$

$$x = 16 \text{ mL/hr}$$

The pump set at 16 mL/hr will deliver 1,620 units/hr.

The client's APTT after 6 hours is reported as 43 seconds. According to the protocol, rebolus with 40 units/kg and increase rate by 2 units/kg/hr.

Step 4: Calculate the dosage (units/hr) of the continuous infusion increase based on the protocol using the client's weight in kg.

Calculate the dosage (units) of heparin rebolus.

$40 \text{ units}/\cancel{\text{kg}} \times 90 \cancel{\text{kg}} = 3{,}600 \text{ units}$

Determine the volume (mL) to administer 3,600 units.

$$100 \text{ units} : 1 \text{ mL} = 3{,}600 \text{ units} : x \text{ mL}$$
$$\frac{100x}{100} = \frac{3{,}600}{100}$$
$$x = 36 \text{ mL bolus}$$

Now determine the infusion rate increase (2 units/kg/hr × kg).

$$2 \text{ units}/\cancel{\text{kg}}/\text{hr} \times 90 \cancel{\text{kg}} = 180 \text{ units/hr}$$

The infusion rate should be increased by 180 units/hr.

Calculate the adjustment in the hourly infusion rate (mL/hr).

$$100 \text{ units} : 1 \text{ mL} = 180 \text{ units} : x \text{ mL}$$
$$\frac{100x}{100} = \frac{180}{100}$$
$$x = 1.8 \text{ mL/hr}$$

Increase rate:

$$\begin{array}{rr} & 16 \text{ mL/hr (current rate)} \\ + & 1.8 \text{ mL/hr (increase)} \\ \hline 17.8 = & 18 \text{ mL/hr (new rate)} \end{array}$$

Increase the rate on the pump to 18 mL/hr.

Remember to get another nurse for independent verification of the adjusted rate.

Note: The rate in mL/hr has been rounded to the nearest whole mL. If the pump is programmed to infuse in tenths, express answers in tenths; if not, round to the nearest whole mL.

PRACTICE **PROBLEMS**

Calculate the units of measure indicated by the problem.

1. Order: Infuse 1,000 units/hr of heparin from a solution of 1,000 mL 0.45% NS with 25,000 units of heparin. Calculate the rate in mL/hr. ________________

2. Order: Infuse D5 0.9% NS 1,000 mL with 25,000 units of heparin at 35 mL/hr. Calculate the dosage in units/hr. ________________

3. Order: Infuse 750 mL D5W with 30,000 units of heparin at 25 mL/hr. Calculate the dosage in units/hr. ______________________

4. Order: Infuse D5W 1,000 mL with 25,000 units of heparin at 100 mL/hr. Determine the dosage in units/hr. ______________________

5. A client weighs 176 lb. Heparin infusion 20,000 units in 1,000 mL 0.9% sodium chloride. Order: Bolus with heparin sodium at 80 units/kg, then initiate drip at 18 units/kg/hr. (Round weight to the nearest tenth as indicated.) Calculate the following:

   a. ______________________ bolus dosage

   b. ______________________ infusion rate (initial)

   c. ______________________ mL/hr

Use the following weight-based heparin protocol for question 6. (Round weight to the nearest tenth as indicated; IV pump is calibrated in whole mL/hr.)

1. Bolus with heparin at 80 units/kg.
2. Begin intravenous infusion of heparin at 18 units/kg/hr using 25,000 units heparin in 500 mL D5W for 50 units per mL.
3. Adjust intravenous heparin daily based on APTT results.
   - APTT less than 35 seconds: Rebolus with 80 units/kg and increase rate by 4 units/kg/hr.
   - APTT 35-45 seconds: Rebolus with 40 units/kg and increase rate by 2 units/kg/hr.
   - APTT 46-70 seconds: **No change.**
   - APTT 71-90 seconds: Decrease rate by 2 units/kg/hr.
   - APTT greater than 90 sec. **Stop heparin** infusion for 1 hour and decrease rate by 3 units/kg/hr.

6. A client weighs 134.2 lb. Determine the bolus dose of heparin, the initial infusion rate, and then adjust the hourly infusion rate up or down based on the APTT results using the above weight-based heparin protocol. APTT is reported as 31 seconds.

Answers on pp. 622-623

POINTS TO REMEMBER

- Heparin is a potent anticoagulant; it is often administered intravenously but can be administered subcutaneously.
- Heparin is measured in USP units. When orders are written, the word *units* is spelled out to prevent misinterpretation.
- Heparin dosages must be accurately calculated to prevent inherent dangers associated with the medication. Discrepancies in dosage should be verified with the prescriber.
- Heparin order, dosage, vial, and the amount to give should be checked by another nurse before administering.
- When subcut heparin is administered, a tuberculin syringe is used (calibrated in tenths and hundredths of a milliliter). Answers are expressed in hundredths.

(continued)

- Read heparin labels carefully because heparin comes in several strengths.
- There are several IV calculations that can be done (mL/hr, units/hr).
- Heparin is commonly ordered in units/hr and infused with an electronic infusion device.
- Heparin sodium for injection and heparin lock solution cannot be used interchangeably.
- The method of calculating IV heparin dosages can also be used to calculate IV dosages for other medications. Ratio and proportion and dimensional analysis can be used as well.
- Heparin dosages are individualized according to the weight of the client in kilograms and adjusted based on the APTT.
- Protocols for IV heparin vary from institution to institution; always know and follow the institution's policy. Heparin protocol consist of three steps in the administration process: (1) bolus, (2) continuous infusion, (3) rebolus and/or adjust infusion rate (increase, decrease, or discontinue).
- Monitoring a client's APTT while they are receiving heparin is a **must.**
- Heparin is a high-alert medication that requires independent double verification by two nurses.
- New heparin labels indicate the strength (amount) per the entire container (vial)and the amount per mL.

CLINICAL **REASONING**

Scenario: A client has an order for heparin 3,500 units in 500 mL D5W to infuse at a rate of 40 mL/hr. The nurse prepares the IV using the heparin labeled 100 units per mL and adds 35 mL of heparin to the IV.

a. What error occurred in the preparation of the IV solution and why? ______________

____

b. What preventive measures should the nurse have taken? ______________

Answers on p. 623

CHAPTER **REVIEW**

For questions 1-12, calculate the dosage of heparin you will administer, and shade the dosage on the syringe provided. For questions 13 through 47, calculate the units as indicated by the problem. Use labels where provided to calculate dosages.

1. Order: Heparin 3,500 units subcut daily.

   Available: Heparin 10,000 units per mL

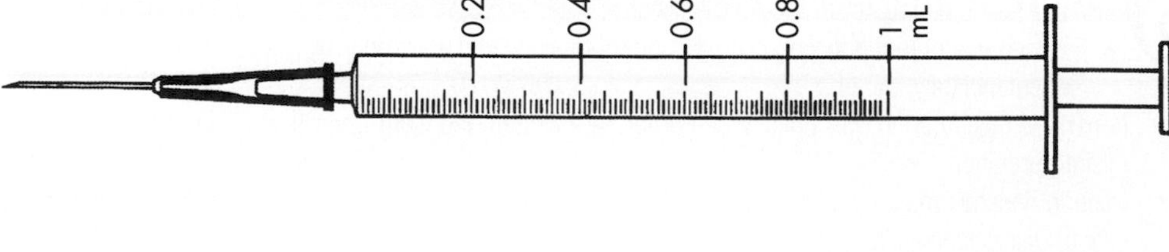

____

2. Order: Heparin 16,000 units subcut stat.

   Available: Heparin labeled 20,000 units per mL.

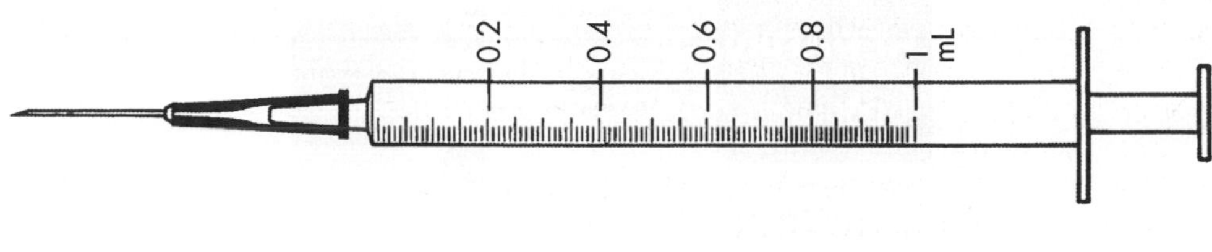

____

3. Order: Heparin 2,000 units subcut daily.

   Available: Heparin labeled 2,500 units per mL.

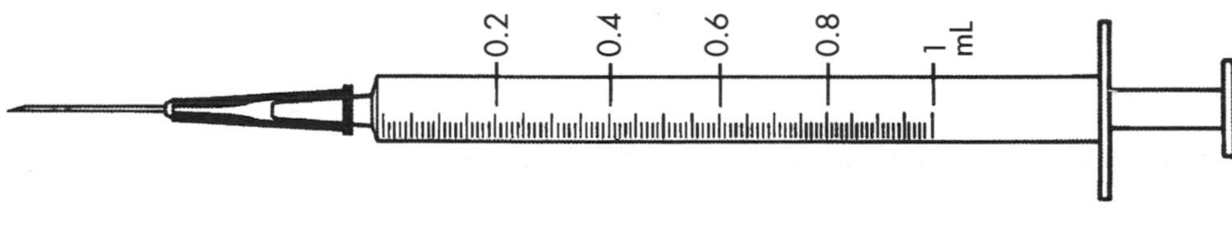

____

4. Order: Heparin 2,000 units subcut daily.

   Available:

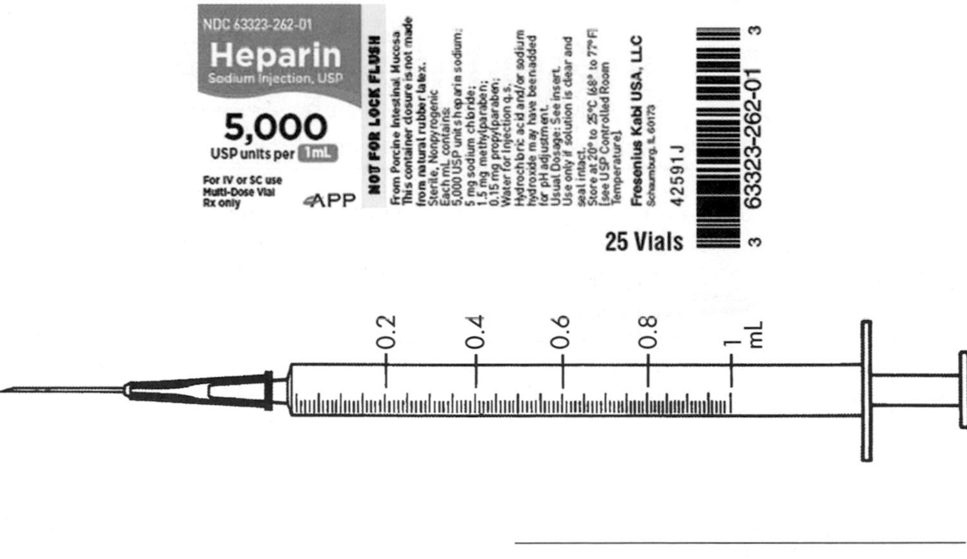

____

5. Order: Heparin 500 units subcut q4h.

   Available:

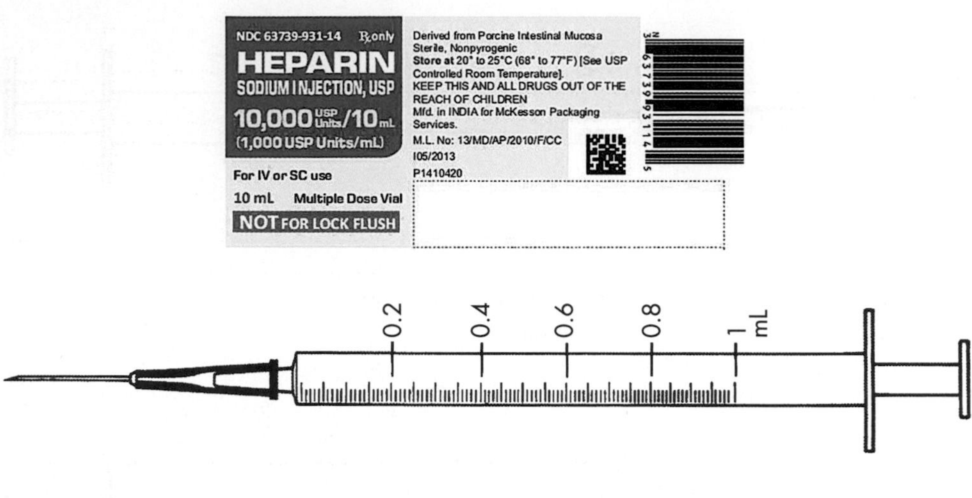

6. Order: Heparin flush 10 units every shift to flush a heparin lock.

   Available:

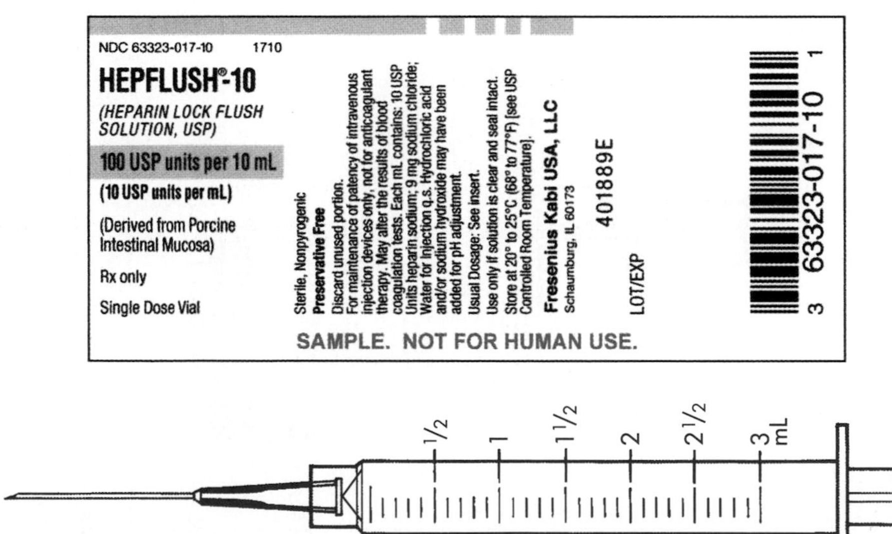

7. Order: Heparin 50,000 units IV in D5W 500 mL.

   Available: 10,000 units per mL.

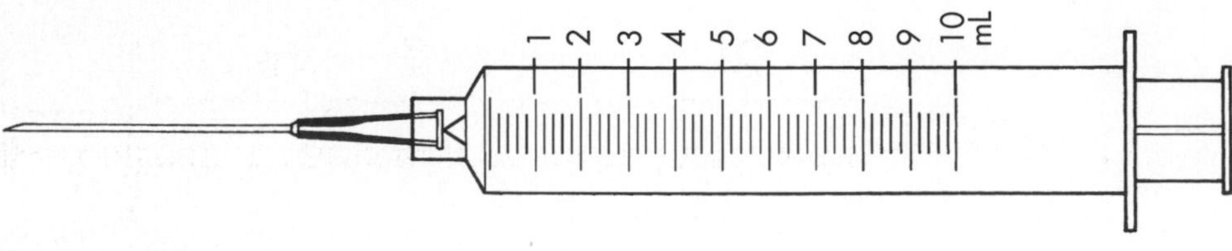

8. Order: Heparin 15,000 units subcut daily.

   Available: Heparin labeled 20,000 units per mL.

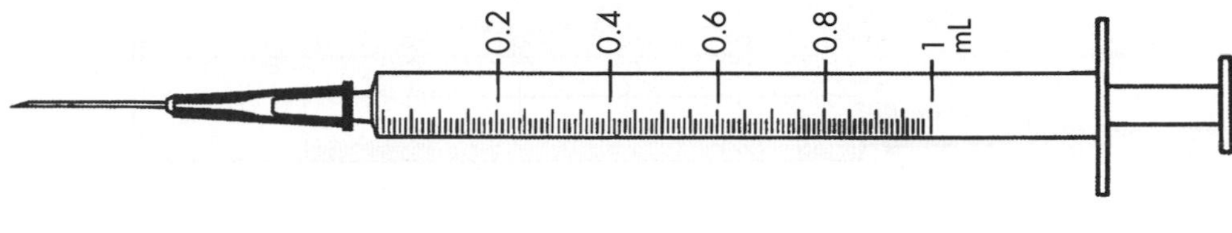

____

9. Order: 3,000 units of heparin to a liter of IV solution.

   Available: 2,500 units per mL.

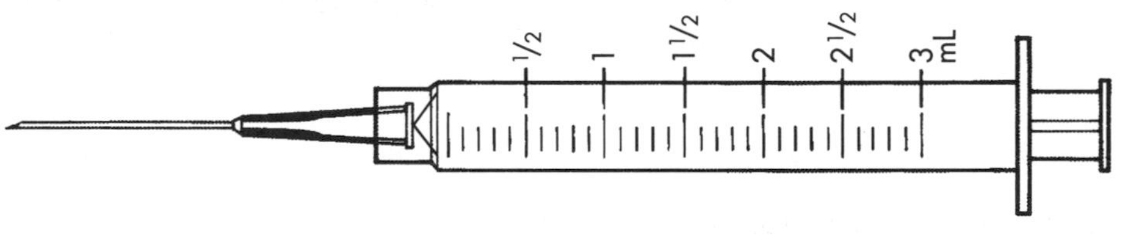

____

10. Order: Heparin 17,000 units subcut daily.

    Available: Heparin labeled 20,000 units per mL.

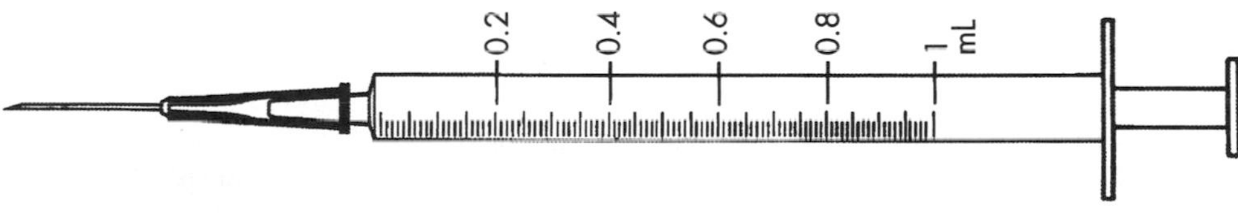

____

11. Order: Heparin bolus of 8,500 units IV stat.

    Available:

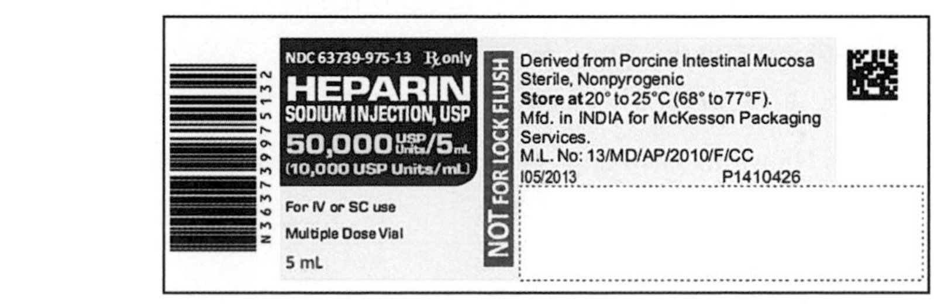

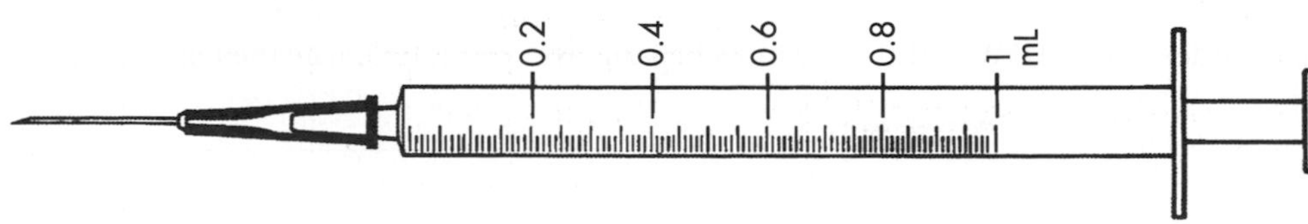

____

12. Order: Heparin 2,500 units subcut q12h.

 Available: Heparin labeled 10,000 units per mL.

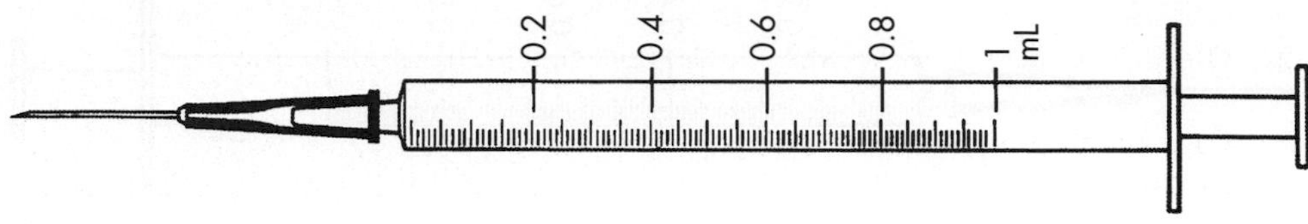

 ____

13. Order: Heparin 2,000 units/hr IV. Available: 25,000 units of heparin in 1,000 mL of 0.9% NS.

 What rate in mL/hr will deliver 2,000 units/hr? ______________________

14. Order: Heparin 1,500 units/hr IV. Available: 25,000 units of heparin in 500 mL D5W.

 What rate in mL/hr will deliver 1,500 units/hr? ______________________

15. Order: Heparin 1,800 units/hr IV. Available: 25,000 units heparin in 250 mL D5W.

 What rate in mL per hr will deliver 1,800 units/hr? ______________________

16. Order: 40,000 units heparin in 1 L 0.9% NaCl to infuse at 25 mL/hr.

 Calculate the hourly heparin dosage (units/hr). ______________________

17. Order: Heparin 25,000 units in 250 mL D5W to infuse at 11 mL/hr.

 Calculate the hourly heparin dosage (units/hr). ______________________

18. Order: Heparin 40,000 units in 500 mL D5W to infuse at 30 mL/hr.

 Calculate the hourly heparin dosage (units/hr). ______________________

19. Order: 1 L of 0.9% NS with 40,000 units heparin over 24 hr. Calculate the following:

 a. mL/hr ______________________

 b. units/hr ______________________

20. Order: 1 L of D5W with 15,000 units heparin over 10 hr. Calculate the following:

 a. mL/hr ______________________

 b. units/hr ______________________

21. Order: 1 L D5W with 35,000 units of heparin at 20 mL/hr.

    Calculate the hourly heparin dosage (units/hr). ____________________

22. Order: 500 mL of 0.9% NS with 10,000 units of heparin at 120 mL/hr.

    Calculate the hourly heparin dosage (units/hr). ____________________

23. Order: Infuse 1,400 units/hr of heparin IV. Available: Heparin 40,000 units in 1,000 mL of D5W.

    Calculate the rate in mL/hr. ____________________

24. Order: Heparin 40,000 units IV in 1 L 0.9% NS at 1,000 units/hr.

    Calculate the rate in mL/hr. ____________________

25. Order: Administer 2,000 units heparin IV every hour. Solution available is 25,000 units of heparin in 1 L 0.9% NS.

    Calculate the rate in mL/hr. ____________________

Calculate the hourly dosage of heparin (units/hr).

26. Order: 50,000 units of heparin in 1,000 mL of D5W to infuse at 60 mL/hr.

    ____

27. Order: 25,000 units of heparin in 500 mL of 0.45% NS to infuse at 20 mL/hr.

    ____

28. Order: 20,000 units of heparin in 500 mL D5W to infuse at 20 mL/hr.

    ____

29. Order: 25,000 units of heparin in 1 L of D5W to infuse at 56 mL/hr.

    ____

30. Order: 20,000 units of heparin in 1,000 mL D5W to infuse at 45 mL/hr.

    ____

31. Order: 30,000 units of heparin in 500 mL of D5W to infuse at 25 mL/hr. ____________________

32. Order: 20,000 units of heparin in 1 L of D5W to infuse at 40 mL/hr. ____________________

33. Order: 40,000 units of heparin in 500 mL 0.45% NS to infuse at 25 mL/hr. ____________________

34. Order: 35,000 units of heparin in 1 L of D5W to infuse at 20 mL/hr. ____________________

35. Order: 25,000 units of heparin in 1 L of D5W to infuse at 30 mL/hr. ____________________

36. Order: 40,000 units of heparin in 1 L of D5W to infuse at 30 mL/hr. ____________________

37. Order: 20,000 units of heparin in 1 L of D5W to infuse at 80 mL/hr. ____________________

38. A central venous line requires flushing with heparin. Which of the two labels shown is appropriate for a heparin flush?

NDC 63739-975-13 ℞ only
HEPARIN
SODIUM INJECTION, USP
50,000 USP Units/5 mL
(10,000 USP Units/mL)
For IV or SC use
Multiple Dose Vial
5 mL
NOT FOR LOCK FLUSH
Derived from Porcine Intestinal Mucosa
Sterile, Nonpyrogenic
Store at 20° to 25°C (68° to 77°F).
Mfd. in INDIA for McKesson Packaging Services.
M.L. No: 13/MD/AP/2010/F/CC
I05/2013 P1410426

A

NDC 63323-017-10 1710
HEPFLUSH®-10
(HEPARIN LOCK FLUSH SOLUTION, USP)
100 USP units per 10 mL
(10 USP units per mL)
(Derived from Porcine Intestinal Mucosa)
Rx only
Single Dose Vial
Sterile, Nonpyrogenic
Preservative Free
Discard unused portion.
For maintenance of patency of intravenous injection devices only, not for anticoagulant therapy. May alter the results of blood coagulation tests. Each mL contains: 10 USP Units heparin sodium; 9 mg sodium chloride; Water for Injection q.s. Hydrochloric acid and/or sodium hydroxide may have been added for pH adjustment.
Usual Dosage: See insert.
Use only if solution is clear and seal intact.
Store at 20° to 25°C (68° to 77°F) [see USP Controlled Room Temperature].
Fresenius Kabi USA, LLC
Schaumburg, IL 60173
401889E
LOT/EXP
3 63323-017-10 1
SAMPLE. NOT FOR HUMAN USE.

B

____

For problems 39-42, round the weight to the nearest tenth.

39. Order: Heparin drip at 18 units/kg/hr.

Available: 25,000 units of heparin sodium in 1,000 mL of D5W. The client weighs 80 kg. At what rate will you set the infusion pump? ____________________

40. A client weighs 200 lb.

Order: Administer a bolus of heparin sodium IV at 80 units/kg. How many units will you administer? ____________________

41. A client weighs 210 lb. Heparin IV infusion: heparin sodium 25,000 units in 1,000 mL of 0.9% NS. Order is to give a bolus with heparin sodium 80 units/kg, then initiate drip at 14 units/kg/hr.

Calculate the following:

a. Heparin bolus dosage ____________________

b. Infusion rate for the IV (initial) ____________________ units/hr

c. At what rate will you set the infusion pump? ____________________

42. A client weighs 154 lb. Heparin IV infusion: heparin sodium 20,000 units in 1,000 mL D5W. The hospital protocol is to give a bolus to the client with 80 units/kg and start drip at 14 units/kg/hr.

    Calculate the following:

    a. Heparin bolus dosage ________________

    b. Infusion rate for the IV ________________ units/hr

    c. Infusion rate in mL/hr ________________

Heparin Protocol for Question 43-44

1. Bolus heparin at 80 units/kg.
2. Begin intravenous infusion of heparin at 18 units/kg/hr using 25,000 units heparin in 250 mL D5W for 100 units per mL.
3. Adjust intravenous heparin daily based on APTT results.
   - APTT less than 35 sec: Rebolus with 80 units/kg and increase rate by 4 units/kg/hr.
   - APTT 35-45 sec: Rebolus with 40 units/kg and increase rate by 2 units/kg/hr.
   - APTT 46-70 sec: **No change.**
   - APTT 71-90 sec: Decrease rate by 2 units/kg/hr.
   - APTT greater than 90 sec: **Stop heparin** infusion for 1 hour and decrease rate by 3 units/kg/hr

43. A client weighs 100 kg. Determine the bolus dose of heparin, the initial infusion rate, and then adjust the hourly infusion rate up or down based on APTT results using the above weight-based heparin protocol. The APTT is reported as 71 seconds. The pump delivers in whole mL/hr.

44. A client weighs 162.8 lb. Determine the bolus dose of heparin, the initial infusion rate, and then adjust the hourly infusion rate up or down based on APTT results using the above weight based protocol. The APTT is reported as 38 sec. The pump delivers in tenths of a mL.

45. **<u>Directions: For Question #45.</u>** Calculate the heparin dose in units/hr and the heparin infusion rate in mL/hr. (The pump is capable of delivering in tenths of a mL.)

    Order: Heparin 20 units/kg/hr. IV infusion for a patient/client who weighs 89 kg.

    Available: Heparin 25,000 units in 500 mL D_5W (50 units per mL)

    a. Calculate dose in units/hr ________________

    b. Determine the rate in mL/hr ________________

Answers on pp. 623-628

evolve

For additional practice problems, refer to the Dosages Measured in Units section of the Elsevier's Interactive Drug Calculation Application, Version 1 on Evolve.

ANSWERS

Chapter 23

Answers to Practice Problems

1. 25,000 units : 1,000 mL = 1,000 units : x mL

or

$$\frac{25{,}000 \text{ units}}{1{,}000 \text{ mL}} = \frac{1{,}000 \text{ units}}{x \text{ mL}}$$

$$25{,}000x = 1{,}000 \times 1{,}000$$

$$\frac{25{,}000x}{25{,}000} = \frac{1{,}000{,}000}{25{,}000}$$

$$x = 40 \text{ mL/hr}$$

Answer: 40 mL/hr

2. 25,000 units : 1,000 mL = x units : 35 mL

$$\frac{1{,}000x}{1{,}000} = \frac{875{,}000}{1{,}000}$$

$$x = 875 \text{ units/hr}$$

Answer: 875 units/hr.

3. 30,000 units : 750 mL = x units : 25 mL

$$\frac{750x}{750} = \frac{750{,}000}{750}$$

$$x = 1{,}000 \text{ units/hr}$$

Answer: 1,000 units/hr

4. Calculate units/hr infusing.

1,000 mL : 25,000 units = 100 mL : x units

$$\frac{1{,}000x}{1{,}000} = \frac{2{,}500{,}000}{1{,}000}$$

$$x = \frac{2{,}500}{1}$$

Answer: 2,500 units/hr

5. Convert the weight to kilograms.

Conversion factor: 2.2 lb = 1 kg

176 lb ÷ 2.2 = 80 kg

a. Calculate the heparin bolus dosage.

80 units/kg × 80 kg = 6,400 units

Answer: 6,400 units

b. Calculate the infusion rate for the IV drip (initial).

80 units/kg/hr × 80 kg = 1,440 units/hr

c. Determine the rate in mL/hr at which to set the infusion rate.

1,000 mL : 20,000 units = x mL : 1,440 units

$$\frac{20{,}000x}{20{,}000} = \frac{1{,}440{,}000}{20{,}000}$$

$$x = \frac{144}{2}$$

$$x = 72 \text{ mL/hr}$$

Answer: 72 mL/hr

6. **Step 1:** Convert the client's weight to kilograms.

Conversion factor: 1 kg = 2.2 lb

134.2 lb ÷ 2.2 = 61 kg

Step 2: Calculate the heparin bolus dosage.

80 units/kg × 61 kg = 4,880 units. The client should receive 4,880 units IV heparin as a bolus.

Determine the volume (mL) the client would receive. The concentration of heparin is stated as 50 units per mL.

50 units : 1 mL = 4,880 units : x mL

$$\frac{50x}{50} = \frac{4{,}880}{50}$$

$$x = \frac{4{,}880}{50} = 97.6$$

x = 98 mL (bolus is 98 mL)

Step 3: Calculate the infusion rate (18 units/kg/hr).

18 units/kg/hr × 61 kg = 1,098 units/hr. Determine the rate in mL/hr at which to set the infusion device (using the concentration of 50 units per mL).

50 units : 1 mL = 1,098 units : x mL

$$\frac{50x}{50} = \frac{1{,}098}{50}$$

$$x = \frac{1{,}098}{50} = 21.9$$

$$x = 22 \text{ mL/hr}$$

The client's APTT is 31 seconds. According to the protocol, rebolus with 80 units/kg and increase the rate by 4 units/kg/hr.

Step 4: Calculate the dosage (units/hr) of the continuous infusion increase based on the protocol using the client's weight in kg.

Calculate the dosage (units) of heparin rebolus.

80 units/kg × 61 kg = 4,880 units

Determine the volume (mL) to administer 4,880 units

50 units : 1 mL = 4,880 units : x mL

$$\frac{50x}{50} = \frac{4{,}880}{50}$$

$$x = \frac{4{,}880}{50} = 97.6$$

x = 98 mL bolus

Now determine the infusion rate increase (4 units/kg/hr × kg).

4 units/kg/hr × 61 kg = 244 units/hr

The infusion rate should be increased by 244 units/hr.

Calculate the adjustment in the hourly infusion rate (mL/hr).

50 units : 1 mL = 244 units : x mL

$$\frac{50x}{50} = \frac{244}{50}$$

$$x = \frac{244}{50} = 4.8$$

x = 5 mL/hr

Increase rate:

22 mL/hr (current rate)
+5 mL/hr (increase)
27 mL/hr (new infusion rate)

Note: This problem could also be done using the dimensional analysis or formula method.

Answers to Clinical Reasoning Questions

a. The nurse used the incorrect concentration of heparin to prepare the IV solution. Heparin concentration of 100 units per mL is used for maintaining the patency of a line and for flushing.

b. The nurse should have read the label carefully because heparin comes in a variety of concentrations. The label indicates what the heparin flush is used for and that it is not for anticoagulant therapy. In addition, heparin is a high alert medication and should have been checked with another nurse. Heparin IV flushes are available in 10 units per mL and 100 units per mL. Heparin for IV flush is never used interchangeably with heparin sodium for injection.

Answers to Chapter Review

Some problems where labels provided for calculation of dose, an alternate solution might be to use the total amount (volume) in the vial and the number of mL to calculate the dose. Problems are shown using the dosage strength per mL.

1. 10,000 units : 1 mL = 3,500 units : x mL

or

$$\frac{3{,}500 \text{ units}}{10{,}000 \text{ units}} \times 1 \text{ mL} = x \text{ mL}$$

x = 0.35 mL. The dosage ordered is less than the available strength; therefore you will need less than 1 mL to administer the dosage.

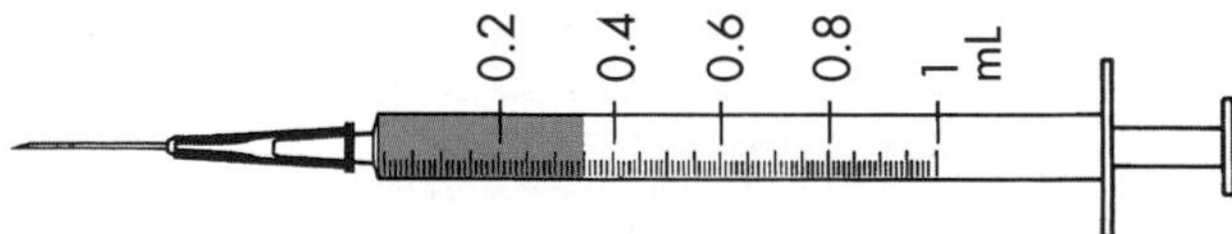

2. 20,000 units : 1 mL = 16,000 units : x mL

or

$$\frac{16{,}000 \text{ units}}{20{,}000 \text{ units}} \times 1 \text{ mL} = x \text{ mL}$$

Answer: 0.8 mL. The dosage ordered is less than the available strength; therefore you will need less than 1 mL to administer the dosage.

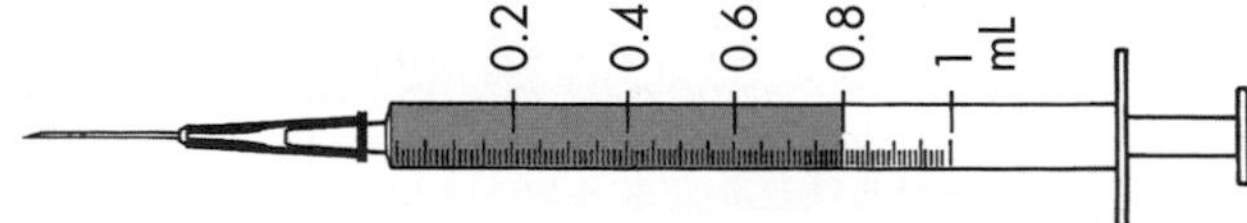

3. 2,500 units : 1 mL = 2,000 units : x mL

or

$$\frac{2{,}000 \text{ units}}{2{,}500 \text{ units}} \times 1 \text{ mL} = x \text{ mL}$$

Answer: 0.8 mL. The dosage ordered is less than the available strength; therefore you will need less than 1 mL to administer the dosage.

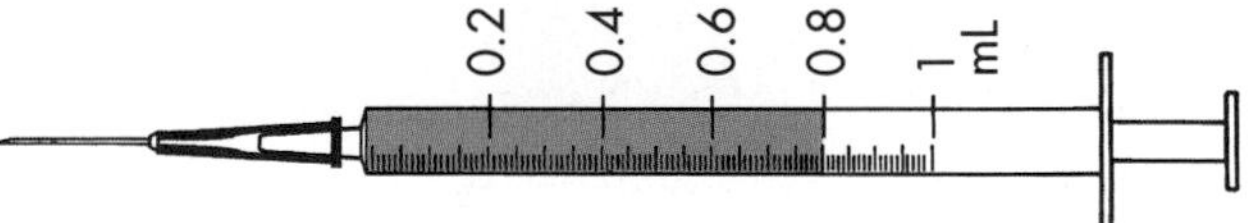

4. 5,000 units : 1 mL = 2,000 units : x mL

or

$$\frac{2{,}000 \text{ units}}{5{,}000 \text{ units}} \times 1 \text{ mL} = x \text{ mL}$$

Answer: 0.4 mL. The dosage ordered is less than the available strength; therefore you will need less than 1 mL to administer the dosage.

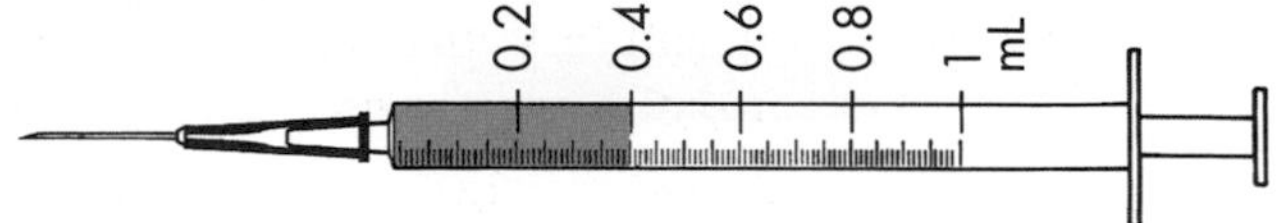

5. 1,000 units : 1 mL = 500 units : x mL

or

$$\frac{500 \text{ units}}{1{,}000 \text{ units}} \times 1 \text{ mL} = x \text{ mL}$$

Answer: 0.5 mL. The dosage ordered is less than the available strength; therefore, you will need less than 1 mL to administer the dosage.

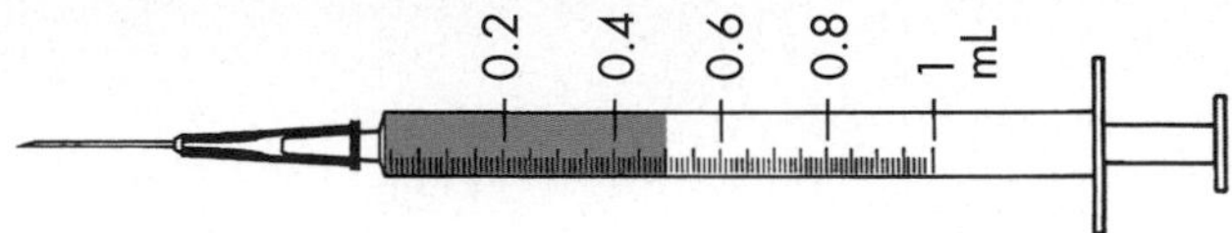

6. 10 units : 1 mL = 10 units : x mL

or

$$\frac{10 \text{ units}}{10 \text{ units}} \times 1 \text{ mL} = x \text{ mL}$$

1 mL contains 10 units, so you will need 1 mL to flush the heparin lock.

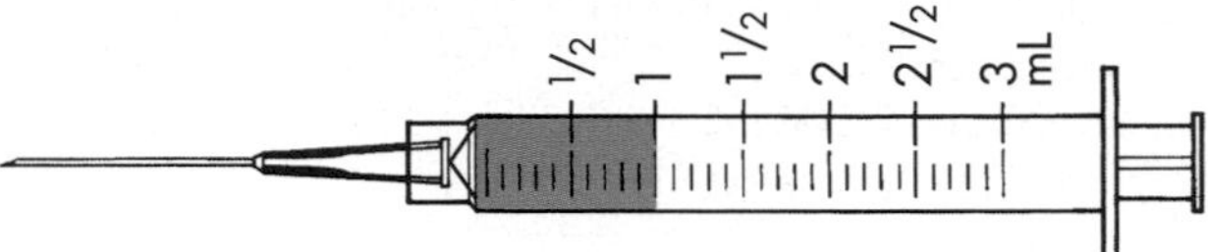

7. 10,000 units : 1 mL = 50,000 units : x mL

or

$$\frac{50{,}000 \text{ units}}{10{,}000 \text{ units}} \times 1 \text{ mL} = x \text{ mL}$$

Answer: 5 mL. The dosage ordered is more than the available strength; therefore you will need more than 1 mL to administer the dosage.

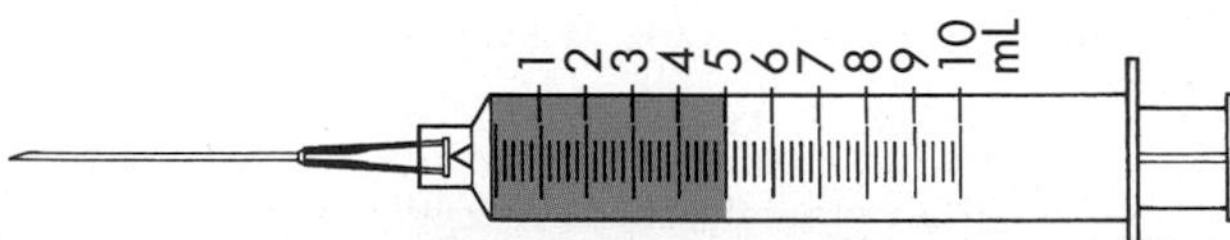

8. 20,000 units : 1 mL = 15,000 units : x mL

or

$$\frac{15{,}000 \text{ units}}{20{,}000 \text{ units}} \times 1 \text{ mL} = x \text{ mL}$$

Answer: 0.75 mL. The dosage ordered is less than the available strength; therefore you will need less than 1 mL to administer the dosage.

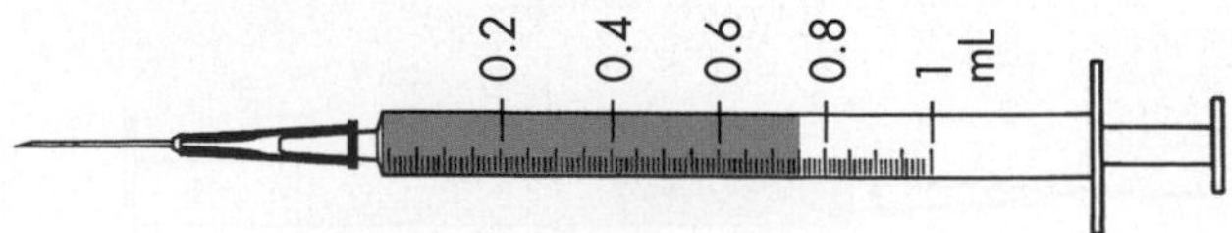

9. 2,500 units : 1 mL = 3,000 units : x mL

or

$$\frac{3{,}000 \text{ units}}{2{,}500 \text{ units}} \times 1 \text{ mL} = x \text{ mL}$$

Answer: 1.2 mL. The dosage ordered is more than the available strength; therefore you will need more than 1 mL to administer the dosage.

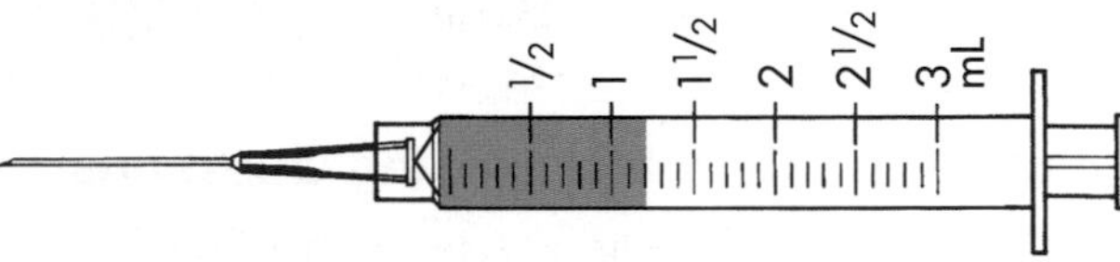

10. 20,000 units : 1 mL = 17,000 units : x mL

or

$$\frac{17{,}000 \text{ units}}{20{,}000 \text{ units}} \times 1 \text{ mL} = x \text{ mL}$$

Answer: 0.85 mL. The dosage ordered is less than the available strength; therefore you will need less than 1 mL to administer the dosage.

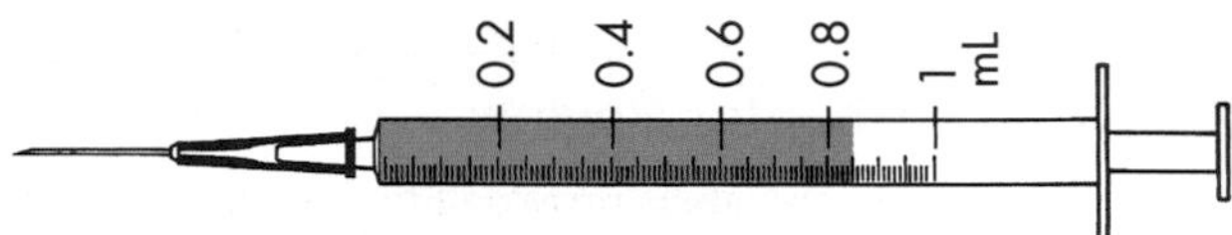

11. 10,000 units : 1 mL = 8,500 units : x mL

or

$$\frac{8{,}500 \text{ units}}{10{,}000 \text{ units}} \times 1 \text{ mL} = x \text{ mL}$$

Answer: 0.85 mL. The dosage ordered is less than the available strength; therefore you will need less than 1 mL to administer the dosage.

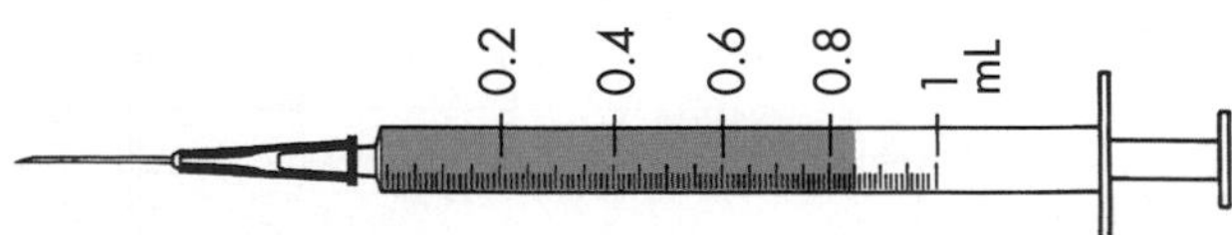

12. 10,000 units : 1 mL = 2,500 units : x mL

or

$$\frac{2{,}500 \text{ units}}{10{,}000 \text{ units}} \times 1 \text{ mL} = x \text{ mL}$$

Answer: 0.25 mL. The dosage ordered is less than the available strength; therefore you will need less than 1 mL to administer the dosage.

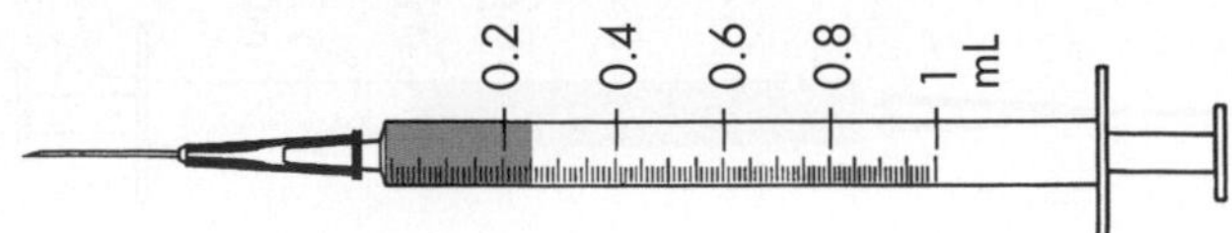

13. 25,000 units : 1,000 mL = 2,000 units : x mL

$$\frac{25{,}000x}{25{,}000} = \frac{2{,}000{,}000}{25{,}000}$$

x = 80 mL/hr. To administer 2,000 units of heparin per hour, 80 mL/hr must be given.

14. 25,000 units : 500 mL = 1,500 units : x mL

$$\frac{25{,}000x}{25{,}000} = \frac{750{,}000}{25{,}000}$$

$$x = \frac{750{,}000}{25{,}000}$$

x = 30 mL/hr. To administer 1,500 units of heparin per hour, 30 mL/hr must be given.

15. 25,000 units : 250 mL = 1,800 units : x mL

$$\frac{25{,}000x}{25{,}000} = \frac{450{,}000}{25{,}000}$$

x = 18 mL/hr. To administer 1,800 units of heparin per hour, 18 mL/hr must be given.

16. 1 L = 1,000 mL

40,000 units : 1,000 mL = x units : 25 mL

$$\frac{1{,}000x}{1{,}000} = \frac{1{,}000{,}000}{1{,}000}$$

$$x = \frac{1{,}000{,}000}{1{,}000}$$

x = 1,000 units/hr

17. 25,000 units : 250 mL = x units : 11 mL

$$\frac{250x}{250} = \frac{275{,}000}{250}$$

x = 1,100 units/hr

18. 40,000 units : 500 mL = x units : 30 mL

$$\frac{500x}{500} = \frac{1{,}200{,}000}{500}$$

x = 2,400 units/hr

19. 1 L = 1,000 mL

a. Calculate mL/hr.

$$\frac{1{,}000 \text{ mL}}{24 \text{ hr}} = 41.6 = 42 \text{ mL/hr}$$

b. Calculate units/hr.

40,000 units : 1,000 mL = x units : 42 mL

$$\frac{1{,}000x}{1{,}000} = \frac{1{,}680{,}000}{1{,}000}$$

$$x = \frac{1{,}680{,}000}{1{,}000}$$

x = 1,680 units/hr

20. 1 L = 1,000 mL

a. Calculate mL/hr.

$$\frac{1{,}000 \text{ mL}}{10 \text{ hr}} = 100 \text{ mL/hr}$$

b. Calculate units/hr.

15,000 units : 1,000 mL = x units : 100 mL

$$\frac{1{,}000x}{1{,}000} = \frac{1{,}500{,}000}{1{,}000}$$

$$x = \frac{1{,}500{,}000}{1{,}000}$$

x = 1,500 units/hr

21. 1 L = 1,000 mL

35,000 units : 1,000 mL = x units : 20 mL

$$\frac{1{,}000x}{1{,}000} = \frac{700{,}000}{1{,}000}$$

$$x = \frac{700{,}000}{1{,}000}$$

x = 700 units/hr

22. 10,000 units : 500 mL = x units : 120 mL

$$\frac{500x}{500} = \frac{1{,}200{,}000}{500}$$

$$x = \frac{1{,}200{,}000}{500}$$

x = 2,400 units/hr

23. Calculate mL/hr to be administered.

40,000 units : 1,000 mL = 1,400 units : x mL

$$\frac{40{,}000x}{40{,}000} = \frac{1{,}400{,}000}{40{,}000}$$

x = 35 mL/hr

24. 1 L = 1,000 mL

40,000 units : 1,000 mL = 1,000 units : x mL

$$\frac{40{,}000x}{40{,}000} = \frac{1{,}000{,}000}{40{,}000}$$

$$x = \frac{1{,}000{,}000}{40{,}000}$$

x = 25 mL/hr

25. 1 L = 1,000 mL

25,000 units : 1,000 mL = 2,000 units : x mL

$$\frac{25{,}000x}{25{,}000} = \frac{2{,}000{,}000}{25{,}000}$$

$$x = \frac{2{,}000{,}000}{25{,}000}$$

x = 80 mL/hr

26. 50,000 units : 1,000 mL = x units : 60 mL

$$\frac{1{,}000x}{1{,}000} = \frac{3{,}000{,}000}{1{,}000}$$
$$x = \frac{3{,}000{,}000}{1{,}000}$$
$$x = 3{,}000 \text{ units/hr}$$

27. 25,000 units : 500 mL = x units : 20 mL

$$\frac{500x}{500} = \frac{500{,}000}{500}$$
$$x = \frac{500{,}000}{500}$$
$$x = 1{,}000 \text{ units/hr}$$

28. 20,000 units : 500 mL = x units : 20 mL

$$\frac{500x}{500} = \frac{400{,}000}{500}$$
$$x = \frac{400{,}000}{500}$$
$$x = 800 \text{ units/hr}$$

29. 1 L = 1,000 mL

25,000 units : 1,000 mL = x units : 56 mL

$$\frac{1{,}000x}{1{,}000} = \frac{1{,}400{,}000}{1{,}000}$$
$$x = \frac{1{,}400{,}000}{1{,}000}$$
$$x = 1{,}400 \text{ units/hr}$$

30. 20,000 units : 1,000 mL = x units : 45 mL

$$\frac{1{,}000x}{1{,}000} = \frac{900{,}000}{1{,}000}$$
$$x = \frac{900{,}000}{1{,}000}$$
$$x = 900 \text{ units/hr}$$

31. 30,000 units : 500 mL = x units : 25 mL

$$\frac{500x}{500} = \frac{750{,}000}{500}$$
$$x = \frac{750{,}000}{500}$$
$$x = 1{,}500 \text{ units/hr}$$

32. 1 L = 1,000 mL

20,000 units : 1,000 mL = x units : 40 mL

$$\frac{1{,}000x}{1{,}000} = \frac{800{,}000}{1{,}000}$$
$$x = \frac{800{,}000}{1{,}000}$$
$$x = 800 \text{ units/hr}$$

33. 40,000 units : 500 mL = x units : 25 mL

$$\frac{500x}{500} = \frac{1{,}000{,}000}{500}$$
$$x = \frac{1{,}000{,}000}{500}$$
$$x = 2{,}000 \text{ units/hr}$$

34. 1 L = 1,000 mL

35,000 units : 1,000 mL = x units : 20 mL

$$\frac{1{,}000x}{1{,}000} = \frac{700{,}000}{1{,}000}$$
$$x = \frac{700{,}000}{1{,}000}$$
$$x = 700 \text{ units/hr}$$

35. 1 L = 1,000 mL

25,000 units : 1,000 mL = x units : 30 mL

$$\frac{1{,}000x}{1{,}000} = \frac{750{,}000}{1{,}000}$$
$$x = \frac{750{,}000}{1{,}000}$$
$$x = 750 \text{ units/hr}$$

36. 1 L = 1,000 mL

40,000 units : 1,000 mL = x units : 30 mL

$$\frac{1{,}000x}{1{,}000} = \frac{1{,}200{,}000}{1{,}000}$$
$$x = \frac{1{,}200{,}000}{1{,}000}$$
$$x = 1{,}200 \text{ units/hr}$$

37. 1 L = 1,000 mL

20,000 units : 1,000 mL = x units : 80 mL

$$\frac{1{,}000x}{1{,}000} = \frac{1{,}600{,}000}{1{,}000}$$
$$x = \frac{1{,}600{,}000}{1{,}000}$$
$$x = 1{,}600 \text{ units/hr}$$

38. Label "B" 10 units per mL is appropriate for flush. Heparin sodium for injection cannot be interchanged with heparin lock solution.

39. a. First determine units/kg the client should receive.

18 units/~~kg~~/hr × 80 ~~kg~~ = 1,400 units/hr

b. 1,000 mL : 25,000 units = x mL : 1,440 units/hr

$$\frac{25{,}000x}{25{,}000} = \frac{1{,}440{,}\cancel{000}}{25{,}\cancel{000}}$$
$$x = \frac{1{,}440}{25} = 57.6$$
$$x = 58 \text{ mL/hr}$$

Answer: 58 mL/hr

40. a. Convert the weight to kilograms.

Conversion factor: 2.2 lb = 1 kg

200 lb ÷ 2.2 = 90.9 kg

b. Calculate the heparin bolus dosage.

80 units/~~kg~~ × 90.9 ~~kg~~ = 7,272 units

Answer: 7,272 units

41. a. Convert the weight to kilograms.

Conversion factor: 2.2 lb = 1 kg

210 lb ÷ 2.2 = 95.45 kg = 95.5 kg

Calculate the heparin bolus dosage.

80 units/~~kg~~ × 95.5 ~~kg~~ = 7,640 units

Answer: 7,640 units

b. Calculate the infusion rate for the heparin drip.

14 units/~~kg~~/hr × 95.5 ~~kg~~ = 1,337 units/hr

c. Calculate the infusion rate in mL/hr.

1,000 units : 25,000 units = x mL : 1,337 units/hr

$$\frac{25{,}000x}{25{,}000} = \frac{1{,}337{,}\cancel{000}}{25{,}\cancel{000}}$$

$$x = \frac{1{,}337}{25} = 53.4$$

$$x = 53 \text{ mL/hr}$$

Answer: 53 mL/hr

42. a. Convert the weight to kilograms.

Conversion factor: 2.2 lb = 1 kg

154 lb ÷ 2.2 = 70 kg

Calculate the heparin bolus dosage.

80 units/~~kg~~ × 70 ~~kg~~ = 5,600 units

Answer: 5,600 units

b. Calculate the infusion rate for the heparin drip.

14 units/~~kg~~/hr × 70 ~~kg~~ = 980 units/hr

Answer: 980 units/hr

c. Calculate the infusion rate in mL/hr.

1,000 mL : 20,000 units = x mL : 980 units

$$\frac{20{,}000x}{20{,}000} = \frac{98\cancel{0}{,}\cancel{000}}{2\cancel{0}{,}\cancel{000}}$$

$$x = \frac{98}{2}$$

$$x = 49 \text{ mL/hr}$$

43. **Step 1:** Calculate the heparin bolus dosage. (No weight conversion required; the weight is in kg.)

80 units/~~kg~~ × 100 ~~kg~~ = 8,000 units. The client should receive 8,000 units IV heparin as a bolus.

Determine the volume (mL) the client would receive. The concentration is indicated as 100 units per mL.

100 units : 1 mL = 8,000 units : x mL

$$\frac{100x}{100} = \frac{8{,}000}{100}$$

$$x = \frac{8{,}000}{100}$$

x = 80 mL (bolus is 80 mL)

Step 2: Calculate the infusion rate (18 units/kg/hr × kg).

18 units/~~kg~~/hr × 100 ~~kg~~ = 1,800 units/hr

Determine the rate in mL/hr at which to set the infusion device (using the concentration of 100 units per mL).

100 units : 1 mL = 1,800 units : x mL

$$\frac{100x}{100} = \frac{1{,}800}{100}$$

$$x = \frac{1{,}800}{100}$$

$$x = 18 \text{ mL/hr}$$

The client's APTT is reported as being 71 sec. (According to the protocol, decrease the rate by 2 units/kg/hr; there's no rebolus.)

Step 3: Determine the infusion decrease rate (2 units/kg/hr × kg).

2 units/~~kg~~/hr × 100 ~~kg~~ = 200 units/hr. The infusion rate should be decreased by 200 units/hr.

Step 4: Calculate the adjustment in the hourly infusion rate (mL/hr).

100 units : 1 mL = 200 units : x mL

$$\frac{100x}{100} = \frac{200}{100}$$

$$x = \frac{200}{100}$$

$$x = 2 \text{ mL/hr}$$

Decrease rate:

18 mL/hr (current rate)
−2 mL/hr (decrease)
16 mL/hr (new infusion rate)

Decrease the rate on the pump to 16 mL/hr.

Note: This problem could also be done using dimensional analysis or formula method.

44. **Step 1:** Calculate the heparin bolus dosage.

Convert the weight to kg. Equivalent: 2.2 lb = 1 kg

162.8 lb ÷ 2.2 = 74 kg

80 units/kg × 74 kg = 5,920 units

The client should receive 5,920 units IV heparin as a bolus.

Determine the volume (mL) the client would receive.

The concentration is indicated as 100 units per mL.

100 units : 1 mL = 5,920 units : x mL

$$\frac{100x}{100} = \frac{5{,}920}{100}$$

$$x = \frac{5{,}920}{100}$$

$x = 59.2$ mL (bolus is 59.2 mL)

Step 2: Calculate the infusion rate (18 units/kg/hr × kg)

18 units/kg/hr × 74 kg = 1,332 units/hr

Determine the rate in mL/hr at which to set the infusion device (using the concentration of 100 units per mL).

100 units : 1 mL = 1,332 units : x mL

$$\frac{100x}{100} = \frac{1{,}332}{100}$$

$$x = \frac{1{,}332}{100}$$

$x = 13.3$ mL/hr (The pump delivers in tenths of a mL)

The client's APTT is reported as being 38 sec (according to the protocol). Rebolus with 40 units/kg and increase rate by 2 units/kg/hr.

Rebolus: 40 units/kg × 74 kg = 2,960 units

100 units : 1 mL = 2,960 units : x mL

$$\frac{100x}{100} = \frac{2{,}960}{100}$$

$x = 29.6$ mL (bolus)

Step 3: Determine the infusion increase rate.

2 units/kg/hr × kg

2 units/kg/hr × 74 kg = 148 units/hr

Step 4: Calculate the adjustment in the hourly infusion rate (mL/hr)

100 units : 1 mL = 148 units : x mL

$$\frac{100x}{100} = \frac{148}{100}$$

$$x = \frac{148}{100}$$

$x = 1.48 = 1.5$ mL/hr

Increase rate:

13.3 mL/hr (current rate)
+1.5 mL/hr (increase)
14.8 mL/hr (new infusion rate)

Increase the rate on the pump to 14.8 mL/hr.

Note: This problem could also be done using dimensional analysis or formula method.

45. No weight conversion required, the weight is in kg.

a. Calculate the dose in units/hr

20 units/kg/hr × 89 kg = 1,780 units/hr

Answer: 1,780 units/hr

b. Determine the rate in mL/hr to deliver 1,780 units/hr

50 units : 1 mL = 1,780 units : x mL

$$\frac{50x}{50} = \frac{1{,}780}{50}$$

$$x = \frac{1{,}780}{50}$$

$x = 35.6$ mL/hr (pump capable of delivering in tenths)

Answer: 35.6 mL/hr. The pump would be set at 35.6 mL/hr to deliver 1,780 units/hr.

CHAPTER 24
Critical Care Calculations

Objectives

After reviewing this chapter, you should be able to:

1. Calculate dosages in mcg/min, mcg/hr, and mg/min
2. Calculate dosages in mg/kg/hr, mg/kg/min, and mcg/kg/min

The content in this chapter may not be required as part of the nursing curriculum. It is included as a reference for nurses working in specialty areas.

This chapter provides basic information on medicated IV drips and titration. The care of clients receiving medications to control vital functions requires continual nursing intervention. In the critical care setting, clients often receive medications that are potent and require close monitoring. These may include medications to maintain the client's blood pressure within normal range and antiarrhythmic medications to regulate the client's heart rate and/or rhythm. When these medications are administered, the nurse continuously monitors the client's vital signs (BP and pulse) to titrate (adjust) the dosage of medications in response to the client's vital signs.

Because of the potency of the medications and their tendency to induce changes in blood pressure and heart rate, accurate calculation of dosages is essential. These medications may be administered at a constant rate or the rate of the IV may be titrated to the client response.

Medications in the critical care area can be ordered by milliliters per hour (mL/hr), drops per minute (gtt/min) using a microdrop set, micrograms per kilogram per minute (mcg/kg/min), or milligrams per hour (mg/hr). Infusion pumps and volume control devices are usually used to administer these medications. Examples of medicated IV drips that require titration include: dopamine, Isuprel, and epinephrine.

Titrated medications are added to a specific volume of fluid and then adjusted to infuse at the rate at which the desired effect is obtained. **The drugs that are titrated are potent antiarrhythmic, vasopressor, and vasodilator medications; they must be monitored very carefully by the nurse.** IV medications that are titrated usually start at the lowest dosage and are increased and decreased as needed. Medications that are titrated are administered according to protocol. Nurses must know the institution's protocol regarding titration of medications. Because of the potency of medications used, minute changes in the infusion can cause an effect on the client.

Although there have been instances in the past in which critical care medications were administered using volume-control tubing that has a microdrop calibration (60 gtt/mL), they should be used only in dire circumstances when an infusion pump is not available. Critical care medications should be administered by electronic infusion pumps. Despite the use of electronic infusion pumps, calculation errors, infusion pump malfunction, or errors in programming an infusion pump can occur. Nurses should never assume; verify calculations and programming of the pump with a second nurse before administering medications.

Like insulin and heparin, many of the medications administered are high-alert medications. Errors in programming infusion pumps or administration of medications at a faster rate than specified or recommended can result in life-threatening effects.

An example of an order that involves titration of medication is, "Titrate Dopamine to maintain systolic blood pressure greater than 90 mm Hg." The nurse may start, for example, at 3 mcg/kg/min, and gradually increase the rate until the systolic blood pressure is maintained above 90 mm Hg. Each time there is a change in rate, the dosage of medication the client receives is changed; therefore, it is essential that the dosage be recalculated each time the nurse changes the rate. Dosages are adjusted until the desired effect is achieved.

SAFETY ALERT!

Electronic infusion devices are routinely used to administer medications that are potent and require close monitoring. If an electronic infusion device, such as a volumetric pump or syringe pump, is not available, a microdrip set calibrated at 60 gtt/mL can be used.

Calculating Rate in mL/hr

Calculating the rate in mL/hr from a medication dosage ordered for IV administration is one of the most common calculations the nurse encounters. Let's look at some examples illustrating this before getting into other calculations that may be done.

Example 1: A solution of Trandate (labetalol) 100 mg in100 mL D5W is to infuse at a rate of 25 mg/hr. Calculate the rate in mL/hr.

Calculate the rate in mL/hr using the solution strength available.

✓ Solution Using Ratio and Proportion

$$100\text{ mg} : 100\text{ mL} = 25\text{ mg} : x\text{ mL}$$

$$100x = 100 \times 25$$

$$\frac{100x}{100} = \frac{2{,}500}{100}$$

$$x = 25\text{ mL/hr}$$

or

✓ Solution Using the Formula Method

$$\frac{25\text{ mg}}{100\text{ mg}} \times 100\text{ mL} = x\text{ mL/hr}$$

$$x = 25\text{ mL/hr}$$

To infuse 25 mg/hr, set the IV rate at 25 mL/hr.

✓ Solution Using Dimensional Analysis

- As shown in previous chapters involving medications in solution, the dimensional analysis equation is set up by first isolating what is being calculated. In this example, it is mL/hr; therefore, mL/hr is placed to the left of the equation.
- The starting fraction will be the information in the problem containing mL. (mL is placed in the numerator.)
- Set up each fraction after the starting fraction to match the previous denominator.
- Cancel the units, reduce if possible, and perform the mathematical operations.

Equation will be as follows:

$$\frac{x\text{ mL}}{\text{hr}} = \frac{100\text{ mL}}{\underset{4}{\cancel{100}}\ \cancel{\text{mg}}} \times \frac{\overset{1}{\cancel{25}}\ \cancel{\text{mg}}}{1\text{ hr}}$$

$$x = \frac{100}{4}$$

$$x = 25\text{ mL/hr}$$

Example 2: A solution of Isuprel 2 mg in 250 mL D5W is to infuse at a rate of 5 mcg/min.

Step 1: Calculate the dose per hour.

$$60 \text{ min} = 1 \text{ hr}$$
$$5 \text{ mcg}/\cancel{\text{min}} \times 60\ \cancel{\text{min}}/\text{hr} = 300 \text{ mcg/hr}$$

Step 2: Convert 300 mcg to mg to match the available strength.

$$1{,}000 \text{ mcg} = 1 \text{ mg}$$
$$300 \text{ mcg} = 0.3 \text{ mg}$$

Step 3: Calculate the rate in mL/hr.

$$2 \text{ mg} : 250 \text{ mL} = 0.3 \text{ mg} : x \text{ mL}$$
$$2x = 250 \times 0.3$$
$$\frac{2x}{2} = \frac{75}{2} = 37.5 = 38$$
$$x = 38 \text{ mL/hr}$$

To infuse 5 mcg/min, set the IV rate at 38 mL/hr.

✔ Solution Using Dimensional Analysis

Note: In this equation, you will need two additional conversion factors, 60 min = 1 hr and 1,000 mcg = 1 mg.

$$\frac{x \text{ mL}}{\text{hr}} = \frac{\overset{125}{\cancel{250}} \text{ mL}}{\underset{1}{\cancel{2}}\ \cancel{\text{mg}}} \times \frac{1\ \cancel{\text{mg}}}{\underset{200}{\cancel{1{,}000}}\ \cancel{\text{mcg}}} \times \frac{\overset{1}{\cancel{5}}\ \cancel{\text{mcg}}}{1\ \cancel{\text{min}}} \times \frac{60\ \cancel{\text{min}}}{1 \text{ hr}}$$
$$x = \frac{125 \times 60}{200}$$
$$x = \frac{7{,}5\cancel{00}}{2\cancel{00}} = 37.5 = 38$$
$$x = 38 \text{ mL/hr}$$

Now that you have seen examples of calculating the rate in mL/hr, let's look at some other calculations.

Calculating Critical Care Dosages per Hour or per Minute

Example: Infuse dopamine 400 mg in 500 mL D5W at 30 mL/hr. Calculate the dosage in mcg/min and mcg/hr.

✔ Solution Using Ratio and Proportion

Step 1:

$$400 \text{ mg} : 500 \text{ mL} = x \text{ mg} : 30 \text{ mL}$$
$$\text{(known)} \qquad \text{(unknown)}$$
$$500x = 400 \times 30$$
$$500x = 12{,}000$$
$$x = \frac{12{,}000}{500}$$
$$x = 24 \text{ mg/hr}$$

Remember, ratio and proportion can be set up using several formats.

Step 2: The next step is to convert 24 mg to mcg because the question asked for mcg/min and mcg/hr. Change mg to mcg by using the equivalent 1,000 mcg = 1 mg. To change mg to mcg, multiply by 1,000 or move the decimal point three places to the right.

$$24 \text{ mg/hr} = 24{,}000 \text{ mcg/hr}$$

Step 3: Now that you have the mcg/hr, the next step is to change mcg/hr to mcg/min. This is done by dividing the number of mcg/hr by 60 (60 minutes = 1 hour).

$$24{,}000 \text{ mcg}/\cancel{\text{hr}} \div 60 \text{ min}/\cancel{\text{hr}} = 400 \text{ mcg/min}$$

(*Note:* This is in mcg/min; however, these meds are usually delivered in mL/hr by pump and you would need to take calculation further. You will see problems later in this chapter changing mcg/min to mL/hr.)

✓ Solution Using Dimensional Analysis

$$\frac{x \text{ mg}}{\text{hr}} = \frac{\overset{4}{\cancel{400}} \text{ mg}}{\underset{5}{\cancel{500}} \text{ mL}} \times \frac{30 \cancel{\text{mL}}}{1 \text{ hr}}$$

$$x = \frac{120}{5}$$

$$x = 24 \text{ mg/hr}$$

To determine mg/min, 24 mg ÷ 60 min/hr = 0.4 mg = 400 mcg/min

SAFETY ALERT!

Accurate math is essential because these medications are extremely potent.

Medications Ordered in Milligrams per Minute

Medications such as lidocaine and Pronestyl are ordered in mg/min.

Example: A client is receiving Pronestyl 60 mL/hr. The solution available is Pronestyl 2 g in 500 mL D5W. Calculate the mg/hr and the mg/min the client will receive.

Step 1: A conversion is necessary; g must be converted to mg. This is what you are being asked for (mg/min, mg/hr).

$$\text{Equivalent: } 1 \text{ g} = 1{,}000 \text{ mg}$$

Therefore, 2 g = 2,000 mg (1,000 × 2), or move decimal three places to right.

Step 2: Now determine the mg/hr by setting up a proportion.

$$2{,}000 \text{ mg} : 500 \text{ mL} = x \text{ mg} : 60 \text{ mL}$$

$$500x = 2{,}000 \times 60$$

$$\frac{500x}{500} = \frac{120{,}000}{500}$$

$$x = 240 \text{ mg/hr}$$

Step 3: Convert mg/hr to mg/min.

$$240 \text{ mg}/\cancel{\text{hr}} \div 60 \text{ min}/\cancel{\text{hr}} = 4 \text{ mg/min}$$

✓ Solution Using Dimensional Analysis

(*Note:* The starting factor here is the conversion factor to match the desired numerator, and mg/min is desired; the solution strength is in grams.)

$$\frac{x \text{ mg}}{\text{hr}} = \frac{\overset{2}{\cancel{1{,}000}} \text{ mg}}{1 \cancel{\text{g}}} \times \frac{2 \cancel{\text{g}}}{\underset{1}{\cancel{500}} \cancel{\text{mL}}} \times \frac{60 \cancel{\text{mL}}}{1 \text{ hr}}$$

$$x = \frac{240}{1}$$

$$x = 240 \text{ mg/hr}$$

To determine mg/min, 240 mg/$\cancel{\text{hr}}$ ÷ 60 min/$\cancel{\text{hr}}$ = 4 mg/min.

Calculating Dosages Based on mcg/kg/min

Medications are also ordered for clients based on dosage per kilogram per minute. These medications include Nipride, dopamine, and dobutamine. In these problems, the weight will be rounded to the nearest tenth for calculation.

Example: Order: Dopamine 2 mcg/kg/min. The solution available is 400 mg in 250 mL D5W. The client weighs 150 lb.

Step 1: Convert the client's weight in pounds to kilograms.

$$2.2 \text{ lb} = 1 \text{ kg}$$

To convert the client's weight, divide 150 lb by 2.2.

$$150 \text{ lb} \div 2.2 = 68.18 \text{ kg} = 68.2 \text{ kg}$$

Note that the conversion could also be done using ratio and proportion or dimensional analysis.

Step 2: Now that you have the client's weight in kilograms, determine the dosage per minute.

$$68.2 \cancel{\text{kg}} \times 2 \text{ mcg}/\cancel{\text{kg}}/\text{min} = 136.4 \text{ mcg/min}$$

Converting mcg/min to mL/hr then would be easy using this example (conversion factor 1,000 mcg = 1 mg).

1. Convert mcg/min to mcg/hr.

$$136.4 \text{ mcg}/\cancel{\text{min}} \times 60 \cancel{\text{min}}/\text{hr} = 8{,}184 \text{ mcg/hr}$$

2. Convert mcg/hr to mg/hr.

$$8{,}184 \div 1{,}000 = 8.18 = 8.2 \text{ mg/hr}$$

3. Determine IV flow rate.

✓ Solution Using Ratio and Proportion

$$400 \text{ mg} : 250 \text{ mL} = 8.2 \text{ mg} : x \text{ mL}$$

$$400x = 250 \times 8.2$$

$$\frac{400x}{400} = \frac{2{,}050}{400} = 5.1$$

$$x = 5 \text{ mL/hr}$$

✓ Solution Using Dimensional Analysis

$$\frac{x \text{ mL}}{\text{hr}} = \frac{\overset{5}{\cancel{250}} \text{ mL}}{\underset{8}{\cancel{400}} \cancel{\text{mg}}} \times \frac{1 \cancel{\text{mg}}}{1{,}000 \cancel{\text{mcg}}} \times \frac{136.4 \cancel{\text{mcg}}}{1 \cancel{\text{min}}} \times \frac{60 \cancel{\text{min}}}{1 \text{ hr}}$$

$$x = \frac{40{,}92\cancel{0}}{8{,}00\cancel{0}} = 5.1$$

$$x = 5 \text{ mL/hr}$$

IV Flow Rates for Titrated Medications

As already mentioned, critical care medications are ordered within parameters to obtain a desirable response in a client. When a solution is titrated, the **lowest dose of the medication is set first and increased or decreased as necessary. The higher dosage should not be exceeded without an order.**

Dosage errors with titrated medications can result in dire consequences. Therefore, the nurse should have knowledge regarding the medication, the proper dosage adjustment, and the frequency of adjustments based on client assessment and the prescribed parameters. Electronic infusion devices (pumps) are used with critical medications that are titrated. As discussed in Chapter 22, knowing how to calculate mL/hr is required for electronic infusion devices such as the pump. It is important to remember that there are pumps used in the critical care area that can accept one decimal place. Always check the equipment you are using before deciding to round flow rates to whole milliliters per hour (mL/hr). There are also IV pumps available in the critical care setting, referred to as *smart pumps.* Smart pumps are computerized infusion pumps that are equipped with medication error prevention software that sets off an alarm when infusion settings exceed best practice guidelines. These pumps also allow health care facilities to create a library of medications, along with medication dosing guidelines. The medication library in the smart pump can be tailored to the specific needs of the organization.

There are some smart pumps that have incorporated calculating IV rates for specific medications. The nurse is able to select the medication from the IV pump "library," enter the desired dose, the concentration of the medication, and the client's weight in kilograms. After the data are entered, the pump displays the IV rate in mL/hr. The increase in technology with pumps, however, does not relieve the nurse from his or her responsibility to think critically. Library features in pumps that have the ability to perform the needed calculations should be used to check calculations and not as a tool for dosage calculation. Smart pumps should be used as a drive to safe practice and used properly to ensure client safety.

Because of the consequences associated with titrated medications, it is a common practice at many institutions to have double or triple checking of medication dosages and the mathematical computations associated with them even in instances where calculators may be used.

SAFETY ALERT!

Know the institution's policy regarding the administration of titrated medications. **Never exceed** the prescribed upper dose limit. Notify the prescriber when the maximum limit is reached for a new order.

Example 1: Nipride has been ordered to titrate at 3 to 6 mcg/kg/min to maintain a client's systolic blood pressure below 140 mm Hg. The solution contains 50 mg Nipride in 250 mL D5W. The client weighs 56 kg. Determine the flow rate setting for a volumetric pump.

1. Convert to **like units.**
   Equivalent: 1,000 mcg = 1 mg
   Therefore 50 mg = 50,000 mcg

2. Calculate the concentration of solution in mcg/mL.

$$50{,}000 \text{ mcg} : 250 \text{ mL} = x \text{ mcg} : 1 \text{ mL}$$
$$\frac{250x}{250} = \frac{50{,}000}{250}$$
$$x = 200 \text{ mcg/mL}$$

The concentration of solution is 200 mcg/mL.

3. Calculate the dosage range using the upper and lower dosages.

$$\text{(Lower dosage) } 3 \text{ mcg/}\cancel{\text{kg}}\text{/min} \times 56\ \cancel{\text{kg}} = 168 \text{ mcg/min}$$
$$\text{(Upper dosage) } 6 \text{ mcg/}\cancel{\text{kg}}\text{/min} \times 56\ \cancel{\text{kg}} = 336 \text{ mcg/min}$$

4. Convert dosage range to mL/min.

$$\text{(Lower dosage) } 200 \text{ mcg} : 1 \text{ mL} - 168 \text{ mcg} : x \text{ mL}$$
$$\frac{200x}{200} = \frac{168}{200}$$
$$x = 0.84 \text{ mL/min}$$
$$\text{(Upper dosage) } 200 \text{ mcg} : 1 \text{ mL} = 336 \text{ mcg} : x \text{ mL}$$
$$\frac{200x}{200} = \frac{336}{200}$$
$$x = 1.68 \text{ mL/min}$$

5. Convert mL/min to mL/hr.

$$\text{(Lower dosage) } 0.84 \text{ mL/}\cancel{\text{min}} \times 60\ \cancel{\text{min}}\text{/hr} = 50.4 = 50 \text{ mL/hr (gtt/min)}$$
$$\text{(Upper dosage) } 1.68 \text{ mL/}\cancel{\text{min}} \times 60\ \cancel{\text{min}}\text{/hr} = 100.8 = 101 \text{ mL/hr (gtt/min)}$$

A dosage range of 3 to 6 mcg/kg/min is equal to a flow rate of 50 to 101 mL/hr (gtt/min).

The client's condition has stabilized, and the flow rate is now maintained at 60 mL/hr. What dosage will be infusing per minute?

$$200 \text{ mcg} : 1 \text{ mL} = x \text{ mcg} : 60 \text{ mL}$$
$$x = 12{,}000 \text{ mcg/hr}$$
$$12{,}000 \text{ mcg/}\cancel{\text{hr}} \div 60 \text{ min/}\cancel{\text{hr}} = 200 \text{ mcg/min}$$

✓ Solution Using Dimensional Analysis

1. Calculate the dosage range first.

$$\text{(Lower dosage) } 3 \text{ mcg/}\cancel{\text{kg}}\text{/min} \times 56\ \cancel{\text{kg}} = 168 \text{ mcg/min}$$
$$\text{(Upper dosage) } 6 \text{ mcg/}\cancel{\text{kg}}\text{/min} \times 56\ \cancel{\text{kg}} = 336 \text{ mcg/min}$$

2. Calculate the IV rate in mL/hr for the lower dosage.

$$\frac{x \text{ mL}}{\text{hr}} = \frac{\overset{5}{\cancel{250}} \text{ mL}}{\underset{1}{\cancel{50}}\ \cancel{\text{mg}}} \times \frac{1\ \cancel{\text{mg}}}{1{,}000\ \cancel{\text{mcg}}} \times \frac{168\ \cancel{\text{mcg}}}{1\ \cancel{\text{min}}} \times \frac{60\ \cancel{\text{min}}}{1 \text{ hr}}$$
$$x = 50.4 = 50 \text{ mL/hr (gtt/min)}$$

3. Calculate the IV rate in mL/hr for the upper dosage.

$$\frac{x \text{ mL}}{\text{hr}} = \frac{\overset{5}{\cancel{250}} \text{ mL}}{\underset{1}{\cancel{50}}\ \cancel{\text{mg}}} \times \frac{1\ \cancel{\text{mg}}}{1{,}000\ \cancel{\text{mcg}}} \times \frac{336\ \cancel{\text{mcg}}}{1\ \cancel{\text{min}}} \times \frac{60\ \cancel{\text{min}}}{1 \text{ hr}}$$
$$x = 100.8 = 101 \text{ mL/hr (gtt/min)}$$

A dosage range of 3 to 6 mcg/kg/min is equal to a flow rate of 50 to 101 mL/hr (gtt/min).

The client's condition has stabilized, and the IV flow rate is now maintained at 60 mL/hr. What dosage will be infusing per minute?

$$\frac{x \text{ mcg}}{\text{min}} = \frac{\overset{4}{\cancel{1{,}000}} \text{ mcg}}{1 \cancel{\text{mg}}} \times \frac{50 \cancel{\text{mg}}}{\underset{1}{\cancel{250}} \cancel{\text{mL}}} \times \frac{60 \cancel{\text{mL}}}{1 \cancel{\text{hr}}} \times \frac{1 \cancel{\text{hr}}}{60 \text{ min}}$$

$$x = 200 \text{ mcg/min}$$

Developing a Titration Table

After calculating an initial IV rate for a medication being titrated, the client is monitored. If the desired response is not achieved, the dosage may have to be increased. This will require the nurse to find the corresponding IV rate in mL/hr for the new dosage. Any time the dosage is changed, recalculation of the corresponding IV rate is required. Rather than performing calculations each time a dosage is modified, the nurse can develop a titration table to provide the IV rate for any possible change in the medication dosage.

Let's look at the previous example (Example 1) and develop a titration table to increase the dosage by 1 mcg/min up to 6 mcg/min. Set up a ratio proportion to develop the titration table; use the minimum rate required to deliver 3 mcg/min to find the incremental flow rate that provides a dosage rate change of 1mcg/min.

The proportion is:

$$\frac{3 \text{ mcg/min}}{50 \text{ mL/hr}} = \frac{1 \text{ mcg/min}}{x \text{ mL/hr}}$$

$$\frac{3x}{3} = \frac{50}{3} = 16.6$$

$$x = 17 \text{ mL/hr}$$

So, for each change of 1 mcg/min, the incremental IV flow rate is 17 mL/hr.

Titration Table

Dosage Rate (mcg/min)	Flow Rate (mL/hr)
3 mcg/min **(minimum)**	50 mL/hr
4 mcg/min	67 mL/hr
5 mcg/min	84 mL/hr
6 mcg/min **(maximum)**	101 mL/hr

Notice in this problem mL/hr was rounded to the nearest whole number. Remember, there are pumps capable of accepting one decimal place.

Example 2: Nitroglycerin has been ordered to titrate at 10 mcg/min to 60 mcg/min, and the rate should be increased by 10 mcg/min every 3-5 minutes for chest pain. The solution contains 50 mg nitroglycerin in 250 mL D5W.

Step 1: Calculate the dose per hour using the upper and lower dosages.

$$10 \text{ mcg}/\cancel{\text{min}} \times 60 \cancel{\text{min}}/\text{hr} = 600 \text{ mcg/hr}$$

$$60 \text{ mcg}/\cancel{\text{min}} \times 60 \cancel{\text{min}}/\text{hr} = 3{,}600 \text{ mcg/hr}$$

Step 2: Convert mcg to mg to match the available strength.

$$1{,}000 \text{ mcg} = 1 \text{ mg}$$

$$600 \text{ mcg} = 0.6 \text{ mg}$$

$$3{,}600 \text{ mcg} = 3.6 \text{ mg}$$

Step 3: Calculate the rate in mL/hr.

$$50 \text{ mg} : 250 \text{ mL} = 0.6 \text{ mg} : x \text{ mL}$$
$$50x = 250 \times 0.6$$
$$\frac{50x}{50} = \frac{150}{50}$$
$$x = 3 \text{ mL/hr}$$

To infuse 10 mcg/min, set the IV rate at 3 mL/hr (minimum).

$$50 \text{ mg} : 250 \text{ mL} = 3.6 \text{ mg} : x \text{ mL}$$
$$50x = 250 \times 3.6$$
$$\frac{50x}{50} = \frac{900}{50}$$
$$x = 18 \text{ mL/hr}$$

To infuse 60 mcg/min, set the IV rate at 18 mL/hr (maximum). A dosage range of 10 to 60 mcg/min is equal to a flow rate of 3 to 18 mL/hr.

Dimensional Analysis Setup

Calculate the lower dosage.

$$\frac{x \text{ mL}}{\text{hr}} = \frac{\overset{5}{\cancel{250}} \text{ mL}}{\underset{1}{\cancel{50}} \cancel{\text{mg}}} \times \frac{1 \cancel{\text{mg}}}{1{,}000 \cancel{\text{mcg}}} \times \frac{10 \cancel{\text{mcg}}}{1 \cancel{\text{min}}} \times \frac{60 \cancel{\text{min}}}{1 \text{ hr}}$$
$$x = 3 \text{ mL/hr}$$

Calculate upper dosage.

$$\frac{x \text{ mL}}{\text{hr}} = \frac{\overset{5}{\cancel{250}} \text{ mL}}{\underset{1}{\cancel{50}} \cancel{\text{mg}}} \times \frac{1 \cancel{\text{mg}}}{1{,}000 \cancel{\text{mcg}}} \times \frac{60 \cancel{\text{mcg}}}{1 \cancel{\text{min}}} \times \frac{60 \cancel{\text{min}}}{1 \text{ hr}}$$
$$x = 18 \text{ mL/hr}$$

A dosage range of 10-60 mcg/min is equal to a flow rate of 3-18 mL/hr.

Develop a titration table using 10 mcg increments. Set up the proportion using the minimum to determine the dosage change of 10 mcg/min.

$$\frac{10 \text{ mcg/min}}{3 \text{ mL/hr}} = \frac{10 \text{ mcg/min}}{x \text{ mL/hr}}$$
$$\frac{10x}{10} = \frac{30}{10}$$
$$x = 3 \text{ mL/hr}$$

So, for each change of 10 mcg/min, the incremental IV flow rate is 3 mL/hr.

Titration Table

Dosage Rate (mcg/min)	Flow Rate (mL/hr)
10 mcg/min **(minimum)**	3 mL/hr
20 mcg/min	6 mL/hr
30 mcg/min	9 mL/hr
40 mcg/min	12 mL/hr
50 mcg/min	15 mL/hr
60 mcg/min **(maximum)**	18 mL/hr

Example 3: Levophed (norepinephrine bitartrate) has been ordered to titrate at 3 mcg/min to 10 mcg/min, and the rate should be increased at 1 mcg/min to maintain blood pressure and keep systolic blood pressure greater than 100 mmHg. The solution contains 2 mg Levophed in 250 mL D_5W. Develop a titration table at 1 mcg increments. The pump delivers in tenths.

Step 1: Calculate the dose per hour using the upper and lower dosages.

$$3 \text{ mcg}/\cancel{\text{min}} \times 60 \cancel{\text{min}}/\text{hr} = 180 \text{ mcg/hr}$$
$$10 \text{ mcg}/\cancel{\text{min}} \times 60 \cancel{\text{min}}/\text{hr} = 600 \text{ mcg/hr}$$

Step 2: Convert mcg to mg to match the available strength.

$$1{,}000 \text{ mcg} = 1 \text{ mg}$$
$$180 \text{ mcg} = 0.18 \text{ mg}$$
$$600 \text{ mcg} = 0.6 \text{ mg}$$

Step 3: Calculate the rate in mL/hr

$$2 \text{ mg} : 250 \text{ mL} = 0.18 \text{ mg} : x \text{ mL}$$
$$2x = 250 \times 0.18$$
$$\frac{2x}{2} = \frac{45}{2}$$
$$x = 22.5 \text{ mL/hr}$$

To infuse 3 mcg/min, set the IV rate at 22.5 mL/hr (minimum)

$$2 \text{ mg} : 250 \text{ mL} = 0.6 \text{ mg} : x \text{ mL}$$
$$2x = 250 \times 0.6$$
$$\frac{2x}{2} = \frac{150}{2}$$
$$x = 75 \text{ mL/hr}$$

To infuse 10 mcg/min, set the IV rate at 75 mL/hr. A dosage range of 3-10 mcg/min is equal to a flow rate of 22.5-75 mL/hr.

Dimensional Analysis Setup

Calculate the lower dosage.

$$\frac{x \text{ mL}}{\text{hr}} = \frac{\overset{125}{\cancel{250}} \text{ mL}}{\underset{1}{\cancel{2}} \cancel{\text{mg}}} \times \frac{1 \cancel{\text{mg}}}{1{,}000 \cancel{\text{mcg}}} \times \frac{3 \cancel{\text{mcg}}}{1 \cancel{\text{min}}} \times \frac{60 \cancel{\text{min}}}{1 \text{ hr}}$$
$$x = 22.5 \text{ mL/hr}$$

Calculate the upper dosage.

$$\frac{x \text{ mL}}{\text{hr}} = \frac{\overset{125}{\cancel{250}} \text{ mL}}{\underset{1}{\cancel{2}} \cancel{\text{mg}}} \times \frac{1 \cancel{\text{mg}}}{1{,}000 \cancel{\text{mcg}}} \times \frac{10 \cancel{\text{mcg}}}{1 \cancel{\text{min}}} \times \frac{60 \cancel{\text{min}}}{1 \text{ hr}}$$
$$x = 75 \text{ mL/hr}$$

A dosage range of 3-10 mcg/min is equal to a flow rate of 22.5-75 mL/hr.

Find the incremental flow rate for a dosage rate change of 1 mcg/min by setting up a ratio proportion.

The proportion is:

$$\frac{3 \text{ mcg/min}}{22.5 \text{ mL/hr}} = \frac{1 \text{ mcg/min}}{x \text{ mL/hr}}$$

$$\frac{3x}{3} = \frac{22.5}{3}$$

$$x = 7.5 \text{ mL/hr}$$

So, for each change of 1 mcg/min, the incremental IV flow rate is 7.5 mL/hr.

Titration Table

Dosage Rate (mcg/min)	Flow Rate (mL/hr)
3 mcg/min **(minimum)**	22.5 mL/hr
4 mcg/min	30 mL/hr
5 mcg/min	37.5 mL/hr
6 mcg/min	45 mL/hr
7 mcg/min	52.5 mL/hr
8 mcg/min	60 mL/hr
9 mcg/min	67.5 mL/hr
10 mcg/min **(maximum)**	75 mL/hr

PRACTICE **PROBLEMS**

1. A client weighing 50 kg is to receive a Dobutrex solution of 250 mg in 500 mL D5W ordered to titrate between 2.5 and 5 mcg/kg/min.

   a. Determine the flow rate setting for a volumetric pump. ______________________

   b. If the IV flow rate is being maintained at 25 mL/hr after several titrations, what is the dosage infusing per minute? ______________________

2. Order: Epinephrine at 30 mL/hr. The solution available is 2 mg of epinephrine in 250 mL D5W. Calculate the following:

   a. mg/hr ______________________

   b. mcg/hr ______________________

   c. mcg/min ______________________

3. Aminophylline 0.25 g is added to 500 mL D5W to infuse at 20 mL/hr. Calculate the following:

   mg/hr ______________________

4. Order: Pitocin at 15 microgtt/min. The solution contains 10 units of Pitocin in 1,000 mL D5W.

   Calculate the number of units per hour the client is receiving. ______________________

5. Order: 3 mcg/kg/min of Nipride.

   Available: 50 mg of Nipride in 250 mL D5W. Client's weight is 60 kg.

   Calculate the flow rate in mL/hr that will deliver this dosage. ______________________

6. A nitroglycerin drip is infusing at 3 mL/hr. The solution available is 50 mg of nitroglycerin in 250 mL D5W. Calculate the following:

   a. mcg/hr ______________________

   b. mcg/min ______________________

7. Order: Procainamide to titrate at 2 mg/min to the maximum of 6 mg/min. The available solution is procainamide 2 g in 250 mL D5W. Develop a titration table in 2 mg/min increments up to the maximum dose.

Answers on pp. 648-649

POINTS TO REMEMBER

- The safest way to administer potent medications that require frequent monitoring is by an electronic infusion device.
- When calculating dosages to be administered without any type of electronic infusion pump, always use microdrop tubing (60 gtt = 1 mL). This is preferred because the drops are smaller, so more accurate titration is possible.
- Calculate dosages accurately. Double-checking math calculations helps ensure a proper dosage.
- Obtain an accurate weight of your client.
- Use a calculator whenever possible.
- Use an infusion pump for titration of IV medications in mL/hr.
- Know the institution's policy relating to titration.
- Do not exceed the upper dose limit.

CLINICAL **REASONING**

Scenario: Isuprel is ordered for a client at the rate of 3 mcg/min with a solution containing Isuprel 1 mg in 250 mL D5W. The nurse performed the following calculation to determine the rate by pump in mL/hr.

- Calculated the dosage per hour:

$$3 \text{ mcg}/\cancel{\text{min}} \times 60 \ \cancel{\text{min}}/\text{hr} = 180 \text{ mcg/hr}$$

- Converted 180 mcg to milligrams to match the units in the solution strength:

$$180 \text{ mcg} = 0.018 \text{ mg}$$

- Calculated the rate in mL/hr:

$$1 \text{ mg} : 250 \text{ mL} = 0.018 \text{ mg} : x \text{ mL}$$
$$x = 250 \times 0.018$$
$$x = 4.5 = 5 \text{ mL/hr}$$

a. What error did the nurse make in her calculation to determine the rate in mL/hr?

____

b. What could be the potential outcome of the error? ______________

c. What should the rate be in mL/hr? ______________

d. What preventive measures could have been taken by the nurse? ______________

Answer on p. 649

CHAPTER **REVIEW**

Calculate the dosages as indicated. Use the labels where provided.

1. Client is receiving Isuprel at 30 mL/hr. The solution available is 2 mg of Isuprel in 250 mL D5W. Calculate the following:

   a. mg/hr ______________

   b. mcg/hr ______________

   c. mcg/min ______________

2. Infuse dopamine 800 mg in 500 mL D5W at 30 mL/hr. Calculate the dosage in mcg/hr and mcg/min.

   a. mcg/hr ______________

   b. mcg/min ______________

   c. Calculate the number of milliliters you will add to the IV for this dosage. ______________

   Available:

EXP. LOT
NDC 0641-**0112-25**
25 x 5 mL *Single Use* Vials
DOPAMINE
HCl INJECTION, USP
200 mg/5 mL
(40 mg/mL)
FOR IV INFUSION ONLY

POTENT DRUG: MUST DILUTE BEFORE USING
Each mL contains dopamine hydrochloride 40 mg (equivalent to 32.3 mg dopamine base) and sodium bisulfite 10 mg in Water for Injection. pH 2.5-5.0. Sealed under nitrogen.
USUAL DOSE: See package insert.
Do not use if solution is discolored.
Store at 15° - 30° C (59° - 86° F).
Caution: Federal law prohibits dispensing without prescription.
B-50112c

esi ELKINS-SINN, INC. Cherry Hill, NJ 08003-4099
A subsidiary of A. H. Robins Company

3. Infuse Nipride at 30 mL/hr. The solution available is 50 mg sodium nitroprusside in D5W 250 mL.

   Available:

   Protect from light.
   Exp.
   Lot
   2 mL Single-dose Fliptop Vial NDC 0074-3024-01
   NITROPRESS®
   Sodium Nitroprusside Injection
   50 mg / 2 mL Vial (25 mg/mL)
   FOR I.V. INFUSION ONLY.
   Monitor blood pressure before and during administration. 06-7378-2/R2-12/93
   ABBOTT LABS, NORTH CHICAGO, IL 60064, USA

   Calculate the following:

   a. mcg/hr ______________________

   b. mcg/min ______________________

   c. Number of milliliters you will add to the IV for this dosage ______________________

4. Order: Lidocaine 2 g in 250 mL D5W to infuse at 60 mL/hr. Calculate the following:

   a. mg/hr ______________________

   b. mg/min ______________________

5. Order: Aminophylline 0.25 g to be added to 250 mL of D5W. The order is to infuse over 6 hr.

   Available:

   20 mL Single-dose Ampul NDC 0074-7386-01
   AMINOPHYLLINE Inj., USP ℞ only
   500 mg (25 mg/mL)
   Protect from light.
   DO NOT USE IF CRYSTALS HAVE SEPARATED FROM SOLUTION.
   Each mL contains aminophylline (calculated as the dihydrate) 25 mg (equivalent to 19.7 mg/mL of anhydrous theophylline). May contain an excess of ethylenediamine for pH adjustment. pH 8.8 (8.6 to 9.0). Discard unused portion. Sterile, nonpyrogenic. For I.V. use. Usual dose: See insert.
   58-3947-2/R12-12/02
   ABBOTT LABORATORIES, NORTH CHICAGO, IL 60064 USA

   a. Calculate the dosage in mg/hr the client will receive. ______________________

   b. Calculate the number of milliliters you will add to the IV for this dosage. ______________________

6. A client is receiving Pronestyl at 30 mL/hr. The solution available is 2 g Pronestyl in 250 mL D5W. Calculate the following:

   a. mg/hr ______________________

   b. mg/min ______________________

7. Order: Pitocin (oxytocin) drip at 45 microgtt/min. The solution available is 20 units of Pitocin in 1,000 mL of D5W. Calculate the following:

   a. units/min ______________________

   b. units/hr ______________________

8. Order: 30 units Pitocin (oxytocin) in 1,000 mL D5W at 40 mL/hr.

   How many units of Pitocin is the client receiving per hour? ______________________ units/hr

9. A client is receiving bretylium at 45 microgtt/min. The solution available is 2 g bretylium in 500 mL D5W. Calculate the following:

   a. mg/hr ______________________

   b. mg/min ______________________

10. A client is receiving nitroglycerin 50 mg in 250 mL D5W. The order is to infuse 500 mcg/min.

    What flow rate in mL/hr would be needed to deliver this amount? ______________________

11. Dopamine has been ordered to maintain a client's blood pressure; 400 mg dopamine has been placed in 500 mL D5W to infuse at 35 mL/hr.

    How many milligrams are being administered per hour? ______________________

12. A client is receiving Isuprel 2 mg in 250 mL D5W. The order is to infuse at 20 mL/hr. Calculate the following:

    a. mg/hr ______________________

    b. mcg/hr ______________________

    c. mcg/min ______________________

13. Order: 1 g of aminophylline in 1,000 mL D5W to infuse over 10 hr.

    Calculate the dosage in mg/hr the client will receive. ______________

14. A client is receiving lidocaine 2 g in 250 mL D5W. The solution is infusing at 22 mL/hr. Calculate the following:

    a. mg/hr ______________

    b. mg/min ______________

15. Order: Esmolol 2.5 g in 250 mL 0.9% NS at 30 mL/hr. Calculate the following:

    a. mg/hr ______________

    b. mg/min ______________

16. Order: Dobutamine 500 mg in 500 mL D5W to infuse at 30 mL/hr.

    Calculate the following:

    a. mcg/hr ______________

    b. mcg/min ______________

17. Order: Dopamine 400 mg in 500 mL 0.9% NS to infuse at 200 mcg/min. A volumetric pump is being used.

    Calculate the rate in mL/hr. ______________

18. Order: Magnesium sulfate 3 g/hr.

    Available: 25 g of 50% magnesium sulfate in 300 mL D5W.

    What rate in mL/hr would be needed to administer the required dose? ______________

19. Order: Nipride 50 mg in 250 mL D5W to infuse at 2 mcg/kg/min. Client's weight is 120 lb.

    Calculate the dosage per minute. ______________________

20. Order: Dobutrex 250 mg in 500 mL of D5W at 3 mcg/kg/min. The client weighs 80 kg.

    What dosage in mcg/min should the client receive? ______________________

21. Order: Infuse 1 g of aminophylline in 1,000 mL of D5W at 0.7 mg/kg/hr. The client weighs 110 lb.

    a. Calculate the dosage in mg/hr. ______________________

    b. Calculate the dosage in mg/min. ______________________

    c. Reference states no more than 20 mg/min. Is the order safe? ______________________

22. Norepinephrine (Levophed) 2 to 6 mcg/min has been ordered to maintain a client's systolic blood pressure at 100 mm Hg. The solution concentration is 2 mg in 500 mL D5W.

    Determine the flow rate setting for a volumetric pump. ______________________

23. Esmolol is to titrate between 50 to 75 mcg/kg/min. The client weighs 60 kg. The solution strength is 5,000 mg of esmolol in 500 mL D5W.

    a. Determine the flow rate for a volumetric pump. ______________________

    b. The titration rate is at 24 mL/hr. What is the dosage infusing per minute? ______________________

24. Order: Dobutamine 500 mg in 250 mL D5W to infuse at 10 mcg/kg/min. The client weighs 65 kg.

    Calculate the flow rate in mL/hr (gtt/min). ______________________

25. Aminophylline 0.25 g is added to 250 mL D5W. The order is to infuse over 6 hr.

    Calculate the dosage in mg/hr the client will receive. ______________________

26. A client is receiving lidocaine 1 g in 500 mL D5W at a rate of 20 mL/hr. Calculate the following:

    a. mg/hr ______________________

    b. mg/min ______________________

27. A client is receiving Septra 300 mg in 500 mL D5W (based on trimethoprim) at a rate of 15 gtt/min (15 microgtt/min). The tubing is microdrop (60 gtt/mL). Calculate the following:

 a. mg/min ________________

 b. mg/hr ________________

28. Esmolol 1.5 g in 250 mL D5W has been ordered at a rate of 100 mcg/kg/min for a client weighing 102.4 kg. Determine the following:

 a. dosage in mcg/min ________________

 b. rate in mL/hr ________________

29. Order: Dopamine 400 mg in 500 mL D5W to infuse at 20 mL/hr. Determine the following:

 a. mg/min ________________

 b. mcg/min ________________

30. A client has an order for inamrinone (previously called amrinone) 250 mg in 250 mL 0.9% NS at 3 mcg/kg/min. Client's weight is 59.1 kg. Determine the flow rate in mL/hr.

____

31. Inocor 250 mg in 250 mL of 0.9% NS to infuse at a rate of 5 mcg/kg/min is ordered for a client weighing 165 lb. Calculate the following:

 a. mcg/min ________________

 b. mcg/hr ________________

 c. mL/hr ________________

32. Order: Cardizem 125 mg in 100 mL D5W to infuse at 20 mg/hr.

Available:

NDC 0088-1790-32
CARDIZEM® Injectable
(diltiazem HCl Injection)
25 mg (5 mg/mL)
FOR DIRECT INTRAVENOUS BOLUS INJECTION AND CONTINUOUS INTRAVENOUS INFUSION
Sterile 5-mL Vial
SINGLE-USE CONTAINER. DISCARD UNUSED PORTION.
Date Removed From Refrigeration______
Date To Be Discarded______
Mfd. for Hoechst Marion Roussel, Inc. Kansas City, MO 64137 USA
50007742 C6

Determine the following:

 a. How many milliliters will you add to the IV? ________________

 b. Determine the rate in mL/hr. (Consider the medication in the volume.) ________________

33. Order: 2 g Pronestyl in 500 mL D5W to infuse at 2 mg/min.

    Determine the rate in mL/hr. ____________________

34. Dopamine is ordered at a rate of 3 mcg/kg/min for a client weighing 95.9 kg. The solution strength is 400 mg dopamine in 250 mL D_5W. Determine the flow rate for an IV pump. The pump is capable of delivering in tenths of a mL. ____________

35. Infuse Dobutamine 250 mg in 500 mL D_5W at 5 mcg/kg/min. The client weighs 143 lb. Concentration of solution is 500 mcg per mL. How many mcg of dobutamine will be infused per minute? ________ per hour? ________

36. A medication has been ordered at 2 to 4 mcg/min to maintain a client's systolic BP greater than 100 mm Hg. The medication being titrated has 8 mg of medication in 250 mL D_5W. Determine the IV rate for 2 to 4 mcg range. Then assume that after several changes in mL/hr have been made, the BP has stabilized at a rate of 5 mL/hr. How many mcg/min is the client receiving at this rate? Determine the flow rate for an IV pump capable of delivering in tenths of a mL.

    ____________________ Flow rate for 2-4 mcg range

    ____________________ mcg per/min at 5 mL /hr

37. Order: Nitroglycerin to titrate at 40 mcg/min for chest pain to a maximum of 100 mcg/min. The solution contains 40 mg of nitroglycerin in 250 mL D5W. Develop a titration table from minimum to maximum dose in 20 mcg/min increments. Assume the pump can deliver in tenths.

38. Order: Levophed 4 mcg/min to maintain BP systolic greater than 100 mm Hg to a maximum of 12 mcg/min. Available solution: Levophed 4 mg in 500 mL D5W. Develop a titration table in 2 mcg/min increments.

Answers on pp. 649-656

evolve

For additional practice problems, refer to the Advanced Calculations section of the Critical Care Dosages section of the Elsevier's Interactive Drug Calculation Application, Version 1 on Evolve.

ANSWERS

Chapter 24

Answers to Practice Problems

1. a. Step 1: Conversion: Equivalent: 1,000 mcg = 1 mg. Therefore 250 mg = 250,000 mcg.

   Step 2: 250,000 mcg : 500 mL = x mcg : 1 mL

   $$\frac{500x}{500} = \frac{250{,}000}{500};\ x = 500 \text{ mcg/mL}$$

   Concentration of solution is 500 mcg/mL.

   Step 3: Calculate dosage range.

   Lower dosage:

   2.5 mcg/$\cancel{\text{kg}}$/min × 50 $\cancel{\text{kg}}$ = 125 mcg/min

   Upper dosage:

   5 mcg/$\cancel{\text{kg}}$/min × 50 $\cancel{\text{kg}}$ = 250 mcg/min

   Step 4: Convert dosage range to mL/min.

   Lower dosage:

   500 mcg : 1 mL = 125 mcg : x mL

   $$\frac{500x}{500} = \frac{125}{500}$$

   $$x = 0.25 \text{ mL/min}$$

   Upper dosage:

   500 mcg : 1 mL = 250 mcg : x mL

   $$\frac{500x}{500} = \frac{250}{500}$$

   $$x = 0.5 \text{ mL/min}$$

   Step 5: Convert mL/min to mL/hr.

   Lower dosage: 0.25 mL/$\cancel{\text{min}}$ × 60 $\cancel{\text{min}}$/hr = 15 mL/hr (gtt/min)

   Upper dosage: 0.5 mL/$\cancel{\text{min}}$ × 60 $\cancel{\text{min}}$/hr = 30 mL/hr (gtt/min)

   A dosage range of 2.5-5 mcg/kg/min is equal to a flow rate of 15-30 mL/hr (gtt/min).

   b. Determine dosage infusing per minute at 25 mL/hr:

   500 mcg : 1 mL = x mcg : 25 mL

   $$x = 12{,}500 \text{ mcg/hr}$$

   12,500 mcg ÷ 60 min = 208.3 mcg/min

2. a. 2 mg : 250 mL = x mg : 30 mL

   $$\frac{250x}{250} = \frac{60}{250}$$

   $$x = 0.24 \text{ mg/hr}$$

   b. Convert milligrams to micrograms (1,000 mcg = 1 mg).

   0.24 mg = 240 mcg/hr

   c. Convert mcg/hr to mcg/min.

   240 mcg/$\cancel{\text{hr}}$ ÷ 60 min/$\cancel{\text{hr}}$ = 4 mcg/min

3. a. Change grams to milligrams. (Note that you were asked to calculate mg/hr.)

   0.25 g = 250 mg (1 g = 1,000 mg)

   b. Calculate mg/hr.

   250 mg : 500 mL = x mg : 20 mL

   $$\frac{500x}{500} = \frac{5{,}000}{500}$$

   $$x = 10 \text{ mg/hr}$$

4. *Note:* Calculate units per hour only.

   Step 1: 60 gtt : 1 mL = 15 gtt : x mL

   $$\frac{60x}{60} = \frac{15}{60}$$

   $$x = 0.25 \text{ mL/min}$$

   Step 2: 0.25 mL/$\cancel{\text{min}}$ × 60 $\cancel{\text{min}}$/hr = 15 mL/hr

   Step 3: 10 units : 1,000 mL = x units : 15 mL

   $$\frac{1{,}000x}{1{,}000} = \frac{150}{1{,}000};\ x = 0.15 \text{ units/hr}$$

5. Step 1: Determine the dosage per minute.

   60 $\cancel{\text{kg}}$ × 3 mcg/$\cancel{\text{kg}}$/min = 180 mcg/min

   Step 2: Convert to dosage per hour.

   180 mcg/$\cancel{\text{min}}$ × 60 $\cancel{\text{min}}$/hr = 10,800 mcg/hr

   Step 3: Convert to like units (1,000 mcg = 1 mg).

   10,800 mcg = 10.8 mg

   Calculate flow rate (mL/hr).

   50 mg : 250 mL = 10.8 mg : x mL

   $$50x = 250 \times 10.8$$

   $$\frac{50x}{50} = \frac{2{,}700}{50}$$

   $$x = 54 \text{ mL/hr}$$

6. a. 50 mg : 250 mL = x mg : 3 mL

   $$\frac{250x}{250} = \frac{150}{250}$$

   $$x = 0.6 \text{ mg/hr}$$

   Convert to micrograms (1,000 mcg = 1 mg).

   0.6 mg/hr = 600 mcg/hr

   b. Convert mcg/hr to mcg/min.

   600 mcg/$\cancel{\text{hr}}$ ÷ 60 min/$\cancel{\text{hr}}$ = 10 mcg/min

7. Step 1: Calculate the dose per hour using the lower and upper dosages.

$2 \text{ mg}/\cancel{\text{min}} \times 60 \cancel{\text{min}}/\text{hr} = 120 \text{ mg/hr}$

$6 \text{ mg}/\cancel{\text{min}} \times 60 \cancel{\text{min}}/\text{hr} = 360 \text{ mg/hr}$

Step 2: Convert mg to g to match the available strength.

1,000 mg = 1 g

120 mg = 0.12 g

360 mg = 0.36 g

Step 3: Calculate the rate in mL/hr

$2 \text{ g} : 250 \text{ mL} = 0.12 \text{ g} : x \text{ mL}$

$2x = 250 \times 0.12$

$$\frac{2x}{2} = \frac{30}{2}$$

$x = 15 \text{ mL/hr}$

To infuse 2 mg/min, set the IV rate at 15 mL/hr (minimum).

$2 \text{ g} : 250 \text{ mL} = 0.36 \text{ g} : x \text{ mL}$

$2x = 250 \times 0.36$

$$\frac{2x}{2} = \frac{90}{2}$$

$x = 45 \text{ mL/hr}$

To infuse 6 mg/min, set the IV rate at 45 mL/hr (maximum).

A dosage range of 2-6 mg/min is equal to a flow rate of 15-45 mL/hr.

Set up proportion to determine the dosage of 2 mg/min.

$$\frac{2 \text{ mg/min}}{15 \text{ mL/hr}} = \frac{2 \text{ mg/min}}{x \text{ mL/hr}}$$

$$\frac{2x}{2} = \frac{30}{2}$$

$x = 15 \text{ mL/hr}$

So for a change of 2 mg/min, the incremental IV flow rate is 15 mL/hr.

Titration Table

Dosage Rate (mcg/min)	Flow Rate (mL/hr)
2 mg/min **(minimum)**	15 mL/hr
4 mg/min	30 mL/hr
6 mg/min **(maximum)**	45 mL/hr

Note: This problem could also be done using dimensional analysis.

Answers to Clinical Reasoning Questions

a. The nurse made the error in the second step (converting 180 mcg to mg to match the units in the solution strength). This led to the error in the mL/hr rate.

$180 \text{ mcg} = 0.18 \text{ mg } (1{,}000 \text{ mcg} = 1 \text{ mg})$

$180 \div 1{,}000 = 0.18 \text{ mg}$

b. The error would result in an incorrect IV rate in mL/hr; the answer obtained is used to determine the rate in mL/hr. Use of 0.018 mg would net an incorrect answer.

$1 \text{ mg} : 250 \text{ mL} = 0.018 \text{ mg} : x \text{ mL}$

$x = 250 \times 0.018$

$x = 4.5 = 5 \text{ mL/hr}$

c. The rate in mL/hr should be 45 mL/hr and not 5 mL/hr.

$1 \text{ mg} : 250 \text{ mL} = 0.18 \text{ mg} : x \text{ mL}$

$x = 250 \times 0.18$

$x = 45 \text{ mL/hr}$

d. The nurse should have double-checked the math at each step. In addition, having another nurse check the calculation may have helped in recognizing the error in calculation.

Answers to Chapter Review

1. a. Calculate the dosage per hr.

$2 \text{ mg} : 250 \text{ mL} = x \text{ mg} : 30 \text{ mL}$

$$\frac{250x}{250} = \frac{60}{250}$$

$$x = \frac{60}{250}$$

$x = 0.24 \text{ mg/hr}$

b. Convert milligrams to micrograms (1,000 mcg = 1 mg).

$1{,}000 \times 0.24 \text{ mg/hr} = 240 \text{ mcg/hr}$

c. Convert mcg/hr to mcg/min.

$240 \text{ mcg/hr} \div 60 \text{ min} = 4 \text{ mcg/min}$

2. Step 1: Determine dosage per hour.

$$800\text{ mg}:500\text{ mL} = x\text{ mg}:30\text{ mL}$$

$$\frac{500x}{500} = \frac{24{,}000}{500}$$

$$x = \frac{24{,}000}{500}$$

$$x = 48\text{ mg/hr}$$

a. Step 2: Convert milligrams to micrograms (1,000 mcg = 1 mg).

$$48\text{ mg/hr} \times 1{,}000 = 48{,}000\text{ mcg/hr}$$

b. Step 3: Convert mcg/hr to mcg/min.

48,000 mcg/~~hr~~ ÷ 60 min/~~hr~~ = 800 mcg/min

c. 200 mg : 5 mL = 800 mg : x mL

or

$$\frac{800\text{ mg}}{200\text{ mg}} \times 5\text{ mL} = x\text{ mL}$$

Answer: 20 mL. The dosage ordered is greater than what is available. Therefore you will need more than 5 mL to administer the dosage.

3. a. Determine dosage per hour.

$$50\text{ mg}:250\text{ mL} = x\text{ mg}:30\text{ mL}$$

$$\frac{250x}{250} = \frac{1{,}500}{250}$$

$$x = \frac{1{,}500}{250}$$

$$x = 6\text{ mg/hr}$$

Convert milligrams to micrograms (1,000 mcg = 1 mg).

$$6\text{ mg/hr} \times 1{,}000 = 6{,}000\text{ mcg/hr}$$

b. Convert mcg/hr to mcg/min.

6,000 mcg/~~hr~~ ÷ 60 min/~~hr~~ = 100 mcg/min

c. 50 mg : 2 mL = 50 mL : x mL

$$\frac{50\text{ mg}}{50\text{ mg}} \times 2\text{ mL} = x\text{ mL}$$

Answer: 2 mL. The dosage ordered is contained in a volume of 2 mL.

Alternate solution: 25 mg : 1 mL = 50 mg : x mL

or

$$\frac{50\text{ mg}}{25\text{ mg}} \times 1\text{ mL} = x\text{ mL}$$

4. a. Convert metric weight to the same as answer requested. Convert grams to milligrams.

1 g = 1,000 mg; therefore 2 g = 2,000 mg

$$2{,}000\text{ mg}:250\text{ mL} = x\text{ mg}:60\text{ mL}$$

$$\frac{250x}{250} = \frac{120{,}000}{250}$$

$$x = \frac{120{,}000}{250}$$

$$x = 480\text{ mg/hr}$$

b. Convert mg/hr to mg/min.

480 mg/~~hr~~ ÷ 60 min/~~hr~~ = 8 mg/min

5. a. Step 1: Convert grams to milligrams (1,000 mg = 1 g).

$$0.25\text{ g} = 250\text{ mg}$$

Step 2: Calculate mg/hr.

$$250\text{ mg}:6\text{ hr} = x\text{ mg}:1\text{ hr}$$

$$\frac{6x}{6} = \frac{250}{6}$$

$$x = \frac{250}{6} = 41.66$$

$$x = 41.7\text{ mg/hr}$$

b. 500 mg : 20 mL = 250 mg : x mL

or

$$\frac{250\text{ mg}}{500\text{ mg}} \times 20\text{ mL} = x\text{ mL}$$

Answer: 10 mL. The dosage ordered is less than the available strength; therefore you will need less than 20 mL to administer the dosage.

Alternate solution: 25 mg : 1 mL = 250 mg : x mL

or

$$\frac{250\text{ mg}}{25\text{ mg}} \times 1\text{ mL} = x\text{ mL}$$

6. a. Convert grams to milligrams (1,000 mg = 1 g).

$$2\text{ g} = 2{,}000\text{ mg}$$

Calculate mg/hr.

$$2{,}000\text{ mg}:250\text{ mL} = x\text{ mg}:30\text{ mL}$$

$$\frac{250x}{250} = \frac{60{,}000}{250}$$

$$x = \frac{60{,}000}{250}$$

$$x = 240\text{ mg/hr}$$

b. Convert mg/hr to mg/min.

240 mg/~~hr~~ ÷ 60 min/~~hr~~ = 4 mg/min

7. a. Step 1: Calculate gtt/min to mL/min.

$60 \text{ gtt} : 1 \text{ mL} = 45 \text{ gtt} : x \text{ mL}$

$$\frac{60x}{60} = \frac{45}{60}$$

$$x = \frac{45}{60}$$

$$x = 0.75 \text{ mL/min}$$

Step 2: Calculate units/min.

$20 \text{ units} : 1{,}000 \text{ mL} = x \text{ units} : 0.75 \text{ mL}$

$$\frac{1{,}000x}{1{,}000} = \frac{15}{1{,}000}$$

$$x = \frac{15}{1{,}000}$$

$$x = 0.015 \text{ units/min}$$

b. Calculate units/hr.

$0.015 \text{ units/}\cancel{\text{min}} \times 60 \text{ }\cancel{\text{min}}\text{/hr} = 0.9 \text{ units/hr}$

8. $30 \text{ units} : 1{,}000 \text{ mL} = x \text{ units} : 40 \text{ mL}$

$$\frac{1{,}000x}{1{,}000} = \frac{1{,}200}{1{,}000}$$

$$x = \frac{1{,}200}{1{,}000}$$

$$x = 1.2 \text{ units/hr}$$

9. a. Change metric measures to same as question.

$2 \text{ g} = 2{,}000 \text{ mg } (1 \text{ g} = 1{,}000 \text{ mg})$

Calculate mg/hr.

$2{,}000 \text{ mg} : 500 \text{ mL} = x \text{ mg} : 45 \text{ mL}$

$$\frac{500x}{500} = \frac{90{,}000}{500}$$

$$x = \frac{90{,}000}{500}$$

$$x = 180 \text{ mg/hr}$$

b. Change mg/hr to mg/min.

$180 \text{ mg/}\cancel{\text{hr}} \div 60 \text{ min/}\cancel{\text{hr}} = 3 \text{ mg/min}$

10. Determine dosage per hour.

$500 \text{ mcg/}\cancel{\text{min}} \times 60 \text{ }\cancel{\text{min}}\text{/hr} = 30{,}000 \text{ mcg/hr}$

Convert micrograms to milligrams to match the available strength.

$1{,}000 \text{ mcg} = 1 \text{ mg}$

$30{,}000 \text{ mcg/hr} = 30 \text{ mg/hr}$

Calculate flow rate in mL/hr.

$50 \text{ mg} : 250 \text{ mL} = 30 \text{ mg} : x \text{ mL}$

$$\frac{50x}{50} = \frac{7{,}500}{50}$$

$$x = 150 \text{ mL/hr}$$

Set at 150 mL/hr to deliver 500 mcg/min.

11. $400 \text{ mg} : 500 \text{ mL} = x \text{ mg} : 35 \text{ mL}$

$$\frac{500x}{500} = \frac{14{,}000}{500}$$

$$x = 28 \text{ mg/hr}$$

12. a. Calculate mg/hr.

$2 \text{ mg} : 250 \text{ mL} = x \text{ mg} : 20 \text{ mL}$

$$\frac{250x}{250} = \frac{40}{250}$$

$$x = \frac{40}{250}$$

$$x = 0.16 \text{ mg/hr}$$

b. Convert milligrams to micrograms (1,000 mcg = 1 mg).

$0.16 \text{ mg} \times 1{,}000 = 160 \text{ mcg/hr}$

c. Convert mcg/hr to mcg/min (60 min = 1 hr).

$160 \text{ mcg/}\cancel{\text{hr}} \div 60 \text{ min/}\cancel{\text{hr}} = 2.66 = 2.7 \text{ mcg/min}$

13. Convert metric weight to same as question.

$1{,}000 \text{ mg} = 1 \text{ g}$

Calculate mg/hr.

$1{,}000 \text{ mg} : 10 \text{ hr} = x \text{ mg} : 1 \text{ hr}$

$$\frac{10x}{10} = \frac{1{,}000}{10}$$

$$x = 100 \text{ mg/hr}$$

14. a. Convert grams to milligrams.

$2 \text{ g} = 2{,}000 \text{ mg } (1{,}000 \text{ mg} = 1 \text{ g})$

$2{,}000 \text{ mg} : 250 \text{ mL} = x \text{ mg} : 22 \text{ mL}$

$$\frac{250x}{250} = \frac{44{,}000}{250}$$

$$x = \frac{44{,}000}{250}$$

$$x = 176 \text{ mg/hr}$$

b. Change mg/hr to mg/min.

$176 \text{ mg/}\cancel{\text{hr}} \div 60 \text{ min/}\cancel{\text{hr}} = 2.93 = 2.9 \text{ mg/min}$

15. Convert g to mg.

$2.5 \text{ g} = 2{,}500 \text{ mg } (1 \text{ g} = 1{,}000 \text{ mg})$

a. $250 \text{ mL} : 2{,}500 \text{ mg} = 30 \text{ mL} : x \text{ mg}$

$$\frac{250x}{250} = \frac{75{,}000}{250}$$

$$x = \frac{75{,}000}{250}$$

$$x = 300 \text{ mg/hr}$$

b. Convert mg/hr to mg/min.

$300 \text{ mg/}\cancel{\text{hr}} \div 60 \text{ min/}\cancel{\text{hr}} = 5 \text{ mg/min}$

16. a. Calculate mg/hr.

$$500 \text{ mg} : 500 \text{ mL} = x \text{ mg} : 30 \text{ mL}$$
$$\frac{500x}{500} = \frac{15{,}000}{500}$$
$$x = \frac{15{,}000}{500}$$
$$x = 30 \text{ mg/hr}$$

Convert milligrams to micrograms (1,000 mcg = 1 mg).

$$30 \text{ mg} = 30{,}000 \text{ mcg/hr}$$

b. Convert mcg/hr to mcg/min.

$$30{,}000 \text{ mcg/}\cancel{\text{hr}} \div 60 \text{ min/}\cancel{\text{hr}} = 500 \text{ mcg/min}$$

17. Determine dosage per hour.

$$200 \text{ mcg/}\cancel{\text{min}} \times 60 \text{ }\cancel{\text{min}}\text{/hr} = 12{,}000 \text{ mcg/hr}$$

Convert micrograms to milligrams (1,000 mcg = 1 mg).

$$12{,}000 \text{ mcg} \div 1{,}000 = 12 \text{ mg/hr}$$

Calculate the mL/hr.

$$400 \text{ mg} : 500 \text{ mL} = 12 \text{ mg} : x \text{ mL}$$
$$\frac{400x}{400} = \frac{6{,}000}{400}$$
$$x = 15 \text{ mL/hr}$$

18. $25 \text{ g} : 300 \text{ mL} = 3 \text{ g} : x \text{ mL}$

$$\frac{25x}{25} = \frac{900}{25}$$
$$x = \frac{900}{25}$$

$x = 36$ mL/hr; would administer 3 g

19. Convert weight in pounds to kilograms (2.2 lb = 1 kg).

$$120 \text{ lb} \div 2.2 = 54.54 = 54.5 \text{ kg}$$

Calculate dosage per minute.

$$54.5 \text{ }\cancel{\text{kg}} \times 2 \text{ mcg/}\cancel{\text{kg}}\text{/min} = 109 \text{ mcg/min}$$

20. No conversion of weight is required.

$$80 \text{ }\cancel{\text{kg}} \times 3 \text{ mcg/}\cancel{\text{kg}}\text{/min} = 240 \text{ mcg/min}$$

21. a. Convert weight in pounds to kilograms (2.2 lb = 1 kg).

$$110 \text{ lb} \div 2.2 = 50 \text{ kg}$$

Calculate the dosage per hour.

$$50 \text{ }\cancel{\text{kg}} \times 0.7 \text{ mg/}\cancel{\text{kg}}\text{/hr} = 35 \text{ mg/hr}$$

b. Calculate the dosage per minute.

$$35 \text{ mg/}\cancel{\text{hr}} \div 60 \text{ min/}\cancel{\text{hr}} = 0.58 \text{ mg/min} = 0.6 \text{ mg/min}$$

c. The dosage is safe; it falls within the safe range.

22. Step 1: Convert to like units.

Equivalent: 1,000 mcg = 1 mg

Therefore 2 mg = 2,000 mcg

Step 2: Calculate the concentration of solution in mcg per mL.

$$2{,}000 \text{ mcg} : 500 \text{ mL} = x \text{ mcg} : 1 \text{ mL}$$
$$\frac{500x}{500} = \frac{2{,}000}{500}$$
$$x = 4 \text{ mcg per mL}$$

Lower dosage: $4 \text{ mcg} : 1 \text{ mL} = 2 \text{ mcg} : x \text{ mL}$

$$\frac{4x}{4} = \frac{2}{4}$$
$$x = 0.5 \text{ mL/min}$$

Upper dosage: $4 \text{ mcg} : 1 \text{ mL} = 6 \text{ mcg} : x \text{ mL}$

$$\frac{4x}{4} = \frac{6}{4}$$
$$x = 1.5 \text{ mL/min}$$

Step 3: Convert mL/min to mL/hr.

Lower dosage: $0.5 \text{ mL/}\cancel{\text{min}} \times 60 \text{ }\cancel{\text{min}}\text{/hr} =$ 30 mL/hr (gtt/min)

Upper dosage: $1.5 \text{ mL/}\cancel{\text{min}} \times 60 \text{ }\cancel{\text{min}}\text{/hr} =$ 90 mL/hr (gtt/min)

A dosage range of 2-6 mcg/min is equal to a flow rate of 30-90 mL/hr (gtt/min).

23. Step 1: Convert to like units of measurement.

Equivalent: 1,000 mcg = 1 mg

Therefore 5,000 mg = 5,000,000 mcg

Step 2: Calculate the concentration of solution in mcg per mL.

$$5{,}000{,}000 \text{ mcg} : 500 \text{ mL} = x \text{ mcg} : 1 \text{ mL}$$
$$\frac{500x}{500} = \frac{5{,}000{,}000}{500}$$
$$x = 10{,}000 \text{ mcg per mL}$$

The concentration of solution is 10,000 mcg per mL.

Step 3: Calculate the dosage range.

Lower dosage: $50 \text{ mcg/}\cancel{\text{kg}}\text{/min} \times 60 \text{ }\cancel{\text{kg}} =$ 3,000 mcg/min

Upper dosage: $75 \text{ mcg/}\cancel{\text{kg}}\text{/min} \times 60 \text{ }\cancel{\text{kg}} =$ 4,500 mcg/min

Step 4: Convert the dosage range to mL/min.

$10{,}000 \text{ mcg}:1 \text{ mL} = 1{,}000 \text{ mcg}:x \text{ mL}$

Lower dosage: $10{,}000 \text{ mcg}:1 \text{ mL} = 3{,}000 \text{ mcg}:x \text{ mL}$

$$\frac{10{,}000x}{10{,}000} = \frac{3{,}000}{10{,}000}$$

$$x = 0.3 \text{ mL/min}$$

Upper dosage: $10{,}000 \text{ mcg}:1 \text{ mL} = 4{,}500 \text{ mcg}:x \text{ mL}$

$$\frac{10{,}000x}{10{,}000} = \frac{4{,}500}{10{,}000}$$

$$x = 0.45 \text{ mL/min}$$

Step 5: Convert mL/min to mL/hr.

Lower dosage: $0.3 \text{ mL/}\cancel{\text{min}} \times 60 \text{ }\cancel{\text{min}}\text{/hr} = 18 \text{ mL/hr (gtt/min)}$

Upper dosage: $0.45 \text{ mL/}\cancel{\text{min}} \times 60 \text{ }\cancel{\text{min}}\text{/hr} = 27 \text{ mL/hr (gtt/min)}$

a. A dosage range of 50-75 mcg is equal to a flow rate of 18-27 mL/hr (gtt/min).

b. Determine the dosage per minute infusing at 24 mL/hr.

$10{,}000 \text{ mcg}:1 \text{ mL} = x \text{ mcg}:24 \text{ mL}$

$x = 10{,}000 \times 24 = 240{,}000 \text{ mcg/hr}$

$240{,}000 \text{ mcg/}\cancel{\text{hr}} \div 60 \text{ min/}\cancel{\text{hr}} = 4{,}000 \text{ mcg/min}$

24. Calculate the dosage per minute for the client.

$65 \text{ }\cancel{\text{kg}} \times 10 \text{ mcg/}\cancel{\text{kg}}\text{/min} = 650 \text{ mcg/min}$

Determine the dosage per hour.

$650 \text{ mcg/}\cancel{\text{min}} \times 60 \text{ }\cancel{\text{min}}\text{/hr} = 39{,}000 \text{ mcg/hr}$

Convert to like units.

$$1{,}000 \text{ mcg} = 1 \text{ mg}$$

$$39{,}000 \text{ mcg/hr} = 39 \text{ mg/hr}$$

Calculate mL/hr flow rate.

$$500 \text{ mg}:250 \text{ mL} = 39 \text{ mg}:x \text{ mL}$$

$$\frac{500x}{500} = \frac{9{,}750}{500} = 19.5$$

$$x = 20 \text{ mL/hr}$$

Answer: To deliver a dosage of 10 mcg/kg/min, set the flow rate at 20 mL/hr (gtt/min).

25. Convert grams to milligrams.

$$1{,}000 \text{ mg} = 1 \text{ g}$$

$$0.25 \text{ g} = 250 \text{ mg}$$

Calculate mg/hr.

$$250 \text{ mg} \div 6 \text{ hr} = 41.6 = 42 \text{ mg/hr}$$

Answer: The client is receiving 42 mg of aminophylline per hour.

26. a. Convert grams to milligrams.

$$1 \text{ g} = 1{,}000 \text{ mg}$$

Calculate mg/hr.

$$1{,}000 \text{ mg}:500 \text{ mL} = x \text{ mg}:20 \text{ mL}$$

$$\frac{500x}{500} = \frac{20{,}000}{500}$$

$$x = \frac{20{,}000}{500}$$

$$x = 40 \text{ mg/hr}$$

b. Convert mg/hr to mg/min.

$40 \text{ mg/}\cancel{\text{hr}} \div 60 \text{ min/}\cancel{\text{hr}} = 0.66 = 0.7 \text{ mg/min}$

Answer: At the rate of 20 mL/hr, the client is receiving a dosage of 40 mg/hr or 0.7 mg/min.

27. a. Convert gtt/min to mL/min.

$$60 \text{ gtt}:1 \text{ mL} = 15 \text{ gtt}:x \text{ mL}$$

$$\frac{60x}{60} = \frac{15}{60} = 0.25$$

$$x = 0.3 \text{ mL/min}$$

Determine mg/min.

$$300 \text{ mg}:500 \text{ mL} = x \text{ mg}:0.3 \text{ mL}$$

$$\frac{500x}{500} = \frac{90}{500} = 0.18$$

$$x = 0.2 \text{ mg/min}$$

b. Calculate mg/hr.

$0.2 \text{ mg/}\cancel{\text{min}} \times 60 \text{ }\cancel{\text{min}}\text{/hr} = 12 \text{ mg/hr}$

Answer: At 15 gtt/min, the client is receiving a dosage of 0.2 mg/min and 12 mg/hr.

28. a. 10,240 mcg/min

b. 102 mL/hr

Calculate the dosage per minute.

$100 \text{ mcg/}\cancel{\text{kg}}\text{/min} \times 102.4 \text{ }\cancel{\text{kg}} = 10{,}240 \text{ mcg/min}$

Convert mcg/min to mg/min.

$10{,}240 \text{ mcg} \div 1{,}000 = 10.24 = 10.2 \text{ mg/min}$

Convert mg/min to mg/hr.

$10.2 \text{ mg/}\cancel{\text{min}} \times 60 \text{ }\cancel{\text{min}}\text{/hr} = 612 \text{ mg/hr}$

Calculate flow rate.

$$1 \text{ g} = 1{,}000 \text{ mg};\ 1.5 \text{ g} = 1{,}500 \text{ mg}$$

$$1{,}500 \text{ mg}:250 \text{ mL} = 612 \text{ mg}:x \text{ mL}$$

$$1{,}500\,x = 250 \times 612$$

$$\frac{1{,}500x}{1{,}500} = \frac{153{,}000}{1{,}500}$$

$$x = 102 \text{ mL/hr}$$

or

$$\frac{1{,}500 \text{ mg}}{250 \text{ mL}} = \frac{612 \text{ mg}}{x \text{ mL}}$$

29. a. 0.27 mg/min
    b. 270 mcg/min

    Calculate the mg/hr infusing.

$$500 \text{ mL} : 400 \text{ mg} = 20 \text{ mL} : x \text{ mg}$$

or

$$\frac{500 \text{ mL}}{400 \text{ mg}} = \frac{20 \text{ mL}}{x \text{ mg}}$$

$$500x = 400 \times 20$$

$$\frac{500x}{500} = \frac{8{,}000}{500}$$

$$x = 16 \text{ mg/hr}$$

Calculate the mg/min infusing.

$$16 \text{ mg/}\cancel{\text{hr}} \div 60 \text{ min/}\cancel{\text{hr}} = 0.266 = 0.27 \text{ mg/min}$$

$$1{,}000 \text{ mcg} = 1 \text{ mg}$$

$$0.27 \text{ mg/min} = 270 \text{ mcg/min}$$

30. 11 mL/hr

    Calculate dosage per minute.

$$3 \text{ mcg/}\cancel{\text{kg}}\text{/min} \times 59.1 \cancel{\text{kg}} = 177.3 \text{ mcg/min}$$

Convert mcg/min to mcg/hr.

$$177.3 \text{ mcg/}\cancel{\text{min}} \times 60 \cancel{\text{min}}\text{/hr} = 10{,}638 \text{ mcg/hr}$$

Convert mcg/hr to mg/hr (1,000 mcg = 1 mg).

$$10{,}638 \text{ mcg/hr} \div 1{,}000 = 10.63 = 10.6 \text{ mg/hr}$$

Calculate the flow rate.

$$250 \text{ mg} : 250 \text{ mL} = 10.6 \text{ mg} : x \text{ mL}$$

or

$$\frac{250 \text{ mg}}{250 \text{ mL}} = \frac{10.6 \text{ mg}}{x \text{ mL}}$$

$$250x = 250 \times 10.6$$

$$\frac{250x}{250} = \frac{2{,}650}{250} = 10.6$$

$$x = 11 \text{ mL/hr}$$

31. a. 375 mcg/min
    b. 22,500 mcg/hr
    c. 23 mL/hr

    Convert client's weight to kilograms (2.2 lb = 1 kg).

$$165 \text{ lb} \div 2.2 = 75 \text{ kg}$$

Calculate dosage per minute.

$$5 \text{ mcg/}\cancel{\text{kg}}\text{/min} \times 75 \cancel{\text{kg}} = 375 \text{ mcg/min}$$

Convert mcg/min to mcg/hr.

$$375 \text{ mcg/}\cancel{\text{min}} \times 60 \cancel{\text{min}}\text{/hr} = 22{,}500 \text{ mcg/hr}$$

Convert mcg/hr to mg/hr (1,000 mcg = 1 mg).

$$22{,}500 \text{ mcg/hr} \div 1{,}000 = 22.5 \text{ mg/hr}$$

Calculate flow rate.

$$250 \text{ mg} : 250 \text{ mL} = 22.5 \text{ mg} : x \text{ mL}$$

or

$$\frac{250 \text{ mg}}{250 \text{ mL}} = \frac{22.5 \text{ mg}}{x \text{ mL}}$$

$$250x = 250 \times 22.5$$

$$\frac{250x}{250} = \frac{5{,}625}{250} = 22.5$$

$$x = 23 \text{ mL/hr}$$

32. a. $5 \text{ mg} : 1 \text{ mL} = 125 \text{ mg} : x \text{ mL}$

or

$$\frac{125 \text{ mg}}{5 \text{ mg}} \times 1 \text{ mL} = x \text{ mL}$$

Answer: 25 mL. The dosage ordered is more than the available strength. Therefore you will need more than 5 mL to administer the dosage.

    b. $125 \text{ mg} : 125 \text{ mL} = 20 \text{ mg} : x \text{ mL}$

$$125x = 125 \times 20$$

$$\frac{125x}{125} = \frac{2{,}500}{125}$$

$$x = 20 \text{ mL/hr}$$

33. Calculate the dosage per hour.

$$2 \text{ mg/}\cancel{\text{min}} \times 60 \cancel{\text{min}}\text{/hr} = 120 \text{ mg/hr}$$

Convert grams to milligrams.

$$1{,}000 \text{ mg} = 1 \text{ g}; 2 \text{ g} = 2{,}000 \text{ mg}$$

Calculate mL/hr.

$$2{,}000 \text{ mg} : 500 \text{ mL} = 120 \text{ mg} : x \text{ mL}$$

$$2{,}000x = 500 \times 120$$

$$\frac{2{,}000x}{2{,}000} = \frac{60{,}0\cancel{00}}{2{,}0\cancel{00}}$$

$$x = 30 \text{ mL/hr}$$

34. Calculate the dosage per minute.

$3 \text{ mcg/}\cancel{\text{kg}}\text{/min} \times 95.9 \cancel{\text{kg}} = 287.7 \text{ mcg/min}$

Convert mcg/min to mcg/hr.

$287.7 \text{ mcg/}\cancel{\text{min}} \times 60 \cancel{\text{min}}\text{/hr} = 17{,}262 \text{ mcg/hr}$

Convert mcg/hr to mg/hr (1,000 mcg = 1 mg).

$17{,}262 \text{ mcg/hr} \div 1{,}000 = 17.26 = 17.3 \text{ mg/hr}$

Calculate the IV flow rate.

$$400 \text{ mg} : 250 \text{ mL} = 17.3 \text{ mg} : x \text{ mL}$$
$$400x = 250 \times 17.3$$
$$\frac{400x}{400} = \frac{4{,}325}{400}$$
$$x = \frac{4{,}325}{400} = 10.81$$
$$x = 10.8 \text{ mL/hr}$$

To infuse 3 mcg/kg/min, set the rate at 10.8 mL/hr. The rate is not rounded to 11 mL/hr because the IV pump is capable of delivering in tenths of a mL.

35. Convert lb to kg (2.2 lb = 1 kg).

$143 \text{ lb} \div 2.2 = 65 \text{ kg}$

Find concentration per minute (mcg/min).

$65 \cancel{\text{kg}} \times 5 \text{ mcg/}\cancel{\text{kg}}\text{/min} = 325 \text{ mcg/min}$

Find concentration per hour.

$325 \text{ mcg/}\cancel{\text{min}} \times 60 \cancel{\text{min}}\text{/hr} = 19{,}500 \text{ mcg/hr}$

The concentration of dobutamine infused per minute is 325 mcg/min and 19,500 mcg/hr.

36. Convert mcg/min to mcg/hr.

$2 \text{ mcg/}\cancel{\text{min}} \times 60 \cancel{\text{min}}\text{/hr} = 120 \text{ mcg/hr}$

Convert mcg/hr to mg/hr (1,000 mcg = 1 mg).

$120 \text{ mcg/hr} \div 1{,}000 = 0.12 \text{ mg/hr}$

Calculate the lower mL/hr flow rate.

$$8 \text{ mg} : 250 \text{ mL} = 0.12 \text{ mg} : x \text{ mL}$$
$$8x = 250 \times 0.12$$
$$\frac{8x}{8} = \frac{30}{8}$$
$$x = \frac{30}{8} = 3.75$$
$$x = 3.8 \text{ mL/hr}$$

The flow rate for the lower 2 mcg/min dosage is 3.8 mL/hr.

Calculate the upper 4 mcg/min flow rate.

Convert mcg/min to mcg/hr.

$4 \text{ mcg/}\cancel{\text{min}} \times 60 \cancel{\text{min}}\text{/hr} = 240 \text{ mcg/hr}$

Convert mcg/hr to mg/hr (1,000 mcg = 1 mg).

$240 \text{ mcg/hr} \div 1{,}000 = 0.24 \text{ mg/hr}$

Calculate the upper mL/hr flow rate.

$$8 \text{ mg} : 250 \text{ mL} = 0.24 \text{ mg} : x \text{ mL}$$
$$8x = 250 \times 0.24$$
$$\frac{8x}{8} = \frac{60}{8}$$
$$x = \frac{60}{8}$$
$$x = 7.5 \text{ mL/hr}$$

The flow rate for the upper 4 mcg/min = 7.5 mL/hr.

The flow rate range to titrate a dosage of 2-4 mcg/min is 3.8-7.5 mL/hr (mL/hr is not rounded; pump capable of delivering in tenths of a mL).

Calculate the dosage infusing at 5 mL/hr.

$$250 \text{ mL} : 8 \text{ mg} = 5 \text{ mL} : x \text{ mg}$$
$$\frac{250x}{250} = \frac{8 \times 5}{250}$$
$$x = \frac{40}{250}$$
$$x = 0.16 \text{ mg/hr}$$

Convert mg/hr to mcg/hr (1,000 mcg = 1 mg).

$0.16 \text{ mg/hr} \times 1{,}000 = 160 \text{ mcg/hr}$

Convert mcg/hr to mcg/min.

$160 \text{ mcg/}\cancel{\text{hr}} \div 60 \text{ min/}\cancel{\text{hr}} = 2.66 = 2.7 \text{ mcg/min}$

At the flow rate of 5 mL/hr, the client is now receiving 2.7 mcg/min.

37. Step 1: Calculate the dose per hour using the lower and upper dosages.

$$40 \text{ mcg}/\cancel{\text{min}} \times 60 \ \cancel{\text{min}}/\text{hr} = 2{,}400 \text{ mcg/hr}$$

$$100 \text{ mcg}/\cancel{\text{min}} \times 60 \ \cancel{\text{min}}/\text{hr} = 6{,}000 \text{ mcg/hr}$$

Step 2: Convert mcg to mg to match the available strength.

1,000 mcg = 1 mg

2,400 mcg = 2.4 mg

6,000 mcg = 6 mg

Step 3: Calculate the rate in mL/hr

$$40 \text{ mg} : 250 \text{ mL} = 2.4 \text{ mg} : x \text{ mL}$$

$$40x = 250 \times 2.4$$

$$\frac{40x}{40} = \frac{600}{40}$$

$$x = 15 \text{ mL/hr}$$

To infuse 40 mcg/min, set the IV rate at 15 mL/hr (minimum)

$$40 \text{ mg} : 250 \text{ mL} = 6 \text{ mg} : x \text{ mL}$$

$$40x = 250 \times 6 =$$

$$\frac{40x}{40} = \frac{1{,}500}{40}$$

$$x = 37.5 \text{ mL/hr}$$

To infuse 100 mcg/min, set the IV rate at 37.5 mL/hr (maximum).

A dosage of 40 to 100 mcg/min is equal to 15 to 37.5 mL/hr.

Set up proportion to determine the dosage change of 20 mcg/min.

$$\frac{40 \text{ mcg/min}}{15 \text{ mL/hr}} = \frac{20 \text{ mcg/min}}{x \text{ mL/hr}}$$

$$\frac{40x}{40} = \frac{300}{40}$$

$$x = 7.5 \text{ mL/hr}$$

So, for each change of 20 mcg/min, the incremental IV flow rate is 7.5 mL/hr.

Titration Table

Dosage Rate (mcg/min)	Flow Rate (mL/hr)
40 mcg/min **(minimum)**	15 mL/hr
60 mcg/min	22.5 mL/hr
80 mcg/min	30 mL/hr
100 mcg/min **(maximum)**	37.5 mL/hr

38. **Step 1:** Calculate the dose per hour using the lower and upper dosages.

$$4 \text{ mcg}/\cancel{\text{min}} \times 60 \ \cancel{\text{min}}/\text{hr} = 240 \text{ mcg/hr}$$

$$12 \text{ mcg}/\cancel{\text{min}} \times 60 \ \cancel{\text{min}}/\text{hr} = 720 \text{ mcg/hr}$$

Step 2: Convert mcg/hr to available strength.

1,000 mcg = 1 mg

240 mcg = 0.24 mg

720 mcg = 0.72 mg

Step 3: Calculate the rate in mL/hr.

$$4 \text{ mg} : 500 \text{ mL} = 0.24 \text{ mg} : x \text{ mL}$$

$$4x = 500 \times 0.24$$

$$\frac{4x}{4} = \frac{120}{4}$$

$$x = 30 \text{ mL/hr}$$

To infuse 4 mcg/min, set the IV rate at 30 mL/hr (minimum).

$$4 \text{ mg} : 500 \text{ mL} = 0.72 \text{ mg} : x \text{ mL}$$

$$4x = 500 \times 0.72$$

$$\frac{4x}{4} = \frac{360}{4}$$

$$x = 90 \text{ mL/hr}$$

To infuse 12 mcg/min, set the IV rate at 90 mL/hr (maximum).

A dosage of 4-12 mcg/min is equal to 30-90 mL/hr.

Set up a proportion to determine the dosage change of 2 mcg/min.

$$\frac{4 \text{ mcg/min}}{30 \text{ mL/hr}} = \frac{2 \text{ mcg/min}}{x \text{ mL/hr}}$$

$$\frac{4x}{4} = \frac{60}{4}$$

$$x = 15 \text{ mL/hr}$$

For each change of 2 mcg/min, the incremental flow rate is 15 mL/hr.

Titration Table

Dosage Rate (mcg/min)	Flow Rate (mL/hr)
4 mcg/min **(minimum)**	30 mL/hr
6 mcg/min	45 mL/hr
8 mcg/min	60 mL/hr
10 mcg/min	75 mL/hr
12 mcg/min **(maximum)**	90 mL/hr

CHAPTER 25
Pediatric and Adult Dosage Calculations Based on Weight

Objectives

After reviewing this chapter, you should be able to:

1. Convert body weight from pounds to kilograms
2. Convert body weight from kilograms to pounds
3. Calculate dosages based on milligram per kilogram
4. Determine whether a dosage is safe
5. Determine body surface area (BSA) using the West nomogram
6. Calculate BSA using formulas according to units of measure
7. Determine dosages using the BSA
8. Calculate the flow rates for pediatric IV therapy
9. Calculate the safe dosage ranges and determine if within normal range for medications administered IV in pediatrics
10. Calculate pediatric IV maintenance fluids

Experts agree that children are a vulnerable population and have a higher potential for experiencing adverse effects of medications and harm from medication errors than adults. Therefore, accuracy in dosage calculation, determining if the dosage is in the safe dose range for the child, validating calculations, being knowledgeable about the medication being administered (i.e., possible adverse reactions, indications for use) before administration of medications, and using appropriate measuring devices to administer medications safely to children becomes even more of a priority. According to the ISMP, Results of Pediatric Medication Safety Survey (Part 2), "Pediatric patients are three times more likely than adults to experience a harmful medication error or adverse drug reaction" (2015).

Causes of medication errors with pediatric clients have been documented in literature and include the following:

- Confusion between adult and pediatric formulations.
- Errors with oral liquid dosage forms that are available in multiple pediatric concentrations
- Incorrect preparation of medications that require dilution
- Improper education of parents or caregivers for child regarding preparation of medications and administration
- Calculation errors due to multiple calculations to individualize dosages on basis of age, weight, mg/kg, or Body Surface Area (BSA)
- Use of inaccurate measuring devices (household teaspoons) as opposed to devices such as oral dosing devices for small volume doses. However, errors have also been reported when parents used standardized instruments according to the American Academy of Pediatrics (AAP) especially when they reported their child's dose using teaspoon or tablespoon units. According to the AAP, parents mix up terms such as milliliter, teaspoon, and tablespoon. These terms are often used interchangeably to describe a child's dose when discussing dosages with parents as well as being shown on medication labels and prescriptions.

The results of a study released recently caused alarm and discussion on the news program Today.com, Channel 4 NBC News on September 12, 2016 by the well-known Dr. Mehmet Oz, who reported that according to a new study, an alarming number of parents are unintentionally giving their children incorrect doses of liquid medications. 85% of parents made errors. The study being referred to, "Liquid Medication Errors and Dosing Tools: A Randomized Controlled Experiment," published in October 2016 *Pediatrics,* found that, "68% of the errors made involved overdosing, and that use of a dosing cup was associated with a four times increased odds of a dosing error compared to when an oral syringe was used. The study, published on line September 12, 2016 found that 85% of parents made at least one dosing error in nine trials; 21% made at least one large error, measuring out more than two times the recommended dose." The study also reinforced that the use of a wide range of measurement units (mL, tsp, tbs) was a factor contributing to the errors. Based on the study's findings and reinforced by Dr. Oz, the oral syringe should be used instead of dosing cups to administer small doses to children. These findings have implications for nurses, health care providers, and for the future making of medication labels as well as dosing devices to ensure safe medication administration to children. The reason for errors in pediatric medication administration that are mentioned are only a few of the reasons.

Multiple factors impact medication dosing for children and make them more susceptible to adverse effects of drugs. Such factors include:

- Size, weight, and Body Surface Area (BSA) of the infant or child
- Higher percentage of water per kg of body weight
- Physiological capabilities (e.g., a lessened ability to metabolize medications, immaturity of systems, differences in rate of medication absorption and excretion) differ in comparison to adults
- Increased metabolism

To maximize drug effects and minimize adverse effects before administering medications to children, the nurse must carefully calculate the dose, and know whether the ordered dose is safe for the individual child. Accuracy is always important when calculating medication dosages. For infants and children, exact and careful mathematics takes on even greater importance. A miscalculation, even small discrepancies, may be dangerous for a child. Nurses must adhere to pediatric protocols and guidelines, and always use a reference to verify medication orders to ensure that medication dosages are correct and safe. In many healthcare institutions, the pharmacy supplies medications in unit dose to reduce the chance of error. This, however, does not alleviate the nurse's responsibility from verifying that the prescribed dose ordered is accurate and safe.

SAFETY ALERT!

Accuracy in dosage calculation becomes even more of a priority when calculating and administering medications to infants and children. Medication errors have been identified as being most common in children, and most preventable errors have been identified as being the most common. Death as a result of medication errors is a higher risk in children than in adults.

Body weight is an important factor used to calculate medication dosages for children and adults, although it is used more frequently with children. Medications may be prescribed based on body weight or body surface area.

The safe administration of medications to infants and children requires knowledge of the methods used in calculating doses. In addition, the nurse must apply the principles of the "six rights" of medication administration (right medication, right dosage, right time, right route, right client, right documentation) when working with pediatric clients and families. Nurses are also responsible for educating the families regarding medication administration.

Dosages for infants and children are based on their unique physiological differences. The prescriber must consider weight, height, body surface area, age, and condition of the child when ordering dosages. As mentioned previously, the two methods used for calculating safe pediatric dosages are body weight (e.g., mg/kg) and body surface area (BSA, measured in square meters [m^2]). The body weight method is more common in pediatrics and is emphasized in this chapter, as well as is the BSA. The BSA method is based on both height and weight. BSA is especially used in pediatric Oncology and critical care. As stated previously, body weight and BSA methods are also used for adults, especially in critical care, and the calculation methods used are the same.

Although the prescriber is responsible for ordering the medication and dosage, **the nurse remains responsible for verifying the dosage to be sure it is correct and safe for administration.**

SAFETY ALERT!

As the nurse administering medications to children, you are legally responsible for recognizing incorrect and unsafe dosages and for alerting the prescriber.

Pediatric Medication Dosages

If a dosage is higher than normal, it may be unsafe, and a dosage lower than normal may not have the desired therapeutic effect, which is also unsafe. The nurse must be able to determine whether a prescribed pediatric dosage is within the recommended safe range. It is imperative that the nurse check reputable medication resources for specific dosage details. The recommended dose or dosage range can be found in the package insert, or on the medication label. Other references that may be checked for more in-depth and additional information on a medication are drug formularies at the institution, the Physician's Desk Reference (PDR), United States Pharmacopeia, medication guide books, and the manufacturer's website prescribing information. Various pocket-size pediatric medication handbooks are also available; one that is widely used is *The Harriette Lane Handbook* (Johns Hopkins Hospital, 2015).

SAFETY ALERT!

To ensure safe practice, when in doubt, consult a reliable source. Always double-check dosages by comparing the prescribed dose with the recommended safe dose.

Determining medication dosages according to body weight and BSA is a means of individualizing medication therapy. Although body weight and BSA are common determinants for medication dosing in children as previously stated, they are also used to calculate adult medication dosages, particularly for those who are very old or grossly underweight.

Principles Relating to Basic Calculations

Before calculating medications for the child or infant, some guidelines are helpful.

1. Calculation of pediatric dosages, as with adult dosages, involves the use of ratio and proportion, the formula method, or dimensional analysis to determine the amount of medication to administer.
2. Pediatric dosages are much smaller than those for an adult. Micrograms are used a great deal. The tuberculin syringe (1-mL capacity) is used to administer very small dosages.
3. Intramuscular (IM) dosages are usually not more than 1 mL for small children and older infants; however, this can vary with the size of the child. The recommended IM dosage for small infants is not more than 0.5 mL.
4. The recommended subcutaneous (subcut) dosage for children is not more than 0.5 mL.
5. Dosages that are less than 1 mL may be measured in tenths of a milliliter or with a tuberculin syringe in hundredths of a milliliter.
6. Medications in pediatrics are not generally rounded off to the nearest tenth but may be administered with a tuberculin syringe (measured in hundredths) to ensure accuracy.
7. All answers must be labeled.
8. Know your institution's policy on the rounding of pediatric dosages.

Calculation of Dosages Based on Body Weight

Let's begin our discussion with the calculation of dosages according to milligrams per kilogram (mg/kg) of body weight. Before calculating dosages according to mg/kg of body weight, it is essential that you be able to convert a child's weight. Most recommendations for medication dosages are based on weight in kilograms. The nurse then compares the child's ordered dosage to the recommended safe dosage from a reputable medication resource before administering any medication to a child. This helps ensure that the dose ordered is safe and effective before calculating the amount to administer and administering the dosage to the child, thereby decreasing the chance of error, which could cause harm.

Therefore, the most common conversion you will encounter involves the conversion from pounds to kilograms. To do this, remember the conversion 1 kg = 2.2 lb. Conversions of weights are presented in Chapter 9. The methods of converting presented in Chapter 8 can also be used. It is, however, essential that we review this again.

RULE

To convert from pounds to kilograms, use the conversion 1 kg = 2.2 lb. To convert from pounds to kilograms, divide by 2.2, and express the weight to the nearest tenth.

Converting Pounds to Kilograms

Let's do some sample problems with the conversion of weights.

Example 1: Convert a child's weight of 30 lb to kilograms.

$$2.2 \text{ lb} = 1 \text{ kg}$$ (conversion factor)

✓ Solution Using Ratio and Proportion

$$2.2 \text{ lb} : 1 \text{ kg} = 30 \text{ lb} : x \text{ kg}$$

$$\frac{\cancel{2.2}x}{\cancel{2.2}} = \frac{30}{2.2}$$

$$x = \frac{30}{2.2} = 13.63$$

$$x = 13.6 \text{ kg}$$

$$\text{Child's weight} = 13.6 \text{ kg}$$

(rounded to the nearest tenth)

✓ Solution Using Dimensional Analysis

$$x \text{ kg} = \frac{1 \text{ kg}}{2.2 \cancel{\text{lb}}} \times \frac{30 \cancel{\text{lb}}}{1}$$

$$x = \frac{30}{2.2} = 13.63$$

$$x = 13.6 \text{ kg}$$

$$\text{Child's weight} = 13.6 \text{ kg}$$

(rounded to the nearest tenth)

Example 2: Convert an infant's weight of 14 lb and 6 oz to kilograms.

1. Convert ounces to parts of a pound.

$$16 \text{ oz} = 1 \text{ lb}$$ (conversion factor)

✓ Solution Using Ratio and Proportion

$$16 \text{ oz} : 1 \text{ lb} = 6 \text{ oz} : x \text{ lb}$$

$$\frac{\cancel{16}x}{\cancel{16}} = \frac{6}{16}$$

$$x = \frac{6}{16} = 0.37$$

$$x = 0.4 \text{ lb}$$

(rounded to the nearest tenth)

Add the computed pounds to the total pounds as follows:

$$14 \text{ lb} + 0.4 \text{ lb} = 14.4 \text{ lb}$$
$$\text{Infant's weight} = 14.4 \text{ lb}$$

SAFETY ALERT!

Use caution when converting ounces to a fraction of a pound. Also, after converting the ounces to pounds, remember to add the answer to the remaining whole pounds to get the total pounds. Then convert the total pounds to kilograms.

2. Convert total pounds to kilograms.

✓ Solution Using Ratio and Proportion

$$2.2 \text{ lb} = 1 \text{ kg} \quad \text{(conversion factor)}$$
$$2.2 \text{ lb} : 1 \text{ kg} = 14.4 \text{ lb} : x \text{ kg}$$
$$\frac{\cancel{2.2}x}{\cancel{2.2}} = \frac{14.4}{2.2}$$
$$x = \frac{14.4}{2.2} = 6.54$$
$$x = 6.5 \text{ kg} \quad \text{(rounded to the nearest tenth)}$$
$$\text{Infant's weight} = 6.5 \text{ kg}$$

✓ Solution Using Dimensional Analysis

$$x \text{ lb} = \frac{1 \text{ lb}}{16 \cancel{\text{oz}}} \times \frac{6 \cancel{\text{oz}}}{1}$$
$$x - \frac{6}{16} = 0.37$$
$$x = 0.4 \text{ lb} \quad \text{(rounded to the nearest tenth)}$$
$$\text{Infant's weight} = 14.4 \text{ lb}$$
$$x \text{ kg} = \frac{1 \text{ kg}}{2.2 \cancel{\text{lb}}} \times \frac{14.4 \cancel{\text{lb}}}{1}$$
$$x = \frac{14.4}{2.2} = 6.54$$
$$x = 6.5 \text{ kg} \quad \text{(rounded to the nearest tenth)}$$
$$\text{Infant's weight} = 6.5 \text{ kg}$$

Example 3: Convert the weight of a 157-lb adult to kilograms.

$$2.2 \text{ lb} = 1 \text{ kg} \quad \text{(conversion factor)}$$

✓ Solution Using Ratio and Proportion

$$2.2 \text{ lb} : 1 \text{ kg} = 157 \text{ lb} : x \text{ kg}$$
$$\frac{\cancel{2.2}x}{\cancel{2.2}} = \frac{157}{2.2}$$
$$x = \frac{157}{2.2} = 71.36$$
$$x = 71.4 \text{ kg} \quad \text{(rounded to the nearest tenth)}$$
$$\text{Adult's weight} = 71.4 \text{ kg}$$

✓ Solution Using Dimensional Analysis

$$x \text{ kg} = \frac{1 \text{ kg}}{2.2 \not{\text{lb}}} \times \frac{157 \not{\text{lb}}}{1}$$

$$x = \frac{157}{2.2} = 71.36$$

$$x = 71.4 \text{ kg} \quad \text{(rounded to the nearest tenth)}$$

$$\text{Adult's weight} = 71.4 \text{ kg}$$

PRACTICE PROBLEMS

Convert the following weights in pounds to kilograms. Round to the nearest tenth.

1. 15 lb = ______________ kg
2. 68 lb = ______________ kg
3. 31 lb = ______________ kg
4. 52 lb = ______________ kg
5. 71 lb = ______________ kg
6. 133 lb = ______________ kg
7. 8 lb 4 oz = ______________ kg
8. 5 lb 12 oz = ______________ kg
9. $100\frac{1}{4}$ lb = ______________ kg
10. $92\frac{3}{4}$ lb = ______________ kg

Answers on p. 710

Converting Kilograms to Pounds

RULE

To convert from kilograms to pounds, use the conversion 1 kg = 2.2 lb. To convert from kilograms to pounds, multiply by 2.2, and express the weight to the nearest tenth.

Example 1: Convert a child's weight of 24.3 kg to pounds.

2.2 lb = 1 kg (conversion factor)

✓ Solution Using Ratio and Proportion

$$2.2 \text{ lb} : 1 \text{ kg} = x \text{ lb} : 24.3 \text{ kg}$$

$$x = 24.3 \times 2.2 = 53.46$$

$$x = 53.5 \text{ lb} \quad \text{(rounded to the nearest tenth)}$$

$$\text{Child's weight} = 53.5 \text{ lb}$$

✓ Solution Using Dimensional Analysis

$$x \text{ lb} = \frac{2.2 \text{ lb}}{1 \not{\text{kg}}} \times \frac{24.3 \not{\text{kg}}}{1}$$

$$x = 2.2 \times 24.3 = 53.46$$

$$x = 53.5 \text{ lb}$$

$$\text{Child's weight} = 53.5 \text{ lb}$$

Example 2: Convert an adult's weight of 70.2 kg to pounds.

2.2 lb = 1 kg (conversion factor)

✓ Solution Using Ratio and Proportion

$$2.2 \text{ lb} : 1 \text{ kg} = x \text{ lb} : 70.2 \text{ kg}$$
$$x = 70.2 \times 2.2 = 154.44$$
$$x = 154.4 \text{ lb} \quad \text{(rounded to the nearest tenth)}$$
$$\text{Adult's weight} = 154.4 \text{ lb}$$

✓ Solution Using Dimensional Analysis

$$x \text{ lb} = \frac{2.2 \text{ lb}}{1 \cancel{\text{kg}}} \times \frac{70.2 \cancel{\text{kg}}}{1}$$
$$x = 2.2 \times 70.2 = 154.44$$
$$x = 154.4 \text{ lb} \quad \text{(rounded to the nearest tenth)}$$
$$\text{Adult's weight} = 154.4 \text{ lb}$$

Example 3: Convert the weight of a 10.2-kg child to pounds.

$$2.2 \text{ lb} = 1 \text{ kg} \quad \text{(conversion factor)}$$

✓ Solution Using Ratio and Proportion

$$2.2 \text{ lb} : 1 \text{ kg} = x \text{ lb} : 10.2 \text{ kg}$$
$$x = 10.2 \times 2.2 = 22.44$$
$$x = 22.4 \text{ lb} \quad \text{(rounded to the nearest tenth)}$$
$$\text{Child's weight} = 22.4 \text{ lb}$$

✓ Solution Using Dimensional Analysis

$$x \text{ lb} = \frac{2.2 \text{ lb}}{1 \cancel{\text{kg}}} \times \frac{10.2 \cancel{\text{kg}}}{1}$$
$$x = 2.2 \times 10.2 = 22.44$$
$$x = 22.4 \text{ lb} \quad \text{(rounded to the nearest tenth)}$$
$$\text{Child's weight} = 22.4 \text{ lb}$$

PRACTICE **PROBLEMS**

Convert the following weights in kilograms to pounds. Round to the nearest tenth.

11. 21.3 kg = ______________ lb
12. 17.7 kg = ______________ lb
13. 22 kg = ______________ lb
14. 15 kg = ______________ lb
15. 34 kg = ______________ lb
16. 71.4 kg = ______________ lb
17. 73 kg = ______________ lb
18. 98.3 kg = ______________ lb
19. 34.9 kg = ______________ lb
20. 28.7 kg = ______________ lb

Answers on p. 710

Infants 0 to 4 weeks old (neonates) and premature infants may also be given medications. The scale will convert the child's weight in grams, or the weight may be reported in grams, rather than kilograms. Therefore, it may be necessary for the nurse to convert the weight in grams to kilograms because most dosage recommendations are commonly given in kilograms.

As discussed in the chapter on metric conversions, 1 kg = 1,000 g; therefore, to convert grams to kilograms, divide by 1,000 or move the decimal point three places to the left.

RULE

To convert grams to kilograms, use the conversion 1 kg = 1,000 g. Divide the number of grams by 1,000, or move the decimal point three places to the left. Round kilograms to the nearest tenth.

Converting Grams to Kilograms

Example 1: Convert an infant's weight of 3,000 g to kilograms.

$$1 \text{ kg} = 1{,}000 \text{ g} \qquad \text{(conversion factor)}$$

✓ Solution Using Ratio and Proportion

$$1 \text{ kg} : 1{,}000 \text{ g} = x \text{ kg} : 3{,}000 \text{ g}$$

$$\frac{\cancel{1{,}000}x}{\cancel{1{,}000}} = \frac{3{,}\cancel{000}}{1{,}\cancel{000}}$$

$$x = 3 \text{ kg}$$

$$\text{Infant's weight} = 3 \text{ kg}$$

$$\text{Decimal movement: } 3\underset{\smile\smile\smile}{000} = 3 \text{ kg}$$

✓ Solution Using Dimensional Analysis

$$x \text{ kg} = \frac{1 \text{ kg}}{1{,}000 \cancel{\text{g}}} \times \frac{3{,}000 \cancel{\text{g}}}{1}$$

$$x = \frac{3{,}\cancel{000}}{1{,}\cancel{000}}$$

$$x = 3 \text{ kg}$$

$$\text{Infant's weight} = 3 \text{ kg}$$

Example 2: Convert an infant's weight of 1,350 g to kilograms.

$$1 \text{ kg} = 1{,}000 \text{ g} \qquad \text{(conversion factor)}$$

✓ Solution Using Ratio and Proportion

$$1 \text{ kg} : 1{,}000 \text{ g} = x \text{ kg} : 1{,}350 \text{ g}$$

$$\frac{1{,}000x}{1{,}000} = \frac{1{,}35\cancel{0}}{1{,}00\cancel{0}} = 1.35$$

$$x = 1.4 \text{ kg} \qquad \text{(rounded to the nearest tenth)}$$

$$\text{Infant's weight} = 1.4 \text{ kg}$$

$$\text{Decimal movement: } 1\underset{\smile\smile\smile}{350} = 1.35 \text{ kg} = 1.4 \text{ kg} \qquad \text{(rounded to the nearest tenth)}$$

✓ Solution Using Dimensional Analysis

$$x \text{ kg} = \frac{1 \text{ kg}}{1{,}000 \cancel{\text{g}}} \times \frac{1{,}350 \cancel{\text{g}}}{1}$$

$$x = \frac{1{,}35\cancel{0}}{1{,}00\cancel{0}} = 1.35$$

$$x = 1.4 \text{ kg} \qquad \text{(rounded to the nearest tenth)}$$

$$\text{Infant's weight} = 1.4 \text{ kg}$$

Example 3: Convert an infant's weight of 2,700 g to kilograms.

$$1 \text{ kg} = 1{,}000 \text{ g} \qquad \text{(conversion factor)}$$

✓ Solution Using Ratio and Proportion

$$1 \text{ kg} : 1{,}000 \text{ g} = x \text{ kg} : 2{,}700 \text{ g}$$

$$\frac{1{,}000x}{1{,}000} = \frac{2{,}7\cancel{00}}{1{,}0\cancel{00}}$$

$$\text{Infant's weight} = 2.7 \text{ kg}$$

$$\text{Decimal movement: } 2700 = 2.7 \text{ kg}$$

✓ Solution Using Dimensional Analysis

$$x \text{ kg} = \frac{1 \text{ kg}}{1{,}000 \cancel{\text{g}}} \times \frac{2{,}700 \cancel{\text{g}}}{1}$$

$$x = \frac{2{,}7\cancel{00}}{1{,}0\cancel{00}}$$

$$x = 2.7 \text{ kg}$$

$$\text{Infant's weight} = 2.7 \text{ kg}$$

PRACTICE **PROBLEMS**

Convert the following weights in grams to kilograms. Round to the nearest tenth.

21. 4,000 g = ______________________ kg
22. 1,450 g = ______________________ kg
23. 2,900 g = ______________________ kg
24. 3,600 g = ______________________ kg
25. 1,875 g = ______________________ kg

Answers on p. 710

Remember

1. 2.2 lb = 1 kg, 1 kg = 1,000 g
2. To convert from pounds to kilograms, divide the number of pounds by 2.2. Carry the division to the hundredths place, and round the weight to the nearest tenth. Calculations based on body weight can be rounded off to the nearest tenth.
3. To convert from kilograms to pounds, multiply the number of kilograms by 2.2 and round the weight to the nearest tenth.
4. If the child's weight is in ounces and pounds, convert the ounces to the nearest tenth of a pound, and then add the answer to pounds to get the total pounds. Convert the total pounds to kilograms, and round to the nearest tenth.
5. To convert from grams to kilograms, divide by 1,000 or move the decimal point three places to the left. Round kilograms to the nearest tenth as indicated.

Before beginning to calculate dosages based on weight, let's review some terms that may be used.

Recommended dosage (also referred to as the safe dosage)—This information comes from a reputable resource, such as a medication reference written especially for pediatrics or another medication reference book. Recommended dosages may also be indicated on the medication label under children's dosages. This is usually expressed in mg/kg for a 24-hour period to be given in one or more divided doses. This may also be seen as mcg/kg and occasionally mg/lb. Recommended dosage can also be stated as a range and referred to as safe dosage range (SDR). This is the upper and lower limits of the dosage as stated by an approved medication reference.

Total daily dosage—Dosage obtained by multiplying the child's weight after it is converted to kilograms with the use of a reputable medication reference: multiply child's weight in kilograms by dosage expressed as mg/kg.

Divided dosage (also referred to as the single dose)—This represents the dosage a child should receive each time the medication is administered. The recommended daily dosage may be stated as mg/kg/day to be divided into a certain number of individual dosages, such as "three divided dosages," q6h, and so on. "Three divided dosages" means that the total daily dosage is divided equally and administered three times per day. q6h means the total daily dosage is divided equally and administered every 6 hours, for a total of four dosages per day (24 hr ÷ 6 hr). This is the dosage for 24 hours divided by the frequency, or the number of times, the child will receive the medication.

Deciding if the dosage is safe—This is done by comparing the ordered dosage with the recommended dosage. In other words, this is decided by comparing and evaluating the 24-hour ordered amount with the recommended dosage.

As stated, the most common method for prescribing and administering the therapeutic amount for a child is to calculate the amount of medication according to the child's body weight in kilograms. Therefore, it is important to be able to convert a child's weight correctly.

Verification of safe pediatric doses recommended by body weight is essential and requires a systematic approach.

- Convert the child's weight in kilograms (rounded to tenths).
- Calculate the safe dose by multiplying the weight in kg by the recommended dose from a reputable medication reference (rounded to tenths). Multiply mg/kg by child's weight in kg.
- Compare the ordered dose with the recommended dosage, and determine if the dosage is safe.
- If the dosage is safe, calculate the amount to give and administer the dosage. If the dosage is unsafe, notify the prescriber before administering the medication.

! SAFETY ALERT!

Before administering any medication to a child, always ask yourself if the dosage is safe. When in doubt, contact the prescriber before administering.

Let's begin by looking at examples:

Single Dose Medications

Sometimes medications may be ordered as a single dose (mg/kg/dose). Single doses are usually intended for one-time administration or prn. The dosage ordered is based on mg/kg/dose, calculated by multiplying the recommended dose in kg by the child's weight in kg for each dose.

Example 1: The prescriber orders Narcan 1.2 mg IV stat for a child who weighs 12 kg. You need to determine if the dosage is safe.

Recommended dosage is 0.1 mg/kg/dose from a reputable medication resource (e.g., *The Harriet Lane Handbook*).

1. No conversion of weight is required. The child's weight is in kg, and the recommended dosage is stated as 0.1 mg/kg.
2. Calculate the mg/kg as recommended by a reputable medication resource.
   - Multiply mg/kg/dose by the child's weight in kg.
     $0.1 \text{ mg}/\cancel{\text{kg}}/\text{dose} \times 12 \cancel{\text{kg}} = 1.2 \text{ mg/dose}$

The calculation of the safe dose could also be done by setting up a ratio and proportion and dimensional analysis.

✓ Solution Using Ratio and Proportion

$$0.1\text{ mg} : 1\text{ kg} = x\text{ mg} : 12\text{ kg}$$
$$x = 1.2\text{ mg/dose}$$

The safe dose for a child weighing 12 kg is 1.2 mg/dose.

Remember that a ratio and a proportion can be written in different formats.

✓ Solution Using Dimensional Analysis

The recommended dose is the starting fraction (in this case, 0.1 mg/kg).

$$\frac{x\text{ mg}}{\text{dose}} = \frac{0.1\text{ mg}}{\cancel{\text{kg}}/\text{dose}} \times \frac{12\ \cancel{\text{kg}}}{1}$$
$$x = 0.1 \times 12$$
$$x = 1.2\text{ mg/dose}$$

The safe dose for a child weighing 12 kg is 1.2 mg/dose.

3. Decide if the dosage is safe by comparing the ordered and recommended dosage. For this child's weight, 1.2 mg is the recommended dosage, and 1.2 mg is the ordered dosage. Yes, the dosage is safe.
4. Calculate the dosage. Use ratio and proportion, the formula method, or dimensional analysis to determine the number of mL to administer.

Order: Narcan 1.2 mg IV stat

Available:

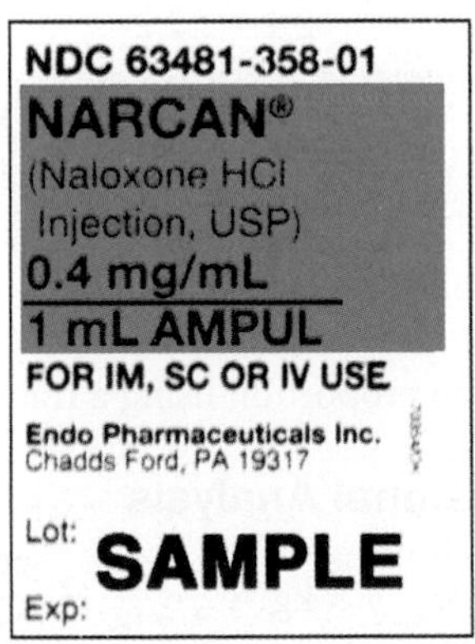

✓ Solution Using Ratio and Proportion

$$0.4\text{ mg} : 1\text{ mL} = 1.2\text{ mg} : x\text{ mL} \quad \text{OR} \quad \frac{0.4\text{ mg}}{1\text{ mL}} = \frac{1.2\text{ mg}}{x\text{ mL}}$$

$$\frac{0.4x}{0.4} = \frac{1.2}{0.4} \qquad x = 3\text{ mL}$$
$$x = 3\text{ mL}$$

✓ Solution Using Formula

$$\frac{1.2\text{ mg}}{0.4\text{ mg}} \times 1\text{ mL} = x\text{ mL}$$
$$x = 3\text{ mL}$$

✓ Solution Using Dimensional Analysis

$$x \text{ mL} = \frac{1 \text{ mL}}{0.4 \cancel{\text{mg}}} \times \frac{1.2 \cancel{\text{mg}}}{1}$$

$$x = \frac{1.2}{0.4}$$

$$x = 3 \text{ mL}$$

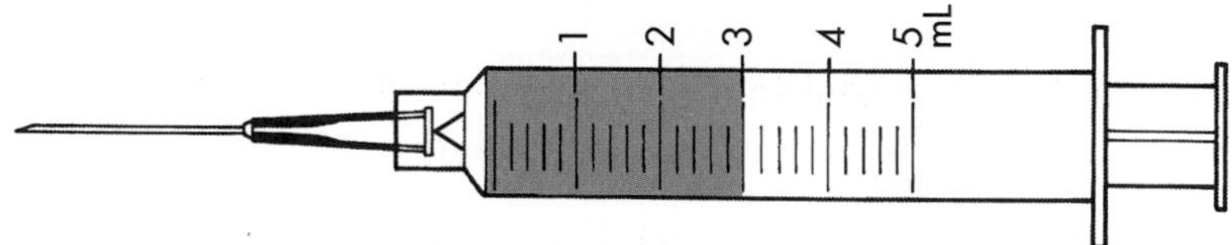

Single Dose Range Medications

Some single dose medications can indicate a minimum and maximum range.

Example 2: The prescriber orders Vistaril 15 mg IM q4h prn for nausea. The child weighs 38 lb. You need to determine if the dosage is safe.

The recommended dosage is 0.5 to 1 mg/kg/dose q4h prn from a reputable medication resource (e.g., *The Harriet Lane Handbook*).

1. Convert the child's weight in lb to kg and round to the nearest tenth of a kilogram.

✓ Solution Using Ratio and Proportion

$$2.2 \text{ lb} : 1 \text{ kg} = 38 \text{ lb} : x \text{ kg}$$

$$\frac{2.2x}{2.2} = \frac{38}{2.2}$$

$$x = \frac{38}{2.2} = 17.27$$

$$x = 17.3 \text{ kg}$$

$$\text{Child's weight} = 17.3 \text{ kg}$$

(rounded to the nearest tenth)

This could also be set up as a ratio proportion using a fraction format (refer to Chapter 4).

✓ Solution Using Dimensional Analysis

$$x \text{ kg} = \frac{1 \text{ kg}}{2.2 \cancel{\text{lb}}} \times \frac{38 \cancel{\text{lb}}}{1}$$

$$x = \frac{38}{2.2} = 17.27$$

$$x = 17.3 \text{ kg}$$

$$\text{Child's weight} = 17.3 \text{ kg}$$

(rounded to the nearest tenth)

2. Calculate the recommended dosage. Note the recommended dosage is stated as a range; 0.5 to 1 mg/kg/dose. Calculate the minimum and maximum safe dosage range. Multiply the mg/kg/dose by the child's weight in kg.

   Minimum per dose: $0.5 \text{ mg}/\cancel{\text{kg}}/\text{dose} \times 17.3 \cancel{\text{kg}} = 8.65 = 8.7 \text{ mg/dose}$ (rounded to nearest tenth)

   Maximum per dose: $1 \text{ mg}/\cancel{\text{kg}}/\text{dose} \times 17.3 \cancel{\text{kg}} = 17.3 \text{ mg/dose}$

This can also be done using ratio proportion and dimensional analysis.

✓ Solution Using Ratio and Proportion

$$0.5 \text{ mg} : 1 \text{ kg} = x \text{ mg} : 17.3 \text{ kg}$$
$$x = 8.65 = 8.7 \text{ mg/dose} \quad \text{(rounded to nearest tenth)}$$
$$\text{Answer} = 8.7 \text{ mg/dose}$$

$$1 \text{ mg} : 1 \text{ kg} = x \text{ mg} : 17.3 \text{ kg}$$
$$x = 17.3 \text{ mg/dose}$$
$$\text{Answer} = 17.3 \text{ mg/dose}$$

The safe dose range for a child weighing 17.3 kg is 8.7 mg to 17.3 mg/dose.

Remember that Ratio and Proportion can be stated in different formats.

✓ Solution Using Dimensional Analysis

Recommended dosages will be starting fraction, in this case (0.5 mg/kg and 1 mg/kg.)

$$\frac{x \text{ mg}}{\text{dose}} = \frac{0.5 \text{ mg}}{\cancel{\text{kg}}/\text{dose}} \times \frac{17.3 \cancel{\text{kg}}}{1}$$
$$x = 17.3 \times 0.5 = 8.65$$
$$x = 8.7 \text{ mg/dose} \quad \text{(rounded to nearest tenth)}$$
$$\text{Answer} = 8.7 \text{ mg/dose}$$

$$\frac{x \text{ mg}}{\text{dose}} \times \frac{1 \text{ mg}}{\cancel{\text{kg}}/\text{dose}} \times \frac{17.3 \cancel{\text{kg}}}{1}$$
$$x = 17.3 \times 1$$
$$x = 17.3 \text{ mg/dose}$$
$$\text{Answer} = 17.3 \text{ mg/dose}$$

The safe dose for a child weighing 17.3 kg is 8.7 mg to 17.3 mg/dose.

3. Decide if the dosage ordered is safe. The recommended dosage range is 8.7 mg to 17.3 mg/dose, and the ordered dosage of 15 mg is within the range. Yes, the ordered dosage is safe.
4. Calculate the dosage.
   Order: Vistaril 15 mg IM q4h prn for nausea.

   Available:

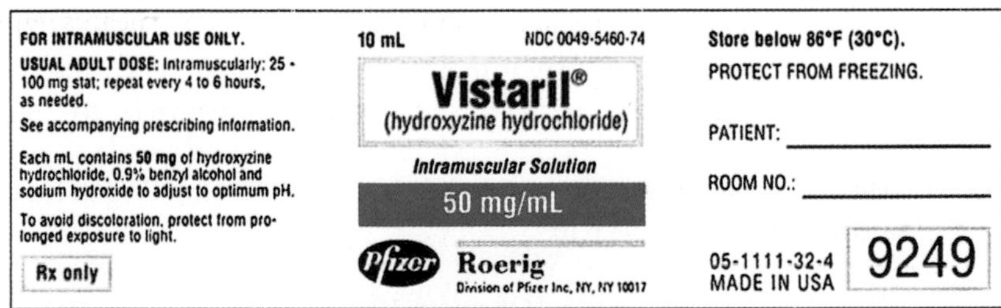

✓ Solution Using Ratio and Proportion

$$50 \text{ mg} : 1 \text{ mL} = 15 \text{ mg} : x \text{ mL}$$
$$\frac{50x}{50} = \frac{15}{50}$$
$$x = \frac{15}{50}$$
$$x = 0.3 \text{ mL}$$

✔ Solution Using Formula Method

$$\frac{15 \text{ mg}}{50 \text{ mg}} \times 1 \text{ mL} = x \text{ mL}$$

$$x = \frac{15}{50}$$

$$x = 0.3 \text{ mL}$$

✔ Solution Using Dimensional Analysis

$$x \text{ mL} = \frac{1 \text{ mL}}{50 \cancel{\text{mg}}} \times \frac{15 \cancel{\text{mg}}}{1}$$

$$x = \frac{15}{50}$$

$$x = 0.3 \text{ mL}$$

Measure dose using a 1 mL syringe.

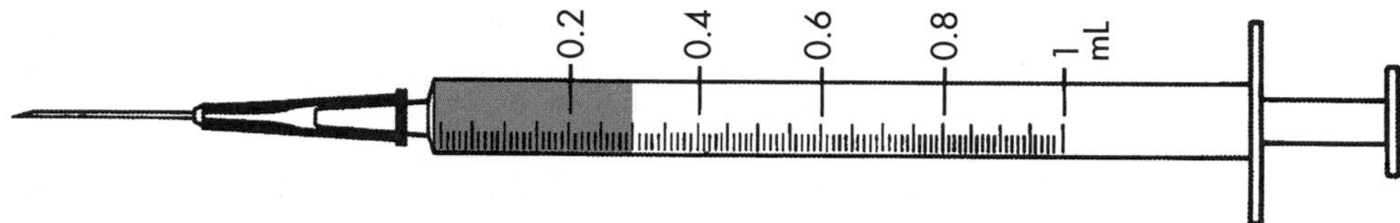

Now let's look at dosages that are around the clock. They are recommended as a total daily dosage, mg/kg/day, and divided into a number of dosages per day, such as "divided doses every 8 hours," "three divided doses," and so on. Three divided doses indicate the total daily dosage is divided equally and administered tid or q8h. If a medication states, for example, "four divided doses," this means the medication (total daily dose) is equally administered four times a day either qid or q6h. As you will see, with some medications, it may specify recommendations that dosage should be divided equally and administered q6h. Attention to time intervals for the day is important in determining whether a dosage is safe.

Example 3: The prescriber orders acetaminophen (Ofirmev) 700 mg IV q6h for pain for a child who weighs 94.6 lb.

Available: Acetaminophen (Ofirmev) 10 mg per mL

Recommended dosage from a reputable medication source (e.g., *The Harriet Lane Handbook*) for a child (age 2-12 years) or adolescent/adult weighing less than 50 kg is 15 mg/kg/dose q6h, or 12.5 mg/kg/dose q4h IV, up to a maximum of 75 mg/kg/24 hr.

Is the dosage ordered safe? If the dosage is safe, calculate the number of milliliters needed to add to the IV.

Step 1: Convert the child's weight in lb to kg; the recommended dosage is stated in kilograms.

This calculation can be done by setting up a ratio and proportion using the format of fractions or colons. Using this example, the setup as a ratio and proportion might be as follows:

✓ Solution Using Ratio and Proportion

$$2.2 \text{ lb} : 1 \text{ kg} = 94.6 \text{ lb} : x \text{ kg}$$
$$\frac{2.2x}{2.2} = \frac{94.6}{2.2}$$
$$x = \frac{94.6}{2.2}$$
$$x = 43 \text{ kg}$$

This calculation could also be done using dimensional analysis.

✓ Solution Using Dimensional Analysis

$$x \text{ kg} = \frac{1 \text{ kg}}{2.2 \cancel{\text{lb}}} \times \frac{94.6 \cancel{\text{lb}}}{1}$$
$$x = \frac{94.6}{2.2}$$
$$x = 43 \text{ kg}$$

Step 2: Calculate the recommended dosage. Note that the recommended dosage you will be using is for q6h and for a weight of less than 50 kg. Multiply the mg/kg/dose × the child's weight in kg. $15 \text{ mg}/\cancel{\text{kg}}/\text{dose} \times 43 \cancel{\text{kg}} = 645 \text{ mg/dose}$

This calculation can also be done by setting up a ratio and proportion or dimensional analysis.

✓ Solution Using Ratio and Proportion

$$15 \text{ mg} : 1 \text{ kg} = x \text{ mg} : 43 \text{ kg}$$
$$x = 645 \text{ mg/dose}$$

The safe dose range for a child weighing 43 kg is 645 mg/dose.

Remember that a ratio and proportion can be written in different formats.

✓ Solution Using Dimensional Analysis

The recommended dose is the starting fraction (in this case, 15 mg/kg/dose).

$$\frac{x \text{ mg}}{\text{dose}} = \frac{15 \text{ mg}}{\cancel{\text{kg}}/\text{dose}} \times \frac{43 \cancel{\text{kg}}}{1}$$
$$x = 15 \times 43$$
$$x = 645 \text{ mg/dose}$$

The safe dose for the child weighing 43 kg is 645 mg/dose.

Step 3: Decide if the dosage is safe by comparing the ordered and the recommended dosage. For this child's weight, 645 mg/dose is the recommended dosage. The dosage is not safe because the ordered dose of 700 mg q6h exceeds the recommended dosage. Remember that there may be factors that warrant a larger dose; call the prescriber to verify the dosage.

Because the dosage ordered is not safe, we will not be calculating the number of milliliters to add to the IV.

When dosages are compared for safety, it may be easiest to calculate how many total milligrams or micrograms are ordered. This way usually involves multiplication rather than division. This requires only one calculation, as opposed to two, and may decrease the chance of errors because fewer errors are usually made with multiplication than with division.

Example 4: Order: Gentamicin 50 mg IVPB q8h for a child weighing 40 lb. The recommended dosage for a child is 6 to 7.5 mg/kg/day divided q8h. Is the dosage ordered safe?

Step 1: First, a weight conversion is necessary because you have the child's weight in pounds and the reference is in kilograms. Convert the child's weight in pounds to kilograms and round to the nearest tenth.

✓ Solution Using Ratio and Proportion

$$2.2\text{ lb} : 1\text{ kg} = 40\text{ lb} : x\text{ kg}$$

$$\frac{\cancel{2.2}x}{\cancel{2.2}} = \frac{40}{2.2} \qquad x = \frac{40}{2.2} = 18.18$$

$$x = 18.2\text{ kg}$$

$$\text{Child's weight} = 18.2\text{ kg}$$

(rounded to the nearest tenth)

✓ Solution Using Dimensional Analysis

$$x\text{ kg} = \frac{1\text{ kg}}{2.2\ \cancel{\text{lb}}} \times \frac{40\ \cancel{\text{lb}}}{1}$$

$$x = \frac{40}{2.2} = 18.18$$

$$x = 18.2\text{ kg}$$

$$\text{Child's weight} = 18.2\text{ kg}$$

(rounded to the nearest tenth)

Step 2: Now that you have converted the weight, you can calculate the safe dosage. You must calculate and obtain a range. (The recommended dosage is 6 to 7.5 mg/kg/day.)

Therefore, calculate the range between the lower (minimum dosage) and upper (maximum dosage):

Minimum total daily dosage: 6 mg/$\cancel{\text{kg}}$/day × 18.2 $\cancel{\text{kg}}$ = 109.2 mg/day

Maximum total daily dosage: 7.5 mg/$\cancel{\text{kg}}$/day × 18.2 $\cancel{\text{kg}}$ = 136.5 mg/day

The safe dosage range for the child weighing 18.2 kg is 109.2-136.5 mg/day.

Note: Per day could be stated as daily or every 24 hours.

✓ Solution Using Ratio and Proportion

$$6\text{ mg} : 1\text{ kg} = x\text{ mg} : 18.2\text{ kg} \qquad 7.5\text{ mg} : 1\text{ kg} = x\text{ mg} : 18.2\text{ kg}$$

$$x = 109.2\text{ mg/day} \qquad x = 136.5\text{ mg/day}$$

The safe dosage range for the child weighing 18.2 kg is 109.2-136.5 mg/day.

✓ Solution Using Dimensional Analysis

$$\frac{x\text{ mg}}{\text{day}} = \frac{6\text{ mg}}{1\ \cancel{\text{kg}}/\text{day}} \times \frac{18.2\ \cancel{\text{kg}}}{1}$$

$$x = 18.2 \times 6$$

$$x = 109.2\text{ mg/day}$$

$$\frac{x\text{ mg}}{\text{day}} = \frac{7.5\text{ mg}}{\cancel{\text{kg}}/\text{day}} \times \frac{18.2\ \cancel{\text{kg}}}{1}$$

$$x = 18.2 \times 7.5$$

$$x = 136.5\text{ mg/day}$$

The safe dosage range for the child weighing 18.2 kg is 109.2 mg-136.5 mg/day.

Step 3: Now divide the total daily dosage by the number of times the medication will be given in a day.

$$q8h = 24 \div 8 = 3$$

Minimum total daily dosage: 109.2 mg ÷ 3 = 36.4 mg per dose

Maximum total daily dosage: 136.5 mg ÷ 3 = 45.5 mg per dose

The single dosage range is 36.4 to 45.5 mg/dose q8h. Now decide if the ordered dosage is safe. The ordered dosage is 50 mg, and the allowable, safe dosage range is 36.4 to 45.5 mg/dose q8h. The ordered dosage of 50 mg q8h exceeds the amount allowed per dose. No, the dosage is too high and not safe. Remember that factors such as the child's medical condition might warrant a larger dose. Contact the prescriber to discuss the order.

As discussed previously, you could eliminate the division to find the amount per dose by using the total daily dosage.

Calculate recommended minimum and maximum daily dosage range for this child.

You know the total daily dosage is divided into 3 doses in 24 hours.

Minimum total daily dosage: 6 mg/~~kg~~/day × 18.2 ~~kg~~ = 109.2 mg/day

Maximum total daily dosage: 7.5 mg/~~kg~~/day × 18.2 ~~kg~~ = 136.5 mg/day

Daily dosage according to this order: In this case
50 mg q8h = 50 mg/~~dose~~ × 3 ~~doses~~/day = 150 mg/day

Decide if the ordered daily dose is safe. The ordered daily dosage is 150 mg, and the allowable safe daily dosage is 109.2 to 136.5 mg/day. No, the dosage ordered is not safe, 150 mg/day exceeds the daily dosage range of 109.2 mg-136.5 mg/day.

Example 5: Order: Penicillin V Potassium 100 mg p.o. q6h for a child weighing 36 lb. According to *The Harriet Lane Handbook*, the recommended dosage of Penicillin V Potassium po for a child is 25-50 mg/kg/day ÷ q6-8 hr.

Is the dosage ordered safe? If the dosage is safe, calculate the number of milliliters needed to administer the dose.

Step 1: First, convert the child's weight in pounds to the nearest tenth of a kilogram.

✓ Solution Using Ratio and Proportion

$$2.2 \text{ lb} : 1 \text{ kg} = 36 \text{ lb} : x \text{ kg}$$

$$\frac{\cancel{2.2}x}{\cancel{2.2}} = \frac{36}{2.2}$$

$$x = \frac{36}{2.2} = 16.36$$

$$x = 16.4 \text{ kg} \quad \text{(rounded to the nearest tenth)}$$

$$\text{Child's weight} = 16.4 \text{ kg}$$

✓ Solution Using Dimensional Analysis

$$x\text{ kg} = \frac{1\text{ kg}}{2.2\not{\text{lb}}} \times \frac{36\not{\text{lb}}}{1}$$

$$x = \frac{36}{2.2} = 16.36$$

$$x = 16.4\text{ kg} \quad \text{(rounded to the nearest tenth)}$$

$$\text{Child's weight} = 16.4\text{ kg}$$

Step 2: Now that you have converted the weight to kilograms, you can calculate the safe dosage for this child. You must calculate and obtain a range. (The recommended dosage range is 25-50 mg/kg/day.)

Therefore, calculate the lower and upper range.

Minimum total daily dosage: 25 mg/~~kg~~/day × 16.4 ~~kg~~ = 410 mg/day

Maximum total daily dosage: 50 mg/~~kg~~/day × 16.4 ~~kg~~ = 820 mg/day

The safe dosage range for a child weighing 16.4 kg is 410 mg-820 mg/day.

✓ Solution Using Ratio and Proportion

$$25\text{ mg} : 1\text{ kg} = x\text{ mg} : 16.4\text{ kg} \qquad 50\text{ mg} : 1\text{ kg} = x\text{ mg} : 16.4\text{ kg}$$

$$x = 410\text{ mg/day} \qquad x = 820\text{ mg/day}$$

The safe dosage range for the child weighing 16.4 kg is 410 mg-820 mg/day.

✓ Solution Using Dimensional Analysis

$$\frac{x\text{ mg}}{\text{day}} = \frac{25\text{ mg}}{\not{\text{kg}}/\text{day}} \times \frac{16.4\not{\text{kg}}}{1}$$

$$x = 25 \times 16.4$$

$$x = 410\text{ mg/day}$$

$$\frac{x\text{ mg}}{\text{day}} = \frac{50\text{ mg}}{\not{\text{kg}}/\text{day}} \times \frac{16.4\not{\text{kg}}}{1}$$

$$x = 50 \times 16.4$$

$$x = 820\text{ mg/day}$$

The safe dosage range for the child weighing 16.4 kg is 410-820 mg/day.

If 100 mg is ordered q6h, is this a safe dosage?

$$24\text{ h} \div 6\text{ h} = 4\text{ doses per day}$$

$$100\text{ mg} \times 4\text{ doses} = 400\text{ mg per day}$$

The ordered dosage is not safe; it is below the recommended dosage. The ordered daily dosage is 400 mg (100 mg × 4 doses = 400 mg/day). The safe daily dosage is 410-820 mg/day.

Note: This could have also been done by finding the amount allowed per dose and then comparing it to what was ordered per dose; in this case, 100 mg per dose or q6h is ordered.

Although the dosage ordered is below the recommended dosage, it would not be considered safe. It is important to realize that even when small discrepancies exist between the safe dosage and what is ordered (e.g., in this problem, the safe minimum dosage is 410 mg, and the child is receiving 400 mg), the difference, although small, can be significant. The allowable dosage is 410-820 mg/day. The dosage ordered may not be sufficient to achieve the therapeutic effect. The prescriber should be notified. Underdosage of an antibiotic may cause a superinfection.

Step 3: Calculate the amount of medication needed to administer the ordered dosage.

Penicillin V Potassium oral solution is available in a dosage strength of 125 mg per 5 mL.

Because the dose ordered is not safe, we will not calculate the dose in this problem.

Example 6: The recommended dosage for neonates receiving Ampicillin is 75-150 mg/kg/day q8h. What is the safe daily dosage for an infant weighing 2,600 g? What is the safe dosage range to be administered q8h?

Step 1: Change the infant's weight in grams to kilograms. Reference expressed as mg/kg.

$$1{,}000 \text{ g} = 1 \text{ kg} \qquad \text{(conversion factor)}$$

$$1{,}000 \text{ g} : 1 \text{ kg} = 2{,}600 \text{ g} : x \text{ kg}$$

$$\frac{1{,}000x}{1{,}000} = \frac{2{,}6\cancel{00}}{1{,}0\cancel{00}}$$

$$\text{Infant's weight} = 2.6 \text{ kg}$$

$$\text{Decimal movement: } 2\underset{\smile\smile\smile}{600} = 2.6 \text{ kg}$$

✓ Solution Using Dimensional Analysis

$$x \text{ kg} = \frac{1 \text{ kg}}{1{,}000 \cancel{\text{g}}} \times \frac{2{,}600 \cancel{\text{g}}}{1}$$

$$x = \frac{2{,}6\cancel{00}}{1{,}0\cancel{00}}$$

$$x = 2.6 \text{ kg}$$

Step 2: Calculate the safe daily dosage.

Minimum total daily dosage: 75 mg/~~kg~~/day × 2.6 ~~kg~~ = 195 mg/day.

Maximum total daily dosage: 150 mg/~~kg~~/day × 2.6 ~~kg~~ = 390 mg/day.

Total daily dose is 195-390 mg/day.

Step 3: Calculate the dosage range to administer q8h.

$$24\text{h} \div \text{q8h} = 3 \text{ doses per day.}$$

Minimum divided dosage (q8h):

$$195 \text{ mg} \div 3 \text{ doses} = 65 \text{ mg/dose.}$$

Maximum divided dosage (q8h):

$$390 \text{ mg} \div 3 \text{ doses} = 130 \text{ mg/dose.}$$

The allowable safe dosage range q8h is 65-130 mg/dose.

The daily dosage could also be calculated using ratio and proportion or dimensional analysis (refer to examples previously given for setup of problem using these methods).

> **SAFETY ALERT!**
>
> Remember to avoid medication errors, it is imperative to calculate a safe dosage for a child and compare it with the dosage that has been ordered. Question dosages that are significantly low and unusually high before proceeding to administer them. Remember that the nurse is legally liable for any medication administered.

Adult Dosages Based on Body Weight

The information that has been provided regarding the calculation of dosages for children based on weight can also be applied to adults. Let's look at an example. Refer to the partial Ticar package insert.

TICAR®
brand of
sterile ticarcillin disodium
for Intramuscular or Intravenous Administration

DOSAGE AND ADMINISTRATION
Clinical experience indicates that in serious urinary tract and systemic infections, intravenous therapy in the higher doses should be used. Intramuscular injections should not exceed 2 grams per injection.
Adults:

Bacterial septicemia Respiratory tract infections Skin and soft-tissue infections Intra-abdominal infections Infections of the female pelvis and genital tract	200 to 300 mg/kg/day by I.V. infusion in divided doses every 4 or 6 hours. (The usual dose is 3 grams given every 4 hours [18 grams/day] or 4 grams given every 6 hours [16 grams/day] depending on weight and the severity of the infection.)
Urinary tract infections	
Complicated:	150 to 200 mg/kg/day by I.V. infusion in divided doses every 4 or 6 hours. (Usual recommended dosage for average [70 kg] adults: 3 grams q.i.d.)
Uncomplicated:	1 gram I.M. or direct I.V. every 6 hours.

Example: Order: Ticar 4 g IV q6h for a client with a respiratory tract infection. Client weighs 175 lb. Notice that the recommended dosage from the package insert for a respiratory tract infection is 200 to 300 mg/kg/day q4-6h. Is the dosage ordered safe?

Step 1: Convert the weight in pounds to kilograms.

$$2.2 \text{ lb} = 1 \text{ kg} \quad \text{(conversion factor)}$$

$$175 \text{ lb} \div 2.2 = 79.54 \text{ kg} = 79.5 \text{ kg} \quad \text{(rounded to the nearest tenth)}$$

Step 2: Calculate the recommended dosage.

Minimum total daily dosage: $200 \text{ mg}/\cancel{\text{kg}}/\text{day} \times 79.5\ \cancel{\text{kg}} = 15{,}900 \text{ mg/day}$.

Maximum total daily dosage: $300 \text{ mg}/\cancel{\text{kg}}/\text{day} \times 79.5\ \cancel{\text{kg}} = 23{,}850 \text{ mg/day}$.

15,900 mg to 23,850 mg/day is the recommended dosage per day.

Step 3: Determine the number of milligrams allowed per dosage.

Minimum dosage for each single dose: 15,900 mg ÷ 4 = 3,975 mg/dose

Maximum dosage for each single dose: 23,850 ÷ 4 = 5,962.5 mg/dose

3,975-5,962.5 mg/dose is allowed.

Step 4: Determine if the dosage is safe.

$$1{,}000 \text{ mg} = 1 \text{ g}$$
$$4 \text{ g} = 4{,}000 \text{ mg } (4 \times 1{,}000) = 4{,}000 \text{ mg}$$
$$4{,}000 \text{ mg} \times 4 \text{ doses} = 16{,}000 \text{ mg/day}$$

The ordered dosage of Ticar 4 g q6h is within the range of 15,900-23,850 mg/day and is safe.

PRACTICE **PROBLEMS**

Round weights and dosages to the nearest tenth where indicated. Use labels where provided to answer the questions.

26. A child weighs 35 lb and has an order for Keflex (cephalexin) 150 mg p.o. q6h.

Available:

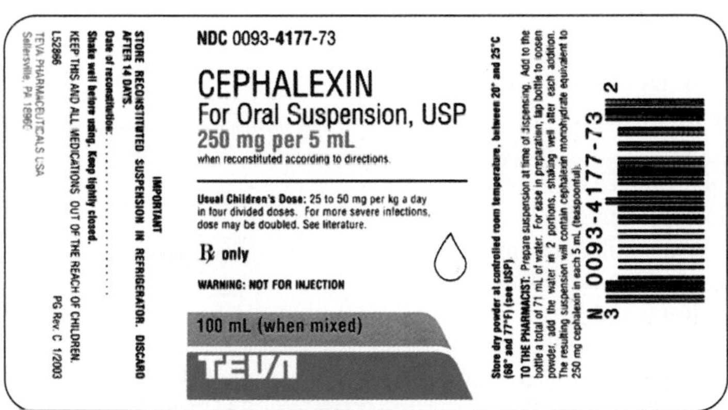

a. What is the recommended dosage in mg/kg/day? ______

b. What is the child's weight in kilograms to nearest tenth? ______

c. What is the safe dosage range for this child? ______

d. Is the dosage ordered safe? (Prove mathematically.) ______

e. How many milliliters will you administer for each dosage? ______

27. According to *The Harriet Lane Handbook*, the recommended dosage of Kanamycin IV for a child is 15-30 mg/kg/day divided q8-12 hr. Kanamycin 200 mg IV q8h is ordered for a child weighing 35 kg.

    a. What is the safe dosage for this child for 24 hours? ______________

    b. What is the divided dosage? ______________

    c. Is the dosage ordered safe? (Prove mathematically.) ______________

28. According to *The Harriet Lane Handbook*, the recommended dosage of clindamycin oral solution is 10-30 mg/kg/24 hr divided q6-8 hr. The child weighs 40 kg. (Base calculations on the medication being administered q6h.)

    a. What is the maximum dosage for this child in 24 hours? ______________

    b. What is the divided dosage range? ______________

29. Phenobarbital 10 mg p.o. q12h is ordered for a child weighing 9 lb. The recommended maintenance dosage is 3 to 5 mg/kg/day q12h.

    a. What is the child's weight in kilograms to the nearest tenth? ______________

    b. What is the safe dosage range for this child? ______________

    c. Is the dosage ordered safe? (Prove mathematically.) ______________

    d. Phenobarbital elixir is available in a dosage strength of 20 mg per 5 mL. What will you administer for one dosage? Calculate the dosage if it is safe. ______________

30. Morphine sulfate 7.5 mg subcut q4h p.r.n. is ordered for a child weighing 84 lb. The recommended maximum dose for a child is 0.1 to 0.2 mg/kg/dose.

    Available:

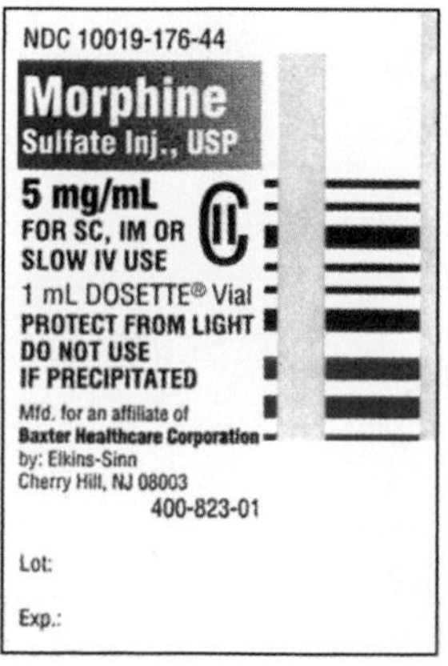

a. What is the child's weight in kilograms to the nearest tenth? ______

b. What is the safe dosage range for this child? ______

c. Is the dosage ordered safe? (Prove mathematically.) ______

d. How many milliliters will you administer for one dosage? ______

31. The recommended initial dosage of mercaptopurine is 2.5–5 mg/kg/day p.o. The child weighs 44 lb.

a. What is the child's weight in kilograms? ______

b. What is the initial safe daily dosage range for this child? ______

32. For a child the recommended dosage of IV vancomycin is 40 mg/kg/day. Vancomycin 200 mg IV q6h is ordered for a child weighing 38 lb.

a. What is the child's weight in kilograms to the nearest tenth? ______

b. What is the safe dosage for this child in 24 hours? ______

c. What is the divided dosage? ______

d. Is the dosage ordered safe? (Prove mathematically.) ______

33. A 44-lb child has an order for Erythromycin oral suspension 250 mg p.o. q6h. The usual dosage for children under 50 lb is 30 to 50 mg/kg/day in divided dosages q6h.

a. What is the child's weight in kilograms? ______

b. What is the safe range of dosage for this child in 24 hours? ______

c. Is the dosage ordered safe? (Prove mathematically.) ______

34. Refer to the Amphotericin B insert to calculate the dosage for an adult weighing 66.3 kg with good cardiorenal function. ______________________

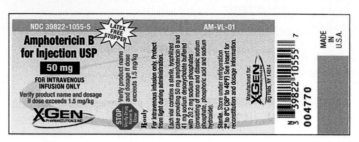

Partial Insert for Fungizone (Amphotericin B)

DOSAGE AND ADMINISTRATION

CAUTION: Under no circumstances should a total daily dose of 1.5 mg/kg be exceeded. Amphotericin B overdoses can result in cardio-respiratory arrest (see OVERDOSAGE).

FUNGIZONE Intravenous should be administered by *slow* intravenous infusion. Intravenous infusion should be given over a period of approximately 2 to 6 hours (depending on the dose) observing the usual precautions for intravenous therapy (see PRECAUTIONS, General). The recommended concentration for intravenous infusion is 0.1 mg/mL (1 mg/10 mL).

Since patient tolerance varies greatly, the dosage of amphotericin B must be individualized and adjusted according to the patient's clinical status (e.g., site and severity of infection, etiologic agent, cardio-renal function, etc.).

A single intravenous **test dose** (1 mg in 20 mL of 5% dextrose solution) administered over 20-30 minutes may be preferred. The patient's temperature, pulse, respiration, and blood pressure should be recorded every 30 minutes for 2 to 4 hours.

In patients with **good cardio-renal function** and a **well tolerated test dose**, therapy is usually initiated with a daily dose of 0.25 mg/kg of body weight. However, in those patients having **severe and rapidly progressive fungal infection**, therapy may be initiated with a daily dose of 0.3 mg/kg of body weight. In patients with **impaired cardio-renal function** or a **severe reaction to the test dose**, therapy should be initiated with smaller daily doses (i.e., 5 to 10 mg).

35. A 200-lb adult is to be treated with Ticar for a complicated urinary tract infection. The recommended dosage is 150 to 200 mg/kg/day IV in divided dosages every 4 or 6 hours.

    a. What is the adult's weight in kilograms to the nearest tenth? ______________________

    b. What is the daily dosage range in grams for this client? ______________________

36. A child with esophageal candidiasis weighs 12 lb, 6 oz. The recommended dose of IV fluconazole is 6 mg/kg on the first day, followed by 3 mg/kg once daily for 2 weeks.

    a. What is the child's weight in kilograms to the nearest tenth? ______________________

    b. What is the first dosage for this child? ______________________

    c. What is the subsequent dosage for this child? ______________________

Answers on pp. 710-711

POINTS TO REMEMBER

- To convert pounds to kilograms, divide by 2.2; express weight to the nearest tenth.
- To convert kilograms to pounds, multiply by 2.2; express weight to the nearest tenth.
- To convert grams to kilograms, divide by 1,000; round to the nearest tenth as indicated.
- To calculate dosages, the weight must be converted to the reference.
- To calculate the dosage based on weight, do the following:
  1. Determine the weight in kilograms if needed.
  2. Multiply the weight in kilograms by the recommended dosage.
  3. Divide the total daily dosage by the number of dosages needed to administer.
  4. Calculate the number of tablets or the volume to administer for each dosage by use of ratio and proportion, the formula method, or dimensional analysis.

- When the recommended dosage is given as a range, calculate based on the low and high values for each dosage.
- Question any discrepancies in dosages ordered and remember that factors such as age, weight, and medical conditions can cause the differences. Ask the prescriber to clarify the order when a discrepancy exists. Small discrepancies can be significant. Dosages that exceed the recommended dosage are not safe, and a dosage less than recommended is also unsafe because it may not achieve the intended therapeutic effect.
- Use appropriate resources to determine the safe range for a child's dosage. Compare the safe dosage with the dosage ordered to decide if the dosage is safe.

Calculating Pediatric Dosages Using Body Surface Area

Body Surface Area (BSA) is used to calculate safe dosages for infants, children, and selected adult populations. Examples of types of medications that may require BSA-based dosing include chemotherapy medications and medications given to clients who have severe burns, receiving radiation treatment, and those with renal disease. BSA is the total surface area of the body expressed in square meters (m^2). BSA is calculated using the height and weight measurements. BSA can be determined using a special BSA slide ruler, BSA calculator, Nomogram chart, or a mathematical formula. Figure 25-1 shows a BSA calculator and the BSA slide ruler. The BSA calculator can also be found on the internet.

We will discuss the use of the nomogram that estimates the BSA and a formula calculation to determine the BSA. The BSA is determined from the height and weight of a child and the use of the West Nomogram (Figure 25-2). This information is then applied to a formula for dosage calculations.

Remember that all children are not the same size at the same age; therefore, the West nomogram can be used to determine the BSA of a child. The West nomogram is not easy to use, although it is still employed in some institutions. The nomogram can be used to calculate the BSA for both children and adults for heights up to 240 cm (95 inches) and

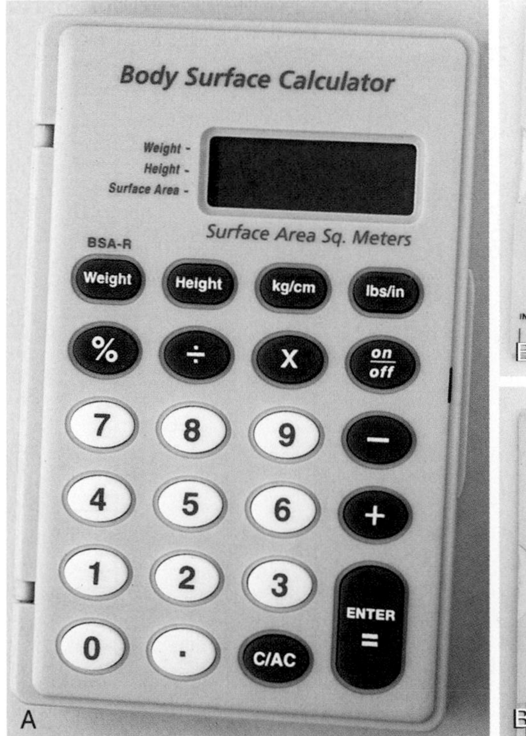

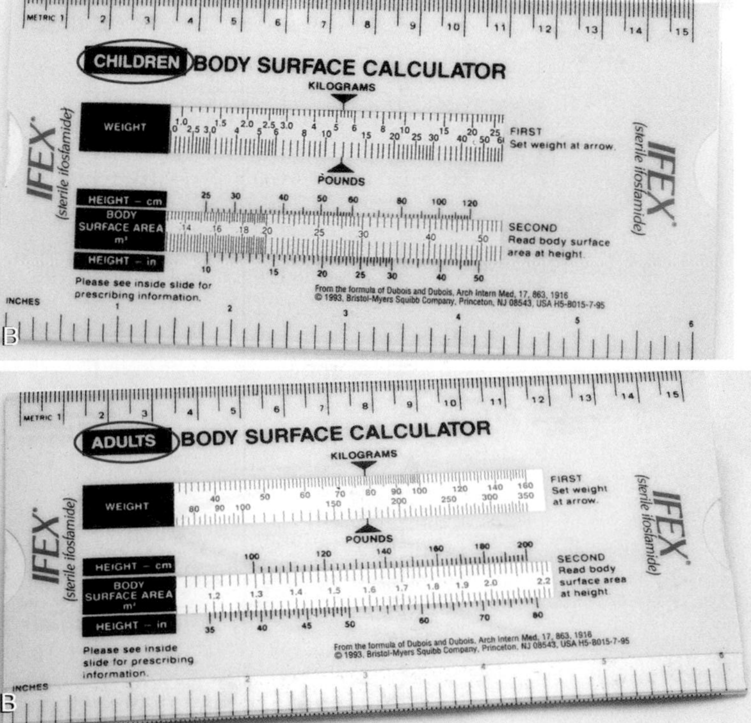

Figure 25-1 **A,** BSA Calculator. **B,** BSA slide ruler showing children's and adult side. (From Macklin D, Chernecky C, Infortuna H: *Math for clinical practice,* ed 2, St. Louis, 2011, Mosby.)

weights up to 80 kg (180 lb). The West Nomogram is the best-known BSA chart (see Figure 25-2). It is possible to determine the BSA from weight alone if the child is of normal height and weight.

> **SAFETY ALERT!**
>
> To use the normal column on the West Nomogram, you must be familiar with the normal height and weight standards for children. Check reliable resources such as a pediatric growth and development chart. Do not guess on the normal height and weight.

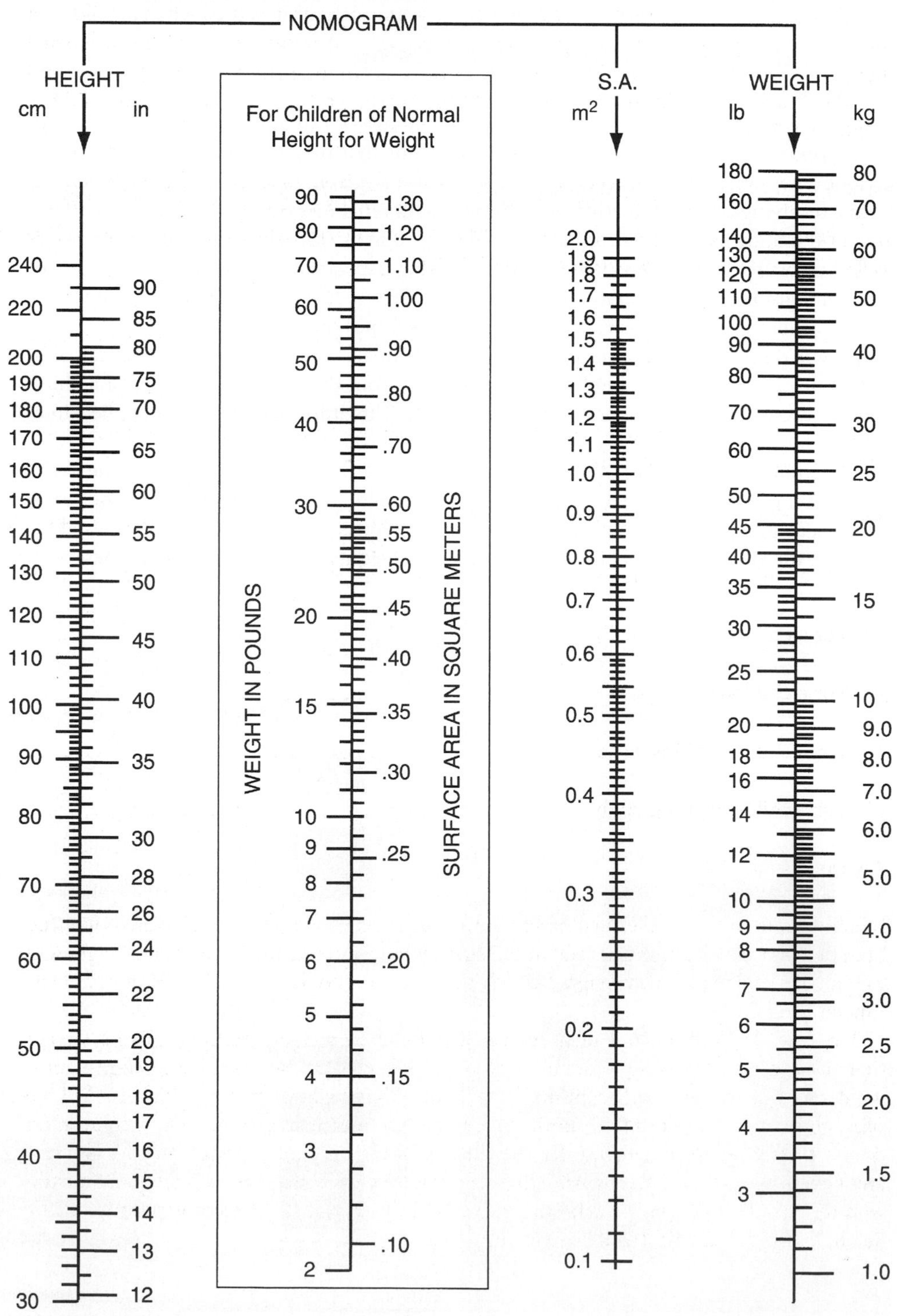

Figure 25-2 West Nomogram for estimation of body surface area. (From Kliegman RM, Stanton BF, St. Geme JW, Schor NF, Behrman RE: *Nelson textbook of pediatrics,* ed 20, Philadelphia, 2016, Saunders.)

Reading the West Nomogram Chart

Refer to Figure 25-2. It is important to note that the increments of measurement and the spaces on the BSA nomogram are not consistent. **Always read the numbers to determine what the calibrations are measuring.** For example, refer to the column for children of normal height and weight (second column from left); the calibrations between 15 and 20 lb are 1-lb increments. However, if you look at the bottom of the scale representing surface area in square meters, there are four calibrations between 0.10 and 0.15. Each line, therefore, is read as 0.11, 0.12, 0.13, etc. If the child is of a normal height and weight for his or her age, the BSA can be determined from weight alone. Notice the boxed column listing weight on the left and surface in square meters on the right; this is used when a child is of normal height for his or her weight. For example, a child weighing 70 lb and of normal height has a BSA of 1.10 m^2. If you look at the nomogram for a child who weighs 10 lb and use the nomogram column of normal height for weight, you will see that a 10-lb child has a BSA of 0.27 m^2.

SAFETY ALERT!

The increments and the spaces on the BSA nomogram are not consistent. Be certain that you read the numbers and the calibration values between them correctly.

PRACTICE PROBLEMS

Refer to the nomogram and determine the BSA (expressed in square meters) for the following children of normal height and weight.

37. For a child weighing 30 lb __________

38. For a child weighing 42 lb __________

39. For a child weighing 52 lb __________

40. For a child weighing 44 lb __________

41. For a child weighing 11 lb __________

42. For a child weighing 20 lb __________

Answers on p. 712

In addition to being determined based on weight, the BSA can also be calculated by using both height and weight. If you refer to the chart, you will notice the columns for height and weight. This chart includes weight in both pounds and kilograms and height in both centimeters and inches.

For children who are not of normal height for their weight, the scales at the far left (height) and far right (weight) are used. Notice that both of these scales have two measurements: centimeters and inches for height and pounds and kilograms for weight. To find the BSA, place a ruler extending from the height column on the left to the weight column on the far right. The estimated BSA for the child is where the line intersects the SA (surface area) column. For example, by using the far right and left scales, you will find that a child who weighs 50 lb and is 36 inches tall has a BSA of 0.8 m^2. If the ruler is slightly off the height or weight, the BSA will be incorrect.

PRACTICE PROBLEMS

Using the nomogram, calculate the following BSAs.

43. A child who is 90 cm long and weighs 50 lb ______________
44. A child who is 60 cm long and weighs 10 lb ______________
45. A child who is 100 cm long and weighs 10 kg ______________
46. A child who is 30 inches long and weighs 20 lb ______________
47. A child who weighs 60 lb and is 39 inches tall ______________
48. A baby who weighs 13 lb and is 19 inches long ______________
49. A child who weighs 30 lb and is 32 inches tall ______________
50. A child who weighs 13 kg and is 65 cm tall ______________
51. A child who is 90 cm long and weighs 40 lb ______________
52. A child who is 19 inches long and weighs 5 lb ______________

Answers on p. 712

Calculating Body Surface Area Using a Formula

As shown, BSA can be calculated using a nomogram; however, it is a tool that requires practice to use and can result in error if the ruler is just slightly offline. The BSA may also be obtained by using a mathematical formula. The height and weight are used (adults and children). There are two formulas used. The formula used is based on the units in which the measurements are obtained. One formula is based on metric measurement of height in centimeters and weight in kilograms. The other is based on household measurement of height in inches and weight in pounds. Common formulas for calculating BSA include:

- Metric BSA $(m^2) = \sqrt{\dfrac{\text{Weight (kg)} \times \text{Height (cm)}}{3{,}600}}$
- Household BSA $(m^2) = \sqrt{\dfrac{\text{Weight (lb)} \times \text{Height (in)}}{3{,}131}}$

Notice the difference in the formulas in addition to metric measures versus household is the difference in the denominators. Either formula is easy to use to calculate the BSA using the square-root function on the calculator. Calculators are increasingly being used for determination of critical care dosages and in pediatric units where extensive calculations may be required. BSA calculators are also available on the internet. It has been determined that the safest and most accurate way to calculate a BSA is to use a formula and a calculator that can perform square roots ($\sqrt{\ }$). Let's begin by looking at how the formulas are used.

Formula for Calculating BSA From Kilograms and Centimeters

Steps

1. Multiply the weight in kilograms by height in centimeters.
2. Divide the product obtained in Step 1 by 3,600.
3. Enter the square root sign into the calculator.
4. Round the final BSA in square meters to the nearest hundredth.

Formula

$$\text{Metric BSA (m}^2\text{)} = \sqrt{\frac{\text{Weight (kg)} \times \text{Height (cm)}}{3{,}600}}$$

Example 1: Calculate the BSA for a child who weighs 23 kg and whose height is 128 cm. Express BSA to the nearest hundredth.

$$(\text{m}^2) = \sqrt{\frac{23\ (\text{kg}) \times 128\ (\text{cm})}{3{,}600}} = \sqrt{0.817}$$

$$\sqrt{0.817} = 0.903 = 0.9\ \text{m}^2$$

The BSA was calculated as follows: 23 × 128 ÷ 3,600 = 0.817, then the square root ($\sqrt{\ }$) was entered. The final BSA in square meters was rounded to the nearest hundredth.

Example 2: Calculate the BSA for an adult who weighs 100 kg and whose height is 180 cm. Express BSA to the nearest hundredth.

$$(\text{m}^2) = \sqrt{\frac{100\ (\text{kg}) \times 180\ (\text{cm})}{3{,}600}} = \sqrt{5}$$

$$\sqrt{5} = 2.236 = 2.24\ \text{m}^2$$

Formula for Calculating Body Surface Area From Pounds and Inches

Steps

1. Multiply the weight in pounds by height in inches.
2. Divide the product obtained in step 1 by 3,131.
3. Enter the square root sign into the calculator.
4. Round the final BSA in square meters to the nearest hundredth.

Formula

$$\text{Household BSA (m}^2\text{)} = \sqrt{\frac{\text{Weight (lb)} \times \text{Height (in)}}{3{,}131}}$$

Example 1: Calculate the BSA for a child who weighs 25 lb and is 32 inches tall. Express the BSA to the nearest hundredth.

$$(\text{m}^2) = \sqrt{\frac{25\ (\text{lb}) \times 32\ (\text{in})}{3{,}131}} = \sqrt{0.255}$$

$$\sqrt{0.255} = 0.504 = 0.5\ \text{m}^2$$

Example 2: Calculate the BSA for an adult who weighs 143.7 lb and is 61.2 inches tall. Express the BSA to the nearest hundredth.

$$(\text{m}^2) = \sqrt{\frac{143.7\ (\text{lb}) \times 61.2\ (\text{in})}{3{,}131}} = \sqrt{2.808}$$

$$\sqrt{2.808} = 1.675 = 1.68\ \text{m}^2$$

SAFETY ALERT!

Round the final answer **only** to the nearest hundredth to obtain a more accurate BSA for medication dosage. When using a calculator, don't forget the last step of pressing the square-root function.

It is important to point out the slight variation in m^2 calculated by the metric and household methods because of rounding used to convert centimeters to inches: 1 inch = 2.54 cm, although it is rounded to 2.5 cm and used. Let's look at an example to illustrate this. Calculate the BSA of an adult whose weight is 95 kg (209 lb) and height is 180 cm (72 in).

Metric BSA

$$(\text{m}^2) = \sqrt{\frac{\text{Weight (kg)} \times \text{Height (cm)}}{3{,}600}} = \sqrt{\frac{95(\text{kg}) \times 180\ (\text{cm})}{3{,}600}} = \sqrt{4.75}$$

$$\sqrt{4.75} = 2.179 = 2.18\ \text{m}^2$$

Household BSA

$$(\text{m}^2) = \sqrt{\frac{\text{Weight (lb)} \times \text{Height (in)}}{3{,}131}} = \sqrt{\frac{209(\text{lb}) \times 72\ (\text{in})}{3{,}131}} = \sqrt{4.806}$$

$$\sqrt{4.806} = 2.192 = 2.19\ \text{m}^2$$

Notice that either metric or household measurement result in essentially the equivalent BSA.

Technological Advances

It is important to note that computer technology is being used more today and has made available applications that can be downloaded onto devices such as IPhones that can calculate the BSA after the data are input. The following are examples of websites that might be used:
http://medical.appdownloadreview.com/online/pasi-bsa-calculator
http://www.halls.md/body-surface-area/bsa.htm
http://www.pharmacologyweekly.com/app/medical-calculators/body-mass-index-bmi-weight-bsa-calculator

PRACTICE **PROBLEMS**

Determine the BSA for each of the following clients using a formula. Express the BSA to the nearest hundredth.

53. An adult whose weight is 95.5 kg and height is 180 cm ____________________

54. A child whose weight is 10 kg and height is 70 cm ____________________

55. A child whose weight is 4.8 lb and height is 21 inches ____________________

56. An adult whose weight is 170 lb and height is 67 inches ____________________

57. A child whose weight is 92 lb and height is 35 inches ____________________

58. A child whose weight is 24 kg and height is 92 cm ____________________

Answers on p. 712

SAFETY ALERT!

Always check a dosage against BSA in square meter recommendations using appropriate resources: for example, the PDR, medication inserts, or a pediatric medication handbook.

Medications, particularly chemotherapy agents, often provide the recommended dosage according to BSA in square meters.

Example: Cisplatin is an antineoplastic agent. The recommended pediatric/adult IV dosage for bladder cancer is 50 to 70 mg/m^2 every 3 to 4 weeks. For carmustine, which is used to treat Hodgkin disease and brain tumors, the recommended IV dosage for an adult is 150 to 200 mg/m^2.

POINTS TO REMEMBER

- The formula method to calculate BSA is more accurate than use of the nomogram.
- The formulas used to calculate BSA are as follows:

$$\text{Metric BSA (m}^2\text{)} = \sqrt{\frac{\text{Weight (kg)} \times \text{Height (cm)}}{3{,}600}}$$

$$\text{Household BSA (m}^2\text{)} = \sqrt{\frac{\text{Weight (lb)} \times \text{Height (in)}}{3{,}131}}$$

Determining BSA with a Formula Requires Use of a Calculator

- Multiply height × weight (cm × kg, or lb × inches).
- Divide by 3,600 or 3,131, depending on the units of measure (divide by 3,600 if measures are in metric units [cm, kg] and by 3,131 if measures are in household units [inches, lb]).
- Enter the ($\sqrt{\ }$) (square root sign) to arrive at BSA in square meters.
- Round square meters to hundredths (two decimal places).
- There are applications available today that can be downloaded onto mobile devices that have computer programs that calculate the BSA.

Dosage Calculation Based on Body Surface Area

If you know the child's BSA, the dosage is calculated by multiplying the recommended dosage by the child's BSA (m^2).

Example 1: The recommended dosage is 3 mg per m^2. The child has a BSA of 1.2 m^2.

$$1.2\ \cancel{m^2} \times \frac{3\text{ mg}}{\cancel{m^2}} = 3.6\text{ mg}$$

✓ Solution Using Dimensional Analysis

$$x\text{ mg} = \frac{3\text{ mg}}{\cancel{m^2}} \times \frac{1.2\ \cancel{m^2}}{1}$$

$$x = 1.2 \times 3$$

$$x = 3.6\text{ mg}$$

Example 2: The recommended dose is 30 mg per m^2. The child has a BSA of 0.75 m^2.

$$0.75\ \cancel{m^2} \times \frac{30\text{ mg}}{\cancel{m^2}} = 22.5\text{ mg}$$

✓ Solution Using Dimensional Analysis

$$x \text{ mg} = \frac{30 \text{ mg}}{\cancel{m^2}} \times \frac{0.75 \cancel{m^2}}{1}$$
$$x = 30 \times 0.75$$
$$x = 22.5 \text{ mg}$$

To do the calculation with dimensional analysis, use the recommended dosage given to convert the BSA to dosage in milligrams, as the first fraction.

Calculating Using a Formula

A child's BSA is expressed in square meters (m^2) and inserted into the formula below.

Formula

$$\frac{\text{BSA of child } (m^2)}{1.7\ (m^2)} \times \text{Adult dosage} = \text{Estimated child's dosage}$$

RULE

If only the recommended dosage for an adult is cited, then the formula is used to calculate the child's dosage. The formula uses the average adult dosage, the average adult BSA (1.7 m^2), and the child's BSA in square meters.

Example 1: The prescriber has ordered a medication for which the average adult dosage is 125 mg. What will the dosage be for a child with a BSA of 1.4 m^2?

$$\frac{1.4 \cancel{m^2}}{1.7\ (\cancel{m^2})} \times 125 \text{ mg} = 102.94 \text{ mg} = 102.9 \text{ mg (round to the nearest tenth)}$$

Example 2: The adult dosage for a medication is 100 to 300 mg. What will the dosage range be for a child with a BSA of 0.5 m^2?

$$\frac{0.5 \cancel{m^2}}{1.7\ (\cancel{m^2})} \times 100 \text{ mg} = 29.41 \text{ mg} = 29.4 \text{ mg (rounded to nearest tenth)}$$
$$\frac{0.5 \cancel{m^2}}{1.7\ (\cancel{m^2})} \times 300 \text{ mg} = 88.23 \text{ mg} = 88.2 \text{ mg (rounded to nearest tenth)}$$

The dosage range is 29.4-88.2 mg.

PRACTICE **PROBLEMS**

Using the West nomogram chart when indicated, calculate the child's dosage for the following medications. Express your answer to the nearest tenth.

59. The child's height is 32 inches, and weight is 25 lb. The recommended adult dosage is 25 mg.

    a. What is the child's BSA? ________________

    b. What is the child's dosage? ________________

60. The child's height is 100 cm and weight is 10 kg. The adult dosage is 200 to 400 mg.

    a. What is the child's BSA? ______________________

    b. What is the child's dosage range? ______________________

61. The normal adult dosage of a medication is 5 to 15 mg. What will the dosage range be for a child whose BSA is 1.5 m^2? ______________________

62. 5 mg of a medication is ordered for a child with a BSA of 0.8 m^2. The average adult dosage is 20 mg. Is this a correct dosage? (Prove mathematically.) ______________________

63. 7 mg of a medication is ordered for a child with a BSA of 0.9 m^2. The average adult dosage is 25 mg. Is this correct? (Prove mathematically.) ______________________

64. An antibiotic for which the average adult dosage is 250 mg is ordered for a child with a BSA of 1.5 m^2. What will the child's dosage be? ______________________

65. The recommended adult dosage of a medication is 20 to 30 mg. The child has a BSA of 0.74 m^2. What will the child's dosage range be? ______________________

66. The child's weight is 20 lb and height is 30 inches. The adult dosage of a medication is 500 mg.

    a. What is the child's BSA? ______________________

    b. What is the child's dosage? ______________________

67. The recommended adult dosage for an antibiotic is 500 mg 4 times a day. The child's BSA is 1.3 m^2. What will the child's dosage be? ______________________

Answers on pp. 712-713

POINTS TO REMEMBER

- BSA is determined from the West nomogram by using the child's height and weight and is expressed in square meters.
- The BSA can also be determined by using a formula and calculator. The formula used depends on the units in which measurements are obtained.

$$\text{Metric BSA (m}^2\text{)} = \sqrt{\frac{\text{Weight (kg)} \times \text{Height (cm)}}{3{,}600}}$$

$$\text{Household BSA (m}^2\text{)} = \sqrt{\frac{\text{Weight (lb)} \times \text{Height (in)}}{3{,}131}}$$

- The normal height and weight column on the West nomogram is used only when the child's height and weight are within normal limits.
- When you know the child's BSA, the dosage is determined by multiplying the BSA by the recommended dosage. (This is used when the recommended dosage is written by using the average dosage per square meter.) Dimensional analysis can also be used with the recommended dosage as the equivalent fraction.
- To determine whether a child's dosage is safe, a comparison must be made between what is ordered and the calculation of the dosage based on BSA.
- If only the recommended dosage for an adult is cited, then the formula is used to calculate the child's dosage. The formula uses the average adult dosage, the average adult BSA (1.7 m^2), and the child's BSA in square meters.

$$\frac{\text{BSA of child (m}^2\text{)}}{1.7\ (\text{m}^2)} \times \text{Adult dosage} = \text{Estimated child's dosage}$$

- If a dosage seems to be unsafe, consult the prescriber before administering the dose.

IV Therapy and Children

Pediatric IV Administration

Administration of IV fluids to children is very specific because of their physiological development. Microdrop sets are used for infants and small children; electronic devices are used to control the rate of delivery. The rate of infusion for infants and children must be carefully monitored. The IV drop rate must be slow for small children to prevent complications such as cardiac failure because of fluid overload. Various IV devices decrease the size of the drop to "mini" or "micro" drop or 1/60 mL, thus delivering 60 minidrops or microdrops per milliliter. IV medications may be administered to a child over a period of time (several hours) or on an intermittent basis. For intermittent medication administration, several methods of delivery are used, including the following:

Small-volume IV bags—These may be used if the child has a primary IV line in place. A secondary tubing set is attached to a small-volume IV bag, and the piggyback method is used.

Volume Control Sets—are used frequently to administer IV fluids hourly and intermittent IV medications to children. These are often referred to by their trade name which include: Buretrol, Volutrol or Soluset. A volume control set consists of a calibrated chamber with a 150 mL capacity that connects to an IV solution. (Figure 25-3 shows a typical system that consists of a calibrated chamber.) When used to regulate IV fluid infusion, the nurse fills the chamber every one to two hours as needed. The chamber is calibrated in small increments. Small, prescribed amounts of fluid are added to the chamber, and the clamp above the chamber is fully closed. This protects the client from receiving more fluid than intended. This is especially important with children.

For the intermittent medication administration, the nurse injects the medication through the injection port at the top of the chamber, and adds an appropriate amount of IV fluid to dilute the medication, and it is infused over a specific period of time (see Figure 25-3). An IV flush (small amount of IV fluid) is administered immediately after the medication is infused.

An electronic controller or pump may also be used to administer intermittent IV medications. When used, the electronic device sounds an alarm when the Buretrol chamber is empty. Volume control devices may also be used in the adult setting for clients with fluid restrictions.

SAFETY ALERT!

IV infusions should be monitored as frequently as every hour. A solution to flush the IV tubing is administered after the medication.

Regardless of the method used for medication administration in children, **a solution to flush the IV tubing is administered after the medication.** The purpose of the flush is to make sure the medication has cleared the tubing and the total dosage has been administered. Most institutions flush with normal saline solution as opposed to heparin. The amount of fluid used varies according to the length of the tubing from the medication source to the infusion site. **When IV medications are diluted for administration, the policy for including medication volume as part of the volume specified for dilution varies from institution to institution, as does the amount of flush. When flow rates (gtt/min, mL/hr) are calculated, it varies from institution to institution as to whether the flush is included. The nurse is responsible for checking the protocol at the institution to ensure that the correct procedure is followed.**

Note: In the sample calculations that follow, a 15-mL volume will be used as a flush unless otherwise specified, and the medication volume will be considered as part of the total dilution volume. The flush will not be considered in the total volume.

SAFETY ALERT!

An excessively high concentration of an IV medication can cause vein irritation and potentially life-threatening effects. Dilution calculation is essential for the nurse.

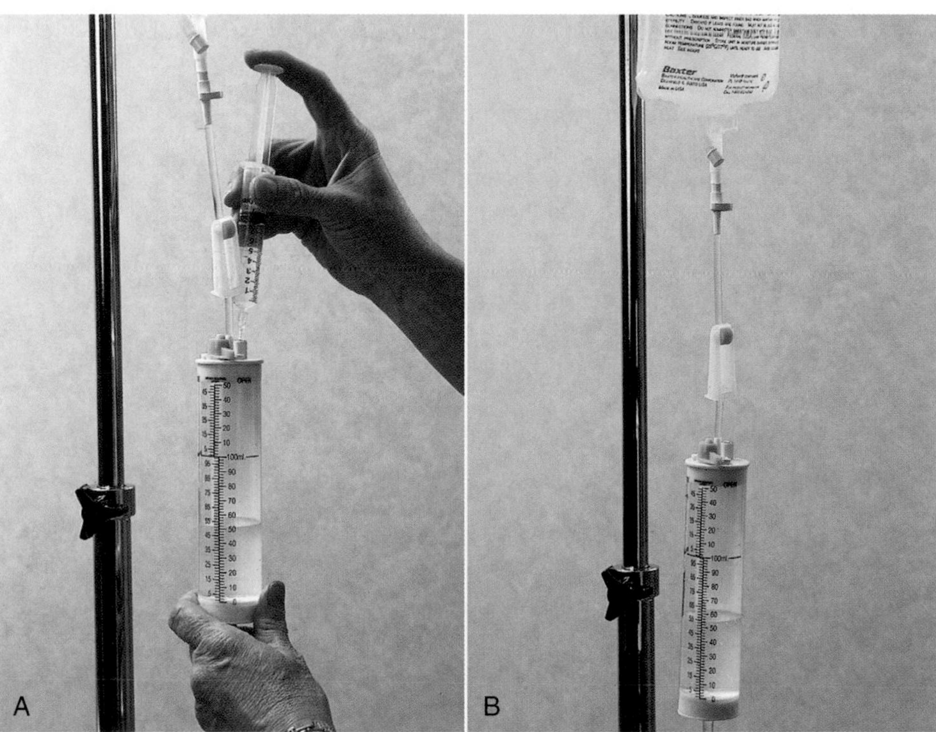

Figure 25-3 Volume-controlled device (buretrol). (From Potter PA, Perry AG, Stockert P, Hall A: *Essentials for Nursing Practice,* ed 8, St Louis, 2015, Mosby.)

Calculating IV Medications Using Volume Control Set

A calibrated buretrol can be used to administer medications by using a roller clamp rather than a pump. In this case, it is necessary to use the formula presented in Chapter 22 or dimensional analysis and calculate gtt/min. Remember, buretrols are volume control devices and have a drop factor of 60 gtt/mL.

$$x \text{ gtt/min} = \frac{\text{Total volume (mL)} \times \text{drop factor (gtt/mL)}}{\text{Time in minutes}}$$

Example: An antibiotic dose of 100 mg in 2 mL is to be diluted in 20 mL of D5W to infuse over 30 minutes. A 15-mL flush follows. The administration set is a microdrop (buretrol). (The policy of the institution is to treat the medication volume as part of the total dilution volume.)

Step 1: Read the medication label, and determine what volume the 100 mg dosage is contained in. This is 2 mL.

Step 2: Allow 18 mL of D5W to run into the buretrol, and then add the 2 mL containing the 100 mg of medication. Roll the buretrol between your hands to allow medication to mix thoroughly. (2 mL + 18 mL = 20 mL for volume.)

Step 3: Determine the flow rate necessary to deliver the medication plus the flush in 30 minutes.

Total volume is 20 mL. Infusion time is 30 minutes.

$$x \text{ gtt/min} = \frac{20 \text{ mL (diluted medication)} \times 60 \text{ gtt/mL}}{30 \text{ min}}$$

$$x = \frac{20 \times \overset{2}{\cancel{60}}}{\underset{1}{\cancel{30}}} = 40 \text{ gtt/min}$$

$$x = 40 \text{ gtt/min}$$

Answer: $x = 40$ gtt/min; 40 microgtt/min

Note: If the flush is considered with the intermittent medication, note that the total volume will be diluted medication + flush, and then proceed with calculation (gtt/min, mL/hr).

✓ Solution Using Dimensional Analysis

To calculate gtt/min (refer to steps in Chapter 22 if necessary):

$$\frac{x \text{ gtt}}{\text{min}} = \frac{\overset{20}{\cancel{60}} \text{ gtt}}{1 \cancel{\text{mL}}} \times \frac{\overset{2}{\cancel{20}} \cancel{\text{mL}}}{\underset{\underset{1}{\cancel{3}}}{\cancel{30}} \text{ min}}$$

$$x = \frac{40}{1}$$

$$x = 40 \text{ gtt/min; } 40 \text{ microgtt/min}$$

Step 4: Adjust the IV flow rate to deliver 40 microgtt/min (40 gtt/min).

Step 5: Label the buretrol with the medication name, dosage, and medication infusing label.

Step 6: When administration of the medication is completed, add the 15-mL flush, and continue to infuse at 40 microgtt/min. Replace the label with a flush infusing label.

Step 7: When the flush is completed, restart the primary line and remove the flush infusing label. Document the medication according to institution policy on the medication administration record (MAR) or in the computer and the volume of fluid on the intake and output (I&O) sheet according to agency policy.

TIPS FOR CLINICAL PRACTICE

To express the volume of gtt/min in mL/hr, remember that a microdrop administration set delivers 60 gtt/mL; therefore, gtt/min = mL/hr. In this case, if the gtt/min = 40, then the mL/hr = 40.

As already mentioned, the buretrol can be used along with an electronic controller or pump. When used as previously stated, the electronic device will sound an alarm each time the buretrol empties. Let's examine the calculation necessary if the buretrol is used along with the pump or a controller. Calculations for which the buretrol is used with a pump or controller are done in mL/hr. Let's use the same example shown previously to illustrate the difference in calculation steps.

Example 1: An antibiotic dose of 100 mg in 2 mL is to be diluted in 20 mL of D5W to infuse over 30 minutes. A 15-mL flush follows. An infusion controller is used, and the tubing is a microdrop buretrol.

The same Steps 1 and 2 as shown in the previous example for buretrol only are followed.

Step 1: Calculate the flow rate for this microdrop.

Total volume is 20 mL; the flush is not considered in the volume.

Step 2: Total volume is 20 mL. Infusion time is 30 minutes. Use a ratio and proportion or dimensional analysis to calculate the rate in mL/hr.

✓ Solution Using Ratio and Proportion

$$20 \text{ mL} : 30 \text{ minutes} = x \text{ mL} : 60 \text{ minutes}$$

$$30x = 60 \times 20$$

$$\frac{30x}{30} = \frac{1{,}20\not{0}}{3\not{0}} = 40 \text{ mL/hr}$$

$$x = 40 \text{ mL/hr}$$

Answer: Set the controller to infuse at 40 mL/hr.

✓ Solution Using Dimensional Analysis

To calculate mL/hr (refer to steps in Chapter 22 if necessary):

$$\frac{x \text{ mL}}{\text{hr}} = \frac{20 \text{ mL}}{\overset{}{\underset{1}{\cancel{30}}} \cancel{\text{min}}} \times \frac{\overset{2}{\cancel{60}} \cancel{\text{min}}}{1 \text{ hr}}$$

$$x = \frac{40}{1}$$

$$x = 40 \text{ mL/hr}$$

Example 2: An antibiotic dose of 150 mg in 1 mL is to be diluted in 35 mL NS to infuse over 45 minutes. A 15-mL flush follows. A volumetric pump will be used.

Total volume is 35 mL. Infusion time is 45 minutes. Calculate mL/hr rate.

✔ Solution Using Ratio and Proportion

$$35 \text{ mL} : 45 \text{ minutes} = x \text{ mL} : 60 \text{ minutes}$$

$$45x = 35 \times 60$$

$$\frac{45x}{45} = \frac{2{,}100}{45} = 46.6$$

$$x = 47 \text{ mL/hr}$$

Answer: Set the pump to infuse at 47 mL/hr.

✔ Solution Using Dimensional Analysis

$$\frac{x \text{ mL}}{\text{hr}} = \frac{35 \text{ mL}}{\cancelto{3}{45} \cancel{\text{min}}} \times \frac{\cancelto{4}{60} \cancel{\text{min}}}{1 \text{ hr}}$$

$$x = \frac{140}{3} = 46.6$$

$$x = 47 \text{ mL/hr}$$

Set the pump to infuse at 47 mL/hr.

PRACTICE **PROBLEMS**

Determine the volume of solution that must be added to the buretrol in the following problems. Then determine the flow rate in gtt/min for each IV using a microdrop, and indicate mL/hr for a controller. (For all problems, use the medication volume as part of the total diluent volume.)

68. An IV medication dosage of 500 mg is ordered to be diluted to 30 mL and infuse over 50 minutes with a 15 mL flush to follow. The dosage of medication is contained in 3 mL. Determine the following:

    a. Dilution volume ____________

    b. Rate in gtt/min ____________

    c. Rate in mL/hr ____________

69. The volume of a 20 mg dosage of medication is 2 mL. Dilute to 15 mL, and administer over 45 minutes with a 15 mL flush to follow. Determine the following:

    a. Dilution volume ____________

    b. Rate in gtt/min ____________

    c. Rate in mL/hr ____________

Answers on p. 713

Determining Whether an IV Dose Is Safe for Children

As seen earlier in this chapter, medications can be calculated based on mg/kg or body surface area (BSA). IV dosages for children are calculated on that basis as well. The IV medication can be assessed to determine if it is within normal range as well. The safe daily dosage is calculated and then compared with the order.

To determine whether an IV dosage for a child is safe, consult an appropriate medication resource for the recommended dosage. Remember to carefully read the reference to determine if the medication is calculated according to BSA in square meters (common with chemotherapy drugs), micrograms, or units per day or per hour. When a dosage is within the normal limits, calculate and administer the dosage. If a dosage is not within the normal limits, consult the prescriber before administering the medication. *Note:* If the order is based on the child's BSA and the BSA is not known, you will need to use the West nomogram or the formula presented and determine the BSA. Let's look at some examples.

Example 1: A child's BSA is 0.8 m^2, and the order is for 1.8 mg of a medication in 100 mL D5W at 10 AM. The recommended dosage is 2 mg/m^2.

Step 1: As previously shown in this chapter, if BSA is known, calculate the dosage for the child by multiplying the recommended dosage by the BSA. The recommended dosage is 2 mg/m^2, and the child's BSA is 0.8 m^2.

$$0.8\ \cancel{m^2} \times 2\ \text{mg}/\cancel{m^2} = 1.6\ \text{mg}$$

Step 2: Determine if the dosage is within the normal range.

The safe dosage is 1.6 mg for this child, but 1.8 mg is ordered. Notify the prescriber before administering the dosage. *Note:* The dosage in this example can also be determined by using dimensional analysis.

✓ Solution Using Dimensional Analysis

$$x\ \text{mg} = \frac{2\ \text{mg}}{\cancel{m^2}} \times \frac{0.8\ \cancel{m^2}}{1}$$

$$x = 1.6\ \text{mg}$$

Example 2: A child weighing 10 kg has an order for IV Solu-Medrol 125 mg IV q6h for 48 hours. The recommended dosage is 30 mg/kg/day IV and can be divided into doses q4-6h for 48 hours.

Step 1: Determine the dosage for the child.

$$10\ \cancel{\text{kg}} \times 30\ \text{mg}/\cancel{\text{kg}}/\text{day} = 300\ \text{mg/day}$$

Step 2: Determine if the dosage ordered is within normal range.

The dosage: 125 mg q6h (4 doses).

$$125\ \text{mg} \times 4 = 500\ \text{mg/day}$$

Check with the prescriber; the dosage is more than what the child should receive. *Note:* The dosage in this example can also be determined by using dimensional analysis.

✓ Solution Using Dimensional Analysis

$$\frac{x\ \text{mg}}{\text{kg}} = \frac{30\ \text{mg}}{1\ \cancel{\text{kg}}/\text{day}} \times \frac{10\ \cancel{\text{kg}}}{1}$$

$$x = 300\ \text{mg/day}$$

PRACTICE PROBLEMS

Determine the normal dosage range for the following problems to the nearest tenth. State your course of action.

70. A child weighing 17 kg has an order for an IV of 250 mL D5W containing 2,500 units of medication, which is to infuse at 50 mL/hr. The recommended dosage for the medication is 10 to 25 units/kg/hr. Determine whether the dosage ordered is within normal limits. ____________________

71. A child with a BSA of 0.75 m^2 has an order for 84 mg IV of a medication in 100 mL D5W q12h. The recommended dosage is 100 to 250 mg/m^2/day in two divided doses. Determine whether the dosage ordered is within normal limits. ____________________

Answers on p. 713

Calculation of Daily Fluid Maintenance

Fluid overload or dehydration can pose a great threat to infants or young children. Nurses, therefore, must monitor not only the amount of medication but also the amount of fluid a child receives. To prevent fluid overload or dehydration, nurses must closely monitor the amount of fluid a child receives. The fluid a child receives over a 24-hour period is referred to as daily fluid maintenance needs (amount of fluid needed to maintain normal hydration). Daily fluid maintenance is also sometimes referred to as daily fluid requirements (DFR). The daily fluid maintenance includes both oral and parenteral fluids. The amount of maintenance fluid required depends on the weight of the child expressed in kilograms (kg). It does not include replacement for losses through vomiting, diarrhea, or fever. (See Table 25-1 for formula used to calculate the daily fluid maintenance.)

TABLE 25-1 Daily Fluid Maintenance Formula

- 100 mL/kg/day for the first 10 kg of body weight
- 50 mL/kg/day for the next 10 kg of body weight
- 20 mL/kg/day for each kg above 20 kg of body weight

Let's look at examples calculating the daily fluid maintenance and the hourly rate. (The IV pump is programmable in whole numbers.)

Example 1: Child who weighs 7 kg

$$100 \text{ mL/}\cancel{\text{kg}}\text{/day} \times 7 \cancel{\text{kg}} = 700 \text{ mL/day or per 24 hr}$$

$$x \text{ mL/hr} = \frac{700 \text{ mg}}{24 \text{ hr}} = 29.1$$

$$x = 29 \text{ mL/hr}$$

Example 2: Child weighs 14 kg

$$100\text{ mL}/\cancel{\text{kg}}/\text{day} \times 10\ \cancel{\text{kg}} = 1{,}000\text{ mL/day (for first 10 kg)}$$
$$50\text{ mL}/\cancel{\text{kg}}/\text{day} \times 4\ \cancel{\text{kg}} = 200\text{ mL/day (for remaining 4 kg)}$$
$$\text{Total: } 1{,}000\text{ mL/day} + 200\text{ mL/day} = 1{,}200\text{ mL/day or per 24 hr}$$
$$x\text{ mL/hr} = \frac{1{,}200\text{ mL}}{24\text{ hr}}$$
$$x = 50\text{ mL/hr}$$

Example 3: A child weighs 35 lb

Step 1: Convert 35 lb to kg

$$\text{Conversion factor: } 2.2\text{ lb} = 1\text{ kg}$$
$$35\text{ lb} \div 2.2 = 15.9\text{ kg}$$

Step 2: Apply formula to calculate the daily fluid maintenance.

$$100\text{ mL}/\cancel{\text{kg}}/\text{day} \times 10\ \cancel{\text{kg}} = 1{,}000\text{ mL/day (for first 10 kg)}$$
$$50\text{ mL}/\cancel{\text{kg}}/\text{day} \times 5.9\ \cancel{\text{kg}} = 295\text{ mL/day (for remaining 5.9 kg)}$$
$$\text{Total: } 1{,}000\text{ mL/day} + 295\text{ mL/day} = 1{,}295\text{ mL/day or per 24 hr}$$
$$x\text{ mL/hr} = \frac{1{,}295\text{ mL}}{24\text{ hr}} = 53.9$$
$$x - 54\text{ mL/hr}$$

Note: In addition to the methods shown, ratio and proportion and Dimensional Analysis may bc uscd to calculate the Daily Fluid Maintenance.

PRACTICE **PROBLEMS**

Determine the Daily Fluid Maintenance and the hourly rate. (IV pump is programmable in whole numbers.)

72. Child weighs 13 kg

 a. Daily fluid maintenance ______________________ mL/day

 b. rate ______________________ mL/hr

73. Infant weighing 3,300 g

 a. Daily fluid maintenance ______________________ mL/day

 b. rate ______________________ mL/hr

Answers on p. 713

POINTS TO REMEMBER

IV Therapy and Children

- Pediatric IV medications are diluted for administration. It is important to know the institution's policy as to whether the medication volume is included as part of the total dilution volume.
- A flush is used after administration of IV medications in children. The volume of the flush will vary depending on the length of the IV tubing from the medication source.
- Check the institution's policy as to whether the volume of the flush is added to the diluted medication volume.
- Pediatric medication administration requires frequent assessment.
- Use an appropriate reference to calculate the normal dosage range for IV administration, and then compare it with the dosage ordered to determine whether it is within normal range.
- Daily Fluid Maintenance sometimes referred to as Daily Fluid Requirements
- The amount of maintenance fluid required is based on the child's weight in kg
- Daily Fluid Maintenance Formula
  - 100 mL/kg/day for first 10 kg of body weight
  - 50 mL/kg/day for next 10 kg of body weight
  - 20 mL/kg/day for each kg above 20 kg of body weight

Pediatric Oral and Parenteral Medications

Several methods have been presented to determine dosages for children in this chapter. It is important, however, to bear in mind that although the dosage may be determined according to weight, BSA, and other methods, the dosage to administer is calculated by using the same methods as for adults (ratio and proportion, the formula method, or dimensional analysis). It is important to remember the following differences with children's dosages.

Remember

1. Dosages are smaller for children than for adults.
2. Most oral medications for infants and small children come in liquid form to facilitate swallowing.
3. The oral route is preferred; however, when necessary, medications are administered by the parenteral route.
4. Not more than 1 mL is injected IM for small children and older infants; small infants should not receive more than 0.5 mL by IM injection.
5. Parenteral dosages are frequently administered with a tuberculin syringe.

SAFETY ALERT!

When in doubt, always double-check pediatric dosages with another nurse to decrease the chance of an error. Never assume! Think before administering.

CLINICAL **REASONING**

Scenario: According to *The Harriet Lane Handbook*, the recommended dosage for a child for ibuprofen as an antipyretic is 5-10 mg/kg/dose q6-8h p.o. The 7-month-old weighs $18\frac{1}{2}$ lb. The prescriber ordered 20 mg p.o. q6h for a temperature above 102° F. The infant's temperature is 102.8° F, and the nurse is preparing to administer the medication. The nurse believes the dosage is low but administers the medication based on the dosage being safe because it is below the safe dosage range. Several hours have passed, and the infant's temperature continues to increase.

a. What is the required single dosage for this infant? ____________

b. What should the nurse's actions have been and why? ____________

c. What preventive measures could have been taken by the nurse in this situation? ____________

Answers on p. 714

CHAPTER REVIEW

Read the dosage information or label given for the following problems. Express body weight conversion to the nearest tenth where indicated and dosages to the nearest tenth.

1. Lasix 10 mg IV stat is ordered for a child weighing 22 lb. The recommended dose is 1–2 mg/kg/dose. Is the dosage ordered safe? (Prove mathematically.) ____________________

2. Furadantin oral suspension 25 mg p.o. q6h is ordered for a child weighing 37.4 lb. Recommended dosage is 5–7 mg/kg/24 hr divided q6h.

   Available: Furadantin oral suspension 25 mg per 5 mL.

   a. What is the child's weight in kilograms to the nearest tenth? ____________________

   b. What is the dosage range for this child? ____________________

   c. Is the dosage ordered safe? (Prove mathematically.) ____________________

   d. How many milliliters must be given per dosage to administer the ordered dosage? Calculate the dose if the order is safe. ____________________

3. Cefaclor 225 mg p.o. q8h is ordered for a child weighing 35 kg. ____________________

   Available:

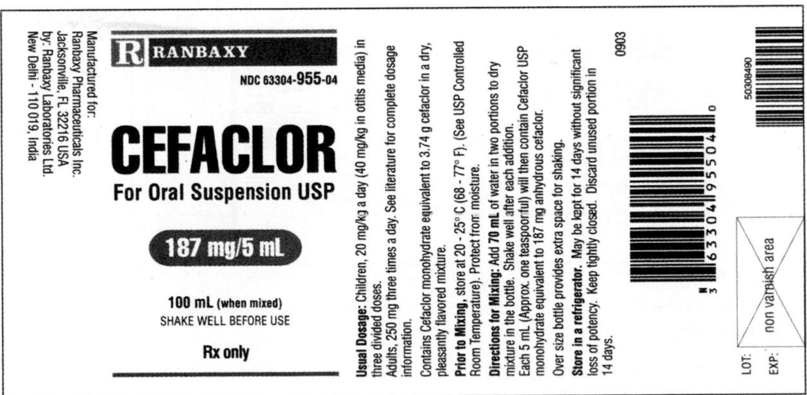

   Is the dosage ordered safe? (Prove mathematically) ____________________

4. Vibramycin 50 mg p.o. q12h is ordered for a child weighing 30 lb. The recommended dosage is 2.2–4.4 mg/kg/day in two divided doses. Is the dose ordered safe? (Prove mathematically) ____________________

5. Cleocin suspension 150 mg p.o. q8h is ordered for a child weighing 36 lb. The recommended dosage is 10 to 30 mg/kg/day divided q6-8h. Is the dosage ordered safe? (Prove mathematically.) __________

6. Keflex (cephalexin) suspension 250 mg p.o. q6h is ordered for a child weighing 66 lb. The usual pediatric dosage is 25 to 50 mg/kg/day in four divided dosages. Available: Keflex suspension 250 mg per 5 mL.

   a. Is the dosage ordered safe? (Prove mathematically.) __________

   b. How many milliliters would you need to administer one dosage? Calculate the dose if the order is safe. __________

7. Streptomycin sulfate 400 mg IM daily is ordered for a child weighing 35 kg. The recommended dosage is 20 to 40 mg/kg/day once daily.

   a. Is the dosage ordered safe? (Prove mathematically.) __________

   b. A 1-g vial of streptomycin sulfate is available in powdered form with the following instructions: Dilution with 1.8 mL of sterile water will yield 400 mg per mL. How many milliliters will you need to administer the ordered dosage? Calculate the dosage if the order is safe. __________

8. A child weighing 46 lb has an order for ranitidine (Zantac) 20 mg IV q8h. Is the dosage ordered safe? (Prove mathematically.)

   Available:

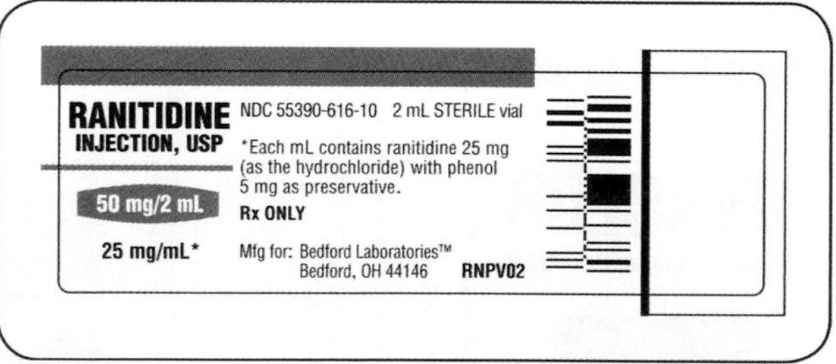

Pediatric Use:

While limited data exist on the administration of IV ranitidine to children, the recommended dose in pediatric patients is for a total daily dose of 2 to 4 mg/kg, to be divided and administered every 6 to 8 hours, up to a maximum of 50 mg given every 6 to 8 hours. This recommendation is derived from adult clinical studies and pharmacokinetic data in pediatric patients. Limited data in neonatal patients (less than one month of age) receiving ECMO have shown that a dose of 2 mg/kg is usually sufficient to increase gastric pH to >4 for at least 15 hours. Therefore, doses of 2 mg/kg given every 12 to 24 hours or as a continuous infusion should be considered.

*Excerpt from package insert for Ranitidine Injection from Bedford Laboratories (www.bedfordlabs.com)

9. The recommended dosage for neonates receiving ceftazidime (Tazidime) is 30 mg/kg q12h. The neonate weighs 3,500 g.

   a. What is the neonate's weight in kilograms to the nearest tenth? ______________________

   b. What is the safe dosage for this neonate? ______________________

10. A 40-lb child who is 5 years old has an order for midazolam 1.5 mg IV stat. The recommended dose for a child 6 months-5 years is 0.05-0.1 mg/kg/dose. Is the dosage ordered safe? ______________________

11. The recommended dosage for Mithracin for the treatment of testicular tumors is 25 to 30 mcg/kg. The client weighs 190 lb.

   a. What is the client's weight in kilograms to the nearest tenth? ______________________

   b. What is the dosage range in milligrams for this client? (Round to the nearest tenth.) ______________________

Using the nomogram on p. 682, determine the BSA and calculate each child's dosage by using the formula. Express dosages to the nearest tenth.

12. The child's height is 30 inches, and weight is 20 lb. The adult dosage of an antibiotic is 500 mg.

   a. What is the BSA? ______________________

   b. What is the child's dosage? ______________________

13. The child's height is 120 cm, and weight is 40 kg. The adult dosage for a medication is 250 mg.

   a. What is the BSA? ______________________

   b. What is the child's dosage? ______________________

14. The child's height is 50 inches, and weight is 70 lb. The adult dosage for a medication is 150 mg.

   a. What is the BSA? ______________________

   b. What is the child's dosage? ______________________

Determine the child's dosage for the following medications. Express answers to the nearest tenth.

15. The adult dosage of a medication is 50 mg. What will the dosage be for a child with a BSA of 0.7 m^2? ______________________

16. The adult dosage of a medication is 10 to 20 mg. What will the dosage range be for a child whose BSA is 0.66 m^2? ________________

17. The adult dosage of a medication is 2,000 units. What will the dosage be for a child with a BSA of 0.55 m^2? ________________

18. The adult dosage of a medication is 200 to 250 mg. What will the dosage range be for a child with a BSA of 0.55 m^2? ________________

Calculate the child's dosage in the following problems. Determine if the prescriber's order is correct. If the order is incorrect, give the correct dosage. Express answers to the nearest tenth.

19. A child with a BSA of 0.49 m^2 has an order for 25 mg of a medication. The adult dosage is 60 mg. ________________

20. A child with a BSA of 0.32 m^2 has an order for 4 mg of a medication. The adult dosage is 10 mg. ________________

21. A child with a BSA of 0.68 m^2 has an order for 50 mg of a medication. The adult dosage is 125 to 150 mg. ________________

Using the formula method for calculating BSA, determine the BSA in the following clients, and express answers to the nearest hundredth.

22. A 15-year-old who weighs 100 lb and is 55 inches tall ________________

23. An adult who weighs 60.9 kg and is 130 cm tall ________________

24. A child who weighs 55 lb and is 45 inches tall ________________

25. An adult who weighs 65 kg and is 132 cm tall ________________

26. An infant who weighs 6 kg and is 55 cm long ________________

27. A child who weighs 42 lb and is 45 inches tall ________________

28. An adult who weighs 74 kg and is 160 cm tall ________________

Calculate the dosages to be given. Use labels where provided.

29. Order: Azidothymidine 7 mg p.o. q6h.

    Available: Azidothymidine 10 mg per mL ________________

30. Order: Digoxin 0.1 mg p.o. daily.

    Available:

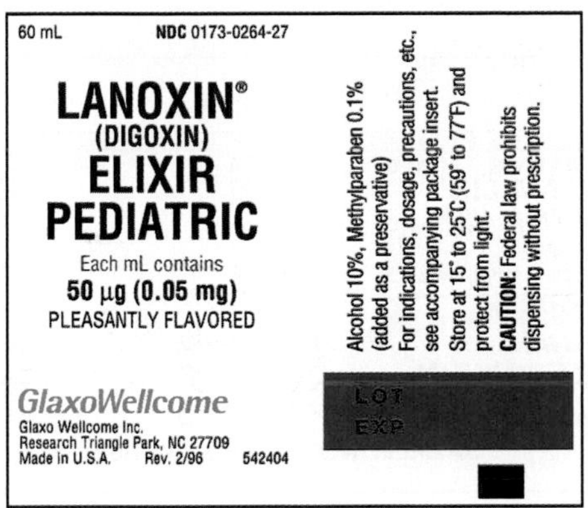

____

31. Order: Retrovir 80 mg p.o. q8h.

    Available: Retrovir syrup labeled 50 mg per 5 mL

____

32. Order: Tegretol 0.25 g p.o. t.i.d.

    Available:

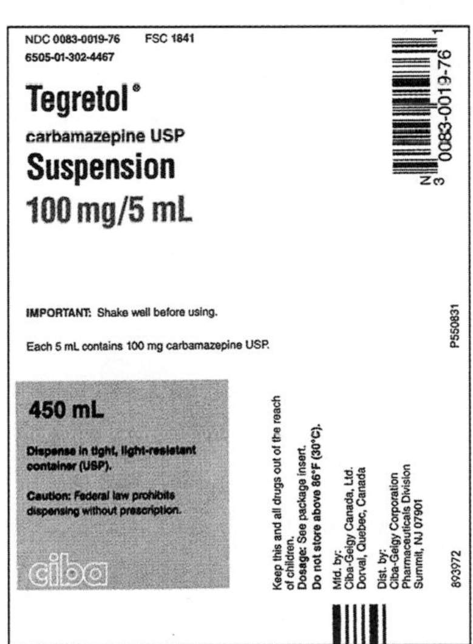

____

33. Order: Amoxicillin 100 mg p.o. t.i.d.

    Available: Amoxicillin oral suspension
    labeled 250 mg per 5 mL ______________________________

Calculate the dosages below. Use the labels where provided. Calculate to the nearest hundredth where necessary.

34. Order: Gentamicin 7.3 mg IM q12h.

    Available: 20 mg per 2 mL

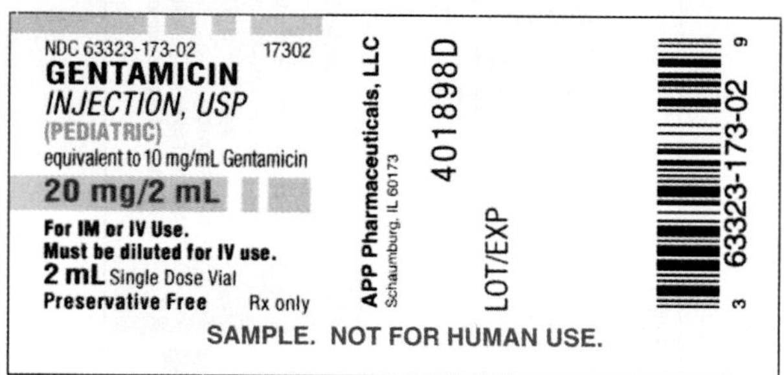

____

35. Order: Atropine 0.1 mg subcut stat.

    Available: Atropine 400 mcg per mL ____________________

36. Order: Nebcin (tobramycin sulfate) 60 mg IV q8h.

    Available:

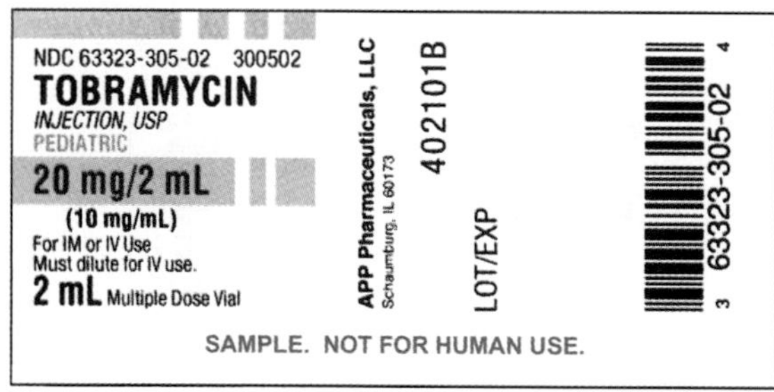

____

Calculate the dosages to be given. Round answers to the nearest tenth as indicated (express answers in milliliters).

37. Order: Tylenol 0.4 g p.o. q4h p.r.n. for temp greater than 101° F.

    Available: Tylenol elixir labeled
    160 mg per 5 mL ____________________

38. Order: Methotrexate 35 mg IM daily once a week (on Tuesdays).

    Available:

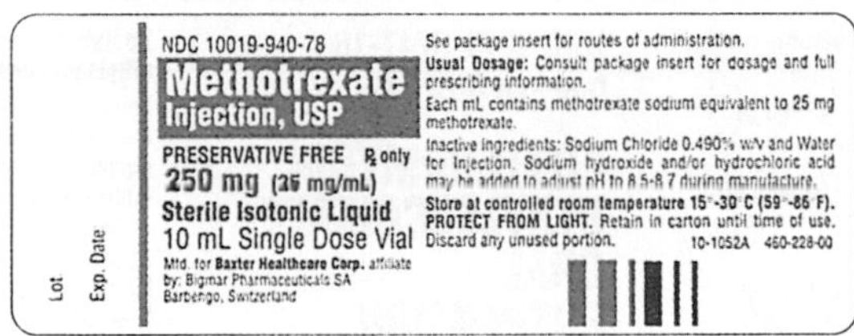

____

39. Order: Clindamycin 100 mg IV q6h.

    Available: Clindamycin labeled 150 mg per mL

____

40. Order: Amikacin 150 mg IV q8h.

    Available:

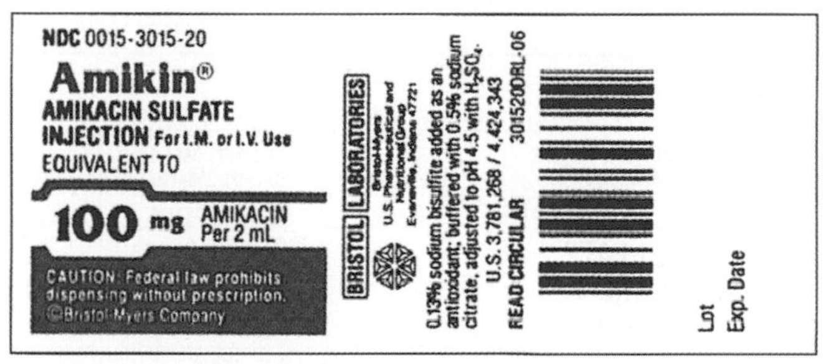

____

41. Order: Dilantin 62.5 mg p.o. b.i.d.

    Available: Dilantin oral suspension labeled 125 mg per 5 mL ______________________

42. Order: Erythromycin 300 mg p.o. q6h.

    Available:

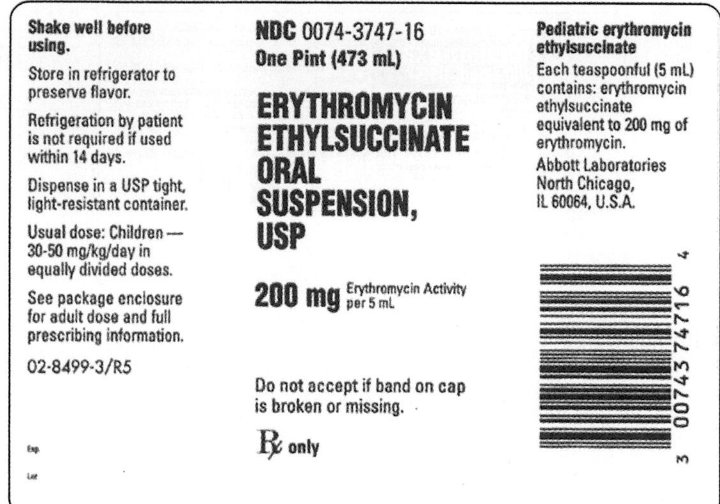

____

43. Order: Albuterol 3 mg p.o. b.i.d.

    Available:

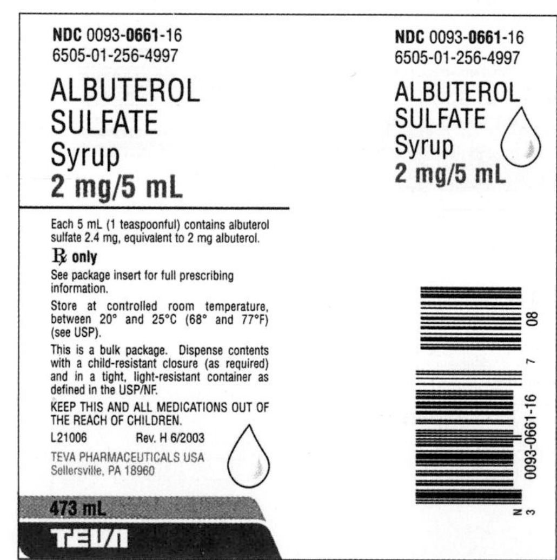

____

44. Order: Ferrous sulfate 45 mg p.o. every day.

    Available: Ferrous sulfate drops
    15 mg per 0.6 mL

____

45. Order: Methylprednisolone 14 mg IV q6h.

Available:

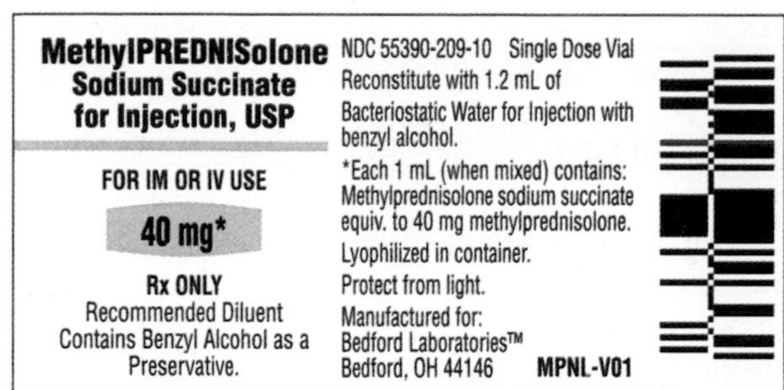

____

46. Order: Famotidine 20 mg p.o. b.i.d.

Available: Famotidine 8 mg per mL. ______________________

Round weights and dosages to the nearest tenth as indicated.

47. Order: Ceclor (cefaclor) 180 mg p.o. q8h. The infant weighs 10 lb. The recommended dosage is 20 mg/kg/day in three divided doses.

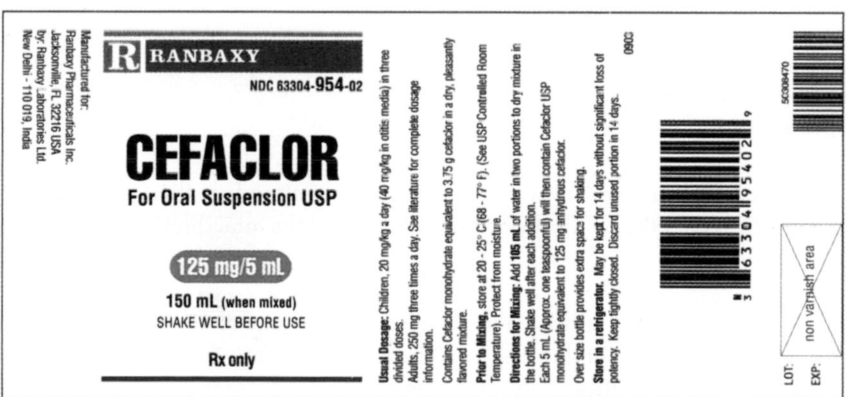

a. Is the dosage ordered safe? ______________________

b. How many milliliters will you need to administer the dosage? Calculate the dose to administer if the dosage is safe. ______________________

48. Order: Amprenavir 650 mg p.o. t.i.d. for a child weighing 66 lb. The recommended dosage is 22.5 mg/kg up to three times a day.

Is the dosage ordered safe? ______________________

49. Acetaminophen (Ofirmev) 525 mg IV q4h is ordered for a child weighing 92.4 lb. According to *The Harriet Lane Handbook,* the dosage for a child (age 2-12 years) or adolescent/adult weighing less than 50 kg is 15 mg/kg/dose q6h, or 12.5 mg/kg/dose q4h IV up to a maximum of 75 mg/kg/24hr.

    a. What is the safe dosage for this child? ______________

    b. Is the dosage ordered safe? ______________

50. Order: Minoxidil for a child weighing 31 lb. The recommended dosage range is 0.25 to 1 mg/kg/day.

    What is the safe dosage range for this child? ______________

Determine the dosage in the following problems. Round dosages to the nearest tenth as indicated.

51. The recommended dose for Oncovin (vincristine) is 2 mg per m^2. The child has a BSA of 0.8 m^2. ______________

52. The recommended dose for acyclovir is 250 mg per m^2. The child has a BSA of 0.82 m^2. ______________

53. The recommended dose for bleomycin in an adult with Hodgkin disease is 10 to 20 units per m^2. The adult has a BSA of 1.83 m^2. Give the dosage range. ______________

Determine the flow rate in gtt/min for each IV using a microdrip, then indicate mL/hr for a controller. (Consider the medication volume as part of the total dilution volume as shown in the chapter.)

54. A child is to receive 10 units of a medication. The dosage of 10 units is contained in 1 mL. Dilute to 30 mL, and infuse in 20 minutes. A 15-mL flush is to follow. Medication is placed in a buretrol. Determine the rate in:

    a. gtt/min ______________

    b. mL/hr ______________

55. A child is to receive 80 mg of a medication. The dosage of 80 mg is contained in 2 mL. Dilute to 80 mL, and infuse in 60 minutes. A 15-mL flush is to follow. Medication is placed in a buretrol. Determine the rate in:

    a. gtt/min ______________

    b. mL/hr ______________

Determine the normal dosage range for the following problems to the nearest tenth. State your course of action.

56. A child weighing 23 kg has an order for 500 mg of a medication in 100 mL D5W q12h. The normal daily dosage range is 40 to 50 mg/kg. Determine if the dosage ordered is within normal range, and state your course of action. ______________________

57. A child weighing 20 kg has an order for 2 mg IV of a medication at 10 AM in 100 mL D5W. The normal daily dosage is 0.05 mg/kg. Determine if the dosage ordered is within normal range, and state your course of action. ______________________

Answers on pp. 714-719

Calculate the Daily Fluid Maintenance and the hourly rate for the following: (Pump is programmed in whole milliliters unless otherwise indicated.)

58. Child weighing 25 kg

   a. Daily fluid maintenance ______________________ mL/day

   b. IV rate ______________________ mL/hr

59. Infant weighing 4,200 g

   a. Daily fluid maintenance ______________________ mL/day

   b. IV rate ______________________ mL/hr (pump capable of delivering in tenths of a mL)

Directions for 60-61: Round the answer in mg to the nearest tenth.

60. A child weighs 21 lb and is 30 inches in height. The recommended dose for vincristine is 1.5-2 mg per m^2 once weekly. Determine the BSA using the formula. What is the dosage range for the child?

   a. BSA ______________________

   b. Dosage range ______________________ mg

61. An adult weighs 75 kg and is 162 cm tall. The recommended dose for Acyclovir is 750 mg per m^2 IV tid. Determine the BSA using the formula. Determine the number of mg the patient/client should receive.

   a. BSA ______________________

   b. Dosage ______________________ mg

Answers on p. 719

evolve

For additional practice problems, refer to the Pediatric Dosages section of the Elsevier's Interactive Drug Calculation Application, Version 1 on Evolve.

ANSWERS

Chapter 25

Answers to Practice Problems

1. 6.8 kg
2. 30.9 kg
3. 14.1 kg
4. 23.6 kg
5. 32.3 kg
6. 60.5 kg
7. 3.8 kg
8. 2.6 kg
9. 45.6 kg
10. 42.2 kg
11. 46.9 lb
12. 38.9 lb
13. 48.4 lb
14. 33 lb
15. 74.8 lb
16. 157.1 lb
17. 160.6 lb
18. 216.3 lb
19. 76.8 lb
20. 63.1 lb
21. 4 kg
22. 1.5 kg
23. 2.9 kg
24. 3.6 kg
25. 1.9 kg

NOTE

Any of the methods presented in Chapter 25 can be used to calculate dosages; not all are shown in the Answer Key.

26. a. 25 to 50 mg/kg/day

b. Convert weight first (2.2 lb = 1 kg).
35 ÷ 2.2 = 15.9 kg

c. 25 mg : 1 kg = x mg : 15.9 kg
x = 397.5 mg/day

50 mg : 1 kg = x mg : 15.9 kg
x = 795 mg/day

or

25 mg/~~kg~~/day × 15.9 ~~kg~~ = 397.5 mg/day
50 mg/~~kg~~/day × 15.9 ~~kg~~ = 795 mg/day
Dosage range is 397.5 to 795 mg/day.

d. The dosage ordered falls within the range that is safe (150 mg × 4 = 600 mg). 600 mg/day falls within the 397.5 to 795 mg/day range.

e. 250 mg:5 mL = 150 mg:x mL

or

$$\frac{150 \text{ mg}}{250 \text{ mg}} \times 5 \text{ mL} = x \text{ mL}$$

x = 3 mL

27. a. 15 mg:1 kg = x mg:35 kg
x = 525 mg/day

30 mg:1 kg = x mg:35 kg
x = 1,050 mg/day

or

15 mg/~~kg~~/day × 35 ~~kg~~ = 525 mg/day
30 mg/~~kg~~/day × 35 ~~kg~~ = 1,050 mg/day
The safe dosage range for this child is 525 − 1,050 mg/day.

b. $$\frac{525 \text{ mg}}{3} = 175 \text{ mg q8h}$$

$$\frac{1{,}050 \text{ mg}}{3} = 350 \text{ mg q8h}$$

The divided dosage range is 175-350 mg q8h.

c. The dosage is safe. 200 mg × 3 = 600 mg.
600 mg/day falls within the range of 525-1,050 mg/day. Also, the dosage q8h falls within the divided dosage range of 175-350 mg q8h.

28. a. 10 mg:1 kg = x mg:40 kg
x = 400 mg/day

or

10 mg/~~kg~~/day × 40 ~~kg~~ = 400 mg/day
30 mg:1 kg = x mg:40 kg
x = 1,200 mg/day

or

30 mg/~~kg~~/day × 40 ~~kg~~ = 1,200 mg/day
Answer: 1,200 mg/day is the maximum dosage.

b. q6h = 24 ÷ 4 = 4 doses per day
400 mg ÷ 4 = 100 mg q6h
1,200 mg ÷ 4 = 300 mg q6h
Answer: 100-300 mg q6h is the divided dosage range (300 mg q6h is maximum divided dose).

29. a. Weight conversion (2.2 lb = 1 kg)
9 ÷ 2.2 = 4.1 kg

b. 3 mg:1 kg = x mg:4.1 kg
x = 12.3 mg/day

or

3 mg/~~kg~~/day × 4.1 ~~kg~~ = 12.3 mg/day
5 mg:1 kg = x mg:4.1 kg
x = 20.5 mg/day

or

5 mg/~~kg~~/day × 4.1 ~~kg~~ = 20.5 mg/day
Safe dosage range for the child for a day is 12.3-20.5 mg/day.

c. The dosage ordered is safe.
10 mg × 2 = 20 mg/day. The maximum dosage per day is 20.5 mg.

d. 20 mg:5 mL = 10 mg:x mL

or

$$\frac{10 \text{ mg}}{20 \text{ mg}} \times 5 \text{ mL} = x \text{ mL}$$

x = 2.5 mL

You need to give 2.5 mL to administer the ordered dosage of 10 mg.

30. a. Convert weight to kilograms (2.2 lb = 1 kg).
    84 lb ÷ 2.2 = 38.2 kg
  b. 0.1 mg : 1 kg = x mg : 38.2 kg
    x = 3.8 mg/dose

    or

    38.2 ~~kg~~ × 0.1 mg/~~kg~~/dose = 3.82 mg = 3.8 mg/dose

    or

    0.2 mg : 1 kg = x mg : 38.2 kg
    x = 7.6 mg/dose

    38.2 ~~kg~~ × 0.2 mg/~~kg~~/dose = 7.64 mg = 7.6 mg/dose

    3.8-7.6 mg/dosage
  c. The dosage ordered is safe. 7.5 mg is less than 7.6 mg.
  d. You would administer 1.5 mL.

    5 mg : 1 mL = 7.5 mg : x mL

    or

$$\frac{7.5 \text{ mg}}{5 \text{ mg}} \times 1 \text{ mL} = x \text{ mL}$$

$$x = 1.5 \text{ mL}$$

31. Convert the child's weight to kilograms (2.2 lb = 1 kg).
  a. 44 lb ÷ 2.2 = 20 kg
  b. 2.5 mg : 1 kg = x mg : 20 kg
    x = 50 mg/day

    or

    5 mg : 1 kg = x mg : 20 kg
    x = 100 mg/day

    or

    5 mg/~~kg~~/day × 20 ~~kg~~ = 100 mg/day

    50-100 mg/day

32. a. Convert weight (2.2 lb = 1 kg).
    38 lb ÷ 2.2 = 17.3 kg
  b. 40 mg : 1 kg = x mg : 17.3 kg
    x = 692 mg/day

    or

    40 mg/~~kg~~/day × 17.3 ~~kg~~ = 692 mg/day
  c. $\frac{692 \text{ mg}}{4} = 173$ mg/dose
  d. The dosage ordered is not safe. 200 mg × 4 = 800 mg/day. 800 mg is greater than 692 mg/day. It also exceeds the dose that should be given q6h. Check with prescriber.

33. Convert weight (2.2 lb = 1 kg).
  a. 44 lb ÷ 2.2 = 20 kg
  b. 30 mg : 1 kg = x mg : 20 kg
    x = 600 mg/day

    or

    30 mg/~~kg~~/day × 20 ~~kg~~ = 600 mg/day

    50 mg : 1 kg = x mg : 20 kg
    x = 1,000 mg/day

    or

    50 mg/~~kg~~/day × 20 ~~kg~~ = 1,000 mg/day

    600-1,000 mg/day
  c. The dosage ordered is safe.
    250 mg × 4 = 1,000 mg. 1,000 mg falls within the safe range.

34. No weight conversion is required.
    0.25 mg : 1 kg = x mg : 66.3 kg
    x = 16.57 = 16.6 mg

    or

    0.25 mg/~~kg~~ × 66.3 ~~kg~~ = 16.57 = 16.6 mg

    Answer: 16.6 mg is the dosage for the adult.

35. Weight conversion is required (2.2 lb = 1 kg).
  a. 200 lb ÷ 2.2 = 90.9 kg
  b. 150 mg : 1 kg = x mg : 90.9 kg
    x = 13,635 mg/day

    or

    150 mg/~~kg~~ × 90.9 ~~kg~~ = 13,635 mg/day

    200 mg : 1 kg = x mg : 90.9 kg
    x = 18,180 mg/day

    or

    200 mg/~~kg~~/day × 90.9 ~~kg~~ = 18,180 mg/day

  To determine the number of grams, convert the milligrams obtained to grams (1,000 mg = 1 g).

    13,635 mg ÷ 1,000 = 13.63 g

    (13.6 g to nearest tenth)

    18,180 mg ÷ 1,000 = 18.18 g

    (18.2 g to nearest tenth)

    The daily dosage range in grams is 13.6-18.2 g/day.

36. Convert weight (2.2. lb = 1 kg, 16 oz = 1 lb).
    6 oz ÷ 16 = 0.37 lb = 0.4 lb (to nearest tenth)
    Total weight in pounds = 12.4 lb
    a. 12.4 lb ÷ 2.2 = 5.63 = (5.6 to nearest tenth)
    b. 6 mg : 1 kg = x mg : 5.6 kg
    x = 33.6 mg
    or
    $6 \text{ mg}/\cancel{\text{kg}} \times 5.6 \cancel{\text{kg}} = 33.6 \text{ mg}$
    Answer: 33.6 mg for the first dose.
    c. 3 mg : 1 kg = x mg : 5.6 kg
    x = 16.8 mg
    or
    $3 \text{ mg}/\cancel{\text{kg}} \times 5.6 \cancel{\text{kg}} = 16.8 \text{ mg}$
    Answer: 16.8 mg daily for the subsequent dose.

37. 0.6 m^2
38. 0.78 m^2
39. 0.9 m^2
40. 0.8 m^2
41. 0.28 m^2
42. 0.44 m^2
43. 0.8 m^2
44. 0.28 m^2
45. 0.52 m^2
46. 0.45 m^2
47. 0.9 m^2
48. 0.3 m^2
49. 0.58 m^2
50. 0.51 m^2
51. 0.68 m^2
52. 0.18 m^2

53. $\sqrt{\dfrac{95.5 \text{ (kg)} \times 180 \text{ (cm)}}{3{,}600}}$
    $\sqrt{4.775} = 2.185 = 2.19 \text{ m}^2$
    Answer: 2.19 m^2

54. $\sqrt{\dfrac{10 \text{ (kg)} \times 70 \text{ (cm)}}{3{,}600}}$
    $\sqrt{0.194} = 0.44 \text{ m}^2$
    Answer: 0.44 m^2

55. $\sqrt{\dfrac{4.8 \text{ (lb)} \times 21 \text{ (in)}}{3{,}131}}$
    $\sqrt{0.032} = 0.178 = 0.18 \text{ m}^2$
    Answer: 0.18 m^2

56. $\sqrt{\dfrac{170 \text{ (lb)} \times 67 \text{ (in)}}{3{,}131}}$
    $\sqrt{3.637} = 1.907 = 1.91 \text{ m}^2$
    Answer: 1.91 m^2

57. $\sqrt{\dfrac{92 \text{ (lb)} \times 35 \text{ (in)}}{3{,}131}}$
    $\sqrt{1.028} = 1.014 = 1.01 \text{ m}^2$
    Answer: 1.01 m^2

58. $\sqrt{\dfrac{24 \text{ (kg)} \times 92 \text{ (cm)}}{3{,}600}}$
    $\sqrt{0.613} = 0.783 = 0.78 \text{ m}^2$
    Answer: 0.78 m^2

59. a. 0.52 m^2
    b. $\dfrac{0.52 \cancel{\text{m}^2}}{1.7 (\cancel{\text{m}^2})} \times 25 \text{ mg} = \dfrac{0.52 \times 25}{1.7} = \dfrac{13}{1.7} = 7.64$
    Answer: 7.6 mg

60. a. 0.53 m^2
    $\dfrac{0.53 \cancel{\text{m}^2}}{1.7 (\cancel{\text{m}^2})} \times 200 \text{ mg} = \dfrac{0.53 \times 200}{1.7} = \dfrac{106}{1.7}$
    $\dfrac{106}{1.7} = 62.35 = 62.4 \text{ mg}$
    $\dfrac{0.53 \cancel{\text{m}^2}}{1.7 (\cancel{\text{m}^2})} \times 400 \text{ mg} = \dfrac{212}{1.7} = 124.7$
    Answer: The child's dosage range is 62.4-124.7 mg.

61. $\dfrac{1.5 \cancel{\text{m}^2}}{1.7 (\cancel{\text{m}^2})} \times 5 \text{ mg} = \dfrac{1.5 \times 5}{1.7} = \dfrac{7.5}{1.7}$
    $\dfrac{7.5}{1.7} = 4.41 = 4.4 \text{ mg}$
    $\dfrac{1.5 \cancel{\text{m}^2}}{1.7 (\cancel{\text{m}^2})} \times 15 \text{ mg} = \dfrac{22.5}{1.7} = 13.23$
    13.23 mg = 13.2 mg
    Answer: 4.4-13.2 mg

62. $\dfrac{0.8 \cancel{\text{m}^2}}{1.7 (\cancel{\text{m}^2})} \times 20 \text{ mg} = \dfrac{0.8 \times 20}{1.7} = \dfrac{16}{1.7}$
    $\dfrac{16}{1.7} = 9.41 \text{ mg} = 9.4 \text{ mg}$
    Answer: The dosage is incorrect. The correct dosage is 9.4 mg.

63. $\dfrac{0.9 \cancel{\text{m}^2}}{1.7 (\cancel{\text{m}^2})} \times 25 \text{ mg} = \dfrac{0.9 \times 25}{1.7} = \dfrac{22.5}{1.7}$
    $\dfrac{22.5}{1.7} = 13.23 \text{ mg} = 13.2 \text{ mg}$
    Answer: The dosage is incorrect. The correct dosage is 13.2 mg.

64. $\dfrac{1.5 \cancel{\text{m}^2}}{1.7 (\cancel{\text{m}^2})} \times 250 \text{ mg} = \dfrac{1.5 \times 250}{1.7} = \dfrac{375}{1.7}$
    $\dfrac{375}{1.7} = 220.58 = 220.6 \text{ mg}$
    Answer: The child's dosage is 220.6 mg.

65. $\frac{0.74\ \cancel{m^2}}{1.7\ (\cancel{m^2})} \times 20 \text{ mg} = \frac{0.74 \times 20}{1.7} = \frac{14.8}{1.7}$

$\frac{14.8}{1.7} = 8.7 \text{ mg}$

$\frac{0.74\ \cancel{m^2}}{1.7\ (\cancel{m^2})} \times 30 \text{ mg} = \frac{0.74 \times 30}{1.7} = \frac{22.2}{1.7}$

$\frac{22.2}{1.7} = 13.05 = 13.1 \text{ mg}$

Answer: The child's dosage range is 8.7-13.1 mg.

66. a. 0.44 m^2

b. $\frac{0.44\ \cancel{m^2}}{1.7\ (\cancel{m^2})} \times 500 \text{ mg} = \frac{220}{1.7} = 129.41$

Answer: The child's dosage is 129.4 mg.

67. $\frac{1.3\ \cancel{m^2}}{1.7\ (\cancel{m^2})} \times 500 \text{ mg} = \frac{1.3 \times 500}{1.7} = \frac{650}{1.7} = 382.35$

Answer: The child's dosage is 382.4 mg.

68. a. Dilution volume: 27 mL

b. $x \text{ gtt/min} = \frac{30 \text{ mL (diluted medication)} \times 60 \text{ gtt/mL}}{50 \text{ min}}$

$x = \frac{30 \times 60}{50} = \frac{1800}{50} = 36 \text{ gtt/min}$

or

Use a ratio and proportion to determine mL/hr first. Remember that with a buretrol when a pump or controller is not used, mL/hr = gtt/min.

$30 \text{ mL} : 50 \text{ min} = x \text{ mL} : 60 \text{ min}$

or

$\frac{30 \text{ mL}}{50 \text{ min}} = \frac{x \text{ mL}}{60 \text{ min}}$

Answer: x = 36 gtt/min; 36 microgtt/min

c. 36 mL/hr

69. a. Dilution volume: 13 mL

b. $x \text{ gtt/min} = \frac{15 \text{ mL (diluted medication)} \times 60 \text{ gtt/mL}}{45 \text{ min}}$

$x = \frac{15 \times 60}{45} = \frac{900}{45} = 20 \text{ gtt/min}$

or

Use a ratio and proportion and determine mL/hr first.

$15 \text{ mL} : 45 \text{ min} = x \text{ mL} : 60 \text{ min}$

or

$\frac{15 \text{ mL}}{45 \text{ min}} = \frac{x \text{ mL}}{60 \text{ min}}$

Answer: x = 20 gtt/min; 20 microgtt/min

c. 20 mL/hr

70. Step 1: Determine the dosage range per hour.

$10 \text{ units}/\cancel{kg}/\text{hr} \times 17\ \cancel{kg} = 170 \text{ units/hr}$

$25 \text{ units}/\cancel{kg}/\text{hr} \times 17\ \cancel{kg} = 425 \text{ units/hr}$

Step 2: Determine dosage infusing per hour.

$2{,}500 \text{ units} : 250 \text{ mL} = x \text{ units} : 50 \text{ mL}$

$250x = 2{,}500 \times 50$

$\frac{250x}{250} = \frac{125{,}000}{250} = 500$

$x = 500 \text{ units/hr}$

Step 3: Compare the dosage ordered to see if it is within the safe range.

The IV is infusing at 50 mL/hr, which is 500 units/hr.
The normal dosage range is 170-425 units/hr.
500 units/hr is greater than the dosage range.
Check with the prescriber before administering.

71. Step 1: Determine the dosage range.

$0.75\ \cancel{m^2} \times 100 \text{ mg}/\cancel{m^2}/\text{day} = 75 \text{ mg/day}$

$0.75\ \cancel{m^2} \times 250 \text{ mg}/\cancel{m^2}/\text{day} = 187.5 \text{ mg/day}$

The dosage range is 75-187.5 mg per day.

Step 2: Determine the dosage the child is receiving.

84 mg q12h (2 dosages)

$84 \text{ mg} \times 2 = 168 \text{ mg/day}$

Step 3: Determine if dosage is within safe range.
The 84 mg q12h (84 mg × 2 = 168 mg/day) is within the safe range of 75-187.5 mg/day, so administer the medication.

72. a. $100 \text{ mL}/\cancel{kg}/\text{day} \times 10\ \cancel{kg} = 1{,}000 \text{ mL/day}$
(for first 10 kg)

$50 \text{ mL}/\cancel{kg}/\text{day} \times 3\ \cancel{kg} = 150 \text{ mL/day}$
(for the remaining 3 kg)

Total: 1,000 mL/day + 150 mL/day = 1,150 mL/day

Answer: 1,150 mL/day or per 24 hr

b. $x \text{ mL/hr} = \frac{1{,}150 \text{ mL}}{24 \text{ hr}} = 47.9$

$x = 48 \text{ mL/hr}$

Answer: 48 mL/hr

73. Convert weight: Equivalent: 1 kg = 1,000 g

$3{,}300 \text{ g} \div 1{,}000 = 3.3 \text{ kg}$

a. $100 \text{ mL}/\cancel{kg}/\text{day} \times 3.3\ \cancel{kg} = 330 \text{ mL/day}$

Answer: 330 mL/day or per 24 hr

b. $x \text{ mL/hr} = \frac{330 \text{ mL}}{24 \text{ hr}} = 13.7$

$x = 14 \text{ mL/hr}$

Answer: 14 mL/hr

Answers to Clinical Reasoning Questions

a. 42-84 mg/dose

b. Contact the prescriber; the dosage is too low. The dose is not safe because it is below the recommended therapeutic dose to decrease the child's temperature.

c. The nurse should have notified the prescriber immediately so that the order could be revised. The child's temperature indicates an underdosage that is not safe. Do not assume it is safe because the dosage is lower than the recommended dosage.

Answers to Chapter Review

1. Convert weight (2.2 lb = 1 kg).
   a. 22 lb ÷ 2.2 = 10 kg
   b. 1 mg/~~kg~~ × 10 ~~kg~~ = 10 mg/dose
      2 mg/~~kg~~ × 10 ~~kg~~ = 20 mg/dose

   The dosage ordered for this child is safe. 10 mg falls within the range of 10-20 mg per dose.

2. Convert child's weight in lb to kg.

   2.2 lb = 1 kg

   a. 37.4 lb ÷ 2.2 = 17 kg
   b. The dosage range is 5-7 mg/day/24 hr.
      5 mg/~~kg~~/24 hr × 17 ~~kg~~ = 85 mg/24 hr (day).
      7 mg/~~kg~~/24 hr × 17 ~~kg~~ = 119 mg/24 hr (day).
      Answer: The dosage range is 85-119 mg/day.
      q6h = 4 dosages
      85 mg ÷ 4 = 21.25 mg = 21.3 mg per dose (q6h)
      119 mg ÷ 4 = 29.75 mg = 29.8 mg per dose (q6h)
      The divided dosage range is 21.3-29.8 mg per dose.
      The dosage ordered is 25 mg q6h.
   c. The dosage ordered is safe because 25 mg × 4 doses = 100 mg/day. It falls within the range of 85-119 mg/day. The dosage q6h also falls within the divided dosage range of 21.3-29.8 mg q6h.
   d. 25 mg : 5 mL = 25 mg : x mL

      or

      $$\frac{25 \text{ mg}}{25 \text{ mg}} \times 5 \text{ mL} = x \text{ mL}$$

      $x = 5$ mL

   Answer: Give 5 mL per dose. The dosage ordered is contained in 5 mL.

3. No conversion of weight is required. The child's weight is in kilograms, and the recommended dosage is expressed in kilograms (20 mg/kg/day).

   20 mg/~~kg~~/day × 35 ~~kg~~ = 700 mg/day

   q8h = 3 dosages

   700 mg ÷ 3 =

   233.33 = 233.3 mg per dosage

   The dosage ordered is not safe. 225 mg × 3 = 675 mg/day. 675 mg/day is less than 700 mg/day and the dose being given q6h is less than 233.3 mg. Check with prescriber. Dose may be too low to be effective.

4. Convert the child's weight in pounds to kilograms. The recommended dosage is expressed in kilograms (2.2-4.4 mg/kg/day) (2.2 lb = 1 kg).

   30 lb = 30 ÷ 2.2 = 13.6 kg.

   2.2 mg/~~kg~~/day × 13.6 ~~kg~~ = 29.9 mg/day.

   4.4 mg/~~kg~~/day × 13.6 ~~kg~~ = 59.8 mg/day.

   q12h = 2 dosages.

   29.9 mg ÷ 2 = 15 mg per dose.

   59.8 mg ÷ 2 = 29.9 mg per dose.

   50 mg × 2 = 100 mg/day. The dosage is too high; notify the prescriber. 100 mg/day is greater than 29.9-59.8 mg/day. Also, the dose being administered q12h exceeds the recommended dosage.

5. Convert the child's weight in pounds to kilograms. The recommended dosage is stated in kilograms (10-30 mg/kg/day) (2.2 lb = 1 kg).

   36 lb = 36 ÷ 2.2 = 16.4 kg

   50 mg/~~kg~~/day × 16.4 ~~kg~~ = 164 mg/day.

   30 mg/~~kg~~/day × 16.4 ~~kg~~ = 492 mg/day.

   The medication is given q6-8h. The dosage in this problem is ordered q8h.

   24 ÷ 8 = 3 dosages

   164 mg ÷ 3 = 54.7 mg per dose.

   492 mg ÷ 3 = 164 mg per dose.

   The dosage ordered is 150 mg q8h.

   150 mg × 3 = 450 mg/day.

   The dosage is safe. 450 mg/day falls within the range of 164-492 mg/day. Also, the dose being administered q8h falls within the range of 54.7-164 mg per dose.

6. a. Convert the child's weight in pounds to kilograms. The recommended dosage is expressed in kilograms (25-50 mg/kg) (2.2 lb = 1 kg).

$$66 \text{ lb} = 66 \div 2.2 = 30 \text{ kg}$$

$$25 \text{ mg/}\cancel{\text{kg}}\text{/day} \times 30\ \cancel{\text{kg}} = 750 \text{ mg/day}$$

$$50 \text{ mg/}\cancel{\text{kg}}\text{/day} \times 30\ \cancel{\text{kg}} = 1{,}500 \text{ mg/day}$$

The safe range is 750-1,500 mg/day.

The medication is given in divided dosages.

The dosage ordered is q6h.

$$24 \div 6 = 4 \text{ dosages}$$

$$750 \text{ mg} \div 4 = 187.5 \text{ mg/per dosage}$$

$$1{,}500 \text{ mg} \div 4 = 375 \text{ mg/per dosage}$$

The dosage range is 187.5-375 mg per dose q6h. 250 mg × 4 = 1,000 mg/day. This is a safe dosage because the total dosage falls within the safe range for 24 hr, and the divided dosage also falls within the safe range.

b. You would give 5 mL for one dosage.

$$250 \text{ mg} : 5 \text{ mL} = 250 \text{ mg} : x \text{ mL}$$

or

$$\frac{250 \text{ mg}}{250 \text{ mg}} \times 5 \text{ mL} = x \text{ mL}$$

$$x = 5 \text{ mL}$$

The dosage ordered is contained in 5 mL; therefore you will need to administer 5 mL.

7. a. No conversion of weight is required. The child's weight is stated in kilograms, and the recommended dosage is 20-40 mg/kg/day.

$$20 \text{ mg/}\cancel{\text{kg}}\text{/day} \times 35\ \cancel{\text{kg}} = 700 \text{ mg/day}$$

$$40 \text{ mg/}\cancel{\text{kg}}\text{/day} \times 35\ \cancel{\text{kg}} = 1{,}400 \text{ mg/day}$$

The safe range is 700-1,400 mg/day.

The prescriber ordered 400 mg IM daily. This dosage is not safe. 400 mg daily falls below the safe range for 24 hr. The dosage ordered may not be effective. Contact the prescriber.

b. The dosage is not calculated; the dosage ordered daily is not safe.

8. Convert the child's weight in pounds to kilograms. The recommended dosage is expressed in kilograms (2-4 mg/kg/day) (2.2 lb = 1 kg).

$$46 \text{ lb} = 46 \div 2.2 = 20.9 \text{ kg}$$

$$2 \text{ mg/}\cancel{\text{kg}}\text{/day} \times 20.9\ \cancel{\text{kg}} = 41.8 \text{ mg/day}$$

$$4 \text{ mg/}\cancel{\text{kg}}\text{/day} \times 20.9\ \cancel{\text{kg}} = 83.6 \text{ mg/day}$$

The safe dosage range is 41.8-83.6 mg/day. The dosage is ordered q8h.

$$24 \div 8 = 3 \text{ doses.}$$

$$41.8 \text{ mg} \div 3 = 13.9 \text{ mg per dose.}$$

$$83.6 \text{ mg} \div 3 = 27.9 \text{ mg per dose.}$$

The dose ordered is safe. 20 mg × 3 = 60 mg/day.

60 mg/day falls within the range of 41.8-83.6 mg/day. The dose administered q8h also falls within the range of 13.9-27.9 mg per dose.

9. Convert the neonate's weight in grams to kilograms (1,000 g = 1 kg).

a. 3,500 g = 3.5 kg

b. $30 \text{ mg/}\cancel{\text{kg}} \times 3.5\ \cancel{\text{kg}} = 105 \text{ mg}$

The safe dosage for the neonate is 105 mg q12h.

10. Convert the child's weight in pounds to kilogram. The recommended dosage is expressed in kilograms.

(0.05-0.1 mg/kg/dose)

40 lb = 40 ÷ 2.2 = 18.2 kg.

$0.05 \text{ mg/}\cancel{\text{kg}}\text{/dose} \times 18.2\ \cancel{\text{kg}} = 0.9 \text{ mg per dose.}$

$0.1 \text{ mg/}\cancel{\text{kg}}\text{/dose} \times 18.2\ \cancel{\text{kg}} = 1.8 \text{ mg per dose.}$

The dose range for this child is 0.9-1.8 mg per dose. The dose ordered is safe. 1.5 mg falls within the range of 0.9-1.8 mg per dose.

11. Weight conversion is required (2.2 lb = 1 kg).

a. 190 lb ÷ 2.2 = 86.4 kg

b. $86.4\ \cancel{\text{kg}} \times 25 \text{ mcg/}\cancel{\text{kg}} = 2{,}160 \text{ mcg}$

$86.4\ \cancel{\text{kg}} \times 30 \text{ mcg/}\cancel{\text{kg}} = 2{,}592 \text{ mcg}$

To determine the number of milligrams, convert the micrograms obtained to milligrams (1,000 mcg = 1 mg).

2,160 mcg ÷ 1,000 = 2.16 mg (2.2 mg, to the nearest tenth)

2,592 mcg ÷ 1,000 = 2.59 (2.6 mg to the nearest tenth)

The daily dosage range in milligrams is 2.2 to 2.6 mg.

12. a. 0.45 m^2

b. $\frac{0.45\ \cancel{\text{m}^2}}{1.7\ (\cancel{\text{m}^2})} \times 500 \text{ mg} = 132.35 = 132.4 \text{ mg}$

13. a. 1.2 m^2

b. $\frac{1.2\ \cancel{\text{m}^2}}{1.7\ (\cancel{\text{m}^2})} \times 250 \text{ mg} = 176.5 \text{ mg}$

14. a. 1.06 m^2

b. $\frac{1.06 \cancel{m^2}}{1.7 (\cancel{m^2})} \times 150 \text{ mg} = 93.52 = 93.5 \text{ mg}$

15. $\frac{0.7 \cancel{m^2}}{1.7 (\cancel{m^2})} \times 50 \text{ mg} = 20.6 \text{ mg}$

16. $\frac{0.66 \cancel{m^2}}{1.7 (\cancel{m^2})} \times 10 \text{ mg} = 3.9 \text{ mg}$

$\frac{0.66 \cancel{m^2}}{1.7 (\cancel{m^2})} \times 20 \text{ mg} = 7.8 \text{ mg}$

The dosage range is 3.9-7.8 mg.

17. $\frac{0.55 \cancel{m^2}}{1.7 (\cancel{m^2})} \times 2{,}000 \text{ units} = 647.1 \text{ units}$

18. $\frac{0.55 \cancel{m^2}}{1.7 (\cancel{m^2})} \times 200 \text{ mg} = 64.7 \text{ mg}$

$\frac{0.55 \cancel{m^2}}{1.7 (\cancel{m^2})} \times 250 \text{ mg} = 80.9 \text{ mg}$

The dosage range is 64.7-80.9 mg.

19. Dosage is incorrect; the child's dosage is 17.3 mg.

$\frac{0.49 \cancel{m^2}}{1.7 (\cancel{m^2})} \times 60 \text{ mg} = 17.3 \text{ mg}$

The dosage of 25 mg is too high.

20. $\frac{0.32 \cancel{m^2}}{1.7 (\cancel{m^2})} \times 10 \text{ mg} = 1.9 \text{ mg}$

The dosage of 4 mg is too high.

21. Dosage is correct.

$\frac{0.68 \cancel{m^2}}{1.7 (\cancel{m^2})} \times 125 \text{ mg} = 50 \text{ mg}$

$\frac{0.68 \cancel{m^2}}{1.7 (\cancel{m^2})} \times 150 \text{ mg} = 60 \text{ mg}$

The dosage of 50 mg falls within the range of 50-60 mg.

22. $\sqrt{\frac{100 \text{ (lb)} \times 55 \text{ (in)}}{3{,}131}} = \sqrt{\frac{5{,}500}{3{,}131}} = \sqrt{1.756}$

$\sqrt{1.756} = 1.325$

Answer: 1.33 m^2

23. $\sqrt{\frac{60.9 \text{ (kg)} \times 130 \text{ (cm)}}{3{,}600}} = \sqrt{\frac{7{,}917}{3{,}600}} = \sqrt{2.199}$

$\sqrt{2.199} = 1.482$

Answer: 1.48 m^2

24. $\sqrt{\frac{55 \text{ (lb)} \times 45 \text{ (in)}}{3{,}131}} = \sqrt{\frac{2{,}475}{3{,}131}} = \sqrt{0.790}$

$\sqrt{0.790} = 0.888$

Answer: 0.89 m^2

25. $\sqrt{\frac{65 \text{ (kg)} \times 132 \text{ (cm)}}{3{,}600}} = \sqrt{\frac{8{,}580}{3{,}600}} = \sqrt{2.383}$

$\sqrt{2.383} = 1.543$

Answer: 1.54 m^2

26. $\sqrt{\frac{6 \text{ (kg)} \times 55 \text{ (cm)}}{3{,}600}} = \sqrt{\frac{330}{3{,}600}} = \sqrt{0.091}$

$\sqrt{0.091} = 0.301$

Answer: 0.3 m^2

27. $\sqrt{\frac{42 \text{ (lb)} \times 45 \text{ (in)}}{3{,}131}} = \sqrt{\frac{1{,}890}{3{,}131}} = \sqrt{0.603}$

$\sqrt{0.603} = 0.776$

Answer: 0.78 m^2

28. $\sqrt{\frac{74 \text{ (kg)} \times 160 \text{ (cm)}}{3{,}600}} = \sqrt{\frac{11{,}840}{3{,}600}} = \sqrt{3.288}$

$\sqrt{3.288} = 1.813$

Answer: 1.81 m^2

29. $10 \text{ mg} : 1 \text{ mL} = 7 \text{ mg} : x \text{ mL}$

or

$\frac{7 \text{ mg}}{10 \text{ mg}} \times 1 \text{ mL} = x \text{ mL}$

Answer: 0.7 mL. The dosage ordered is less than the available strength; therefore you will need less than 1 mL to administer the dosage.

30. $0.05 \text{ mg} : 1 \text{ mL} = 0.1 \text{ mg} : x \text{ mL}$

or

$\frac{0.1 \text{ mg}}{0.05 \text{ mg}} \times 1 \text{ mL} = x \text{ mL}$

Answer: 2 mL. The dosage ordered is more than the available strength; therefore you will need more than 1 mL to administer the dosage.

31. $50 \text{ mg} : 5 \text{ mL} = 80 \text{ mg} : x \text{ mL}$

or

$\frac{80 \text{ mg}}{50 \text{ mg}} \times 5 \text{ mL} = x \text{ mL}$

Answer: 8 mL. The dosage ordered is greater than the available strength; therefore you will need more than 5 mL to administer the dosage.

32. Conversion required. Equivalent: 1,000 mg = 1 g. Therefore 0.25 g = 250 mg.

$100 \text{ mg} : 5 \text{ mL} = 250 \text{ mg} : x \text{ mL}$

or

$\frac{250 \text{ mg}}{100 \text{ mg}} \times 5 \text{ mL} = x \text{ mL}$

Answer: 12.5 mL. The dosage ordered is greater than the available strength; therefore you will need more than 5 mL to administer the dosage.

33. $250 \text{ mg} : 5 \text{ mL} = 100 \text{ mg} : x \text{ mL}$

or

$\frac{100 \text{ mg}}{250 \text{ mg}} \times 5 \text{ mL} = x \text{ mL}$

Answer: 2 mL. The dosage ordered is less than the available strength; therefore you will need less than 5 mL to administer the dosage.

34. $20 \text{ mg} : 2 \text{ mL} = 7.3 \text{ mg} : x \text{ mL}$

or

$\frac{7.3 \text{ mg}}{20 \text{ mg}} \times 2 \text{ mL} = x \text{ mL}$

Answer: 0.73 mL. The dosage ordered is less than the available strength; therefore you will need less than 2 mL to administer the dosage.

35. A conversion is required. Equivalent: 1,000 mcg = 1 mg. Therefore 0.1 mg = 100 mcg.

$400 \text{ mcg} : 1 \text{ mL} = 100 \text{ mcg} : x \text{ mL}$

or

$\frac{100 \text{ mcg}}{400 \text{ mcg}} \times 1 \text{ mL} = x \text{ mL}$

Answer: 0.25 mL. The dosage ordered is less than the available strength; therefore you will need less than 1 mL to administer the dosage.

36. $20 \text{ mg} : 2 \text{ mL} = 60 \text{ mg} : x \text{ mL}$

or

$\frac{60 \text{ mg}}{20 \text{ mg}} \times 2 \text{ mL} = x \text{ mL}$

Answer: 6 mL. The dosage ordered is more than the available strength; therefore you will need more than 2 mL to administer the dosage.

37. Conversion required. Equivalent: 1,000 mg = 1 g.

Therefore 0.4 g = 400 mg.

$160 \text{ mg} : 5 \text{ mL} = 400 \text{ mg} : x \text{ mL}$

or

$\frac{400 \text{ mg}}{160 \text{ mg}} \times 5 \text{ mL} = x \text{ mL}$

Answer: 12.5 mL. The dosage ordered is more than the available strength; therefore you will need more than 5 mL to administer the dosage.

38. $25 \text{ mg} : 1 \text{ mL} = 35 \text{ mg} : x \text{ mL}$

or

$\frac{35 \text{ mg}}{25 \text{ mg}} \times 1 \text{ mL} = x \text{ mL}$

Answer: 1.4 mL. The dosage ordered is more than the available strength; therefore you will need more than 1 mL to administer the dosage.

39. $150 \text{ mg} : 1 \text{ mL} = 100 \text{ mg} : x \text{ mL}$

or

$\frac{100 \text{ mg}}{150 \text{ mg}} \times 1 \text{ mL} = x \text{ mL}$

Answer: 0.66 = 0.7 mL. The dosage ordered is less than the available strength; therefore you will need less than 1 mL to administer the dosage.

40. $100 \text{ mg} : 2 \text{ mL} = 150 \text{ mg} : x \text{ mL}$

or

$\frac{150 \text{ mg}}{100 \text{ mg}} \times 2 \text{ mL} = x \text{ mL}$

Answer: 3 mL. The dosage ordered is more than the available strength; therefore you will need more than 2 mL to administer the dosage.

41. $125 \text{ mg} : 5 \text{ mL} = 62.5 \text{ mg} : x \text{ mL}$

or

$\frac{62.5 \text{ mg}}{125 \text{ mg}} \times 5 \text{ mL} = x \text{ mL}$

Answer: 2.5 mL. The dosage ordered is less than the available strength; therefore you will need less than 5 mL to administer the dosage.

42. $200 \text{ mg} : 5 \text{ mL} = 300 \text{ mg} : x \text{ mL}$

or

$\frac{300 \text{ mg}}{200 \text{ mg}} \times 5 \text{ mL} = x \text{ mL}$

Answer: 7.5 mL. The dosage ordered is more than the available strength; therefore you will need more than 5 mL to administer the dosage.

43. $2 \text{ mg} : 5 \text{ mL} = 3 \text{ mg} : x \text{ mL}$

or

$\frac{3 \text{ mg}}{2 \text{ mg}} \times 5 \text{ mL} = x \text{ mL}$

Answer: 7.5 mL. The dosage ordered is more than the available strength; therefore you will need more than 5 mL to administer the dosage.

44. $15 \text{ mg} : 0.6 \text{ mL} = 45 \text{ mg} : x \text{ mL}$

or

$\frac{45 \text{ mg}}{15 \text{ mg}} \times 0.6 \text{ mL} = x \text{ mL}$

Answer: 1.8 mL. The dosage ordered is greater than the available strength; therefore you will need more than 0.6 mL to administer the dosage.

45. 40 mg : 1 mL = 14 mg : x mL

or

$$\frac{14 \text{ mg}}{40 \text{ mg}} \times 1 \text{ mL} = x \text{ mL}$$

Answer: 0.35 = 0.4 mL rounded to the nearest tenth. The dosage ordered is less than the available strength; therefore you will need less than 1 mL to administer the dosage.

46. 8 mg : 1 mL = 20 mg : x mL

or

$$\frac{20 \text{ mg}}{8 \text{ mg}} \times 1 \text{ mL} = x \text{ mL}$$

Answer: 2.5 mL. The dosage ordered is more than the available strength; therefore you will need more than 1 mL to administer the dosage.

47. a. Convert the child's weight in pounds to kilograms. The recommended dosage is expressed in kilograms (20 mg/kg/day) (2.2 lb = 1 kg).

10 lb = 10 ÷ 2.2 = 4.5 kg

20 mg/~~kg~~/day × 4.5 ~~kg~~ = 90 mg/day

The medication is given in three divided doses. The dosage for the child is ordered q8h.

24 ÷ 8 = 3 doses.

90 mg ÷ 3 = 30 mg per dose

180 mg × 3 = 540 mg/day

Notify the prescriber; the dosage is too high (not safe).

540 mg/day is greater than 90 mg/day. In addition, the dose the child is receiving q8h exceeds the dose recommended.

b. The volume to be administered is not calculated because the dosage ordered is not safe.

48. Convert the child's weight in pounds to kilograms. The recommended dosage is in kilograms (22.5 mg/kg) (2.2 lb = 1 kg).

66 lb = 66 ÷ 2.2 = 30 kg

22.5 mg/~~kg~~ × 30 ~~kg~~ = 675 mg/dose

The medication is given up to three times a day. The dosage for the child is ordered tid. The dosage ordered is not safe. The child is receiving 650 mg/dose, which is less than the recommended dosage and may not be effective. Notify the prescriber.

49. a. Convert the child's weight in pounds to kilograms (2.2 lb = 1 kg). The recommended dosage is in kilograms, and the dosage is ordered q4h. The dosage is determined using 12.5 mg/kg/dose.

92.4 lb = 92.4 ÷ 2.2 = 42 kg

12.5 mg/~~kg~~/dose × 42 ~~kg~~ = 525 mg/dose

The safe dosage for this child is 525 mg/dose

b. The dosage ordered for the child is safe. For this child's weight, 525 mg/dose is the recommended dosage, and 525 mg is the ordered dosage.

50. Convert the child's weight in pounds to kilograms. The recommended dosage is in kilograms (0.25-1 mg/kg) (2.2 lb = 1 kg).

31 lb = 31 ÷ 2.2 = 14.1 kg

0.25 mg/~~kg~~/day × 14.1 ~~kg~~ = 3.5 mg/day

1 mg/~~kg~~/day × 14.1 ~~kg~~ = 14.1 mg/day

The safe dosage range for this child is 3.5-14.1 mg/day.

51. $0.8 \cancel{m^2} \times \frac{2 \text{ mg}}{\cancel{m^2}} = 1.6 \text{ mg}$

52. $0.82 \cancel{m^2} \times \frac{250 \text{ mg}}{\cancel{m^2}} = 205 \text{ mg}$

53. $1.83 \cancel{m^2} \times \frac{10 \text{ units}}{\cancel{m^2}} = 18.3 \text{ units}$

$1.83 \cancel{m^2} \times \frac{20 \text{ units}}{\cancel{m^2}} = 36.6 \text{ units}$

Dosage range is 18.3 to 36.6 units

NOTE

For problems 54-55, a ratio and proportion could be set up and mL/hr determined first, which, when a burette is used without a pump or controller, is the same as gtt/min. If gtt/min is determined first, remember that it is the same as mL/hr.

54. $x \text{ gtt/min} = \dfrac{30 \text{ mL} \times 60 \text{ gtt/mL}}{20 \text{ min}}$

$x = \dfrac{1{,}800}{20}$; $x = 90$ gtt/min

or

mL /hr determined with ratio and proportion

$30 \text{ mL} : 20 \text{ min} = x \text{ mL} : 60 \text{ min}$

or

$\dfrac{30 \text{ mL}}{20 \text{ min}} = \dfrac{x \text{ mL}}{60 \text{ min}}$

a. 90 gtt/min; 90 microgtt/min

b. 90 mL /hr

55. $x \text{ gtt/min} = \dfrac{80 \text{ mL} \times 60 \text{ gtt/mL}}{60 \text{ min}}$

$x = \dfrac{4{,}800}{60}$; $x = 80$ gtt/min

or

Determine mL /hr

$80 \text{ mL} : 60 \text{ min} = x \text{ mL} : 60 \text{ min}$

$\dfrac{80 \text{ mL}}{60 \text{ min}} = \dfrac{x \text{ mL}}{60 \text{ min}}$

a. 80 gtt/min; 80 microgtt/min

b. 80 mL /hr

56. Step 1: Calculate the safe dosage range for child.

$23 \cancel{\text{kg}} \times 40 \text{ mg}/\cancel{\text{kg}} = 920$ mg

$23 \cancel{\text{kg}} \times 50 \text{ mg}/\cancel{\text{kg}} = 1{,}150$ mg

Step 2: Calculate the dosage the child receives in 24 hours.

500 mg q12hr (2 dosages) $500 \times 2 = 1{,}000$ mg

Step 3: Compare dosage ordered with safe range.

The dosage ordered is 1,000 mg; it is within the safe range of 920-1,150 mg/day.

57. Step 1: Calculate the safe dosage range for the child.

$20 \cancel{\text{kg}} \times 0.05 \text{ mg}/\cancel{\text{kg}} = 1$ mg

Step 2: Child receives 2 mg of medication at 10 AM.

Step 3: The dosage ordered is 2 mg. 1 mg is the safe dosage; notify the prescriber that 2 mg is not a safe dose.

58. a. $100 \text{ mL}/\cancel{\text{kg}}/\text{day} \times 10 \cancel{\text{kg}} = 1{,}000$ mL/day (for the first 10 kg)

$50 \text{ mL}/\cancel{\text{kg}}/\text{day} \times 10 \cancel{\text{kg}} = 500$ mL/day (for next 10 kg)

$20 \text{ mL}/\cancel{\text{kg}}/\text{day} \times 5 \cancel{\text{kg}} = 100$ mL/day (for remaining 5 kg)

Total: 1,000 mL/day + 500 mL/day = 100 mL/day = 1,600 mL/day

Answer: 1,600 mL/day or per 24 hr

b. $x \text{ mL/hr} = \dfrac{1{,}600 \text{ mL}}{24 \text{ hr}} = 66.6$

$x = 67$ mL/hr

Answer: 67 mL/hr

59. Convert weight:

Equivalent: 1 kg = 1,000 g

$4{,}200 \text{ g} \div 1{,}000 = 4.2$ kg

a. $100 \text{ mL}/\cancel{\text{kg}}/\text{day} \times 4.2 \cancel{\text{kg}} = 420$ mL/day

Answer: 420 mL/day

b. $x \text{ mL/hr} = \dfrac{420 \text{ mL}}{24 \text{ hr}} = 17.5$

$x = 17.5$ mL/hr

Answer: 17.5 mL/hr (pump capable of delivering in tenths of a mL)

60. a. $\text{m}^2 = \sqrt{\dfrac{21 \text{ (lb)} \times 30 \text{ (in)}}{3{,}131}} = 0.448 = 0.45 \text{ m}^2$

Answer: 0.45 m^2

b. $0.45 \cancel{\text{m}^2} \times \dfrac{1.5 \text{ mg}}{\cancel{\text{m}^2}} = 0.67 = 0.7$ mg

$0.45 \cancel{\text{m}^2} \times \dfrac{2 \text{ mg}}{\cancel{\text{m}^2}} = 0.9$ mg

Dosage range is 0.7-0.9 mg

61. a. $\text{m}^2 = \sqrt{\dfrac{75 \text{ (kg)} \times 162 \text{ (cm)}}{3{,}600}} = 1.837 = 1.84 \text{ m}^2$

Answer: 1.84 m^2

b. $1.84 \cancel{\text{m}^2} \times \dfrac{750 \text{ mg}}{\cancel{\text{m}^2}} = 1{,}380$ mg

Answer: 1,380 mg

Comprehensive Post-Test

Solve the following calculation problems. Remember to apply the principles learned in the text relating to dosages. Use labels where provided. Shade in the dosage on the syringe where indicated.

1. Order: Amoxicillin and clavulanate potassium 300 mg p.o. q8h (ordered according to dose of amoxicillin).

   Available:

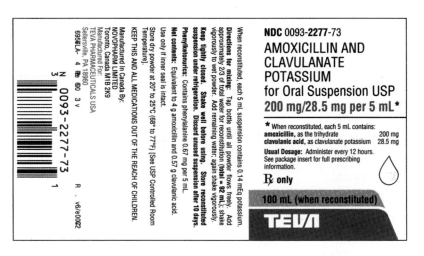

   ____

2. Order: Campral DR (delayed-release) 666 mg p.o. t.i.d.

   Available:

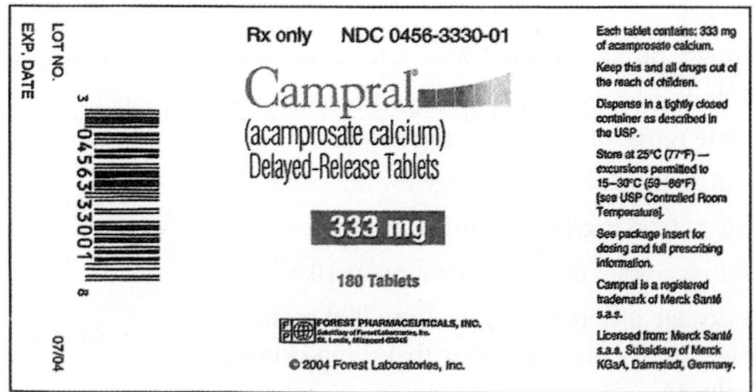

   ____

3. Order: Septra DS 1 tab p.o. q12h for 14 days.

   Available:

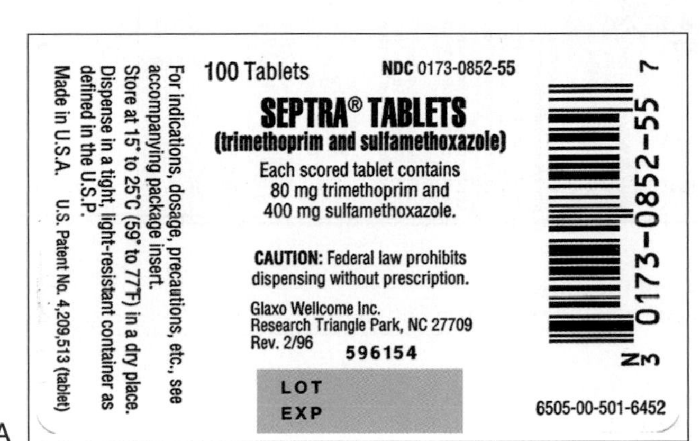

A

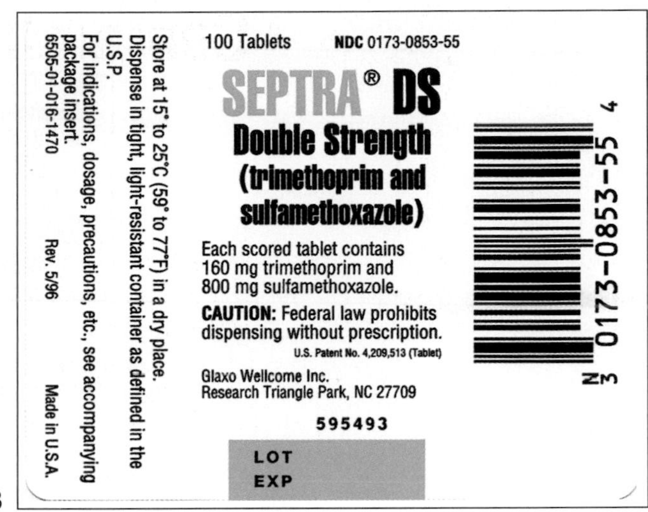

B

   a. Indicate by letter which tablets the nurse would choose to administer to the client based on the order. ________________

   b. State why. ________________

4. Order: Heparin 6,500 units subcut daily. (Express your answer in hundredths.)

   Available:

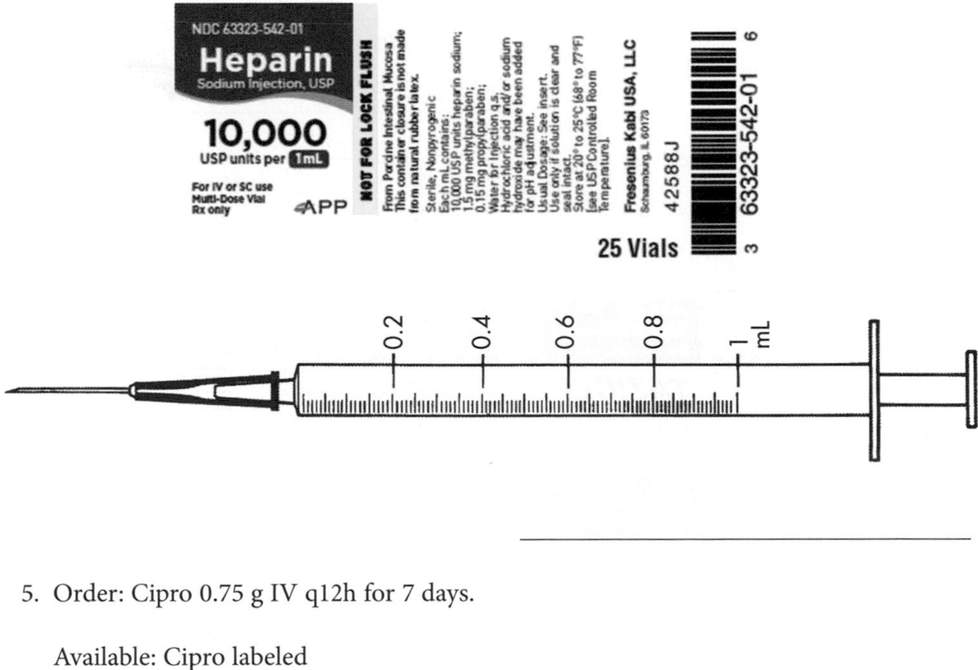

____

5. Order: Cipro 0.75 g IV q12h for 7 days.

   Available: Cipro labeled
   400 mg per 40 mL ________________

6. Order: Amphotericin B 75 mg in 1,000 mL D5W to infuse over 6 hr daily. The reconstituted solution contains 50 mg per 10 mL.

   Available:

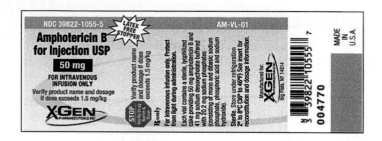

   a. How many milliliters will the nurse add to the IV solution? ____________

   b. The IV is to infuse in 6 hr. The administration set delivers 10 gtt/mL. At what rate in gtt/min should the IV infuse? ____________

7. The recommended dose of Retrovir for adults with symptomatic HIV infection is 1 mg/kg infused over 1 hour q4h. Determine dosage for a client weighing 110 lb. ____________

8. Order: Epivir 0.3 g p.o. every day.

   Available: Epivir tablets labeled 150 mg

   How many tablets will the nurse administer? ____________

9. Order: Tazicef 0.25 g IV q12h.

   Available:

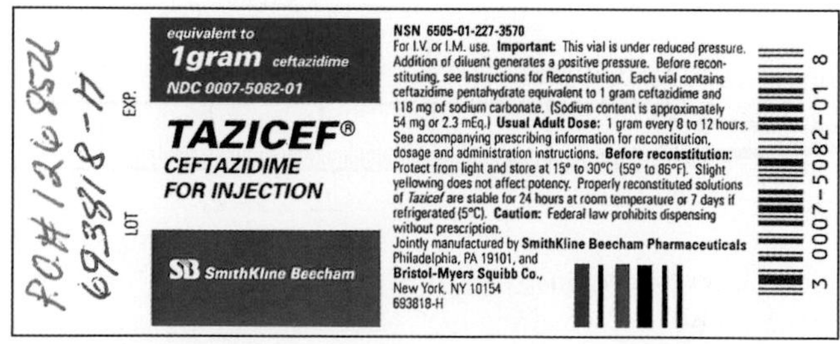

Directions for reconstitution state the following for IV infusion: 1-g vial, add 10 mL sterile water to provide 95 mg per mL; 2-g vial, add 10 mL sterile water to provide 180 mg per mL.

   a. Using the information provided, what concentration will the nurse prepare? ____________

b. How many milliliters will the nurse administer? ______________________

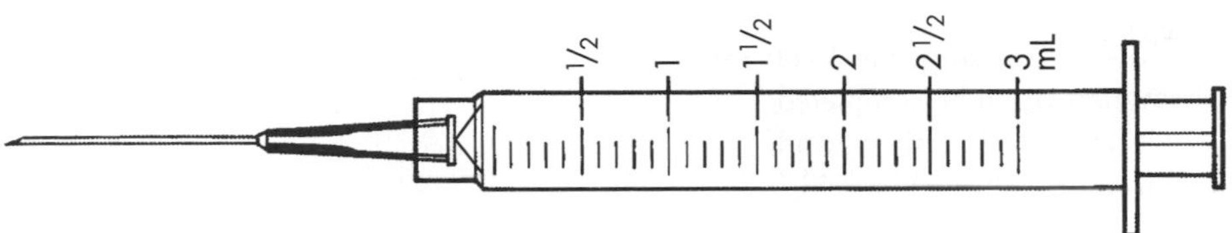

10. Order: Prandin 3 mg p.o. b.i.d.

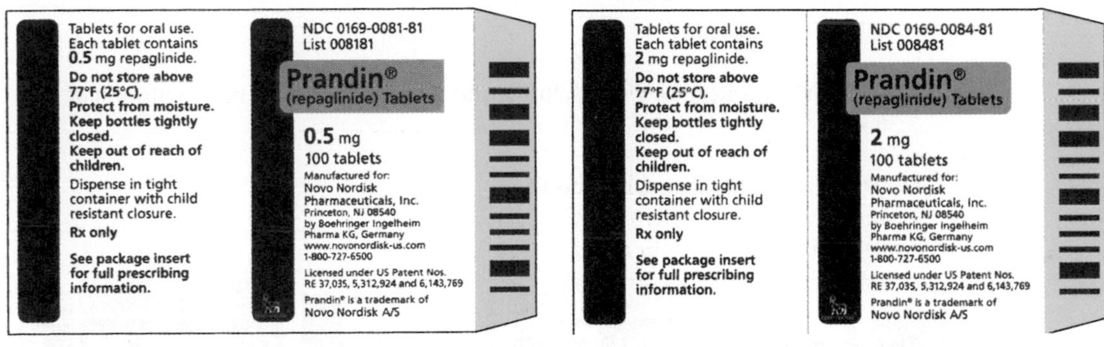

How many of which tablets would be best to administer to the client? ______________________

11. Order: Transfuse 1 unit packed red blood cells (250 mL) over 3 hr. The administration set delivers 20 gtt/mL. At what rate in gtt/min should the IV infuse? ______________________

12. A client is receiving 500 mg of Flagyl IVPB q8h. The Flagyl has been placed in 100 mL D5W to infuse over 45 minutes. The administration set delivers 10 gtt/mL. At what rate in gtt/min should the IV infuse? ______________________

13. Calculate the infusion time for an IV of 1,000 mL of D5NS infusing at 60 mL/hr. Express time in hours and minutes. ______________________

14. The prescriber orders Septra Suspension 60 mg p.o. q12h for a child weighing 12 kg. The pediatric medication reference states that Septra Suspension contains trimethoprim (TMP) 40 mg and sulfamethoxazole (SMZ) 200 mg in 5 mL oral suspension, and the safe dosage of the medication is based on trimethoprim. The safe dosage is 6 to 12 mg/kg/day of TMP given q12h. Is the dosage ordered safe? ______________________

15. A medicated IV of 100 mL is to infuse at a rate of 50 mL/hr.

    a. Determine the infusion time. ______________________

    b. The IV was started at 10:00 AM. When will it be completed? (State time in military and traditional time.) ______________________

16. A client is to receive 10 mcg/min nitroglycerin IV. The concentration of solution is 50 mg in 250 mL D5W. What should the flow rate be (in mL/hr) to deliver 10 mcg/min? ______________________

17. Order: Humulin Regular U-100 6 units and Humulin NPH U-100 16 units subcut at 7:30 AM.

    What is the total units the nurse will administer? ______________________

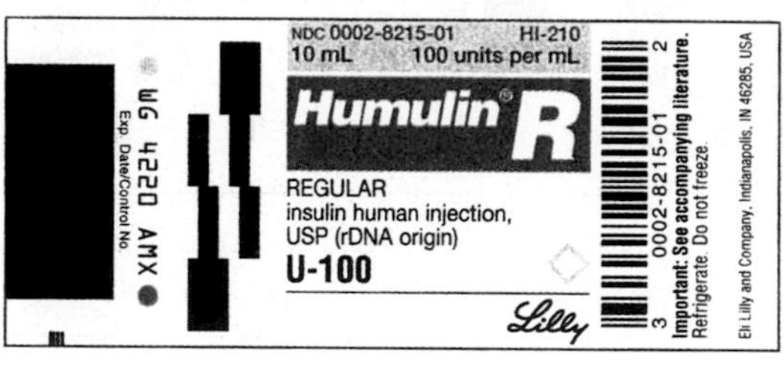

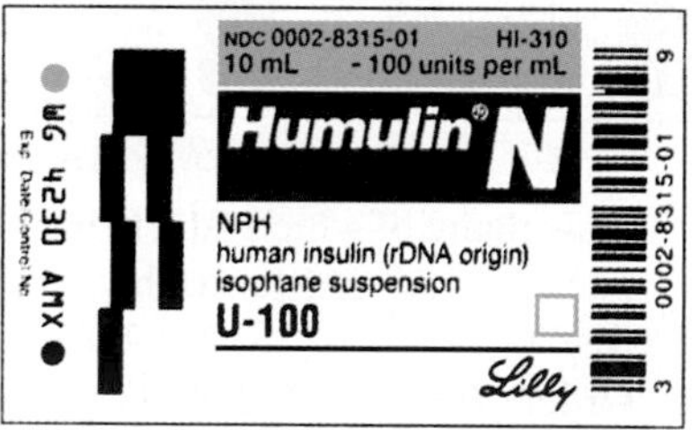

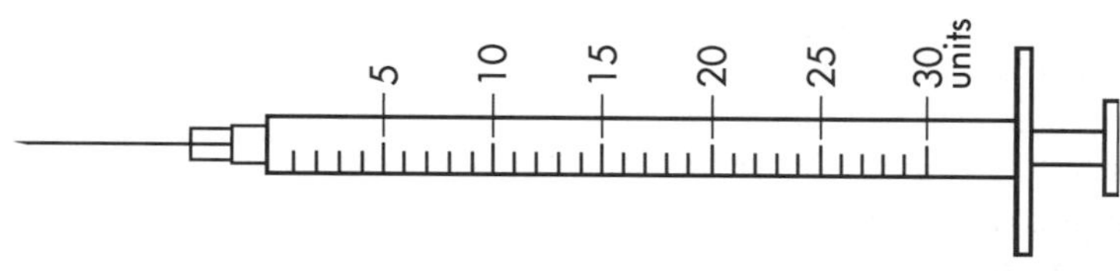

18. A dosage of 500 mg in a volume of 3 mL is to be diluted to 55 mL to infuse over 50 minutes. A 20-mL flush is to follow.

    a. What is the dilution volume? ______________________

    b. At what rate in gtt/min should the IV infuse? (Administration set is a microdrop.) ______________________

    c. Indicate the rate in mL/hr. ______________________

19. Calculate the body surface area (BSA), using the formula, for a child who weighs 102 lb and is 51 inches tall. Calculate the BSA to the nearest hundredth. ______________________

20. Acyclovir IV is to be administered to a child who has herpes simplex encephalitis. The child weighs 13.6 kg and is 60 cm tall. The recommended dosage is 500 mg/m^2. Use the formula to calculate the BSA.

Available:

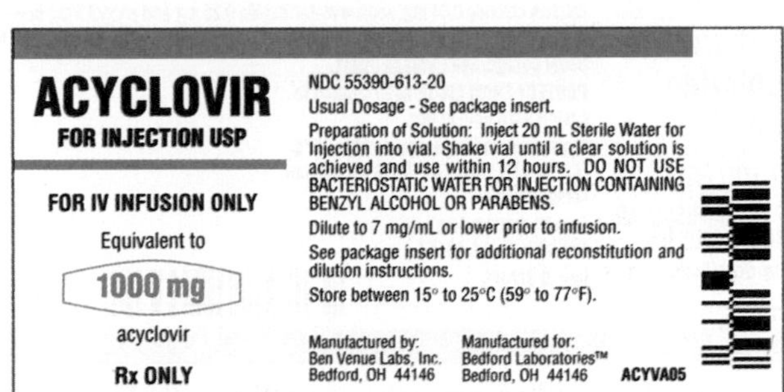
ACYCLOVIR
FOR INJECTION USP
FOR IV INFUSION ONLY
Equivalent to
1000 mg
acyclovir
Rx ONLY
NDC 55390-613-20
Usual Dosage - See package insert.
Preparation of Solution: Inject 20 mL Sterile Water for Injection into vial. Shake vial until a clear solution is achieved and use within 12 hours. DO NOT USE BACTERIOSTATIC WATER FOR INJECTION CONTAINING BENZYL ALCOHOL OR PARABENS.
Dilute to 7 mg/mL or lower prior to infusion.
See package insert for additional reconstitution and dilution instructions.
Store between 15° to 25°C (59° to 77°F).
Manufactured by: Ben Venue Labs, Inc. Bedford, OH 44146
Manufactured for: Bedford Laboratories™ Bedford, OH 44146
ACYVA05

a. What is the BSA? (Express your answer to the nearest hundredth.) ______________

b. What will the dosage be? ______________

c. The reconstituted Zovirax provides 50 mg per mL. Calculate the number of milliliters to administer. ______________

21. Prepare the following strength solution: 2/5 strength Ensure Plus 250 mL. ______________

22. A child weighing 21.4 kg has an order for 500 mg of a medication in 100 mL D5W q12h. The normal daily dosage range is 40 to 50 mg/kg. Determine if the dosage is within normal range, and state the course of action. ______________

23. Calculate the amount of dextrose and NaCl in 2 L of D5 ¼ NS.

a. Dextrose ______________ g

b. Sodium chloride ______________ g

24. 500 mL D5W was to infuse in 3 hours at 28 gtt/min (28 macrogtt/min). The drop factor is 10 gtt/mL. After 1½ hours, you notice 175 mL has infused.

a. Recalculate the IV flow rate. ______________

b. Determine the percentage of change. ______________

c. State the course of action. ______________

25. Order: Infuse D5W 500 mL with 20,000 units heparin at 25 mL/hr. Determine the following:

______________ units/hr

26. Order: Phenergan (promethazine hydrochloride) 25 mg IV push before surgery. The literature states: Do not give at a rate above 25 mg/min.

    Available:

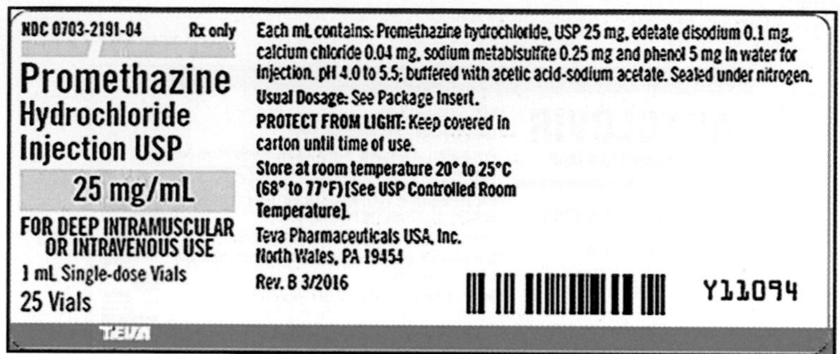

    a. How many milliliters will the nurse prepare? ______________

    b. What is the number of minutes the medication should be administered? ______________

27. Order: Morphine sulfate 80 mg in 250 mL of IV fluid to infuse at a rate of 20 mL/hr.

    Determine the dosage in mg/hr the client is receiving. ______________

28. Order: Diltiazem HCl (cardizem) 25 mg IV over 2 minutes.

    Available:

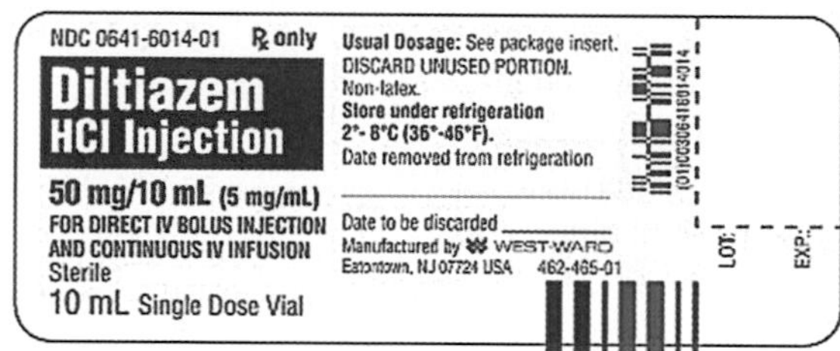

    a. How many milliliters will the nurse add to the IV? ______________

    b. How many milliliters will the nurse infuse per minute? ______________

29. Order: Cipro 0.5 g p.o. q12h.

    Available: Cipro tablets labeled 250 mg

    How many tablets will be needed for 10 days of therapy? ______________

30. Order: Lanoxin (digoxin) tablets 0.375 mg p.o. stat.

    Available: Scored tablets labeled 125 mcg, 250 mcg, and 500 mcg.

    a. Which Lanoxin tablet(s) will the nurse use to prepare the dosage? ______________

    b. How many tablets should the client receive? ______________

31. Order: Infergen 12 mcg subcut stat.

    Available: Infergen 15 mcg per 0.5 mL.

    How many milliliters will the nurse administer? ________________

32. Order: Digoxin 0.125 mg IV daily for 7 days.

    Available:

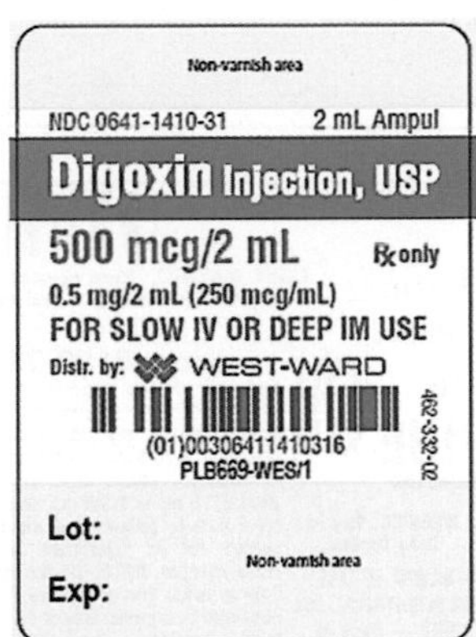

a. How many milliliters will the nurse administer? ________________

b. Shade the dosage in on the syringe provided.

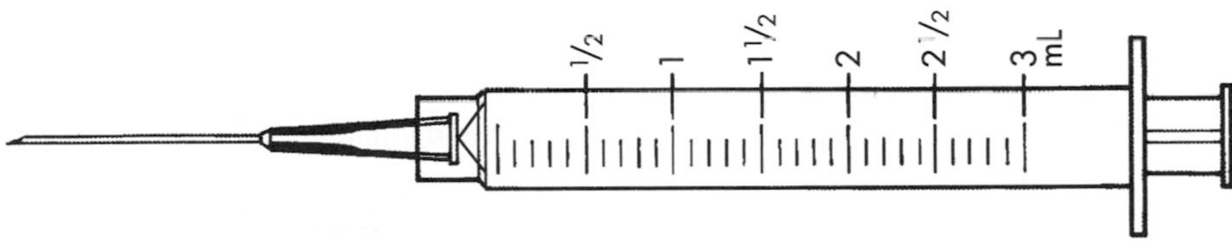

For problems 33-34, round weight to the nearest tenth as indicated.

33. The heparin protocol at an institution is: Bolus client with 80 units/kg of body weight and start drip at 14 unit/kg/hr. Using the heparin protocol, determine the following for a client weighing 242 lb.

    a. Heparin bolus dosage ________________

    b. Infusion rate for the heparin IV drip ________________

34. Order: 20 units/kg/hr heparin IV. The client weighs 88 kg.

    How many units will the client receive per hour? ________________

35. Order: Digoxin 0.375 mg IV push (infused slowly over 5 minutes).

    Available: Digoxin 0.25 mg per mL

    a. How many milliliters should the nurse administer? ______________________

    b. At what rate in mL/min should the IV infuse? ______________________

36. Order: Morphine 8 mg IV q4h p.r.n. (infusion not to exceed 10 mg/4 min).

    Available:

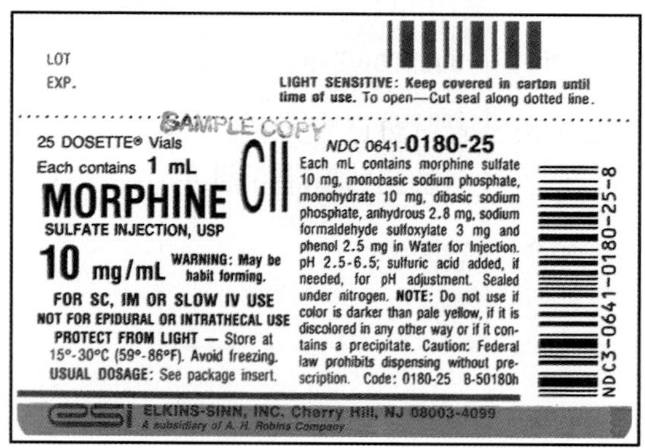
LOT
EXP.
LIGHT SENSITIVE: Keep covered in carton until time of use. To open—Cut seal along dotted line.
SAMPLE COPY
25 DOSETTE® Vials
Each contains 1 mL
MORPHINE
CII
SULFATE INJECTION, USP
10 mg/mL
WARNING: May be habit forming.
FOR SC, IM OR SLOW IV USE
NOT FOR EPIDURAL OR INTRATHECAL USE
PROTECT FROM LIGHT — Store at 15°-30°C (59°-86°F). Avoid freezing.
USUAL DOSAGE: See package insert.
NDC 0641-0180-25
Each mL contains morphine sulfate 10 mg, monobasic sodium phosphate, monohydrate 10 mg, dibasic sodium phosphate, anhydrous 2.8 mg, sodium formaldehyde sulfoxylate 3 mg and phenol 2.5 mg in Water for Injection. pH 2.5-6.5; sulfuric acid added, if needed, for pH adjustment. Sealed under nitrogen. NOTE: Do not use if color is darker than pale yellow, if it is discolored in any other way or if it contains a precipitate. Caution: Federal law prohibits dispensing without prescription. Code: 0180-25 B-50180h
NDC3-0641-0180-25-8
ELKINS-SINN, INC. Cherry Hill, NJ 08003-4099
A subsidiary of A. H. Robins Company

    a. How many milliliters will the nurse administer? ______________________

    b. How many minutes will it take for the IV to infuse? ______________________

37. Refer to the chart below and calculate the client's fluid intake in milliliters.

ORAL INTAKE	IV INTAKE
4 oz gelatin 2 oz water 12 oz apple juice	100 mL

What is the client's intake in mL? ______________

Refer to the Heparin Weight-Based Protocol provided below to answer question 38.

1. Bolus heparin at 80 units/kg.
2. Begin intravenous infusion of heparin at 18 units/kg/hr using 25,000 units heparin in 250 mL D5W for 1,000 units per mL.
3. Adjust intravenous heparin daily based on APTT results.
   - APTT less than 35 sec: Rebolus with 80 units/kg and increase rate by 4 units/kg/hr.
   - APTT 35-45 sec: Rebolus with 40 units/kg and increase rate by 2 units/kg/hr.
   - APTT 46-70 sec: **No change.**
   - APTT 71-90 sec: Decrease rate by 2 units/kg/hr.
   - APTT greater than 90 sec: **Stop heparin** infusion for 1 hour and decrease rate by 3 units/kg/hr.

38. Client weighs 187 lb. Determine the bolus dose of heparin and the initial intravenous rate of heparin. The APTT is reported as being 43 seconds. Determine the rebolus and adjust the intravenous rate based on the APTT results.

39. A client is ordered to begin Levophed (norepinephrine bitartrate) at 4 mcg/min to maintain blood pressure and titrate to maintain systolic blood pressure greater than 100 mm Hg to a maximum of 12 mcg/min. Available solution is Levophed 8 mg in 1,000 mL D5W. Develop a titration table from minimum to maximum dose in 2 mcg/min increments. (The IV pump is calibrated in whole mL.)

40. Versed (midazolam) 10 mcg/kg IV is ordered for sedation of a client. The client weighs 127.2 lb. How many mcg should the client receive? ____________

41. Order: Kantrex 32 mg IV q8h for an infant.

Available: Kantrex labeled 75 mg per 2 mL

a. How many mL will the nurse add to the IV? ____________

b. Shade the dosage in on the syringe provided.

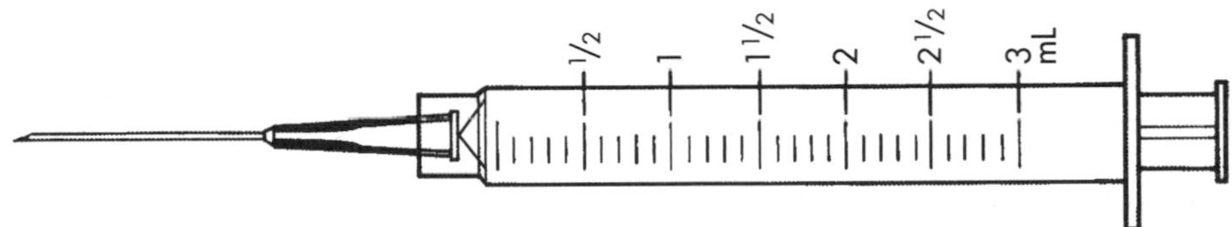

42. Order: Gemzar 900 mg IV weekly

Available:

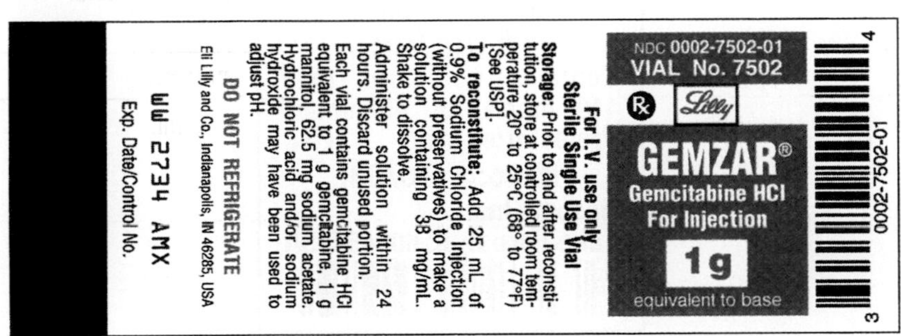
NDC 0002-7502-01
VIAL No. 7502
Rx Lilly
GEMZAR®
Gemcitabine HCl
For Injection
1 g
equivalent to base
For I.V. use only
Sterile Single Use Vial
Storage: Prior to and after reconstitution, store at controlled room temperature 20° to 25°C (68° to 77°F) [See USP].
To reconstitute: Add 25 mL of 0.9% Sodium Chloride Injection (without preservatives) to make a solution containing 38 mg/mL. Shake to dissolve.
Administer solution within 24 hours. Discard unused portion.
Each vial contains gemcitabine HCl equivalent to 1 g gemcitabine, 1 g mannitol, 62.5 mg sodium acetate. Hydrochloric acid and/or sodium hydroxide may have been used to adjust pH.
DO NOT REFRIGERATE
Eli Lilly and Co., Indianapolis, IN 46285, USA
Exp. Date/Control No.
0002-7502-01

How many mL will the nurse add to the IV? ____________

43. Using a full strength hydrogen peroxide (3%) solution, prepare 180 mL of 1/3 strength hydrogen peroxide solution for wound care, using normal saline as the diluent.
Answer ____________

44. Refer to the following medication orders and correct them according to the ISMP published list of Error Prone Abbreviations and Symbols.

    a. MS 4 mg sc q4h prn pain ______________________

    b. Digoxin .375 mg p.o. qd ______________________

45. Order: Ultram 0.1 g po q6h prn for pain.

    Available:

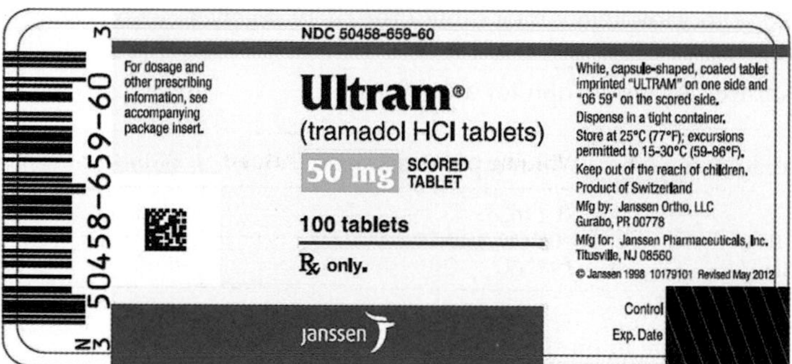

    How many tab(s) will the nurse administer? ______________________

46. Order: Vitamin K 2.5 mg subcut stat.

    Available:

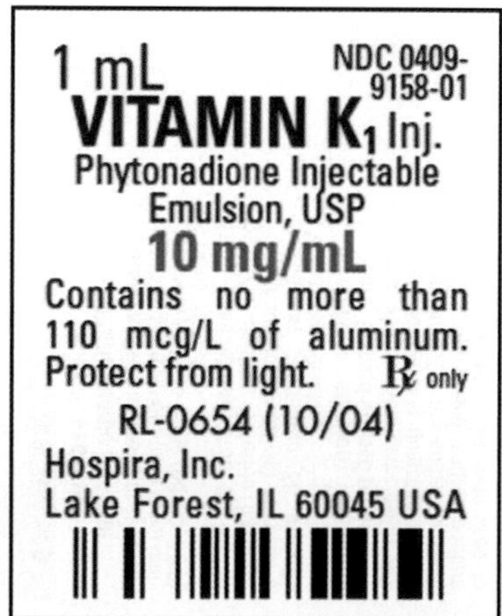

    a. How many mL will the nurse administer? ______________________

    b. Shade the dosage on the syringe provided.

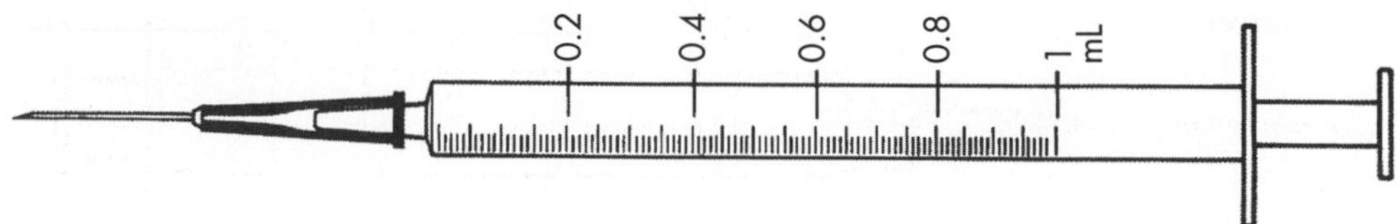

47. Order: Unasyn 1,550 mg IV q6h

Available: Refer to label and portion of the package insert.

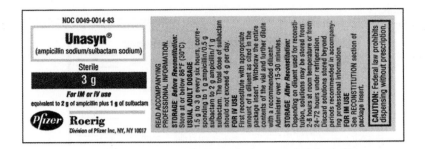

Unasyn Vial Size	Volume of Diluent to Be Added	Withdrawal Volume
1.5 g	3.2 mL	4 mL
3 g	6.4 mL	8 mL

How many mL will the nurse administer? ___________________________

48. Order: Morphine Sulfate 6 mg IM and Phenergan (promethazine HCl). 20 mg IM q6h prn for pain post operatively.

Available:

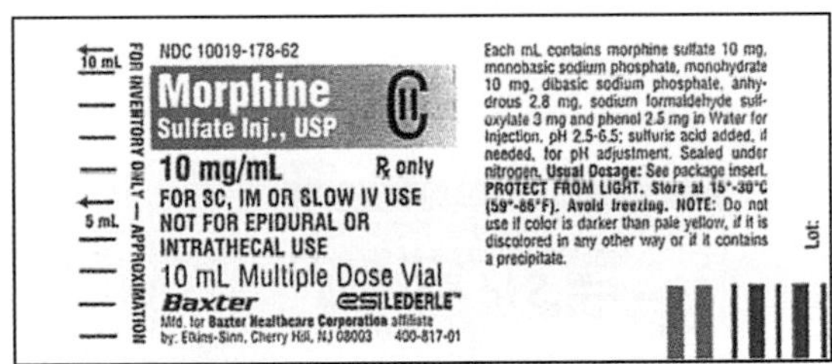

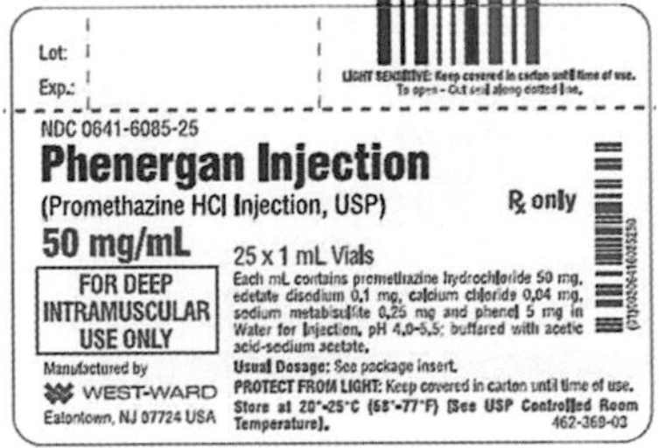

a. What is the total dose in mL the nurse will administer? ___________________

b. Shade the dosage on the syringe provided.

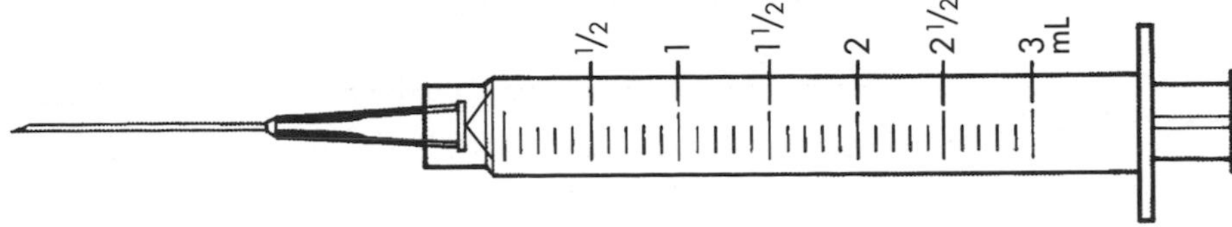

49. Order: Zantac (ranitidine) 15 mg IV q8h for a child weighing 33 lb. According to *The Harriet Lane Handbook,* the recommended dosage of ranitidine is 2-4 mg/kg/24hr ÷ q6-8hr.

Available:

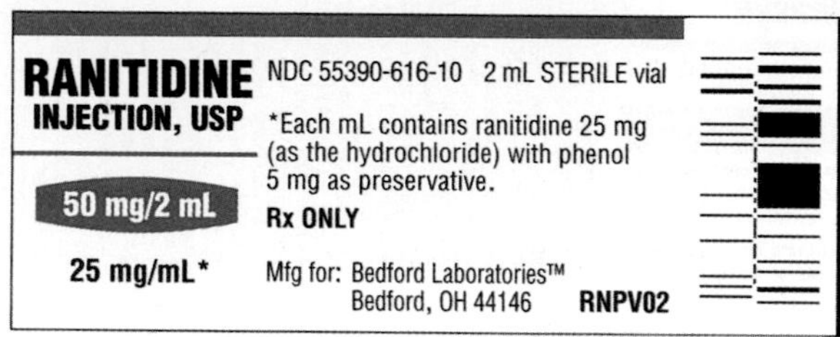

a. Is the dosage ordered safe? (prove mathematically)

b. If the dosage ordered is safe, calculate the mL the nurse would administer ______.

If not safe, explain why and describe what the nurse should do. ______________

____.

50. Order: Vincristine 4 mg IV q Thursday for a child who weighs 45 kg and is 155 cm. The recommended dose of Vincristine is 1.5-2 mg/m² in a single dose weekly. (Use the BSA Formula.) Round dosage to nearest tenth.

Available:

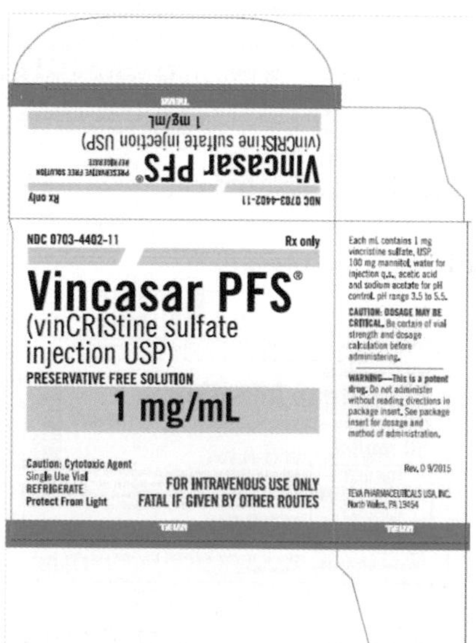

a. Is the dose ordered safe? (Prove mathematically)

b. If the dosage ordered is safe, calculate the mL you would administer __________.

If not safe, explain why and describe what you should do. ______________

____.

51. Calculate the I & O from 7 am–3 pm

A client has IV fluids D_5 ½ NS with 20 meq potassium chloride (KCl) infusing at 75 mL/hr at 7 am. An order is received to increase the IV fluid to 100 mL/hr at 10 am. The IV fluids are held for 1 hour while Ampicillin 1 g in 100 mL of 0.9% NS is infused from 12pm to 1pm. The client consumes the following:

Breakfast: 1½ glasses of cranberry juice (glass = 6oz)

2½ cups of tea (cup = 8oz)

Lunch: ¾ can of gingerale (can = 12oz)

½ bowl of broth (bowl = 6oz)

4oz ice cream

The client voids four times during the shift for 375 mL, 250 mL, 400 mL, and 300 mL of urine.

Intake ______________ mL

Output ______________ mL

52. A continuous heparin infusion is to begin at 15 units/kg/hr for a client weighing 82 kg. Available: 25,000 units in 250 mL D_5W. Calculate the mL/hr (the pump is capable of delivering in tenths of a mL).

______________________________ mL/hr

For questions 53-55, calculate the daily fluid maintenance and hourly IV rate using the following formula:

100 mL/kg/day for the first 10 kg of body weight

50 mL/kg/day for next 10 kg of body weight

20 mL/kg/day for each kg of body weight above 20 kg

53. Child weighs 32 kg

Infuse __________ mL of __________ mL/hr (pump delivers in tenths of a mL).

54. Infant weighs 2,500 g

Infuse ______________ mL at ____________ mL/hr (pump delivers in tenths of a mL)

55. Child weighs 78 lb (round weight to the nearest tenth)

Infuse ______________ mL at ______________ mL/hr (pump delivers in whole mL)

Answers on pp. 734-741

ANSWERS

NOTE
Calculations may be performed using formula method, ratio and proportion, or dimensional analysis.

1. 200 mg : 5 mL = 300 mg : x mL

or

$$\frac{300 \text{ mg}}{200 \text{ mg}} \times 5 \text{ mL} = x \text{ mL}$$

Answer: 7.5 mL

2. 333 mg : 1 tab = 666 mg : x tab

or

$$\frac{666 \text{ mg}}{333 \text{ mg}} \times 1 \text{ tab} = x \text{ tab}$$

Answer: 2 delayed-release tabs

3. a. Tablets B: Septra DS.
   b. The prescriber's order indicates DS, which means double strength; therefore the client should be given the tabs that are labeled DS.

4. 10,000 units : 1 mL = 6,500 units : x mL

or

$$\frac{6{,}500 \text{ units}}{10{,}000 \text{ units}} \times 1 \text{ mL} = x \text{ mL}$$

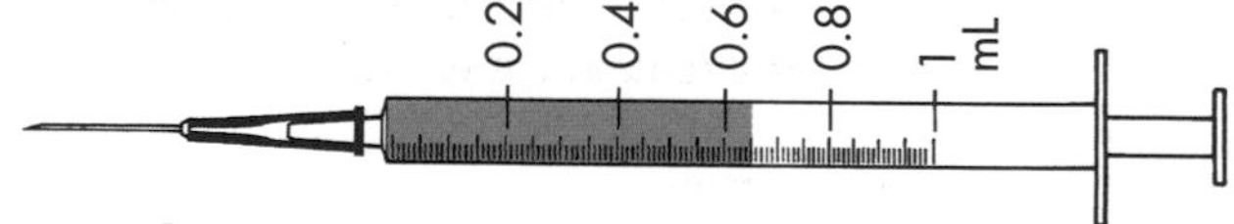

Answer: 0.65 mL

5. Conversion is required. Equivalent: 1,000 mg = 1 g
Therefore 0.75 g = 750 mg
400 mg : 40 mL = 750 mg : x mL

or

$$\frac{750 \text{ mg}}{400 \text{ mg}} \times 40 \text{ mL} = x \text{ mL}$$

Answer: 75 mL

6. a. 50 mg : 10 mL = 75 mg : x mL

or

$$\frac{75 \text{ mg}}{50 \text{ mg}} \times 10 \text{ mL} = x \text{ mL}$$

Answer: 15 mL

b. 1. Determine mL/hr.

$$x \text{ mL/hr} = \frac{1{,}000 \text{ mL}}{6 \text{ hr}}; x = 166.6 = 167 \text{ mL/hr}$$

2. Use formula and determine gtt/min.

$$x \text{ gtt/min} = \frac{167 \text{ mL} \times 10 \text{ gtt/mL}}{60 \text{ min}};$$

$x = 27.8 = 28$ gtt/min; 28 macrogtt/min

NOTE
Problem 6 could also be done by using the shortcut method illustrated in Chapter 22.

7. Convert weight in pounds to kilograms. Equivalent: 2.2 lb = 1 kg
Therefore 110 lb ÷ 2.2 = 50 kg
50 ~~kg~~ × 1 mg/~~kg~~ = 50 mg
Answer: 50 mg

8. Conversion is required. Equivalent: 1,000 mg = 1 g
Therefore 0.3 g = 300 mg
150 mg : 1 tab = 300 mg : x tab

or

$$\frac{300 \text{ mg}}{150 \text{ mg}} \times 1 \text{ tab} = x \text{ tab}$$

Answer: 2 tabs

9. a. 95 mg per mL (Vial is 1 g.)
   b. Conversion is required. 1,000 mg = 1 g
Therefore 0.25 g = 250 mg
95 mg : 1 mL = 250 mg : x mL

or

$$\frac{250 \text{ mg}}{95 \text{ mg}} \times 1 \text{ mL} = x \text{ mL}$$

Answer: 2.63 mL = 2.6 mL

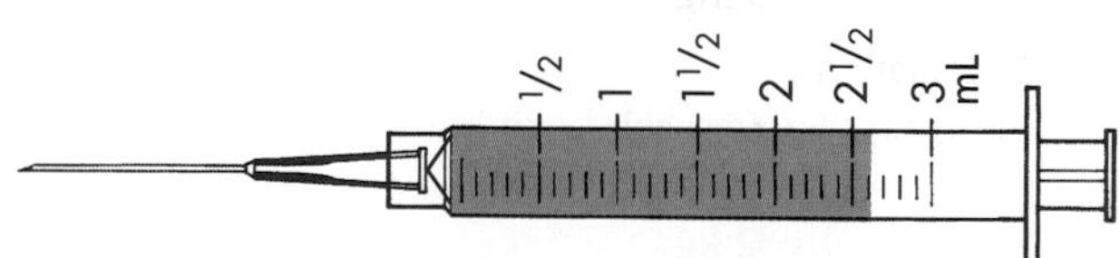

10. Answer: 3 tabs (one 2 mg tab and two 0.5 mg tabs)
Total = 3 mg (2 mg tab + 1 mg = 3 mg)
Administer the least number of tablets to the client.

11. Step 1: Determine mL/hr.

$$x \text{ mL/hr} = \frac{250 \text{ mL}}{3 \text{ hr}}; x = 83.3 = 83 \text{ mL/hr}$$

Step 2: Calculate gtt/min.

$$x \text{ gtt/min} = \frac{83 \text{ mL} \times 20 \text{ gtt/mL}}{60 \text{ min}}$$

$$x = 27.6 = 28 \text{ gtt/min}$$

Answer: 28 macrogtt/min; 28 gtt/min
The shortcut method could also have been used to do the problem.

12. $x \text{ gtt/min} = \dfrac{100 \text{ mL} \times 10 \text{ gtt/mL}}{45 \text{ min}}$

$x = 22.2 = 22 \text{ gtt/min}$

Answer: 22 macrogtt/min; 22 gtt/min

13. $\dfrac{1{,}000 \cancel{\text{mL}}}{60 \cancel{\text{mL}}/\text{hr}} = 16.66$

60 min = 1 hr

$60 \text{ min}/\cancel{\text{hr}} \times 0.66 \cancel{\text{hr}} = 39.6 = 40 \text{ min}$

Answer: 16 hr + 40 min

14. No weight conversion required. Weight is stated in kg.

$6 \text{ mg}/\cancel{\text{kg}}/\text{day} \times 12 \cancel{\text{kg}} = 72 \text{ mg/day}$

$12 \text{ mg}/\cancel{\text{kg}}/\text{day} \times 12 \cancel{\text{kg}} = 144 \text{ mg/day}$

Divided dosage: 72 mg/day ÷ 2 = 36 mg q12h

144 mg/day ÷ 2 = 72 mg q12h

The safe dosage range is 72-144 mg/day.

The divided dosage is 36-72 mg q12h.

Answer: The prescriber ordered 60 mg q12h. The dosage is safe (60 mg × 2 = 120 mg); it falls within the safe dosage range.

15. $\dfrac{100 \cancel{\text{mL}}}{50 \cancel{\text{mL}}/\text{hr}} = 2 \text{ hr}$

a. 2 hr

b. 12 noon or 12 PM (10:00 AM and 2 hours); military time: 1200

16. Determine the dosage per hour.

$10 \text{ mcg}/\cancel{\text{min}} \times 60 \cancel{\text{min}} = 600 \text{ mcg/hr}$

Convert mcg to mg to match solution.

1,000 mcg = 1 mg, therefore

600 mcg = 0.6 mg

Calculate mL/hr.

50 mg : 250 mL = 0.6 mg : x mL

or

$\dfrac{50 \text{ mg}}{250 \text{ mL}} = \dfrac{0.6 \text{ mg}}{x \text{ mL}}$

$x = 3 \text{ mL/hr}$

Answer: To deliver 10 mcg/min, set the flow rate at 3 mL/hr (gtt/min).

17. 22 units (Humulin Regular 6 units + Humulin NPH 16 units)

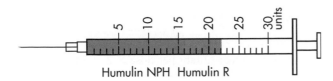

18. a. 52 mL

b. $x \text{ gtt/min} = \dfrac{55 \text{ mL} \times 60 \text{ gtt/mL}}{50 \text{ min}}$

$x = 66 \text{ gtt/min}$

Answer: 66 microgtt/min; 66 gtt/min. The shortcut method could also have been used to do this problem.

c. 66 mL/hr (gtt/min with a microdrop = mL/hr)

19. $\sqrt{\dfrac{102 \text{ (lb)} \times 51 \text{ (in)}}{3{,}131}} = \sqrt{1.66} = 1.288 = 1.29 \text{ m}^2$

Answer: 1.29 m^2

20. a. $\sqrt{\dfrac{13.6 \text{ (kg)} \times 60 \text{ (cm)}}{3{,}600}} = \sqrt{0.226} = 0.475$

$= 0.48 \text{ m}^2$

Answer: 0.48 m^2.

b. $0.48 \cancel{\text{m}^2} \times 500 \text{ mg}/\cancel{\text{m}^2} = 240 \text{ mg}$

Answer: 240 mg

c. 50 mg : 1 mL = 240 mg : x mL

or

$\dfrac{240 \text{ mg}}{50 \text{ mg}} \times 1 \text{ mL} = x \text{ mL}$

Answer: 4.8 mL. The dosage ordered is greater than the available strength; therefore you will need more than 1 mL to administer the dosage.

21. $\dfrac{2}{5} \times 250 \text{ mL} = x \text{ mL}$

$\dfrac{500}{5} = x$

$x = 100$ mL of Ensure Plus

250 mL − 100 mL = 150 mL (water)

Therefore, you would add 150 mL of water to 100 mL of Ensure Plus to make 250 mL 2/5-strength Ensure Plus.

22. Step 1: Calculate the normal daily dosage range.

$40 \text{ mg}/\cancel{\text{kg}}/\text{day} \times 21.4 \cancel{\text{kg}} = 856 \text{ mg}$

$50 \text{ mg}/\cancel{\text{kg}}/\text{day} \times 21.4 \cancel{\text{kg}} = 1{,}070 \text{ mg}$

The safe dosage range is 856-1,070 mg/day.

Step 2: Calculate the dosage infusing in 24 hr.

500 mg q12h = (2 dosages)

500 mg × 2 = 1,000 mg in 24 hr

Step 3: Assess the accuracy of the dosage ordered.

500 mg q12h (1,000 mg) falls within the 856-1,070 mg/day dosage range. Administer the medication as ordered.

23. 1 L = 1,000 mL; therefore 2 L = 2,000 mL

a. Dextrose: 5 g : 100 mL = x g : 2,000 mL

$$\frac{100x}{100} = \frac{10,000}{100}$$

or

$$\frac{5\text{ g}}{100\text{ mL}} = \frac{x\text{ g}}{2,000\text{ mL}}$$

$x = 100$ g dextrose

b. NaCl: 0.225 g : 100 mL = x g : 2,000 mL

$$\frac{100x}{100} = \frac{450}{100}$$

or

$$\frac{0.225\text{ g}}{100\text{ mL}} = \frac{x\text{ g}}{2,000\text{ mL}}$$

$x = 4.5$ g NaCl

NOTE

Remember, ¼ NS (sodium chloride) is written as 0.225.

24. Time remaining: 3 hr − 1.5 hr = 1.5 hr (1½)

Volume remaining: 500 mL − 175 mL = 325 mL

a. Step 1: Calculate mL/hr.

325 mL ÷ 1.5 hr = 216.6 = 217 mL/hr

Step 2: Calculate the gtt/min.

$$x\text{ gtt/min} = \frac{217\text{ mL} \times 10\text{ gtt/mL}}{60\text{ min}}$$

$$x = \frac{217 \times 1}{6} = \frac{217}{6}$$

$x = 36$ gtt/min; 36 macrogtt/min

The IV rate would have to be changed to 36 gtt/min (36 macrogtt/min).

b. Step 3: Determine the percentage of change.

$$\frac{36 - 28}{28} = \frac{8}{28} = 0.285 = 29\%$$

c. Course of action: Assess the client, and notify the prescriber. This increase is greater than 25%. The order may have to be revised.

Alternate calculation without percents:

Ordered rate ± (ordered rate ÷ 4) = acceptable IV readjustment rate

28 (28 macrogtt/min) + (28 ÷ 4) = 28 + 7 = 35 gtt/min; 35 macrodrop per min

28 (28 macrogtt/min) − (28 ÷ 4) = 28 − 7 = 21 gtt/min; 21 macrodrop per min

The safe range is 21 gtt/min (21 macrogtt/min) to 35 gtt/min (35 macrogtt/min). 36 macrogtt/min (36 gtt/min) is more than the acceptable range.

NOTE

In problem 24, in addition to determining mL/hr, another method could be used to determine the drop factor constant and then gtt/min calculated using the drop factor constant

25. Calculate the units/hr infusing.

500 mL : 20,000 units = 25 mL : x units

$$\frac{500x}{500} = \frac{500,000}{500}$$

$x = 1,000$ units/hr

An IV of 500 mL containing 20,000 units of heparin infusing at 25 mL/hr is administering 1,000 units /hr.

26. a. 50 mg : 1 mL = 25 mg : x mL

or

$$\frac{25\text{ mg}}{50\text{ mg}} \times 1\text{ mL} = x\text{ mL}$$

$x = 0.5$ mL

b. 25 mg : 1 min = 25 mg : x min

$$\frac{25x}{25} = \frac{25}{25} = 1$$

$x = 1$ min

27. 80 mg : 250 mL = x mg : 20 mL

$$\frac{250x}{250} = \frac{1,600}{250} = 6.4$$

$x = 6.4$ mg/hr

28. a. 5 mg : 1 mL = 25 mg : x mL

$$\frac{25\text{ mg}}{5\text{ mg}} \times 1\text{ mL} = x\text{ mL}$$

$x = 5$ mL

Alternate Solution

50 mg : 10 mL = 25 mg : x mL

or

$$\frac{25\text{ mg}}{50\text{ mg}} \times 10\text{ mL} = x\text{ mL}$$

$x = 5$ mL

This setup would yield the same answer of 5 mL

b. $\frac{5\text{ mL}}{2\text{ min}} = 2.5$ mL/min

29. 1,000 mg = 1 g

0.5 g = 500 mg

Answer: 40 tabs (2 tabs per dose × 2 = 4 tabs; 4 tabs × 10 days = 40 tabs)

30. 1,000 mcg = 1 mg   0.375 mg = 375 mcg

a. Give the client one 250-mcg tab and one 125-mcg tab.

250-mcg tab
+ 125-mcg tab
375 mcg

b. 2 tabs (one 250-mcg tab and one 125-mcg tab) Give the least number of tablets without scoring.

31. $15 \text{ mcg} : 0.5 \text{ mL} = 12 \text{ mcg} : x \text{ mL}$

or

$$\frac{12 \text{ mcg}}{15 \text{ mcg}} \times 0.5 \text{ mL} = x \text{ mL}$$

$$x = 0.4 \text{ mL}$$

32. a. No conversion necessary; use the dosage strength indicated on the label in mg (0.5 mg per 2 mL)

$$0.5 \text{ mg} : 2 \text{ mL} = 0.125 \text{ mg} : x \text{ mL}$$

or

$$\frac{0.125 \text{ mg}}{0.5 \text{ mg}} \times 2 \text{ mL} = x \text{ mL}$$

$$x = 0.5 \text{ mL}$$

b.

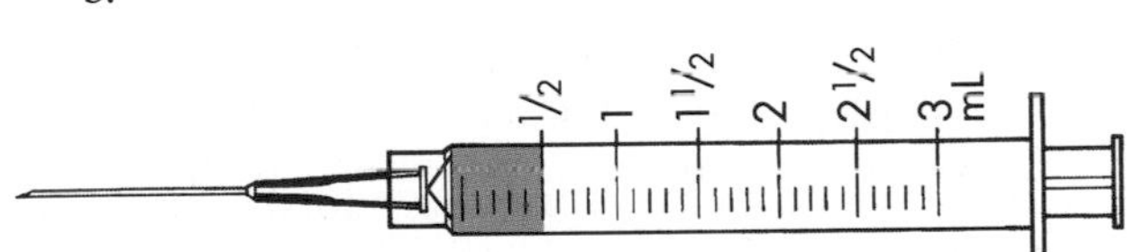

33. Convert weight: 2.2 lb = 1 kg

242 lb ÷ 2.2 = 110 kg

a. 80 units/~~kg~~ × 110 ~~kg~~ = 8,800 units (bolus)

b. 14 units/~~kg~~/hr × 110 ~~kg~~ = 1,540 units/hr

34. 20 units/~~kg~~/hr × 88 ~~kg~~ = 1,760 units/hr

35. a. $0.25 \text{ mg} : 1 \text{ mL} = 0.375 \text{ mg} : x \text{ mL}$

or

$$\frac{0.375 \text{ mg}}{0.25 \text{ mg}} \times 1 \text{ mL} = x \text{ mL}$$

Answer: 1.5 mL

b. $1.5 \text{ mL} : 5 \text{ min} = x \text{ mL} : 1 \text{ min}$

$5x = 1.5$

$x = 0.3 \text{ mL/min}$

36. a. $10 \text{ mg} : 1 \text{ mL} = 8 \text{ mg} : x \text{ mL}$

or

$$\frac{8 \text{ mg}}{10 \text{ mg}} \times 1 \text{ mL} = x \text{ mL}$$

Answer: 0.8 mL

b. $10 \text{ mg} : 4 \text{ min} = 8 \text{ mg} : x \text{ min}$

$$\frac{10x}{10} = \frac{32}{10}$$

$$x = 3.2 \text{ min}$$

NOTE

Any of the problems could also be done using the dimensional analysis or formula method.

37. Conversion is required. Equivalent: 30 mL = 1 oz

Total oz = 18 oz

18 oz × 30 = 540 mL

540 mL (p.o.) + 100 mL (IV) = 640 mL

Answer: 640 mL

38. Step 1: Convert the client's weight to kilograms.

Equivalent: 1 kg = 2.2 lb

187 lb ÷ 2.2 = 85 kg

Step 2: Calculate the heparin bolus dosage.

80 units/~~kg~~ × 85 ~~kg~~ = 6,800 units. The client should receive 6,800 units IV heparin as a bolus.

Determine the volume (mL) the client would receive. The concentration of heparin is 1,000 units per mL.

$1{,}000 \text{ units} : 1 \text{ mL} = 6{,}800 \text{ units} : x \text{ mL}$

$$\frac{1{,}000x}{1{,}000} = \frac{6{,}800}{1{,}000}$$

$$x = \frac{6{,}800}{1{,}000}$$

$x = 6.8$ mL (bolus is 6.8 mL)

Step 3: Calculate the infusion rate (18 units/kg/hr).

18 units/~~kg~~/hr × 85 ~~kg~~ = 1,530 units/hr. Determine the rate in mL/hr at which to set the infusion device using the concentration of 1,000 units per mL.

$1{,}000 \text{ units} : 1 \text{ mL} = 1{,}530 \text{ units} : x \text{ mL}$

$$\frac{1{,}000x}{1{,}000} = \frac{1{,}530}{1{,}000}$$

$$x = \frac{1{,}530}{1{,}000}$$

$x = 1.53 = 1.5$ mL/hr (not rounded to a whole number because the pump is capable of delivering in tenths of a mL)

The client's APTT is 43 sec. According to the protocol, rebolus with 40 units/kg, and increase the rate by 2 units/kg/hr.

Step 4: Calculate the dosage of heparin rebolus and the continuous infusion increase based on the APTT according to the protocol.

Calculate the dosage (units) of heparin rebolus.

40 units/~~kg~~ × 85 ~~kg~~ = 3,400 units

Determine the volume (mL) to administer 3,400 units.

$1{,}000 \text{ units} : 1 \text{ mL} = 3{,}400 \text{ units} : x \text{ mL}$

$\frac{1{,}000x}{1{,}000} = \frac{3{,}400}{1{,}000}$

$x = \frac{3{,}400}{1{,}000}$

$x = 3.4$ mL (bolus)

Now determine the infusion rate increase (2 units/kg/hr × kg.)

2 units/~~kg~~/hr × 85 ~~kg~~ = 170 units/hr

The infusion rate should be increased by 170 units/hr.

Calculate the adjustment in hourly infusion rate (mL/hr).

$1{,}000 \text{ units} : 1 \text{ mL} = 170 \text{ units} : x \text{ mL}$

$\frac{1{,}000x}{1{,}000} = \frac{170}{1{,}000}$

$x = \frac{170}{1{,}000}$

$x = 0.17 = 0.2$ mL/hr

The rate should be increased by 0.2 mL/hr.

Increase rate:

1.5 mL/hr (current rate)
+ 0.2 mL/hr (increase)

1.7 mL/hr (new infusion rate; not rounded to a whole number because pump is capable of delivering in tenths of a mL)

39. Calculate the dosage per hour using the upper and lower dosages.

4 mcg/~~min~~ × 60 ~~min~~/hr = 240 mcg/hr

12 mcg/~~min~~ × 60 ~~min~~/hr = 720 mcg/hr

Convert mcg/hr to match the available strength.

Equivalent: 1,000 mcg = 1 mg

240 mcg = 0.24 mg

720 mcg = 0.72 mg

Calculate rate in mL/hr for upper and lower dosage.

$8 \text{ mg} : 1{,}000 \text{ mL} = 0.24 \text{ mg} : x \text{ mL}$

$\frac{8x}{8} = \frac{1{,}000 \times 0.24}{8}$

$\frac{8x}{8} = \frac{240}{8}$

$x = \frac{240}{8}$

$x = 30$ mL/hr

To infuse 4 mcg/min, set the infusion pump at 30 mL/hr.

$8 \text{ mg} : 1{,}000 \text{ mL} = 0.72 \text{ mg} : x \text{ mL}$

$\frac{8x}{8} = \frac{1{,}000 \times 0.72}{8}$

$\frac{8x}{8} = \frac{720}{8}$

$x = \frac{720}{8}$

$x = 90$ mL/hr

To infuse 12 mcg/min, set the infusion pump at 90 mL/hr.

Dosage range of 4-12 mcg/min is equal to a IV flow rate of 30-90 mL/hr.

Set up a proportion to determine the incremental flow rate for a dosage rate change of 2 mcg/min

$\frac{4 \text{ mcg/min}}{30 \text{ mL/hr}} = \frac{2 \text{ mcg/min}}{x \text{ mL/hr}}$

$\frac{4x}{4} = \frac{60}{4}$

$x = \frac{60}{4}$

$x = 15$ mL/hr

For each dosage change of 2 mcg/min, the incremental flow rate is 15 mL/hr.

Set up titration table.

Titration Table

Dosage Rate (mcg/min)	Flow Rate (mL/hr)
4 mcg/min **(minimum)**	30 mL/hr
6 mcg/min	45 mL/hr
8 mcg/min	60 mL/hr
10 mcg/min	75 mL/hr
12 mcg/min **(maximum)**	90 mL/hr

40. 1. Convert weight: Equivalent: 2.2 lb = 1 kg

127.2 lb ÷ 2.2 = 57.8 kg

2. 10 mcg/~~kg~~ × 57.8 ~~kg~~ = 578 mcg

Answer: 578 mcg

41. a. 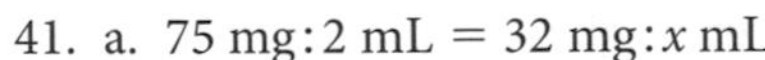75 mg : 2 mL = 32 mg : x mL

or

$$\frac{32 \text{ mg}}{75 \text{ mg}} \times 2 \text{ mL} = x \text{ mL}$$

$x = 0.85 = 0.9$ mL

Answer: 0.9 mL

b.

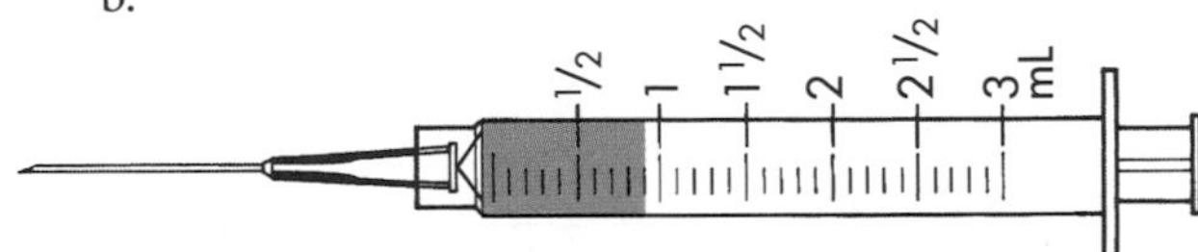

42. 38 mg : 1 mL = 900 mg : x mL

or

$$\frac{900 \text{ mg}}{38 \text{ mg}} \times 1 \text{ mL} = x \text{ mL}$$

$x = 23.68 = 23.7$ mL

Answer: 23.7 mL

43. No conversion required.

$$\frac{1}{3} \times 180 \text{ mL} = x \text{ mL}$$

$$x = \frac{180}{3}$$

$x = 60$ mL

Answer: You need 60 mL of solute (hydrogen peroxide) to prepare the desired solution (180 mL of 1/3 strength). The total to make is 180 mL. The amount of solvent needed, therefore, is:
180 mL − 60 mL = 120 mL (solvent/ normal saline).
To make 180 mL of 1/3 strength hydrogen peroxide, mix 60 mL of full strength hydrogen peroxide and 120 mL of normal saline.

44. a. Morphine Sulfate 4 mg subcut q4h prn pain

b. Digoxin 0.375 mg p.o. daily (every day)

45. A conversion is required. Equivalent: 1,000 mg = 1 g

0.1 g = 100 mg

50 mg : 1 tab = 100 mg : x tab

or

$$\frac{100 \text{ mg}}{50 \text{ mg}} \times 1 \text{ tab} = x \text{ tab}$$

Answer: 2 tabs

46. 10 mg : 1 mL = 2.5 mg : x mL

or

$$\frac{2.5 \text{ mg}}{10 \text{ mg}} \times 1 \text{ mL} = x \text{ mL}$$

a. Answer: 0.25 mL. The available dosage strength is more than the ordered dosage. Therefore the nurse would need less than 1 mL to administer the ordered dosage.

b.

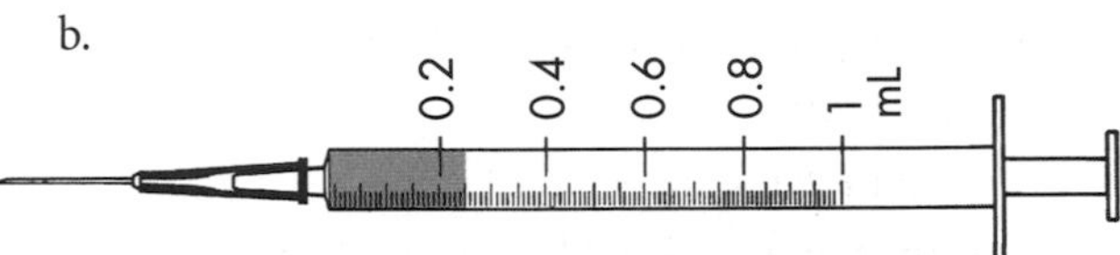

47. Conversion is required. Equivalent: 1 g = 1,000 mg

1,550 mg = 1.55 g

3 g : 8 mL = 1.55 g : x mL

or

$$\frac{1.55 \text{ g}}{3 \text{ g}} \times 8 \text{ mL} = x \text{ mL}$$

$$x = \frac{12.4}{3} = 4.13 = 4.1 \text{ mL}$$

Answer: 4.1 mL; 4.13 rounded to the nearest tenth. The available dosage strength is more than the ordered dosage. Therefore the nurse will need less than 8 mL to administer the ordered dosage.

48. **Step 1:** Calculate each medication:

Morphine: 10 mg : 1 mL = 6 mg : x mL

or

$$\frac{6 \text{ mg}}{10 \text{ mg}} \times 1 \text{ mL} = x \text{ mL}$$

Answer: 0.6 mL (Morphine)

Phenergan: 50 mg : 1 mL = 20 mg : x mL

or

$$\frac{20 \text{ mg}}{50 \text{ mg}} \times 1 \text{ mL} = x \text{ mL}$$

Answer: 0.4 mL (Phenergan)

a. Answer: 0.6 mL of Morphine is needed and 0.4 mL of Phenergan. The available strengths for both medications is more than the dosage ordered. Therefore the nurse would need less than 1 mL to administer each medication.

Step 2: Add the two medications together to obtain the total volume.

Morphine 0.6 mL + Phenergan 0.4 mL = 1 mL.

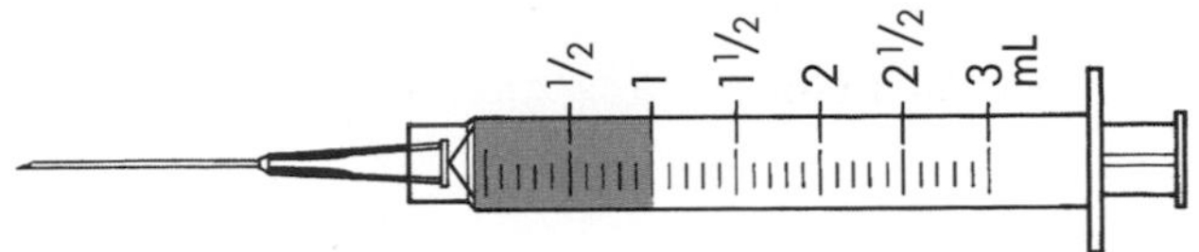

49. a. First convert the weight. Equivalent: 2.2 lb = 1 kg

$33 \text{ lb} \div 2.2 = 15 \text{ kg}$

$2 \text{ mg}/\cancel{\text{kg}}/24 \text{ hr} \times 15 \cancel{\text{kg}} = 30 \text{ mg}/24 \text{ hr}$

$4 \text{ mg}/\cancel{\text{kg}}/24 \text{ hr} \times 15 \cancel{\text{kg}} = 60 \text{ mg}/24 \text{ hr}$

Answer: The dose ordered is safe:
$15 \text{ mg} \times 3 = 45 \text{ mg}/24 \text{ hr}$
45 mg/24 hr falls within the safe dosage range of 30 to 60 mg/24 hr.

b. $25 \text{ mg} : 1 \text{ mL} = 15 \text{ mg} : x \text{ mL}$

or

$$\frac{15 \text{ mg}}{25 \text{ mg}} \times 1 \text{ mL} = x \text{ mL}$$

Answer: 0.6 mL. The available dosage strength is more than the ordered dosage. Therefore the nurse will need less than 1 mL to administer the ordered dosage.

Alternate Solution

$50 \text{ mg} : 2 \text{ mL} = 15 \text{ mg} : x \text{ mL}$

or

$$\frac{15 \text{ mg}}{50 \text{ mg}} \times 2 \text{ mL} = x \text{ mL}$$

This setup would net the same answer (0.6 mL).

50. **Step 1:** Determine the BSA

$$\text{m}^2 = \sqrt{\frac{45 \text{ (kg)} \times 155 \text{ (cm)}}{3{,}600}} = \sqrt{\frac{6{,}975}{3{,}600}} = \sqrt{1.937}$$

$$\sqrt{1.937} = 1.391 = 1.39 \text{ m}^2$$

$$1.38 \text{ m}^2 \times \frac{1.5 \text{ mg}}{\cancel{\text{m}^2}} = 2.08 = 2.1 \text{ mg}$$

$$1.39 \text{ m}^2 \times \frac{2 \text{ mg}}{\cancel{\text{m}^2}} = 2.78 = 2.8 \text{ mg}$$

a. Dosage not safe. 4 mg falls outside the range of 2.1 to 2.8 mg per (weekly) dose.

b. Because the dosage is not safe, the milliliters to administer is not calculated, and the prescriber would be notified.

51. **Step 1:** Determine IV intake

$75 \text{ mL/hr (7a-10a)} = 75 \text{ mL}/\cancel{\text{hr}} \times 3 \cancel{\text{hr}} = 225 \text{ mL}$

100 mL/hr (10a–12p and 1p–3p) =

$100 \text{ mL}/\cancel{\text{hr}} \times 4 \cancel{\text{hr}} = 400 \text{ mL}$

Ampicillin 100 mL (12p–1p) =

$100 \text{ mL} \times 1 \text{ hr} = 100 \text{ mL}$

Total IV intake = 725 mL

Step 2: Determine p.o. intake

Cranberry juice $6 \text{ oz} \times 1\tfrac{1}{2} = 9 \text{ oz}$

Tea $8 \text{ oz} \times 2\tfrac{1}{2} = 20 \text{ oz}$

Gingerale $12 \text{ oz} \times \tfrac{3}{4} = 9 \text{ oz}$

Broth $6 \text{ oz} \times \tfrac{1}{2} = 3 \text{ oz}$

Ice cream 4 oz

Total oz = 45 oz

Convert oz to mL: Equivalent 1 oz = 30 mL

$45 \text{ oz} \times 30 = 1{,}350 \text{ mL}$

Step 3: IV intake 725 mL + p.o. intake 1,350 mL = 2,075 mL

Answer: Total intake = 2,075 mL

Step 4: Total output: 375 mL + 250 mL + 400 mL + 300 mL = 1,325 mL

Answer: Total output: 1,325 mL

52. **Step 1:**

No weight conversion required; weight is in kilograms.

Determine the number of units/hr based on client's weight in kilograms.

$15 \text{ units}/\cancel{\text{kg}}/\text{hr} \times 82 \cancel{\text{kg}}$ requires 1,230 units/hr of heparin.

Step 2:

Calculate the IV rate in mL/hr that delivers the client's hourly dose of heparin.

$25{,}000 \text{ units} : 250 \text{ mL} = 1{,}230 \text{ units} : x \text{ mL}$

$$\frac{25{,}000x}{25{,}000} = \frac{307{,}500}{25{,}000}$$

$$x = \frac{307{,}500}{25{,}000}$$

$x = 12.3 \text{ mL/hr}$

Answer: 12.3 mL/hr will deliver the client's hourly dose of 1,230 units. The rate is stated in tenths; the pump is capable of delivering in tenths of a milliliter.

53. No weight conversion required; child's weight is in kilograms.

Child's weight = 32 kg

Step 1: Determine the mL/day using the formula.

$$100 \text{ mL/}\cancel{\text{kg}}\text{/day} \times 10 \cancel{\text{kg}} = 1{,}000 \text{ mL/day for first 10 kg}$$
$$50 \text{ mL/}\cancel{\text{kg}}\text{/day} \times 10 \cancel{\text{kg}} = 500 \text{ mL/day for next 10 kg}$$
$$20 \text{ mL/}\cancel{\text{kg}}\text{/day} \times 12 \cancel{\text{kg}} = \underline{240 \text{ mL/day}} \text{ for remaining 12 kg}$$
$$\text{Total} = 1{,}740 \text{ mL/day or per 24 hr}$$

Answer: 1,740 mL/day or per 24 hr

Step 2: Determine ml/hr.

$$x \text{ mL/hr} = \frac{1{,}740 \text{ mL}}{24 \text{ hr}} = 72.5 \text{ mL/hr}$$

Answer: 72.5 mL/hr will deliver 1,740 mL/24 hr or per day. Pump capable of delivering in tenths of a milliliter.

54. **Step 1:** Weight conversion required. Convert weight to kilograms. Equivalent: 1 kg = 1,000 g

$$2{,}500 \text{ g} \div 1{,}000 = 2.5 \text{ kg}$$

Step 2: Select and apply appropriate formula.

$$100 \text{ mL/}\cancel{\text{kg}}\text{/day} \times 2.5 \cancel{\text{kg}} = 250 \text{ mL/day or per 24 hr}$$

Answer: 250 mL/day or per 24 hr

Step 3: Determine mL/hr.

$$x \text{ mL/hr} = \frac{250 \text{ mL}}{24 \text{ hr}} = 10.41 = 10.4 \text{ mL/hr}$$

Answer: 10.4 mL/hr; 10.41 rounded to the nearest tenth of a milliliter. The pump is capable of delivering in tenths of a milliliter.

55. Weight conversion is required. Convert weight to kilograms. Equivalent: 2.2 lb = 1 kg

$78 \text{ lb} \div 2.2 = 35.45 = 35.5 \text{ kg}$

Step 1: Determine the mL/day using the formula.

$$100 \text{ mL/}\cancel{\text{kg}}\text{/day} \times 10 \cancel{\text{kg}} = 1{,}000 \text{ mL/day for the first 10 kg}$$
$$50 \text{ mL/}\cancel{\text{kg}}\text{/day} \times 10 \cancel{\text{kg}} = 500 \text{ mL/day for the next 10 kg}$$
$$20 \text{ mL/}\cancel{\text{kg}}\text{/day} \times 15.5 \cancel{\text{kg}} = \underline{310 \text{ mL/day}} \text{ for the remaining 15.5 kg}$$
$$\text{Total} = 1{,}810 \text{ mL/day or per 24 hr}$$

Step 2: Determine mL/hr

$$x \text{ mL/hr} = \frac{1{,}810 \text{ mL}}{24 \text{ hr}} = 75.4 \text{ mL/hr} = 75 \text{ mL/hr}$$

The pump is capable of delivering in whole mL; therefore mL/hr is rounded to a whole number.

References

Administration on Aging: Aging statistics. Retrieved from http://www.aoa.acl.gov/Aging_Statistics/index.aspx.

As U-500 Insulin Safety Concerns Mount, It's Time To Rethink Safe Use of Strengths Above U-100 (October 31, 2013). Retrieved from https://www.ismp.org/newsletters/acute care/show article.aspx? id =62

Clayton BD, Willihnganz M: *Basic pharmacology for nurses,* ed 17, St. Louis, 2017, Mosby.

Cohen, MR (editor): *Medication errors, abridged edition,* Washington, DC, 2010, American Pharmacists Association.

DeYoung J, Bauer R, Brady C, Eley, S: Controlling blood glucose levels in hospital patients: current recommendations, *American Nurse Today.* Retrieved from www.americannursetoday.com/assets/0/434/436/440/7770/7772/7776/7802/1d02b00b-9a5b-40ce-9192-d4d123514a7b.pdf.

FDA Drug Safety Communication: Important change to heparin container labels to clearly state the total drug strength. (Posted 12/6/2012). Retrieved from www.fda.gov/drugs/drugsafety/ucm330695.htm

Institute of Medicine: Report brief: preventing medication errors, 2006. Retrieved from www.iom.edu/~/media/Files/Report%20Files/2006/Preventing-Medication-Errors-Quality-Chasm-Series/medicationerrorsnew.pdf.

Institute for Safe Medication Practices: Guidance on the interdisciplinary safe use of automated dispensing cabinets, 2008. Retrieved from www.ismp.org/tools/guidelines/ADC_Guidelines_final.pdf.

Institute for Safe Medication Practices (2013a). Important change with heparin labels. Retrieved from http://www.ismp.org/NAN/files/NAN-20130610.pdf

Institute for Safe Medication Practices: ISMP's list of error-prone abbreviations, symbols, and dose designations, 2015. Retrieved from www.ismp.org/Tools/errorproneabbreviations.pdf.

ISMP Medication Safety Alert. Side tracks on the safety express. Interruptions lead to errors and unfinished.... Wait, what was I doing? November 29, 2012. Retrieved from https://psnet.ahrq.gov/resources/resources/25472.

Johns Hopkins Hospital: *The Harriet Lane handbook,* ed 20, St. Louis, 2015, Mosby.

The Joint Commission: Official "do not use" list, 2017. Retrieved from http://www.jointcommission.org/assets/1/18/Do_Not_Use_List.pdf.

The Joint Commission: Preventing pediatric medication errors, *Sentinel Event Alert,* issue 39, April 11, 2008. Retrieved from www.jointcommission.org/assets/1/18/SEA_39.pdf.

McBride S, Delaney J, Tietze M: Health information technology and nursing, *American Journal of Nursing,* 112(8), 36-42, August 2012.

National Coordinating Council for Medication Error Reporting and Prevention: Move toward full use of metric dosing: Eliminate dosage cups that measure liquids in fluid drams. Use cups that measure mL, *NAN Alert,* June 30, 2015. Retrieved from http://www.nccmerp.org.

National Quality Forum: Serious reportable events in health care—2011 update: a consensus report, Washington, DC, 2011, NQF. Retrieved from www.qualityforum.org.

Perry AG, Potter PA, Elkin MK, Ostendorf WR: *Nursing interventions and clinical skills,* ed 6, St. Louis, 2016, Mosby.

Potter PA, Perry AG, Stockert PA, Hall A: *Fundamentals of nursing,* ed 9, St. Louis, 2016, Mosby.

Quality and Safety in Nursing, A Competency Approach to Improving Outcomes. Second edition, copyright 2017. Wiley Blackwell. Edited by Gwen Sherwood and Jane Barnsteiner.

Sherwood G, Barnsteiner J (editors): *Quality and safety in nursing: a competency approach to improving outcomes,* ed 2, Hoboken, NJ, 2017, Wiley-Blackwell.

The "rights" of Medication Administration. Jennifer Olin. Retrieved from http://www.rncentral.com/blog/2012/the-rights-of-medication-administration.

Verrue, C., Mehuys, E., Boussery, K., Remon, J., & Petrovic, M (2011). Tablet-Splitting: A common yet not so innocent practice. Journal of Advanced Nursing 67 (1), 26-32.

Viscusi E, Singla N, Gonzalez A, Saad N, Stepanian J: *Special report: IV acetaminophen improves pain management and reduces opioid requirements in surgical patients,* New York, 2012, McMahon Publishing.

Appendix Table of Contents

Appendix A: Apothecary System, 744

Appendix B: FDA and ISMP Lists of Look-Alike Drug Names with Recommended Tall Man Letters, 745

Appendix C: TJC's "Do Not Use" List of Abbreviations, 751

Appendix D: ISMP's List of *Error-Prone Abbreviations, Symbols,* and *Dose Designations,* 752

Appendix E: ISMP List of *High-Alert Medications in Acute Care Settings,* 754

Appendix F: ISMP List of *High-Alert Medications* in Community/ Ambulatory Healthcare, 755

As noted in Chapter 7, the **apothecary system** is an antiquated system of measurement. The system is sometimes referred to as the fraction system because parts of a unit are expressed by using fractions, with the exception of the fraction one-half, which is expressed as *ss* or $\overline{ss}$. The notations in this system are unusual and confusing.

Because of the unusual notations, the use of fractions and roman numerals, and inaccuracies, the apothecary system is no longer recommended for safe practice. Some of the medication dosing cups used to administer liquid medications still have the apothecary measure drams (approximately the size of a teaspoon) indicated on them. The apothecary measures and symbols have been included on the TJC's "Do Not Use" list, as well as ISMP. The brief discussion of apothecary system appears here so that they can be differentiated from acceptable units of measure. Remember use metric.

Apothecary Units:

- The grain is the basic unit for weight.
- Volume measures include: minim (approximately the size of a drop), dram (approximately the size of a teaspoon), and ounce (which is the same as the household ounce).
- Many of the household measures originated from the apothecary system, for example ounce, which is still in use.

Apothecary Units Abbreviation/Symbols

Unit	Abbreviation	Symbol
grain	gr	N/A
ounce	oz	℥
dram	dr	ʒ
minim	m	N/A

*ss, $\overline{ss}$–Apothecary symbol for ½

Below is a partial listing of some of the common Apothecary–Metric Approximate Equivalents

Volume	Weight
1 oz = 30 mL	15 gr = 1 g (1,000 mg)
15-16 m = 1 mL	1 gr = 60-65 mg
1 dr = 4-5 mL	gr ½ or $\overline{ss}$ = 30 mg gr ¼ = 15 mg
1 m = 1 gtt	gr ⅙ = 10 mg gr 1/100 = 0.6 mg gr 1/150 = 0.4 mg

Apothecary/Metric Approximate Equivalent Clock

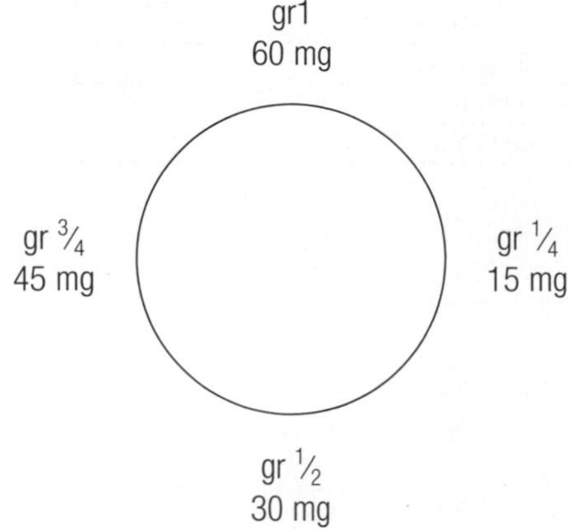

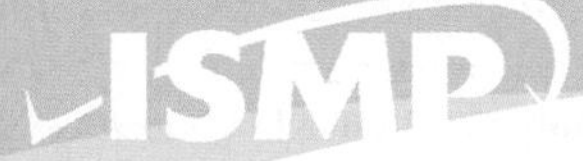

Institute for Safe Medication Practices

FDA and ISMP Lists of Look-Alike Drug Names with Recommended Tall Man Letters

Since 2008, ISMP has maintained a list of drug name pairs and trios with recommended, **bolded** tall man (uppercase) letters to help draw attention to the dissimilarities in look-alike drug names. The list includes mostly generic-generic drug name pairs, although a few brand-brand or brand-generic name pairs are included. The US Food and Drug Administration (FDA) list of drug names with recommended tall man letters was initiated in 2001 with the agency's Name Differentiation Project (www.ismp.org/sc?id=520).

While numerous studies between 2000 and 2016 have demonstrated the ability of tall man letters alone or in conjunction with other text enhancements to improve the accuracy of drug name perception and reduce errors due to drug name similarity,[1-9] some studies have suggested that the strategy is ineffective.[10-12] The evidence is mixed due in large part to methodological differences and significant study limitations. Nevertheless, while gaps still exist in our full understanding of the role of tall man lettering in the clinical setting, there is sufficient evidence to suggest that this simple and straightforward technique is worth implementing as one among numerous strategies to mitigate the risk of errors due to similar drug names. To await irrefutable, scientific proof of effectiveness minimizes and undervalues the study findings and anecdotal evidence available today[13] that support this important risk-reduction strategy. As such, the use of tall man letters has been endorsed by ISMP, The Joint Commission (recommended but not required), the US Food and Drug Administration (as part of its Name Differentiation Project), as well as other national and international organizations, including the World Health Organization and the International Medication Safety Network (IMSN).[14]

Table 1 provides an alphabetized list of FDA-approved established drug names with recommended tall man letters.

Table 2 provides an alphabetized list of additional drug names with recommendations from ISMP regarding the use and placement of tall man letters. This is not an official list approved by FDA. It is intended for voluntary use by healthcare practitioners, drug information vendors, and medication technology vendors. Any product label changes by manufacturers require FDA approval.

To promote standardization regarding which letters to present in uppercase, ISMP follows a tested methodology whenever possible called the CD3 rule.[15] The methodology suggests working from the left of the drug name first by capitalizing all the characters to the right once 2 or more dissimilar letters are encountered, and then, working from the right, returning 2 or more letters common to both words to lowercase letters. When the rule cannot be applied because there are no common letters on the right side of the name, the methodology suggests capitalizing the central part of the word only. When application of this rule fails to lead to the best tall man lettering option (e.g., makes names appear too similar, makes names hard to read based on pronunciation), an alternative option is considered.

ISMP suggests that the **bolded**, tall man lettering scheme provided by FDA and ISMP for the drug name pairs listed in **Tables 1** and **2** be followed to promote consistency.

continued on next page >

Table 1. FDA-Approved List of Generic Drug Names with Tall Man Letters

Drug Name With Tall Man Letters	Confused With
aceta**ZOLAMIDE**	aceto**HEXAMIDE**
aceto**HEXAMIDE**	aceta**ZOLAMIDE**
bu**PROP**ion	bus**PIR**one
bus**PIR**one	bu**PROP**ion
chlorpro**MAZINE**	chlorpro**PAMIDE**
chlorpro**PAMIDE**	chlorpro**MAZINE**
clomi**PHENE**	clomi**PRAMINE**
clomi**PRAMINE**	clomi**PHENE**
cyclo**SERINE**	cyclo**SPORINE**
cyclo**SPORINE**	cyclo**SERINE**
DAUNOrubicin	**DOXO**rubicin
dimenhy**DRINATE**	diphenhydr**AMINE**
diphenhydr**AMINE**	dimenhy**DRINATE**
DOBUTamine	**DOP**amine
DOPamine	**DOBUT**amine
DOXOrubicin	**DAUNO**rubicin

continued on next page >

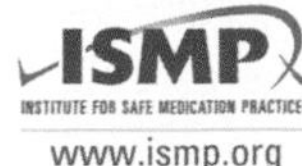

Institute for Safe Medication Practices

FDA and ISMP Lists of Look-Alike Drug Names with Recommended Tall Man Letters

Table 1. FDA-Approved List of Generic Drug Names with Tall Man Letters (continued)

Drug Name With Tall Man Letters	Confused With
glipiZIDE	glyBURIDE
glyBURIDE	glipiZIDE
hydrALAZINE	hydrOXYzine – HYDROmorphone
HYDROmorphone	hydrOXYzine – hydrALAZINE
hydrOXYzine	hydrALAZINE – HYDROmorphone
medroxyPROGESTERone	methylPREDNISolone - methylTESTOSTERone
methylPREDNISolone	medroxyPROGESTERone - methylTESTOSTERone
methylTESTOSTERone	medroxyPROGESTERone - methylPREDNISolone
mitoXANTRONE	Not specified
niCARdipine	NIFEdipine
NIFEdipine	niCARdipine
prednisoLONE	predniSONE
predniSONE	prednisoLONE
risperiDONE	rOPINIRole
rOPINIRole	risperiDONE
sulfADIAZINE	sulfiSOXAZOLE
sulfiSOXAZOLE	sulfADIAZINE
TOLAZamide	TOLBUTamide
TOLBUTamide	TOLAZamide
vinBLAStine	vinCRIStine
vinCRIStine	vinBLAStine

Table 2. ISMP List of Additional Drug Names with Tall Man Letters***

Drug Name With Tall Man Letters	Confused With
ALPRAZolam	LORazepam – clonazePAM
aMILoride	amLODIPine
amLODIPine	aMILoride
ARIPiprazole	RABEprazole
AVINza*	INVanz*
azaCITIDine	azaTHIOprine
azaTHIOprine	azaCITIDine
carBAMazepine	OXcarbazepine
CARBOplatin	CISplatin
ceFAZolin	cefoTEtan – cefOXitin – cefTAZidime – cefTRIAXone
cefoTEtan	ceFAZolin – cefOXitin – cefTAZidime – cefTRIAXone
cefOXitin	ceFAZolin – cefoTEtan – cefTAZidime – cefTRIAXone
cefTAZidime	ceFAZolin – cefoTEtan – cefOXitin – cefTRIAXone
cefTRIAXone	ceFAZolin - cefoTEtan – cefOXitin – cefTAZidime
CeleBREX*	CeleXA*
CeleXA*	CeleBREX*
chlordiazePOXIDE	chlorproMAZINE**

continued on next page >

* *Brand names always start with an uppercase letter. Some brand names incorporate tall man letters in initial characters and may not be readily recognized as brand names. An asterisk follows all brand names on the ISMP list.*
** *These drug names are also on the FDA list.*
*** *The ISMP list is not an official list approved by FDA. It is intended for voluntary use by healthcare practitioners and drug information and technology vendors. Any manufacturers' product label changes require FDA approval.*

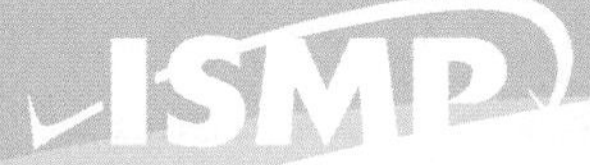

Institute for Safe Medication Practices

FDA and ISMP Lists of Look-Alike Drug Names with Recommended Tall Man Letters

Table 2. ISMP List of Additional Drug Names with Tall Man Letters*** (continued)

Drug Name With Tall Man Letters	Confused With
chlorproMAZINE**	chlordiazePOXIDE
CISplatin	CARBOplatin
cloBAZam	clonazePAM
clonazePAM	cloNIDine – cloZAPine – cloBAZam – LORazepam
cloNIDine	clonazePAM – cloZAPine – KlonoPIN*
cloZAPine	clonazePAM – cloNIDine
DACTINomycin	DAPTOmycin
DAPTOmycin	DACTINomycin
DEPO-Medrol*	SOLU-Medrol*
diazePAM	dilTIAZem
dilTIAZem	diazePAM
DOCEtaxel	PACLitaxel
DOXOrubicin**	IDArubicin
DULoxetine	FLUoxetine – PARoxetine
ePHEDrine	EPINEPHrine
EPINEPHrine	ePHEDrine
epiRUBicin	eriBULin
eriBULin	epiRUBicin
fentaNYL	SUFentanil
flavoxATE	fluvoxaMINE
FLUoxetine	DULoxetine – PARoxetine
fluPHENAZine	fluvoxaMINE
fluvoxaMINE	fluPHENAZine - flavoxATE
guaiFENesin	guanFACINE
guanFACINE	guaiFENesin
HumaLOG*	HumuLIN*
HumuLIN*	HumaLOG*
hydrALAZINE**	hydroCHLOROthiazide – hydrOXYzine**
hydroCHLOROthiazide	hydrOXYzine** – hydrALAZINE**
HYDROcodone	oxyCODONE
HYDROmorphone**	morphine – oxyMORphone
HYDROXYprogesterone	medroxyPROGESTERone**
hydrOXYzine**	hydrALAZINE** – hydroCHLOROthiazide
IDArubicin	DOXOrubicin** – idaruCIZUmab
idaruCIZUmab	IDArubicin
inFLIXimab	riTUXimab
INVanz*	AVINza*
ISOtretinoin	tretinoin
KlonoPIN*	cloNIDine
LaMICtal*	LamISIL*
LamISIL*	LaMICtal*

* Brand names always start with an uppercase letter. Some brand names incorporate tall man letters in initial characters and may not be readily recognized as brand names. An asterisk follows all brand names on the ISMP list.
** These drug names are also on the FDA list.
*** The ISMP list is not an official list approved by FDA. It is intended for voluntary use by healthcare practitioners and drug information and technology vendors. Any manufacturers' product label changes require FDA approval.

continued on next page >

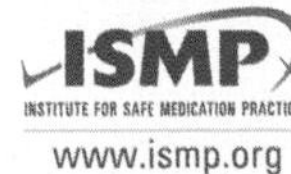

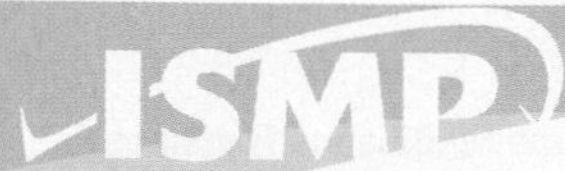

Institute for Safe Medication Practices

FDA and ISMP Lists of Look-Alike Drug Names with Recommended Tall Man Letters

Table 2. ISMP List of Additional Drug Names with Tall Man Letters* (continued)**

Drug Name With Tall Man Letters	Confused With
lamiVUDine	lamoTRIgine
lamoTRIgine	lamiVUDine
levETIRAcetam	levOCARNitine – levoFLOXacin
levOCARNitine	levETIRAcetam
levoFLOXacin	levETIRAcetam
LEVOleucovorin	leucovorin
LORazepam	ALPRAZolam – clonazePAM
medroxyPROGESTERone**	HYDROXYprogesterone
metFORMIN	metroNIDAZOLE
methazolAMIDE	methIMAzole – metOLazone
methIMAzole	metOLazone – methazolAMIDE
metOLazone	methIMAzole – methazolAMIDE
metroNIDAZOLE	metFORMIN
metyraPONE	metyroSINE
metyroSINE	metyraPONE
miFEPRIStone	miSOPROStol
miSOPROStol	miFEPRIStone
mitoMYcin	mitoXANTRONE**
mitoXANTRONE**	mitoMYcin
NexAVAR*	NexIUM*
NexIUM*	NexAVAR*
niCARdipine**	niMODipine – NIFEdipine**
NIFEdipine**	niMODipine – niCARdipine**
niMODipine	NIFEdipine** – niCARdipine**
NovoLIN*	NovoLOG*
NovoLOG*	NovoLIN*
OLANZapine	QUEtiapine
OXcarbazepine	carBAMazepine
oxyCODONE	HYDROcodone – OxyCONTIN*– oxyMORphone
OxyCONTIN*	oxyCODONE – oxyMORphone
oxyMORphone	HYDROmorphone** – oxyCODONE – OxyCONTIN*
PACLitaxel	DOCEtaxel
PARoxetine	FLUoxetine – DULoxetine
PAZOPanib	PONATinib
PEMEtrexed	PRALAtrexate
penicillAMINE	penicillin
PENTobarbital	PHENobarbital
PHENobarbital	PENTobarbital
PONATinib	PAZOPanib
PRALAtrexate	PEMEtrexed
PriLOSEC*	PROzac*

* Brand names always start with an uppercase letter. Some brand names incorporate tall man letters in initial characters and may not be readily recognized as brand names. An asterisk follows all brand names on the ISMP list.
** These drug names are also on the FDA list.
*** The ISMP list is not an official list approved by FDA. It is intended for voluntary use by healthcare practitioners and drug information and technology vendors. Any manufacturers' product label changes require FDA approval.

continued on next page >

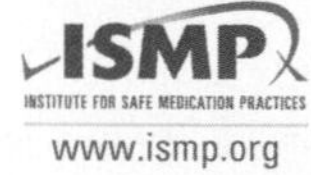

www.ismp.org

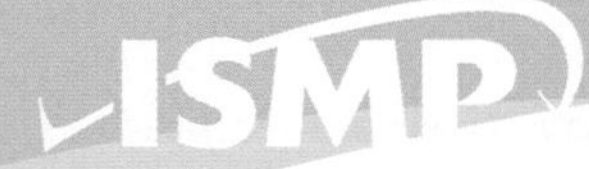

Institute for Safe Medication Practices

FDA and ISMP Lists of Look-Alike Drug Names with Recommended Tall Man Letters

Table 2. ISMP List of Additional Drug Names with Tall Man Letters*** (continued)

Drug Name With Tall Man Letters	Confused With
PROzac*	PriLOSEC*
QUEtiapine	OLANZapine
quiNIDine	quiNINE
quiNINE	quiNIDine
RABEprazole	ARIPiprazole
raNITIdine	riMANTAdine
rifAMPin	rifAXIMin
rifAXIMin	rifAMPin
riMANTAdine	raNITIdine
RisperDAL*	rOPINIRole**
risperiDONE**	rOPINIRole**
riTUXimab	inFLIXimab
romiDEPsin	romiPLOStim
romiPLOStim	romiDEPsin
rOPINIRole**	RisperDAL*– risperiDONE**
SandIMMUNE*	SandoSTATIN*
SandoSTATIN*	SandIMMUNE*
sAXagliptin	SITagliptin
SEROquel*	SINEquan*
SINEquan*	SEROqucl*
SITagliptin	sAXagliptin – SUMAtriptan
Solu-CORTEF*	SOLU-Medrol*
SOLU-Medrol*	Solu-CORTEF* – DEPO-Medrol*
SORAfenib	SUNItinib
SUFentanil	fentaNYL
sulfADIAZINE**	sulfaSALAzine
sulfaSALAzine	sulfADIAZINE**
SUMAtriptan	SITagliptin – ZOLMitriptan
SUNItinib	SORAfenib
TEGretol*	TRENtal*
tiaGABine	tiZANidine
tiZANidine	tiaGABine
traMADol	traZODone
traZODone	traMADol
TRENtal*	TEGretol*
valACYclovir	valGANciclovir
valGANciclovir	valACYclovir
ZOLMitriptan	SUMAtriptan
ZyPREXA*	ZyrTEC*
ZyrTEC*	ZyPREXA*

* Brand names always start with an uppercase letter. Some brand names incorporate tall man letters in initial characters and may not be readily recognized as brand names. An asterisk follows all brand names on the ISMP list.
** These drug names are also on the FDA list.
*** The ISMP list is not an official list approved by FDA. It is intended for voluntary use by healthcare practitioners and drug information and technology vendors. Any manufacturers' product label changes require FDA approval.

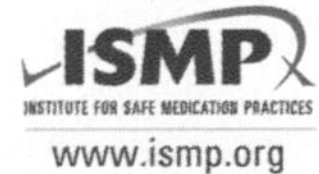

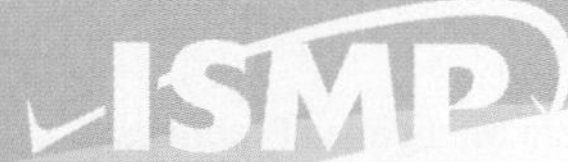

Institute for Safe Medication Practices

FDA and ISMP Lists of Look-Alike Drug Names with Recommended Tall Man Letters

References

1) DeHenau C, Becker MW, Bello NM, Liu S, Bix L. Tallman lettering as a strategy for differentiation in look-alike, sound-alike drug names: the role of familiarity in differentiating drug doppelgangers. *Appl Ergon.* 2016;52:77-84.
2) Filik R, Purdy K, Gale A, Gerrett D. Drug name confusion: evaluating the effectiveness of capital ("tall man") letters using eye movement data. *Soc Sci Med.* 2004;59(12):2597-601.
3) Filik R, Purdy K, Gale A, Gerrett D. Labeling of medicines and patient safety: evaluating methods of reducing drug name confusion. *Hum Factors.* 2006;48(1):39-47.
4) Grasha A. Cognitive systems perspective on human performance in the pharmacy: implications for accuracy, effectiveness, and job satisfaction (Report No. 062100). Alexandria (VA): NACDS. 2000.
5) Darker IT, Gerret D, Filik R, Purdy KJ, Gale AG. The influence of 'tall man' lettering on errors of visual perception in the recognition of written drug names. *Ergonomics.* 2011;54(1):21–33.
6) Or CK, Chan AH. Effects of text enhancements on the differentiation performance of orthographically similar drug names. *Work.* 2014;48(4):521–8.
7) Or CK, Wang H. A comparison of the effects of different typographical methods on the recognizability of printed drug names. *Drug Saf.* 2014;37(5):351–9.
8) Filik R, Price J, Darker I, Gerrett D, Purdy K, Gale A. The influence of tall man lettering on drug name confusion: a laboratory-based investigation in the UK using younger and older adults and healthcare practitioners. *Drug Saf.* 2010;33(8):677–87.
9) Gabriele S. The role of typography in differentiating look-alike/sound-alike drug names. *Healthc Q.* 2006; 9(Spec No):88-95.
10) Schell KL. Using enhanced text to facilitate recognition of drug names: evidence from two experimental studies. *Appl Ergon.* 2009;40(1):82–90.
11) Irwin A, Mearns K, Watson M, Urquhart J. The effect of proximity, tall man lettering, and time pressure on accurate visual perception of drug names. *Hum Factors.* 2013;55(2):253–66.
12) Zhong W, Feinstein JA, Patel NS, Dai D, Feudtner C. Tall man lettering and potential prescription errors: a time series analysis of 42 children's hospitals in the USA over 9 years. *BMJ Qual Saf.* Published Online First: November 3, 2015.
13) Leape LL, Berwick MB, Bates DW. What practices will most improve safety? Evidence-based medicine meets patient safety. *JAMA.* 2002;288(4):501-7.
14) Position statement on improving the safety of international non-proprietary names of medicines (INNs). Horsham (PA): International Medication Safety Network; November 2011.
15) Gerrett D, Gale AG, Darker IT, Filik R, Purdy KJ. Tall man lettering. Final report of the use of tall man lettering to minimise selection errors of medicine names in computer prescribing and dispensing systems. Loughborough University Enterprises Ltd; 2009.

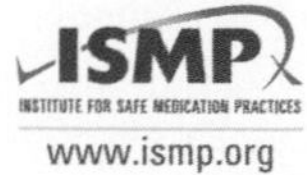

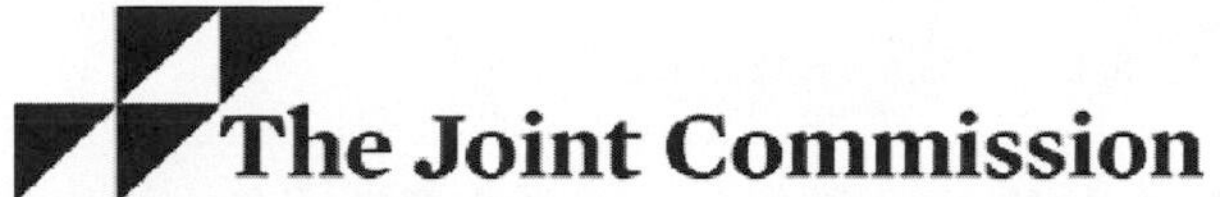

Official "Do Not Use" List[1]

Do Not Use	Potential Problem	Use Instead
U (unit)	Mistaken for "0" (zero), the number "4" (four) or "cc"	Write "unit"
IU (International Unit)	Mistaken for IV (intravenous) or the number 10 (ten)	Write "International Unit"
Q.D., QD, q.d., qd (daily)	Mistaken for each other	Write "daily"
Q.O.D., QOD, q.o.d, qod (every other day)	Period after the Q mistaken for "I" and the "O" mistaken for "I"	Write "every other day"
Trailing zero (X.0 mg)* Lack of leading zero (.X mg)	Decimal point is missed	Write X mg Write 0.X mg
MS	Can mean morphine sulfate or magnesium sulfate	Write "morphine sulfate" Write "magnesium sulfate"
MSO_4 and $MgSO_4$	Confused for one another	

[1] Applies to all orders and all medication-related documentation that is handwritten (including free-text computer entry) or on pre-printed forms.

***Exception:** A "trailing zero" may be used only where required to demonstrate the level of precision of the value being reported, such as for laboratory results, imaging studies that report size of lesions, or catheter/tube sizes. It may not be used in medication orders or other medication-related documentation.

Updated 3/5/09

Institute for Safe Medication Practices

ISMP's List of *Error-Prone Abbreviations, Symbols,* and *Dose Designations*

The abbreviations, symbols, and dose designations found in this table have been reported to ISMP through the ISMP National Medication Errors Reporting Program (ISMP MERP) as being frequently misinterpreted and involved in harmful medication errors. They should **NEVER** be used when communicating medical information. This includes internal communications, telephone/verbal prescriptions, computer-generated labels, labels for drug storage bins, medication administration records, as well as pharmacy and prescriber computer order entry screens.

Abbreviations	Intended Meaning	Misinterpretation	Correction
µg	Microgram	Mistaken as "mg"	Use "mcg"
AD, AS, AU	Right ear, left ear, each ear	Mistaken as OD, OS, OU (right eye, left eye, each eye)	Use "right ear," "left ear," or "each ear"
OD, OS, OU	Right eye, left eye, each eye	Mistaken as AD, AS, AU (right ear, left ear, each ear)	Use "right eye," "left eye," or "each eye"
BT	Bedtime	Mistaken as "BID" (twice daily)	Use "bedtime"
cc	Cubic centimeters	Mistaken as "u" (units)	Use "mL"
D/C	Discharge or discontinue	Premature discontinuation of medications if D/C (intended to mean "discharge") has been misinterpreted as "discontinued" when followed by a list of discharge medications	Use "discharge" and "discontinue"
IJ	Injection	Mistaken as "IV" or "intrajugular"	Use "injection"
IN	Intranasal	Mistaken as "IM" or "IV"	Use "intranasal" or "NAS"
HS **hs**	Half-strength At bedtime, hours of sleep	Mistaken as bedtime Mistaken as half-strength	Use "half-strength" or "bedtime"
IU**	International unit	Mistaken as IV (intravenous) or 10 (ten)	Use "units"
o.d. or OD	Once daily	Mistaken as "right eye" (OD-oculus dexter), leading to oral liquid medications administered in the eye	Use "daily"
OJ	Orange juice	Mistaken as OD or OS (right or left eye); drugs meant to be diluted in orange juice may be given in the eye	Use "orange juice"
Per os	By mouth, orally	The "os" can be mistaken as "left eye" (OS-oculus sinister)	Use "PO," "by mouth," or "orally"
q.d. or QD**	Every day	Mistaken as q.i.d., especially if the period after the "q" or the tail of the "q" is misunderstood as an "i"	Use "daily"
qhs	Nightly at bedtime	Mistaken as "qhr" or every hour	Use "nightly"
qn	Nightly or at bedtime	Mistaken as "qh" (every hour)	Use "nightly" or "at bedtime"
q.o.d. or QOD**	Every other day	Mistaken as "q.d." (daily) or "q.i.d. (four times daily) if the "o" is poorly written	Use "every other day"
q1d	Daily	Mistaken as q.i.d. (four times daily)	Use "daily"
q6PM, etc.	Every evening at 6 PM	Mistaken as every 6 hours	Use "daily at 6 PM" or "6 PM daily"
SC, SQ, sub q	Subcutaneous	SC mistaken as SL (sublingual); SQ mistaken as "5 every;" the "q" in "sub q" has been mistaken as "every" (e.g., a heparin dose ordered "sub q 2 hours before surgery" misunderstood as every 2 hours before surgery)	Use "subcut" or "subcutaneously"
ss	Sliding scale (insulin) or ½ (apothecary)	Mistaken as "55"	Spell out "sliding scale;" use "one-half" or "½"
SSRI **SSI**	Sliding scale regular insulin Sliding scale insulin	Mistaken as selective-serotonin reuptake inhibitor Mistaken as Strong Solution of Iodine (Lugol's)	Spell out "sliding scale (insulin)"
i/d	One daily	Mistaken as "tid"	Use "1 daily"
TIW or tiw	3 times a week	Mistaken as "3 times a day" or "twice in a week"	Use "3 times weekly"
U or u**	Unit	Mistaken as the number 0 or 4, causing a 10-fold overdose or greater (e.g., 4U seen as "40" or 4u seen as "44"); mistaken as "cc" so dose given in volume instead of units (e.g., 4u seen as 4cc)	Use "unit"
UD	As directed ("ut dictum")	Mistaken as unit dose (e.g., diltiazem 125 mg IV infusion "UD" misinterpreted as meaning to give the entire infusion as a unit [bolus] dose)	Use "as directed"
Dose Designations and Other Information	**Intended Meaning**	**Misinterpretation**	**Correction**
Trailing zero after decimal point (e.g., 1.0 mg)**	1 mg	Mistaken as 10 mg if the decimal point is not seen	Do not use trailing zeros for doses expressed in whole numbers
"Naked" decimal point (e.g., .5 mg)**	0.5 mg	Mistaken as 5 mg if the decimal point is not seen	Use zero before a decimal point when the dose is less than a whole unit
Abbreviations such as mg. or mL. with a period following the abbreviation	mg mL	The period is unnecessary and could be mistaken as the number 1 if written poorly	Use mg, mL, etc. without a terminal period

Institute for Safe Medication Practices

ISMP's List of *Error-Prone Abbreviations, Symbols,* and *Dose Designations* (continued)

Dose Designations and Other Information	Intended Meaning	Misinterpretation	Correction
Drug name and dose run together (especially problematic for drug names that end in "l" such as Inderal40 mg; Tegretol300 mg)	Inderal 40 mg Tegretol 300 mg	Mistaken as Inderal 140 mg Mistaken as Tegretol 1300 mg	Place adequate space between the drug name, dose, and unit of measure
Numerical dose and unit of measure run together (e.g., 10mg, 100mL)	10 mg 100 mL	The "m" is sometimes mistaken as a zero or two zeros, risking a 10- to 100-fold overdose	Place adequate space between the dose and unit of measure
Large doses without properly placed commas (e.g., 100000 units; 1000000 units)	100,000 units 1,000,000 units	100000 has been mistaken as 10,000 or 1,000,000; 1000000 has been mistaken as 100,000	Use commas for dosing units at or above 1,000, or use words such as 100 "thousand" or 1 "million" to improve readability
Drug Name Abbreviations	**Intended Meaning**	**Misinterpretation**	**Correction**
To avoid confusion, do not abbreviate drug names when communicating medical information. Examples of drug name abbreviations involved in medication errors include:			
APAP	acetaminophen	Not recognized as acetaminophen	Use complete drug name
ARA A	vidarabine	Mistaken as cytarabine (ARA C)	Use complete drug name
AZT	zidovudine (Retrovir)	Mistaken as azathioprine or aztreonam	Use complete drug name
CPZ	Compazine (prochlorperazine)	Mistaken as chlorpromazine	Use complete drug name
DPT	Demerol-Phenergan-Thorazine	Mistaken as diphtheria-pertussis-tetanus (vaccine)	Use complete drug name
DTO	Diluted tincture of opium, or deodorized tincture of opium (Paregoric)	Mistaken as tincture of opium	Use complete drug name
HCl	hydrochloric acid or hydrochloride	Mistaken as potassium chloride (The "H" is misinterpreted as "K")	Use complete drug name unless expressed as a salt of a drug
HCT	hydrocortisone	Mistaken as hydrochlorothiazide	Use complete drug name
HCTZ	hydrochlorothiazide	Mistaken as hydrocortisone (seen as HCT250 mg)	Use complete drug name
MgSO4**	magnesium sulfate	Mistaken as morphine sulfate	Use complete drug name
MS, MSO4**	morphine sulfate	Mistaken as magnesium sulfate	Use complete drug name
MTX	methotrexate	Mistaken as mitoxantrone	Use complete drug name
NoAC	novel/new oral anticoagulant	No anticoagulant	Use complete drug name
PCA	procainamide	Mistaken as patient controlled analgesia	Use complete drug name
PTU	propylthiouracil	Mistaken as mercaptopurine	Use complete drug name
T3	Tylenol with codeine No. 3	Mistaken as liothyronine	Use complete drug name
TAC	triamcinolone	Mistaken as tetracaine, Adrenalin, cocaine	Use complete drug name
TNK	TNKase	Mistaken as "TPA"	Use complete drug name
TPA or tPA	tissue plasminogen activator, Activase (alteplase)	Mistaken as TNKase (tenecteplase), or less often as another tissue plasminogen activator, Retavase (retaplase)	Use complete drug names
ZnSO4	zinc sulfate	Mistaken as morphine sulfate	Use complete drug name
Stemmed Drug Names	**Intended Meaning**	**Misinterpretation**	**Correction**
"Nitro" drip	nitroglycerin infusion	Mistaken as sodium nitroprusside infusion	Use complete drug name
"Norflox"	norfloxacin	Mistaken as Norflex	Use complete drug name
"IV Vanc"	intravenous vancomycin	Mistaken as Invanz	Use complete drug name
Symbols	**Intended Meaning**	**Misinterpretation**	**Correction**
ʒ ♍	Dram Minim	Symbol for dram mistaken as "3" Symbol for minim mistaken as "mL"	Use the metric system
x3d	For three days	Mistaken as "3 doses"	Use "for three days"
> and <	More than and less than	Mistaken as opposite of intended; mistakenly use incorrect symbol; "< 10" mistaken as "40"	Use "more than" or "less than"
/ (slash mark)	Separates two doses or indicates "per"	Mistaken as the number 1 (e.g., "25 units/10 units" misread as "25 units and 110" units)	Use "per" rather than a slash mark to separate doses
@	At	Mistaken as "2"	Use "at"
&	And	Mistaken as "2"	Use "and"
+	Plus or and	Mistaken as "4"	Use "and"
°	Hour	Mistaken as a zero (e.g., q2° seen as q 20)	Use "hr," "h," or "hour"
Φ or ⊘	zero, null sign	Mistaken as numerals 4, 6, 8, and 9	Use 0 or zero, or describe intent using whole words

**These abbreviations are included on The Joint Commission's "minimum list" of dangerous abbreviations, acronyms, and symbols that must be included on an organization's "Do Not Use" list, effective January 1, 2004. Visit www.jointcommission.org for more information about this Joint Commission requirement.

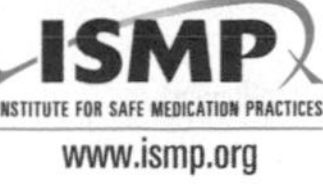

www.ismp.org

Institute for Safe Medication Practices (ISMP)

ISMP List of *High-Alert Medications in Acute Care Settings*

High-alert medications are drugs that bear a heightened risk of causing significant patient harm when they are used in error. Although mistakes may or may not be more common with these drugs, the consequences of an error are clearly more devastating to patients. We hope you will use this list to determine which medications require special safeguards to reduce the risk of errors. This may include strategies such as standardizing the ordering, storage, preparation, and administration of these products; improving access to information about these drugs; limiting access to high-alert medications; using auxiliary labels and automated alerts; and employing redundancies such as automated or independent double-checks when necessary. (Note: manual independent double-checks are not always the optimal error- reduction strategy and may not be practical for all of the medications on the list.)

Classes/Categories of Medications
adrenergic agonists, IV (e.g., **EPINEPH**rine, phenylephrine, norepinephrine)
adrenergic antagonists, IV (e.g., propranolol, metoprolol, labetalol)
anesthetic agents, general, inhaled and IV (e.g., propofol, ketamine)
antiarrhythmics, IV (e.g., lidocaine, amiodarone)
antithrombotic agents, including: ■ anticoagulants (e.g., warfarin, low molecular weight heparin, IV unfractionated heparin) ■ Factor Xa inhibitors (e.g., fondaparinux, apixaban, rivaroxaban) ■ direct thrombin inhibitors (e.g., argatroban, bivalirudin, dabigatran etexilate) ■ thrombolytics (e.g., alteplase, reteplase, tenecteplase) ■ glycoprotein IIb/IIIa inhibitors (e.g., eptifibatide)
cardioplegic solutions
chemotherapeutic agents, parenteral and oral
dextrose, hypertonic, 20% or greater
dialysis solutions, peritoneal and hemodialysis
epidural or intrathecal medications
hypoglycemics, oral
inotropic medications, IV (e.g., digoxin, milrinone)
insulin, subcutaneous and IV
liposomal forms of drugs (e.g., liposomal amphotericin B) and conventional counterparts (e.g., amphotericin B desoxycholate)
moderate sedation agents, IV (e.g., dexmedetomidine, midazolam)
moderate sedation agents, oral, for children (e.g., chloral hydrate)
narcotics/opioids ■ IV ■ transdermal ■ oral (including liquid concentrates, immediate and sustained-release formulations)
neuromuscular blocking agents (e.g., succinylcholine, rocuronium, vecuronium)
parenteral nutrition preparations
radiocontrast agents, IV
sterile water for injection, inhalation, and irrigation (excluding pour bottles) in containers of 100 mL or more
sodium chloride for injection, hypertonic, greater than 0.9% concentration

Specific Medications
EPINEPHrine, subcutaneous
epoprostenol (Flolan), IV
insulin U-500 (special emphasis)*
magnesium sulfate injection
methotrexate, oral, non-oncologic use
opium tincture
oxytocin, IV
nitroprusside sodium for injection
potassium chloride for injection concentrate
potassium phosphates injection
promethazine, IV
vasopressin, IV or intraosseous

*All forms of insulin, subcutaneous and IV, are considered a class of high-alert medications. Insulin U-500 has been singled out for special emphasis to bring attention to the need for distinct strategies to prevent the types of errors that occur with this concentrated form of insulin.

Background
Based on error reports submitted to the ISMP National Medication Errors Reporting Program, reports of harmful errors in the literature, studies that identify the drugs most often involved in harmful errors, and input from practitioners and safety experts, ISMP created and periodically updates a list of potential high-alert medications. During May and June 2014, practitioners responded to an ISMP survey designed to identify which medications were most frequently considered high-alert drugs by individuals and organizations. Further, to assure relevance and completeness, the clinical staff at ISMP, members of the ISMP advisory board, and safety experts throughout the US were asked to review the potential list. This list of drugs and drug categories reflects the collective thinking of all who provided input.

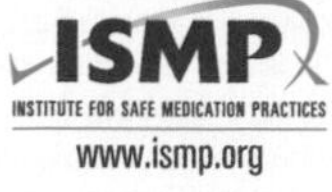

www.ismp.org

ISMP List of *High-Alert Medications* in Community/Ambulatory Healthcare

High-alert medications are drugs that bear a heightened risk of causing significant patient harm when they are used in error. Although mistakes may or may not be more common with these drugs, the consequences of an error are clearly more devastating to patients. We hope you will use this list to determine which medications require special safeguards to reduce the risk of errors and minimize harm. This may include strategies like providing mandatory patient education; improving access to information about these drugs; using auxiliary labels and automated alerts; employing automated or independent double checks when necessary; and standardizing the prescribing, storage, dispensing, and administration of these products.

Classes/Categories of Medications
antiretroviral agents (e.g., efavirenz, lami**VUD**ine, raltegravir, ritonavir, combination antiretroviral products)
chemotherapeutic agents, oral (excluding hormonal agents) (e.g., cyclophosphamide, mercaptopurine, temozolomide)
hypoglycemic agents, oral
immunosuppressant agents (e.g., aza**THIO**prine, cyclo**SPORINE**, tacrolimus)
insulin, all formulations
opioids, all formulations
pediatric liquid medications that require measurement
pregnancy category X drugs (e.g., bosentan, **ISO**tretinoin)

Specific Medications
car**BAM**azepine
chloral hydrate liquid, for sedation of children
heparin, including unfractionated and low molecular weight heparin
met**FORMIN**
methotrexate, non-oncologic use
midazolam liquid, for sedation of children
propylthiouracil
warfarin

Background
Based on error reports submitted to the ISMP Medication Errors Reporting Program (ISMP MERP), reports of harmful errors in the literature, and input from practitioners and safety experts, ISMP created a list of potential high-alert medications. During June-August 2006, 463 practitioners responded to an ISMP survey designed to identify which medications were most frequently considered high-alert drugs by individuals and organizations. In 2008, the preliminary list and survey data as well as data about preventable adverse drug events from the ISMP MERP, the Pennsylvania Patient Safety Reporting System, the FDA MedWatch database, databases from participating pharmacies, public litigation data, literature review, and a small focus group of ambulatory care pharmacists and medication safety experts were evaluated as part of a research study funded by an Agency for Healthcare Research and Quality (AHRQ) grant. This list of drugs and drug categories reflects the collective thinking of all who provided input. This list was created as part of the AHRQ funded project "Using risk models to identify and prioritize outpatient high-alert medications" (Grant # 1P20HS017107-01).

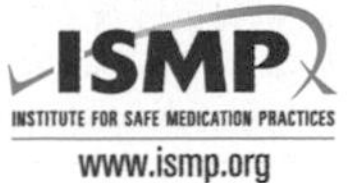

www.ismp.org

Index

A

- ā, 152*t*
- aa, 152*t*
- Abbreviations
  - in apothecary system, 86
  - on medication labels, 181, 188-189
  - in medication orders, 151, 151*b*
    - commonly used, 152*t*
    - "Do Not Use" List for, 151
    - of medication names, 154
    - for units of measure, 151*t*
  - for scheduling medications, 174*t*
  - U and IU, 89
  - for units of measure in metric system, 76-77, 77*b*
- a.c. (ac), 152*t*
- Access devices, intermittent venous, 525, 525*f,* 526
- Acetic acid solution, using household measures, 88
- Acronyms, on medication orders, 151*b,* 154
- Activated partial thromboplastin time (APTT), 609
- AcuDose Rx, 171
- Acute Care Guidelines for Timely Administration of Scheduled Medications, 135
- ad lib, 152*t*
- ADC. *see* Automated dispensing cabinets
- ADD-Vantage system, 524, 524*f*
- Addition
  - of decimals, 32-33
  - of fractions, 16-17, 16*b*
- Administration
  - medication, 126-148, 145*b*-146*b*
    - "30 minute rule" for, 135
    - chapter review for, 146-148
    - client education about, 138-139
    - critical thinking and, 130
    - documentation of, 165, 168
    - in elderly, 131-132
    - equipment used for, 142-144
    - factors that influence medication dosages and action in, 130
    - home care considerations for, 139-140
    - on medication labels, route of, 184-185, 184*f,* 185*f*
    - for mentally ill persons, 137
    - military time for, 174
    - practice problems for, 145, 148
    - rights of, 132-137, 133*b*
    - scheduled medications in, time-critical *vs.* non-time-critical, 135
    - scheduling medication times in, 174, 174*t*
    - technology in, 173
    - time and frequency, errors due to, 135
    - use of computers in, 169-170
  - methods of, 125-289
  - route of, 140-141
    - on medication labels, 184-185, 184*f,* 185*f*
    - in medication orders, 155
- Adult dosages, based on body weight, 676-677
- Alerts, on medication labels, 187, 188*f*
- American Recovery and Reinvestment Act of 2009, 169
- amp, 152*t*
- Ampule, 360, 360*f*
- Ante meridian (am, AM), 117, 152*t*
- AOT. *see* Assisted outpatient treatment, court-ordered
- Apidra (glulisine), 483
- Apothecary system, 85-91, 86*b,* 86*f,* 89*b,* 250
  - abbreviations and symbols for, 86
  - chapter review for, 90-91
    - answers to, 91
  - medication errors in, 85
  - metric system *vs.,* 74, 85
  - one half, 85, 86
  - practice problems for, 89-90
    - answers to, 91
  - Roman numerals in, 7
- APTT. *see* Activated partial thromboplastin time
- aq, 152*t*
- Arabic numbers
  - equivalents for Roman numerals, 6, 6*b*
  - in metric system, 78*b*
- Aspart (NovoLog), 483
- Assisted outpatient treatment (AOT), court-ordered, 137
- Automated dispensing cabinets (ADC), 129, 170-171
- AZT, 154

B

- Bar-code medication delivery, 172-173, 172*f*
  - eMAR and, 173
- Barcoding
  - for prevention of medication errors, 127
  - symbols, on medication labels, 184
- Barrel, of syringe, 362, 363*f*
- Basal/bolus insulin therapy, 497
- Baxter Mini-Bag Plus, 524, 525*f*
- b.i.d. (bid), 152*t*
- b.i.w., 152*t*
- "Black box" warning, 127
- Blood administration tubing, 523, 523*f*
- Body surface area (BSA)
  - for burn assessment, percentage and, 55-56
  - dosage calculation based on, 687-688
  - pediatric dosage calculation using, 681*f,* 682*b*
  - using a formula, 684-686, 685*b*
- Body weight
  - conversion relating to, 120
  - dosage calculation based on. *see* Weight, dosage calculation based on
- Boiling point, 111
- Bolus
  - insulin therapy, 497
  - intravenous, 526, 576
- Borrowing, subtracting fractions using, 18-19, 18*b*
- Brand name, on medication labels, 181, 181*f*
- BSA. *see* Body surface area
- Buccal tablets, 294*f,* 295
  - administration of, 141
- Burn, percentage of, 55-56

C

- ºC. *see* Celsius
- c̄, 152*t*
- Calculation, methods of, 125-289
- Calibrated dropper, 142, 142*f,* 318-319, 318*f*
- Calibrated spoons, 320, 320*f*
- Caplets, 293
- caps, 152*t*
- Capsules, 295-296
  - calculating dosages involving, 296-302, 297*b*-298*b,* 303*b*
    - with divided doses, 303
    - dosage strength in, 296-297
    - maximum number in, 297
    - practice problems for, 304-316, 352-357
  - gelatin, 296, 296*f*
  - opening, 296
  - problems, variation of, 302-303
  - ratio and proportion in, 48
  - sprinkle, 296
  - timed-release, 296*f*
- Carpuject, 361, 362*f*
- Cartridge, 361, 362*f*
- CBDA. *see* Computer-based drug administration
- CD, 152*t*
- Celsius, converting between Fahrenheit, 111, 112*f,* 120
  - formulas for, 112-113
- Centi, 75, 76*t*
- Centigrade, converting between Fahrenheit, 111, 112*f,* 120
  - formulas for, 112-113
- Centimeters (cm), 79*b,* 113
- Central line, 521
- Change, percent of, 63-64, 65
- Chart, for medication administration, 136
- Charting
  - of I&O, 105*b*
  - of IV fluids, 103*f*
  - of IV solutions, 518, 519*f*
  - of IV therapy, 575
- Chemical name, on medication orders, 153*f,* 154, 154*f*
- Chest circumference, 113
- Chewable tablets, 295, 296*f*
- Children
  - administering oral medications to, 144-145, 144*f*
  - dosage calculation for. *see* Pediatric dosage calculation
  - IV therapy and, 690-691, 691*b,* 691*f*
  - medication errors in, 131
  - safe IV dose for, 695-697
- Client, right, 133
- Client education, 138-139
- Client identifiers, 133
- Client's full name, in medication orders, 153
- Clock, traditional *vs.* military, 117-118, 117*f,* 121
- Clotting factors, Roman numerals for, 8
- cm (centimeters), 113-114
- Cohen, Michael, 169

Combined medications, medication labels for, 189-191, 189*f*, 190*f*, 191*f*
Comparison
of decimals, 31-32
of fractions, 13-15, 13*b*, 14*b*
of percents and ratios, 60
Completion times, 119-120
Complex fraction, 12
Computer-based drug administration (CBDA), 173
Computer-controlled dispensing system, 170-171, 172*f*
Computerized MAR, 170
Computerized physician/prescriber order entry (CPOE), 151, 169-170
medication errors and, 129
medication orders and, 164
Computers
for medication administration, 169-170
for medication orders, 150-151
Concentration, after reconstitution, 429, 429*f*, 438-439, 439*b*
"Consumers watchdog." *see* Food and Drug Administration
Continuous IV infusions, 515
Continuous subcutaneous insulin infusion (CSII pump), 488
Control numbers, on medication labels, 188
Controlled substances
medication labels for, 189
Roman numerals for, 7, 8, 8*f*
Conversion, 92-93, 93*b*, 106*b*
between Celsius and Fahrenheit, 111, 112*f*, 120
formulas for, 112-113
chapter review for, 106-109, 121-123
answers to, 110, 124
of decimal to percent, 57 58, 57*b*, 58*b*
defined, 92
equivalents to remember in, 92*t*
of fractions, 13
to percent, 57, 57*b*
methods of, 93-95
conversion factor, 93
dimensional analysis as, 96, 98-99
moving decimal points as, 93-94
using ratio and proportion as, 94-95
for military time, 117-119, 117*f*, 121
of percentages to fraction, decimals, and ratios, 56-58
practice problems for, 94, 96-97, 105-106, 113, 114-115, 116, 117, 118-119, 120
answers to, 110, 123
of ratio to percent, 58, 58*b*
relating to length, 113-114, 114*b*, 120
relating to weight, 115-117, 120
within same system, 79, 79*b*, 80-81, 96
between systems, 97-99
using dimensional analysis, 271-272
Conversion factor(s)
for converting between systems, 97, 98, 99
for dimensional analysis, 96
equivalents as, 93
for input and output, 101-103
for moving decimal point, 93-94
Coumadin, 11, 12*f*
Court-ordered assisted outpatient treatment, 137
CPOE. *see* Computerized physician/prescriber order entry
CR, 152*t*
Cranial nerves, Roman numerals for, 8
Creams, in percentage, 55, 60
Critical care calculation, 629-656, 640*b*
chapter review for, 641-647
answers to, 649-656
clinical reasoning for, 640-641
answers to, 640-641
for developing titration table, 636-639, 637*t*, 639*t*
Critical care calculation *(Continued)*
for dosages based on mcg/kg/min, 633-634
for dosages per hour or per minute, 631-632
of IV flow rates for titrated medications, 634-636
for medications ordered in milligrams per minute, 632-633
practice problems for, 639-640
answers to, 648-649
for rate in mL/hr, 630-631
Critical thinking, medication administration and, 130
Cross-cancellation, 19
Crushing tablets, 296
Cubic centimeter (cc), 77, 79
for intake and output calculations, 100
Cup (c, C), 86
household/metric equivalents of, 86*f*, 87, 87*b*
in medication orders, 151*t*, 152*t*
metric equivalent of, 101
ounces in, 101

D

Daily fluid maintenance, calculation of, 696-697, 696*t*
Dalteparin sodium (Fragmin), 604, 604*f*
Date
in medication administration records, 167
order was written, in medication order, 153
Deci, 75, 76*t*
Deciliter (dL), 77*b*
Decimal points
medication errors and, 28, 30
movement of
conversion by, 93-95
division by, 37
multiplication by, 35, 35*b*
use of, 28-29
zeros after, 31*b*
zeros before, 31*b*
Decimals, 28-43, 40*b*
adding and subtracting, 32-33
changing
to fractions, 39
fractions to, 39
chapter review for, 40-43
answers to, 43
comparing value of, 31-32
definition of, 28
dividing, 35-36
by decimal, 36-37
by decimal movement, 37
by whole number, 36
in metric system, 78*b*
multiplying, 34-35
by decimal movement, 35, 35*b*
to percentage, conversion of, 57-58, 57*b*, 58*b*, 65
percentage to, conversion of, 56-58, 56*b*, 64
place values for, 29, 29*b*
practice problems for, 31, 32, 33, 35, 38, 39-40
answers to, 43
in proportion, solving for *x*, 47
reading and writing, 29-31
rounding off, 37-38, 37*b*
Deka, 76*t*
Denominator
of fraction, 11, 12*f*
lowest common, 13
of ratio, 44
Depo-Provera label, 372, 372*f*
Detemir (Levemir), 483
dil., 152*t*
Diluent, 427-428
Dimensional analysis
in calculating injectable medications, 381, 382, 383
conversions in
intake and output calculations, 101, 102
within same system, 96
steps for, 96*b*
between systems, 98, 99
for medications in units, 385, 386
Dimensional analysis method
basics of, 271-272, 271*b*, 272*b*
practice problems for, 272, 286
dosage calculation using, 270-289, 276*b*
chapter review for, 278-285, 286-289
practice problems for, 272, 276-278, 286
understanding the basics of, 270-272
Disintegrating tablets, 295
Displacement factor, 430, 430*b*
Distractions, medication errors and, 129
Distribution systems, medication, 164-178, 175*b*
bar-code medication delivery in, 172-173, 172*f*
chapter review for, 176-178
answers to, 178
computer-controlled dispensing system in, 170-171, 172*f*
practice problems for, 175-176
answers to, 178
unit-dose system in, 170, 171*f*
Divided dosage, 666
Dividend, 36
Division
of decimals, 35-36
by decimal, 36-37
by decimal movement, 37
by whole number, 36
of fractions, 20-21, 20*b*
Division factor, 550, 550*b*
Divisor, 36
"Do Not Use" List, 151
Doctor's order. *see* Medication orders
Documentation
in medication administration, 165, 168
right, 136
Dosage(s)
body weight and, 115, 120
calculating, for parenteral medications, 379-387, 387*b*
according to the syringe, 380-383
clinical reasoning for, 392, 419
guidelines for, 379-380
maximum volume to administer, in single intramuscular site, 380
with mixing medications, in same syringe, 386
practice problems for, 387-391, 417-418
in units, 374-386
calculation of, with reconstitution, for injectable solutions, 443-445
divided, 666
expressed as ratio or percent, 182, 182*f*
factors that influence, 130
for heparin
based on weight, 604, 609-612, 609*b*, 609*f*
for IV solutions, 607-609
subcutaneous, 606-607, 607*f*
medication, Roman numerals in, 8, 9
in medications order, 155
recommended, 665-666
right, 134
safe, 666
total daily, 666
usual, on medication labels, 189
Dosage calculation
dimensional analysis for, 270-289, 276*b*
chapter review for, 278-289
practice problems for, 276-278, 286
errors, avoiding of, 248*b*, 249*b*, 252*b*
formula method for, 248-269, 252*b*
chapter review for, 254-267, 269
formula for, 248-249
practice problems for, 253-254, 268-269
with rule for different units or systems of measure, 250*b*
setup for, 250
steps for use of, 249-252, 249*b*

Dosage calculation *(Continued)*
involving tablets and capsules, 296-302, 297*b*-298*b*, 303*b*
with divided doses, 303
dosage strength in, 296-297
maximum number in, 297
practice problems for, 304-316, 352-357
of liquid oral medications, 317-318
other medication measurements used in, 88-89, 88*f*
ratio and proportion in, 48-49, 49*b*, 219-221, 221*b*
chapter review for, 225-243, 247
practice problems for, 222-225, 243-246
Dosage strengths
after reconstitution, for injectable solution, 429, 429*f*, 438
for heparin, 604, 604*b*, 604*f*
on medication labels, 181-182, 181*f*, 182*f*
in parenteral labels, 371-372, 371*t*
Dram, 85, 86
Drop (gtt), in medication orders, 151*t*, 152*t*
Drop chamber, 540, 541*f*
Drop factor, 539-540, 541*f*
Drop factor constant, 550, 550*b*
Droppers, calibrated, 318-319, 318*f*
Drops, 87
DS, 152*t*
Dual-channel infusion pump, 527*f*
Dual-scale version, of insulin syringe, 370, 370*f*

E

EC, 152*t*
EHR. *see* Electronic health records
Elderly, medication administration in, 131-132
Electric infusions devices, 630*b*
Electronic health records (EHRs), 169
Electronic infusion devices, 526-528, 527*f*, 528*b*, 529*f*
Electronic medication administration records (eMARs), 165, 166, 166*b*
bar-code medication system and, 173
documentation of, 168
right documentation and, 136
Electronic volumetric pumps, 527*f*, 528
elix, 152*t*
Elixir, 317
eMAR. *see* Electronic medication administration records
Enoxaparin (Lovenox), 604, 604*f*
Enteral feeding, reconstitution of solutions for, 445-447, 446*f*, 447*b*
Enteral medications, 292
Enteric-coated tablets/capsules, 141, 294
Equipments, intravenous, 514-535, 530*b*
ADD-Vantage system as, 524, 524*f*
Baxter Mini-Bag Plus as, 524, 525*f*
chapter review for, 532-533
answers to, 535
clinical reasoning for, 531
answer to, 534
electronic infusion devices as, 526-528, 527*f*, 528*b*, 529*f*
infusion devices for home care setting as, 530, 530*b*
infusion set as, 521, 521*f*
IV piggyback as, 515, 522, 522*f*, 524*b*
needleless system as, 526, 526*b*, 526*f*
practice problems for, 530-531
answers on, 534
primary and secondary lines as, 522, 522*f*
saline and heparin IV locks as, 525-526, 525*f*-526*f*, 526*b*
tandem piggyback setup as, 522*f*, 523
volume control devices as, 524, 525*f*
Equivalents
among metric and household systems, 92
in dimensional analysis, 271
Errors, medication, 126-129
causes of, 128
consequences of, 126
Errors, medication *(Continued)*
contributing factors to, 128-129
decimal points and, 28, 30
due to documentation, 136
due to dosage errors, 134
due to incorrect transcription, 151
due to look-alike/sound-alike (LASA) medications, 133
due to route of administration, 134-135
due to time and frequency of administration, 135
error-prone abbreviations and, 151
with heparin, 603-604
in high-alert medications, 129
incorrect transcription in, of original prescriber's order, 169
with infusion pumps, 134
with insulin, 482-483
miscommunication of, 128
outcomes from, 126
polypharmacy and, 131
prevention of
in elderly, 131-132
medication reconciliation for, 137-138
nurse's role in, 139-140, 140*f*
organizations involved in, 127-129
Roman numerals and, 8*b*, 9
technological advances in, 128
Expiration date, on medication labels, 187-189, 188*f*
Extended-release tablets, 295, 301*f*
Extremes, of proportions, 45-46

F

°F. *see* Fahrenheit
Facsimile, of medication orders, 151
Factor-label method, 270
Fahrenheit, converting between Celsius and, 111, 112*f*, 120
formulas for, 112-113
FDA. *see* Food and Drug Administration
Feeding, enteral, reconstitution of solutions for, 445-447, 446*f*, 447*b*
50 unit Lo-Dose, 369
Film tab, 295
Filter needle, 360
fl, 152*t*
fld, 152*t*
Flow rate, intravenous calculations of, 536-556
in drops per minute using a formula, 543-546
in drops per minute with large volumes of fluid, 546-550
for infusion pumps in mL/hr, 536-538
in manually regulated IVs, 539-543, 540*f*, 541*f*
recalculation of, 565-569
shortcut method for, 550-554, 550*b*
using dial-flow controller, 556, 556*f*
when several solutions are ordered, 554-556
Food and Drug Administration (FDA), in medication errors prevention, 85-86, 127
Form of preparation, on medication labels, 183-184, 183*f*
Formula, calculating using, 688, 688*b*
Formula method
calculating a problem with an unknown with, 562-565
for calculating flow rates, 543-544
in calculating injectable medications, 381, 382, 383
for dosage calculation, 248-269, 252*b*
chapter review for, 254-267, 269
formula for, 248-249
practice problems for, 253-254, 268-269
with rule for different units or systems of measure, 250*b*
setup for, 250
steps for use of, 249-252, 249*b*
for medications in units, 384, 385
Fraction system, 85. *see also* Apothecary system
Fractions, 11-27
adding, 16-17, 16*b*
changing, to decimals, 39
changing decimals to, 39
chapter review for, 22-25
answers on, 27
comparing, 13, 13*b*, 14*b*
complex, 12
converting, 13
denominator of, 11, 12*f*, 61
lowest common, 13
dividing, 20-21, 20*b*
fundamental rules of, 14*b*
improper, 12
changed to mixed number of, 13
mixed number, 12
changed to improper fraction of, 13
multiplying, 19-20, 19*b*
numerator of, 11, 12*f*, 61
to percentage, conversion of, 57, 57*b*, 64
percentage to, conversion of, 56-58, 56*b*, 64
practice problems for, 14-15, 16, 21-22
answers on, 26
to prevent medication errors, 11, 12*f*
proper, 12
proportion as, 45, 46
solving for *x*, 47
ratios as, 44, 46
reducing, 15, 15*b*
subtracting, 17-19, 17*b*
using borrowing, 18-19, 18*b*
from whole number, 18, 18*b*
types of, 12
of whole number, 11, 12, 12*f*
subtracting fractions from, 18, 18*b*
Fragmin (dalteparin sodium), 604, 604*f*
Freezing point, 111
Frequency, of administration, on medication orders, 155

G

Gastrostomy tube (GT), 152*t*
medications administered via, 296
Gauze, measurement of, 113
Gelcaps, 296, 296*f*
Generic name
on medication labels, 179-181, 180*b*, 180*f*
on medication orders, 153*f*, 154, 154*b*, 154*f*
Glass, ounces in, 101
Glulisine (Apidra), 483
Glycemic control, 496
Grains, 9*b*, 86
grams vs., *85, 86f*
Gram (g), 76, 77*b*, 78, 79*b*
grains *vs.*, 85, 86*f*
to kilogram, converting, 664-665
in medication orders, 151*t*
gtt (drops), in medication orders, 151*t*, 152*t*

H

h, 152*t*
Handwritten medication administration record, 165, 165*f*, 166*b*
documentation of, 168
errors and, 169
HDC. *see* Hypodermoclysis
Head circumference, 113, 114
Health Information Technology for Economic and Clinical Health Act (HITECH Act) of 2009, 169
Hecto, 76*t*
Heparin
errors on, 603-604
as high-alert medication, 603
labels for
new, 603-604
reading, 605, 605*b*, 605*f*
low molecular weight, 604, 604*f*

Heparin calculations, 603-628, 614*b*-615*b*
chapter review for, 614-621
answers to, 623-628
clinical reasoning for, 614
answers to, 623
of dosage
based on weight, 604, 609-612, 609*b*, 609*f*
IV solution, 607-609
subcutaneous, 606-607, 607*f*
dosage strengths for, 604, 604*b*, 604*f*
practice problems for, 612-613
answers to, 622-623
Heparin flush solution, dosage strengths for, 604, 604*b*
Heparin IV locks, 525-526, 525*f*-526*f*, 526*b*
Heparin protocols, 609-610, 609*b*, 609*f*
Heparin sodium for injection
dosage strength for, 604*b*
reading, labels for, 605, 605*f*
Heplocks, 525
Herbal medications, 138-139
High-alert medications, 129
heparin as, 603
insulin as, 482
HITECH Act. *see* Health Information Technology for Economic and Clinical Health Act (HITECH Act) of 2009
Home care setting
infusion devices for, 530, 530*b*
medication administration in, 139-140
Hour marks, Roman numerals for, 7
Household system, 85-91, 86*f*, 89*b*
abbreviation errors in, 87
chapter review for, 90-91
answers to, 91
equivalents among, 92
medication errors in, 88
metric equivalents of, 87, 87*b*
metric system *vs.*, 74
particulars of, 87-88
practice problems for, 89-90
answers to, 91
Household utensils, for medication dosages, 87
hr, 152*t*
Humalog insulin (lispro), 483
Hydrogen peroxide (H_2O_2), dilution of, 449-450
Hypodermic syringes, 364-368
large-capacity, 367, 368*f*
small, 364-365, 364*f*, 365*f*
Hypodermoclysis (HDC), 515

I

ID route. *see* Intradermal (ID) route
IM route. *see* Intramuscular (IM) route
Improper fraction, 12
changed to mixed number of, 13
mixed number changed to, 13
Inch (in), metric equivalent of, 114
Incision, measurement of, 113
Infusion pumps, 527*f*
calculating flow rates for, in mL/hr, 536-538
medication errors with, 134
problems with, 527
Infusion times, intravenous calculations of
for large volumes of fluid, 572-574
for small volumes of fluid, 574-575
total, 570-572
from volume and hourly rate ordered, 570-572
volumes and, 562
Infusions, intravenous
administration by IV push, 576-579
injection ports, 521
intermittent, 515, 521, 521*f*
intermittent venous access devices and, 525, 525*f*, 526
IV push and, 515, 526
sites for, 521
volumes of, 562
Inhalation, medication administration via, 141
Initials, in medication administration records, 165*f*, 167*f*, 168
Insertion, medication administration via, 141
Instillation, medication administration via, 141
Institute for Safe Medication Practices (ISMP)
fractions and, 11
list of error-prone abbreviations, 151
metric measurement of medication, 85
in prevention of medication errors, 127
Institute of Medicine (IOM), in prevention of medication errors, 127
Insulin, 482-512, 501*b*
action times for, 484, 485*f*
practice problems for, 486, 509
appearance of, 487-488
basal/bolus, 497
chapter review for, 502-509
answers to, 510-512
clinical reasoning for, 501
answers to, 510
dosages, measured, 483
errors with, 482-483
as high-alert medication, 482
labels for, 483-484, 484*f*
measuring two types of, in same syringe, 498-500, 499*f*
orders for, 496-497
premixed, fixed, and combination, 487-488, 487*f*
preparing single dosage of, in insulin syringe, 497-498
regular, 483
sliding scale protocol and, 497
types of, 483
U-100, 483
label for, 484, 484*f*
U-500, 483
label for, 484, 484*f*
Insulin administration, 488-495
in double-scale 1-mL syringe, 489, 490*f*, 492
in Lo Dose syringe, 489, 490, 490*f*
practice problems for, 491, 492-493, 510
in single-scale 1-mL syringe, 489, 490*f*, 491
in U-100 syringe, 489-492, 490*f*
for U-500 insulin, 493-495
via insulin pen, 488*f*, 489
via insulin pumps, 488, 488*f*
Insulin coverage, 496-497
Insulin glargine (Lantus), 483
Insulin pen, 488*f*, 489
Insulin pumps, 488, 488*f*
Insulin syringes, 144*f*, 369-370, 370*f*
1-mL double-scale, 489, 490*f*, 492
1-mL single-scale, 489, 490*f*, 491
Lo-Dose, 369-370, 370*f*, 489, 490, 490*f*
measuring, two types of insulin in same, 498-500, 499*f*
practice problems for, 491, 492-493, 510
preparing single dosage in, 497-498
U-100, 489-492, 490*f*
U-500, 493-495
Intake and output (I&O)
calculation of, 100-106
conversion factors in, 101-103
dimensional analysis for, 101
in charting, of intravenous (IV) solutions, 518, 519*f*
defined, 100
flow sheet for, 100*f*, 104*f*
Intermittent IV infusions, 515, 521, 521*f*
Intermittent peripheral infusion devices (IPIDs), 525
Intermittent venous access devices, 525, 525*f*, 526
International System of Units (SI), 74. *see also* Metric system
International time, conversion between traditional and, 117-118, 117*f*, 121
International unit, 88
Interruptions, medication errors and, 129
Intradermal (ID) route, 141
of parenteral medications, 359
Intramuscular (IM) route, 141
maximum volume to administer, in single intramuscular site, 380
of parenteral medications, 359
Intranasal administration, 141
Intravenous (IV) bag, height of, 521
Intravenous (IV) bolus, 526
Intravenous calculations, 536-602
for administration of medications by IV push, 576-579
of amount of medication in a specific amount of solution, 560-562
chapter review for, 580-587
answers to, 595-602
clinical reasoning for, 580
answers to, 595
of flow rate, 536-556
in drops per minute using a formula, 543-546
in drops per minute with large volumes of fluid, 546-550
for infusion pumps in mL/hr, 536-538
in manually regulated IVs, 539-543, 540*f*, 541*f*
recalculation of, 565-569
shortcut method for, 550-554, 550*b*
using dial-flow controller, 556, 556*f*
when several solutions are ordered, 554-556
of infusion times
for large volumes of fluid, 572-574
for small volumes of fluid, 574-575
total, 570-572
from volume and hourly rate ordered, 570-572
volumes and, 562
of intermittent IV infusions piggyback, 556-559
Intravenous (IV) equipments, 514-535, 530*b*
ADD-Vantage system as, 524, 524*f*
Baxter Mini-Bag Plus as, 524, 525*f*
chapter review for, 532-533
answers to, 535
clinical reasoning for, 531
answer to, 534
electronic infusion devices as, 526-528, 527*f*, 528*b*, 529*f*
infusion devices for home care setting as, 530, 530*b*
infusion set as, 521, 521*f*
IV piggyback as, 515, 522, 522*f*, 524*b*
needleless system as, 526, 526*b*, 526*f*
practice problems for, 530-531
answers on, 534
primary and secondary lines as, 522, 522*f*
saline and heparin IV locks as, 525-526, 525*f*-526*f*, 526*b*
tandem piggyback setup as, 522*f*, 523
volume control devices as, 524, 525*f*
Intravenous flow rate, 521
calculation of
in drops per minute using a formula, 543-546
in drops per minute with large volumes of fluid, 546-550
for infusion pumps in mL/hr, 536-538
with intermittent IV infusions piggyback, 556-559
in manually regulated IVs, 539-543, 540*f*, 541*f*
recalculation of, 565-569
shortcut method for, 550-554, 550*b*
for titrated medications, 634-636
using dial-flow controller, 556, 556*f*
when several solutions are ordered, 554-556
Intravenous (IV) fluids
administration of, 521-530
calculating percentage of solute in, 519-521
charting of, 103*f*, 518, 519*f*
flow rate. *see* Intravenous (IV) flow rate
systems for administering. *see* Intravenous (IV) equipments
types of, 515, 515*b*

Intravenous (IV) heparin solutions, dosage, calculation of, 607-609
Intravenous (IV) infusion pumps, 527*f*
calculation of flow rates for, in mL/hr, 536-538
problems with, 527
Intravenous (IV) infusion set, 521, 521*f*
Intravenous infusion times, calculation of
for large volumes of fluid, 572-574
for small volumes of fluid, 574-575
total, 570-572
from volume and hourly rate ordered, 570-572
volumes and, 562
Intravenous infusions
administration by IV push, 576-579
injection ports, 521
intermittent, 515, 521, 521*f*
intermittent venous access devices and, 525, 525*f*, 526
IV push and, 515, 526
sites for, 521
volumes of, 562
Intravenous infusions piggyback, intermittent, calculation of, 556-559
Intravenous (IV) injection ports, 521
Intravenous (IV) lines
central, 521
peripheral, 521
peripherally inserted central catheter (PICC), 521
primary and secondary, 522, 522*f*
Intravenous (IV) locks, saline and heparin, 525-526, 525*f*-526*f*, 526*b*
Intravenous (IV) medications, calculation using volume control set, 692-694, 693*b*
Intravenous (IV) orders, 518, 518*b*, 518*f*
Intravenous piggyback (IVPB), 152*t*, 515, 522, 522*f*, 524*b*
Intravenous push, 515, 526
administration of medications by, 576-579
Intravenous (IV) route, 141
maximum volume to administer, in single intramuscular site, 380
of parenteral medications, 359
Intravenous (IV) sites, 521
Intravenous (IV) solutions, 514-535, 530*b*
abbreviations for, 515, 515*b*, 516*b*
additives to, 518, 518*b*
chapter review for, 532-533
answers to, 535
charting of, 103*f*, 518, 519*f*
clinical reasoning for, 531
answer to, 534
delivery methods, 515, 515*b*
heparin, 607-609
labels for, 516-517, 516*f*, 517*f*
in percentage, 55, 59, 60
practice problems for, 530-531
answers on, 534
strength of, 516-517, 516*b*, 516*f*, 517*f*
Intravenous syringes, 367
Intravenous (IV) therapy, 530*b*
chapter review for, 532-533
answers to, 535
charting of, 518, 519*f*, 575
children and, 690-691, 691*b*, 691*f*
clinical reasoning for, 531
answer to, 534
delivery methods, 515, 515*b*
intake and output (I&O) in, charting of, 518, 519*f*
orders for, 518, 518*b*, 518*f*
practice problems for, 530-531
answers on, 534
Intravenous tubing
calculation of IV flow rates and, 539-543
calibration of, 539-540, 540*f*
drop chamber, 540, 541*f*
drop factor, 539-540, 541*f*
Intravenous tubing *(Continued)*
macrodrop, 540, 540*f*
microdrop, 540*f*, 542
Irrigation, of solutions and soaks, 449-450, 450*b*
ISMP. *see* Institute for Safe Medication Practices
IV medication protocols, 514
IV route. *see* Intravenous (IV) route
IVPB. *see* Intravenous piggyback
IVSS, 152*t*

K

Kangaroo pump, 445-446, 446*f*
Kendra's Law, 136, 137
Kilo, 75, 76*t*
Kilograms (kg), 77*b*, 79, 79*b*
conversion of
grams to, 664-665
to pounds, 116, 662-663, 662*b*
pounds to, 115-116, 660-662, 661*b*
household equivalent of, 96
in medication orders, 151*t*
KVO, 152*t*

L

L (liter), in medication orders, 151*t*
LA, 152*t*
Labels, medication, 179-218, 197*b*
abbreviations such as USP or NF on, 188-189
barcoding symbols on, 184
chapter review for, 201-215
answers to, 216-218
for combined medications, 189-191, 189*f*, 190*f*, 191*f*
for controlled substances, 189
directions for mixing or reconstituting a medication on, 186, 187*f*
dosage expressed as ratio or percent on, 182, 182*f*
dosage strength on, 181-182, 181*f*, 182*f*
expiration date on, 187-189, 188*f*
form of preparation on, 183-184, 183*f*
generic name on, 179-181, 180*b*, 180*f*
for insulin, 483-484, 484*f*
for intravenous (IV) solutions, 516-517, 516*f*, 517*f*
lot/control numbers on, 188
manufacturer's name on, 188
medication information on, 191, 192*f*-193*f*
on multidose packaging, 191
National Drug Code (NDC) number on, 188
for over-the-counter medications, 193-197, 193*f*
parenteral, 371-372
dosage strengths in, 371-372, 371*t*
measured in units, 377
milliequivalents in, 378
percentage strengths in, 376
practice problems for, 372-376, 378-379, 417
ratio strength in, 377
total volume in, 371
practice problems for, 198-200
answers to, 215-216
precautions on, 187, 188*f*
review of, 194-197, 194*f*, 195*f*, 196*f*, 197*f*
route of administration on, 184-185, 184*f*, 185*f*
showing apothecary and metric measures, 86*f*
showing milliequivalents and units, 88*f*
storage directions on, 188
total amount in container on, 186
total volume on, 185-186, 186*f*
trade name on, 181, 181*f*
on unit-dose packaging, 191, 191*f*
usual dosage on, 189
Lantus (insulin glargine), 483
Layered tablets, 295, 295*f*
Leading zero
before decimal point, 31*b*
in metric system, 77-78
Length
metric measures relating to, 113-114, 114*b*, 120
units of measure in metric system for, 74-75, 75*t*, 79*b*
Length of stay (LOS), 152*t*, 153
Levemir (detemir), 483
LIB (left in bag or bottle), 103, 103*f*, 104*f*
Lidocaine, for reconstitution, 428
Linear measurement, units of measure in metric system, 74-75, 75*t*, 79*b*
Liquid (volume), units of measure in metric system for, 75*t*, 79, 79*b*
Liquid medication, ratio and proportion in, 48
Liquid oral medications, 323*b*
calculating, 317-318
dosage strength *vs.* total volume of, 320
dosing errors with, 318
forms of, 317
measuring, 318-323, 318*f*, 319*f*, 320*f*
medication label on, 317, 317*f*
practice problems for, 323-332, 352-357
problem setup on, 320-323
Lispro (Humalog), 483
Liter (L), 76, 77*b*, 79, 79*b*
in medication orders, 151*t*
Lo-Dose insulin syringes, 369-370, 370*f*, 489, 490, 490*f*
Look-alike/sound-alike (LASA) medications, 133
LOS. *see* Length of stay
Lot number, on medication labels, 188
Lotion, in percentage, 55, 60
Lovenox (enoxaparin), 604, 604*f*
Low molecular weight heparin, 604, 604*f*
Lowest common denominator (LCD), 13
Luer-Lok syringe, 144*f*, 362, 363*f*

M

Macrodrop tubing, 540, 540*f*
Maintenance fluids, 514
Manufacturer's name, on medication labels, 188
MAR. *see* Medication administration records
Math review, 1-72
of fractions, 11-27
of percentage, 55-68
post-test for, 69-71
answers to, 72
pre-test for, 2-4
answers to, 5
of ratio and proportion, 44-54, 49*b*
of Roman numerals, 6-10
MDI. *see* Metered-dose inhaler
Means, of proportions, 45-46
Measurement systems
additional conversions in health care setting for, 111-124, 120*b*-121*b*
apothecary and household, 85-91
converting within and between, 92-110, 97-99
calculating intake and output, 100-105
methods of, 93-95
same, 96
metric, 74-84
for strength or potency of medications, 88
used in dosage calculation, 88-89, 88*f*
Measuring cup, 86
household/metric equivalents of, 86*f*, 87, 87*b*
syringe-type device *vs.*, 87
Medibottle, 144*f*
Medication administration, 126-148, 145*b*-146*b*
chapter review for, 146-148
answers to, 148
client education on, 138-139
critical thinking and, 130
documentation of, 165, 168
in elderly, 131-132

Medication administration *(Continued)*
equipment used for, 142-144
administering oral medications to child, 144-145, 144*f*
calibrated dropper as, 142, 142*f*
medicine cup as, 142, 142*f*
nipple as, 143, 143*f*
oral syringe as, 143, 143*f*
parenteral syringe as, 143-144, 144*f*
soufflé cup as, 142, 142*f*
factors that influence medication dosages and action in, 130
home care considerations for, 139-140
for mentally ill persons, 137
military time for, 174
practice problems for, 145
answers to, 148
rights of, 132-137, 133*b*
right client in, 133
right documentation in, 136
right dose in, 134
right indication in, 136
right medication in, 133-134
right response in, 137
right route in, 134-135
right time in, 135
right to know in, 136
right to refuse in, 136-137
routes of, 140-141
on medication labels, 184-185, 184*f*, 185*f*
scheduling medication times in, 174
abbreviations for, 174*t*
time-critical *vs.* non-time-critical, 135
technology in, 173
advantages and disadvantages of, 173-174
"30 minute rule" for, 135
time and frequency, errors due to, 135
use of computers in, 169-170
Medication administration records (MAR), 164-178, 166*b*, 175*b*
chapter review for, 176-178
answers to, 178
computerized, 170
dates in, 167
electronic, 165, 166*b*, 166*f*, 168
right documentation and, 136
essential components of, 167-168, 168*b*
explanation of, 169
handwritten, 165, 165*f*, 166*b*, 168, 169
initials in, 168
medication information in, 167
medication orders as, 164
practice problems for, 175-176
answers to, 178
prn medications in, 166, 167*f*
right documentation and, 136
right medications and, 133
special instructions (parameters) in, 168
time of administration in, 167-168
Medication container, 131-132, 132*f*
Medication distribution systems, 164-178, 175*b*
bar-code medication delivery in, 172-173, 172*f*
chapter review for, 176-178
answers to, 178
computer-controlled dispensing system in, 170-171, 172*f*
practice problems for, 175-176
answers to, 178
unit-dose system in, 170, 171*f*
Medication errors, 126-129
causes of, 128
consequences of, 126
contributing factors to, 128-129
decimal points and, 28, 30
due to documentation, 136
due to dosage errors, 134
Medication errors *(Continued)*
due to incorrect transcription, 151
due to look-alike/sound-alike (LASA) medications, 133
due to route of administration, 134-135
due to time and frequency of administration, 135
error-prone abbreviations and, 151
in high-alert medications, 129
incorrect transcription in, of original prescriber's order, 169
with infusion pumps, 134
with insulin, 482-483
miscommunication of, 128
outcomes from, 126
polypharmacy and, 131
prevention of
in elderly, 131-132
medication reconciliation for, 137-138
nurse's role in, 139-140, 140*f*
organizations involved in, 127-129
Roman numerals and, 8*b*, 9
technological advances in, 128
Medication information
in medication administration records, 167
on medication labels, 191, 192*f*-193*f*
Medication labels, 179-218, 197*b*
abbreviations such as USP or NF on, 188-189
barcoding symbols on, 184
chapter review for, 201-215
answers to, 216-218
for combined medications, 189-191, 189*f*, 190*f*, 191*f*
for controlled substances, 189
directions for mixing or reconstituting a medication on, 186, 187*f*
dosage expressed as ratio or percent on, 182, 182*f*
dosage strength on, 181-182, 181*f*, 182*f*
expiration date on, 187-189, 188*f*
form of preparation on, 183-184, 183*f*
generic name on, 179-181, 180*b*, 180*f*
for intravenous (IV) solutions, 516-517, 516*f*, 517*f*
lot/control numbers on, 188
manufacturer's name on, 188
medication information on, 191, 192*f*-193*f*
on multidose packaging, 191
National Drug Code (NDC) number on, 188
for over-the-counter medications, 193-197, 193*f*
parenteral, 371-372
dosage strengths in, 371-372, 371*t*
measured in units, 377
milliequivalents in, 378
percentage strengths in, 376
practice problems for, 372-376, 378-379, 417
ratio strength in, 377
total volume in, 371
practice problems for, 198-200
answers to, 215-216
precautions on, 187, 188*f*
review of, 194-197, 194*f*, 195*f*, 196*f*, 197*f*
Roman numerals on, 7, 8*f*
route of administration on, 184-185, 184*f*, 185*f*
showing apothecary and metric measures, 86*f*
showing milliequivalents and units, 88*f*
storage directions on, 188
total amount in container on, 186
total volume on, 185-186, 186*f*
trade name on, 181, 181*f*
on unit-dose packaging, 191, 191*f*
usual dosage on, 189
Medication orders, 149-163, 158*b*, 164
abbreviation in, 151, 151*b*
commonly used, 152*t*
"Do Not Use" List for, 151
error-prone, 151
of medication names, 154
units of measure in, 151*t*
Medication orders *(Continued)*
chapter review for, 159
answers to, 162
components of, 153-156
client's full name as, 153
date and time the order was written as, 153
dosage of medication as, 155
name of medication as, 153-154, 153*f*, 154*f*
route of administration as, 155
signature of the person writing the order as, 155-156
time and frequency of administration as, 155
computers for, 150-151
fax (facsimile) transmission of, 151
for insulin, 496-497
interpretation of, 156-158
for intravenous (IV) therapy, 518, 518*b*, 518*f*
practice problems for, 158-159
answers to, 162
transcription of, 151, 152
verbal, 150-151
writing, 152
Medication reconciliation, 137-138
Medication regimen, 138
Medications
dosages and action, factors that influence, 130
herbal, 138-139
high-alert, 129
heparin as, 603
insulin as, 482
liquid oral, 323*b*
calculating, 317-318
dosage strength *vs.* total volume of, 320
dosing errors with, 318
forms of, 317
measuring, 318-323, 318*f*, 319*f*, 320*f*
medication label on, 317, 317*f*
practice problems for, 323-332, 352-357
problem setup on, 320-323
look-alike/sound-alike (LASA), 133
name of, in medication orders, 153-154, 153*f*, 154*f*
oral, 292-358
chapter review for, 333-351, 358
clinical reasoning for, 332-333, 358
unit-dose packaging for, 292
over-the-counter, 138-139
parenteral, 359-426
administration of, 141, 359
chapter review for, 392-416
dosages for, calculating, 379-387, 387*b*
indications for, 359
labels for, 371-372
packaging of, 359-362, 360*f*, 361*f*, 362*f*
syringes for, 362-371, 365*b*, 371*b*
ratio and proportion for, 44
capsule form, 48
liquid, 48
tablet form, 48
right, 133-134
right to refuse, 136
route of, in medication orders, 155
solid oral, 297*b*-298*b*, 303*b*
forms of, 292-303, 296*f*
practice problems for, 304-316, 352-357
problem setup on, 298-302
time and frequency of, in medication orders, 155
time-critical scheduled *vs.* non-time-critical schedules, 135
Medicine cup, 318, 318*f*
medication administration via, 142, 142*f*
volume measures on, metric, 79, 79*f*
Medicine droppers, 142*f*, 318-319, 318*f*
Medicine spoon, 144*f*
Medlocks, 525
Meniscus, 318, 318*f*
Meter (m), 74, 76, 79*b*

Metered-dose inhaler (MDI), 141
Metric system, 74-84, 81*b*, 251*b*
apothecary system *vs.*, 85
benefit of, 74
chapter review for, 81- 83
answers to, 84
definition of, 74
equivalents among, 92
household equivalents of, 86*f*, 87, 87*b*
leading and trailing zeroes in, 77-78, 78*b*
particulars of, 74-76
practice problems for, 78, 81
answers to, 84
prefixes in, 75-76, 76*t*
to prevent medication error, 74
rules of, 77-78, 78*b*
larger unit to smaller unit, 93*b*
smaller unit to larger unit, 93*b*
units of measure in, 74, 75*t*, 78-79
abbreviations for, 76-77, 77*b*
conversions between, 79, 79*b*, 80-81, 97
for length, 74-75, 75*t*, 79*b*, 113-114, 114*b*, 120
for volume, 75*t*, 79, 79*b*
for weight, 75*t*, 78-79, 79*b*
Micro, 75, 76*t*
Microdrop tubing, 540*f*, 542
Microgram (mcg), 76, 77*b*, 78*b*, 79, 79*b*
in medication orders, 151*t*
Micrograms/kilogram/minute (mcg/kg/min), calculating dosages based on, 633-634
Military time, 174-175
calculations, 119
conversion for, 117-118, 117*f*, 121
Milli, 75, 76*t*
Milliequivalents (mEq), 88, 88*f*
in medication orders, 151*t*
parenteral medications in, 378
Milligram (mg), 76, 77*b*, 78, 79*b*
grains *vs.*, 85, 86*f*
in medication orders, 151*t*
Milligram/minute (mg/min), medications ordered in, 632-633
Milliliter (mL)
abbreviation for, 76, 77*b*
for intake and output calculations, 100
in medication orders, 151*t*
medicine cup showing volume measure in, 79*f*
metric equivalents of, 79, 79*b*
Milliliters/hour (mL/hr)
calculating rate in, 630-631
calculation of flow rates in, for infusion pumps, 536-538
Millimeter (mm), 79*b*, 113
Milliunits (mU), 88, 155
min, 152*t*
Mini-Bag Plus, Baxter, 524, 525*f*
Minim (m), 85, 86
mix, 152*t*
Mix-o-vial, 361, 361*f*
Mixed number, 12
changed to improper fraction of, 13
improper fraction changed to, 13
Mixing directions, on medication labels, 186, 187*f*
Multi-dose vials, 360
Multidose packaging, 191
Multiple-dose vial, 430, 430*b*
Multiple-strength solution, 431, 438-439, 438*b*, 439*b*
Multiplication
of decimals, 34-35
by decimal movement, 35, 35*b*
of fractions, 19-20, 19*b*

N

Name
of client, in medication orders, 153
generic, 153*f*, 154, 154*b*, 154*f*
on medication labels, 179-181, 180*b*, 180*f*
Name *(Continued)*
of medication, in medication orders, 153-154, 153*f*, 154*f*
trade, 153, 153*f*, 154*b*, 154*f*
on medication labels, 181, 181*f*
NAS, 152*t*
National Drug Code (NDC)
in barcoding, 127
number, on medication labels, 188
National Formulary (NF), on medication labels, 181, 188-189
National Patient Safety Goals (NPSG)
on medication administration, 127, 137
on medication orders, 150
National Quality Forum (NQF), 128
NDC. *see* National Drug Code
Needleless syringe, 363, 363*f*
Needleless system, as intravenous (IV) equipments, 526, 526*b*, 526*f*
Needles
filter, 360
safety, 363, 363*f*
NG, 152*t*
NGT, 152*t*
Nipple, medication administration via, 143, 143*f*
noc, 152*t*
noct, 152*t*
Non-Luer-Lok syringe, 362
Non-time-critical scheduled medications, 135
Noncompliance, in client education, 138
Nonproprietary name, on medication order, 153*f*, 154, 154*f*
Normal saline solutions
for reconstitution, 428
using household measures, 88
NovoLog (aspart), 483
n.p.o (NPO), 152*t*
NPSG. *see* National Patient Safety Goals
NQF. *see* National Quality Forum
NS (N/S), 152*t*
Numerator
of fraction, 11, 12*f*, 61
of ratio, 44

O

oint, 152*t*
Ointments, in percentage, 55, 60
Omnicell Omni Rx, 171
Omnicell system, 171, 172*f*
One half (ss), in apothecary system, 85, 86
Oral medications, 292-358
administration of, 140
equipment for, to children, 144-145, 144*f*
chapter review for, 333-351
answers to, 358
clinical reasoning for, 332-333
answers to, 358
liquid, 323*b*
calculating, 317-318
dosage strength *vs.* total volume of, 320
dosing errors with, 318
forms of, 317
measuring, 318-323, 318*f*, 319*f*, 320*f*
medication label on, 317, 317*f*
practice problems for, 323-332, 352-357
problem setup on, 320-323
solid, 297*b*-298*b*, 303*b*
forms of, 292-303, 296*f*
practice problems for, 304-316, 352-357
problem setup on, 298-302
unit-dose packaging for, 292
Oral syringe, 143, 143*f*, 319, 319*f*
Order sheets, 152
Ounces (oz)
in apothecary system, 85, 86
conversion of weight from, to kilograms, 115-116
in cup, 101
in glass, 101
household/metric equivalents of, 87*b*
household system, metric equivalent of, 101
in medication orders, 151*t*
in pint, 101
Output
calculation of, 100-106
dimensional analysis for, 101
in charting, of intravenous (IV) solutions, 518, 519*f*
defined, 100
flow sheet for, 100*f*
Over-the-counter medications, 138-139
medication labels for, 193-197, 193*f*
OxyFast, 142, 143*f*

P

p̄, 152*t*
Package inserts
on prescription medications, 191, 192*f*-193*f*
for reconstitution, 441-442, 442*f*
Parenteral medications, 359-426
administration of, 141, 359
chapter review for, 392-416
answers to, 419-426
dosages for, calculating, 379-387, 387*b*
according to the syringe, 380-383
clinical reasoning for, 392, 419
guidelines for, 379-380
maximum volume to administer, in single intramuscular site, 380
with mixing medications, in same syringe, 386-387
practice problems for, 387-391, 417-418
in units, 384-386
indications for, 359
labels for, 371-372
dosage strength in, 371, 371*t*
measured in units, 377
milliequivalents in, 378
percentage strengths in, 376
practice problems for, 372-376, 378-379, 417
ratio strength in, 377
total volume in, 371
packaging of, 359-362, 360*f*, 361*f*, 362*f*
syringes for, 362-371, 365*b*, 371*b*
calculating injectable medications according to, 380-383
clinical reasoning for, 371, 419
insulin, 369-370, 370*f*
intravenous, 367
large hypodermics, 367, 368*f*
Luer-Lok, 362, 363*f*
mixing medications in, 386
needleless, 363, 363*f*
non-Luer-Lok, 362
parts of, 362, 363*f*
practice problems for, 366-367, 416-417
prefilled, 362, 362*f*
safety needles, 363, 363*f*
SafetyGlide™ needle, 363*f*
small hypodermics, 364-365, 364*f*, 365*f*
tuberculin, 369, 369*f*
types of, 364-371
Parenteral nutrition solutions, 521
Parenteral syringe, 143-144, 144*f*
Patient-controlled analgesia devices, 528, 529*f*
p.c (pc), 152*t*
Pediatric dosage calculation, based on weight, 657-719, 658*b*, 680*b*-681*b*, 687*b*, 690*b*, 698*b*
basic calculations, principles relating to, 659
body weight, 659-660, 660*b*
chapter review for, 699-709
answers to, 714-719
clinical reasoning for, 698
answers to, 714
grams to kilograms conversion, 664-665
IV therapy and, 690-691, 691*b*, 691*f*

Pediatric dosage calculation *(Continued)*
kilograms to pounds conversion, 662-663, 662*b*
oral and parental medications, 698, 698*b*
pediatric medication dosages in, 659, 659*b*
pounds to kilograms conversion, 660-662, 661*b*
practice problems for, 662, 663-664, 664*b*, 665-666, 666*b*, 677-680, 683-684, 686-687, 687*b*, 688-689, 694, 696-697
answers to, 710-713
for single dose medications, 666-676, 676*b*
for total daily dosage, 666
using body surface area, 681-682, 681*f*, 682*b*, 684-688, 685*b*
per, 152*t*
Percentage(s), 55-72, 64*b*
of burns, 55-56
of change, 63-64, 63*b*, 65
chapter review for, 65-67
answers to, 68
of concentration, of solution, 55
conversion of
decimal to, 57-58, 57*b*, 58*b*
to fraction, decimals, and ratios, 56-58, 56*b*
fraction to, 57, 57*b*
ratio to, 58, 58*b*
definition of, 55
dosage expressed as, 182, 182*f*
in IV fluids, ointments, creams, and lotions, 60
measures, 59
of one number is of another, 61-62, 61*b*
of partial quantities, 55
practice problems for, 58-61, 63, 64
answers to, 68
of quantity, 61, 61*b*
ratios and, comparing, 60, 60*b*
symbol for, 55
Percentage solutions, 55, 59, 376
Percentage strengths, in parenteral medications, 376
Percents, 55
Percutaneous endoscopic gastrostomy, medications administered via, 296
Percutaneous medication administration, 141
Periodic table, Roman numerals for, 8
Peripheral line, 521
Peripherally inserted central catheter (PICC) line, 521
Personal digital assistants (PDAs), for prevention of medication errors, 140
Pill cutter, 293, 294*f*
Pill Timer, 132*f*
Pint (pt)
household/metric equivalents of, 87*b*
in medication orders, 151*t*
metric equivalent of, 79, 101
Plunger, of syringe, 362, 363*f*
pm (post meridian), 117, 152*t*
Polypharmacy, medication errors and, 131
Pounds
converting kilograms to, 662-663, 662*b*
household/metric equivalents of, 87*b*
to kilograms, conversion of, 115-116, 660-662, 661*b*
p.r., 152*t*
Precautions, on medication labels, 187, 188*f*
Prefilled syringe, 362, 362*f*
Prefixes, in metric system, 75-76, 76*t*
Prescription Medication Package Inserts, 191, 192*f*-193*f*
Primary line, 522, 522*f*
p.r.n (prn), 152*t*
Prn medications, MAR showing, 166, 167*f*
Proper fraction, 12
Proportion, 44-54, 49*b*
in calculating injectable medications, 381, 382, 383
chapter review for, 50-53
answers to, 53-54
defined, 45
Proportion *(Continued)*
dosage calculation and, 48-49, 49*b*, 219-221, 221*b*
chapter review for, 225-243, 247
practice problems for, 222-225, 243-246
extremes of, 45
format for, 45
to make conversions, 94-95
for intake and output calculations, 101, 102
rules of, 94*b*
between systems, 97, 98, 99
means of, 45
for medications in units, 384, 385
practice problems for, 50
answers to, 53
proving equality of ratios in, 45, 46, 49
reading of, 45
solving for *x* in, 46-48
in weight of medication
capsule form, 48
liquid, 48
tablet form, 48
Proprietary name
on medication labels, 181, 181*f*
on medication orders, 153, 153*f*, 154*f*
Pulvules, 296
Pupillary size, 113
Pyxis Med Station system, 171, 172*f*

Q

q., 152*t*
q2h, 152*t*
q4h, 152*t*
q6h, 152*t*
q8h, 152*t*
q12h, 152*t*
q.a.m., 152*t*
q.h. (qh), 152*t*
q.i.d (qid), 152*t*, 155
q.s., 152*t*
Quality and Safety Education for Nurses, 127-128, 140
Quantity, percent of, 61
Quart (qt)
household/metric equivalents of, 86, 87*b*
in medication orders, 151*t*
metric equivalent of, 79
Quotient, 36

R

Ratio(s), 44-54, 49*b*
chapter review for, 50-53
answers to, 53-54
dosage calculation and, 48-49, 49*b*, 219-221, 221*b*
chapter review for, 225-243, 247
practice problems for, 222-225, 243-246
dosage expressed as, 182, 182*f*
to make conversions, 94-95
for intake and output calculations, 101, 102
rules of, 94*b*
between systems, 97, 98, 99
numerator and denominator of, 44
to percentage, conversion of, 58, 58*b*, 65
percentage to, conversion of, 56-58, 56*b*, 64
percents and, comparing, 60
practice problems for, 50
answers to, 53
proving equality in proportions of, 46, 49
solving for *x* in, 46-48
use of, 44
in weight of medication
capsule form, 48
liquid, 48
tablet form, 48
Ratio measures, in solutions, 45, 45*b*
Ratio solutions, 377
in calculating injectable medications, 381, 382, 383
for medications in units, 384, 385
Ratio strengths, 45
in parenteral medications, 377
Recombinant DNA insulin, 483
Recommended dosage, 665-666
Reconstitution, of solutions, 427-481, 445*b*
basic principles for, 428-431, 428*b*, 429*f*, 430*b*
practice problems for, 431-437, 473
chapter review for, 452-472
answers to, 475-481
clinical reasoning for, 451
answers to, 474, 475*b*
with different directions depending on route of administration, 441, 441*b*, 441*f*
diluent for, 427-428
directions on medication labels for, 186, 187*f*
displacement factor with, 430, 430*b*
dosage strength or concentration after, 429, 429*f*, 438-439
dosages, calculation of, 443-445
with more than one direction for mixing (multiple strength), 438-439, 438*b*, 439*b*
practice problems for, 440-441, 473
noninjectable, 445-450, 447*b*, 450*b*
calculation of, 447-448
for enteral feeding, 445-447, 446*f*, 447*b*
irrigating, 449-450, 450*b*
practice problems for, 447, 450, 473-474, 474*b*
strength of, determining, 447
package insert for, 441-442, 442*f*
in single-dose or multiple-dose vial, 430, 430*b*
storage after, 430
terminology relating to, 427-428
when final concentration (dosage strength) is not stated, 438
rect, 152*t*
Reduction, of fractions, 15, 15*b*
Refusal of medications, 137
Replacement fluids, 514
Roman numerals, 6-10
in apothecary system, 7
Arabic equivalents for, 6, 6*b*
chapter review for, 10
answers to, 10
for clotting factors, 8
controlled substances for, 7, 8, 8*f*
with grains, 9
hour marks for, 7
labels of medications on, 7, 8*f*
medication errors and, 8*b*, 9
mnemonic device for, 6, 6*b*
for periodic table for, 8
practice problems for, 9
answers to, 10
system of notation, 7
Rounding off decimals, 37-38, 37*b*
Route of administration, 140-141
on medication labels, 184-185, 184*f*, 185*f*
in medication orders, 155
right, 134-135
Rule of nines, for burn assessment, 55-56

S

s̄, 152*t*
Safe dosage, 666
Safe dosage range (SDR), pediatrics, 666
Safety needles, 363, 363*f*
SafetyGlide™ needle, 363*f*
Saline IV locks, 525-526, 525*f*-526*f*, 526*b*
Saline solutions
for reconstitution, 428
using household measures, 88
Scheduling medication times, 174
abbreviation for, 174t
Scored tablets, 293, 293*f*, 296*f*
Secondary line, 521, 522, 522*f*
Serious Reportable Events (SREs), 128
Signature, of the person writing the order, 155-156

Single dose medications, pediatric, 666-676
Single dose range medications, pediatrics, 668-676, 676*b*
Single-dose vials, 360, 430
Single-strength solution, 429*f*, 431
sl (SL), 152*t*
Slash mark (/), on medication labels, 183*b*
Sliding scale insulin (SSI), 496-497
Smart pumps, 528
Soaks, irrigation of, 449-450, 450*b*
sol, 152*t*
Solid oral medications, 297*b*-298*b*, 303*b*
  forms of, 292-303, 296*f*
  practice problems for, 304-316, 352-357
  problem setup on, 298-302
soln, 152*t*
Solute, 427
    in intravenous (IV) fluids, 519-521
Solution bags, labeling of, 575
Solutions
  calculation of, 447-448
  defined, 428
  determining the amount of medication in a specific amount of, 560-562
  intravenous, 514-535, 530*b*
    abbreviations for, 515, 515*b*, 516*b*
    additives to, 518, 518*b*
    chapter review for, 532-533, 535
    charting of, 103*f*, 518, 519*f*
    clinical reasoning for, 531, 534
    delivery methods, 515, 515*b*
    labels for, 516-517, 516*f*, 517*f*
    in percentage, 55, 59, 60
    practice problems for, 530-531, 534
    strength of, 516-517, 516*b*, 516*f*, 517*f*
  irrigation of, 449-450, 450*b*
  multiple-strength, 431, 438-439, 438*b*, 439*b*
  percentage, 55, 59, 376
  ratio, 377
  ratio measures in, 45
  single-strength, 429*f*, 431
  strength of, determining, 447
  using household measures, 87-88
Solvent, 427-428
  universal, 447
s.o.s (SOS), 152*t*
Soufflé cup, 142, 142*f*
Speak Up™ campaign, 139, 140*f*
Special instructions (parameters), in medication administration records, 167*f*, 168
Sprinkle capsules, 296
SR (sustained release), 152*t*
S&S, 152*t*
Standard U-100 syringe, 370, 370*f*
stat (STAT), 152*t*
Sterile water, for reconstitution, 428, 428*b*
Storage
  after reconstitution, 430
  directions, on medication labels, 188
Strength
  of medication, ratio and proportion in, liquid, 48
  of solutions, ratio measures in, 45
Subcut route. *see* Subcutaneous (subcut) route
Subcutaneous (subcut) route, 141
  maximum volume to administer, in single intramuscular site, 380
  of parenteral medications, 359
Sublingual medications, 140-141
Sublingual tablets, 294, 294*f*, 296*f*, 301*f*
Subtraction
  of decimals, 32-33
  of fractions, 17-19, 17*b*
    using borrowing, 18-19, 18*b*
    from whole number, 18, 18*b*
supp, 152*t*
susp, 152*t*
Suspension, 317, 317*f*
Symbols, in apothecary system, 86
syp, 152*t*
syr, 152*t*
Syringe pumps, 528, 529*f*
Syringe-type device, measuring cup *vs.*, 87
Syringes, 362-371, 365*b*, 371*b*
  calculating injectable medications according to, 380-383
  clinical reasoning for, 371
    answers to, 419
  hypodermic, 364-368
    large-capacity, 367, 368*f*
    small, 364-365, 364*f*, 365*f*
  insulin, 144*f*, 369-370, 370*f*
    1-mL double-scale, 489, 490*f*, 492
    1-mL single-scale, 489, 490*f*, 491
    Lo-Dose, 369-370, 370f, 489, 490, 490*f*
    measuring, two types of insulin in same, 498-500, 499*f*
    practice problems for, 491, 492-493, 510
    preparing single dosage in, 497-498
    U-100, 489-492, 490*f*
    U-500, 493-495
  intravenous, 367
  Luer-Lok, 362, 363*f*
  mixing medications in, 386
  needleless, 363, 363*f*
  non-Luer-Lok, 362
  oral, 319, 319*f*
  parts of, 362, 363*f*
  practice problems for, 366-367
    answers to, 416-417
  prefilled, 362, 362*f*
  safety needles for, 363, 363*f*
  SafetyGlide™ needle, 363*f*
  small hypodermics, 364-365, 364*f*, 365*f*
  tuberculin, 369, 369*f*
  types of, 364-371
Syrup, 317
Système international d'unités (SI), 74
Systems of measurement, 73-124
  rules for different, 250*b*

T

tab, 152*t*
Tablespoon (T, tbs)
  household/metric equivalents of, 87, 87*b*
  in medication orders, 151*t*
Tablet cutter, 293, 294*f*
Tablets, 292-296
  buccal, 294*f*, 295
  calculating dosages involving, 296-302, 297*b*-298*b*, 303*b*
    with divided doses, 303
    dosage strength in, 296-297
    maximum number in, 297
    practice problems for, 304-316, 352-357
  chewable, 295, 296*f*
  crushing, 296
  disintegrating, 295
  enteric-coated, 294
  extended-release, 295, 301*f*
  layered, 295, 295*f*
  opening, 296
  problems, variation of, 302-303
  ratio and proportion in, 48
  scored, 293, 293*f*, 296*f*
  sublingual, 294, 294*f*, 296*f*, 301*f*
  timed-release, 295, 296*f*
  types of, 293
Tall Man lettering
  for look-alike/sound-alike (LASA) medications, 133-134
  on medication labels, 180
Tandem piggyback setup, 522*f*, 523
Teaspoon (t, tsp)
  household/metric equivalents of, 87, 87*b*
  in medication orders, 151*t*
Technological advances, in prevention of medication errors, 128
Technology, advantages and disadvantages of, 173-174
Telephone, medication orders through, 150, 150*b*
Temperature scales, conversions between Celsius and Fahrenheit, 111, 112*f*, 120
  formulas for, 112-113
The Joint Commission (TJC)
  "Do Not Use" List of, 151
  in prevention of medication errors, 127
Thermometers, conversions between Celsius and Fahrenheit scales on, 111, 112*f*, 120
    formulas for, 112-113
"30 minute rule," 135
30 unit Lo-Dose, 369
t.i.d (tid), 152*t*
Time
  of administration
    documentation of, 168
    in medication administration records, 167-168
    on medication orders, 155
  completion, 119-120
  military, 174-175
    calculations, 119
    conversion for, 117-118, 117*f*, 121
  order was written, in medication order, 153
  scheduling medication, 174
    abbreviations for, 174*t*
Time-critical scheduled medications, 135
Timed-release capsule, 296*f*
Timed-release tablets, 295, 296*f*
tinct, 152*t*
Tip, of syringe, 362, 363*f*
Titrated medications, 629
  IV flow rates for, 634-636
  titration table for, 636-639, 637*t*, 639*t*
Titration table, developing a, 636-639, 637*t*, 639*t*
Topical medications, 141
Total amount in container, 186
Total daily dosage, 666
Total parenteral nutrition (TPN), 521
Total volume
  on medication labels, 185-186, 186*f*
  parenteral, 371
tr, 152*t*
Trade name
  on medication labels, 181, 181*f*
  on medication orders, 153, 153*f*, 154*b*, 154*f*
Trademark, 181
Traditional time
  calculations, 119-120
  conversion from military time to, 118
Trailing zero
  after decimal point, 30*b*
  in metric system, 77-78
Transcription, of medication orders, 151, 152
Transdermal medication, 141
Tresiba (insulin degludec injection), 483
Tuberculin syringe, 144*f*, 369, 369*f*
Tubex, 361

U

ung, 152*t*
Unit-dose cabinet, 170, 171*f*
Unit dose drug dispensing system, 170
Unit-dose packaging
  medication labels for, 191, 191*f*
  for oral medications, 292
Unit-dose system, 170
United States Pharmacopeia (USP)
  on apothecary system, 85-86
  on medication labels, 181, 188-189
  in prevention of medication errors, 127

Units, 88, 155
international, 88
medications in, calculating dosages for, 384-386
parenteral medications measured in, 377
Units of measure
in medication orders, 151*t*
in metric system, 74, 75*t*, 78-79
abbreviations for, 76-77, 77*b*
conversions between, 79, 79*b*, 80-81, 97
for length, 74-75, 75*t*, 79*b*, 113-114, 114*b*, 120
for volume, 75*t*, 79, 79*b*
for weight, 75*t*, 78-79, 79*b*
for ratio and proportion in dosage calculation, 49
rules for different, 250*b*
Universal solvent, 447
USP. *see* United States Pharmacopeia
Usual dosage, on medication labels, 189
Utensils, for medication dosages, 87

V

v, 152*t*
vag, 152*t*
Valium, 8*f*
Verbal orders, of medication order, 150-151, 150*b*
Vials, 360, 360*f*, 361*f*
single-dose *vs.* multiple-dose, 430, 430*b*
Vicodin, 8*f*
Volume, units of measure in metric system for, 75*t*, 79, 79*b*
Volume control devices, as intravenous (IV) equipments, 524, 525*f*
Volume control set, 692-694, 693*b*

W

Warnings, on medication labels, 187, 188*f*
Weight
conversion relating to, 115-117, 120
dosage calculation based on, 657-719, 658*b*, 680*b*-681*b*, 687*b*, 690*b*, 698*b*
for adult, 676-677
basic calculations, principles relating to, 659
body weight, 659-660, 660*b*
converting grams to kilograms for, 664-665
converting kilograms to pounds for, 662-663, 662*b*
converting pounds to kilograms for, 660-662, 661*b*
pediatric medication dosages in, 659, 659*b*
practice problems for, 662, 663-664, 664b, 665-666, 666*b*, 677-680, 683-684, 686-687, 687*b*, 688-689, 694, 696-697, 710-713
for single dose medications, 666-676, 676*b*
using body surface area, 681-682, 681*f*, 682*b*, 684-688, 685*b*
Weight *(Continued)*
of medication, ratio and proportion in
capsule form, 48
liquid, 48
tablet form, 48
units of measure in metric system for, 75*t*, 78-79, 79*b*
Weight-based protocol, for heparin calculations, 604, 609-612, 609*b*, 609*f*
West nomogram chart, 682*f*, 683, 683*b*
Whole number
dividing, by a decimal, 36-37
dividing a decimal by, 36
fractions and, 11, 12, 12*f*
subtracting fractions from, 18, 18*b*

X

x, in ratio and proportion, solving for, 46-48

Z

Zeros
after decimal point, 31*b*
before decimal point, 31*b*
leading, in metric system, 77
trailing, in metric system, 77
Zyprexa, prescribing information for, 192*f*-193*f*

Drug Label Index

Boldface indicates generic drug name.

A

Abacavir sulfate (Ziagen), 309
Acetaminophen (Cherry), 337
Acetaminophen (Tylenol), 255
Acyclovir, 203, 435, 460
Acyclovir (Zovirax), 331
Adalimumab (Humira), 374
Aerobid (**flunisolide**), 185
Albuterol sulfate, 706
Aleve (**naproxen sodium**), 193
Allopurinol (Zyloprim), 344
Alprazolam oral solution, 242
Alprazolam (Xanax), 230, 338
Amikacin sulfate injection (Amikin), 705
Amikin (**amikacin sulfate injection**), 705
Aminophylline injection, 260, 410, 642
Amiodarone HCl injection, 206, 376
Amlodipine besylate and benazepril HCl (Lotrel), 230
Amoxicillin, 187, 198, 237, 434, 453
Amoxicillin and clavulanate potassium, 209, 229, 315
Amoxicillin and clavulanate potassium oral suspension, 330, 455
Amoxicillin oral suspension, 258, 329, 336
Amphotericin B, 468, 559, 680
Ampicillin, 275, 453
Ampicillin sodium/sulbactam sodium (Unasyn), 465
Antivert (**meclizine HCl**), 278
Apidra® (**insulin glulisine rDNA origin**), 485
Apixaban (Eliquis), 306, 342
Aquamephyton (**phytonadione**), 397
Aranesp (**darbepoetin alfa**), 285, 402
Aricept (**donepezil HCl**), 266
Ativan injection (**Lorazepam**), 372, 405
Atomoxetine HCl (Strattera), 284, 304, 345
Atorvastatin calcium (lipitor), 153, 341
Atropine sulfate injection, 180, 237
Azithromycin (Zithromax), 243, 335, 436, 465
Azulfidine (**sulfasalazine**), 313

B

Baclofen (Lioresal), 306
Benztropine mesylate (Cogentin), 256, 310
Betamethasone (Celestone, Soluspan), 409
Bexarotene (Targretin), 265
Biaxin (**clarithromycin**), 266, 281, 324, 456
Bicillin C-R (**penicillin G benzathine/penicillin G procaine**), 395
Bosulif (**bosutinib**), 204
Bosutinib (Bosulif), 204
Brexpiprazole (Rexulti), 308, 338
Bumetanide injection, 209, 408
Buprenorphine and naloxone (Suboxone®) sublingual film, 184, 295, 346
Buprenorphine hydrochloride injection, 415
Bupropion (**Welbutrin**), 348
Butorphanol tartrate injection, 414

C

Calcium gluconate injection, 213, 376
Canagliflozin (Invokana), 214, 339
Capoten (**captopril**), 314
Captopril (Capoten), 314
Carbamazepine (Tegretol), 307, 703
Cardizem (**diltiazem HCL injection**), 646
Cardizem LA (**diltiazem hydrochloride**), 210
Carvedilol, 334
Cefaclor oral suspension, 241, 283, 699, 707
Cefazolin, 461
Cefdinir (Omnicef), 469
Cefepime hydrochloride (Maxipime), 462
Cefotan (**cefotetan**), 456
Cefotetan (Cefotan), 456
Cefpodoxmine proxetil (Vantin), 461
Cefprozil, 342, 464
Ceftazidime (Tazicef), 441, 451
Ceftazidime (Tazidime), 457
Ceftriaxone, 429, 436, 470
Ceftriaxone sodium (Rocephin), 361, 433, 467
Celestone, Soluspan (**betamethasone**), 409
CellCept oral suspension, 317
Cephalexin, 228, 677
Cherry (**acetaminophen**), 337
Chlordiazepoxide HCl (Librium), 257
Chlorpromazine HCl (Thorazine), 301, 309, 372
Cialis (**tadalafil**), 201, 335
Cimetidine HCl injection (Tagamet), 262, 407, 558
Clarinex (**desloratadine**), 308
Clarithromycin (Biaxin), 266, 281, 324, 456
Clindamycin injection, 186, 392, 558
Clonazepam, 314
Clonazepam (Klonopin), 281, 293, 295
Clorazepate dipotassium (Tranxene), 198, 227
Clozapine (Clozaril), 263, 341
Clozaril (**clozapine**), 263, 341
Cogentin (**benztropine mesylate**), 256, 310
Compazine (**prochlorperazine**), 241, 343, 387
Coumadin (**crystalline warfarin sodium**), 11, 12, 305
Crixivan (**indinavir sulfate**), 210
Cyanocobalamin injection, 236
Cymbalta (**duloxetine**), 313
Cytarabine, 187, 195, 454, 458
Cytotec (**misoprostol**), 349

D

Dabigatran etexilate (Pradaxa), 213
Dalteparin sodium injection (Fragmin), 604
Darbepoetin alfa (Aranesp), 285, 402
Demerol (**meperidine HCl injection**), 180, 188, 386, 390, 403, 411, 418, 425
Denosumab (Prolia), 215
Depakene (**valproic acid**), 317, 328
Depakote ER (**divalproex sodium**), 310
Depakote® Sprinkle, 183, 184
Depo-Provera (**medroxyprogesterone acetate**), 205, 240, 372, 405
Desloratadine (Clarinex), 308
Dexamethasone elixir, 349
Dexamethasone sodium phosphate, 210, 284, 412, 415
Dextrose 5% injection, 516, 533
Dextrose 5% injection and **0.9% sodium chloride,** 517, 533
Dextrose 5% injection and **0.45% sodium chloride,** 517, 532
DiaBeta (**glyburide**), 227
Diazepam injection, 408
Diflucan (**fluconazole injection**), 375
Diflucan (**fluconazole oral suspension**), 437
Digoxin injection, 201, 394, 404
Digoxin (Lanoxin), 227, 255, 277, 298, 305
Digoxin (Lanoxin) elixir pediatric, 325, 703
Dilantin, 207
Dilantin-125 (**phenytoin oral suspension**), 241
Dilantin (**phenytoin sodium injection**), 396
Dilatrate-SR (**isosorbide dinitrate**), 226
Dilaudid-HP (**hydromorphone HCl**), 195, 394
Diltiazem HCl, 199
Diltiazem HCl injection, 257
Diltiazem HCl injection (Cardizem), 210, 646
Dimethyl fumarate (Tecfidera), 214, 311, 347
Dinoprostone (Prepidil Gel), 202
Diphenhydramine HCl injection, 240, 399
Dipyridamole (Persantine), 226
Divalproex sodium (Depakote ER), 310
Donepezil HCl (Aricept), 266
Dopamine HCl injection, 641
Doxycycline injection, 263
Doxycycline monohydrate (Vibramycin), 235
Duloxetine (Cymbalta), 313
Duragesic (**fentanyl transdermal system**), 196
Duramorph (**morphine sulfate injection**), 375

E

Effient (**prasugrel**), 233
Eliquis (**apixaban**), 306, 342
Enalapril maleate (Vasotec), 263
Enoxaparin sodium (Lovenox injection), 407, 604
Epinephrine injection, 182, 242, 377
Epivir oral solution (**lamivudine**), 329
Epoetin alfa (Epogen), 207, 378, 406
Epogen (**epoetin alfa**), 207, 378, 406
Ery-Tab (**Erythromycin**), 183, 225, 339, 350
Erythromycin, 225, 339, 350
Erythromycin (Ery-Tab), 183, 225, 339, 350
Erythromycin ethylsuccinate oral suspension, 327, 435, 706
Escitalopram oxalate (Lexapro), 279
Esomeprazole magnesium (Nexium), 343
Ethosuximide (Zarontin), 233
Evista (**Raloxifene HCl**), 234

F

Famciclovir (Famvir), 348
Famotidine injection, 397

Famotidine (Pepcid), 466
Famvir (**famciclovir**), 348
Feldene (**piroxicam**), 254
Fenofibrate (TriCor→), 181, 261
Fentanyl citrate injection, 412
Fentanyl transdermal system (Duragesic), 196
Filgrastim (Neupogen), 413
Flagyl (**metronidazole**), 231, 255
Fluconazole injection (Diflucan), 375
Fluconazole oral suspension (Diflucan), 437
Flunisolide (Aerobid), 185
Fluoxetine hydrochlride oral solution (Prozac liquid), 331
Fortovase (**saquinavir**), 202
Fragmin (**dalteparin sodium injection),** 604
Furosemide, 180, 188, 204, 345, 391
Furosemide injection, 374, 391
Furosemide (Lasix), 180, 232, 265, 273, 391
Furosemide oral solution, 142

G

Garamycin (**gentamicin**), 409
Gemcitabine HCl (Gemzar), 431
Gemfibrozil (Lopid), 261
Gemzar (**Gemcitabine HCl**), 431
Gentamicin, 274
Gentamicin (Garamycin), 409
Gentamicin injection, 235, 259, 704
Geodon (**ziprasidone HCl**), 233, 344
Gleevec (**imatinib mesylate**), 199
Glucophage (**metformin hydrochloride**), 154
Glyburide (DiaBeta), 227
Glycopyrrolate injection, 401
Glyset (**miglitol**), 312
Granisetron HCl (Kytril), 204

H

Halcion (**triazolam**), 194
Haloperidol decanoate injection, 283, 390
Heparin Lock Flush, 605, 616, 620
Heparin sodium injection, 236, 258, 377, 396, 605, 615, 616, 617, 620
Humalog (**insulin lispro injection**), 485, 486, 506
Human insulin injection/rDNA (Novolin R), 503
Human insulin isophane suspension (Humulin 70/30), 506
Human insulin isophane suspension/rDNA (Novolin N), 485, 505
Human insulin rDNA origin (Humulin N), 484, 502
Humira (**adalimumab**), 374
Humulin 70/30 (**human insulin isophane suspension**), 506
Humulin N (**human insulin rDNA origin**), 484, 485, 486, 502
Humulin R (**insulin human injection**), 88, 377, 379, 484, 485, 486, 502
Hydrochlorothiazide (Hydrodiuril), 254, 337
Hydrocodone bitartrate and acetaminophen (Lortab 5/500), 212
Hydrocodone bitartrate and acetaminophen (Vicodin), 8
Hydrocodone bitartrate and acetaminophen (VicodinES), 196
Hydrocortisone sodium succinate (Solu-Cortef), 400
Hydrodiuril (**hydrochlorothiazide**), 254, 337
Hydromorphone HCl (Dilaudid-HP), 195, 394
Hydromorphone hydrochloride injection, 206, 373
Hydroxyzine hydrochloride (Vistaril), 238, 402, 669

I

Ibuprofen (Motrin), 316
Imatinib mesylate (Gleevec), 199
Inderal® LA (propranolol hydrochloride), 183, 195, 316
Inderal® (propranolol hydrochloride), 264
Indinavir sulfate (Crixivan), 210
Indocin (**indomethacin**), 312
Indomethacin (Indocin), 312
Insulin aspart injection (NovoLog), 485, 507
Insulin detemir (Levemir), 485
Insulin glargine injection (Lantus®), 485
Insulin glulisine rDNA origin (Apidra®), 485
Insulin human injection (Humulin R), 377, 484, 485, 502
Insulin lispro injection (Humalog), 485, 506
Invokana (**canagliflozin**), 214, 339
Isentress™ (**raltegravir**), 181
Isoniazid injection, 416
Isosorbide dinitrate (Dilatrate-SR), 226

J

Janumet (**sitagliptin/metformin HCl**), 205, 265, 334

K

K-Tab (**potassium chloride**), 232
Kaletra (**lopinavir/ritonavir oral solution**), 197
Kanamycin sulfate (Kantrex), 340
Kantrex (**Kanamycin sulfate**), 340
Ketorolac (**tromethamine injection**), 393
Klonopin (**clonazepam**), 281, 293, 295
Kytril (**granisetron HCl**), 204

L

Lactated Ringer's and **5% dextrose injection,** 516
Lactated Ringer's injection, 532
Lactulose, 340
Lamivudine (epivir oral solution), 329
Lanoxin (**digoxin**), 227, 255, 277, 298, 305
Lanoxin (**digoxin**) elixir pediatric, 325, 703
Lantus® (**insulin glargine injection**), 485, 486
Lasix (**furosemide**), 180, 232, 265, 273, 391
Latuda (**lurasidone HCl**), 344
Leucovorin calcium, 432
Levemir (**insulin detemir**), 485
Levothroid (**levothyroxine sodium**), 234
Levothyroxine sodium, 460
Levothyroxine sodium (Levothroid), 234
Levothyroxine sodium (Synthroid), 202, 304, 314
Lexapro (**escitalopram oxalate**), 279
Librium (**chlordiazepoxide HCl**), 257
Lidocaine HCl injection, 182, 376, 428, 632
Linaclotide (Linzess), 213, 337
Lincocin (**lincomycin injection**), 404
Lincomycin hydrochloride injection, 260
Lincomycin injection (Lincocin), 404
Linezolid (Zyvox), 311
Linzess (**linaclotide**), 213, 337
Lioresal (**baclofen**), 306
Lipitor (**atorvastatin calcium**), 153, 341
Loperamide hydrochloride oral solution, 325
Lopid (**gemfibrozil**), 261
Lopinavir/ritonavir oral solution (Kaletra), 197
Lorazepam injection, 238
Lortab 5/500 (**hydrocodone bitartrate and acetaminophen**), 212
Lotrel (**amlodipine besylate and benazepril HCl**), 230
Lovenox (**enoxaparin sodium injection),** 407, 604
Lurasidone HCl (Latuda), 344
Lyrica (**pregabalin**), 315, 323, 351

M

Maxipime (**cefepime hydrochloride**), 462
Meclizine HCl (Antivert), 278
Medroxyprogesterone acetate (Depo-Provera), 205, 240, 372
Memantine HCl oral solution (Namenda), 182, 186
Meperidine HCl injection (Demerol), 180, 188, 386, 390, 403, 411, 418, 425
Metformin hydrochloride, 183, 186, 208
Metformin hydrochloride (extended release), 264
Metformin hydrochloride (glucophage), 154
Methotrexate injection, 194, 282, 705
Methylphenidate hydrochloride, 209
Methylprednisolone sodium succinate, 395, 432, 452, 455, 707
Metoclopramide injection, 406
Metoprolol succinate (TOPROL-XL), 267
Metronidazole (Flagyl), 231, 255
Miglitol (Glyset), 312
Minoxidil, 316
Misoprostol (Cytotec), 349
Morphine sulfate, 180, 203, 256, 678
Morphine sulfate injection, 259, 279, 375, 391
Morphine sulfate (MS Contin), 207
Motrin (**ibuprofen**), 316
MS Contin (**morphine sulfate**), 207

N

Nabumetone (Relafen), 304
Nalbuphine HCl (Nubain), 413
Naloxone HCl injection, 401
Naloxone HCL injection (Narcan), 667
Namenda (**memantine HCl oral solution**), 182, 186
Naproxen sodium (Aleve), 193
Narcan (**naloxone HCL injection),** 667
Neulasta (**pegfilgrastim**), 214
Neupogen (**Filgrastim**), 413
Nexium (**esomeprazole magnesium**), 343
Nitroglycerin, 211, 301
Nitroglycerin (Nitrostat®), 85, 86, 140, 166, 184, 250, 294, 301, 636
Nitropress (**sodium nitroprusside injection),** 642
Nitrostat® (**nitroglycerin**), 85, 86, 140, 166, 184, 250, 294, 301, 636
Norvir® (**ritonavir**), 200
Norvir® (**ritonavir oral solution**), 185, 188, 330
Novolin N (**human insulin isophane suspension/rDNA),** 485, 505
Novolin R (**human insulin injection/rDNA**), 503
NovoLog (**insulin aspart injection**), 485, 507
Nubain (**Nalbuphine HCl**), 413

O

Octreotide acetate (Sandostatin®), 238, 389, 393
Olanzapine (Zyprexa), 192, 347, 442
Omnicef (**cefdinir**), 469
Ondansetron injection, 400
Orphenadrine citrate injection, 414
Oseltamivir phosphate (Tamiflu), 214, 328, 333
Oxacillin, 471
Oxbutynin chloride, 351
Oxcarbazepine (Trileptal), 239, 349
Oxycodone and acetaminophen (Percocet), 190, 212, 333
Oxycodone and aspirin (percodan), 212, 333
Oxycodone hydrochloride, 332
Oxycodone hydrochloride oral solution, 200
Oxycodone hydrochloride (Oxycontin), 310
Oxycodone hydrochloride (OxyFast), 142, 143
Oxycontin (**oxycodone hydrochloride**), 310
OxyFast (**oxycodone hydrochloride**), 142, 143
Oxytocin injection, 379

P

Paricalcitol (Zemplar), 201
Pegfilgrastim (Neulasta), 214
Penicillin G benzathine/penicillin G procaine (Bicillin C-R), 395
Penicillin G potassium (Pfizerpen), 439, 440, 454, 457
Penicillin G Sodium, 463
Penicillin V Potassium oral solution (Veetids), 182, 327, 673, 675
Pepcid (**famotidine**), 466
Percocet (**oxycodone and acetaminophen**), 190, 212, 333
Percodan (**oxycodone and aspirin**), 212, 333

Persantine (**dipyridamole**), 226
Pfizerpen (**penicillin G potassium**), 439, 440, 454, 457
Phenazopyridine HCl (Pyridium), 311
Phenobarbital sodium injection, 388
Phenytoin oral suspension (Dilantin-125), 241
Phenytoin sodium injection (Dilantin), 396
Phytonadione (Aquamephyton), 397
Piperacillin sodium and tazobactam sodium (Zosyn), 464
Piroxicam (Feldene), 254
Potassium chloride, 88, 278, 378, 517
Potassium chloride (K-Tab), 232
Potassium chloride oral solution, 236
Pradaxa (**dabigatran etexilate**), 213
Prandin (**repaglinide**), 231
Prasugrel (Effient), 233
Prednisone, 262
Pregabalin (Lyrica), 315, 323, 351
Prepidil Gel (**dinoprostone**), 202
Procainamide HCl (Procanbid) extended release, 339
Procainamide hydrochloride injection (Pronestyl), 410
Procanbid (**procainamide HCl**) extended release, 339
Prochlorperazine (Compazine), 241, 343, 387
Prolia **(Denosumab),** 215
Promethazine HCl injection, 398, 411
Promethazine hydrochloride oral solution, 326
Pronestyl (**procainamide hydrochloride injection**), 410
Protamine sulfate injection, 282
Prozac liquid (**fluoxetine hydrochlride oral solution**), 331
Pyridium (**phenazopyridine HCl**), 311

R

Raloxifene HCl (Evista), 234
Raltegravir (Isentress™), 181
Ranitidine injection, 239, 277, 403, 700
Relafen (**nabumetone**), 304
Repaglinide (Prandin), 231
Rexulti (**brexpiprazole**), 308, 338
Rifadin (**rifampin**), 229
Rifampin (Rifadin), 229
Rifaximin (Xifaxan), 334
Risperdal, 231
Ritonavir oral solution (Norvir®), 185, 188, 330
Rivaroxaban (Xarelto), 215
Rocephin (**ceftriaxone sodium**), 361, 433, 467

S

Sandostatin® (**octreotide acetate**), 238, 389, 393
Saquinavir (Fortovase), 202
Septra® DS (**trimethoprim and sulfamethoxazole**), 190, 230
Septra® (**trimethoprim and sulfamethoxazole**), 190
Sertraline Hcl (Zoloft), 209, 348
Sildenafil citrate (Viagra), 346
Simvastatin (Zocor), 206
Sinemet® 10-100 (**Carbidopa-Levodopa**), 189
Sinemet® 25-100 (**Carbidopa-Levodopa**), 189, 261
Sinemet® CR 50-200 (**Carbidopa-Levodopa**), 189
Sitagliptin/metformin HCl (Janumet), 205, 265, 334
Sodium chloride 0.9% injection, 517
Sodium nitroprusside injection (Nitropress), 642
Solu-Cortef (**hydrocortisone sodium succinate**), 400
Solu-Medrol (**methylprednisolone sodium succinate**), 452
Spironolactone (Aldactone), 336
Strattera (**atomoxetine HCl**), 284, 304, 345
Streptomycin, 471
Streptozocin (Zanosar), 211
Suboxone® (**buprenorphine and naloxone**) sublingual film, 184, 295, 346
Sulfamethoxazole and trimethoprim injection, 191, 559
Sulfasalazine (Azulfidine), 313
Synthroid (**levothyroxine sodium**), 202, 304, 314

T

Tadalafil (Cialis), 201, 335
Tagamet (**cimetidine HCl injection**), 262, 407, 558
Tamiflu (**oseltamivir phosphate**), 214, 328, 333
Targretin (**bexarotene**), 265
Tarka® (**trandolapril/verapamil HCl ER**), 191
Tazicef (**ceftazidime**), 441, 451
Tazidime (**ceftazidime**), 457
Tecfidera (**dimethyl fumarate**), 214, 311, 347
Tegretol (**carbamazepine**), 307, 703
Terbutaline sulfate, 280, 350
Theophylline, anhydrous (Uniphyl), 282, 307
Thiamine hydrochloride injection, 242, 280, 388
Thorazine (**chlorpromazine HCl**), 301, 309, 372
Ticar (**ticarcilin disodium**), 676
Ticarcilin disodium (Ticar), 676
Tigan (**Trimethobenzamide HCl**), 228, 373, 411
Tobramycin injection, 704
Tobramycin sulfate injection, 399
Topamax (**topiramate**), 203
Topiramate (Topamax), 203
TOPROL-XL (**metoprolol succinate**), 267
Tramadol HCl (Ultram), 200
Trandolapril/verapamil HCl ER (Tarka®), 191
Tranxene (**clorazepate dipotassium**), 227
Triazolam (Halcion), 194
TriCor→ (**fenofibrate**), 181, 186, 261
Trileptal (**oxcarbazepine**), 239, 349
Trimethobenzamide HCl (Tigan), 228, 373, 411
Trimethoprim and sulfamethoxazole (Septra®), 190
Trimethoprim and sulfamethoxazole (Septra® DS), 190, 230
Tromethamine injection (Ketorolac), 393
Tylenol (**acetaminophen**), 255, 333

U

Ultram (**tramadol HCl**), 200
Unasyn (**ampicillin sodium/sulbactam sodium**), 465
Uniphyl (**theophylline, anhydrous**), 282, 307

V

Valium (**diazepam**), 8, 208, 389, 408
Valproic acid (Depakene), 317, 328
Vancomycin hydrochloride, 459
Vantin (**cefpodoxmine proxetil**), 461
Vasotec (**enalapril maleate**), 263
Veetids (**Penicillin V Potassium oral solution**), 182, 327, 673, 675
Verteporfin (Visudyne), 472
Vfend (**voriconazole**), 463
Viagra (**sildenafil citrate**), 346
Vibramycin (**doxycycline monohydrate**), 235
Vicodin (**hydrocodone bitartrate and acetaminophen**), 8
VicodinES (**hydrocodone bitartrate and acetaminophen**), 196
Vistaril (**hydroxyzine hydrochloride**), 238, 402, 669
Visudyne (**verteporfin**), 472
Voriconazole (Vfend), 463

W

Welbutrin (bupropion), 348

X

Xanax (**alprazolam**), 230, 338
Xarelto (**rivaroxaban**), 215
Xifaxan (**rifaximin**), 334

Z

Zanosar (**streptozocin**), 211
Zarontin (**ethosuximide**), 233
Zemplar (**paricalcitol**), 201
Ziagen (**abacavir sulfate**), 309
Ziprasidone HCl (Geodon), 233
Zithromax (**azithromycin**), 243, 335, 436, 465
Zocor (**simvastatin**), 206
Zoloft (**Sertraline Hcl**), 209, 348
Zosyn (**piperacillin sodium and tazobactam sodium**), 464
Zovirax (**acyclovir**), 331
Zyloprim (**allopurinol**), 344
Zyprexa (**olanzapine**), 192, 347, 442
Zyvox (**linezolid**), 311